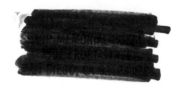

PLASTIC SURGERY

Indications, Operations, and Outcomes

Bruce M. Achauer, MD, FACS
Professor of Surgery,
Division of Plastic Surgery,
University of California Irvine,
California College of Medicine,
Orange, California

Elof Eriksson, MD, PhD, FACS
Joseph E. Murray Professor of Plastic and Reconstructive Surgery,
Harvard Medical School;
Chief, Division of Plastic Surgery,
Brigham and Women's Hospital;
Chief, Division of Plastic Surgery,
Children's Hospital,
Boston, Massachusetts

Bahman Guyuron, MD, FACS
Clinical Professor of Plastic Surgery,
Case Western Reserve University,
Cleveland, Ohio;
Medical Director,
Zeeba Medical Campus,
Lyndhurst, Ohio

John J. Coleman III, MD, FACS
Professor of Surgery;
Chief of Plastic Surgery;
Staff Physician,
Indiana University Medical Center;
Director, Pediatric Burn Unit;
Staff Physician,
Riley Children's Hospital;
Staff Physician,
Wishard Memorial Hospital,
Indianapolis, Indiana

Robert C. Russell, MD, FRACS, FACS
Clinical Professor of Surgery,
Division of Plastic Surgery,
Southern Illinois University School of Medicine,
Springfield, Illinois

Craig A. Vander Kolk, MD, FACS
Associate Professor of Plastic Surgery;
Director, Cleft and Craniofacial Center,
Johns Hopkins University School of Medicine,
Baltimore, Maryland

PLASTIC SURGERY

Indications, Operations, and Outcomes

Volume One

Part I *Principles and Techniques*
Part II *General Reconstructive Surgery*

EDITORS

Bruce M. Achauer, MD, FACS
Professor of Surgery,
Division of Plastic Surgery,
University of California Irvine,
California College of Medicine,
Orange, California

Elof Eriksson, MD, PhD, FACS
Joseph E. Murray Professor of Plastic and Reconstructive Surgery,
Harvard Medical School;
Chief, Division of Plastic Surgery,
Brigham and Women's Hospital;
Chief, Division of Plastic Surgery,
Children's Hospital,
Boston, Massachusetts

OUTCOMES EDITOR

Edwin G. Wilkins, MD, MS
Associate Professor of Plastic Surgery,
University of Michigan Health Systems,
Ann Arbor, Michigan

MANAGING EDITOR

Victoria M. VanderKam, RN, BS, CPSN
Clinical Nurse, Division of Plastic Surgery,
University of California Irvine Medical Center,
Orange, California

ILLUSTRATIONS BY

Min Li, MD
Indiana University School of Medicine,
Department of Surgery, Section of Plastic Surgery,
Indianapolis, Indiana

with 6279 illustrations, including 963 in color, and 18 color plates

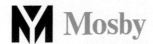

Mosby

A Harcourt Health Sciences Company

St. Louis   London   Philadelphia   Sydney   Toronto

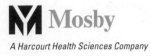

Mosby

A Harcourt Health Sciences Company

Acquisitions Editor: Richard Zorab
Developmental Editor: Dolores Meloni
Project Manager: Carol Sullivan Weis
Senior Production Editor: Florence Achenbach
Designers: Dave Zielinski/Mark Oberkrom

Mosby, Inc.
A Harcourt Health Sciences Company
11830 Westline Industrial Drive
St. Louis, Missouri 63146

Printed in the United States of America

Volume 1 ISBN 0-8151-1019-7
Set ISBN 0-8151-0984-9

00 01 02 03 04 GW/MVY 9 8 7 6 5 4 3 2 1

Contributors

BRUCE M. ACHAUER, MD, FACS
Professor of Surgery,
Division of Plastic Surgery,
University of California Irvine,
California College of Medicine,
Orange, California

GREGORY J. ADAMSON, MD
Clinical Instructor of Orthopedics,
University of Illinois College of Medicine at Peoria;
Staff, St. Francis Medical Center,
Peoria, Illinois

GHADA Y. AFIFI, MD
Clinical Assistant Professor,
Division of Plastic Surgery,
Department of Surgery,
Loma Linda University Medical Center and Children's
    Hospital;
Attending Surgeon, Plastic Surgery,
Jerry L. Pettis Memorial Veterans Affairs Medical Center,
Loma Linda, California;
Private Practice,
Newport Beach, California

RICHARD D. ANDERSON, MD
Plastic Surgery Staff,
Scottsdale Healthcare Hospitals;
Private Practice,
Scottsdale, Arizona

JAMES P. ANTHONY, MD
Associate Professor of Surgery,
Division of Plastic Surgery,
University of California–San Francisco,
San Francisco, California

HÉCTOR ARÁMBULA, MD
Professor of Plastic Surgery,
Postgraduate Division of Medicine,
Universidad Nacional Autonoma de Mexico;
Chairman, Plastic Surgery Service,
Hospital de Traumatologia Magdalena de las Salinas,
Instituto Mexicano del Seguro Social, IMSS,
Mexico City, Mexico

LOUIS C. ARGENTA, MD
Julius A. Howell Professor and Chairman,
Department of Plastic Surgery,
Wake Forest University School of Medicine;
Professor and Chairman,
Department of Plastic and Reconstructive Surgery,
North Carolina Baptist Hospital,
Winston-Salem, North Carolina

DUFFIELD ASHMEAD IV, MD
Assistant Clinical Professor of Plastic Surgery and
    Orthopedics,
University of Connecticut School of Medicine,
Farmington, Connecticut;
Director, Division of Hand Surgery,
Connecticut Children's Medical Center,
Hartford, Connecticut

CHRISTOPHER J. ASSAD, BS, MD, FRCSC
Plastic and Reconstructive Surgeon;
Associate Staff,
Halton Health Care Services Corporation,
Milton District Hospital,
Milton, Ontario, Canada

THOMAS J. BAKER, MD
Professor of Plastic Surgery–Voluntary,
University of Miami School of Medicine;
Senior Attending Physician,
Mercy Hospital,
Miami, Florida

TRACY M. BAKER, MD
Instructor in Plastic Surgery,
University of Miami School of Medicine,
Miami, Florida

JUAN P. BARRET, MD
Professor, Rijksuniversiteit Groningen;
Plastic and Reconstructive Surgeon,
University Hospital Groningen,
Groningen, The Netherlands

MUNISH K. BATRA, MD
Assistant Clinical Instructor–Voluntary,
Division of Plastic Surgery,
University of California–San Diego Medical Center,
San Diego, California;
Private Practice,
Del Mar, California

BRUCE S. BAUER, MD, FACS
Associate Professor of Surgery,
Northwestern University Medical School;
Head, Division of Plastic Surgery,
The Children's Memorial Hospital,
Chicago, Illinois

STEPHEN P. BEALS, MD, FACS, FAAP,
Assistant Professor of Plastic Surgery,
Mayo Medical School;
Adjunct Professor,
Department of Speech and Hearing Science,
Arizona State University;
Craniofacial Consultant,
Barrow Neurological Institute
Phoenix, Arizona

MICHAEL S. BEDNAR, MD
Associate Professor,
Department of Orthopedic Surgery and Rehabilitation,
Stritch School of Medicine,
Loyola University–Chicago,
Maywood, Illinois

RAMIN A. BEHMAND, MD
Chief Resident,
Division of Plastic and Reconstructive Surgery,
University of Michigan Hospitals,
Ann Arbor, Michigan

RUSSELL W. BESSETTE, DDS, MD
Clinical Professor of Plastic Surgery,
State University of New York–Buffalo,
School of Medicine;
Executive Director of Research,
Sisters Hospital,
Buffalo, New York

MARINA D. BIZZARRI-SCHMID, MD
Instructor in Anesthesia,
Harvard Medical School;
Anesthesiologist,
Brigham and Women's Hospital,
Boston, Massachusetts

GREG BORSCHEL, MD
Plastic Surgery Resident,
University of Michigan Hospitals,
Ann Arbor, Michigan

MARK T. BOSCHERT, MS, MD
Attending Physician,
St. Joseph Health Center;
Private Practice,
St. Charles, Missouri,
Attending Physician,
Barnes-St. Peters Hospital,
St. Peters, Missouri

JOHN BOSTWICK, MD, FACS
Professor and Chairman of Plastic Surgery,
Emory University School of Medicine;
Chief of Plastic Surgery,
Emory University Hospital,
Atlanta, Georgia

J. BRIAN BOYD, MB, ChB, MD, FRCSC, FACS
Professor of Surgery,
The Ohio State University College of Medicine,
Columbus, Ohio;
Chairman of Plastic Surgery,
Cleveland Clinic–Florida,
Fort Lauderdale, Florida

WILLIAM R. BOYDSTON, MD, PhD
Pediatric Neurosurgeon,
Children's Healthcare of Atlanta,
Scottish Rite Children's Hospital,
Atlanta, Georgia

KARL H. BREUING, MD
Instructor in Surgery,
Harvard Medical School;
Attending Physician, Plastic Surgery,
Brigham and Women's Hospital;
Attending Physician, Plastic Surgery,
Children's Hospital;
Attending Physician, Plastic Surgery,
Faulkner Hospital;
Attending Physician, Plastic Surgery,
Dana Farber Cancer Institute,
Boston, Massachusetts

FORST E. BROWN, MD
Emeritus Professor of Plastic Surgery,
Dartmouth Medical School,
Hanover, New Hampshire;
Consultant,
Veterans Administration Hospital,
White River Junction, Vermont

RICHARD E. BROWN, MD, FACS
Clinical Associate Professor;
Hand Fellowship Director,
Division of Plastic Surgery,
Southern Illinois University School of Medicine,
Springfield, Illinois

MARIE-CLAIRE BUCKLEY, MD
Plastic Surgery Fellow,
University of Minnesota Medical School,
Division of Plastic and Reconstructive Surgery,
Minneapolis, Minnesota

GREGORY M. BUNCKE, MD, FACS
Clinical Assistant Professor of Surgery,
University of California–San Francisco,
San Francisco, California;
Clinical Assistant Professor of Surgery,
Stanford University,
Stanford, California;
Co-Director, Division of Microsurgery,
California Pacific Medical Center,
San Francisco, California

HARRY J. BUNCKE, MD
Clinical Professor of Surgery,
University of California–San Francisco,
San Francisco, California;
Associate Clinical Professor of Surgery,
Stanford Medical School,
Stanford, California;
Director, Microsurgical Transplantation–Replantation
    Service,
California Pacific Medical Center–Davies,
San Francisco, California

RUDOLF BUNTIC, MD
Clinical Instructor,
Division of Plastic Surgery,
Stanford University,
Stanford, California;
Attending Microsurgeon,
California Pacific Medical Center,
San Francisco, California

ELISA A. BURGESS, MD
Resident in Plastic Surgery,
Oregon Health Sciences University,
Portland, Oregon

FERNANDO D. BURSTEIN, MD
Clinical Associate Professor,
Plastic and Reconstructive Surgery,
Emory University School of Medicine;
Chief, Plastic and Reconstructive Surgery;
Co-Director, Center for Craniofacial Disorders,
Scottish Rite Children's Medical Center,
Atlanta, Georgia

GRANT W. CARLSON, MD
Professor of Surgery,
Emory University School of Medicine;
Chief of Surgical Services,
Crawford Long Hospital;
Chief of Surgical Oncology,
Emory Clinic,
Atlanta, Georgia

JAMES CARRAWAY, MD, AB
Professor of Plastic Surgery;
Chairman, Division of Plastic Surgery,
Eastern Virginia Medical School,
Norfolk, Virginia

STANLEY A. CASTOR, MD
Plastic Surgery Staff Physician,
The Watson Clinic,
Lakeland, Florida

BERNARD CHANG, MD
Director, Plastic and Reconstructive Surgery,
Mercy Medical Center,
Baltimore, Maryland

YU-RAY CHEN, MD
Professor, Department of Plastic Surgery,
Chang Gung University Medical School
Tao-Yuan, Taiwan;
Superintendent and Attending Surgeon,
Department of Plastic Surgery,
Chang Gung Memorial Hospital,
Taipei, Taiwan

ANDREAS CHIMONIDES, BS, MD
Staff Physician,
Butler Memorial Hospital,
Butler, Pennsylvania;
Staff Physician,
St. Francis Medical Center;
Staff Physician,
University of Pennsylvania Medical Center–St. Margaret's
    Hospital,
Pittsburgh, Pennsylvania

MARK A. CODNER, MD
Clinical Assistant Professor,
Emory University School of Medicine;
Private Practice,
Atlanta, Georgia

I. KELMAN COHEN, MD
Professor of Surgery;
Director, Wound Healing Center,
Medical College of Virginia,
Virginia Commonwealth University,
Richmond, Virginia

MYLES J. COHEN, MD
Clinical Assistant Professor of Surgery,
University of Southern California School of Medicine;
Attending Physician,
Cedars Sinai Medical Center,
Los Angeles, California

STEVEN R. COHEN, MD
Associate Clinical Professor,
Division of Plastic and Reconstructive Surgery,
University of California Medical Center–San Diego;
Chief, Craniofacial Surgery,
Children's Hospital of San Diego,
San Diego, California

VICTOR COHEN, MD
Resident Physician,
McGill University Health Center,
McGill University School of Medicine,
Montreal, Quebec, Canada

JOHN J. COLEMAN III, MD, FACS
Professor of Surgery;
Chief of Plastic Surgery;
Staff Physician,
Indiana University Medical Center;
Director, Pediatric Burn Unit;
Staff Physician,
Riley Children's Hospital;
Staff Physician,
Wishard Memorial Hospital,
Indianapolis, Indiana

LAWRENCE B. COLEN, MD
Associate Professor of Plastic and Reconstructive Surgery,
Eastern Virginia Medical School,
Norfolk, Virginia

E. DALE COLLINS, MD, MS
Assistant Professor of Surgery,
Dartmouth Medical School,
Hanover, New Hampshire;
Medical Director, Comprehensive Breast Program,
Dartmouth-Hitchcock Medical Center,
Lebanon, New Hampshire

MATTHEW J. CONCANNON, MD, FACS
Assistant Professor;
Director of Hand and Microsurgery,
University of Missouri,
Columbia, Missouri

BRUCE F. CONNELL, MD
Clinical Professor of Surgery,
University of California Irvine,
California College of Medicine,
Orange, California

AISLING CONRAN, MD
Assistant Professor, Clinical Anesthesia,
University of Chicago,
Chicago, Illinois

PAUL C. COTTERILL, BS, MD, ABHRS,
Honorary Lecturer,
Sunnybrook Hospital,
Department of Dermatology,
University of Toronto,
Toronto, Ontario, Canada

KIMBALL MAURICE CROFTS, MD
Staff Physician,
Utah Valley Regional Medical Center,
Provo, Utah;
Staff Physician,
Timpanogos Regional Hospital,
Orem, Utah;
Staff Physician,
Mt. View Hospital,
Payson, Utah;
Staff Physician,
Sevier Valley Hospital,
Richfield, Utah

LISA R. DAVID, MD
Assistant Professor,
Department of Plastic and Reconstructive Surgery,
Wake Forest University School of Medicine;
Attending Physician,
North Carolina Baptist Hospital,
Winston-Salem, North Carolina

WILLIAM M. DAVIDSON, AB, DMD, PhD
Professor and Chairman,
Department of Orthodontics,
University of Maryland Dental School;
Associate Staff, Dentistry,
Johns Hopkins Hospital,
Baltimore, Maryland

MARK A. DEITCH, MD
Assistant Professor of Surgery,
Division of Orthopedic Surgery,
University of Maryland School of Medicine,
Baltimore, Maryland

MARK D. DeLACURE, MD, FACS
Chief, Division of Head and Neck Surgery and Oncology;
Associate Professor of Otolaryngology–Head and Neck
    Surgery,
Department of Otolaryngology;
Associate Professor of Reconstructive Plastic Surgery,
Institute of Reconstructive Plastic Surgery,
Department of Surgery,
New York University School of Medicine,
New York, New York

VALERIE BURKE DeLEON, MA,
Department of Cell Biology and Anatomy,
Johns Hopkins University School of Medicine,
Baltimore, Maryland

JOHN Di SAIA, MD
Assistant Clinical Professor,
Division of Plastic Surgery,
University of California Irvine,
California College of Medicine,
Orange, California

RICHARD V. DOWDEN, MD
Clinical Assistant Professor,
Case Western Reserve University,
Cleveland, Ohio

CRAIG R. DUFRESNE, MD, FACS
Clinical Professor of Plastic Surgery,
Georgetown University,
Washington, DC;
Plastic Surgery Section Chief;
Co-Director, Center for Facial Rehabilitation,
Fairfax Hospital,
Inova Hospital System,
Fairfax, Virginia

FELMONT F. EAVES III, MD, FACS
Assistant Clinical Professor,
University of North Carolina,
Chapel Hill, North Carolina;
Attending Physician,
Charlotte Plastic Surgery Center;
Attending Physician,
Carolinas Medical Center;
Attending Physician,
Presbyterian Hospital;
Attending Physician,
Mercy Hospital,
Charlotte, North Carolina

PHILIP EDELMAN, MD
Associate Professor of Medicine;
Director, Toxicology and Clinical Services,
Division of Occupational and Environmental Medicine,
George Washington University School of Medicine,
Washington, DC

ERIC T. EMERSON, MD
Private Practice,
Gastonia, North Carolina

TODD B. ENGEN, MD
Clinical Faculty,
University of Utah School of Medicine,
Salt Lake City, Utah;
Clinical Director,
Excel Cosmetic Surgery Center,
Orem, Utah

BARRY L. EPPLEY, MD, DMD
Assistant Professor of Plastic Surgery,
Indiana University School of Medicine,
Indianapolis, Indiana

ELOF ERIKSSON, MD, PhD, FACS
Joseph E. Murray Professor of Plastic and Reconstructive
  Surgery,
Harvard Medical School;
Chief, Division of Plastic Surgery,
Brigham and Women's Hospital;
Chief, Division of Plastic Surgery,
Children's Hospital,
Boston, Massachusetts

GREGORY R.D. EVANS, MD, FACS
Professor of Surgery;
Chair, Division of Plastic Surgery,
University of California Irvine,
California College of Medicine
Orange, California

JEFFREY A. FEARON, MD, FACS, FAAP
Director, The Craniofacial Center,
North Texas Hospital for Children at Medical City Dallas,
Dallas, Texas

LYNNE M. FEEHAN, MS, PT
Senior Hand Therapist,
Hand Program,
Workers' Compensation Board of British Columbia,
Richmond, British Columbia, Canada

RANDALL S. FEINGOLD, MD, FACS
Assistant Clinical Professor, Plastic and Reconstructive
  Surgery,
Albert Einstein College of Medicine,
Bronx, New York;
Attending Surgeon,
Long Island Jewish Medical Center,
New Hyde Park, New York;
Chief, Division of Plastic Surgery,
North Shore University Hospital at Forest Hills,
Forest Hills, New York

ROBERT D. FOSTER, MD
Assistant Professor in Residence,
Division of Plastic and Reconstructive Surgery,
University of California–San Francisco,
San Francisco, California

FRANK J. FRASSICA, MD
Professor of Orthopedic Surgery and Oncology,
Johns Hopkins University School of Medicine,
Baltimore, Maryland

ALAN E. FREELAND, MD
Professor, Department of Orthopedic Surgery;
Director, Hand Surgery Service,
The University of Mississippi Medical Center,
Jackson, Mississippi

MENNEN T. GALLAS, MD
Junior Faculty Associate,
University of Texas M.D. Anderson Cancer Center,
Houston, Texas

BING SIANG GAN, MD, PhD, FRCSC
Assistant Professor,
Departments of Surgery and Pharmacology-Toxicology,
University of Western Ontario;
Staff Surgeon,
Hand and Upper Limb Centre;
Staff Surgeon,
St. Joseph's Health Centre,
London, Ontario, Canada

WARREN L. GARNER, MD
Associate Professor of Surgery,
University of Southern California;
Associate Professor of Plastic Surgery;
Director, LAC & USC Burn Center,
Los Angeles, California

DAVID G. GENECOV, MD
Attending Surgeon,
International Craniofacial Institute,
Dallas, Texas

GEORGE K. GITTES, MD
Associate Professor,
Department of Surgery,
University of Missouri–Kansas City;
Holder and Ashcraft Chair of Pediatric Surgical Research,
Children's Mercy Hospital,
Kansas City, Missouri

JEFFREY A. GOLDSTEIN, MD
Associate Professor of Surgery,
Case Western Reserve University;
Medical Director, Craniofacial Center;
Chief of Plastic and Reconstructive Surgery,
Rainbow Babies and Children's Hospital,
Cleveland, Ohio

HECTOR GONZALEZ-MIRAMONTES, MD
Private Practice,
Guadalajara, Mexico

LAWRENCE J. GOTTLIEB, MD
Professor of Clinical Surgery,
University of Chicago,
Pritzker School of Medicine,
Chicago, Illinois

MARK S. GRANICK, MD
Professor of Surgery;
Chief of Plastic Surgery,
MCP-Hahnemann University,
Philadelphia, Pennsylvania

FREDERICK M. GRAZER, MD, FACS
Associate Clinical Professor,
Division of Plastic Surgery,
University of California Irvine,
California College of Medicine;
Staff Physician,
University of California Irvine Medical Center,
Orange, California;
Clinical Professor of Surgery,
The Pennsylvania State University Milton S. Hershey
    Medical Center College of Medicine,
Hershey, Pennsylvania;
Staff Physician,
Hoag Memorial Hospital Presbyterian,
Newport Beach, California

JON M. GRAZER, MD, MPH
Staff Physician,
Hoag Memorial Hospital Presbyterian,
Newport Beach, California;
Staff Physician,
Western Medical Center,
Santa Ana, California

JUDITH M. GURLEY, MD
Assistant Professor of Surgery,
Division of Plastic and Reconstructive Surgery,
Washington University School of Medicine;
Attending Physician,
St. Louis Children's Hospital;
Attending Physician,
Shriner's Hospital for Children,
St. Louis, Missouri

BAHMAN GUYURON, MD, FACS
Clinical Professor of Plastic Surgery,
Case Western Reserve University,
Cleveland, Ohio;
Medical Director,
Zeeba Medical Campus,
Lyndhurst, Ohio

HONGSHIK HAN, MD
Plastic Surgery Resident,
Division of Plastic Surgery,
Northwestern University Medical School,
Chicago, Illinois

ROBERT A. HARDESTY, MD
Professor,
Loma Linda University School of Medicine;
Medical Staff President;
Chief of Plastic Surgery,
Loma Linda University Medical Center,
Loma Linda, California

MAUREEN HARDY, PT, MS, CHT
Clinical Assistant Professor,
University of Mississippi Medical Center;
Director, Hand Management Center,
St. Dominic Hospital,
Jackson, Mississippi

ALAN SCOTT HARMATZ, BS, MD
Assistant Professor of Surgery,
University of Vermont College of Medicine,
Burlington, Vermont;
Attending Physician,
Maine Medical Center,
Portland, Maine

STEPHEN U. HARRIS, MD
Staff Physician,
Nassau County Medical Center,
East Meadow, New York;
Staff Physician,
North Shore Hospital,
Manhasset, New York;
Staff Physician,
Winthrop University Hospital,
Mineola, New York;
Plastic Surgeon,
Long Island Plastic Surgical Group,
Garden City, New York

ROBERT J. HAVLIK, MD
Associate Professor of Surgery,
Indiana University School of Medicine,
Indianapolis, Indiana

DETLEV HEBEBRAND, MD, PhD
Attending Physician,
Hand and Burn Center,
Bergmannsheil Clinic,
Ruhr University,
Bochum, Germany

MARC H. HEDRICK, MD
Assistant Professor of Surgery and Pediatrics,
Division of Plastic and Reconstructive Surgery,
University of California–Los Angeles School of Medicine,
Los Angeles, California

DOMINIC F. HEFFEL, MD
Resident, General Surgery,
University of California–Los Angeles Center for Health
    Sciences,
Los Angeles, California

CHRIS S. HELMSTEDTER, MD
Director of Orthopedic Oncology–Southern California,
Kaiser Permanente,
Baldwin Park, California;
Assistant Clinical Professor, Orthopedics and Surgery,
University of Southern California School of Medicine,
Los Angeles, California

VINCENT R. HENTZ, MD
Professor of Functional Restoration (Hand Surgery),
Stanford University School of Medicine,
Stanford, California

JEFFREY HOLLINGER, DDS, PhD
Professor, Biology and Biomedical Health Engineering;
Director, Center for Bone Tissue Engineering,
Carnegie Mellon University,
Pittsburgh, Pennsylvania

HEINZ-HERBERT HOMANN, MD
Attending Physician,
Hand and Burn Center,
Bergmannsheil Clinic,
Ruhr University,
Bochum, Germany

CHARLES E. HORTON, MD, FACS, FRCSC
Professor of Plastic Surgery,
Eastern Virginia Medical School,
Norfolk, Virginia;
Clinical Professor of Surgery,
Medical College of Virginia,
Richmond, Virginia

CHARLES E. HORTON, Jr., MD
Assistant Professor of Urology,
Eastern Virginia Medical School;
Chief, Department of Urology,
Children's Hospital of the King's Daughters,
Norfolk, Virginia

ERIC H. HUBLI, MD, FACS, FAAP
Craniomaxillofacial Surgeon,
International Craniofacial Institute,
Dallas, Texas

ROGER J. HUDGINS, MD
Assistant Professor,
Morehouse University School of Medicine;
Chief of Pediatric Neurosurgery,
Children's Healthcare of Atlanta,
Scottish Rite Children's Hospital,
Atlanta, Georgia

LAWRENCE N. HURST, MD, FRCSC
Professor and Chairman,
Division of Plastic Surgery,
The University of Western Ontario;
Chief, Division of Plastic Surgery
London Health Sciences Centre, University Campus,
London, Ontario, Canada

ETHYLIN WANG JABS, MD
Dr. Frank V. Sutland Professor of Pediatric Genetics;
Professor of Pediatrics, Medicine, and Plastic Surgery,
John Hopkins University School of Medicine,
Baltimore, Maryland

MOULTON K. JOHNSON, MD
Associate Professor of Orthopedic Surgery,
University of California–Los Angeles,
Los Angeles, California

GLYN JONES, MD, FRCS, FCS
Associate Professor of Plastic Surgery;
Chief of Plastic Surgery,
Crawford Long Hospital,
Emory Clinic,
Atlanta, Georgia

NEIL F. JONES, MD
Professor, Division of Plastic and Reconstructive Surgery,
Department of Orthopedic Surgery,
University of California–Los Angeles;
Chief of Hand Surgery,
University of California–Los Angeles Medical Center,
Los Angeles, California

JESSE B. JUPITER, MD
Professor of Orthopedic Surgery,
Harvard Medical School;
Head, Orthopedic Hand Service,
Massachusetts General Hospital,
Boston, Massachusetts

M.J. JURKIEWICZ, MD, DDS
Professor of Surgery, Emeritus,
Emory University School of Medicine,
Atlanta, Georgia

MADELYN D. KAHANA, MD
Associate Professor of Anesthesiology and Pediatrics,
The University of Chicago Hospital,
Chicago, Illinois

CHIA CHI KAO, MD
Fellow, Department of Reconstructive and Plastic Surgery,
University of Southern California,
Los Angeles, California

AJAYA KASHYAP, MD
Assistant Professor,
University of Massachusetts Medical Center,
Worcester, Massachusetts;
Attending Plastic Surgeon,
Metrowest Medical Center,
Framingham, Massachusetts

JULIA A. KATARINCIC, MD
Consultant, Department of Orthopedic Surgery,
Mayo Clinic,
Rochester, Minnesota

DANIEL J. KELLEY, MD
Assistant Professor;
Director, Head and Neck Oncology/Skull Base Surgery,
Department of Otolaryngology and Bronchoesophagology,
Temple University School of Medicine,
Philadelphia, Pennsylvania

KEVIN J. KELLY, DDS, MD
Associate Professor,
Department of Plastic Surgery,
Vanderbilt University School of Medicine;
Director, Craniofacial Surgery,
Department of Plastic Surgery,
Vanderbilt Medical Center,
Nashville, Tennessee

PRASAD G. KILARU, MD
Clinical Assistant Professor of Surgery,
University of Southern California–Los Angeles,
Los Angeles, California;
Staff Physician,
City of Hope National Medical Center,
Duarte, California

GABRIEL M. KIND, MD
Assistant Clinical Professor,
Department of Surgery,
Division of Plastic and Reconstructive Surgery,
University of California–San Francisco;
Assistant Director of Research;
Assistant Fellowship Director,
The Buncke Clinic,
San Francisco, California

BRIAN M. KINNEY, MD, FACS, MSME
Clinical Assistant Professor of Plastic Surgery,
University of Southern California–Los Angeles;
Former Chief,
Century City Hospital,
Los Angeles, California

ELIZABETH M. KIRALY, MD
Fellow, Hand and Microvascular Surgery,
University of Nevada School of Medicine,
Department of Surgery,
Division of Plastic Surgery,
Las Vegas, Nevada

JOHN O. KUCAN, MD
Professor of Surgery,
Institute of Plastic Surgery,
Southern Illinois University School of Medicine,
Springfield, Illinois

M. ABRAHAM KURIAKOSE, MD, DDS, FACS
Assistant Professor of Otolaryngology,
Division of Head and Neck Surgery,
Department of Otolaryngology,
New York University School of Medicine;
Attending Surgeon,
New York University Medical Center,
New York, New York

AMY L. LADD, MD
Associate Professor,
Division of Hand and Upper Extremity,
Department of Functional Restoration,
Stanford University;
Chief, Hand and Upper Extremity Clinic,
Lucile Salter Packard Children's Hospital,
Stanford, California

PATRICK W. LAPPERT, MD
Assistant Professor of Surgery,
Uniformed Services University of the Health Sciences,
Bethesda, Maryland;
Chief, Department of Plastic Surgery,
Naval Medical Center,
Portsmouth, Virginia

DON LaROSSA, MD
Professor of Plastic Surgery,
The University of Pennsylvania School of Medicine;
Staff Physician,
Hospital of The University of Pennsylvania;
Senior Surgeon,
Children's Hospital of Philadelphia,
Philadelphia, Pennsylvania

DAVID L. LARSON, MD
Professor and Chair of Plastic and Reconstructive Surgery,
Medical College of Wisconsin,
Milwaukee, Wisconsin

DONALD R. LAUB, Jr., MS, MD
Assistant Professor,
Departments of Surgery and Orthopedics,
University of Vermont;
Attending Plastic and Hand Surgeon,
Fletcher Allen Health Care,
Burlington, Vermont

MICHAEL LAW, MD
Fellow, Microsurgery,
University of Southern California–Los Angeles,
Division of Plastic Surgery,
Los Angeles, California

W. THOMAS LAWRENCE, MPH, MD
Professor and Chief,
Section of Plastic Surgery,
University of Kansas Medical Center,
Kansas City, Kansas

W.P. ANDREW LEE, MD, FACS
Assistant Professor of Surgery,
Harvard Medical School;
Chief of Hand Service,
Department of Surgery,
Massachusetts General Hospital,
Boston, Massachusetts

SALVATORE LETTIERI, MD
Senior Associate Consultant,
Mayo Clinic,
Division of Plastic and Reconstructive Surgery,
Rochester, Minnesota

JAN S. LEWIN, PhD
Assistant Professor and Director,
Speech Pathology and Audiology Section,
University of Texas M.D. Anderson Cancer Center,
Houston, Texas

TERRY R. LIGHT, MD
Dr. William M. Scholl Professor;
Chairman, Department of Orthopedic Surgery and
    Rehabilitation,
Stritch School of Medicine,
Loyola University–Chicago,
Maywood, Illinois

SEAN LILLE, MD
Research Professor,
Department of Chemistry and Biochemistry,
Arizona State University,
Tempe, Arizona;
Research Scientist,
Mayo Clinic–Scottsdale,
Scottsdale, Arizona;
Private Practice,
Phoenix, Arizona

TED LOCKWOOD, MD
Associate Clinical Professor,
University of Kansas Medical School;
Assistant Clinical Professor,
University of Missouri–Kansas City Medical School,
Kansas City, Missouri

MICHAEL T. LONGAKER, MD, FACS
John Marquis Converse Professor of Plastic Surgery Research;
Director of Surgical Research,
New York University School of Medicine;
Attending Plastic Surgeon,
New York University Medical Center,
New York, New York

H. PETER LORENZ, MD
Assistant Professor of Plastic Surgery,
University of California–Los Angeles School of Medicine,
Los Angeles, California

GEORGE L. LUCAS, MD
Professor and Chairman,
Orthopedic Surgery;
Program Director,
University of Kansas–Wichita;
Orthopedic Surgeon,
Via Christi Hospital;
Orthopedic Surgeon,
Wesley Medical Center,
Wichita, Kansas

PETER J. LUND, BS, MD
Orthopedic/Hand Surgery,
Methodist Volunteer General Hospital,
Martin, Tennessee

STEVEN D. MACHT, MD, DDS
Clinical Professor of Plastic Surgery,
George Washington University,
Washington, DC

JOHN S. MANCOLL, MD
Private Practice,
Fort Wayne, Indiana

GREGORY A. MANTOOTH, MD
Chief Resident,
Division of Plastic and Reconstructive Surgery,
Indiana University,
Indianapolis, Indiana

BENJAMIN M. MASER, MD
Community Physician,
Department of Functional Restoration,
Stanford University,
Stanford, California

BRUCE A. MAST, MD
Assistant Professor,
Department of Surgery,
Division of Plastic and Reconstructive Surgery,
University of Florida;
Chief, Section of Plastic Surgery,
Malcolm Randall Gainesville Veterans Administration
    Medical Center,
Gainesville, Florida

ALAN MATARASSO, MD
Clinical Associate Professor of Plastic Surgery,
Albert Einstein College of Medicine;
Surgeon,
Manhattan Eye, Ear, Throat Hospital,
New York, New York

G. PATRICK MAXWELL, MD
Assistant Professor of Plastic Surgery,
Vanderbilt University;
Director, Institute for Aesthetic Surgery,
Baptist Hospital,
Nashville, Tennessee

MICHAEL H. MAYER, MD
Physician and Surgeon,
Plastic and Reconstructive Surgery,
Portland, Oregon

TRACY E. McCALL, MD
Chief Plastic Surgery Resident,
State University of New York,
Health Science Center at Brooklyn,
Brooklyn, New York

ROBERT L. McCAULEY, MD
Chief, Plastic and Reconstructive Surgery,
Shriners Burns Hospital Galveston;
Professor of Surgery and Pediatrics,
University of Texas Medical Branch,
Galveston, Texas

LAWRENCE R. MENENDEZ, MD
Associate Professor, Clinical Orthopedics;
Associate Professor, Department of Surgery,
Division of Tumor and Endocrine,
University of Southern California;
Chief of Orthopedics,
Kenneth Norris Jr. Cancer Hospital,
Los Angeles, California

FREDERICK J. MENICK, MD
Private Practice,
Tucson, Arizona

WYNDELL H. MERRITT, MD, FACS
Clinical Assistant Professor of Surgery,
Medical College of Virginia,
Richmond, Virginia

BRYAN J. MICHELOW, MBBCh, FRCS
Clinical Assistant Professor,
Case Western Reserve University,
Cleveland, Ohio

SCOTT R. MILLER, MD
Clinical Instructor of Plastic Surgery,
University of California–San Diego,
San Diego, California;
Attending Surgeon,
Scripps Memorial Hospital,
La Jolla, California

TIMOTHY A. MILLER, MD
Professor,
University of California–Los Angeles;
Chief, Plastic Surgery,
Wadsworth Veterans Administration Medical Center,
Los Angeles, California

FERNANDO MOLINA, MD
Professor, Plastic, Aesthetic, and Reconstructive Surgery;
Head, Division of Plastic and Reconstructive Surgery,
Hospital General Dr. Manual Gea Gonzalez,
Mexico City, Mexico

ROBERT E. MONTROY, MD
Associate Clinical Professor,
Division of Plastic Surgery,
University of California Irvine,
California College of Medicine,
Orange, California;
Chief, Plastic Surgery Section;
Assistant Chief, Spinal Cord Injury/Disease Health Care
    Group,
Department of Veterans Affairs Medical Center,
Long Beach, California

THOMAS S. MOORE, MD
Clinical Professor of Plastic Surgery,
Indiana University School of Medicine;
Chairman, Department of Plastic Surgery,
St. Vincent Hospital,
Indianapolis, Indiana

FARAMARZ MOVAGHARNIA, DO
Plastic Surgeon;
Staff Physician,
Emory Northlake Regional Medical Center,
Atlanta, Georgia

ARIAN MOWLAVI, MD
Plastic Surgery Resident,
Southern Illinois University School of Medicine,
Springfield, Illinois

JOSEPH E. MURRAY, MD
Emeritus Professor of Surgery,
Harvard Medical School,
Boston, Massachusetts

THOMAS A. MUSTOE, MD
Professor and Chief, Division of Plastic Surgery,
Northwestern University Medical School,
Chicago, Illinois

ARSHAD R. MUZAFFAR, MD
Chief Resident,
Department of Plastic Surgery,
University of Texas Southwestern Medical Center,
Parkland Memorial Hospital,
Dallas, Texas

NASH H. NAAM, MD, FACS
Clinical Professor,
Department of Plastic and Reconstructive Surgery,
Southern Illinois University School of Medicine,
Springfield, Illinois;
Director, Southern Illinois Hand Center,
Effingham, Illinois

SATORU NAGATA, MD, PhD
Visiting Professor,
Division of Plastic Surgery,
University of California Irvine,
California College of Medicine,
Orange, California;
Department Director,
Reconstructive Plastic Surgery,
Chiba Tokushukai Hospital,
Narashinodai, Funabashi, Chiba, Japan

DANIEL J. NAGLE, MD
Associate Clinical Professor of Orthopedic Surgery,
Northwestern University Medical School;
Attending Hand and Microsurgeon,
Northwestern Memorial Hospital,
Chicago, Illinois

FOAD NAHAI, MD, FACS
Private Practice,
Atlanta, Georgia

DAVID T. NETSCHER, MD, FACS
Associate Professor,
Division of Plastic Surgery,
Baylor College of Medicine;
Chief, Plastic Surgery,
Veterans Affairs Medical Center,
Houston, Texas

MICHAEL W. NEUMEISTER, MD
Assistant Professor;
Plastic Surgery Program Director;
Chief, Microsurgery and Research,
Southern Illinois University School of Medicine;
Director, Hyperbaric Oxygen Unit,
Co-Director, Regional Burn Unit,
Memorial Medical Center,
Springfield, Illinois

RONALD E. PALMER, MD
Clinical Assistant Professor,
University of Illinois College of Medicine at Peoria,
Peoria, Illinois

FRANK A. PAPAY, MS, MD, FACS, FAAP
Assistant Clinical Professor,
The Ohio State University College of Medicine,
Columbus, Ohio;
Staff Surgeon;
Head, Section of Craniofacial and Pediatric Plastic Surgery,
The Cleveland Clinic Foundation,
Department of Plastic and Reconstructive Surgery,
Cleveland, Ohio

ROBERT W. PARSONS, MD
Professor Emeritus in Plastic Surgery and Pediatrics,
University of Chicago,
Pritzker School of Medicine,
Chicago, Illinois

WILLIAM C. PEDERSON, MD, FACS
Clinical Associate Professor,
Department of Surgery and Orthopedic Surgery,
University of Texas Health Science Center–San Antonio,
San Antonio, Texas

LINDA G. PHILLIPS, MD
Professor of Plastic Surgery;
Chief, Division of Plastic Surgery,
University of Texas Medical Branch,
Galveston, Texas

GEORGE J. PICHA, MD, PhD, FACS
Clinical Assistant Professor,
Division of Plastic Surgery,
Case Western Reserve University,
Cleveland, Ohio;
Private Practice,
Lyndhurst, Ohio

JEFFREY C. POSNICK, DMD, MD, FRCSC, FACS
Clinical Professor, Plastic Surgery, Pediatrics, Oral and
    Maxillofacial Surgery, and Otolaryngology/Head and Neck
    Surgery,
Georgetown University,
Washington, DC;
Director, Posnick Center for Facial Plastic Surgery,
Chevy Chase, Maryland

JASON N. POZNER, MD
Private Practice,
Boca Raton, Florida

STEFAN PREUSS, MD
Fellow, Plastic and Reconstructive Surgery,
Harvard Medical School;
Staff Physician,
Brigham and Women's Hospital;
Staff Physician,
Children's Hospital,
Boston, Massachusetts

JULIAN J. PRIBAZ, MD
Associate Professor of Surgery;
Program Director,
Harvard Plastic Surgery Residency Training Program,
Harvard Medical School;
Associate Surgeon,
Brigham and Women's Hospital;
Associate Surgeon,
Children's Hospital,
Boston, Massachusetts

C. LIN PUCKETT, MD, FACS
Professor and Head, Division of Plastic Surgery,
University of Missouri,
Columbia, Missouri

OSCAR M. RAMIREZ, MD
Clinical Assistant Professor,
Johns Hopkins University School of Medicine;
Clinical Assistant Professor,
University of Maryland,
Baltimore, Maryland;
Director,
Esthétique International,
Plastic Surgical Center,
Timonium, Maryland

GERALD V. RAYMOND, MD
Assistant Professor,
John Hopkins University School of Medicine;
Neurologist,
Kennedy Krieger Institute,
Baltimore, Maryland

RILEY REES, MD
Professor of Plastic and Reconstructive Surgery,
University of Michigan Medical Center;
Chief, Plastic Surgeon Section,
Veterans Administration Medical Center,
Ann Arbor, Michigan,
Associate,
Chelsea Community Hospital,
Chelsea, Michigan

DANIEL REICHNER, MD
Plastic Surgery Resident,
University of California Irvine,
California College of Medicine,
Orange, California

JOAN RICHTSMEIER, MA, PhD
Professor, Department of Cell Biology and Anatomy,
Department of Plastic Surgery,
Johns Hopkins University School of Medicine,
Baltimore, Maryland

DAVID RING, MD
Fellow, Orthopedic Hand Service,
Massachusetts General Hospital,
Boston, Massachusetts

THOMAS L. ROBERTS III, MD
Associate Clinical Professor of Surgery,
Medical University of South Carolina at Spartanburg,
Spartanburg, South Carolina

ROD J. ROHRICH, MD, FACS
Professor and Chairman,
Department of Plastic Surgery,
University of Texas Medical Center at Dallas,
Dallas, Texas

LORNE E. ROTSTEIN, MD, FRCSC, FACS
Associate Professor,
Department of Surgery,
University of Toronto;
Staff Surgeon,
Princess Margaret Hospital,
The Toronto General Hospital University Health Network,
Toronto, Ontario, Canada

J. PETER RUBIN, MD
Fellow in Plastic Surgery,
Harvard Medical School,
Boston, Massachusetts

ROBERT C. RUSSELL, MD, FRACS, FACS
Clinical Professor of Surgery,
Division of Plastic Surgery,
Southern Illinois University School of Medicine,
Springfield, Illinois

A. MICHAEL SADOVE, MD
Professor of Surgery (Plastics),
Indiana University School of Medicine;
Chief, Plastic Surgery,
James Whitcomb Riley Hospital for Children,
Indianapolis, Indiana

KENNETH E. SALYER, MD
Adjunct Professor, Department of Orthodontics,
Baylor College of Dentistry,
Baylor University,
Dallas, Texas;
Clinical Professor, Department of Surgery,
Division of Plastic and Reconstructive Surgery,
University of Texas Health Science Center at San Antonio,
San Antonio, Texas;
Founding Director,
International Craniofacial Institute,
Cleft Lip and Palate Treatment Center,
Dallas, Texas

NICOLAS SASTRE, MD
Professor of Plastic Surgery,
Postgraduate Division of Medical Faculty,
Universidad Nacional Autonoma de Mexico;
Chairman, Plastic Surgery Department,
Hospital General de Mexico,
Mexico City, Mexico

STEPHEN A. SCHENDEL, MD, DDS
Professor and Head, Division of Plastic and Reconstructive
    Surgery;
Chairman, Department of Functional Restoration,
Stanford University,
Stanford, California

STEPHEN B. SCHNALL, MD
Associate Professor of Clinical Orthopedics,
University of Southern California School of Medicine,
Los Angeles, California

ALAN E. SEYFER, MD
Chief, Plastic Surgery,
Professor of Surgery, Anatomy, and Cell Developmental
    Biology,
Oregon Health Sciences University;
Chief, Plastic Surgery,
Doernbecher Childrens Hospital;
Staff Surgeon,
Shriners' Hospital for Crippled Children;
Portland Veterans Administration Medical Center,
Portland, Oregon

JATIN P. SHAH, MD, FACS, FRCS, FDSRCS
Professor of Surgery,
Weill Medical College,
Cornell University;
E.W. Strong Chair in Head and Neck Oncology;
Chief, Head and Neck Service,
Memorial Sloan-Kettering Cancer Center,
New York, New York

ARTHUR SHEKTMAN, MD
Attending Surgeon,
Newton-Wellesley Hospital,
Newton, Massachusetts;
Attending Surgeon,
St. Elizabeth's Medical Center,
Boston, Massachusetts

RANDY SHERMAN, MD
Professor and Chief,
Division of Plastic and Reconstructive Surgery,
University of Southern California–Los Angeles;
Chief, Plastic Surgery,
University of Southern California University Hospital;
Chief, Plastic Surgery,
Los Angeles County Hospital,
Los Angeles, California

PETER P. SIKO, MD
Research Manager,
The Buncke Clinic,
San Francisco, California

CARL E. SILVER, MD
Professor of Surgery,
Albert Einstein College of Medicine;
Chief, Head and Neck Surgery,
Montefiore Medical Center,
Bronx, New York

JEFFREY D. SMITH, MD
Clinical Fellow in Surgery,
Harvard Medical School;
Chief Resident, Plastic Surgery,
Brigham and Women's Hospital;
Chief Resident, Plastic Surgery,
Children's Hospital,
Boston, Massachusetts

NICOLE ZOOK SOMMER, MD
Plastic Surgery Resident,
Southern Illinois University School of Medicine,
Springfield, Illinois

RAJIV SOOD, MD
Associate Professor of Plastic Surgery,
Indiana University Medical Center;
Chief, Plastic Surgery Section,
Wishard Memorial Hospital,
Indianapolis, Indiana

CAROL L. SORENSEN, PsyD
Adjunct Professor of Psychology,
Concordia University,
Irvine, California

PANAYOTIS N. SOUCACOS, MD, FACS
Professor and Chairman,
Department of Orthopedics,
University of Ioannina School of Medicine,
Ioannina, Greece

MYRON SPECTOR, BS, MS, PhD
Professor of Orthopedic Surgery (Biomaterials),
Harvard Medical School;
Director of Orthopedic Research,
Department of Orthopedic Surgery,
Brigham and Women's Hospital,
Boston, Massachusetts

MELVIN SPIRA, MD, DDS
Professor of Surgery,
Division of Plastic Surgery,
Baylor College of Medicine,
Houston, Texas

HANS U. STEINAU, MD
Professor, Department of Plastic Surgery,
Director, Clinic for Plastic Surgery,
Hand and Burn Center,
Bergmannsheil Clinic,
Ruhr University,
Bochum, Germany

PETER J. STERN, MD
Professor and Chairman,
Department of Orthopedic Surgery,
University of Cincinnati College of Medicine,
Cincinnati, Ohio

BERISH STRAUCH, MD
Professor and Chairman,
Department of Plastic Surgery,
Albert Einstein College of Medicine,
Montefiore Medical Center,
Bronx, New York

JAMES M. STUZIN, MD
Clinical Assistant Professor of Plastic Surgery–Voluntary,
University of Miami School of Medicine;
Senior Attending Physician,
Mercy Hospital,
Miami, Florida

MARK R. SULTAN, MD
Associate Clinical Professor of Surgery,
Columbia University;
Chief, Division of Plastic Surgery,
Beth Israel Medical Center,
New York, New York

WILLIAM M. SWARTZ, MD, FACS
Clinical Associate Professor,
Department of Surgery,
University of Pittsburgh,
Pittsburgh, Pennsylvania

JULIA K. TERZIS, MD, PhD, FRCSC
Professor, Department of Surgery,
Division of Plastic and Reconstructive Surgery;
Director, Microsurgery Program,
Eastern Virginia Medical School,
Microsurgical Research Center,
Norfolk, Virginia

VIVIAN TING, MD
Resident in General Surgery,
University of Rochester Medical Center,
Strong Memorial Hospital,
Rochester, New York

BRYANT A. TOTH, MD, FACS
Assistant Clinical Professor of Surgery,
Department of Surgery,
University of California–San Francisco;
Attending Surgeon,
California Pacific Medical Center,
San Francisco, California;
Chief, Division of Plastic Surgery,
Children's Hospital of Northern California,
Oakland, California

LAWRENCE C. TSEN, MD
Assistant Professor of Anesthesia,
Harvard Medical School;
Attending Anesthesiologist,
Department of Anesthesiology,
Perioperative and Pain Medicine,
Brigham and Women's Hospital,
Boston, Massachusetts

MARTIN G. UNGER, MD, FRCSC, ABCS, ABHRS
Clinical Teacher and Lecturer,
University of Toronto;
Chief of Plastic Surgery,
One Medical Place Hospital,
Toronto, Ontario, Canada

ALLEN L. van BEEK, BS, MD
Clinical Associate Professor,
University of Minnesota,
Department of Surgery,
Minneapolis, Minnesota

VICTORIA M. VANDERKAM, RN, BS, CPSN
Clinical Nurse, Division of Plastic Surgery,
University of California Irvine Medical Center,
Orange, California

CRAIG A. VANDER KOLK, MD, FACS
Associate Professor of Plastic Surgery,
Director, Cleft and Craniofacial Center,
Johns Hopkins University School of Medicine,
Baltimore, Maryland

NICHOLAS VEDDER, MD
Associate Professor,
University of Washington,
Seattle, Washington

MARIOS D. VEKRIS, MD
Orthopedic Attending Surgeon,
Ioannina University Hospital,
Ioannina Medical School,
Ioannina, Greece

PETER M. VOGT, MD, PhD
Associate Professor;
Attending Physician,
Hand and Burn Center,
Bergmannsheil Clinic,
Ruhr University,
Bochum, Germany

JEFFREY D. WAGNER, MD
Associate Professor of Surgery,
Department of Surgery,
Division of Plastic and Reconstructive Surgery,
Indiana University School of Medicine,
Indianapolis, Indiana

ROBERT L. WALTON, MD, FACS
Professor of Surgery,
University of Chicago School of Medicine;
Chief, Section of Plastic Surgery,
University of Chicago Hospitals,
Chicago, Illinois

BERNADETTE WANG, MD
Fellow, Hand and Microsurgery,
Curtis National Hand Center,
Union Memorial Hospital,
Baltimore, Maryland

H. KIRK WATSON, MD
Director, Connecticut Combined Hand Surgery Fellowship;
Assistant Clinical Professor of Orthopedics, Rehabilitation,
   and Plastic Surgery,
Yale University School of Medicine,
New Haven, Connecticut;
Clinical Professor, Department of Orthopedics,
University of Connecticut School of Medicine,
Farmington, Connecticut;
Senior Staff,
Hartford Hospital;
Connecticut Children's Medical Center,
Hartford, Connecticut

M. SHARON WEBB, MD, PhD, JD
Attorney-at-Law,
Boston, Massachusetts

DENTON D. WEISS, LCDR, MC, USNR
Department of Plastic Surgery,
Naval Medical Center Portsmouth,
Portsmouth, Virginia

KATHLEEN J. WELCH, MD, MPH
Instructor in Anesthesia,
Harvard Medical School;
Director of Plastic Surgical Anesthesia,
Brigham and Women's Hospital,
Boston, Massachusetts

DEBORAH J. WHITE, MD
Staff Physician,
Scottsdale Healthcare,
Scottsdale, Arizona

GORDON H. WILKES, BS, MD, FRCSC
Clinical Professor of Surgery,
University of Alberta;
Chief of Surgery,
Misericordia Hospital,
Edmonton, Alberta, Canada

J. KERWIN WILLIAMS, MD
Clinical Associate Professor,
Division of Plastic Surgery,
Emory University School of Medicine;
Attending Physician,
Pediatric and Craniofacial Associates,
Atlanta Plastic Surgery,
Atlanta, Georgia

TODD WILLIAMS, MD
Chief Plastic Surgery Fellow,
Southern Illinois University School of Medicine,
Institute for Plastic and Reconstructive Surgery,
Springfield, Illinois

PETER D. WITT, MD, FACS
Associate Professor of Plastic Surgery;
Director, Pediatric Plastic Surgery,
Sutherland Institute,
University of Kansas School of Medicine,
Kansas City, Kansas

JOHN F. WOLFAARDT, BDS, MDent, PhD
Professor,
Faculty of Medicine and Dentistry,
University of Alberta;
Director, Craniofacial Osseointegration and Maxillofacial
   Prosthetic Rehabilitation Unit,
Misericordia Hospital,
Edmonton, Alberta, Canada

WILLIAM A. ZAMBONI, MD
Professor and Chief,
Division of Plastic Surgery,
University of Nevada School of Medicine,
Las Vegas, Nevada

JAMES E. ZINS, MD
Chairman, Department of Plastic Surgery,
The Cleveland Clinic Foundation,
Cleveland, Ohio

ELVIN G. ZOOK, MD
Professor of Plastic Surgery,
Southern Illinois University School of Medicine;
Chairman, Department of Plastic Surgery,
Memorial Medical Center,
Springfield, Illinois

**RONALD M. ZUKER, MD, FRCSC,
    FACS, FAAP**
Professor of Surgery,
University of Toronto;
Head, Division of Plastic Surgery,
The Hospital for Sick Children,
Toronto, Ontario, Canada

To my parents, Reynolds and Maurine Achauer
BMA

To Gudrun, Carl, Anna, Emma,
and Charlotta
EE

General Preface

This large project is dedicated to our colleagues who have contributed individual chapters to this textbook. Those who write chapters for books know that they are the unsung heroes of the medical publishing business. The chapter authors are recognized experts in their fields who have given their time in an effort to communicate their knowledge to the rest of the world. This unselfish work involves a long time commitment and a multistaged process. We would not have plastic surgery textbooks if it were not for the many people who give so freely of their time and expertise. We thank each of our chapter authors; this project is by you and for you, and we hope that you are proud of the finished product.

Plastic Surgery: Indications, Operations, and Outcomes was envisioned as a comprehensive overview of the entire discipline of plastic surgery. The concept was to create a practical book that would be useful for plastic surgeons in practice and for those in training. Each clinical chapter follows a standard format as closely as possible; the chapters first describe the indications for surgery, then discuss the operation of choice, including procedural details, and finally present outcomes information when available.

A project such as this has a history of its own. Bruce Achauer started the process in 1992 by talking to publishers and potential coeditors. He has provided leadership throughout the project. Working together, Achauer, Elof Eriksson, and Bahman Guyuron determined the title, focus, outline, and editors. In the fall of 1995, Achauer, Eriksson, and Guyuron signed a contract with Mosby, agreeing that they would edit the textbook. Jack Coleman, Bob Russell, and Craig Vander Kolk agreed to serve as volume editors.

Early on it was decided that the authors would focus on outcomes as much as possible, although we knew full well that there was little information on outcomes in plastic surgery. The goal was to increase awareness of this need and guide readers to begin thinking toward measuring outcomes. Ed Wilkins accepted the challenge of serving as outcomes editor.

The actual writing of the text began in 1996. The entire process of writing and editing took several years and involved a long-term commitment. The publishing business, like many others, has undergone tremendous change, including consolidation and the creation of larger firms from several companies. There was also an inevitable change of personnel during the process. Although Mosby started the project, Harcourt Health Sciences completed it. Throughout the years, our editorial staff has been extremely helpful.

Many individuals have been involved with this project. We extend our gratitude to the following people: John DeCarville and Bob Hurley, who captured our vision from the start and fully embraced it; Richard Zorab, Senior Editor, and Dolores Meloni, Senior Developmental Editor, of Harcourt Health Sciences, who saw the project through to its fruition; our tireless production staff of Carol Weis, Project Manager, and Florence Achenbach, Rick Dudley, Karen Rehwinkel, Christine Schwepker, and David Stein, Production Editors; and finally, Victoria VanderKam, who was willing to do anything necessary to see this project through.

It has been a fabulous experience, and we are grateful for the opportunity to participate. We thank everybody (authors, illustrators, and editors) for their commitment, hard work, and friendship and for creating this excellent textbook for plastic surgery.

BRUCE M. ACHAUER
ELOF ERIKSSON
BAHMAN GUYURON
JOHN J. COLEMAN
ROBERT C. RUSSELL
CRAIG A. VANDER KOLK

Preface to the First Volume

Plastic surgery is a wonderful specialty in which innovative surgery performed with great precision is the norm. The areas of transplantation, craniofacial surgery, and microsurgery have been discovered and developed by plastic surgeons and form a tribute to the innovations of the specialty. As plastic surgeons, we must constantly try to make advances within our profession; otherwise our specialty may whither away and eventually disappear. Few of us will match the major contributions of Joseph Murray, Paul Tessier, and Harry Bunke. However, we should all strive to make such an impact. In this volume a select group of plastic surgeons and their collaborators have generously shared their knowledge and experience, with the goal of improving the plastic surgery specialty. It would be presumptuous to compare the incremental improvements outlined in this book to the landmark contributions made by the surgeons listed earlier, but the spirit of the authors' dedication and contributions to the field of plastic surgery remains as high.

The authors are recognized experts in their respective fields. Much of the material is new, and I hope that the readers will have as much fun reading it as I have had. I trust that the readers of this book—plastic surgery residents, general surgery residents, medical students, and fellow practicing surgeons—will be able to apply the ideas about which we have written to their practice.

Special thanks to Laura Freeman for editing and typing large parts of this volume.

ELOF ERIKSSON

Outcomes Preface

At the dawn of a new millennium, we are witnessing the most dramatic overhaul of the American health care system in more than a century. Health care reform is well underway, driven by economic and political forces within both the public and private sectors. The watchwords of this not-so-quiet revolution, terms such as *efficiency, cost-effectiveness,* and *value,* reflect the new demand by payers that health care interventions deliver measurable benefit at reasonable costs. Contrary to long-standing traditions in the United States, exactly what constitutes a "reasonable" cost is determined not by those who provide health care but rather by those who foot the bill. The growing emphasis on cost-effectiveness, or "value" for every dollar spent, is forcing providers to fundamentally rethink traditional patterns of care. In this brave new world, medical decisions are made only after the perceived benefits have been weighed against the risks *and* costs of treatment.

Recent reforms also reflect changes in the traditional standards by which we have assessed the effectiveness of care. Treatment options are no longer being judged simply in terms of morbidity and mortality. Instead, interventions are evaluated by studying their impacts on long-term functioning, well-being, and quality of life. This new emphasis on measurement of outcomes from the "patient's viewpoint" is of particular interest to plastic surgeons. Unlike cardiac or transplant surgeries, aesthetic and reconstructive procedures usually do not produce life-saving results. Instead, plastic surgeons endeavor to bestow more subtle benefits on their clientele, improving their body image, psychosocial well-being, and physical functioning. Lest plastic surgeons downplay the significance of their work, it is important to note that health services researchers and payers now evaluate the value of health care interventions in terms of quality-adjusted life years (QALYs) contributed. Interventions that substantially improve quality of life may be viewed as comparable (or superior) to treatment options that increase longevity.

Clearly, assessment of patient-centered outcomes is of critical importance not only to plastic surgeons but to all health care providers. Outcomes data are playing increasingly important roles in determining which treatment modalities are supported by payers and managed care providers. Research assessing the results and costs of care also may determine where and by whom that care is delivered. Outcomes studies also provide key information to patients and providers to assist in medical decision-making. In managing health care delivery systems, outcomes data (such as patient satisfaction) identify potential targets for quality improvement efforts and provide meaningful yardsticks with which to assess progress.

Given the growing importance of assessing and reporting patient-centered results of care, the chapter authors of this textbook have included "Outcomes" sections where appropriate. Available data on a diverse array of outcomes parameters are referenced. However, as the reader will note, considerable gaps still exist in our knowledge of surgical outcomes, particularly in the areas of quality of life and cost analyses. While we attempt to summarize existing outcomes data in each chapter, we also have endeavored to highlight some areas in which more research is needed. For many aesthetic and reconstructive problems and procedures, the quantity of unanswered research questions dwarfs our current body of knowledge. It is the hope of the volume authors and editors that some of the issues raised in these chapters will stimulate new outcomes studies to answer these questions.

EDWIN G. WILKINS

Contents

VOLUME TWO CRANIOMAXILLOFACIAL, CLEFT, AND PEDIATRIC SURGERY
Craig A. Vander Kolk, Editor

VOLUME THREE   HEAD AND NECK SURGERY
John J. Coleman III, Editor

VOLUME FOUR HAND SURGERY
Robert C. Russell, Editor

PART I

PRINCIPLES AND TECHNIQUES

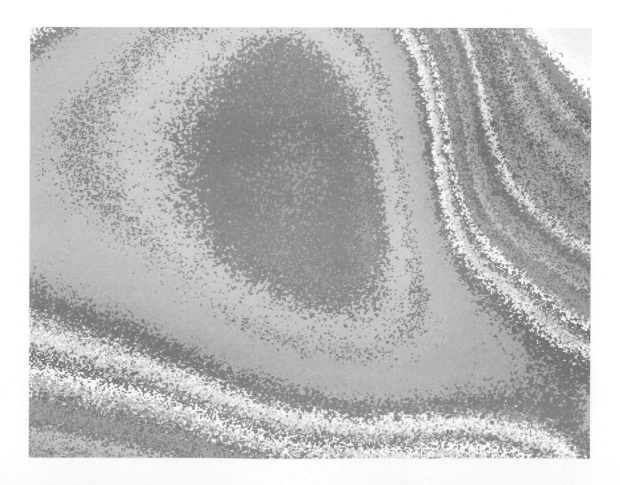

CHAPTER

Evolution and Philosophy

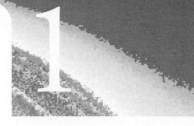

Joseph E. Murray

While auditing a course with first-year medical students recently, I noted their diligence, intelligence, and good manners. The first-year class of medical students is a clean slate, a selected group facing the future, with injury and disease as their only recognized foes. They have chosen their profession primarily as an opportunity for service; their other aims, to obtain material benefits sufficient to educate a family and to enjoy a reasonable standard of living, are secondary.

The essence of any profession is service to others. For a physician to contrast a profession to a business is neither pejorative nor self-laudatory; it is merely recognition of facts. The prime purpose of the medical profession is to give trustworthy service of the highest quality in matters of health, whereas the prime purpose of business is to make money for the owners and stockholders. A well-run business may, as a byproduct, provide more services than does its medical counterpart, but this does not negate the difference in their purposes. First-year business students have different goals and adversaries than do first-year medical students.

During our intern and residency days, most of our energies were spent caring for the sickest patients. We triaged in the emergency ward, resuscitated hearts, intubated guts and bladders and blood vessels, pierced peritoneal and thoracic and cranial cavities, all in the hopes of saving a life. No one will ever forget the deaths of some of these patients, over whom we had struggled so long and hard. Our rewards were immeasurable.

We who selected plastic surgery as a specialty were lured, perhaps, by the requirements for that extra finesse and skill needed to keep marginal tissues alive. Maybe we appreciated more than our fellow residents the aesthetic values of life. Probably we were more aware that disease and injury were not the only conditions requiring treatment, because we noted that natural processes such as aging could be devastating to some individuals. Possibly we saw more clearly that scars, birthmarks, or asymmetric ears and noses were handicaps worthy of correction.

During our plastic surgical residency programs we cared for a variety of problems: patients with congenital deformities from head to toes, head and neck cancer patients, those with military or industrial or domestic injuries, and patients with severe burns. The variety was so great that we became confused about the essence of our specialty when we tried to define or explain plastic surgery. It was not merely reconstructive surgery or a specialty based on an anatomic region; it varied from program to program.

GUIDING PRINCIPLES

The central theme and common bond in plastic surgery is an appreciation of the aesthetic outcome. For the plastic surgeon the total value of life must include personal appearance, whether in the child with a cleft lip, the person who was burned, the cancer patient, or the victim of a serious accident. Plastic surgeons also care about form and function, and many perform no cosmetic surgery at all. The essence of the specialty, however, is an appreciation of and interest in cosmetic surgery.

Given these premises, cosmetic surgery must not be exploited. Cosmetic surgery is too grand, noble, and important. The rapid acceptance by the public of cosmetic surgery confirms its value and the need for it. Cosmetic surgery brings immediate gratification to the patient and surgeon; it also brings an immediate infusion to the surgeon's bank account.

Another danger is the sequestering of patients and plastic surgeons from the mainstream of medicine and surgery. Rees,[4] in a 1978 address at the program director's meeting of the American Association of Plastic Surgeons, analyzed the adverse effects of isolation from the mainstream of surgery as follows:

I believe isolation is already a major problem within plastic surgery. Some of our fellow surgeons perform a limited repertoire of technical maneuvers and tend to become isolated from the mainstream of plastic surgery, to say nothing of the mainstream of surgery, and to say nothing of the mainstream of medicine. Such channelization eventually must lead to *isolation,* and isolation can only lead to *fragmentation*—the ultimate form of superspecialization. This one-way path of channelization, isolation, fragmentation, and invasion could well spell in the end *dissolution* and the end of our impact in the field of surgery.

Another current danger leading to exploitation in cosmetic surgery is the effect of prepayment. The value of prepayment for aesthetic surgery has been proved beyond doubt, because it does minimize patient dissatisfaction. Nevertheless, prepayment has a subtle adverse effect on the surgeon's attitude, because the surgeon can more easily forget obligations to society and ignore unfortunate, time-consuming patients, such as those with pressure sores, recalcitrant leg ulcers, and massive injuries.

Plastic surgery is not the only specialty sometimes guilty of charging excessive fees. The lucrative nature of any medical or surgical practice can be debilitating. Alton Ochsner has commented that when young persons contemplating a medical career state that it will give them a chance to make a great deal of money, he counters, "Whereas the physician can make a good living in medicine, the individual who becomes rich in medicine is a poor physician in that he is doing unnecessary medicine or charging too much or both." He adds, "In medicine we have a compensation far beyond the monetary one, and that is the opportunity and ability to serve people."

If plastic surgeons choose to restrict themselves to nonemergency, lucrative cosmetic surgery, they have a right to do so. It is indefensible for them, however, to consider this the mainstream of plastic surgery or to maintain that these standards also apply to those who still teach with sick patients in hospitals and emergency rooms.

Plastic surgery has gained a distinguished reputation. As with political freedom, however, it must be renewed with each generation. Every plastic surgeon should project the highest possible image in the community, the hospital, and the medical schools. It is not difficult to distinguish what is a proper image. Monroe,[2] in his presidential address, regretfully quoted the impression one of the other national meetings made on *Newsweek* magazine: "The proceedings have [had] . . . more the air of a fashion show than that of a gathering of skilled professionals."

The public and its elected representatives are currently increasing their involvement in the technical matters of education, certification, and related aspects of medical membership. The days of leaving such matters to the exclusive management of the medical profession are over. Nevertheless, surgery is still that "vital and unifying force in medicine." We can collectively use this force constructively if we love and respect our profession and are not swept away by the fads of the day.

No matter what their practice profile, plastic surgeons should strive to upgrade the residency programs in their area. They should become involved in the entire fabric of surgical practice and contribute significant time and money to medical schools, hospitals, and specialty programs. They should repay their debt to the society that educated them as its privileged members. Plastic surgeons should not forget the reasons they selected their profession and specialty. They are not engaged in a commercial enterprise with patients as customers to serve; they are professionals who care for fellow humans.

A PERSONAL PERSPECTIVE

After finishing medical school on Dec. 31, 1943, I completed a 9-month surgical internship at the Peter Bent Brigham Hospital and was called to active duty by the Army Medical Corps. During basic training at Carlisle, Pa, I met Andy Moore (alphabetically assigned in the platoon, Mo, Mu), the start of a lifelong close and dear friendship. Then I was randomly assigned to Valley Forge General Hospital in Phoenixville, Pa, to await overseas assignment.

During medical school and internship, my exposure to plastic surgery was minuscule. I had never seen a skin graft. I had scrubbed on cleft lip and palate surgeries at Children's Hospital. Doctor William Ladd, a founding member of the American Board of Plastic Surgery and the father of American pediatric surgery, did present a patient with esophageal stricture for whom he had constructed an antethoracic esophagus using a tubular pedicle. I still remember the happy little girl running up and down the hospital stairways. In retrospect, this must have made a subliminal impression on my future career.

Formal plastic surgery was nonexistent in Boston. Doctor V.H. Kazanjian, although recognized worldwide for his work during World War I, was dismissed by the Boston surgical establishment as "merely a dentist working at the Massachusetts Eye and Ear Infirmary."

Imagine my amazement, therefore, when I first appeared at Valley Forge Army Hospital, where Lt.-Col. James B. Brown was chief of plastic surgery and 1st Lt. Bradford Cannon was assistant chief. Literally thousands of battle casualty patients were under treatment. While awaiting an overseas assignment (which never came), I immersed myself in dressings and wound care, volunteered to monitor an epidemic of scarlet fever on the Plastic Surgery Service, scrubbed whenever I could, and in general pitched in whenever an extra pair of hands was needed. I was having an epiphany of reconstructive surgery. It was heaven!

Brown and Cannon had molded a group of general surgeons into a cohesive, efficient service. At Valley Forge Army Hospital I worked with such prominent surgeons as Milt Edgerton, Steve Lewis, Bill Littler, Dan Riordan, Bow Davis, Carl Lisher, Gene Bricker, Allen MacDowell, and future leaders of the Hand Society, Walt Graham, Ben Fowler, and Don Eyler. For the first time in my career, I met plastic surgeons who were part of the general mainstream of surgery and could converse with men such as Evarts Graham, Eliot Cutler, and Alfred Blalock as peers.

The skill in planning and executing multistage surgical reconstruction enthralled me. Removing dressings to see the postoperative result was like opening a present, always exciting even when disappointing. I will never forget running into Barrett Brown on the corridor one day after I had just removed the dressing on a "perfect" skin graft. I was overflowing with enthusiasm. He commented in typical Midwestern style, "Looking at a well-healed skin graft is like looking at a field of corn. You never get tired of looking at it."

Returning to the Brigham, I found resectional surgery, although challenging and demanding, less attractive than the reconstructions done at Valley Forge Army Hospital. A renal transplant program was in progress at the Brigham. I had become interested in transplantation biology at Valley Forge when we were forced to use skin allografts as temporary dressings on severely burned patients. Barrett Brown and I used to talk about the problem while scrubbing or during surgery. He had described in 1937 successful skin allografts exchanged between identical twins. He was pessimistic about the future possibility of human allografts, undoubtedly influenced by Leo Loeb of his own Washington University in St. Louis. Loeb had written a widely read book, *The Basis of Individuality,* in which he categorically stated that grafts between humans would never be possible because individual differences existed even at the cellular level.

Today I reflect on the varieties of surgical reparative procedures used in my lifetime and try to establish a hierarchy of concepts. The *reconstructive* element of surgery while I was at Valley Forge offered the most excitement and challenge. Later, back at the Brigham, the ultimate in reconstruction seemed to be *transplantation* (i.e., "spare parts" surgery), replacing a worn-out organ with a new one (Figure 1-1). In

1991 my surgical "dream" was *regeneration,* growing the missing tissue or organ in situ, obviating the need for human donors. Currently, several laboratories are busy studying organ and tissue regeneration. If I were granted another lifetime of surgical research, I would join some interdisciplinary program in genetics, embryology, and biochemistry.

Although I have been recognized by the Nobel Committee, I am well aware that no one person is responsible for medical progress (Figure 1-2). We all "have drunk from wells we did not dig and been warmed by fires we did not build." We all benefit from the dreams and work of our predecessors. The Peter Bent Brigham Hospital, now the Brigham and Women's Hospital, is one of the five major teaching hospitals of the Harvard Medical School. It was built as the University Hospital for the medical school when Harvard Medical School moved physically in 1906 from downtown Boston to its present location on Longwood Ave. The Johns Hopkins

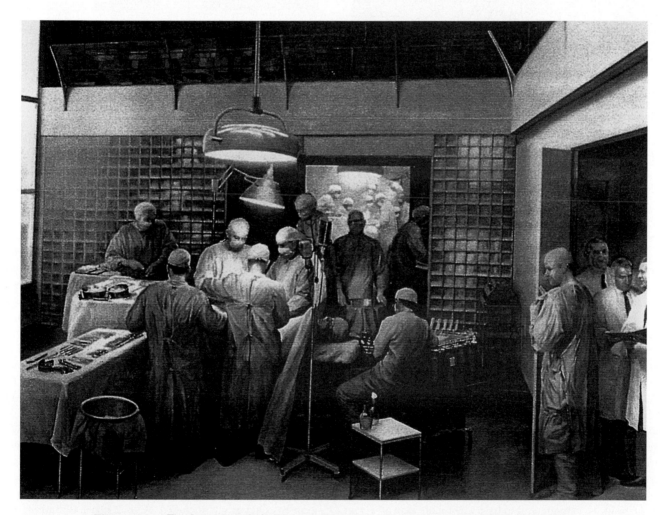

Figure 1-1. The first successful kidney transplantation as depicted by artist Joel Babb. *Left to right:* Miss Rhodes, scrub nurse; Daniel L. Pugh, assistant surgeon; Joseph E. Murray, surgeon; John L. Rowbotham, assistant surgeon; Edward B. Gray, assistant surgeon; Edith Comiskey, circulating nurse; Francis D. Moore, (bringing in donor kidney); Leroy D. Vandam, anesthetist (seated); J. Hartwell Harrison, donor surgeon (in doorway); Gustave J. Dammin, pathologist; John P. Merrill, physician, dialysis; and George W. Thorne, physician-in-chief. Richard Herrick, the patient receiving the new kidney, is shown on the operating table; his twin brother, Ronald Herrick, is the donor whose operation is seen in the next room *(center).*

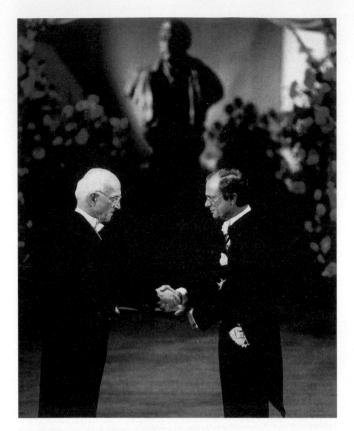

Figure 1-2. Joseph E. Murray *(left)* receiving the Nobel Prize from King Karl Gustaf of Sweden on Dec. 10, 1990.

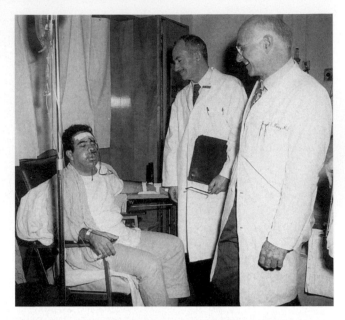

Figure 1-3. Joseph E. Murray *(right)* and Doctor Paul Tessier making rounds at Peter Bent Brigham Hospital, Boston, in 1970s.

tradition of full-time chiefs of service with associated laboratory space came to Boston via the Brigham.

The Brigham's first surgeon-in-chief, Harvey Cushing, demanded that the Brigham surgical research laboratory be located physically in the medical school, which was just across Shattuck St. The close relationship of the surgical laboratory to the medical school, and to the Children's Hospital as well, has been extremely valuable. Neurosurgery started with Cushing at the Brigham and Dandy at Johns Hopkins. The first canine and human mitral valve procedures were done at the Brigham in 1920s. Other pioneering approaches to patient care were developed in part or whole at these institutions. Doctor Robert E. Gross on patent ductus anteriosus, aortic coarctation, and vascular grafts; Francis D. Moore's monumental studies on body composition in animals and humans; and Doctors Thorn and Harrison on evaluation and treatment of endocrine disease. Not surprisingly, therefore, organ transplantation was born at the Brigham. The chiefs of service, administration, nursing, social services, and laboratories were all involved. It remains a vibrant institution continually alert to and supportive of new ideas. I am grateful to have spent more than 50 years there as a student, resident, or staff member (Figure 1-3).

As mentioned, no formal plastic surgery existed in Boston in the 1950s. Cannon at Massachusetts General and I at the Brigham worked with residents from general surgery to cover plastic surgical problems. Doctor Robert Goldwyn was the first Brigham surgical resident to go into plastic surgery, and Doctor George Gifford was the second. Both entered plastic

surgical programs headed by members of my travel club, Goldwyn to Pittsburgh under Willie White and Gifford to Rochester, NY, under Bob McCormack. Goldwyn became the editor of our journal and established the National Archives of Plastic Surgery in 1972 (see Box 1-1). My surgical chief, Francis D. Moore, although completely supportive of my work, always listed me as a general surgeon, never as a plastic surgeon, in the Brigham staff listing.

The first plastic surgical residency program in Boston started in 1966, a combined program of the Brigham and the Children's Hospital, with Doctor John Woods as my first resident. Meanwhile, I stayed in touch with our specialty in various ways: as a member of the original plastic surgical travel club organized by Milton Edgerton (members were Edgerton, Willie White, Dave Robinson, Steve Lewis, Reed Dingham, Bob McCormack, Dick Stark, Sam Paletta, and myself), as plastic surgical representative on the Forum Committee of the American College of Surgeons (ACS), and as a founding member of the Plastic Surgery Research Council, which I erroneously feared would harm plastic surgical participation in the ACS forum programs.

My first plastic surgical experience overseas was with Doctor Paul Brand at the Christian Medical College in Vellore, India. Willie White arranged for 10 plastic surgeons to train, for 2 or 3 months sequentially, an Indian surgeon selected by Paul to become head of plastic surgery after 24 months. Our group included White, Dave Robinson, Erle Peacock, Peter Randall, Jim Hendrix, Milt Edgerton, Frank Masters, Bob Chase, and Biff Bevan. It was a pivotal experience in my life, professionally and sociologically. The needs were overwhelming and the rewards far greater than we deserved. We learned much more than we taught. I am pleased to learn of similar programs by the American Society of Plastic and Reconstructive Surgeons (ASPRS) and of the many

Box I-I.
Preserving Plastic Surgery's History

The National Archives of Plastic Surgery was established in the Francis A. Countway Library of Medicine in 1972, sponsored by the Plastic Surgery Educational Foundation, the American Society of Plastic and Reconstructive Surgeons, the American Association of Plastic Surgeons, the American Society for Aesthetic Plastic Surgery, and the American Society of Maxillofacial Surgeons, to serve as a repository of the archives of the constituent societies, as well as of the manuscript papers, correspondence, iconography, film collections, historic instrument collections, artifacts, and memorabilia of these societies and of eminent American plastic surgeons. Doctor Robert M. Goldwyn, a plastic surgeon of Boston and currently editor of *Plastic and Reconstructive Surgery*, has served as unofficial honorary curator of the collection from the beginning and has acted as liaison between the Countway Library and the supporting national groups.

In addition to the large collection of Doctor Varaztad H. Kazanjian's papers, which include records of most of the patients he treated from World War I through the close of his career in the 1960s, the Archives has received correspondence files, manuscript papers, and other materials of many prominent plastic and reconstructive surgeons. Materials range from a few pieces, including letters, films, and photographs, to many dozens of cartons or transfiles of records. The Archives also has received archival files, consisting mainly of correspondence and manuscript records, of various organizations in the plastic surgery field: the American Society of Plastic and Reconstructive Surgeons (ASPRS), the Educational Foundation of the ASPRS, the American Associa-tion of Plastic Surgeons, the American Society for Aesthetic Plastic Surgery, the American Society of Maxillofacial Surgeons, the Plastic Surgery Research Council, the American Board of Plastic Surgery, and several regional societies.

The Archives has received more than 300 training films of the ASPRS Educational Foundation, as well as slides and other visual materials. In addition, the oral history video collection of prominent plastic surgeons consists of over 70 audio and video tapes. The Archives now contains a large collection of portraits of individual plastic surgeons and group photographs taken at meetings of the constituent societies.

Many historic instruments have come into the Archives along with the personal collections of plastic surgeons. Included in this category is Earl C. Padgett's original dermatome, splints and devices developed by Kazanjian, and instruments owned or developed by Vilray P. Blair, Joseph Safian, Jerome P. Webster, James Barrett Brown, Herbert N. Conway, and Caspar Epsteen.

More than 100 feet of vertical files contain biographic information on plastic surgeons in the United States and the world, as well as materials on the history of plastic surgery. The Archives provides reference service to plastic surgeons and others who may be working on books, historic projects, films, television programs, and exhibits in the field of plastic surgery.

Information from National Archives of Plastic Surgery, The Francis A. Countway Library of Medicine, 10 Shattuck St, Boston.

---

individual plastic surgeons who have organized to give service to developing countries. They enrich everyone.

My first surgical contributions were in the areas of head and neck cancer and transplantation. The major boost to my confidence was participating in a Boston surgical society program in 1954 on the radical surgical treatment of cancer. Sponsored by Grantley Taylor, my assignment was head and neck cancer, on a program with the giants of Massachusetts General Hospital, Richard Sweet, Joe Meigs, Wyland Leadbetter, and E.D. Churchill. Doctor Cannon and Doctor Kazanjian sat in the back of the hall, and I recall gazing at them at times for reassurance. I presented several patients with radical excisions and immediate bone and soft tissue repair. After the talk, Doctor Kazanjian was most encouraging. I poignantly recall him saying that he would never have been allowed to do such procedures.

EDUCATION AND RESEARCH

Sir Archibald McIndoe, renowned for his skillful surgery, headed one of the world's largest plastic surgical centers from World War II until his death in 1960. Primarily a clinician, he foresaw the urgent need for research facilities in his own institution to train fully the successive waves of young plastic surgeons under his guidance. Although McIndoe's concern was the problems of wound healing, surgical reconstruction, and transplantation of tissues, when the East Grinstead Trust was established, the primary purpose of the new unit was to encourage surgical research, "even if of an academic nature without immediate clinical application."

In the pursuit of knowledge, research may at times be an overworked tool. A more acceptable method of learning is the large scientific meeting. In the nineteenth century Cardinal Newman described the "university nature" of the annual meeting as follows[1]:

A fine time of year is chosen, when days are long, skies are bright, the earth smiles and all nature rejoices; a city or town is taken by turns, of ancient name or modern opulence, where buildings are spacious and hospitality hearty. The novelty of place and circumstance, the excitement of strange or the refreshment of well-known faces, . . . the amiable charities of men pleased both with themselves and each other; the elevated spirits, the circulation of thought, the curiosity; the morning sections, the outdoor exercise, the well-furnished, well-earned board, the not ungraceful hilarity, the evening circle; the brilliant lecture . . . the narratives of scientific processes, of hopes, disappointments, conflicts and successes, the splendid eulogistic orations; these and the like constituents of the annual celebration are considered to do something real and substantial for the advancement of knowledge which can be done in no other way.

The annual meeting of the American Association of Plastic Surgeons by definition performs a "university function" because it "organizes the teaching and study of a higher branch of learning." I propose to synthesize the attitude of basic research as outlined by McIndoe with the spirit of the university as embodied by the Association.

Doctor Cronin succinctly stressed "excellence in plastic surgery" in his presidential address in 1964. Technical mastery has always been and always will be the sine qua non for success in plastic surgery. As Rank[3] stated, "[T]he moving and handling of tissues with impaired viability calls for an order of technical exactitude beyond that practiced in the general run of excisional surgery."

After achievement of surgical excellence, the teaching of our skills becomes the predominant urge. We glow as we observe the resident maneuver the Z-plasty, critically weigh the bulky cancer, or finally grasp the psychology behind the nasal hump. Teaching also forces us to keep abreast of developments in wider fields.

The third rung of learning, research, is a more elusive pursuit. True research must always be wholly unpredictable; we cannot know in advance the paths to be trod or the new ideas to be weighed. Whether called basic, fundamental, applied, or clinical (all relatively meaningless terms), research may appear haphazard or improvised because wholly original observations cannot be anticipated. To do so, the observations would have to be surmised on the basis of previously known facts. This is why most original leads are accidental findings made by individuals with a talent for noticing the unexpected. It is impractical and unrealistic to ask what value the results will have. The question can never be answered. We study, we muse, we seek gold but may find oil. Research is a marvelous gamble that makes good sense.

Research is a frame of mind, an ability to see new relationships in familiar surroundings. Expensive laboratories and equipment are not necessary, even in this era of electronic gadgetry. When the first president of the British College of General Practitioners, Doctor William Pickles, celebrated his eightieth birthday in March 1965, a memorial book containing the signatures of almost all his rural patients was presented to him to mark his 50 years of service.

During these years, in addition to his busy practice, he had found time to achieve an international reputation as an epidemiologist. He was the first practitioner in Britain to recognize and describe Bornholm disease; he had studied the slow but steady spread of infectious hepatitis from village to village, by fête or wedding, to define the period of incubation and infectiousness of this disease. He has lectured on five continents. His alert mind saw new relationships in familiar surroundings.

Each specialty has reasons for its inception and continuing existence. However, justification for the inception of a specialty does not ensure its permanence. No surgical specialty has an inherent right to a permanent existence. There is a natural selection and survival of all scientific specialties. The analogy to self-renewal for society may be applied. A specialty "that has reached the heights of excellence may already be caught in the rigidities which will bring it down. An institution may hold itself up to the highest standards and yet already be entombed in the complacency that will eventually spell its decline."

Just as the birth of new specialties such as cardiac surgery is obvious, it is possible to envision new coalitions of existing specialties such as orthopedic and plastic surgery or the demise or radical constriction of others such as otolaryngology. Highly principled workers in every division of surgery will keep looking for new and better ways of doing things. This trait of superior men and women can lead only to more and better new branches of medicine. "No specialty of medicine can be formed merely by a desire for one. A specialty grows in response to research, study, perfection of techniques and popular demand. Specialties made up to satisfy the egos of inferior men are bound to fall by the wayside."

REFERENCES

1. Blehl VF: *The Essential Newman,* pp. 164, 165, New York, 1963, Mentor. (Quoted by Dunphy JE: *New Engl J Med* 271:1245, 1964.

2. Monroe CW: A plea for balance, presidential address, *Plast Reconstr Surg* 52:471-475, 1973.

3. Rank B: Training of plastic surgeons, *Brit J Plast Surg* 17:217, 1964.

4. Rees: Personal communication.

Organizations and Education

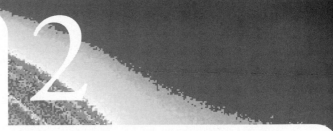

M. J. Jurkiewicz

DEVELOPMENT OF ORGANIZATIONAL STRUCTURE

Organizations in the field of plastic surgery vary in their specific focus (Box 2-1). In general, however, they are established to foster competence in practitioners and thus improve patient care and reassure the public.

This American system contrasts sharply with that in the United Kingdom, where governance of the surgical profession is delegated by the Crown to the Royal College of Surgeons. The Royal College determines the number of surgical registrars and consultants in plastic surgery, whereas the American College of Surgeons has neither sought nor been given such authority. The American system is pluralistic, consisting of voluntary organizations, and adheres to the principle of checks and balances inherent in the three branches of U.S. civic government: executive, legislative, and judicial.

American Surgical Association and American College of Surgeons

The first national organization of surgeons was the American Surgical Association (ASA), established in 1880 by Samuel D. Gross of Philadelphia. Gross stated, "The object of both of these societies [Philadelphia Academy of Surgeons in 1879 and ASA], as expressed in their respective constitutions, prepared by myself and afterwards adopted with certain modifications, is the improvement of the art and science of surgery, and the promotion of the interest not only of their Fellows but of the medical profession at large."[5]

The ASA's creation was prompted to some extent by dissatisfaction with the American Medical Association (AMA) and its surgical section. As E.M. More noted in his 1884 ASA presidential address, "We need a consultation of surgeons. . . . I desire to see the men who practice surgery in its truly comprehensive sense come together for consultation and social intercourse from every part of our great country—the men that represent the art of the nation."[5] Although national in concept, the ASA was dominated by Philadelphia surgeons and the Eastern seaboard.

The first journal devoted to surgery was *Surgery, Gynecology and Obstetrics,* established in Chicago in 1900 by Franklin Martin and edited by Alan Knavel. Ten years later the Clinical Congress of the Surgeons of North America was organized in Chicago under the journal's aegis, which led 3 years later to the establishment of the American College of Surgeons (ACS) in 1913. The ACS, a purely voluntary organization of surgeons, was established to improve the surgical care of patients in North America. The patient care emphasis was explicit, rather than implicit as in the establishment of the ASA, where the focus was on consultation of the surgeons with one another and thereby directed toward patient care. The ACS is rank and file; the ASA is elite by invitation only.

The ACS set standards not only for fellowship but also for minimum training requirements and hospital standards. The standards, probably right for that time, were not so stringent as to exclude any large body of surgeons. The requirements were a medical degree, a 1-year internship, and 2 years as a surgical assistant. Candidates were required to present case reports on 50 of their surgical patients and an additional 50 brief reports. The ACS also examined the candidate's ethical and moral standing in the community.

American Board of Surgery

In 1935, Edward Archibald of Montreal, then ASA president, called attention to the growth of surgery and the only existing standards for surgical practice, those of the College. Archibald called for higher standards and the establishment of the American Board of Surgery (ABS). Evarts A. Graham of St. Louis chaired the enabling committee, whose recommendations included 1 year of internship, 3 years of surgical training, and the establishment of the ABS to evaluate and certify candidates through examination. The ABS was established in 1937 with Graham as chairman.

American Board of Plastic Surgery

Vilray P. Blair, the chief of the plastic surgery division at Washington University and Barnes Hospital in St. Louis, is widely credited as the father of plastic surgery in the United States. A general surgeon by training, he established his career and reputation in the management of patients with maxillofacial diseases and other conditions. Plastic surgical and reconstruction techniques were needed to rehabilitate these patients deformed by ablation of cancer, the ravages of inspection trauma, and congenital malformations. Blair's chief of surgery was Evarts Graham, chairman of the newly established ABS. In 1937 Blair, on his own initiative but undoubtedly approved by Graham as department head, toured the United States at his own expense to enlist support for establishment of a board of plastic surgery. He identified individuals who devoted a major part of their practice to plastic surgery and persuaded them that the time was opportune to establish such a board.

In 1938, prominent plastic surgeons attended an organizational meeting in St. Louis. Later that year the American Board of Plastic Surgery (ABPS) was established as a subsidiary board of the ABS. The ABPS became an independent board in 1941.

Box 2-1.
Organizations for Education Research and Governance in Plastic Surgery

EDUCATION AND RESEARCH
University/health centers
American Medical Association
American Surgical Association
American College of Surgeons
American Association of Plastic Surgeons
American Society of Plastic and Reconstructive
    Surgeons
American Society of Maxillofacial Surgeons
Canadian Society of Plastic and Reconstructive
    Surgeons
Plastic Surgery Educational Foundation
Regional and local societies in surgery and plastic
    surgery
Subspecialty societies
    Aesthetic Society
    Hand Association
    Hand Society
    Society of Head and Neck Surgeons
Plastic Surgery Section of American Academy
    of Pediatrics
Plastic Surgery Research Council
The Surgical Forum
National Endowment for Plastic Surgery

PROFESSIONAL GOVERNANCE
National Board of Medical Examiners
State boards of medical examiners
Medical center committees
    Privileges
    Peer review
    Ethics
    Behavior
    Competence
Regional societies
American Medical Association
American College of Surgeons
American Board of Plastic Surgery
Residency Review Committee
American Board of Medical Specialties
Association of Academic Chairmen in Plastic Surgery

Blair's speeches help explain the original subsidiary status of the ABPS. "It took a World War to awaken a rather unprepared profession to the need and the opportunity of this work [plastic surgery] well performed. This war need was met partly by a few general surgeons . . . but chiefly by individuals among the rhinologists, the gynecologists, the oral surgeons and from a few other specialties . . . working in *close association with the general teams* [emphasis added]. They quickly learned and many have remained outstanding figures in post war practice."[2] Training of plastic surgeons practicing in 1938 was disparate, and some had no formal surgical training before their war experience.

In a 1939 address to the ABS, at Graham's invitation, Blair requested "cooperation in bringing recognition to a very poorly organized group that is seeking to bring order into the practice of a very old specialty." He asked for ABS support in (1) the selection of candidates from general surgical services to represent plastic surgery and (2) the "underwriting or supplementing of possibly deficient formal basic qualification . . . by making provision whereby such men can be made eligible to work in first class hospitals where an efficient surgical housestaff is available."[2]

Blair was an essential pragmatist. He recognized the great difficulties that might be encountered by individuals certified by the fledgling ABPS but without "basic" formal surgical training in their credentials. He therefore reasoned that an initial subsidiary status to the ABS was necessary to make the ABPS viable and to give validity to its certificate. Graham was also a realist, and the collaboration of these two men was instrumental to the success of the ABPS.

Evolution of Standards
A firm grounding in the principles of surgery was essential in Blair's recommendation for standards of training in plastic surgery. Thus the 1 year of internship requisite for all practicing physicians was to be followed by 3 years of general surgical training and then 2 years of plastic surgery. The standards then established, in principle, that the candidate should have full general surgical training before training as a plastic surgeon.

After World War II the ABS increased its standards from 3 to 4 years of training after internship. Subsequently, the rotating internship was replaced by a straight surgical internship. More recently, semantics has dictated replacement of the term *intern* to *postgraduate resident year 1* (PGY-1).

Plastic surgery did not increase its minimum training requirements to 4 years after internship but maintained 5 years of minimum training. Although the de jure requirements for plastic surgery did not keep pace with the principle of complete training in general surgery, the de facto requirements did. Most training programs from 1955 usually have accepted candidates who were board qualified in general surgery. In the 1970s and through the present, the APBS has deemed board qualification in other surgical specialties as acceptable.

The current renewed thrust in curriculum reform has affected education at all levels, including postgraduate plastic surgical education. A growing interest has emerged in increasing training in plastic surgery from 2 to 3 years while still requiring only 3 years of general surgery (PGY-1, PGY-2, and PGY-3). Thus the general training requirement, in a sense, reverts to the original standard established in 1913 by the ACS: an internship and 2 years of surgical training. The required period of training for plastic surgery would not be lengthened overall but would be shortened by a year to 2 years.

American Association of Plastic Surgeons

In 1914, William Sherer of Omaha, Neb, stated that "surgeons with a special interest in plastic surgery should join together to form an organization in which they might exchange ideas and experiences and help educate others."[4] Truman W. Brophy of Chicago supported Sherer's idea of an association of plastic surgeons, which came to fruition in 1921 after World War I. The organization was incorporated in Illinois and originally named the American Association of Oral Surgeons. A condition for membership was both a dental degree and a medical degree, but at the third annual meeting in 1923 the association dropped the dental requirement and adopted the requirement of "fellowship in the American College of Surgeons for those who had distinguished themselves in the field of oral and plastic surgery."[4] The organization's name was subsequently changed to the American Association of Plastic Surgeons (AAPS).

Meetings originally were didactic and in 1924 included " 'wet' operative clinics . . . when members would observe operations and examine patients together."[4] The wet clinics were discontinued in 1947 because the group enlarged beyond the capacity of operating rooms. Meetings were then designed to improve patient care and to facilitate consultation among plastic surgeons. The AAPS was a clinical society that gave its members the opportunity to visit colleagues' clinics and observe surgical procedures.

From the beginning the AAPS emphasized papers on teaching and education. In 1937 the meeting in St. Louis focused on plans for establishment of the ABPS. Subsequently and until recent times, ABPS certifying examinations were always just antecedent to and in conjunction with the meetings of AAPS. In 1964 the AAPS sponsored the first meeting of the program directors in plastic surgery and continued to do so until the program directors recently elected to hold independent meetings. The AAPS also has offered 3-year funding for promising young academic surgeons in their research.

American Society of Plastic and Reconstructive Surgeons

Since membership in the AAPS was restricted, the need for a more inclusive society became apparent. In 1951 the American Society of Plastic and Reconstructive Surgeons (ASPRS) was established. For the past 25 years the purely educational aspects of the ASPRS has been largely assumed by its Educational Foundation. The short courses complement the symposia organized by the Foundation. The ASPRS has increasingly fulfilled the guild functions of organized plastic surgery.

AMERICAN BOARD OF PLASTIC SURGERY

The ABPS is essentially an autonomous organization and elects 18 directors from names submitted by various sponsoring organizations (Box 2-2). These organizations nominate directors, but the ABPS elects directors to replace those who have completed their 6-year tenure. The ABPS also elects its officers and sets its own rules. Once elected, the director's primary responsibility is to the ABPS and not the sponsoring organization.

Certification

The ABPS is responsible for certifying individuals who have completed the training requirements. After successfully passing a written qualifying examination, candidates submit case reports for a practice requirement, then take an oral certifying examination. The certificate states that the candidate has completed the requisite training in an accredited institution and has successfully passed examination by the APBS. This does not directly certify competence; the training program director is responsible for certifying competence through a letter to the ABPS.

Recently the ABPS appointed an executive director to assist directors in managing administrative duties.

Box 2-2.
American Board of Plastic Surgery:
Sponsoring Organizations

Aesthetic Surgery Education & Research Foundation, Inc.
American Association for Accreditation of Ambulatory Surgery Facilities, Inc.
Association of Academic Chairmen of Plastic Surgery
American Association for Hand Surgery
American Head and Neck Society
American Association of Pediatric Plastic Surgeons
American Association of Plastic Surgeons
American Burn Association
American Cleft-Palate Craniofacial Association
American College of Surgeons
American Society for the Peripheral Nerve
American Society for Aesthetic Plastic Surgery, Inc.
American Society for Reconstructive Microsurgery
American Society for Surgery of the Hand
American Society of Maxillofacial Surgeons
American Society of Plastic and Reconstructive Surgeons, Inc.
American Surgical Association
Canadian Society of Plastic Surgeons
Council of State Societies of Plastic and Reconstructive Surgery
Plastic Surgery Research Council
Plastic Surgery Educational Foundation

Residency Review Committee

The Residency Review Committee (RRC) is also essentially autonomous. Its parent bodies are the AMA, ACS, and ABPS, which nominate individuals to serve on the committee. The RRC accredits training institutions through periodic inspections. Site visits are conducted by plastic surgeons or physicians designated by the Accreditation Council for Graduate Medical Education (ACGME) and recognized for expertise in graduate education. These inspectors do not make recommendations but rather present data on the faculty and the institution. The RRC then makes a decision of approval, probation, or withdrawal of accreditation, which is reviewed by ACGME. The parent bodies to ACGME are the AMA, Association of American Medical Colleges (AAMC), American Board of Medical Specialties (ABMS), Coordinational Council on Medical Education (CCME), and American Hospital Association. The ACGME is ultimately responsible for the conduct of graduate medical education but clearly depends heavily on a properly functioning RRC within the specialty.

The RRC in plastic surgery determines whether a training program director, the faculty, and the institution are not only capable but do provide the training and education leading to a competent plastic surgeon. The RRC accredits the institution, whereas the ABPS certifies the candidate. The ABPS determines minimum training requirements and the curriculum in broad terms; the RRC determines the particulars and content of the curriculum; and the ACGME oversees.

Surgical Societies and Associations

Societies and associations within surgery are established in response to actual and perceived needs of its members. In general, they exist to foster dialogue among surgeons, who share experiences, data, research, and outcomes in patient care. They also serve a guild function to foster discussion and action on political, social, and economic issues. They are nonprofit entities that provide a forum for the educational needs of its members, thereby fostering improved patient care.

Regional and local societies also have both educational and guild functions. Many actively promote and foster resident education. They give young surgeons a forum for presentation of research in plastic surgery and often stimulate research by "seed money" grants to fledgling investigators. They serve the guild function at regional and local levels.

As with national organizations, subspecialty societies exist to meet their members' educational and guild needs. The difference is not only the much narrower focus of the educational content, but also heightened emphasis and concentration on a discrete segment of practice. The focus is inherent in the title of the organization (e.g., aesthetic, hand, head, neck). Although fragmentation of the specialty is an unintended consequence, education and thus patient care benefit within the field of concentration.

Universities and medical centers exist to educate medical students, physicians, nurses, and allied health personnel. They are the bedrock on which undergraduate and graduate education is based. They embody the future of plastic surgery and therefore must be supported and nurtured. In addition, physicians' continuing education, while originating with each patient contact, is stimulated and fostered by grand rounds, practical courses, and symposia.

Journals

Journals exist to further the education of their readers and "to build and support research communities among readers: and thereby improve our understanding of the science upon which patient care is built."[1] Education and research within the fields of medicine, surgery, and plastic surgery are published to enhance patient care and to create new knowledge through both practical and theoretic information. Journals also publish and often comment on papers presented at the meetings of organizations and societies. Thus their influence is profound for both progress and stability in plastic surgery.

TRAINING STANDARDS

As discussed earlier, the ABPS was established largely through the efforts of Vilray Blair with the assistance of Evarts Graham. As Blair had envisioned, the plastic surgeons in practice in 1938 and recognized by the ABPS were credentialed and accepted by their peers in surgery. Training programs were established, and graduates were credentialed after satisfactory completion of requisite training. In 1937, 99 individuals were certified from the initial cohort of applicants from diverse surgical backgrounds. Since then, more than 5500 individuals have been certified by the ABPS.

This educational process in plastic surgery and all the specialty fields represented by the 24 member boards of the ABMS has clearly benefited the public. Completion of the requisite training program and success in examinations are positively correlated with peer and program directors' rating of clinical competence. Successful completion of the process of certification by an ABMS member board is a useful index of a physician's ability. It is not a guarantee of excellence or even competence, however, just as lack of such certification is not, by itself, evidence of the lack of physician skill and competence. The public and society clearly regard board certification as a very positive credential. The benefits of board certification by an ABMS member board include recognition by the Federal Government, status in hospitals and managed care organizations, greater compensation and insurance reimbursement, recognition by colleagues, and requirements for fellowship in most specialty societies.[4] The ASPRS, AAPS, and ACS, for example, all require ABPS certification as a condition for membership. It is important to note, however, that evidence from experimental research is insufficient to establish an absolute, positive link between certification and competence (Box 2-3).

Alternate Pathways to Certification

Because the meaning of certification may be vague and medical organizations may be more concerned about members lack without ABMS certification being denied desirable employment, some organizations are developing accreditation pro-

---

Box 2-3
Studies on Board Certification and Competence

Anderson GM, Brook R, Williams A: Board certification and practice style: an analysis of office-based care, *J Fam Pract* 33:395-400, 1991.

Arnold DJ: 28,621 colecystectomies in Ohio, *Am J Surg* 119:714-717, 1970.

Ayanian JZ, Hauptman PJ, Guadagnoli E, et al: Knowledge and practices of generalist and specialist physicians regarding drug therapy for acute myocardial infarction, *N Engl J Med* 331:1136-1142, 1994.

Burg GD, Lloyd JS: Definitions of competence: a conceptual framework. In Lloyd JS, Langsley DG, editors: *Evaluating the skills of medical specialists,* Evanston, Ill, 1983, American Board of Medical Specialties.

Cooper JK, editor: *Medical malpractice claims: a synopsis of the HEW/industry study of medical malpractice insurance claims,* Washington, DC, 1978, US Department of Health, Education and Welfare.

Entman SS, Glass CA, Hickson GB, et al: The relationship between malpractice claims history and subsequent obstetric care, *JAMA* 272:1588-1591, 1994.

Flood AB, Scott WR, Ewy W, et al: Effectiveness in professional organizations: the impact of surgeons and surgical staff organizations on the quality of care in hospitals, *Health Serv Res* 17:341-366, 1982.

Hass JS, Orav EJ, Goldmans L: The relationship between physicians' qualifications and experience and the adequacy of prenatal care and low birthweight, *Am J Public Health,* 85:1087-1091, 1995.

Hickson GB, Clayton EW, Entman SS, et al: Obstetricians' prior malpractice experience and patients' satisfaction with care, *JAMA* 272:1583-1587, 1994.

Kisch AI, Reeder LG: Client evaluation of physician performance, *J Health Soc Behav* 10:51-58, 1969.

Lunz ME, Castleberry BM, James K: Laboratory staff qualifications and accuracy of proficiency test results, *Arch Pathol Lab Med* 116:820-824, 1992.

Lunz ME, Castleberry BM, James K, Stahl J: The impact of the quality of laboratory staff on the accuracy of laboratory results, *JAMA* 258:361-363, 1987.

Maatsch JL, Huang R, Downing SM, Barker D: Predictive validity of medial specialty examinations. Report submitted to National Center of Health Services Research, 1983.

National Academy of Sciences, National Research Council: Study of health care for American veterans. Report submitted to Committee on Veteran's Affairs, US Senate, 1977.

Ramsey PG, Caroline J, Inui TS, et al: Predictive validity of certification by the American Board of Internal Medicine, *Ann Intern Med* 110:719-726, 1989.

Rhee SO, Lyons TF, Payne BC, Moskowitz SE: USMGs versus FMGs: are there performance differences in the ambulatory care setting? *Med Care* 24:248-258, 1986.

Rudov MH, Myers TI, Mirabella A: Medical malpractice insurance claims files closed in 1970. In *Report of the Secretary's Commission on Medical Malpractice,* Washington, DC, 1979, US Department of Health, Education and Welfare.

Sanazaro PJ, Worth RM: Measuring clinical performance of individual internists in office and hospital practice, *Med Care* 23:1097-1114, 1985.

Schubert Associates, Ramachandran D, North American Health Management Service: Development of complaint classification and risk ranking system. Report submitted to Medical Board of California, 1994.

Scott WR, Flood AB, Ewy W: Organizational determinants of services, quality and cost of care in hospitals, *Milbank Memorial Fund Q/Health Society* 47:234-264, 1979.

Shapiro S, Jacobziner H, Densen PM, et al: Further observations on prematurity and perinatal mortality in a general populations of a prepaid group practice medical care plan, *Am J Public Health* 50:1304-1317, 1960.

Shortell SM, LoGerfo JP: Hospital medical staff organization and quality of care: results for myocardial infarction and appendectomy, *Med Care* 19:1041-1053, 1981.

Silbert JH, Williams SV, Krakauer H, Schwartz JS: Hospital and patient characteristics associated with death after surgery: a study of adverse occurrence and failure to rescue, *Med Care* 30:615-627, 1992.

Slogoff S, Hughes FP, Hug CC, et al: A demonstration of validity for certification by the American Board of Anesthesiology, *Acad Med* 69:740-746, 1994.

Taragin M, Sonnenbert FA, Karns ME, et al: Does physician performance explain interspecialty differences in malpractice claim rates? *Med Care* 32:661-667, 1994.

Williamson JW: Validation by performance measures. In Lloyd JS, Langsley DG, editors: *Evaluating the skills of medical specialists,* Evanston, Ill, 1983, American Board of Medical Specialists.

From Bashook PG: Personal communication, 1998.

---

grams to offset the competitive disadvantage with managed care programs. The American Medical Accreditation Program (AMAP) offered by the AMA is potentially the most far-reaching of such programs. Although still not finalized, the initial plan itself is problematic.[3] The AMAP lacks the rigor built into ABMS accreditation and appears to be self-serving to its members, not the public. Similarly, a number of accreditation plans circumvent the ABMS process and face the same problems with the AMAP.

These alternate pathways to certification have undoubtedly confused the public. They do provide some recognition to the physician who chooses such an alternative to ABMS certification, but the impact on the public and the profession is largely negative.

Role of Journals

The major journals have had a phenomenal impact on plastic surgery. Since World War II, plastic surgery has emerged from largely an empirically based art form to a surgical practice based on sound science. Journals have played the major part in the dissemination of the information necessary to develop new knowledge essential to modern plastic surgical practice worldwide.

Horton[1] recently stated, "Editors are the mediators and critics of a conversation among readers. Yet how do these interpretive communities form and develop? How can they be nourished?" These and other questions are very important: how, why, and when does the publication of new information influence a physician's practice? Such questions should serve to stimulate editorial research by journal editors in plastic surgery.

CURRENT ISSUES AND FUTURE RAMIFICATIONS

The principles that formed the basis for education and organization in medicine and therefore plastic surgery are rooted in voluntary participation in the establishment and adherence to standards set by voluntary organizations, beginning with the report by Abraham Flexner to the Carnegie Foundation in 1910. A system of checks and balances in such a voluntary system has served the profession well. As rightly stated, surgery in the United States is the envy of the world in the modern era.

The individuals who framed and established the standards in plastic surgery based those standards on parity of education, training, and experience. Blair and his ABPS colleagues in 1938 established the minimum requirement in plastic surgery as 3 years of training in surgery followed by 2 years of plastic surgery for a total of 6 years, since a rotating internship was required of all physicians at that time for licensure. The minimum requirement in general surgery was 3 years after an internship.

After World War II, educators recognized that 3 years in surgical training was insufficient and made 4 years the minimum. Some of these 4-year programs allowed 1 year of basic science or research. Because the program directors in surgery were uncomfortable with less than 4 years of clinical training, 5 years of clinical training has become the minimum standard since 1950.

The ABPS did not alter the minimum standard, although it has allowed board certification in other specialties (e.g., otolaryngology) also as a minimum standard before entry into plastic surgery. Program directors and plastic surgery residents, however, raised the de facto standard to the historic standard, that is, parity of training, education, and experience in general surgery. Five years of surgical training before entry into plastic surgery has been the overwhelming choice.

Consensus favors a 3-year plastic surgery requirement, largely because the requisite knowledge necessary for competence in plastic surgery has more than doubled. The amount of prior training in general surgery is undecided, but support is growing for a 3-year/3-year integrated concept of plastic surgery education among its leaders, most of whom were born in the immediate post–World War II period. Parity of training has been discarded in favor of training integrated by the director of plastic surgery. The current directors also believe that access to recruitment of medical students similar to approaches in orthopedics and otolaryngology is essential. Finally, funding looms large as an issue.

It is not coincidental that the training of plastic surgeons based on the principle of parity has produced individuals who have transformed plastic surgery. The myocutaneous flap was developed by McCraw as a resident in such a program. The transverse rectus abdominis myocutaneous (TRAM) flap was developed by Hartramph, Black, and Scheflan. All were products of full training in general surgery. The double-opposing Z-plasty for repair of cleft palate, the most significant advance in palate repair since the von Langenbach repair 150 years ago, was developed by Furlow, who was fully trained in general surgery.

A shift to the proposed and now partly implemented 3-year/3-year integrated program may have adverse effects. Less than full training in general surgery before entry in plastic surgery inevitably leads to a difficult transition from resident in training to surgeon capable of independent judgment in intraoperative decisions and subsequent patient management. The curriculum in surgery is the patient. Successful management of sick patients is the crux of a surgeon's competence. The patient base in plastic surgery primarily consists of well patients, all seeking amelioration of real or perceived somatic deformity. Some are extremely sick, with burns, head and neck cancer, septic pressure sores, trauma, sternal wounds, and infections.

The educational program in plastic surgery may produce surgeons, but the product may not be surgeons in the true sense but rather technicians selling their skills in the marketplace. The program director is responsible for choosing those who enter the specialty and validating the trainee's clinical competence and ethical suitability for the practice of plastic surgery. Will the public have the same sense of reassurance they now have with board-certified plastic surgeons? Will peers in surgery and in medicine have the same confidence in plastic surgeons' abilities in patient management? The answers will determine how well the program director's responsibility is met.

REFERENCES

1. Horton R: Prague, the birth of the reader, *Lancet* 350:898-899, 1997.
2. Ivy RH: Some circumstances leading to organization of the American Board of Plastic Surgery, *Plastic Reconstr Surg* 16, 1955.
3. Kassiner JP: The new surrogates for board certification, *N Engl J Med* 337:43-44, 1997.
4. Randall P, McCarthy JG, Wray RC: History of the American Association of Plastic Surgery. Presented at the 75th Annual Meeting of the American Association of Plastic Surgeons, Hilton Head, SC, 1996.
5. Ravitch M: *A century of surgery,* Philadelphia, 1981, Lippincott.

CHAPTER

Ethics: Theory and Practice

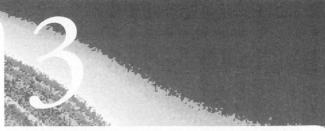

M. Sharon Webb

"We are physicians primarily, surgeons by choice and plastic surgeons for the joy of living. Our foes are disease and injury. The future is interesting."[35] Joseph Murray, the Nobel Prize–winning plastic surgeon, made these comments on the ethical orientation of plastic surgery more than 20 years ago. His observations remain true today. Any discussion of medical ethics in plastic surgery must not only acknowledge the traditions of medical ethics but also recognize the special issues in plastic surgery. Understanding the nature of the specialty is a prerequisite for useful ethical analysis, and plastic surgeons possess the necessary first-hand knowledge.

This chapter first discusses the general methodologies used in medical ethics, evaluating the ethical dimensions of familiar and novel problems that surgeons encounter in day-to-day practice. The chapter then identifies specific ethical problems that plastic surgery faces today and will face in the future.

MORAL PHILOSOPHY AND MEDICINE: ROLE OF NORMATIVE ETHICS

Medical ethics involves the application of ethical theory and moral reasoning to medicine. *Ethics* is defined as the philosophical inquiry into the nature and ground of morality.[7] In straightforward situations, we know what moral choice to make. Lying, stealing, and murder are morally wrong; it is therefore morally right to avoid them. Other situations, such as those often found in medicine, are more complex. Right and wrong may not be clearly evident, or there may be no choice that seems the right one. Ethical theory can be useful in both straightforward and complex situations: in cases where we already know what is right and wrong, ethical theory helps us explain how we reached our conclusions; in cases where right and wrong are not easily identifiable, ethical theory helps us sort through the facts and arrive at a decision that is morally defensible.

The branch of ethics that focuses on the hands-on reasoning we use to analyze moral problems is called *normative ethics.*[13] This is the type of ethics with which people are most familiar. General normative ethics seeks to formulate a system of principles that is adequate to deal with the widest possible range of moral problems. When these principles are applied

specifically to problems in medicine, the inquiry is termed *applied normative ethics,* or more generally, *medical ethics.* Other branches of ethics are termed *nonnormative* because they do not directly address what a person should or should not do in a moral sense. Types of nonnormative ethics includes *metaethics,* which examines the language, concepts, and reasoning of normative ethics in philosophical terms; *social ethics,* which investigates connections between normative ethics and sociology, politics, and economics; and *descriptive ethics,* which is the factual investigation of moral belief and behavior.

This chapter focuses on general and applied normative ethics. General theories of normative ethics are divided into two categories: teleological and deontological.[15] *Teleological* theories (from the Greek *telos,* "end") assess the rightness and wrongness of actions in terms of their consequences. These theories are therefore also known as "consequentialist."[5] The most prominent teleological theory is utilitarianism. By contrast, *deontological* theories (from the Greek *deon,* "duty") hold that an act has inherent features that make it right or wrong independent of its consequences. These theories focus on what is in itself right or wrong, whereas teleological theories often allow the ends to justify the means.

Teleology: Utilitarianism

Utilitarianism, the most familiar form of a teleological theory, originated in the writings of David Hume[30] (1711-1776), Jeremy Bentham[9] (1748-1832), and John Stuart Mill[33] (1806-1873). Utilitarianism claims that the moral rightness of an action can be measured in terms of a particular good that it produces, such as pleasure, friendship, wealth, or health. The good that is produced for the utilitarian is a nonmoral good, that is, a good that has no intrinsic moral component. Health, for example, is not usually evaluated in terms of moral rightness or wrongness; health is a good in itself, desirable on its own terms. The utilitarian evaluates the morality of an action in terms of (1) the amount of a particular nonmoral good that the action produces or (2) the amount of a nonmoral evil (e.g., pain, illness) that the action avoids. This is the central principle of utilitarianism, the *principle of utility,* which assesses morality by balancing the positive and negative nonmoral goods that the action achieves.

The catch phrase for many utilitarians is "the greatest good for the greatest number." This is the social outcome of utilitarian calculation. The utilitarian universe is much more complicated, however, than this simple formula indicates. Although all utilitarians seek to produce the maximum quantifiable amount of a foundational nonmoral good, differences within utilitarianism arise with the type of nonmoral good to be sought. A major distinction in utilitarian thought can be drawn between those theorists who conceive utility only in terms of happiness or pleasure (the hedonists) and those who argue that other values (e.g., knowledge, health, friendship, beauty) represent worthwhile goods (the pluralists).

Another significant distinction within utilitarian thought separates act and rule utilitarians. All these thinkers accept that the principle of utility is the criterion for morally right actions, but they differ in whether they believe that this principle should be applied (1) on an act-by-act basis or (2) to general rules of behavior. Those justifying each particular act by looking at its consequences are called *act utilitarians*. Those who focus on whether a general type of action or rule is most likely to maximize social utility are called *rule utilitarians*. For a rule utilitarian, since the conformity of a particular act to an ethically valid rule makes the act moral, the consequences of each act need not be appraised individually, and beneficial consequences alone do not suffice to make the act right.

Utilitarian theories in medicine justify decisions by referring to the amount of a medical good the action brings about. A decision is right, for example, if it maximizes health and minimizes illness, if it prolongs life and avoids untimely death, if it supports wholeness and decreases disability, or if it maximizes well-being and minimizes suffering.[8] All these rationales are utilitarian in their structure; the action's morality is determined by its outcome. Each justification, however, depends on a different medical value. Prolonging life, for example, is a different nonmoral good than maximizing human wholeness. Here we can see a limit of utilitarian reasoning: how are we to determine which set of nonmoral goals to pursue when two sets conflict with each other? A utilitarian may try to break each value down into other utilitarian terms (e.g., pleasure or happiness), but this just begs the question. Utilitarianism does not itself provide a basis for justifying the choice of a nonmoral value for grounding moral decisions.

Utilitarianism is further limited when the moral decision maker must determine whose interests make an ethical difference. Even if all moral agents were to agree that a certain value (e.g., pleasure) is to be maximized in all situations, does it matter *whose* pleasure is at issue? Is all pleasure morally interchangeable, so that mine is no more important than yours in my ethical decision making? Or is the only available reference point that of the actor, a doctrine known as ethical egoism? Larger circles of moral referents move the actor from considering only the consequences to self to considering the consequences to family, community, nation, or humankind. This raises a practical difficulty for utilitarianism: the more diffuse the reference group, the more difficult it is to predict the consequences.

The choice of a moral reference group poses a more profound problem for utilitarianism. Utilitarianism itself cannot guide us in deciding which reference group has moral significance. We must apply other reasons to identify the person or group for whom consequences morally count. In medicine, for example, the patient often is identified as the relevant referent whose nonmoral goods determine medical morality, but the patient is determined to be morally relevant by referring to principles outside utilitarianism.

Moral philosophers who oppose utilitarianism argue that this theory is deficient because it contains no unchangeable principles of right and wrong. For the utilitarian, consequences are all that matter; since only the principle of utility determines right and wrong, no moral action is absolutely wrong in itself. Thus, for the utilitarian, all normative systems are subject to revision based on their consequences. If adverse consequences do not occur, as measured by their impact on maximizing a particular aspect of social welfare, an act cannot be termed morally wrong.

For example, if no adverse effects, as measured on the chosen nonmoral scale, result from euthanasia, either in a particular case (act utilitarianism) or in general (rule utilitarianism), no reason exists for calling the practice morally wrong. Likewise, the decision to preserve the life of a seriously impaired infant is evaluated by its social, economic, physical, or emotional consequences. This type of thinking is inherently limited because it has no bedrock moral principles; nothing is, absolutely, right or wrong. For the utilitarian, if the amount of a desired value that emanates from a particular course of action outweighs its negatives, the action is morally justified.

Deontology

The deontologist identifies certain features of behavior that are wrong in and of themselves, apart from their consequences. The life of the impaired infant has moral worth in a deontological system for intrinsically moral reasons: it is life and thus worthy in itself, or it is innocent life and thus does not deserve to be harmed. Deontological theories rest on various grounds, some secular and some explicitly theological.

The ethical thought of Immanuel Kant[31] (1724-1804) has influenced most subsequent formulations of deontology. Kant identified reason as the source of morality. Both the capacity to act rationally and the freedom to do so are essential to human nature. From this essential nature arises Kant's moral requirement that we always treat other persons as ends in themselves and never exclusively as means to our ends. This doctrine leads to the principle of respect for persons, which many modern moral philosophers have used to examine decision making in medicine.[22,41] Kant tested the morality of an action by referring to the "categorical imperative." This test first requires that a person view an action in general, or categorical, terms and propose it as a hypothetical rule. Then the person must ask whether this rule could be made into a universal law, equally applicable to everyone.[31] A rule, or "maxim" in Kant's language, that passes this test is considered moral.

Kant believed that universalizability is both necessary and sufficient to identify an action as moral. Other philosophers have affirmed other basic moral criteria, however, which serve as foundations for deontological ethical theories. Ross,[46] for example, considers the principles of fidelity, benificence, and justice to be markers for morality. Rawls,[42] in his Kantian version of a social contract theory, emphasizes the principle of justice. Nozick[36] concentrates on the rights of the person as moral landmarks. Veatch[48] builds his theory of medical ethics around the principle of respect for autonomy. Beauchamp and Childress[7] propose the principles of autonomy, nonmalificence, benificence, and justice as ways to evaluate morality in the medical setting. Although deontological theories vary greatly, they all seek to identify the morality of an action in terms of its inherent characteristics rather than its consequences.

As in utilitarianism, deontology has its limits. First, all deontological theories wrestle with the problem of justification. Why does a particular theory rest on one set of central moral principles rather than others? In medical ethics, for example, certain authors uphold the *principle of benificence* as the primary criterion for assessing the morality of a medical transaction. Various grounds may be given to justify this principle: a covenant of benevolence between physician and patient, a duty inherent in the physician's character, or a theological command "to love one's neighbors." If the justification is challenged or undermined, however, the principle can lose its moral authority.

A second, related issue for deontologists is the relative ordering of different moral principles and the reasoning used to resolve conflicts among them. For example, a person can endorse both the principle of benificence and the principle of patient autonomy in medical decision making. In medical practice, however, the two typically come into conflict: a physician may recommend a particular intervention as being in the patient's best interest, but the patient, exercising autonomy, may refuse the treatment. How can a person reconcile these two principles when they oppose each other in this way?

A third problem for deontologists is related to the first two and involves the limits of the ethical principles. If we accept that a particular moral principle is important, do we then have to make it absolute? The importance of human life is unquestioned, for example, as is the importance of autonomy. Should either principle take on absolute status, however, so that it always determines the moral choice even when other moral factors are involved? Debates among deontologists regarding abortion and euthanasia offer examples of ethical arguments that differ in their analysis of the grounding, priority, and absolutism of moral principles.

Moral Problem Solving

Medical ethics has not been able to reconcile deontological and teleological theories or to settle the controversies within each theory. Ethicists considering moral problems within medicine have relied on a variety of philosophical theories, with the expected plurality of outcomes. What is important for practitioners is not that they determine which theory is intellectually superior, but rather that they understand the strengths and weaknesses of each as applied to concrete problems. The two strands of moral reasoning are often found together in argumentation. Being familiar with each type of theory allows the practitioner to dissect its logic and implications. Understanding the structure of the arguments in moral problem solving allows the practitioner to view them critically, assess their adequacy in the particular situation, and explore their unintended consequences. As a result, the practitioner's strategies for dealing with moral complexity become more effective and more sophisticated.

CODES OF ETHICS AND THE MEDICAL PROFESSION: ROLE OF SOCIAL ETHICS

Ethical reasoning for the physician does not occur in a social vacuum. Understanding the social system within which ethical reasoning takes place is the general task of social ethics. In medicine, social ethics has an additional task. Beyond the received body of moral philosophy just outlined, the physician relies on the ethical norms inherent in the profession of medicine. Social ethics adumbrates these ethical norms and seeks to identify their function in relevant social organizations. The specific ethical norms of medicine have functions within its social structure, and these norms also connect the profession of medicine to the larger social order.

Self-Regulation and Norms

One characteristic of a profession is the power granted by society for self-regulation.[34] Codes of medical ethics are part of the structure of this self-regulation.[24] For many, these professional norms, rather than general principles of moral philosophy, constitute medical ethics. Society and physicians have always shared a concern for the moral aspects of medicine. These publicly espoused moral principles make the profession's rules for self-regulation accessible to the larger society and defensible in terms of shared presuppositions about the physician's role.

Principles that relate the physician's duties to persons outside the medical profession are termed *external norms.* These norms emanate from the physician-patient relationship.[38] Characteristics of this relationship are derived from the physician's obligations to help vulnerable sick people regain their health.[32] External normative obligations for physicians flow from the altruistic premise that the physician is committed to fostering the patient's good.[39]

Unfortunately for the practitioner, there is neither a universally accepted definition of what comprises "the patient's good" nor agreement within the profession or society on who should make this determination.[18] A paternalistic model allows the physician not only to identify the patient's good but also to actualize that good.[28] *Paternalism* generally involves the physician overriding a patient's wishes in order to bring about a benefit or avoid a harm. Contrasting with the paternalistic model in medicine is a focus on the patient's *autonomy.* Ethical theorists defending autonomy, from Kant and Mill through modern ethicists, contend that the person must identify a harm or a benefit and must make decisions accordingly. This emphasis on autonomy as a medical good to be upheld in the physician-patient relationship has gained ascendancy in medical ethics, although with controversy.[16,19] Current legal doctrines of informed consent tend to support the importance of the patient's autonomy in decision making, undercutting traditional medical notions of paternalism.[11] Both autonomy and paternalism, however, are compatible with the external norm of medicine that makes the patient's good paramount.

In addition to external norms, another set of norms involves relationships among members within the profession. These *internal norms* are also part of the profession's self-regulation. During the process of professional socialization, members of the profession are taught internal norms for intraprofessional relationships simultaneously with external, more traditional moral norms.[12] The Hippocratic Oath, considered the cornerstone of medical ethics, illustrates the intertwining of these two types of norms. Although teaching that "whatever houses I may visit, I will come for the benefit of the sick," the Hippocratic Oath also contains this provision: "to hold him who has taught me this art as equal to my parents and to live my life in partnership with him, and if he is in need of money to give him a share of mine, and to regard his offspring as equal to my brothers in male lineage and to teach them this art—if they desire to learn it—without fee and covenant."[29]

Codes of medical ethics in the United States reflect this Hippocratic legacy that combines internal and external norms. The code of ethics promulgated at the first meeting of the American Medical Association (AMA) in 1847 drew from the core of the Hippocratic Oath, professing the external norm that the physician will "minister to the sick with due impressions of the importance of their office, reflecting that the ease, the health, and the lives of those committed to their charge, depend on their skill, attention and fidelity."[3] Along with such external norms, this earliest AMA document incorporated internal norms drawn from the approaches to intraprofessional relations set forth by British physicians' organizations. The 1847 AMA code relied on sources that included the Royal College of Physicians' 1520 ethical code, Samuel Bard's 1769 treatise "A Discourse upon the Duties of the Physician," and Thomas Percival's famous 1794 essay "Medical Ethics, or A Code of Institutes and Precepts Adapted to the Professional Conduct of Physicians and Surgeons."[2]

The AMA Code of Medical Ethics was substantially revised in 1957 to shift its emphasis from intraprofessional etiquette to physicians' duties to patients. In 1980 the revised AMA Principles of Medical Ethics recognized the physician's responsibilities to the larger society.[4] Contemporary versions of these codes promulgated by medical specialties detail both the external norms of the profession and the specialty and their internal norms. For example, the American College of Physicians *Ethics Manual,* after detailing the physician's obligations to the patient, also offers guidelines on such intraprofessional issues as fee splitting, postgraduate medical education, impaired colleagues, advertising, and enticements of patients. The *Ethics Manual* reflects the concerns specific to practitioners of internal medicine. The American Society of Plastic and Reconstructive Surgeons (ASPRS) Code of Ethics addresses similar issues but concentrates on problems typically found within the practice of plastic surgery.* This code contains both AMA-type external norms and "specific principles" that consider such issues as advertising and publicity, solicitations for surgery, exorbitant fees, and unjustified surgical procedures. These specific principles reflect an acute awareness of the temptations that plastic surgeons may encounter, using a combination of general and particular internal and external norms.

Conflicts with Norms

Problems arise when the internal norms of the medical profession are seen as conflicting with the physician's external obligations, or when different external obligations conflict with each other. These problems are not limited to modern medicine. In the eighteenth century, Thomas Percival and John Gregory set out two conflicting paradigms of medical practice that retain vitality today. Thomas Percival,[40] a retired British physician, was asked to resolve a dispute that arose during an epidemic in 1789 about the division of medical labor at the Manchester Infirmary. The outcome of his intervention was an elaborate description of how doctors should interact with each other. Percival's Codes set forth a guildlike fraternal notion of the profession that emphasized its solidarity, altruism, and elitism.[50] A major focus of Percival's Codes was the need to minimize competition among practitioners and to present a united front to those outside the profession. Percival's vision of medicine was attacked by the more liberal John Gregory, who challenged the profession's autonomy and hegemony. He argued that the profession's desire to minimize competition interfered with the public's ability to compare physicians and thus choose who was best.[10,26]

The Percival-Gregory debate echoes in more recent disputes about the ethics of advertising. If medicine is like other businesses, in that the customer needs information to compare competitors in the marketplace, then advertising is part of this model. In this view the traditional notions of collegial and cooperative practice have the economic consequence of interfering with consumers' ability to compare professional services and make direct choices. This critique of tradition would be consistent with Gregory's position. Modern law regarding regulation of advertising also conforms to this view.[49] Specifically, professional medical codes prohibiting advertising have been struck down by the Supreme Court.[1] As a result of these legal trends, advertising has become part of the landscape of medical practice, clearly seen in areas related to aesthetic surgery.

The notion of medicine as commerce that underlies the Supreme Court's reasoning conflicts with both external norms that emphasize medicine's altruism and internal norms that encourage fraternal cooperation. Current Supreme Court doctrine is at odds with Percival's traditional image of medicine. Many practitioners, however, believe that Percival's vision is a more noble one. In this time-honored view,

---

*Available from the ASPRS Executive Office, Arlington Heights, Ill 60005.

self-promotion is not a seemly trait in a competent physician. Instead, providing quality patient care is likely to attract consumers and is unlikely to be perceived as direct competition with colleagues. John Owlsley's following articulation[37] of this position resonates with Percival's codes:

The ethical reason that physicians should not advertise is that medicine is a profession requiring special education and carrying with it special responsibility with standards and traditions of dignity that would be demeaned by something as intemperate as overtly selling services. Doctors are doctors because they want to make a contribution to the health of their fellow man, and only incidentally to make a buck.

The example of advertising shows how the traditional paradigm of the altruistic but autonomous profession setting its own terms for interaction with its consumers comes into direct conflict with the view of medical professionals as economically rational service providers in the health care marketplace. The collision of these two models has ramifications that extend far beyond this limited example. One set of arguments exemplifying this conflict sets forth a global challenge to medicine's traditional commitment to the patient, maintaining that the traditional ideals are inconsistent with the fee structure of medical practice.[44] From this perspective, physicians are criticized as self-deceiving or hypocritical in their ethical pronouncements, since the inevitable conflicts of interest arising in the profession seem to be consistently resolved by physicians in the direction of self-interest.[45] Another set of comprehensive arguments reflecting this conflict in paradigms reduces medicine to a set of business transactions that should be restrained by the same market forces as any other type of commerce.[23,27]

From these two perspectives arise various combinations of internal and external regulatory schemes for the profession as society grapples with the challenges of health care reform and managed care.[14] On one hand, a consistent theme in this literature is that the traditional understanding of the profession is undergoing drastic change, some of which may be positive.[43] On the other hand, even as the physician's commitment to the individual patient has been questioned, the profession retains enough societal support that the traditional focus on the physician-patient relationship remains viable.[17,21]

As the nature of the medical profession changes, so must the internal and external norms that regulate it. Current sociological literature confirms that the profession has lost some of its societally granted power to regulate itself.[52] This has resulted in a loss of social solidarity within the profession, allowing intraprofessional competition to become more prominent. As the internal professional norms weaken and as market-driven competition strengthens, the need for external regulation increases. Arguably, this process is a self-perpetuating one, with professional ethics diminishing in importance as government imposes more controls. A central sociological problem for physicians arises, however, when external structures or regulations impinge on the primacy of the physician-patient relationship. When this line is crossed, the core of professional self-definition is undercut. Balancing the need for new health

care structures with the highly normative professional traditions in medicine will continue to raise ethical issues along with social and economic ones.

In medical practice the interdigitation of ethical issues with economic ones is most clearly seen in plastic surgery. The recent silicone implant controversy highlights how vulnerable the specialty can be to attack on economic/ethical grounds.[47] In part this vulnerability relates to the nature of aesthetic surgery services. Aesthetic surgery, unlike much of medicine, is entirely elective and paid for on a cash basis. These services, then, fall more readily into the marketplace model. Consumers can regard these services as commodities to be bought and sold rather than as health care; surgeons providing these services may come to identify themselves more with businesspeople than with their fellow physicians.[25]

Reconstructive surgery also may be defined as "outside" the territory of health care delivery when these procedures address abnormalities of appearance that do not impose discrete physiological impairments.[20] The forces that tend to push plastic surgery beyond the purview of traditional medical care, however, make it even more important that these services be subjected to the strict scrutiny of medical ethics. Analyzing the practices in this specialty using the tools of moral philosophy and medical sociology will allow its practitioners to preserve its highest ethical traditions in the face of internal and external critiques.

MEDICAL ETHICS AND THE PLASTIC SURGEON: ROLE OF APPLIED ETHICS

Moral philosophy and medical sociology offer methodologies for problem solving, but identifying the problems is the first step toward their solution. Most physicians are familiar with the standard questions in medical ethics, which often involve life-and-death situations. How and when should life support be terminated? What rights do parents have in regard to withholding treatment from a severely impaired newborn? When can a mother refuse lifesaving intervention for herself or her child? Such issues are not usually the province of the plastic surgeon. Questions about allocating scarce resources are also common in medical ethics. How will it be decided who receives the donor organ or the rare, lifesaving drug? Again, the plastic surgeon usually does not have to confront these issues directly.

The plastic surgeon does encounter particular problems that arise from the special nature of the field. Gaspar Tagliacozzi, in the sixteenth century, is credited with describing some of the ideals that form the specialty's foundations: "We restore, repair and make whole those parts of the face which Nature has given but which fortune has taken away, not so much that they may delight the eye but that they may buoy up the spirit and help the mind of the afflicted."[6] Plastic surgeons have moved beyond the face that Tagliacozzi mentions, but they continue to emphasize this melding of form, function, and human well-being.[51] Recognizing the psychological importance of appearance to the patient distinguishes the plastic surgeon's role from that of other physicians, and gives rise to some of the particular ethical issues within the specialty. At the same time, the plastic surgeon must also deal with the more routine matters in medical ethics, including questions about autonomy, conflicts of interest, and physician-patient relationships. Sorting out how the methodologies of ethics can address these various concerns is the task of applied ethics.

Specific Approach

Christopher Ward[51] addresses the applied ethics of plastic surgery and offers a model on how to catalog the specialty's ethical problems. His model uses "bedside ethics" for plastic surgeons, "armchair ethics," and "ethics of the technological imperative." Ward considers bedside ethics to be those norms that pertain to direct encounters with the patient, whether at the bedside or in the consulting room. Armchair ethics is what plastic surgeons discuss when they are trying to solve the larger social problems. Ward finds the armchair role to be a relatively comfortable one, "where plastic surgeons are at their most relaxed and reflective, in an atmosphere where the problems of the world are easily resolved."

The armchair ethics I propose is more strenuous than Ward's but also more wide ranging in scope. This type of ethics can refer to all those situations where plastic surgeons are sitting in metaphorical armchairs instead of standing at the bedside or in the operating room. Armchair ethics then comes to encompass the larger role of plastic surgeons within medical, economic, or political organizations.

Ward's third type, ethics of the technological imperative, is not well developed in his writing; for Ward, this category seems to encompass all the problems that accompany burgeoning technology. Plastic surgery will have its own interpretation of ethics of the technological imperative that pertains to the specialty's discrete technological problems.

I offer this version of Ward's typology as a way to organize the applied ethics of plastic surgery. By examining the various roles plastic surgeons assume in their professional lives, we can better appreciate the contributions that ethical reasoning might make.

"Bedside Ethics"

Bedside ethics applies to day-to-day matters of patient care. For example, autonomy and the physician-patient relationship are among the issues that arise for practitioners as they structure a consultation, determine the patient's surgical goals, weighs their feasibility, and assists the patient in making an appropriate decision about surgical options. Confidentiality issues are another element of this day-to-day practice, as are relations with referring physicians, competing specialties, and third-party payers.

The special problems that emanate from the social context of human appearance also fall under the rubric of bedside ethics. How is the practitioner to communicate with the patient about aesthetic ideals? How is the physician to decide whether these ideals are realistic and attainable? How does the surgeon deal with the limits that biology and technology

impose on surgical optimism? These types of questions, although not traditional ethical ones, are part of the plastic surgeon's bedside ethics.

"Armchair Ethics"

In cosmetic practice the surgeon is more directly involved in the world of commerce, providing services in return for fees. As businesspeople, plastic surgeons use armchair ethics when, for example, they sit in an armchair with their accountant or business manager. Armchair ethics, according to this metaphor, comes to include the ethics that pertains to business transactions between physician and patient. The ethics of business dealings blends with the legal doctrines, as demonstrated by ethical/legal problems in marketing, fair and unfair competition, and conflicts of interest. The physician seeking to resolve these difficulties in a responsible manner may draw from resources in both law and ethics.

The armchair metaphor also extends to situations where the plastic surgeon is meeting with others to work on matters of health care delivery or health care access. Negotiations with third-party payers or with managers in health maintenance organizations thus involve armchair ethics. In these situations the physician must balance devotion to patient care with responsibilities to a larger society in which health care resources must be distributed justly. A physician occupying this "armchair" negotiates with others who have different perspectives and priorities for patient care. Political principles of justice at times may contradict the individualistic ethos of the physician-patient relationship. Those who work together to balance individual needs with communal ones must resolve the ethical conflicts entailed in a way that is satisfactory to all participants if a negotiated agreement is to endure. At the same time, physicians must be careful that their commitment to patient care is not co-opted by those who would impose more economically driven solutions to resource allocation problems.

A separate area for armchair ethics applies to formal encounters with other physicians in peer review organizations or in disciplinary organizations, where ethics again merges with law. Another area of armchair ethics is even more specialized: ethics ends and law takes over in those circumstances where the physician is accused of transgressing legal norms, whether in malpractice or in less familiar domains such as Medicare fraud, racial discrimination, or sexual harassment. In these situations the physician must seek the guidance of legal professionals and cannot rely on medical ethics.

All these environments share a common theme: the plastic surgeon has stepped out of the clinical "bedside ethics" context to assume another role where clinical proficiency loses its dominant importance. In these settings the plastic surgeon participates in transactions that may include nonphysicians as well as physicians and where physicians are likely not to control the course and scope of the encounter. These features may be disconcerting to the physician who is used to controlling the environment to achieve patient care goals. Although this environment and the resulting real-world problems may be less familiar, the physician's role is vital: the physician brings to the table the clinical perspective that would otherwise be lacking.

In these transactions, the physician is able to present the profession's perspective and more importantly to act as the patient's advocate. Part of the physician's ethical obligation includes a willingness to participate in these sorts of situations, and a willingness to become familiar with how to handle this role ethically.

The armchair metaphor extends even further, to those interactions that are entirely nonmedical. Physicians, still governed by armchair ethics, can have an important voice in larger political discussions. For example, plastic surgeons have made significant contributions to legislation about breast reconstruction and malpractice reform, where their voices were heard clearly from among the many interest groups affected by the legislation. If surgeons want to sit at the table in this "armchair," they must educate themselves in the methods of the organizations that dominate this discourse. At the same time, they must keep faith to their own specifically medical norms. Plastic surgeons will find that politicians and lobbyists have their own ethos, often quite dissonant with the precepts of medical ethics. If they are willing to occupy this armchair—often a quite uncomfortable one—it is they may be able to help shape policies in directions more favorable for patient care.

"Ethics of the Technological Imperative"

Ward's ethics of the technological imperative is his most open-ended category, one that he only sketches in his essay. The technological imperative is a well-known issue in the philosophy of science. It dictates that what can be done (technologically) should be done (ethically). The philosopher of science might question this assumption or seek to draw boundaries around it. Ward seems to be advocating the same approach.

Technology is of great interest to plastic surgeons; many practitioners and researchers are prolific innovators, whether in the laboratory or in the operating room. Discussions about the ethics of technology overlap with issues in traditional medical ethics and bioethics. For example, general questions about risky technologies, cost-benefit analysis, and proper informed consent have been analyzed by ethicists over the years in an extensive literature that extends beyond the scope of this chapter. Plastic surgery, however, raises its own technological ethical questions as it develops its own technology, whether it be the conflict of maternal-fetal rights implicated in fetal surgery or the parameters for clinical testing of novel technologies that new forms of breast implants raise for consideration. The ethics of technology, as applied to plastic surgery, is an area where the practitioner's special familiarity with the field and its developing frontiers becomes paramount.

Moral Dimensions

Of greatest importance to the plastic surgeon concerned about ethical issues is a sensitivity to the moral dimensions of medical encounters. Ward's typology helps identify arenas in which this moral dimension will manifest itself. Recognizing a problem as a moral one can then trigger the application of the tools of medical ethics. This chapter attempts to familiarize the practitioner with some of these tools.

TOWARD AN APPLIED ETHIC OF PLASTIC SURGERY

Medical ethics does not propose, of itself, to provide ready-made solutions to moral problems. This chapter provides few, if any, "canned" answers. Instead, familiarity with the methodologies of ethical analysis will allow practitioners to begin to solve problems. On discerning that a given situation in practice has a moral component, plastic surgeons can use the methods of ethical reasoning to help them delineate the moral issues that confront them. Each situation, however, may call for fresh analysis. Medical ethics only becomes useful only when it can be fruitfully applied to what practitioners face in real life. This day-to-day effectiveness in real-life situations is the hallmark of a successful system of applied ethics.

In developing an applied ethic for plastic surgery, physicians have access to a number of resources, some of which have been outlined in this chapter. Moral philosophy has pervasively influenced the field of medical ethics, as has the sociological analysis of the medical profession. Medicine, surgery, and medical ethics are best understood in a historical context; following the historical development of these disciplines allows plastic surgeons to appreciate better their contemporary position. A consistent theme in applying ethics to plastic surgery has been the need for intimate familiarity with the specialty's unique aspects. Practitioners have the advantage of this inside knowledge. This enables them to make focused use of the resources medical ethics provides to identify and analyze their particular problems.

Applied medical ethics is only relevant to practitioners if it addresses their concerns and experiences. The intersection between theories of medical ethics and actual clinical practice, however, allows a vital body of principles to arise that are particular to the specialty of plastic surgery. The forces at work in changing all of health care are especially powerful in plastic surgery. A well-articulated framework of clinically relevant ethical principles will serve the specialty well as it faces the challenges the new century will bring.

REFERENCES

1. *AMA v. FTC.* 638 F.2d 443 (2d Cir), 1980, affirmed by an equally divided Court 455 US 676 (1982), rehearing denied 456 US 666 (1982).
2. American College of Physicians, Ad Hoc Committee on Medical Ethics: American College of Physicians ethics manual, *Ann Intern Med* 101:129, 1984.
3. American Medical Association: *Code of medical ethics,* New York, 1848, H Ludig.
4. American Medical Association: Principles of medical ethics. In Areen J, King P, Goldberg S, et al, editors: *Law, science and medicine,* Westbury, NY, 1996, Foundation Press.
5. Anscombe GEM: Modern moral philosophy, *Philosophy* 33:1, 1958.
6. Barron JN, Saad MN: *Operative plastic and reconstructive surgery,* vol 1, New York, 1980, Churchill Livingstone.

7. Beauchamp TL, Childress JF: *Principles of biomedical ethics,* New York, 1989, Oxford University Press.

8. Beauchamp TL, McCullough LB: *Medical ethics: the moral responsibilities of physicians,* Englewood Cliffs, NJ, 1984, Prentice-Hall.

9. Bentham J: *An introduction to the principles of morals and legislation,* New York, 1948, Hafner.

10. Berlant J: Profession and monopoly: a study of medicine in the United States and Great Britain. In Havinghurst C, Blumstein J, Brennan TA, editors: *Health care law and policy,* Westbury, NY, 1998, Foundation Press.

11. Bianco EA: Consent to treatment. In American College of Legal Medicine: *Legal medicine,* ed 4, St Louis, 1998, Mosby.

12. Bosk C: *Forgive and remember,* Chicago, 1979, Chicago University Press.

13. Brandt RB: Ethical theory: its nature and purpose. In *Ethical theory: the problems of normative and critical ethics,* Englewood Cliffs, NJ, 1959, Prentice-Hall.

14. Brennan TA: *Just doctoring,* Berkeley, Calif, 1991, University of California Press.

15. Broad CD: *Five types of ethical theory,* London, 1930, Routledge and Kegan Paul.

16. Cassell EJ: Autonomy and ethics in action, *N Engl J Med* 297:444, 1977 (editorial).

17. Chervenak FA, McCullough LB, Chez RA: Responding to the ethical challenges posed by the business tools of managed care in the practice of obstetrics and gynecology, *Am J Obstet Gynecol* 175:523, 1996.

18. Childress JF, Siegler M: Metaphors and models of doctor-patient relationships: their implications for autonomy, *Theor Med* 5:17, 1984.

19. Clements CD, Sider RC: Medical ethics assault on medical values, *JAMA* 250:2011, 1983.

20. De Chalain TM: Ethical resource allocation and the quest for normalcy: is pediatric reconstructive surgery justified? *Plast Reconstr Surg* 99:1184, 1997.

21. Emanuel EJ, Dobler NN: Preserving the doctor-patient relationship in the era of managed care, *JAMA* 273:323, 1995.

22. Engelhardt HT: *The foundations of bioethics,* New York, 1996, Oxford University Press.

23. Ervin FR: Strategic business planning for internal medicine, *Am J Med* 101:95, 1996.

24. Friedson E: *Profession of medicine: a study in the sociology of applied knowledge,* New York, 1970, Dodd and Mead.

25. Goldwyn RM: What people think of plastic surgeons, *Plast Reconstr Surg* 80:294, 1987.

26. Gregory J: *Lectures on the duties and qualifications of a physician,* London, 1772, Strahan & Cadell.

27. Havinghurst C: The changing locus of decision making in the health care sector, *J Health Polit Policy Law* 11:697, 1986.

28. Henderson LJ: Physician and patient as a social system, *N Engl J Med* 212:819, 1935.

29. The Hippocratic Oath. In Areen J, King P, Goldberg S, et al, editors: *Law, science and medicine,* Westbury, NY, 1996, Foundation Press.

30. Hume D: *A treatise of human nature,* Oxford, 1888, Oxford University Press (edited by LA Selby-Bigge).

31. Kant I: *Groundwork of the metaphysic of morals,* New York, 1964, Harper & Row (translated by HJ Paton).

32. Kass LR: Professing ethically: on the place of ethics in defining medicine, *JAMA* 249:1305, 1983.

33. Mill JS: *Utilitarianism, On liberty, and Essay on Bentham,* New York, 1974, New American Library (edited by Mary Warnock).

34. Mirvis D: Physicians' autonomy—the relation between public and professional expectations, *N Engl J Med* 328:1346, 1993.

35. Murray JE: On ethics and the training of the plastic surgeon, *Plast Reconstr Surg* 61:270, 1978.

36. Nozick R: Moral complications and moral structures, *Nat Law Forum* 13:1, 1968.

37. Owlsley JQ: Some current trends in the ethics of medical practice, *Plast Reconstr Surg* 56:567, 1975.

38. Pellegrino ED: Toward a reconstruction of medical morality: the primacy of the act of profession and the fact of illness, *J Med Philos* 4:32, 1979.

39. Pellegrino E, Thomasma D: *For the patient's good: the restoration of beneficence in health care,* New York, 1988, Oxford University Press.

40. Percival T: *Medical ethics, or a code of institutes and precepts adapted to the professional conduct of physicians and surgeons,* Manchester, England, 1803, S Russell.

41. Ramsey P: *The patient as person,* New Haven, Conn, 1970, Yale University Press.

42. Rawls J: *A theory of justice,* Cambridge, Mass, 1971, Harvard University Press.

43. Reed RR, Evans D: The deprofessionalization of medicine: causes, effects and responses, *JAMA* 258:3279, 1987.

44. Relman A: Dealing with conflicts of interest, *N Engl J Med* 313:749, 1985.

45. Rodwin M: *Morals and medicine,* New York, 1993, Oxford University Press.

46. Ross WD: *The foundations of ethics,* Oxford, 1939, Clarendon.

47. Vanderford ML, Smith DH, Olive T: The image of plastic surgeons in news media coverage of the silicone breast implant controversy, *Plast Reconstr Surg* 96:521, 1995.

48. Veatch R: *A theory of medical ethics,* New York, 1981, Basic Books.

49. *Virginia State Board of Pharmacy v. Virginia Citizens Consumer Council,* 425 US 748, 1976.

50. Waddington I: The development of medical ethics—a sociological analysis, *Med Hist* 19:36, 1975.

51. Ward C: *Essays on ethics relating to the practice of plastic surgery,* New York, 1995, Churchill Livingstone.

52. Webb MS: Medical ethics under managed care: how can the patient survive? *Ann Plast Surg* 37:233, 1996.

Structure and Function of Skin

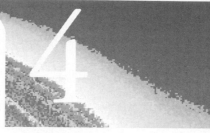

Hongshik Han
Thomas A. Mustoe

The skin (integument, integumentary system) may be the most abused organ system in the human body. Besides the many insults from the harsh extremes of the environment, such as cold, heat, wind, and the sun's ultraviolet (UV) radiation, the skin must withstand exposures from bacteria, viruses, fungi, and harmful chemicals, as well as numerous scratches, abrasions, and lacerations. The skin usually shows remarkable resilience and ability to repair and regenerate.

Although the skin is a forgotten organ whose function is often taken for granted, any breach in its function and integrity is painfully obvious. Death would result if the skin did not regulate and maintain the optimal body temperature for the life-sustaining enzyme reactions and did not prevent the loss of fluid and entry of pathogens.

ANATOMY

Skin is traditionally divided into three anatomic layers: epidermis, dermis, and subcutaneous tissue. Its characteristics vary over different areas. The skin over the dorsal and extensor surfaces is usually thicker than on the ventral and flexor surfaces. Also, the dorsal surface of extremities typically has the thicker hair, whereas the ventral surface of the male trunk has the thicker hair (Figure 4-1).

Epidermis

Epidermis is the outermost layer of skin and consists of stratified squamous epithelium with minimal extracellular matrix. The thickness of epidermis ranges from 0.05 mm on the eyelids to 1.5 mm on the soles. The ultimate goal of epidermis is to produce and maintain the waterproof, semipermeable *stratum corneum*. This is achieved by producing a pool of proliferative cells, which migrate from a basal regenerating layer to the environment in about 40 days.

The innermost layer of epidermis consists of a single layer of cells called *basal cells*. Malignant transformation of these cells produce basal cell carcinoma, the most common form of cancer in humans. Basal cells are columnar in shape, with the long axis perpendicular to the skin surface. These mitotically active cells divide to form *keratinocytes*, whose main function is

to provide a mechanical barrier. The cells in this layer are attached to one another by the intercellular structures known as *desmosomes* (Figure 4-2).

Keratinocytes synthesize water-insoluble keratin, which eventually becomes a major component of stratum corneum and functions as the effective water barrier. Keratinocytes also produce several cytokines that are involved in inflammatory reactions. These cells migrate outward to form the next squamous cell layer, called *stratum spinosum*. It is about five to 12 cells thick, and each cell is polygonal in shape. The daughter cells from the basal layer migrate individually, not as a unit, breaking and re-forming the intercellular desmosome bonds numerous times as they move upward. Malignant transformation of the cells in this layer results in squamous cell carcinoma.

The cells continue to flatten as they migrate outward, and their cytoplasm becomes condensed and filled with irregularly shaped keratohyaline granules, forming *stratum granulosum*. All discernible cellular components have disappeared by this layer, leaving only the protein-filled granules. The water content in the cytoplasm gradually diminishes, leaving the thin, homogenous, flattened, water-insoluble components that form *stratum lucidum*. When the cells finally reach the surface to form stratum corneum, the keratinocytes age and die. The remaining keratin forms a water-insoluble protective barrier against the environment until it is shed away.

Stratum corneum varies in thickness from 10 to 20 μm and is thickest in palms and soles. The squamous cells in the bottom of stratum corneum are arranged in orderly stacks of 10 to 20 cells that are highly interdigitated. As they move through the layer in about 14 days, however, they lose their intercellular organization and desquamate on the surface. Using radioactive and fluorescent labeling techniques, the keratinocytes transit time from the basal layer to the surface is an estimated 40 to 56 days.

Within epidermis there are melanocytes, Merkel cells, and Langerhans' cells. *Melanocytes* are within the basal layer and are wedged between keratinocytes in a ratio of approximately 1:30. They are not connected to the adjacent keratinocytes by desmosomes. Melanocytes function to provide a radiation barrier by producing and packaging melanin in distinctive granules called *melanosomes*. These melanosomes are then

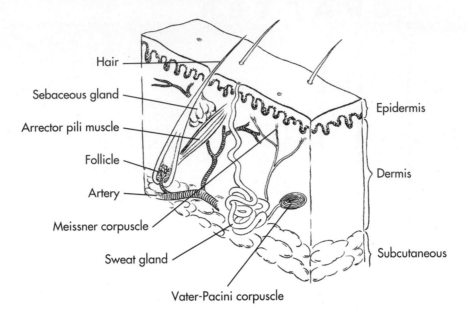

Figure 4-1. Cross-section of normal skin. Skin is anatomically divided into epidermis and dermis. Epidermis provides water-resistant physical barrier, and dermis the tissue mechanical strength with its abundant collagen fibers.

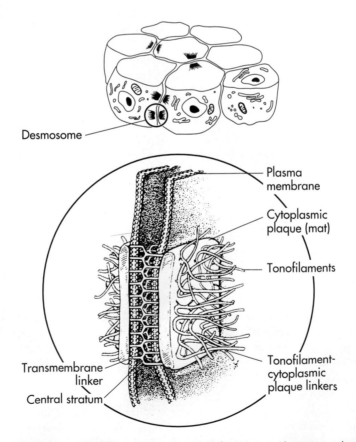

Figure 4-2. Desmosome-tonofilament complex. Each keratinocyte is connected to adjacent ones via desmosomes. The extracellular central stratum is the continuation of the transmembrane linker that is attached to the intracellular cytoplasmic plaque and its associated tonofilaments. These structures form a strong link between keratinocytes, providing a cellular mechanical barrier in the epidermis.

transferred from melanocytes to keratinocytes by the active pinocytosis of the melanocytic dendritic processes. They are subsequently sheared off by a process called *apocopation* and phagocytized by the local keratinocytes. Once within the keratinocytes, they aggregate and fan around the nucleus on the superficial side.

Melanin is found principally in the basal layer in Caucasians (whites), whereas it is found throughout the epidermis in blacks, including the stratum corneum. The density of melanocytes does not vary much among people with different skin color. The differences in the rate of melanin production and melanosome degradation determine the degree of skin pigmentation.

The purpose of melanin is to protect skin from the deleterious effects of UV radiation by absorbing UV light and trapping photochemically activated free radicals. Malignant transformation of melanocytes results in malignant melanoma. Its rarity in blacks is indicative of melanin's protective effect against UV radiation.

Merkel cells (tactile meniscus) are also found within the basal layer and are thought to be pressure receptors. They are very rare and are usually seen only by electron microscopy. Unlike melanocytes, they are connected to the neighboring keratinocytes by desmosomes and are thought to be of neural crest origin.

Langerhans' cells are located within stratum spinosum, or the prickle cell layer, and serve as the front line of skin immune reaction by identifying and processing the antigens for other local immunocompetent cells. These bone marrow-derived cells have numerous dendritic processes, similar to melanocytes. Langerhans' cells process the foreign antigens bound to the Fc portion of immunoglobulin G (IgG) and present them as class II major histocompatibility (MHC) antigens on its surface to the specifically sensitized T lymphocytes. Langerhans' cells also have surface receptors for the C3 component of complement and can carry antigens directly to the regional lymph nodes through dermal lymphatics. They are crucial in skin immunosurveillance against viral infections and cancer and are thought to play a major role in skin allograft rejection.

Dermis

Located underneath epidermis, dermis is the second layer of the skin and represents more than 90% of total skin thickness. The functions of dermis are as follows:
1. Provide the collagen matrix to support the epidermis
2. Maintain the dermal appendages
3. Provide the conduit for nutrients

The epidermal-dermal junction is an undulating boundary layer that increases the area of surface contact, thus increasing the volume of mass transport between two layers and decreasing the shearing potential along their junction. The basal cells of epidermis are firmly attached to the basal lamina by the anchoring proteins of the lamina lucida. The basal lamina, in turn, is fixed to the dermal sublaminar connective tissues (Figure 4-3). This *basement membrane* functions as a barrier to molecules greater than 40 kilodaltons. Mobile inflammatory and neoplastic cells, however, as well as many

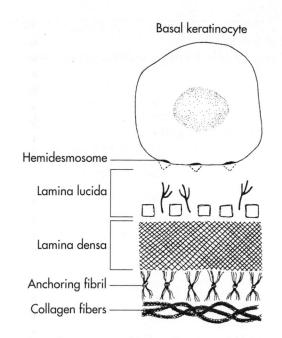

Figure 4-3. Basement membrane. The basal keratinocyte is attached to basal lamina (lamina lucida and lamina densa), which in turn is attached to the thick, underlying collagen fibers. Together, they form the basement membrane of the dermal-epidermal junction, providing an additional mechanical and chemical barrier of the skin.

species of bacteria, are capable of migrating through this structure. The basement membrane is also the site of immune complex deposition, causing various skin pathologies.

Blister Formation

The pathogenesis of skin blisters has an important relationship to the dermal anatomy. *Blister* is defined as the pathologic extracellular fluid (ECF) collection within skin. The dermal inflammation by neoplastic, chemical, or autoimmune causes, as well as the impairment of skin cohesion by traumatic shear stress, may result in the influx of ECF between the skin cleavage plane.

Blisters are divided into the two categories based on their anatomic locations: intraepidermal space and dermal-epidermal junction[4] (Table 4-1). The intraepidermal vesicles are further divided into the following three general categories, with considerable overlap, based on their pathophysiology:
1. The *spongiosis* type is characterized by intercellular edema with widening of intercellular spaces and stretching of "intercellular bridges," producing a spongelike appearance.
2. The *acantholysis* type is characterized by loss of intercellular cohesion with or without prior cellular damage, with subsequent cleft formation.
3. The *cytolysis* type is characterized by necrosis of cells causing disruption of epidermal continuity.

The blisters at the dermal-epidermal junction are also subdivided, but by anatomy, not pathology, as follows:
1. *Junctional blisters* within the lamina lucida are capped with full-thickness epidermis over intact lamina densa.

Table 4-1.
Types of Skin Blisters at Different Anatomic Layers

LAYER	BLISTER/CONDITION
INTRAEPIDERMAL SPACE	
Granular	Pemphigus foliaceus
	Bullous impetigo
	Subcutaneous pustular dermatosis
	Frictional blisters
Spinous	Eczematous dermatitis
	Herpes virus infection
	Mild heat and cold injury
Suprabasal	Pemphigus vulgaris
	Pemphigus vegetans
	Transient acantholytic dermatitis
Basal	Erythema multiforme
	Stevens-Johnson syndrome
	Toxic epidermal necrolysis
	Lupus erythematosus
	Lichen planus
	Epidermolysis bullosa simplex
DERMAL-EPIDERMAL JUNCTION	
Lamina lucida	Bullous pemphigoid
	Herpes gestations
	Cicatricial pemphigoid
	Suction blisters
	Heat and cold injury
Infrabasal lamina	Dermatitis herpetiformis
	Epidermolysis bullosa dystrophica
	Epidermolysis bullosa acquisita
	Porphyria cutanea tarda
	Lichen sclerosus

2. *Dermatolytic blisters* beneath the lamina densa result from connective tissue destruction in the upper papillary dermis.

Bullous pemphigoid is a junctional blister caused by the autoimmune IgG antibodies against the bullous pemphigoid antigen on the surface of the basal keratinocytes. The fine laminin filaments of the lamina lucida connect the hemidesmosomes on epidermal basal cells to the lamina densa, which in turn is connected to the sublaminar collagen fibers by a complex system of microfibril anchoring bundles consisting of type VII collagen.[3]

The compartment of this cutaneous basement membrane is identified as the target of IgG autoantibodies in blistering autoimmune disease. The resulting autoimmune inflammation causes abrogation of affinities among various extracellular matrix molecules. The antibody-antigen binding initiates the classic complement activation, with subsequent formation of the C5b-9 membrane attack complex leading to cell lysis. Also, the C5a chemotactic complement fragment and C3a, C4a, and C5a anaphylatoxins are formed, activating mast cells and basophils to degranulate. The resulting inflammatory vasodilation and influx of ECF into the lamina lucida result in the formation of blisters characteristic of bullous pemphigoid.

Collagen

The thickness of dermis ranges from 0.3 mm over the eyelids to 3 mm on the back. The thin, outer layer of dermis is called the *papillary layer* and consists of randomly arranged thin collagen fibers, abundant ground substance, and fine elastic fibers. The thick inner layer is called the *reticular layer* and extends from the base of papillary layer to the subcutaneous tissue. It consists of coarse elastic fibers and thick collagen bundles that are arranged parallel to the skin surface.

The structural base of dermis is based on the strength of its collagen. Collagen fibers can withstand a static load of up to 20 kg per single fiber of 1 mm in diameter. Postfetal dermal collagen fibers are mainly type I. Early fetal dermis contains mainly type III collagen, which is soon replaced by the more durable type I and remains only in the basement membrane and perivascular region. Constituting 70% of the dry weight of dermis, collagen is the most abundant protein in the body (Figure 4-4).

Fibroblasts synthesize procollagen molecules that wrap around each other in triple-helix conformation to form collagen. Each chain is approximately 1000 amino acids long, with glycine placed at every third unit. Its fibers contain hydroxyproline and hydroxylysine, two modified amino acids that are unique to collagen. Interfibril cross-linking occurs in the extracellular space between collagen side chains and is responsible for collagen's high tensile strength.

Elastin

Fibroblasts also synthesize elastin, a highly branching protein making up about 2% of the dry weight of dermis. Elastin fibers are composed of microfibril bundles and dense elastic matrix. They can be reversibly stretched to twice their

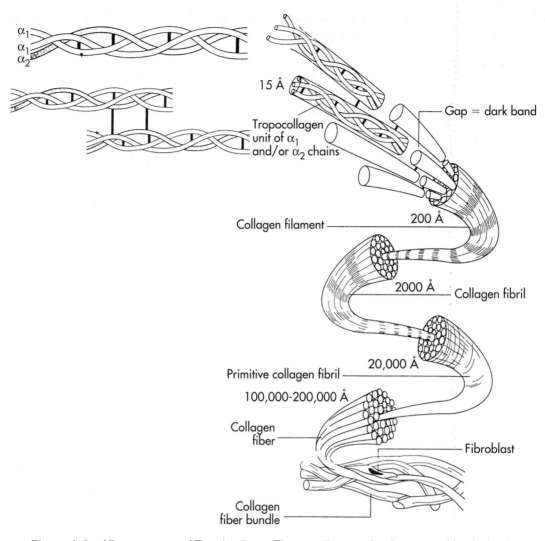

Figure 4-4. Ultra structure of Type I collagen. The procollagen molecules secreted by the local fibroblast wrap around each other in triple-helix conformation to form tropocollagen. The tropocollagen then forms collagen filament, which in turn forms collagen fibril and fibers.

resting length and thus function to return the skin to its resting conformation when stretched. Unlike collagen, elastin fibers contain end-to-side junctions, enabling contraction in two dimensions.

Ground Substance

Ground substance fills the remaining dermal space and functions to provide an aqueous environment for cell migration and integration as well as dermal protein modifications and collagen synthesis. The mucopolysaccharide ground substance is capable of holding water 1000 times its own volume. Also synthesized by the fibroblasts, ground substance is composed primarily of three glycosaminoglycans: hyaluronic acid, dermatan sulfate, and chondroitin-6-sulfate.

Histiocytes and Mast Cells

Histiocytes and mast cells are located within dermis. Histiocytes are mobile macrophages that clear up the debris created by local inflammation. Mast cells manufacture and release histamine and heparin.

Sensory Nerves

Various sensory nerves are within dermis, along with the intricate blood vessels regulating body temperature. Sensory innervation follows the dermatomal distribution of spinal cord segments.

The sensations of touch and pressure are detected by Meissner's and Pacini's (pacinian) corpuscles. *Meissner's corpuscles* are located exclusively in the papillae of palms and soles and mediate tactile sensation. *Pacinian corpuscles* are found primarily in the subcutaneous regions of palms and soles and detect pressure.

The unmyelinated nerve endings in papillary dermis receive the sensations of pain, itch, and temperature. Low-intensity inflammation creates the sensation of itching, whereas high-intensity inflammation causes the sensation of pain. Thus scratching may convert the intolerable sensation of itching into the more tolerable sensation of mild pain and eliminate pruritus.

Hair Follicles

Hair follicles are another important dermal appendage. They develop from the primary epithelial germ cells. The patterns of hair growth on the different parts of body vary greatly. Hairs on the scalp are programmed to grow long, whereas those on the chest or arms are rarely longer than an inch.

Newly grafted skin takes on the hair growth characteristics of the donor site, including the direction of hair follicles. The amount and type of melanin gives hair its color.

Each hair follicle has a smooth muscle called the *arrector pili* attached to its base near the dermal–subcutaneous fat junction at an obtuse angle (Figure 4-5). Arrectores pilorum are innervated by the adrenergic sympathetic fibers and contract to raise the hair on its end as well as to stimulate the secretion of sebum. Although important in many animal species, they are virtually vestigial in humans.

Sweat and Sebaceous Glands

Apocrine sweat glands are activated by the adrenergic sympathetic fibers and are found primarily in axillae and the anogenital region. They do not become active until puberty. In lower mammals they function to produce pheromones. In humans, however, the odor is from the bacterial decomposition. Apocrine glands open into the pilosebaceous follicle, not directly to the skin surface.

Eccrine sweat glands are supplied by the autonomic cholinergic fibers. They are concentrated on the palms, soles, axillae, and forehead but are present throughout the skin, except on the vermilion of lips, labia minora, glans penis, and inner aspects of the prepuce. Eccrine glands help to control body temperature by the production and evaporation of hypotonic solution.

Sebaceous glands are appendages of the hair follicles and drain into the pilosebaceous canal. They are not innervated by the autonomic fibers and are under the control of endocrine system. They are found over all parts of the body, except the palms and soles, and are especially prevalent over the forehead, nose, and cheek. They function to produce *sebum*, a mixture of fatty acids. Sebum's low pH and hydrophobic property function to suppress bacterial growth over the skin surface.

Sebaceous glands also lubricate hair and protect skin against friction while providing additional water-impermeable properties to the epidermis.

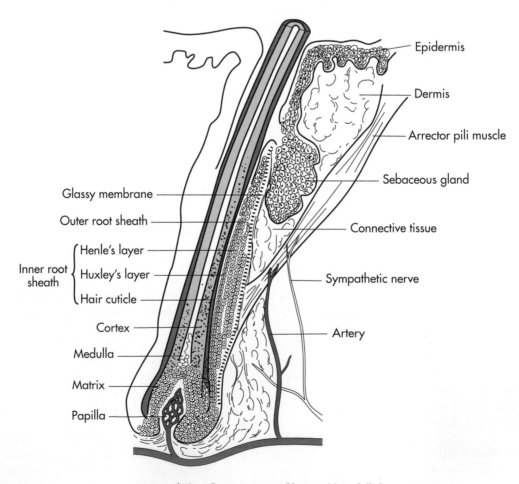

Figure 4-5. Cross-section of hair and hair follicle.

Blood Vessels

Adrenergic sympathetic fibers innervate the blood vessels to regulate vasoconstriction. Dermal arteries originate from the subcutaneous fat and form two horizontal plexuses, one at the dermal-subcutaneous junction and the other in the papillary dermis, interconnected by vertical vascular channels. Individual arterioles rise straight up to supply each dermal papilla (Figure 4-6).

The course of dermal veins inversely correlates with the arteries. The rate of blood flow through these vessels is regulated through both centrally mediated adrenergic afferent fibers and locally released histamine from the resident mast cells.

Glomus bodies are tortuous arteriovenous shunts (anastomoses) that permit great increases in blood flow through the skin when open. This allows a vast amount of body heat to dissipate. Glomus bodies play a crucial role in controlling body temperature.

The next section discusses the physiology of skin thermoregulation and its biomechanical properties.

EMBRYOLOGY

Skin is derived from both ectoderm and mesoderm. The epidermis, pilosebaceous glands, apocrine and eccrine sweat glands, hair follicles, and nail units are derived from the surface *ectoderm.* The ectodermal skin appendages develop with the formation of epidermis at 11 weeks of gestation and complete their development at 5 months. Melanocytes, nerves, and specialized sensory units originate from the *neuroectoderm.*

As early as 5 weeks of human gestation, the neuroectodermal components from the neural crest cells can be detected.

The epidermis initially consists of a single layer of ectodermal cells. Soon they differentiate and form a second layer of squamous epithelium, called *periderm,* over the surface. Peridermal cells are eventually replaced by the cells arising from the basal layer.

The keratinized peridermal cells desquamate and form a part of the *vernix caseosa,* which covers fetal skin throughout pregnancy. It is the greasy white substance enveloping the baby at birth and functions to protect the fetal skin from uremic amniotic fluid and to act as a lubricant during birth.

All components of epidermis are present at birth, and the peridermal cells are completely replaced by stratum corneum within a few months after birth. The mesoderm-derived skin elements form the structural components of dermis: macrophages, mast cells, Langerhans' cells, Merkel cells, fibroblasts, blood and lymphatic vessels, and fat cells. By 11 weeks of gestation the mesoderm-derived mesenchymal cells begin to produce collagenous and elastic connective tissue fibers.

The dermis projects into the epidermal ridges and forms dermal papillae. In some dermal papillae, capillary loops from the subdermal plexus develop to provide nutrients to the epidermis, whereas sensory nerve endings form in other papillae. The initial, simple, endothelium-lined capillaries in dermis acquire a muscular layer from the surrounding mesoderm-derived myoblasts and, as more simple single-layered vessels grow out from them, become arterioles and venules.

The embryology of skin has profound implications for tumor genesis, prognosis, and treatment.

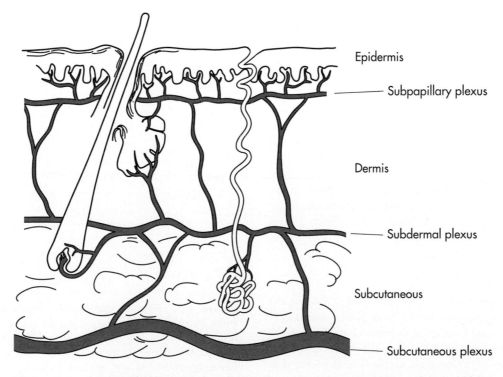

Epidermis

Subpapillary plexus

Dermis

Subdermal plexus

Subcutaneous

Subcutaneous plexus

Figure 4-6. Subdermal plexus and dermal vasculature. Note horizontal layers of dermal blood vessels, each interconnected by vertical vascular channels.

FUNCTIONS

Skin serves to protect the underlying structures from the environmental trauma by preventing the entry of pathogens and potentially toxic substances. Many resident bacterial species exist on the skin surface. Up to 10^3 colony-forming units of *Streptococcus* and *Staphylococcus* are normally present per gram of skin tissue. Further increases in the resident bacterial concentration on intact skin are inhibited by sebum. Highly acidic sebum is directly bactericidal to *Streptococcus* and *Staphylococcus* and bacteriostatic to many other species of pathogenic bacteria.

While functioning to protect its internal structures, skin must allow considerable compressions and extensions. Skin needs to be not only flexible and elastic, but also tough and durable. The biophysical properties of human skin to accommodate these functions are discussed later.

Other important skin functions are passive regulation of intercellular fluid balance and active regulation of body temperature. Water is transported from the dermal glycosaminoglycans to the surface by simple diffusion and by neurally mediated secretions from sweat glands. This fluid transport is a function of the skin's blood supply. Its water barrier property is provided mainly by the lower stratum corneum just above the granular layer.

At environmental temperatures above 36° C (96.8° F), heat is lost almost exclusively by evaporation. Below 36° C, heat is lost mainly through conduction and radiation. Normal physiologic water loss through skin is 0.002 ml/cm²/hr but may increase to 10 to 12 ml after loss of stratum corneum. The evaporation of 1 L of water causes a heat loss of 2428 kJ, or 580 kcal. Thus, in an average adult with a body surface area of 1.5 m², the daily normal physiologic water loss through skin evaporation is approximately 500 to 800 ml, with a corresponding heat loss of 1200 to 2000 kJ.[2]

The significance of the skin's water barrier and temperature regulation functions becomes especially apparent in burn patients.

PHYSICAL PROPERTIES

Skin is anisotropic and time dependent, as well as orientation dependent. The mechanical properties of any given area of skin are the functions of how fast and in which direction the tissue is undergoing the particular test, as determined by its inhomogenous components. The results from tests on skin in one direction may be greatly different from those obtained on skin tested in different direction.

Biphasic Load Deformation

The strength of dermis is directly proportional to the amount of polymeric collagen, since results from similar mechanical properties are obtained from collagen alone. Elastic tissue probably does not contribute significantly to the bulk properties of skin and may be partly responsible for the natural, resting skin tension. When the skin is stressed by a load, rapid extension occurs at first, followed by much less extension.[20]

This biphasic load deformation property of skin is based on the resting conformation of the collagen fibers (Figure 4-7). Each phase of the skin deformation curve is elastic. The collagen fibers are convoluted and relaxed at rest, but when stretched, these fibers straighten and become parallel. This biphasic property of the skin explains why, after a certain amount of initial stretching, the skin suddenly becomes very "stiff" and requires a considerably higher tension for minimal extension.

The extension of the straightened collagen fibers at failure is less than 10%, and this property gives skin its durability, or "toughness." The extension in each phase is directly proportional to the load applied because collagen fibers alone have no power of retraction. When the load is removed, it returns to its original length by the contraction of dermal elastin.

Viscoelasticity

The time-dependent property of skin adds another level of complexity in the second phase of the deformation curve. If a given load is maintained for a period, further irreversible extension gradually occurs. If a series of stresses are cycled, a slightly different curve is obtained for each cycle, and the curves converge as the number of cycles increases.[18] This is referred to as *creep* or *viscous extension*. This viscoelasticity of skin is the fundamental property to address in understanding its mechanical characteristics.

Another way to understand creep is to stretch a piece of skin with isotonic force. The skin expands rapidly at first, then slows down yet continues slow expansion.

Creep's counterpart, *stress relaxation*, occurs when a piece of skin is held at isometric length. In this case the force required to keep the constant length decreases gradually.

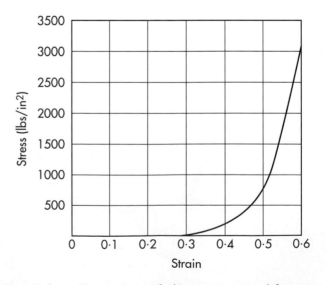

Figure 4-7. Elastic phase of skin stress-strain deformation curve. Note biphasic property of normal skin under tensile stress. As skin is pulled apart, initially, collagen fibers are convoluted and relaxed, thus permitting stretch with little force. However, once fibers straighten out and become parallel, much more force is necessary to stretch skin the same amount due to strength of the collagen fibers.

What happens during creep is unclear, but a gradual change in collagen fiber bonding occurs, or some other form of molecular rearrangement. One hypothesis is that when skin is placed under tension, the water is progressively displaced from the dermal ground substance as a function of loaded tension and time. This delayed efflux of fluid is partly responsible for the time-dependent characteristics of skin.

Even though the creep property of skin has yet to be elucidated, plastic surgeons use it daily in the form of skin flaps and tissue expansion.

CLINICAL IMPLICATIONS

The importance of skin tension in wound healing is immediately obvious when one examines scars in different parts of the body. The resting skin tension varies at different anatomic locations and is particularly high in all directions on skin over the sternum and shoulder, which partly explains the higher incidence of wound stretching and hypertrophic scars over such locations. When closing incisions in these areas, the surgeon should ensure that skin tension is minimized by undermining a wide margin of adjacent skin.

Wrinkles

Although the mechanisms responsible for the formation of wrinkles are not completely understood, they are thought to be related to the repetitive mechanical forces as well as the reduced mass of collagen and altered elastic network associated with aging. Mechanical forces play a significant role, especially for the expression wrinkles. The iterative facial muscle contractions over the dermal collagen matrix stimulate the resident fibroblasts and result in increased thickness of the connective tissue surrounding the muscle, forming the tension lines orthogonal to the direction of its contraction.[1]

The constant force of gravity also contributes to wrinkle formation. The gravity applied to the connective tissue straightens and pulls down the fibrils of the collagen fibers, in effect simulating the isotonic stretching of skin. The dermal collagen matrices are then remodeled permanently by the local fibroblasts.

Chronic Aging Skin

With increasing age the number of collagen cross-links increases, and the proportion of "soluble" to "insoluble" collagen decreases, as does the synthesizing capacity of dermal fibroblasts.[19] Skin becomes stiffer and thinner, with the resting tension of dermal elastin fibers diminishing. Dermal collagen turnover is slower and amount of collagen per unit area of skin is reduced in older skin.[14]

The conformation of collagen fibers also changes with age. In younger persons, fibers in the relaxed state are extremely convoluted secondary to high elastin content. As a person ages, however, fibers become less convoluted. In vitro, fibroblasts age and display a defined life span and potential for division. Human embryonic fibroblast undergoes about 40 to 60 mitotic activities, then terminates division.[5]

Collagen polymers can also be shown to "age" in vitro. The mature collagen polymers form numerous covalent cross-links among them by the condensation of lysyl aldehydes. The collagen cross-linking by lysyl oxidase is initially reversible but soon becomes stable. Other types of collagen cross-linking also increase with age, such as interpolymeric pyridinoline, histidinoalanine, and collagen glycosylation.

In normal individuals a linear decline occurs in dermal thickness after age 20 in both sexes[17] (Figure 4-8). The mean normal forearm dermal thickness of a 20-year-old white male is 1.1 mm, and that of a 70-year-old male is 0.8 mm. For white females the comparable values are 0.85 and 0.75 mm, respectively.

With aging the epidermis also thins, and the dermal-epidermal junction flattens out as well. The binding force between superficial corneocytes decreases,[11] but the rate of skin desquamation also decreases. This contradictory finding could be explained by the decreased number of desquamating epithelial cells in elderly persons. Torsional extensibility and elastic recovery both diminish in aged skin,[8] whereas skin flaccidity, or "slackness," increases.

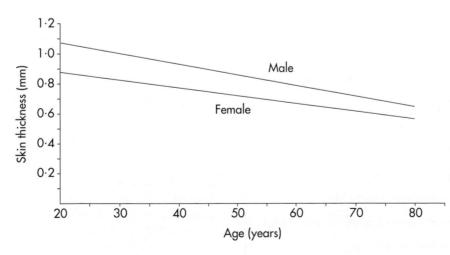

Figure 4-8. Average skin thickness as a function of age.

Besides the reduced density and modified organization of collagen bundles and the altered elastic fiber network, the absolute amount of glycosaminoglycan ground substance, especially hyaluronic acid, is also reduced.[9] These ground substances are responsible for skin turgescence because of their capacity to retain water. Also, water content is decreased in older stratum corneum. This may result from the primary changes in its water-holding capacity or from other alterations in the dermal layer, with less water being provided to the epidermis.

Another interesting phenomenon is that not only do the number of epidermal cells decrease in old age, but the individual cells decrease in size as well.[10] The thinner the skin, the less mechanically protective it becomes, making the aged skin much more susceptible to external damage.

Photoaging Skin

Skin is divided into six types based on the acute effects of sun exposure. Tolerance of sun exposure is a function of skin pigmentation and epidermal–melanin unit efficiency, from pale type I skin, which always burns and never tans, to dark type VI skin, which always tans and never burns[13] (Table 4-2).

The major component of solar radiation responsible for skin redness and erythema in humans is the ultraviolet B (UVB) spectrum, with a wavelength of 290 to 320 nm. UVB light is a complete carcinogen, able to both initiate and promote tumor induction. The potentially more destructive, smaller wavelength UV light is absorbed by stratospheric ozone and does not reach the earth. The visible wavelength of 400 to 700 nm is the familiar white light and is not capable of damaging human skin without the presence of photosensitizing chemicals. The wavelength over 700 nm is infrared light, which evokes heat.

Photosensitivity occurs when dermal photon-absorbing chemicals, called *chromophores,* absorb photons, move to an unstable higher energy state, and release the absorbed energy into the nearby structures and oxygen molecules. The oxygen molecules then become highly unstable free radicals that can destroy the local cellular constituents by transferring the unpaired electrons. More than 90% of UVB light transmission through the untanned skin is impeded by the stratum corneum, but the 10% that penetrates and reaches the basal layer is absorbed, mainly by the intracellular proteins and nucleic acids. UVB light absorption by deoxyribonucleic acid (DNA) forms thymine dimers, which are usually repaired efficiently.

When the efficiency of these repair processes is impaired, however, as in patients with xeroderma pigmentosum, the risk of cutaneous cancer sharply increases. These patients develop the xerotic appearance of photoaging, as well as basal cell and squamous cell carcinoma and melanoma, within the first two decades of life.

Two theories explain the acute effects of excessive sun exposure on skin.[12] One theory is based on the lag time of 4 to 12 hours between initial sun exposure and visible redness, possibly indicative of the delayed release of some vasoactive mediator from epidermal chromophores causing local vasodilation. The other theory states that a small amount of UV radiation may penetrate the dermis and be absorbed directly by vascular endothelial cells, damaging them and thus causing local vasodilation.

Plastic surgeons manage the chronic effects of sun exposure daily. The chronically sun-exposed skin is superficially wrinkled and roughened. Most cases occur in fair-skinned individuals of Northern European descent with a history of substantial sun exposure on the face, back of the neck, and dorsal surface of the upper extremities. The changes observed in long-term sun-exposed skin are largely irreversible, suggesting that the damage occurs at the DNA level as a result of interaction of UV light with the nucleotide base pairs.

In epidermis, thickened acanthotic changes and increased morphologic heterogeneity are seen in the basal layer. The leathery texture and blotchy discoloration of sun-damaged skin may be caused by the increased keratocyte melanosome content and its resident period within the basal layer. In dermis, accumulation of thickened irregular masses of tangled elastin fibers and clumped collagen fibers are seen, as well as increased fibroblasts with morphologic signs of greater metabolic activity.

Histologic studies indicate large losses of collagen secondary to the increased degradation in the dermis of chronically sun-damaged skin. The total collagen content of sun-damaged skin in one study showed a 20% decline compared with the non-sun-exposed skin in the same anatomic area.[16] The septa in the subcutaneous fat are contracted, forming wrinkles and deep furrows, characteristic of the photoaged skin. The fibroblasts cultured from chronically sun-exposed skin have slower growth rates and shorter life spans than the control cells from nonexposed sites of the same donor.

Clinically, these changes translate into slower wound healing and loss of immune responsiveness.

Racial Differences

Any study attempting to elucidate the racial differences in skin characteristics confronts the problem of separating the true racial dissimilarity and the effect of solar-induced skin changes. Clinical dissimilitudes exist, however, that are not attributable to mere differences in the cutaneous effect of solar radiation.

Table 4-2.
Skin Types and Sunburn Sensitivity

TYPE	DESCRIPTION
I	Always burns, never tans
II	Almost always burns, almost never tans
III	Usually burns, sometimes tans
IV	Sometimes burns, usually tans
V	Almost never burns, almost always tans
VI	Never burns, always tans

Black persons have less anatomic regional variations in skin characteristics than fair-skinned individuals because of the decreased effects of long-term UVB light exposure. No statistically significant difference exists in the thickness of stratum corneum between blacks and whites. Black skin has more corneocyte layers, however, and thus is more compactly bundled and requires more tape strips to remove the stratum corneum layer than white skin. About 20 corneocyte layers are observed in stratum corneum of blacks and about 16 in whites. Along with the data indicating greater electrical resistance in black skin, these findings implicate more intercellular cohesion and increased lipid content in black than in white skin. However, up to 2.5 times increased desquamation is noted in black skin compared with that of Caucasians and Asians.

Transepithelial water loss is greater in blacks than whites. Differences in skin permeability and barrier function have also been observed.[6] Decreased transcutaneous permeability to various chemicals has been noted in black skin. A significantly lower penetration of fluocinolone acetonide, dipyrithione, sodium lauryl sulfate, and propylene glycol is observed in black skin compared with white skin.

The shielding effect of melanin against UVB radiation is well known. The incidence of skin cancer in blacks is a fraction of that seen in fair-skinned Caucasians. Blacks have skin that is at least three to four times more photoprotective than white skin at all wavelengths.[7] The mean UVB protection factor for black epidermis is 13.4 and only 3.4 for white skin. The UVB transmission through black epidermis is 7.4%, compared with 29.4% for white epidermis. Thus the black epidermis is much less transparent to UVB radiation. Findings are similar for visible wavelengths.

An even more impressive salutary effect of increased melanin in black skin against UVB light is evident when comparing the minimum erythema dose of UVB radiation on intact skin of blacks and whites. The minimum dose on intact black skin is 10 to 30 times higher than on white skin, greatly exceeding that expected from mere differences in UVB protection factor and transmission efficacy.

Absolute amount of melanosome per unit area of epidermis is no different between blacks and whites. In blacks, however, the melanosomes are individually dispersed in the keratinocyte, whereas in whites they are grouped in membrane-bound aggregates.

Other than the increased number of corneocyte layers and more scattered distribution of melanosomes, few differences in microscopic skin structures exist between blacks and whites. No statistically significant difference exists in epidermal and dermal appendageal density, and variations among individuals correlate more with climatic changes than racial differences as a group. Therefore, with any racial variability, different topical and environmental conditions should also be considered.

Most of the differences in black and white skin characteristics are duplicated when the studies are done not to compare racial variations but to compare between different skin types based on sunburn and tanning properties.[15] Various studies have found that skin type V/VI has a more resistant barrier against UVB light and tape stripping of the stratum corneum, as well as quicker recovery once the perturbation occurs, than skin type II/III, regardless of the race.

Langer's Lines

The clinical implications of skin characteristics thus far have focused on the *intrinsic* variables of wound maturation, such as patient age, body region, skin type, wound size, associated illness (e.g., diabetes, chronic smoking), and postoperative complications (e.g., hematoma, infection). *Extrinsic* variables, on the other hand, include atraumatic surgical techniques, wound edge eversion, and direction of scar placement. The direction of scar placement deserves further elaboration.

German anatomist Karl Langer described the existence of natural skin tension lines in the eighteenth century. He observed that the stabbing wounds from a round-bodied awl produced *linear* clefts, not circular wounds as predicted. By making a series of such wounds across cadavers, he was able to discern that the long axis of such linear clefts align to form a linear pattern across skin. When Langer incised the skin perpendicular to these tension lines in the anterior thigh, the cut section showed the fibers in a transverse array. When cut parallel, however, the section showed fibers running alongside the incision. These observations led him to discover natural tension lines in human skin by the directional arrangement of dermal collagen fibers (Figure 4-9).

Langer's lines are not genetically determined and are probably caused by the tension from the underlying muscles and joint movements. They are generally perpendicular to the direction of muscles' pull. Any secondarily acquired tension over skin, such as from pregnancy, tumor, and wound or joint contracture, can readily change Langer's lines in the adult.

The direction of scar placement with resultant scar formation is most apparent in thyroidectomy incisions. The *vertical* incision perpendicular to the Langer's line results in a prominent, tight, contracted scar that is prone to dehiscence and takes longer to heal. The *horizontal* thyroidectomy incision over or parallel to the Langer's line results in a thin, linear scar that leaves little trace and heals quickly.

Over the upper sternum the Langer's line does not exist, and isometric tension pulls the skin in all directions. Any incision on this area is prone to develop wound dehiscence and prominent hypertrophic scar. This is more pronounced in female patients, whose vertical sternal incisions often turn into conspicuous, butterfly-shaped hypertrophic scars. The added pull of the breast tissue may increase the pull in an inferiolateral direction, thus widening the scar in the same direction, forming "butterfly wings."

Wound Healing and Tension

Most skin tension is borne by the dermal collagen matrix of the reticular layer. Therefore, when placing sutures to close any skin wound, the surgeon should place them through the dermis. The time-dependent viscoelastic property of dermal collagen allows slow yet persistent scar stretching if there is any underlying tension.

Wound support with sutures in place as long as possible

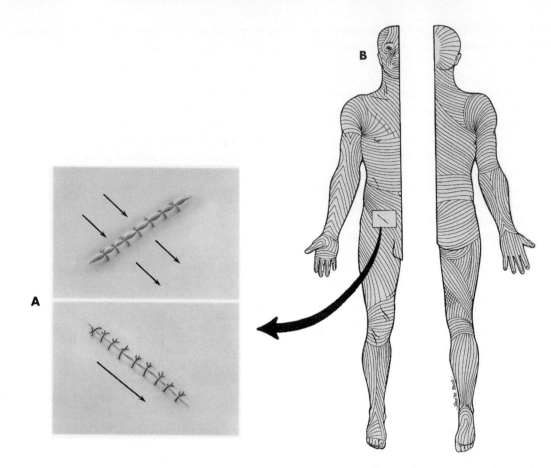

Figure 4-9. Langer's lines. **A,** When an incision is cut across cleavage lines, stress tends to pull the cut edges apart and may retard healing. **B,** Surgical incisions that are parallel to cleavage lines are subjected to less stress and tend to heal more rapidly. (From Thibodeau CA, Patton KT: *Anatomy & Physiology,* ed. 4, St. Louis, 2000, Mosby.)

improves the final scar appearance minimally, if at all. Additional scars would result from inflammatory reactions against the suture materials if they are not removed in timely fashion. Minimizing the underlying tension is more crucial to improve final scar appearance than keeping the sutures as long as possible in hopes of maintaining minimal wound tension. Wound tension is a function of the surrounding skin tension, not the degree of tightness or the length of time the wound is sutured together.

In general, the appearance of a scar is expected to improve for at least a year, and throughout wound maturation, its tensile strength gradually increases. When the normal maturation phase is extended by as yet unknown mechanisms, hypertrophic and keloid scars form.

Wound Contraction and Scar Formation

Uncontrolled wound contraction by overactive myofibroblasts is a major problem in skin grafting and wound healing. The contraction is not simply a function of tissue collagen content. Neither the suppression of collagen synthesis nor the inhibition of its cross-linking prevents wounds from undergoing contraction. Although initially beneficial in wound healing to reduce the wound size by counteracting the natural skin tension pulling the wound apart, severe wound contraction

creates excess tension in the neighboring healthy skin and distorts limb function.

The only definitive method to reduce significantly the amount of wound contraction is to cover the open wound with a skin graft or flap. Children have less excess skin over their face and extremities than adults. Thus the effect of wound contraction is much more devastating in children, resulting in significant distortions and permanent deformities. In children, burn wounds may contract to 15% to 20% of its original wound size without skin graft coverage.

The sequence of wound maturation is largely an unpredictable process. Great individual variations occur in scar formation and maturation, which are the function of many intrinsic and extrinsic variables. Immature scars tend to be red with indurated adjacent areas. As they mature, however, the redness and induration diminish, leaving scars softer and paler than the surrounding skin. In infants up to 3 months of age, wounds heal quickly with minimal resultant scars. In older infants and children, however, scars tend to be more conspicuous and likely will turn hypertrophic secondary to the increased skin elastic recoil. In mature, wrinkled skin of elderly persons with little elastic tension, scars settle sooner, with a better cosmetic appearance.

Scars heal differently at different body regions. Scars on the face and neck tend to be less conspicuous than those on the trunk and extremities, probably because of the more abundant blood supply and less directional pull in face and neck regions. Even within the same region, however, different local skin properties result in different scar characteristics. The coarse, oily skin over the tip of nose with numerous sebaceous glands causes more tissue reactions to injury and thus more prominent scars than the thin, hairless skin over the lip's vermilion border.

Healing Phases

The process of wound healing is not a simple sequence of disjointed events but a continuum of metabolic and physiologic changes lasting long after the superficial coverage of epithelium (see Chapters 5 and 7). The basic processes, however, are divided into three overlapping phases , as follows:

1. During the *inflammatory phase* the basal epithelial cells rapidly divide, migrate across the defect using fibrin strands as supporting structures, and fill the wound to epithelialize the surface by 48 hours.

2. About the third to fourth day after injury the *proliferative phase* begins. The fibroblasts migrate into the wound and begin to multiply rapidly and produce extracellular matrix. Some fibroblasts differentiate into myofibroblasts, whose smooth muscle–like contractile fibers pull the surrounding tissues together to contract the wound.

3. The fibroblasts and macrophages gradually disappear from the wounds in about 3 weeks, marking the beginning of the *remodeling phase.* By 6 weeks, the rate of collagen synthesis and degradation is increased but balanced, progressively organizing the collagen fibers. This is clinically manifested as the gradual flattening of the red, raised scar of the proliferative phase.

The process of scar remodeling continues after the initial violation of skin integrity and indeed persists throughout life. Herman Melville's account of the sailors suffering from the reopening of old wounds in *Moby Dick* illustrates the dynamic equilibrium of the collagen turnover.

REFERENCES

1. Balin AK, Kligman AM, editors: *Aging and the skin,* New York, 1989, Raven.

2. Despopoulos A, Silbernagl S: *Color atlas of physiology,* ed 4, New York, 1991, Thieme.

3. Fine JD: The skin basement membrane zone, *Adv Dermatol* 2:283, 1987.

4. Fritsch PO et al: Mechanics of vesicle formations and classifications. In Fitzpatrick TB et al, editors: *Dermatology in general medicine,* ed 4, New York, 1993, McGraw-Hill.

5. Hayflick L et al: The serial cultivation of human diploid cell strains, *Exp Cell Res* 25:585, 1961.

6. Kompaore F et al: In vivo evaluation of the stratum corneum barrier function in blacks, Caucasians and Asians with two non-invasive methods, *Skin Pharmacol* 6:200, 1993.

7. La Ruche G, Cesarini JP: Histology and physiology of black skin, *Ann Dermatol* 119:567, 1992.

8. Leveque JL et al: In vivo studies of the evolution of physical properties of the human skin with age, *Int J Dermatol* 23:322, 1984.

9. Longas MO: Evidence for structural changes in dermatan sulfate and hyaluronic acid with aging, *Carbohydr Res* 159:127, 1987.

10. Marks R: Alterations of physical function of the skin with aging. In Kligman AM, Takase Y, editors: *Cutaneous aging,* Tokyo, 1988, University of Tokyo Press.

11. Marks R et al: Age related changes in stratum corneum structure and function. In Marks R, Plewig G, editors: *Stratum corneum,* Berlin, 1983, Springer-Verlag.

12. Morrison WL et al: Photobiology, *J Am Acad Dermatol* 25:327, 1991.

13. Pathak MA et al: Preventive treatment of sunburn, dermatoheliosis, and skin cancer with sun-protective agents. In Fitzpatrick TB et al, editors: *Dermatology in general medicine,* ed 4, New York, 1993, McGraw-Hill.

14. Pieraggi MT et al: Fibroblast changes in cutaneous aging, *Virchows Arch* 402:275, 1984.

15. Reed JT et al: Skin type, but neither race nor gender, influence epidermal permeability barrier function, *Arch Dermatol* 131:1134, 1995.

16. Schwartz E et al: Collagen alterations in chronically sun-damaged human skin, *Photochem Photobiol* 58:841, 1993.

17. Tan CY et al: Skin thickness measurement by pulsed ultrasound: its reproducibility, validation and variability, *Br J Dermatol* 106:657, 1982.

18. Vincent JFV: *Structural biomaterials,* rev ed, Princeton, NJ, 1990, Princeton University Press.

19. Vogel HG: Influence of maturation and age and of desmotropic compounds on the mechanical properties of rat skin in vivo, *Bioeng Skin J* 1:35, 1985.

20. Wainwright SA et al: *Mechanical design in organisms,* Princeton, NJ, 1982, Princeton University Press.

CHAPTER

Normal Wound Healing

5

Bruce A. Mast

I. Kelman Cohen

Successful wound healing is fundamental for the practice of all surgery. The biologic processes that result in the restoration of disrupted tissue allow surgeons to treat their patients. Although physicians often take the healing process for granted, plastic surgeons are keenly aware of the wounds being closed, created, or revised. The entire craft of plastic surgery is a surgical struggle with the forces of tissue repair and attempts to combat the formation of excessive scar tissue. Plastic surgeons, as much and perhaps more than physicians in any other discipline, have contributed to the clinical and basic scientific advances in tissue repair over the past decades.

This chapter reviews the molecular, biochemical, and cellular processes of normal wound healing. The specific processes of matrix deposition, epithelialization, angiogenesis, and wound contraction are also presented. Common conditions that adversely affect healing are discussed. The chapter concludes with the future of wound healing research and its impact on plastic surgery.

THE SKIN

Cellular Elements

The skin has a pivotal role in plastic surgery. The same basic biologic processes occur in all human organs and tissues, such that healing is an equal challenge to all surgeons. Skin is the largest organ in the human and has multiple purposes, including fluid maintenance, thermoregulation, and prevention of bacterial infections. The skin is composed of two layers: epidermis and dermis. The most superficial layer is composed of keratinocytes that arise from a germinal basal layer juxtaposed to the dermis. These basal cells mature until they reach the surface as dead cells, thus forming a keratinized, stratified squamous epithelium (see later discussion of epithelialization).

The epidermis and dermis interface through an undulating, alternating weave of epidermal rete pegs and papillary dermis. The reticular dermis is the main structural subunit of the skin, containing the collagenous and noncollagenous extracellular matrix. The dermis also contains blood vessels, nerve endings, hair follicles, and pilosebaceous glands. Therefore the matrix is populated by fibroblasts, smooth muscle cells, endothelial cells, and neurons. The bases of the hair follicles and the pilosebaceous glands contain a layer of basal epithelium that is contiguous with the basal epithelium of the epidermis. The dermis is also important in immunity because of Langerhans' cells, which are extremely important in antigen presentation. The subcutaneous fat contains adipocytes and components of blood vessels and nerves.

Extracellular Matrix

The extracellular matrix (ECM) is a complex portion of the dermis and all other tissues. The ECM undergoes profound and dynamic changes during the healing process and has classically been viewed as a structural foundation for the skin's cellular components. Advances in the understanding of the numerous ECM components have demonstrated that the matrix is also a potent modulator of cellular function. The ECM is traditionally thought to consist of a collagenous portion and a noncollagenous "ground substance." As discussed later, both these components are important for the structural integrity of the skin and wound and have interactive roles in the healing process.

Thirteen types of collagen have been identified (Table 5-1); types I, III, IV, and VII are most involved in the skin and wound healing.[30] Type I collagen is present in virtually all connective tissues except for hyaline cartilage and basement membrane. This is the most prevalent form in dermis and is the predominant component of scar. Type III collagen is also primarily found in skin, with higher proportions during fetal development and during early phases of collagen deposition during wound repair. Collagen types IV and VII are part of the basement membrane complex that anchors the epidermis to the dermis.

Collagen production is a complex process integrating multiple intracellular and extracellular processes.[30] Type I collagen is a fiber-forming collagen that is trimeric, consisting of two identical chains and a third different chain. The timeric molecule is organized into a triple helical pattern that is stabilized by a series of interchain hydrogen bonds, in which hydroxyproline plays an important role. Intermolecular cross-linking and bonding that depend on the hydroxylation of

Table 5-1.
Types of Collagen Found in Vertebrate Species

TYPE	LOCATION	FUNCTIONS
I	Connective tissues No hyaline cartilage or basement membrane	Structural support of tissue through fiber formation
II	Hyaline cartilage (ear) and tissues such as vitreous humor	Structural support of tissue through fiber formation (fibers smaller than type I)
III	Pliable or distensible tissues such as blood vessels Fetal skin	Structural support through small-fiber formation
IV	Basement membranes	Scaffoldlike support
V	All tissues	Comparable to type III
VI	All tissues	Microfibrillar elements
VII	Basement membrane complex in epidermal-dermal junction	Anchoring fibrils
VIII	Descemet's membrane, produced by endothelial cells	Unknown
IX	Hyaline cartilage	Structural support by forming aggregates with type II
X	Hypertrophic cartilage	Unknown
XI	Hyaline cartilage	Unknown
XII	Probably similar to type I	Unknown
XIII	Produced by cells of some tumors	Unknown

Modified from Cohen IK, Diegelmann RF, Lindblad WL, editors: *Wound healing: biochemical and clinical aspects,* Philadelphia, 1993, Saunders.

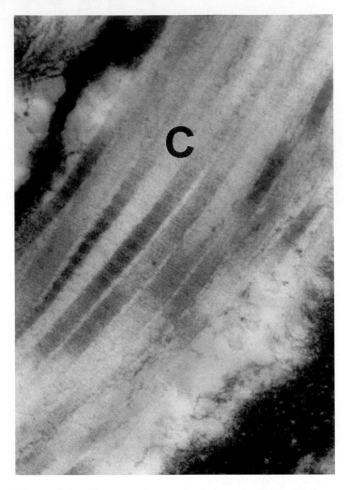

Figure 5-1. Electron micrograph of dermal collagen *(C)* from adult rabbit. (Magnification 140,000×.)

lysine and proline are also vital in providing strength to collagen.

The physiologic roles of collagen largely depend on its extracellular organization into aggregates. The most common aggregate is the *fiber,* which forms as collagen monomers are linearly organized in a staggered manner to yield a large polymer. Further aggregation leads to ultimate fiber and fibril formation (Figure 5-1). Fibrils further aggregate to form bundles, thereby providing structural strength to the tissue. The inability of a healing wound to regenerate the normal organization of collagen is the primary cause of diminished strength of scars compared with wounds. This reduced strength of scars is a matter of quality (matrix organization) rather than quantity (amount of collagen).

Several noncollagenous proteins exist within the ECM. Some proteins, such as elastin, have structural roles, imparting physical properties to the skin. Particular polypeptide hydrophobic domains and conformational structures confer properties that make elastin an elastomer, thereby imparting flexible qualities to tissue.[8] Other proteins have important roles in cellular function by acting as adhesion ligands to

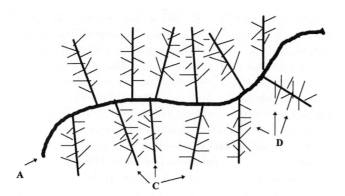

Figure 5-2. Schematic representation of proteoglycan aggregate contained within extracellular matrix. *A,* Hyaluronic acid; *C,* core proteins; *D,* glycosaminoglycans (e.g., chondroitin sulfate, dematan sulfate).

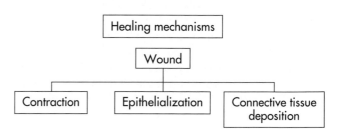

Figure 5-3. Three predominant mechanisms of wound healing.

Table 5-2.
Mechanisms of Healing

	TYPE OF WOUND		
HEALING MECHANISM	**SUTURED REPAIR (PRIMARY INTENTION)**	**OPEN (SECONDARY INTENTION)**	**PARTIAL THICKNESS**
Contraction	0	+++	0
Epithelialization	+	+	+++
Connective tissue deposition	+++	++	0

certain cells. Fibroblasts and keratinocytes have been shown to adhere to proteins such as fibronectin, vitronectin, laminin, fibrinogen, fibrin, and thrombospondin, as well as collagen types I to V.[14]

A large portion of the noncollagenous ECM consists of glycosaminoglycans and their associated proteoglycans. A *glycosaminoglycan* (GAG) is a large polysaccharide composed of a repeating disaccharide. Hyaluronic acid, heparan sulfate, chondroitin sulfate, and keratan sulfate are the most prevalent GAGs in skin. A *proteoglycan* consists of proteins covalently bound to a GAG core by means of a core protein. These molecules are found in intracellular secretory granules as cell membrane–based complexes and as integral components of the ECM. Hyaluronic acid also combines with proteoglycans to form large proteoglycan aggregates within the matrix (Figure 5-2). As such, GAGs and proteoglycans play important roles in cell-matrix interactions, the immune response, basement membrane physiology, and the imparting of physical properties (e.g., hydrational status, compressibility) to the ECM.[49]

NORMAL WOUND HEALING

Observational Descriptions

Wound healing can be described on the basis of clinical observations and the cellular and biochemical events responsible for such observations. Clinically or grossly, wounds heal by a combination of three processes: (1) epithelialization, (2) connective tissue deposition, and (3) contraction (Figure 5-3). In reality, all wounds are repaired by the concurrence of these processes, but depending on the type of wound, one process usually predominates (Table 5-2). For example, healing of a split-thickness skin graft donor site occurs through epithelialization, and connective tissue deposition and contraction are virtually nonexistent. Similarly, the healing that occurs after chemical peels, laser resurfacing, or a partial-thickness burn depends on epithelialization. On the other hand, a 1-cm^2 soft tissue defect on the fingertip, if allowed to heal spontaneously, will do so by contraction, and granulation tissue formation and epithelialization occur to a lesser degree. ECM formation with collagen deposition and cross-linking is the predominant mechanism of healing for surgically closed wounds.

Wound healing can also be described on the basis of the surgical intervention undertaken to facilitate tissue repair. Wounds with edges that are mechanically coapted (sutured or stapled) shortly after injury heal by *primary intention,* whereas wounds that are allowed to heal without coaptation and thus heal mainly by contraction heal by *secondary intention.* Contaminated open wounds that are closed surgically after a period of wound care heal by *delayed primary closure.*

Cellular and Biochemical Processes

The precise mechanisms responsible for the above processes are best described by the complex interaction of the cellular and extracellular matrix components that act in concert to restore the integrity of injured tissue (Figure 5-4). For descriptive purposes the biologic processes of wound healing can be divided into four phases: hemostasis, inflammation, proliferation, and remodeling.[27] Although these processes are described as distinct phases, significant overlap occurs.

HEMOSTASIS. Wound healing begins at the moment that tissue integrity is traumatically disrupted. The same processes are set into motion regardless of the type of injury, so that a planned surgical incision and a ragged traumatic laceration initiate the same repair response. Epidermal, dermal, and vascular elements of the skin or other deeper tissues are disturbed, leaving a gap within the tissue. The initial physiologic response is hemostasis. The exposed collagen of disrupted blood vessels and dermis act as a nidus for platelet aggregation and degranulation. The clotting cascade is activated, and fibrin polymerization occurs as a mature clot is formed in conjunction with the aggregated platelets. Clot and thrombus formation combine with reactive vasospasm, resulting in hemostasis. The clot and thrombus also act as a sealant for the wound, thereby providing a physical barrier that prevents further bacterial contamination and fluid loss.

Coincident with thrombus formation is the deposition of an early, provisional ECM within the wound site. Fibrin, fibronectin, and hyaluronic acid are present and are thought to facilitate cellular infiltration into the wound.[15] Such facilitation most likely occurs as a physical phenomenon because this provisional matrix serves as a scaffold spanning the wound gap.[8,30,48] These ECM components also play roles in cellular adhesion and thus actively assist in cellular entry into the wound site.[15]

Platelets are not merely passive hemostatic components. They are the first cells to enter the wound and provide the first burst of soluble molecules that modulate and mediate healing. These cytokines and polypeptide growth factors act by attaching to specific receptors on the surfaces of specific cells. They are, in fact, hormones, in that they direct specific cells to proliferate, suppress division, or make particular proteins.

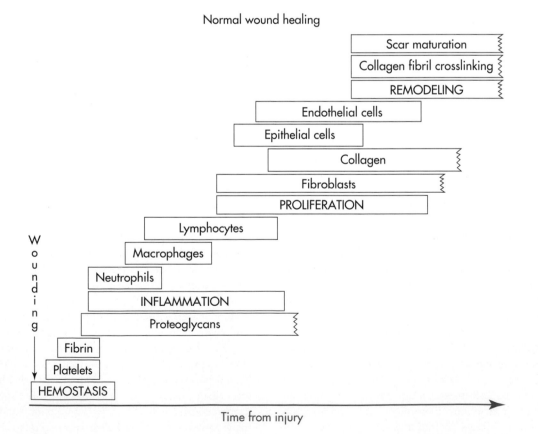

Normal wound healing

Figure 5-4. Main "phases" of wound healing and associated cellular and extracellular components responsible for tissue repair.

Contained within the alpha granules of platelets are several growth factors, including platelet-derived growth factor (PDGF), insulin-like growth factor I (IGF-I), epidermal growth factor (EGF), and transforming growth factor beta (TGF-β).[29] The depot of growth factors released from platelets quickly diffuses from the wound into the surrounding tissue. These growth factors affect various wound cells to initiate and promote healing. Their actions are further amplified by overlapping function and multiple cellular sources. For example, PDGF is a chemoattractant for smooth muscle cells[16] and fibroblasts,[39] thereby influencing angiogenesis and matrix deposition. TGF-β is also a mitogenic factor for fibroblasts and positively affects matrix protein production by these cells.

This initial hemostatic phase of healing also sets the stage for the upcoming inflammatory stage. Among many factors, TGF-β released from platelets and tumor necrosis factor alpha (TNF-α) produced by injured vascular endothelial cells, keratinocytes, and fibroblasts chemotactically draw inflammatory cells into the injured area.[47]

INFLAMMATION. As hemostasis ensues secondary to vasoconstriction, platelet aggregation, and activation of the clotting cascade, various substances are present in the wound site that subsequently result in secondary vasodilation, increased capillary permeability, and chemoattraction and activation of leukocytes. Substances such as C5a (a byproduct of the complement cascade), bacterial proteins with the peptide N-formyl-methionyl-leucyl-phenylalanine (FMLP), and leukotriene B$_4$ are chemoattractants for neutrophils and increase neutrophil adherence to endothelial cells.[47]

Neutrophils are the first leukocytes to enter the wound and thereby establish acute inflammation. They also help to amplify the inflammatory response by virtue of their secretion of more proinflammatory cytokines such as TNF-α and interleukins. By virtue of their bactericidal and phagocytic mechanisms, neutrophils have an immunologic role, controlling local bacterial contamination and preventing infection. Furthermore, neutrophils release proteases (e.g., elastase, collagenase) that remove damaged and denatured ECM components and aid in debridement of devitalized tissue.[28] The insignificant role neutrophils play in collagen deposition and ultimate healing has been demonstrated by multiple studies in which healed wounds of neutropenic animals had similar hydroxyproline contents and breaking strengths as wounds from normal animals.[1,40] Clinical observations also suggest that neutropenic patients seldom have a primary deficiency of wound healing. Rather, these patients have a significantly higher incidence of wound infection, which secondarily results in impaired healing. Neutrophil infiltration peaks at about 24 hours postwounding and slowly recedes as monocytes enter the wound site.[47]

Similar to neutrophils, *monocytes* are attracted to the wound site by bacterial products and C5a. Furthermore, breakdown products of early provisional matrix proteins (e.g., fibronectin) also attract monocytes.[29] One of the most potent chemoattractants for monocytes is TGF-β, which is secreted by platelets

and neutrophils, as well as by monocytes. Therefore, by secreting a monocyte chemoattractant, these cells act to amplify and control the inflammatory response. As circulating monocytes enter the wound site, they become activated and converted into macrophages, which continue to destroy bacteria and debride the wound.

Similar to platelets, *macrophages* also have an integral function related to subsequent healing events. For instance, wounds from guinea pigs rendered monocytopenic by administration of hydrocortisone and antimonocyte serum demonstrate a significant delay in fibroblast recruitment and collagen deposition.[23] The importance of the macrophage lies in its secretion of multiple soluble factors (cytokines and growth factors) that mediate various cellular and biochemical events responsible for healing. For example, TGF-β is mitogenic for fibroblasts and enhances collagen deposition by increasing collagen synthesis and inhibiting collagen degradation.[34] Although other sources of TGF-β are present, macrophages, because of their prolonged presence in the wound (several days), may be the most important and abundant source. Macrophages synthesize and secrete additional growth factors, including TGF-α, leukocyte-derived growth factor (LDGF, a PDGF-like protein), basic fibroblast growth factor (bFGF), and heparin-binding epidermal growth factor (HB-EGF).[29] These factors broaden the effect of macrophages, influencing the behavior of keratinocytes for epithelialization, fibroblasts for matrix production, and smooth muscle cells and endothelial cells necessary for angiognesis. Macrophages also provide a further source of TNF-α and interleukin-1 (IL-1) such that they play a role in the control of the inflammatory response. Macrophages also affect the deposition and organization of collagen by the secretion of collagenase.[47]

Other inflammatory cells implicated in normal wound healing are lymphocytes, plasma cells, and mast cells. The role of lymphocytes is not fully understood. Although they have a significant function in control of inflammation as a result of cytokine production, conflicting data exist regarding the effect of lymphocytes on connective tissue deposition and breaking strength of wounds.[3,47]

The composition of the wound matrix changes during the inflammatory phase. Fibrin is the initial, predominant component of the matrix resulting from hemostatic clot formation. As vascular permeability increases during the onset of acute inflammation, transudation of plasma components ensues, leading to the entry of complement, antibodies, and other plasma components into the wound. During this transudation a provisional ECM is created in the skin wound tract and consists predominantly of fibrin, fibronectin, and GAGs (e.g., hyaluronic acid). Importantly, uninjured fibroblasts in the dermis adjacent to the wound are stimulated by cytokines and growth factors to begin expressing integrin receptors that specifically recognize fibrin. These fibroblasts then can recognize and migrate into the provisional matrix of the fibrin clot. Furthermore, cellular migration is guided by the provisional matrix that exists within the wound, as well as by anatomic tissue planes and planes aligned according to the tension across the wound. This early matrix is influenced by the action of

PDGF and TGF-β on fibroblasts. Hyaluronic acid and sulfated GAGs are secreted by fibroblasts in response to PDGF. Early fibronectin production and subsequent synthesis of type I collagen, elastin, and proteoglycans is stimulated by TGF-β.[27,45,48]

PROLIFERATION. The hemostatic and inflammatory phases of healing set the stage for the migration and proliferation of several cell types, leading directly to restored tissue integrity. The cytokines and growth factors released into the wound site act on various cells, stimulating their proliferation, migration, and synthesis of cellular products. As the fibroblasts and vascular endothelial cells migrate into the provisional matrix of the injury site, they begin to proliferate and cellularity of the wound increases. The proliferative, or repair, phase often lasts several weeks.

As the number of macrophages in the wound begins to decrease, other cells in the wound (e.g., fibroblasts, endothelial cells, keratinocytes) begin to synthesize and secrete growth factors. Fibroblasts secrete IGF-I, bFGF, TGF-β, PDGF, and keratinocyte growth factor (KGF). Endothelial cells produce vascular endothelial growth factor (VEGF), bFGF, and PDGF. Keratinocytes synthesize TGF-β, TGF-α, and keratinocyte-derived autocrine factor (KDAF). These growth factors continue to stimulate proliferation, synthesis of extracellular matrix proteins, and angiogenesis[29] (Table 5-3).

During the repair phase the early provisional matrix is replaced by a more permanent matrix consisting primarily of collagen, although the noncollagenous matrix is retained composed of GAGs and proteoglycans (e.g., chondroitin sulfate, dermatan sulfate). Neovascularization is vital to provide oxygen and nutrients to the healing wound site. Angiogenesis results from endothelial cell migration and proliferation and from budding of existing capillaries. Neovascularization is affected by multiple cellular types and growth factors and tends to proceed along an oxygen gradient toward hypoxic regions within the wound.[35] Epithelialization is prominent and rapid beginning very soon following injury, as basal keratinocytes migrate and then proliferate, restoring the multilayered squamous epithelium (see following sections on angiogenesis and epithelialization).[43]

The entry of fibroblasts into the wound is crucial to the healing process because these cells synthesize collagen, the primary structural component of the repaired tissue. The production of collagen is an elaborate mechanism in which multiple intracellular and extracellular events result in the deposition of collagen fibrils. As collagen is deposited, the early provisional matrix, consisting primarily of fibrin, fibronectin, and proteoglycans, is degraded by serine proteases (e.g., neutrophil elastase).[29] Collagen synthesis and deposition are directly related to fibroblast influx into the wounds, beginning at 2 to 3 days postwounding and lasting up to 14 days. Among the many growth factors that affect collagen flux, TGF-β is the most influential. It not only induces production of type I collagen by fibroblasts, but also effectively diminishes collagen degradation by inhibiting collagenase gene transcription and stimulating the production of tissue inhibitors of metalloproteinases (TIMPs).[45] Initial collagen deposition is exuberant; the quantity of collagen deposited at a wound site is greater than that being synthesized and deposited in normal, uninjured skin. Although the collagen quantity within the wound gradually decreases, the content remains greater than that of normal skin, even when measured 10 weeks after wounding in animals.[9]

In addition to fibroblasts, collagen is produced by smooth muscle cells, epithelial cells, and endothelial cells. Depending on the tissue, these cells may be the primary source of collagen.[44] For example, smooth muscle cells are thought to produce collagen normally, as well as in response to trauma, in the intestinal tract, where few fibroblasts are in continuity with structural collagen.[14] Numerous collagen types differ by their component chains. Type III collagen is synthesized and deposited as the initial form of collagen in healing wounds, but it is quickly replaced by type I, the predominant collagen of skin. Since collagen is the main structural protein of connective tissue, it provides the tensile strength for organs such as skin and bone and for healed wounds. Increasing tensile strength has been correlated with increased collagen content (measured by hydroxyproline content) in animal wounds.[38]

REMODELING. The last and longest phase in healing is remodeling. Proliferation of the various cellular elements that make up the healed wound recedes during this time. The principal process is dynamic remodeling of collagen and formation of a mature scar (i.e., the healed wound). The net deposition of collagen in virtually all tissues, including wounds, is a balance between collagenolytic activity and collagen synthesis, such that production and degradation are ongoing, opposing processes. The ongoing nature of remodeling is perhaps best exemplified by the demonstration of collagenolytic activity in wounds as long as 20 years after wounding.[33]

During remodeling, wound tensile strength continues to increase despite a reduction in the rate of collagen synthesis and an overall reduction in the collagen content of the wound. This gain in strength is a result of structural modification of the newly deposited collagen. Histologically, early unorganized collagen fibrils become thicker and form fascicles that eventually become compact fibers.[26] The increase in fiber diameter is associated with an increase in wound tensile strength.[10] Cross-linking of collagen fibrils is largely responsible for these morphologic changes and the increase in wound strength. These cross-links are covalent bonds that form between collagen molecules, initiated by the deamination of lysine and hydroxylysine residues through the enzyme lysl oxidase, a product of fibroblasts. As maturation continues, cross-linking becomes more complex, thus providing the molecules with greater strength and stability.

Fibroblasts are primarily responsible for the synthesis of ECM components, including collagen, elastin, and proteoglycans. In addition, they also are an important source of the matrix metalloproteinases (MMPs) that degrade the matrix.[20] These proteases all share a need for calcium and for zinc as a

Table 5-3.
Cellular and Matrix Effects of Major Growth Factors and Cytokines

CHEMOTAXIS			PROLIFERATION		STIMULATION		
NEUTROPHILS	MACROPHAGES	FIBROBLASTS	EPITHELIAL CELLS	FIBROBLASTS	ANGIOGENESIS	GRANULATION TISSUE	COLLAGEN METABOLISM
PDGF	PDGF	PDGF		PDGF	PDGF		PDGF
	TGF-β	TGF-β		TGF-β	TGF-β		TGF-β
			EGF	EGF		EGF	
			TGF-α	TGF-α		TGF-α	
			FGF	FGF	FGF	FGF*	
			KGFs				
				IGF-I			IGF-I
					VEGF		
ILs	ILs			ILs			
TNF-α	TNF-α			TNF-α			TNF-α

PDGF, Platelet-derived growth factor; TGF-β, transforming growth factor beta; EGF, epidermal growth factor; TGF-α, transforming growth factor alpha; FGF, fibroblast growth factor; KGFs, keratinocyte growth factors; IGF-I, insulin-like growth factor I; VEGF, vascular endothelial growth factor; TNF-α, tumor necrosis factor alpha; ILs, interleukins.
*Wound contraction.

cofactor for activity. Interstitial collagenase (MMP-1) acts on a single cleavage site on the tightly wound, triple helical collagen molecule within fibrils. This results in partial denaturation of collagen so that other MMPs, such as gelatinase A (MMP-2) and gelatinase B (MMP-9), can further degrade the molecule. Gelatinases also degrade collagen types IV and V. Stromolysin, another MMP, is also active against type IV collagen but degrades noncollagenous matrix proteins as well (e.g., fibronectin, laminin). Fibroblasts also secrete TIMPs, which act to block tissue destruction by MMPs. The intricate control of protease activity resulting in effective and appropriate matrix remodeling is not yet fully understood.

Remodeling is a dynamic process in which scar maturation occurs for months to years after the initial synthesis of collagen by fibroblasts. This is an imperfect process, however, since wound collagen does not achieve the bundled, highly organized pattern seen in normal, uninjured dermis. The strength of healed tissue never equals that of uninjured skin. The increase in tensile strength of rat wounds plateaus approximately 3 months after injury, reaching an apparent maximum strength at 1 year postwounding that is only 80% of the tensile strength of normal skin.[26]

EPITHELIALIZATION

Reconstitution of the disrupted epithelial covering is a vital component of successful wound healing that allows functions related to thermoregulation, fluid balance, protein retention, and inhibition of bacterial infection to be restored. The stratified epithelium is normally active, with regular slough of superficial cells and renewal by the cuboidal basal cells. The basal layer of cells attaches the epidermis to the dermis through the basement membrane zone, where hemidesmosomes are abundant (Figure 5-5). The basement membrane zone is a complex biochemical aggregate consisting of laminin, heparan sulfate, and types IV and VII collagen. For wound epithelialization to occur, the complex attachment of cells to the basement membrane zone must be altered.[43]

Soon after wounding the normally cuboidal basal cells flatten and begin to extend cytoplasmic projections toward the wound site. Tight hemidesmosomal attachments are lost, and basal cell migration begins beneath the overlying thrombus and clot. Such migration is entirely independent of cellular proliferation. As migration proceeds, the leading epithelial cells attain phagocytic capabilities, thereby debriding the migrating path of erythrocytes and devitalized tissue. Migration proceeds in layers one cell or two cells thick and ceases on contact with another advancing front of epithelial cells or when the defect is completely covered. Proliferation of basal cells usually occurs within 1 to 2 days after wounding, with eventual renewal of a stratified epithelium. A complete stratified epithelium can be restored within 4 days in wounds with an intact basement membrane complex. The primary sources of migrating epithelium are the intact epithelial edge juxtaposed to the wound and the basal cells contained within hair follicles and residual pilosebaceous and eccrine glands.[43]

The actual processes of epithelial cell migration are not completely understood. The migrating cells develop multiple gap junctions and contain the contractile protein actin, suggesting intercellular communication and motility. If the basement membrane has been eliminated by the injury, this structure must be reconstituted as migration occurs. A provisional matrix and basement membrane develop from fibronectin in wound fluid. As migration proceeds, the epithelial cells secrete proteases to facilitate their movement

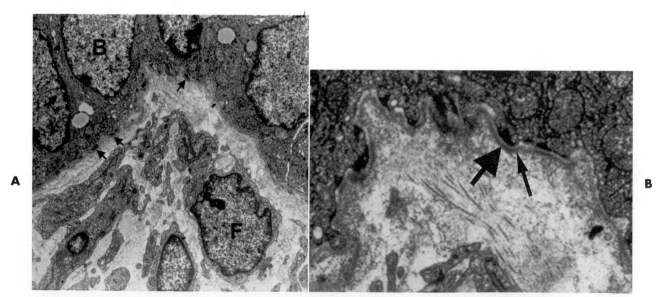

Figure 5-5. **A,** Electron micrograph of epidermal-dermal junction in fetal rabbit. Note multiple hemidesmosomes *(arrows)* anchoring basal epithelial cells *(B)* to dermis. Several fibroblasts *(F)* are seen within dermis. (Magnification 16,600×.) **B,** Magnified view of epidermal-dermal junction in **A** shows hemidesmosome *(large arrow)* and basement membrane *(small arrow).*

through the wound matrix. The wound fibronectin is replaced by epithelial cell–derived fibronectin, laminin, and collagen type IV as the basement membrane is reconstituted.[43]

Migration is influenced by multiple factors (Table 5-4). ECM components are vital for cellular adhesion. Fibronectin and vitronectin support and promote epithelial cell adhesion and migration. Cultured epithelial cells demonstrate expression of fibronectin receptors during growth until confluence is reached, at which time receptor expression ceases. Collagen types I and IV also facilitate epithelial spreading and attachment. Various soluble mediators also affect epithelial cells (Table 5-5). IL-I, bFGF, EGF, PDGF, and TGF-α all

---

Table 5-4.
Matrix Components Affecting Epithelialization

COMPONENT	SOURCE	LOCATION: ACTION
Collagen type I	Fibroblasts	Dermis: supports epithelial cell attachment and migration
Collagen type IV	Epithelial cells Fibroblasts	Basement membrane: supports epithelial cell attachment and migration
Collagen type V	Epithelial cells	Basement membrane: unknown function
Fibronectin	Fibroblasts Macrophages Diffusion from serum	Basement membrane area in wounds: supports cell adhesion and migration
Laminin	Epithelial cells	Basement membrane: epithelial cell adhesion with inhibition of migration
Vitronectin	Serum	Unclear: involved in cell adhesion and migration

Modified from Cohen IK, Diegelmann RF, Lindblad WL, editors: *Wound healing: biochemical and clinical aspects,* Philadelphia, 1992, Saunders.

Table 5-5.
Soluble Mediators of Epithelialization

MEDIATOR	SOURCE	SUBSTANCE/ACTION
Epidermal growth factor	Salivary gland Platelets (?)	Epithelial cell mitogen
Platelet-derived growth factor	Platelets Endothelium	Epithelial cell mitogen
Transforming growth factor alpha	Platelets Epithelial cells Macrophages (?)	Epithelial cell mitogen
Basic fibroblast growth factor	Keratinocytes Fibroblasts Macrophages Endothelium	Epithelial cell mitogen
Interleukin-I	Macrophages Epithelial cells Lymphocytes	Epithelial cell mitogen Stimulates motility
Transforming growth factor beta	Platelets Macrophages Fibroblasts Neutrophils Lymphocytes	Inhibits epithelial cell proliferation Stimulates motility

stimulate or promote epithelial cell migration, growth, or proliferation. Conversely, TGF-β inhibits proliferation.[43]

ANGIOGENESIS

New blood vessel formation, or angiogenesis, is a key element of healing in both wounds closed primarily and open wounds allowed to heal secondarily. The processes of neovascularization are complex and have been elucidated by histologic observations in wounds and by more controlled studies in chick embryo membranes, rabbit corneas, and endothelial cell cultures.[50]

Angiogenesis occurs in response to various stimuli, leading to formation of new capillaries that originate as outgrowths from venules. Dissolution of the basement membrane occurs within the venule in the portion directed toward the stimulus. Endothelial cell migration then proceeds, with specific collagenases creating a path through the tissue. Simultaneously, cellular proliferation and eventual formation of a tubular lumen occur. Vascular connections are created with other newly formed capillaries emerging from neighboring areas within the wound. After establishment of vascular flow, regression and remodeling cause many vessels to dissipate completely and others to differentiate into arteries and veins. These basic steps occur in wounds closed primarily, in wounds healing secondarily, in surgical flaps at the interface with the reconstructed wound bed, and to some degree during neoplasia.[50]

Numerous stimuli and mediators of neovascularization exist (Box 5-1). These angiogenic factors are described as direct acting or indirect acting. Direct-acting factors have been demonstrated to have a direct effect on endothelial cell migration, as demonstrated in cell culture. Such factors include bFGF, aFGF, TGF-α, TNF-α, and vascular endothelial growth factor (VEGF). Indirect-acting angiogenic factors have no documented effect on endothelial cells in culture but have been shown to stimulate angiogenesis in chick embryo membranes and rabbit corneas. These factors include TGF-β, PDGF, prostaglandins, and angiogenin and are thought to exert their actions by recruiting cellular components (e.g., macrophages) that release direct angiogenic factors.[50] Oxygen tension within the wound is also thought to be a potent stimulus and director of angiogenesis. New blood vessel formation has been shown to be directed toward regions of the wound with the lowest oxygen tension. Furthermore, angiogenic factors elicited from macrophages are affected by wound oxygen tension.[22,50]

The term "granulation tissue" is frequently used incorrectly to describe angiogenesis in a wound closed primarily. This is a misnomer coined by those who have no or little experience with clinical wounds. Clinicians described granulation tissue many decades ago on observing the healing tissue that developed within an open wound. Angiogenesis in the open wound creates tissue rich with capillary loops that appear "granular" to the naked eye, much as one would describe "granulated sugar." Such tissue is never

---

Box 5-1.
Angiogenic Factors

DIRECT FACTORS
Basic fibroblast growth factor
Acidic fibroblast growth factor
Transforming growth factor-beta
Tumor necrosis factor-alpha
Vascular endothelial growth factor

INDIRECT FACTORS
Transforming growth factor-beta
Platelet-derived growth factor (? direct)
Prostaglandins
Angiogenin

---

found in a primarily closed wound that heals without infection or in a partial wound disruption. Propagation of the incorrect use of this term must be discouraged because it only confuses our understanding of the healing process.

OPEN WOUND CONTRACTION

Contraction is the process by which the area of an open wound decreases by a concentric reduction in the size of the wound (Fig. 5-6). Contraction is the active biologic process that usually leads to wound closure. When inadequate skin is present, the process of contraction results in a scar deformity called a *contracture*. In addition, a contracture may develop when no tissue loss occurs but contraction of a linear wound scar results in a shortened, deforming scar. Such contractures often occur perpendicular to the movement axis of joints (Figure 5-7).[36]

In open wound closure the process of contraction is secondary to actual movement of the wound edges. *Myofibroblasts* are the cells thought to be responsible for this phenomenon. These specialized fibroblasts contain the contractile protein actin[13] and other features that indicate that these cells may participate in unified movement.[12] In further support of their role in wound contraction, myofibroblasts have been found in a variety of human tissues in which scar contraction is a key pathologic component, such as breast implant capsules, liver biopsies from patients with hepatic cirrhosis, and nodules of Dupuytren's contracture. The risk of recurrence after surgical excision of a Dupuytren's contracture has been correlated with the presence of active myofibroblasts within the skin nodule.[36]

An alternative theory suggests that a dynamic interaction between fibroblasts and the collagenous matrix of the uninjured tissue results in reorganization of the matrix and closure of the wound. Support for this hypothesis is the observation of wound contraction in some animals before the presence of myofibroblasts. Also, in vitro assays using collagen

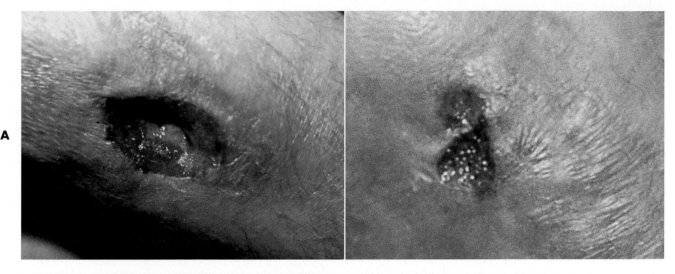

Figure 5-6. A, Deep open wound in leg resulting from partial flap loss due to postoperative hematoma. **B,** Marked reduction in size and volume of wound due to contraction.

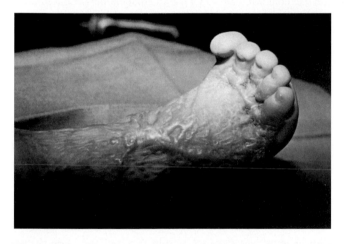

Figure 5-7. Contracture arising in bed of split-thickness skin graft to dorsum of foot and resulting in fixed extension of toes and difficulty with ambulation.

lattices have demonstrated fibroblast-mediated conformational changes in the matrix. This hypothesis suggests that myofibroblasts are merely quiescent fibroblasts rather than contractile cells.[11] Any in vitro study of matrix changes is only a model, however, and may be misleading in regard to the human, in vivo, biologic process.

EFFECTS OF AGING

One of the earliest attempts to delineate the effect of aging on wound healing was the work of Carrell and DuNouy during World War I, who found that increasing age was correlated with a slower rate of closure of open traumatic wounds. The differences in age groups were impressive: 20-year-old patients closed their wounds in 40 days, compared with 56 days for 30-year-old and 76 days for 40-year-old patients. Better

controlled experiments in young and old rats corroborated these findings.[27]

Connective tissue deposition appears to be diminished with increasing age. Primarily closed, linear cutaneous wounds in young rats were found to be thicker and have greater breaking strengths compared with those from older animals. Other investigators have found that hydroxyproline accumulation in human wound sites similarly diminishes with increasing age. Furthermore, young rats exhibit a greater rate of collagen synthesis. Such findings may be related to changes in growth factor physiology in young versus older animals. For example, an age-related reduction in expression of PDGF receptor–β has been observed in older rabbits versus young rabbits.[5]

Similar to differences in matrix deposition, cellular activity in wounds from older animals is reduced. The deoxyribonucleic acid (DNA) and ribonucleic acid (RNA) ribose content of young rat wounds is higher than in older wounds. More specifically, a significantly greater number of fibroblasts have been observed in young rodent wounds at 3 days postwounding. These findings hold true in humans as well. Monocyte and macrophage infiltration occurs earlier in wounds of younger versus older children. Also, the fibroblast outgrowth rate was reduced from punch biopsies taken from skin of older patients. Epithelialization has also been observed to occur at a diminished rate in older humans.[27]

Fibroblasts cultured from children (up to 15 years old) demonstrated greater contractility in collagen gel matrices compared with fibroblasts from early (16 to 40 years), middle (41 to 60 years), and late (61 years and older) adulthood. Fibroblasts respond to TGF-β by the production of ECM components, particularly collagen. Systemic administration of TGF-β has been shown to improve the diminished breaking strength observed in elderly rats and in glucocorticoid, healing-impaired young rats. Newborn human fibroblasts have increased EGF receptor number and affinity compared with fibroblasts from young and old adults. Another study evaluated the effect on healing of age-related regional changes in the tissues being injured by creating an ischemic tissue model. Young rats demonstrated a significantly lesser reduction in healing parameters compared with old rats in this model.[28]

All these data present a real challenge to clinicians, who must discover pharmacologic means to reverse the deleterious effects of aging on connective tissue metabolism. For example, topical use of cytokines or retinoids may be able to diminish skin fragility in elderly patients and thus prevent skin breakdown and pressure ulcer formation.

SYSTEMIC CONDITIONS

Because wound healing is a complex, multiply integrated process, many conditions can impair it. The following are perhaps the most frequently seen in plastic surgical practices: bacterial infection, malnutrition, effects of pharmacologic agents, diabetes, peripheral vascular disease, and tissue irradiation (Table 5-6). These conditions can seriously retard the acute healing process and ultimately lead to the chronic wound state. An entire category of factitious wounds also exists. These self-inflicted wounds created for psychologic secondary gains are probably more common than the average practitioner would think.

Bacterial Infection

Bacterial infection of a wound delays or even reverses the healing process. Bacterial growth, subsequent bacterial enzymatic action, and prolongation of the inflammatory phase of healing are responsible for local tissue destruction and resultant impairment of healing. The abundance of normal bacterial flora of the skin suggests that virtually all wounds are contaminated to a certain degree, but contamination does not always lead to infection or deficient healing. This may be best exemplified by burn wounds, in which a bacterial count of as much as 100,000 per gram of tissue is acceptable for skin grafting. Furthermore, controlled bacterial contamination may actually accelerate healing. Such effects may be species specific; *Staphylococcus aureus,* but not *Staphylococcus epidermidis,* has been shown to accelerate healing without overt wound infection. This effect may be caused by specific components of the bacterial cell wall.[25] Also, abnormal exuberant granulation tissue formation has been linked to insidious bacterial infection. For example, some believe that capsular contractures around mammary implants are caused by low-grade bacterial burden from the products of *S. epidermidis* normally found in breast tissue.

The presence of bacteria in a wound is a normal event. Wound infection results from several different circumstances: the bacterial colony count is greater than what the host can control; the bacterial strain is so virulent that a small bacterial load impedes healing; or the host is immunologically compromised and cannot kill a bacterial burden that would be controlled by a normal host. The host's overall condition is an essential factor. Any type of compromise of host defense mechanisms can lead to a wound infection. Immunosuppression in transplant patients, steroid therapy, and malnutrition are examples of potential systemic alterations that may lead to wound infection.

Malnutrition

Patients with malnutrition have long been observed to have difficulties healing their wounds because of multiple effects on the healing processes.[24] Plastic surgical patients often have large chronic wounds. The appreciable protein loss through these wounds combined with dietary deficiencies worsens protein malnutrition. Such documented protein malnutrition is associated with impaired strength of cutaneous, abdominal, and colonic wounds in animals.[7,18] Severe protein malnutrition affects body protein metabolism and thus may exert adverse effects on collagen synthesis and connective tissue deposition. The malnourished patient may also have deficiencies in vitamins and trace elements.

Depletion of ascorbate (vitamin C) alters tissue repair so that healing fails to occur or healed scars dehisce. The absence of ascorbate, a cofactor needed for proline and lysine hydroxylation, results in an abnormal amino acid sequence in procollagen such that the molecules are rapidly degraded within the cell. Abnormal collagen synthesis in this condition

Table 5-6.
Conditions that Adversely Affect Healing

CONDITION	ADVERSE EFFECT
Wound infection	Prolonged inflammation Proteolysis
Malnutrition	Inflammation Collagen synthesis Cellular proliferation
Effects of immuno-suppressive agents	Inflammation Infection
Effects of antineoplastic agents	Inflammation Infection Cellular proliferation
Radiation	Tissue hypoxia Epithelial damage Impaired fibroblast function
Diabetes	Inflammation Repeated trauma Infection Tissue hypoxia Reduced connective tissue deposition
Peripheral vascular disease	Tissue hypoxia

results in impaired wound healing and the disruption of old wounds as collagenolytic activity continues unabated despite improper collagen synthesis.[35] Several other vitamins, including riboflavin, pyridoxine, and thiamine, are involved in healing, probably as cofactors in cross-linking of collagen.[27] Zinc is required for DNA and RNA polymerase, and a deficiency of this element may retard epithelialization and fibroblast proliferation. Ferrous iron is a cofactor in the hydroxylation step of collagen synthesis, and copper is needed for the oxidative deamination of lysine, which is necessary for cross-linking.[19] Therefore, iron deficiencies may lead to impaired matrix synthesis. These effects can be compounded by an impaired inflammatory response.

Severe malnutrition leads to immunosuppression with diminished effectiveness of inflammatory cells and their soluble products. This could result in elevated risk of wound infections as well as impaired healing from deficiencies of normally elicited cytokines and growth factors.

Pharmacologic Agents

Various medications impart a negative effect on wound healing, including corticosteroids, cytotoxic agents, and immunosuppressive agents. Systemic corticosteroid therapy may blunt the inflammatory response necessary for healing. This antiinflammatory effect is thought to be mediated by stabilization of lysosomal membranes, thereby preventing the secretion of various enzymes and cytokines.[17] The blunted inflammatory response in turn may result in the observed impairment in capillary budding, inhibition of fibroblast proliferation, decreased protein synthesis, and diminished epithelialization.[44]

Vitamin A has been shown in animals to counteract the impairment in wound healing due to steroid administration, presumably by labilization of lysosomes within inflammatory cells, thereby restoring the efficiency of the early healing response.[37] Clinical use of vitamin A is variable because definite improvements in healing have not been conclusively demonstrated in humans. Since steroids' primary effect on healing results from a deficiency in the inflammatory response, administration of these drugs after establishment of the inflammatory phase of healing should have little adverse effect on healing. This has been demonstrated in animals using healing parameters of tensile strength and hydroxyproline content of wounds.[37]

The effect of chemotherapeutic agents used to treat cancer is of particular interest to surgeons, since these drugs are often used in combination with surgical ablation of tumors. A variety of antineoplastic medications have been shown to reduce the breaking strength of cutaneous wounds in experimental animals when administered at therapeutic levels.[6] These cytotoxic agents render their therapeutic effect by interfering with DNA or RNA synthesis, cell division, or protein synthesis. Consequently, their effect on healing occurs primarily during the proliferative phase of healing. Many patients receiving chemotherapy are systemically neutropenic and more prone to wound infection, which further impairs healing.

Immunosuppressive drugs such as prednisone, azathio-prine, cyclosporine, and FK-506 are used in the treatment of a variety of conditions, most often as prevention of rejection after organ transplantation. The therapeutic effect of these drugs results from a blunting of the normal immune response, and cells involved in the inflammatory response of healing are likewise affected, causing a potential deficiency in tissue repair. When surgery is undertaken in patients receiving these medications, physicians must be cognizant of the potential effects on wound healing. If a reconstructive procedure is being performed on a patient after surgical ablation of a neoplasm, the surgeon must know the course of preoperative or postoperative chemotherapy. Wound management then can be modified according to the potential for impaired healing. Likewise, if intralesional corticosteroids are injected during a keloid excision, the sutures may remain in place for a longer time than required for simple excision in the same region.

Diabetes and Peripheral Vascular Disease

Diabetes mellitus is a serious medical condition in which insufficient insulin is produced or diminished tissue sensitivity to insulin results in hyperglycemia. More than 10 million people in the United States have diabetes; half will undergo one or more surgical interventions during their lifetime.[24] The adverse effects on wound healing are multiple, including increased susceptibility to wound infections, direct effects on healing mechanisms, and coexistent peripheral vascular disease.

Most knowledge of the healing deficiencies associated with diabetes stems from animal research. Most frequently, rats are rendered "diabetic" by treatment with streptozocin, which induces a hyperglycemic state. Although this model does not fully imitate the chronic diabetic state encountered in patients, much useful information has been gained. Other animal models less widely used employ naturally hyperglycemic strains of rats and may provide a more appropriate model for the chronic diabetic state. Findings in both these models indicate that diabetic rats have diminished wound tensile strength that is directly correlated with reduced hydroxyproline content, suggesting altered connective tissue deposition. Other studies have also found blunted epithelialization and possibly impaired neovascularization. Results from animal studies are less consistent regarding improvement in healing correlated with control of hyperglycemia.[24,27]

Diabetes is also known to alter leukocyte function, with impaired chemotaxis, phagocytosis, and intracellular bacterial killing. These effects should lead to deficient healing because of a blunted or less efficient inflammatory response, causing diminished modulation of the proliferative phase of healing. Therefore, fibroblast recruitment and connective tissue deposition could be significantly altered. Moreover, these changes in leukocyte function are implicated in the observed higher incidence of wound infection in diabetic patients.[27]

High levels of glucose are thought to interfere with cell membrane transport of a variety of compounds, including ascorbic acid, thereby affecting wound cells such as leukocytes and fibroblasts. In support of this concept, ascorbic acid dietary supplementation of diabetic rats results in increased dermal collagen production.[24] Longstanding hyperglycemia leads to glycosylated protein products that are circulatory as well as contained within cells. Glycosylation of various tissues may explain some of the end-organ damage caused by longstanding diabetes. For example, basement membrane thickening in kidney glomeruli may be an etiologic factor for renal disease. Similarly, glycosylation of nerves may contribute to the peripheral neuropathy often seen in longstanding diabetes. Diabetic ulceration in the feet is a common healing ramification of this disease process (Figure 5-8). Etiologies of these chronic wounds include impaired ability to fight infection, altered sensation from peripheral neuropathy leading to repeated unrecognized trauma, and diminished connective tissue deposition.

Peripheral vascular disease is a relatively common process that most often leads to healing aberrations in the lower extremities. Frequently, arterial insufficiency coexists with diabetes, compounding the impaired wound healing. The presence of significant peripheral vascular disease is best indicated by the absence of palpable pulses in the extremity. The absence of pulses, along with a nonhealing wound in the extremity distal to the region where the vascular examination is abnormal, strongly suggests an ischemic wound. The absence of sufficient arterial blood supply impairs wound healing because of deficient delivery of oxygen and metabolic substrates to support cellular activity. Although some wounds from arterial ischemia occur "spontaneously," most result from a minor or major traumatic injury. Accurate diagnosis of the arterial occlusion, followed by surgical or angiographic revascularization, is almost always required to ensure healing.

Tissue Irradiation

Radiation therapy is a common treatment for malignancy. Radiation has both acute and chronic effects on skin that may result in impaired healing or breakdown of healed tissue. Acute effects include erythema, inflammation, edema, desquamation, and ulceration. Late or chronic effects include change in pigmentation, atrophy of the epithelium and dermis, decreased local vascularity associated with fibrosis, telangiectasia, sebaceous and sweat gland dysfunction, necrosis, and neoplasia.[4,31] The early changes seen after radiation therapy are best treated supportively and symptomatically. Local trauma (e.g., sun exposure) should be avoided, and if open wounds develop, cleansing with mild soaps or saline, followed by application of a thin coat of antibiotic ointment or moisturizer, usually suffices.

The late effects on skin can be more challenging to treat. Simple intervention such as protection of hypopigmented areas may be all that is required, whereas ulcerated skin frequently requires grafting or flaps for reconstruction. Physical therapy may be needed to prevent joint contractures if dermal thickening and fibrosis occur across joints. Careful examination of the irradiated areas must be continued to detect secondary neoplastic formation.[4]

The radiation damage to skin has profound effects on

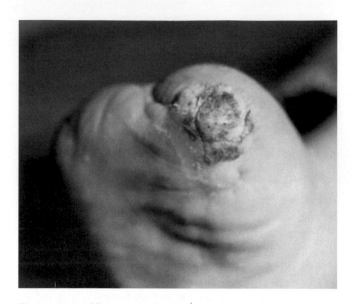

Figure 5-8. Ulceration at site of transmetatarsal amputation of foot in diabetic patient with significant peripheral neuropathy and blunted sensation. Surgical revision was required for removal of pressure point caused by first metatarsal bone stump.

wound healing. Postoperative radiation therapy can lead to delayed healing in a surgical site or even breakdown of an apparently healed wound. In addition, healing complications often occur long after radiation therapy. Most animal studies have used models that mimic these problems poorly because of time constraints and inability to duplicate accurately the irradiation given to humans.[4] The accumulated evidence, however, indicates that irradiation-mediated impairment of wound healing is multifactorial. Fibrosis and decreased vascularity result in a local wound environment that is hypoxic and unsupportive of optimal healing because of impaired angiogenesis and greater susceptibility to wound infection.

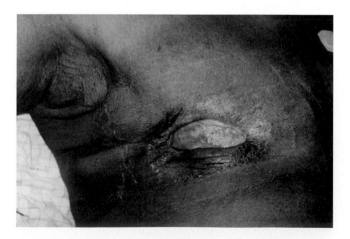

Figure 5-9. Chronic radiation wound of chest wall after mastectomy and postoperative irradiation. Excision and latissimus dorsi flap reconstruction were required. (Axilla is at left upper corner.)

ECM deposition is also diminished, largely from fibroblast depletion but also from impaired proliferation caused by radiation damage. Similarly, epithelial cell replication is blunted, with insufficient or absent epithelialization.[31]

One of the most frustrating and challenging problems facing plastic surgeons is the treatment of these radiation wounds (Figure 5-9). In addition to local wound care and the use of flaps taken from outside the radiated field, newer methods of hyperbaric oxygen[21] and administration of growth factors[31] may facilitate treatment of these wounds.

RESEARCH AND THE FUTURE

Plastic surgeons are keenly aware of the need for both function and aesthetic quality. They are always searching for a means to improve the quality of the wounds being treated or created. Ongoing research in the biology of wound healing will undoubtedly lead to improvements. The finding of regenerative, scarless healing in the mammalian fetus has led to continuing efforts to define key causative elements in scarless healing. The prospect of discovering what causes fetal healing without scar formation and applying it to postnatal conditions is intriguing.

The problems of nonhealing chronic wounds are receiving much attention (Box 5-2). Increased understanding of the interactions among cellular components, cytokines, growth factors, and proteases is providing improved insight into the pathophysiology of the chronic wound site.[29,46] Particular attention has been given to the use of growth factors to improve the healing of such wounds. Clinical studies have documented the successful use of growth factors in accelerating the healing of pressure ulcers and diabetic foot ulcers. Although such studies are promising, the durability of such closed wounds is the same as wounds that heal without exogenous growth factors, as exemplified by similar recurrence rates.[42] Moreover, growth factors alone may be a mere "quick fix." Recent work suggests that excessive proinflammatory cytokines and matrix proteases may be among the major factors leading to chronic wound states. Counteracting these deleterious molecules may be more important to correct the healing process than addition of exogenous growth factors.

Further research is underway investigating "alternative" means of controlling or ameliorating healing, including electrical stimulation of wounds,[2] hyperbaric oxygen therapy,[41] systemic administration of drugs and hormones, and gene therapy.[32] As further work continues, effective and improved means of controlling or treating abnormal healing should become readily available in the near future.

REFERENCES

1. Andersen L, Attstrom R, Feferskov O: Effect of experimental neutropenia on oral wound healing in guinea pigs, *Scand J Dent Res* 86:237-247, 1978.
2. Baker LL, Rubayi S, Villar F, et al: Effect of electrical stimulation waveform on healing of ulcers in human beings with spinal cord injury, *Wound Rep Reg* 4:21-28, 1996.
3. Barbul A, Sisto D, Tettura G, et al: Thymic inhibition of wound healing: abrogation by adult thymectomy, *J Surg Res* 32:332-342, 1982.
4. Bernstein EF, Sullivan FJ, Mitchell JB, et al: Biology of chronic radiation effect on tissues and wound healing, *Clin Plast Surg* 20:435-453, 1993.
5. Brucker MJ, Gruskin E, Farrel C, et al: Differential expression of platelet-derived growth factor receptor-β in an aging model of wound repair, *Wound Rep Reg* 4:219-223, 1996.
6. Cohen SC, Gabelnick HL, Johnson RK, et al: Effects of antineoplastic agents on wound healing in mice, *Surgery* 78:238-244, 1975.
7. Daly JM, Vars HM, Dudrick SJ: Effects of protein depletion on colonic anastomoses, *Surg Gynecol Obstet* 134:15-21, 1972.
8. Davidson JM, Giro G, Quaglino D: Elastin repair. In Cohen IK, Diegelmann RF, Lindblad WL, editors: *Wound healing: biochemical and clinical aspects,* Philadelphia, 1993, Saunders.
9. Diegelmann RF, Rothkipf LC, Cohen IK: Measurement of collagen biosynthesis during wound healing, *J Surg Res* 19:239-243, 1975.
10. Doillon CJ, Dunn MG, Bender E, et al: Collagen fiber formation in repair tissue: development of strength and toughness, *Coll Rel Res* 5:481-492, 1985.
11. Ehrlich HP: Wound closure: evidence of cooperation between fibroblasts and collagen matrix, *Eye* 2:149-157, 1988.
12. Gabbiani G, Runngger-Brandle I: The fibroblast. In Glynn LE, editor: *Tissue repair and regeneration,* New York, 1981, Elsevier Science.
13. Gabbiani G, Hirschel BJ, Ryan B, et al: Granulation tissue as a contractile organ, *J Exp Med* 135:719-734, 1972.
14. Graham MF, Blomquist P, Zederfeldt B: The alimentary tract. In Cohen IK, Diegelmann RF, Lindblad WL, editors: *Wound healing: biochemical and clinical aspects,* Philadelphia, 1993, WB Saunders.
15. Grinnell F. Cell adhesion. In Cohen IK, Diegelmann RF, Lindbald WL, editors: *Wound healing: biochemical and clinical aspects,* Philadelphia, 1993, Saunders.

Box 5-2.
Chronic Wounds

Pressure ulcer
Diabetic foot ulcer
Venous stasis ulcer
Ischemic ulcer
Radiation ulcer

16. Grotendorst GR, Chang T, Seppa HEJ, et al: Platelet-derived growth factor is a chemoattractant for vascular smooth muscle cells, *J Cell Physiol* 113:261-266, 1983.

17. Hunt TK, Ehrlich HP, Garcia JA, et al: Effects of vitamin A on reversing the inhibitory effect of cortisone on healing of open wounds in animals and man, *Ann Surg* 170:633-641, 1969.

18. Irvin TT: Effects of malnutrition and hyperalimentation on wound healing, *Surg Gynecol Obstet* 146:33-37, 1978.

19. Jackson DS: Development of fibrosis: cell proliferation and collagen biosynthesis, *Ann Rheum Dis* 36(suppl):2-4, 1977.

20. Jeffrey JJ: Collagen degradation. In Cohen IK, Diegelmann RF, Lindblad WL, editors: *Wound healing: biochemical and clinical aspects,* Philadelphia, 1993, WB Saunders.

21. Kindwall EP: Hyperbaric oxygen's effect on radiation necrosis, *Clin Plast Surg* 20:473-483, 1993.

22. Knighton DR, Hunt TK, Scheunstuhl H, et al: Oxygen tension regulates expression of angiogenesis factor by macrophages, *Science* 221:1283-1285, 1983.

23. Leibovich SJ, Ross R: The role of the macrophage in wound repair: a study with hydrocortisone and antimacrophage serum, *Am J Pathol* 78:71-100, 1975.

24. Levenson SM, Demetriou AA: Metabolic factors. In Cohen IK, Diegelmann RF, Lindblad WL, editors: *Wound healing: biochemical and clinical aspects,* Philadelphia, 1993, WB Saunders.

25. Levenson SM, Chang TH, Kan-Gruber D, et al: Accelerating effects of nonviable *Staphylococcus aureus,* its cell wall and cell wall peptidoglycan, *Wound Rep Reg* 4:467-469, 1996.

26. Levenson SM, Geever EF, Crowley LV, et al: The healing of rat skin wounds, *Ann Surg* 161:293-308, 1965.

27. Mast BA: The skin. In Cohen IK, Diegelmann RF, Lindblad WL, editors: *Wound healing: biochemical and clinical aspects,* Philadelphia, 1993, WB Saunders.

28. Mast BA, Cohen IK: Pediatric and fetal wound healing. In Benz M, editor: *Pediatric plastic surgery,* New York, 1998, Appleton-Lange.

29. Mast BA, Schultz GS: Interaction of cytokines, proteases and growth factors in acute and chronic wounds, *Wound Rep Reg* 4:411-420, 1996.

30. Miller EJ, Gay S: Collagen structure and function. In Cohen IK, Diegelmann RF, Lindblad WL, editors: *Wound healing: biochemical and clinical aspects,* Philadelphia, 1993, WB Saunders.

31. Mustoe TA, Porras-Reyes BH: Modulation of wound healing in chronic irradiated tissues, *Clin Plast Surg* 20:465-472, 1993.

32. Papadakis MA, Hamon G, Stotts N, et al: Effect of growth hormone replacement on wound healing in healthy older men, *Wound Rep Reg* 4:421-425, 1996.

33. Peacock EE: Collagenolysis: the other side of the equation, *World J Surg* 4:297-302, 1980.

34. Roberts AB, Sporn MR, Assoian RK, et al: Transforming growth factor type β: rapid induction of fibrosis and angiogenesis in vivo and stimulation of collagen formation in vitro, *Proc Natl Acad Sci USA* 83:4167-4171, 1986.

35. Ruberg RL: Role of nutrition in wound healing, *Surg Clin North Am* 64:705-714, 1984.

36. Rudolph R, Vande Berg J, Ehrlich HP: Wound contraction and scar contracture. In Cohen IK, Diegelmann RF, Lindblad WL, editors: *Wound healing: biochemical and clinical aspects,* Philadelphia, 1993, WB Saunders.

37. Sandberg N: Time relationship between administration of cortisone and wound healing in rats, *Acta Chir Scand* 127:445-446, 1964.

38. Sandberg N, Zederfeldt B: The tensile strength of healing wounds and collagen formation in rats and rabbits, *Acta Chir Scand* 126:187-196, 1963.

39. Seppa HEJ, Grotendorst GR, Seppa SI, et al: The platelet-derived growth factor is a chemoattractant for fibroblasts, *J Cell Biol* 92:584-588, 1982.

40. Simpson DM, Ross R: The neutrophilic leukocyte in wound repair: a study with antineutrophilic serum, *J Clin Invest* 51:2009-2023, 1972.

41. Smith BM, Desvigne LD, Slade B, et al: Transcutaneous oxygen measurements predict healing of leg wounds with hyperbaric therapy, *Wound Rep Reg* 4:224-229, 1996.

42. Steed DL, Edington HD, Webster MW: Recurrence rate of diabetic neurotrophic foot ulcers healed using topical application of growth factors released from platelets, *Wound Rep Reg* 4:230-233, 1996.

43. Stenn KS, Malhotra R: Epithelialization. In Cohen IK, Diegelmann RF, Lindblad WL, editors: *Wound healing: biochemical and clinical aspects,* Philadelphia, 1993, WB Saunders.

44. Stevenson TR, Mathes SJ: Wound healing. In Mill TA, Rowlands BJ, editors: *Physiologic basis of modern surgical care,* St Louis, 1988, Mosby.

45. Stocum DL: Tissue restoration: approaches and prospects, *Wound Rep Reg* 4:3-15, 1996.

46. Trengrove NJ, Langton SR, Stacey MC: Biochemical analysis of wound fluid from nonhealing and healing chronic leg ulcers, *Wound Rep Reg* 4:234-239, 1996.

47. Wahl LM, Wahl SM. Inflammation. In Cohen IK, Diegelmann RF, Lindblad WL, editors: *Wound healing: biochemical and clinical aspects,* Philadelphia, 1992, WB Saunders.

48. Weigel PH, Fuller GM, LeBoeuf RD: A model for the role of hyaluronic acid and fibrin in the early events during the inflammatory response and wound healing, *J Theor Biol* 119:219-234, 1986.

49. Weitzhandler M, Bernfield MR: Proteoglycan glycoconjugates. In Cohen IK, Diegelmann RF, Lindblad WL, editors: *Wound healing: biochemical and clinical aspects,* Philadelphia, 1993, WB Saunders.

50. Whalen GF, Zetter BR: Angiogenesis. In Cohen IK, Diegelmann RF, Lindblad WL, editors: *Wound healing: biochemical and clinical aspects,* Philadelphia, 1993, WB Saunders.

Wound Management in the Military

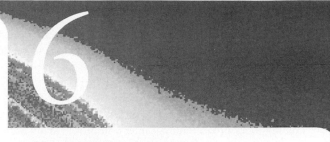

Patrick W. Lappert
Denton D. Weiss
Elof Eriksson

"He who wishes to be a surgeon should go to war."

These words of Hippocrates illustrate the historic relationship between war fighting and advances in surgical knowledge and technique. Surgical history shows that warriors and surgeons have always enjoyed a mutually beneficial relationship; one of General Washington's closest friends was Dr. Benjamin Rush. Many of the greatest warriors, from Alexander to Schwartzkopf, developed such a professional fraternity with a surgeon.

Today's military men have not forgotten this basic lesson of history, which probably accounts for their generosity in supporting surgeons' professional education. Many readers can count themselves among those who have served in the past. It is a worthwhile endeavor, therefore, to examine those issues of wound care peculiar to the military, since war is an unfortunately recurring theme in human affairs, and surgeons are often involved.

FALLACY OF MODERNISM

The technology of war fighting has greatly affected the scale of battle, having progressed from prehistoric tribal melee to the contemporary level of potential intercontinental annihilation. On the other hand, the nature of wound types has not changed. Surgeons today face the same types of wounds that Paré managed in the sixteenth century, differing only in source and not character. Greek fire has merely been replaced with napalm and grapeshot with antipersonnel mines. One new dimension might be radiation-induced contamination.

Military leaders make diligent plans to fight the war just ended. With these plans in hand, they join the battle only to discover that the nature of war is now quite different. Cavalry charges into the teeth of machine gun fire and Maginot defenses in the face of German Blitzkrieg are characteristic of the early days of most wars.

Whereas the warriors appear to be looking backward as they march to battle, historically the medical department has not been as farsighted. Physicians in garrison may believe that what applies in Detroit will readily apply in Damascus. Therefore they tend to arrive at the battle largely unprepared.

A classic example is America's involvement in Vietnam. Surgeons came ashore in Indochina vaguely ready to manage combat wounds, only to discover that more casualties resulted from malaria. Only 20 years had passed since Americans left Indochina after the World War II, having learned to manage this scourge. Within the span of one generation, however, physicians had forgotten that malaria was even an issue.

With the advent of the Uniformed Services University of the Health Sciences, the military now has a large cadre of career military physicians who have been schooled in the historic problems of planning and deployment. The university also has extensive institutional connection to deployed and foreign medical organizations, enabling it to provide current information that is pertinent to the care of military forces throughout the world.

In the case of war wound management, surgeons in garrison are prepared to apply those principles from their training in level I trauma centers and university hospitals. They may fully expect that the greatest problems will be scheduling the spiral computed tomography (CT) scanner or calibrating the operating microscope for the next free flap.

War often surprises even the most diligent planner, however, and sudden unexpected strength in the enemy can turn a state-of-the-art rear-area hospital into a Bronze Age charnel house. What began as a twenty-first-century limb salvage can suddenly degenerate into a Civil War amputation.

Therefore surgeons should not consign the problems of their forefathers to the dusty shelves of libraries. They must occasionally examine how they would manage these problems if they were on some foreign shore and could not rely on turbine-powered helicopters and clean, well-lighted places.

PEACETIME STRATEGY

As Hippocrates contends, a surgeon's professional development is aided by war, but in peacetime the lessons of war also are extended and developed.

Military and Civilian Hospitals

The distinction between peace and war has blurred, as any evening in an urban trauma center will prove. Many military surgeons keep current in their wound management skills by rotating at intervals through these trauma centers, with their unending stream of gunshot wounds, stabbings, burns, and vehicular trauma.

Wound management strategies are much the same in military hospitals as in civilian hospitals. Both are subject to the same professional and institutional certification processes. As with modern civilian hospitals, military hospitals are moving in the direction of centralized, standardized wound management principles, with particular attention paid to information technology. The ability to keep complete, standardized, and easily accessed patient records, including images of the wound, allows the modern wound care center to do the following:

1. Evaluate results of therapy.
2. Standardize therapy.
3. Test new therapies and products.
4. Contain costs.

This becomes particularly important as the technology of wound care broadens, now including an array of topical therapies, hyperbaric oxygen, growth factors, autologous cellular derivatives, autologous cells, low-output lasers, and vacuum dressings. In addition, the military wound care center can employ the military's worldwide information network to serve as consultant to deployed forces.

Medics and Corpsmen

Distinctions arise between military and civilian wound care when considering the care of the deployed forces. Forces in the field or afloat, whether for training, peacekeeping, or patrol, are accompanied by medical personnel of varying expertise.

The basic element of this medical support is the *hospital corpsman,* or *aidman* (medic). These are young men and women, typically with a high school diploma and often working on a college degree, who are specially trained in rendering aid at the scene of injury. They have about the same qualifications as paramedics. They know how to (1) establish and protect airways, (2) stop life-threatening bleeding, (3) relieve pneumothoraces, (4) protect suspected spinal injuries, (5) administer pain medications and antibiotics, (6) dress burn wounds, (7) suture lacerations, (8) stabilize fractures, and (9) generally assess patients and transmit the information to the responsible physicians.

What distinguishes corpsmen from paramedics is that they live among their patients. On board combatant ships, ashore with a squad of Marines, or encamped with a platoon of soldiers, the "Doc" is called to the scene whenever there is injury and usually knows the victim by name before arriving. This produces great diligence and enthusiasm in the corpsman and provides tremendous reassurance to the soldiers.

In time of war this intimacy with the fighting force tends to elicit in the corpsman a sense of urgency that is the embodiment of self-sacrifice. This is why the medics and corpsmen are overrepresented among recipients of the Congressional Medal of Honor, with most of these awarded posthumously.

"Flying Ambulances"

The origin of this close association of soldier and medic is usually attributed to Baron Dominique-Jean Larrey, surgeon to Napoleon. He is credited with having developed the "flying ambulances" (carriages equipped with basic supplies and medical personnel) that would roam on the field of battle, rendering assistance on the scene and evacuating surgical patients back to the field hospital. This arrangement acknowledges the need to have both basic medical personnel on the scene and a means of evacuation to definitive care.

This was a revolutionary development. Before Larrey, standard practice was to wait until the battle had subsided, then wander among the fallen soldiers, looking for those still breathing. Evidence indicates that Larrey's idea may have been an adaptation of the "ambulancias" deployed by Queen Isabella at the battle of Málaga in 1487.

WOUND CARE IN BATTLE

First Echelon: Medic

Most combat units have at least an enlisted hospital corpsman or medic who is the first echelon of response. The medics are responsible for the following:

1. Urgent stabilization of the victim
2. Initial assessment
3. Application of dressings
4. Administration of first-line medications
5. Initiation of evacuation process

ASSESSMENT. They have at their disposal a modest pack that includes a variety of field-ready bandages, pneumatic splints, cravats, tourniquets, basic medications, and a simple suture kit. Corpsmen generally have ready access to communications by which they can obtain consultation or, more importantly, arrange for transport.

If traveling with a special warfare team (e.g., SEAL team, Marine reconnaissance unit, Army Rangers), medics are likely to come in frequent contact with enemy forces and to place themselves in danger to treat wounded soldiers. They may be prevented from requesting help or evacuation if the safety of the team requires radio silence.

The general strategy at this initial level of care is to stabilize patients and establish protective measures until they are delivered to the next echelon. The tempo of battle, the safety of the evacuation route, the availability of ambulance service, and the order of evacuation dictate how long the patient will be kept at this lower echelon. Therefore improvements in this level of care depend on improvements in (1) communication, (2) evacuation, and (3) simple portable therapies that can be applied under adverse conditions and effectively protect the injured part.

COMMUNICATION. Medical personnel today have access to small, portable communication and positioning devices that allow for precise determination of location and for secure communication. Using these devices, the medic can obtain immediate consultation, as well as call into action the next element of care, the ambulance.

It should be understood, however, that the modern battlefield will likely have severe degradation of radio communication. Electronic warfare has become integral to modern war fighting. Arm waving and signal fires may still need to be used.

EVACUATION. As stated earlier, the ambulance is a military development that has had a profound effect on battlefield survival. The contemporary field ambulance includes specially converted trucks that are robust versions of civilian vehicles. They may be specially equipped armored personnel carriers (APCs) that can provide victims and their rescuers with a greater level of protection.

The most favored version of the combat ambulance now truly is the "flying ambulance." Contemporary air ambulance helicopters have made rapid evacuation of victims possible under most circumstances. Routine aerial evacuation, which was introduced in the Korean War, has seen steady improvement over the past 50 years. The benefit to wounded soldiers has been clearly documented by combat experience in Southeast Asia, as well as in the care of civilian trauma in the United States.

The more widespread availability of portable, shoulder-fired antiaircraft missiles may make this reliance on vulnerable helicopters problematic. Nations that do not have air superiority will undergo additional losses in the battlefield[1] (Table 6-1).

PORTABLE THERAPIES. Simple portable therapies, the third component in first-echelon care, include basic splints, tourniquets, and bandages. Newer therapies include military antishock trousers (MAST), the lightweight traction splint, hypertonic saline for resuscitation, the dry fibrin-impregnated battle dressing, and tissue adhesives for simplified wound closure.

With the exception of the fibrin-impregnated battle dressing, civilian surgeons are familiar with these therapies, and their application does not differ in combat.

Second Echelon: Aid Station

The nature of the injury, safety of the evacuation route, and availability of medical support guide the patient's movement to the next echelon. General medical officers represent this next level of care. Their primary function is more advanced patient stabilization, including advanced trauma and cardiac life support (ATLS/ACLS) protocols, triage and communication, and interventions that can return minor casualties to duty.

This level of care is usually referred to as the *aid station,* or *battle dressing station.* The physician usually has a small cadre of corpsmen, airway management equipment, intravenous (IV) solutions, simple wound closure supplies, and basic medications. Decisions concerning triage and evacuation are again made here. This level of care may be bypassed depending on the patient's needs and ambulance resources.

Table 6-1.
Distribution of Wounds in Various Conflicts (%)

BODY PARTS	WORLD WAR II	VIETNAM	FALKLANDS	AFGHANISTAN*
Head and neck	17	8	14	1.8
Thorax, back, and buttocks	7	13	7	4.0
Abdomen and genitalia	8	12	11.5	0.6
Upper extremity	25	25	26.5	35.2
Lower extremity	40	41	41	56.3
Other	3	1		2

From Bhatnagar MK, Smith MB: *Surgery* 105:699, 1988.
*Disproportionate number of extremity injuries seen in Afghan soldiers results from near absence of survivors who had head and trunk injuries, largely because air superiority and evacuation capabilities were lacking.

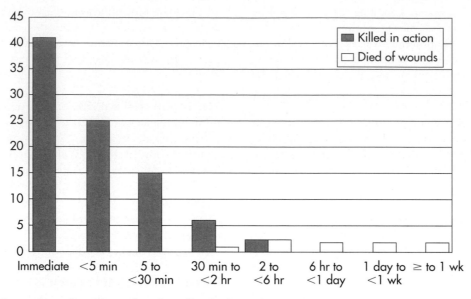

Figure 6-1. Percentage of total combat deaths in Vietnam demonstrating those killed in action versus those who died of wounds. (Courtesy Ronald F. Bellamy, Colonel, USA, retired. From *Textbook of military medicine,* Washington, DC, 1995, TMM Publications.)

"GOLDEN HOUR" VERSUS "GOLDEN MINUTES". With on-scene care and triage an important distinction must be made between civilian and combat casualties. The urban trauma center has the guiding principle, established by Blaisdell, Trunkey, and others, that there is a "golden hour" during which critical interventions can be lifesaving.

As Figure 6-1 shows, no such hour occurs on the battlefield. Experience shows that 40% of battle deaths occur immediately, 65% in less than 5 minutes, and 80% or more within 30 minutes. Furthermore, rapid evacuation and optimal care in transport have only an incremental effect on overall mortality and the paradoxic effect of increased numbers of casualties listed as "died of wounds." This is the result of the different effects of military versus civilian munitions. The devastating wounds caused by high-velocity rifle rounds, the tendency for multiple wounds, and the abundance of exploding munitions define the military effects. Those not killed outright by these devastating wounds die of rapid exsanguination. Within the time the helicopter is dispatched and picks up the victim, hypovolemic shock is established, and evacuation only serves to allow many victims to die in a medical facility instead of on the field of battle.

Knowing this, surgeons are obliged to rethink what they are taught in the civilian trauma center and to shift their first interventions as close to the moment of wounding as possible. Therefore it is more accurate to speak of the "golden minutes." The most critical interventions with the greatest hope for saving lives are those that the victim or fellow soldier can apply and that are available in their own packs. The fibrin-impregnated battle dressing can be carried by each combatant and can dramatically reduce the volume of blood loss. Therefore it may have a significant effect on overall mortality.

Third Echelon: Treatment Facility

In the U.S. armed forces, patients who survive their injuries and cannot be promptly returned to duty are moved to more capable treatment facilities in theater. Such facilities include Air Force air-mobile hospitals, Navy fleet hospitals, Army surgical hospitals, hospital ships, and amphibious assault ships.

The term *amphibious assault ship* refers to several types of warships whose purpose is to deliver landing forces ashore, either by helicopter or landing craft. Because of their mission, these ships have onboard surgical support personnel. This includes general surgeons, anesthesiology services, critical care nursing, radiology, and dental services. Because these vessels have their own transport helicopters and surface craft, they can manage the evacuation of patients without outside assistance.

These vessels possess considerable self-defense capability and typically operate in the company of other airborne and seaborne elements capable of defending the ship. This makes them a safe destination in the scheme of evacuation. Amphibious assault ships can manage blunt and penetrating trauma, treat burn wounds, stabilize fractures, and provide perioperative critical care. Patients requiring more advanced neurosurgical intervention or limb salvage procedures and patients with extensive facial fractures are taken to in-theater facilities with these capabilities (Fig. 6-2).

The U.S. Navy operates two *hospital ships,* which are capable of delivering all forms of surgical support short of cardiopulmonary bypass and organ transplantation. They can

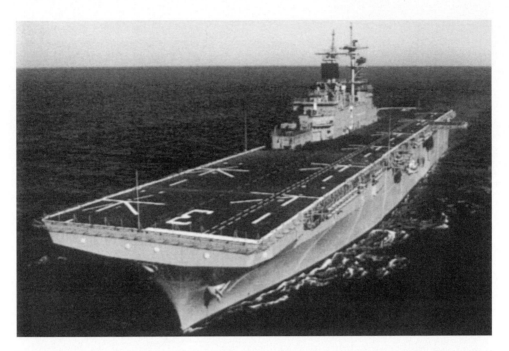

Figure 6-2. Amphibious assault ship U.S.S. Bataan. (Courtesy Tim Hogan, LCDR, CHC, USN.)

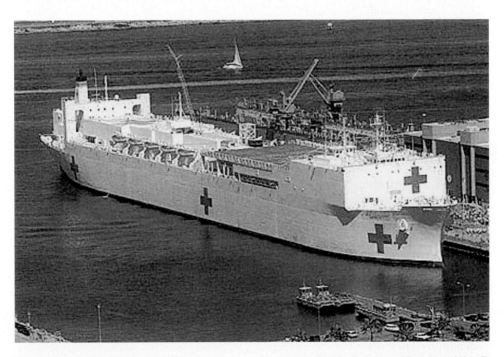

Figure 6-3. One of the U.S. Navy's two hospital ships, U.S.N.S. Comfort. (Courtesy John D. Zarkowsky, Captain, MSC, USN.)

receive casualties by sea or by air and, if stationed at a pier, also by land. They have comprehensive diagnostic radiology, pathology, and other laboratories, including microbiology, chemistry and hematology; full blood-banking services; a large casualty receiving area; fully equipped intensive care unit; physical therapy; and oral surgery. All forms of plastic surgery can be performed aboard one of these ships (Fig. 6-3).

The U.S. Air Force's *air-mobile hospital* and the U.S.

Army's *mobile surgical hospital* (corps hospital) are equipped and staffed similar to the hospital ship. They are highly flexible, modular facilities that can be expanded and upgraded depending on the combat requirements and the policy of evacuation. In rare circumstances, upgrades can include plastic surgical services when necessary and when evacuation is prolonged.

Figure 6-4 shows one model of the flow of casualties from battle.

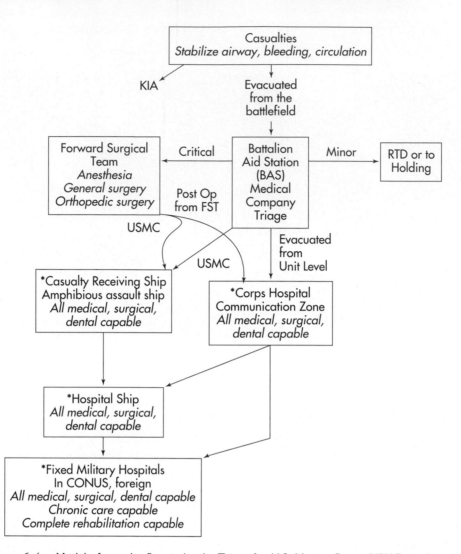

Figure 6-4. Model of casualty flow in battle. Triage for U.S. Marine Corps *(USMC)* tends to be more variable, since they are a more compact and mobile force operating at forward edge of battle. If available, corps hospitals are used in addition to amphibious assault ships that quarter these combatants. Plastic surgeons can be employed at four distinct locations, indicated by asterisks.* Most likely locations are fixed military hospitals in communication zone or aboard hospital ships. *KIA,* Killed in action; *FST,* Forward surgical team; *RTD,* Return to duty; *CONUS,* Continental United States.

NATURE OF MILITARY WOUNDS

Because humans seem predisposed to warfare, they have shown an unrelenting will to develop more effective engines of war. The acceleration of technologic advancement and the capacity for destruction have been unprecedented in the twentieth century. This technology includes the usual low-velocity and high-velocity missiles from side arms and rifles; blast weapons, ranging from grenades and mines to fuel-air explosives and nuclear weapons; incendiary weapons; chemical weapons; and biologic weapons.

As stated, however, with the exception of radioactive injury, all the wounding mechanisms are ancient. The low-velocity missile wound caused by a 9-mm side arm today is similar to the wound caused by a fourteenth-century crossbow. The burn wounds caused by a modern incendiary bomb dropped from a high-speed aircraft are exactly the same as the burn wounds caused by Greek fire from a ninth-century warship. The regional devastation caused by modern biologic weapons delivered by a ballistic missile is no different from the devastation caused by the smallpox intentionally delivered to the Indian natives around the Great Lakes in the seventeenth century. To complete the comparison, the use of nuclear weapons (though unlike anything the world has previously seen) would make the entire world much like the uncivilized portions of the ancient world.

Wound statistics based on the body areas injured reveal the bias induced by the use of body armor. Most nonfatal wounds seen in Vietnam were superficial wounds, followed closely by extremity wounds[8] (Fig. 6-5). The use of body armor by modern soldiers has greatly decreased the incidence of penetrating thoracoabdominal wounds caused by common

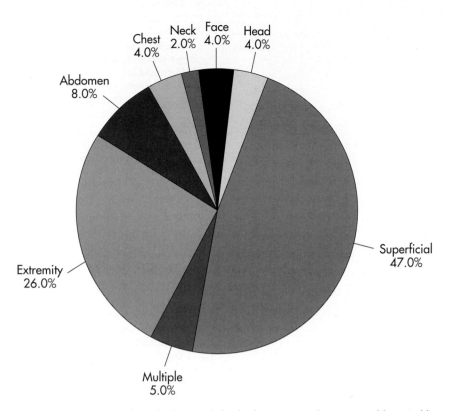

Figure 6-5. Distribution of nonfatal wounds by body region in American soldiers in Vietnam. (Courtesy Ronald F. Bellamy, Colonel, USA, retired. From *Textbook of military medicine,* Washington, DC, 1995, TMM Publications.)

munitions. During the 1982 Lebanon war the Israeli mortality rate was 3% lower than seen in other modern conflicts. All Israeli soldiers were required to wear body armor. The wound statistics among World War II air crews who were required to wear flak vests showed 75% extremity and 16% head wounds.[2]

As the use of body armor becomes more widespread, surgeons can expect to see the percentages shift away from thoracoabdominal wounds to extremity and facial/head wounds. Also, just as chain mail was overcome by the crossbow bolts, body armor will largely be nullified by teflon-coated munitions.

Traumatic Wounds

In the initial evaluation, patients are triaged and the basic ABCs (airway, bleeding, circulation) of trauma care followed. The traumatic wound patient is transferred to an operative setting, where the wound is explored and initial wound care instituted. Gram-positive antibiotics coverage is begun.

After 24 to 48 hours the wound is reexplored and debrided. At this level the wound is evaluated for probable need for major reconstruction. Those patients requiring reconstruction are transferred to fixed military hospitals.

All attempts are made to place the soldier in a position to have reconstruction begun within the first 6 days. After this period, major reconstructions requiring free tissue transfer are delayed for up to 6 weeks (Fig. 6-6).

EXTREMITIES AND GENITALIA. Unlike the single large penetrating wounds seen in World Wars I and II, with the wider use of cluster-type munitions today, patients tend to arrive with multiple wounds (Fig. 6-7). Although controversy has surrounded the merit of debridement for patients with numerous small penetrating wounds caused by fragmentation weapons, lack of debridement undoubtedly can lead to catastrophic results. The problems are mediated by fulminant bacterial necrosis from clostridial and streptococcal organisms (Fig. 6-8). Current management dictates aggressive and meticulous debridement, judicious use of antibiotics, and daily wound care (Fig. 6-9).

Antipersonnel mines, with their lower extremity–mutilating wound patterns, have become a major source of casualties. Today an epidemic of wounds from land mines has resulted from widespread application of these weapons against refugee populations (Fig. 6-10). These patients require debridement, hemorrhage control, emergent long-bone stabilization, and simple wound coverage. Early decisions relating to evacuation issues result in many field amputations. External fixation devices and vascular repair help salvage the limbs of many patients, who must be evacuated to in-theater hospitals or major U.S. military hospitals.

The genital injuries caused by land mines also require urinary diversion interventions at the field hospital, followed by evacuation to a major hospital.

HEAD AND NECK. Patients who sustain head wounds and survive the initial trauma require urgent airway management, hemorrhage control, and expedited evacuation to hospital ship, augmented fleet or air-mobile hospital (corps hospital), or

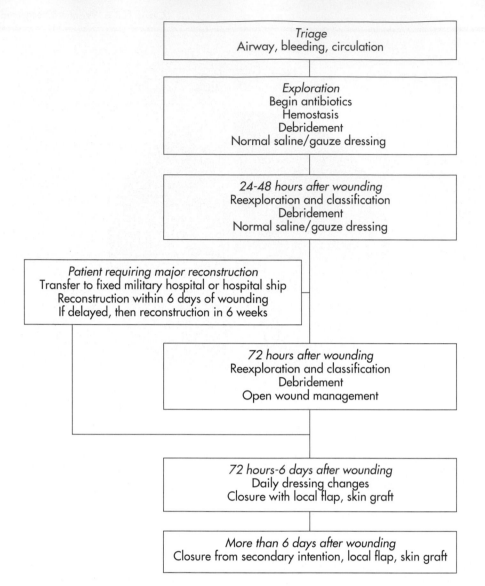

Figure 6-6. Traumatic wound management.

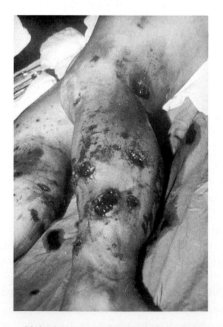

Figure 6-7. Multiple penetrating wounds to lower extremities from cluster munitions.

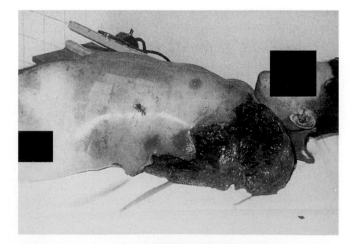

Figure 6-8. This soldier initially sustained high-velocity bullet wound to left shoulder. Severed axillary artery was repaired, but patient developed gas gangrene. Forequarter amputation was performed, but patient died within 36 hours of initial injury.

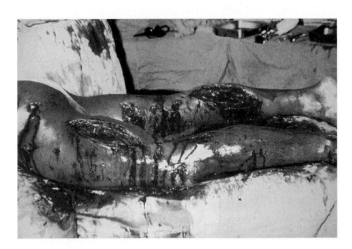

Figure 6-9. Immediate postoperative photo demonstrates aggressive debridement used today to manage multiple soft tissue wounds.

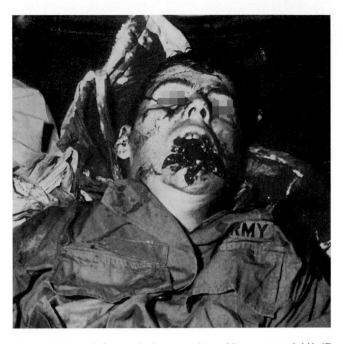

Figure 6-11. A forward observer, this soldier sustained AK-47 bullet wound of oral cavity.

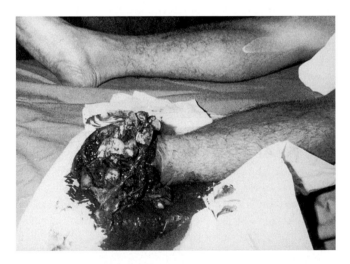

Figure 6-10. Patient with traumatic amputation after triggering antipersonnel mine.

Table 6-2.
Chemical Agents and Treatments

AGENT	TREATMENT
Mustard gas	Dilute hypochlorite/H_2O irrigation
Phosgene oxime	H_2O irrigation
Lewisite	Dilute hypochlorite irrigation
White phosphorus	H_2O/1% copper sulfate irrigation
Hydrochloric acid	H_2O irrigation
Lyes	H_2O irrigation

in-theater hospital (Fig. 6-11). Once stabilized through the initial time-critical steps, reconstruction can be addressed.

Unlike the extremity and soft tissue wounds in other areas of the body, aggressive debridement is not warranted with head and neck wounds. Conservation of the tissues is the goal.

Chemical Weapons

The effects of chemical as well as biologic weapons first require urgent decontamination, both for the patient's benefit and for the protection of medical personnel (Table 6-2).

Mustard gas, initially seen in World War I, is still the most frequently used chemical agent despite the Geneva conven-

tions ban on such weapons. Decontamination of the wound site 1 to 2 minutes after exposure is the only means of stopping or decreasing the effects of mustard gas. Irrigation with dilute hypochlorite and water is the treatment of choice. After this period, patients are treated similar to burn victims. Erythema develops at 4 to 8 hours and vesiculation 2 to 18 hours after initial exposure. Large bullae are opened, and the site is copiously irrigated and then covered with an antimicrobial ointment. Airway management is supportive[4,7] (Fig. 6-12).

Lewisite is an arsenical vesicant similar to mustard gas in terms of its wounding properties. Unlike mustard gas, lewisite's effects are evident within seconds of exposure. Within

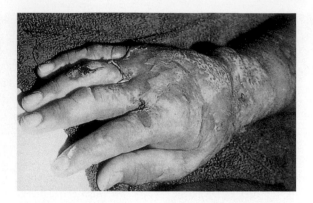

Figure 6-12. Hand of Iranian soldier who was exposed to mustard gas. These wounds are 5 days old and show characteristic bullae and erythema. (Courtesy JL Willems.)

5 minutes of exposure, lewisite is absorbed by the skin. Erythema is present 20 to 30 minutes after exposure, and blisters develop 2 to 3 hours later. Skin decontamination is achieved by irrigating the site with dilute hypochlorite and water.[4]

Phosgene oxime is a corrosive agent that causes severe pain. Erythema, urticaria, and ulceration quickly develop. The effects are immediate because of the rapid absorption of this agent. Treatment is copious irrigation with water, although much of the damage will be irreversible at initial management.[4]

White phosphorus is used in many antipersonnel weapons and ignites when exposed to air. Most patients develop wounds from ignited clothing. These wounds are treated as standard burn wounds. Patients with white phosphorus embedded in their skin must undergo immediate irrigation and debridement of identifiable particles. The wound is furthered evaluated at a corps hospital or casualty receiving ship, where 1% copper sulfate solution is used to irrigate contaminated wounds. This turns white phosphorus a blue-black color (cupric phosphite), which is benign and easy to identify. In managing these patients, the surgeon must be aware that hypocalcemia and hyperphosphatemia may develop. Cardiac monitoring is advised.[6]

Biologic Weapons
Particular biologic weapons may be associated with diverse cutaneous manifestations of infection, as well as bacteriologic contamination of other traumatic wounds. These weapons also increase the requirements for intensive care support, which can easily overwhelm the capacity of even the most well-provided medical facility.

Nuclear Weapons
The application of nuclear weaponry in warfare presents many philosophic and doctrinal problems to the medical department. Size of the casualty population will range from severe with smaller tactical weapons to incomprehensible with larger weapons. Types of injury will include penetrating and blast wounds, followed by many burn wounds. Management of these wounds will be severely compromised by the gastrointestinal and immunologic consequences of high-dose radiation.

Medical personnel, particularly the corpsmen, will be placing themselves in great danger as they work to save lives and comfort victims, dying largely because of radiation exposure. Efforts will be made to control exposure, but many corpsmen will become casualties themselves.

In triage the patient's symptoms are evaluated, and based on this the patient is categorized. Airway management and circulatory support are the priorities. Unlike radiation exposure on the battlefield, loss of airway and circulation will have immediate life-threatening effect. The process of triage at this point must recognize the enormity of the numbers of casualties, the paucity of resources, and the immunologic effects of radiation exposure.

Therefore surgical intervention will likely be offered only to patients with a single problem that can be treated with brief surgery. Casualties with numerous wounds requiring prolonged surgeries will be treated expectantly. Surgery must be performed within 36 hours after radiation exposure because of the immunologic effects. If this is not possible, surgery must be delayed 6 weeks, until immunocompetence can be regained. Infection control will be difficult, and only those patients with low-dose exposure and local infections should be treated with antibiotics.

Hemodynamic support by the administration of IV fluids can be offered only to those treated with antibiotics. The use of salt tablets and potable water can save many lives. The fluid resuscitation requirements of the great numbers of burn victims will rely on the oral route, since it will be a logistical and technical impossibility to manage all victims intravenously.

In 1965 Sorensen and Sejrsen[5] presented a paper that investigated saline solution as a potential means of managing mass burn catastrophes such as a nuclear incident. They tested the viability of oral saline and, if necessary, IV saline on 32 burn victims. Normal saline alone was a viable treatment for patients with burns on 40% or less of their body surface. Those patients with burns on greater than 40% had an initial rise in hemoglobin and hematocrit but within 48 to 72 hours had normalized. Eight patients died from pulmonary complications, none of whom had edema on autopsy.

The authors noted and we agree that in a mass catastrophe, oral saline solution is probably the only treatment available on a large scale. Patients who have received burns should drink 15% to 20% of their body weight in saline solution every 24 hours. The solution consists of 1 teaspoon of salt for each liter of water; 50 L of water and 200 g of salt per person should be the available reserve for a week of therapy.[5]

The use of bone marrow banks to salvage victims from the hematologic effects of radiation will be the newest combat-related therapy. The benefit of this therapy will be profound in individual cases but will likely have little effect on mass mortality[3] (Fig. 6-13).

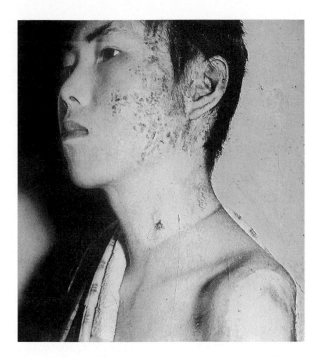

Figure 6-13. Radiation burns on face and neck of Hiroshima victim are typical of patient who would receive supportive and potentially curative care, depending on resources available.

FUTURE WOUNDS AND POPULATIONS

The increasing use of laser devices for targeting and communication can be compared to the early military use of aircraft. In World War I the aircraft was first used as a targeting device and high-speed communication tool. Likewise, with their increasing portability and power, lasers can be expected to graduate from targeting and communications duty to progressively more powerful weapons. Cases have already been reported of military personnel who had eye injuries with wound patterns suggesting intentional use of high-energy lasers. Physicians will probably begin to see focal burn wounds of varying depths caused by directed energy weapons such as lasers.

Over the centuries, war-fighting ethics have fluctuated in the desire to avoid injury to noncombatants. Although some cultures emphasize the need to protect innocent human life, others show no interest in this moral standard. Usually this lack of interest begins with a redefinition of a particular class of humanity, usually along ethnic or religious lines, and more recently on the basis of the "fitness" of a particular segment of humanity. Even cultures that once manifested chivalric heroism now seem willing to slaughter innocent civilians.

We raise this issue because the modern combat surgeon may confront a rush of pediatric wounds and must be prepared for the issues of size and disposition unique to children. Airway management, plating systems, external fixation devices, intensive care, and rehabilitation services will need adaptation to serve these innocent victims of war.

REFERENCES

1. Bhatnagar MK, Smith MB: Trauma in the Afghan guerrilla war: effects of lack of access to care, *Surgery* 105:699, 1988.
2. Coates JB, Beyer JC, editors: *Wound ballistics,* Washington, DC, 1962, US Army Publications.
3. Dons RF, Cerveny TJ, Zajtchuk R, et al, editors: *Textbook of military medicine: medical consequences of nuclear warfare,* Washington, DC, 1989, TMM Publications.
4. Sidell FR, Urbanetti JS, Smith WJ, et al, editors: *Textbook of military medicine: medical aspects of chemical and biological warfare,* Washington, DC, 1997, TMM Publications.
5. Sorensen B, Sejrsen P: Saline solutions in the treatment of burn shock, *Acta Chir Scand* 129:239, 1965.
6. Whelan TJ, editor: *Emergency war surgery,* Washington, DC, 1975, US Government Printing Office.
7. Willems JL: Clinical management of mustard gas casualties, *Ann Med Milit Belg* 3S:1, 1989.
8. Zajtchuk R, Beam T, Bellamy RF, editors: *Textbook of military medicine: anesthesia and perioperative care of the combat casualty,* Washington, DC, 1995, TMM Publications.

CHAPTER 7

Delayed Wound Healing

John S. Mancoll
Linda G. Phillips

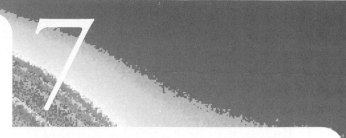

The management of wounds, their complications, and delays in wound healing has always been a focus of surgeons. The Edwin Smith Papyrus is the oldest known surgical treatise, with 142 different references to the management of wounds, pustules, and sores. Although this text was written more than 5000 years ago, some of the same basic surgical tenets regarding "infection," wound care, and nutrition are still practiced today.

Wound healing is a complex process of cellular, immunologic, and hormonal components interacting to result in a healed wound. For most patients this proceeds unabated and without sequelae, but for millions of others, wound healing is not so simple. These patients demand frequent medical attention, use substantial medical and financial resources, and have a lower quality of life as a result of their chronic wounds. Therefore wound healing is a unique problem facing all physicians and surgeons today just as it was five millennia ago. Few other physiologic processes are as fundamental as wound healing in the daily care of patients. Most often, wound healing will progress regardless of the physician's intervention.

Over the past 50 years, plastic surgeons have led the way in the research of wound healing. As a result of this interest in healing, medical peers generally call them when wounds fail. Therefore plastic surgeons not only must be well versed in normal healing processes but also must understand why some patients do not heal properly. They must communicate these wound healing concerns to their consultants and help to prevent situations that may create more chronic wounds in the future.

This chapter reviews the major factors contributing to wound healing difficulties typically seen in plastic surgery.[29,72] Delayed wound healing results from interference with one of the major steps in healing, including collagen synthesis, the inflammatory stage, and the immune response. For organizational purposes, common factors that can directly or indirectly interfere with wound healing may be considered intrinsic or extrinsic, as well as local or systemic (Box 7-1). None of these factors exists alone, however, and many are only clinically significant if they occur in conjunction with one or more of the other elements.

INFECTION

Many of the patients referred to plastic surgeons have nonhealing wounds that are infected. Almost all the factors that can interfere with wound healing do so by increasing the risk of infection. Infection is a common cause of wound healing delays. Many factors can increase a patient's susceptibility to a wound infection (Box 7-2).

Regardless of whether a wound is created in the surgical suite or in the field, a balance exists between the body's defenses and the number of bacteria present. For most bacterial organisms, wound healing will still occur without delays as long as the bacteria counts are less than 10^5 bacteria/gram of tissue.[82,111] French army surgeons in World War I first recognized the relationship between bacterial load in a wound and healing. In 1956 Elek[30] demonstrated that pustule formation occurred only if greater than 10^6 staphylococcal organisms were injected. This study was one of the first to show that the amount of bacteria present in a wound can affect the rate of healing. Since then, numerous clinical and animal experiments have confirmed these results.[61,62,112,115,143] The exception is the more virulent β-hemolytic streptococci; as few as 10^2 organisms per gram of tissue may infect a wound.[114]

Many techniques are available today to assess the bacterial status of a wound (Box 7-3). Subjective findings on physical examination, including pain, swelling, purulent drainage, erythema, and tissue breakdown, are not reliable. Of the many objective techniques described, swab culture and quantitative biopsies are most often used. Although swabbing of the wound is readily performed with little training needed, it should be discouraged in chronic wounds. The results may represent only surface contaminants and thus may not be as reliable. The reported accuracy rate for swabbing is 65% to 98%. Quantitative biopsies, on the other hand, are very accurate if performed correctly.[112] The accuracy rates for tissue biopsies range from 90% to 100%.[115] To address the need for fast and accurate results, Heggers et al[62] developed a rapid slide technique in which a 1-g specimen is diluted and homogenized and a small 0.02-ml aliquot is plated. After Gram staining, the presence of any bacteria on the slide

Box 7-1.
Factors that Interfere with Wound Healing

LOCAL
Infection
Foreign bodies
Ischemia
Smoking
Radiation
Trauma
Cancer
Local toxins
Arterial insufficiency
Venous insufficiency
Hyperthermia

SYSTEMIC
Inherited disorders
Nutritional deficiencies
Aging
Diabetes
Liver disease
Alcoholism
Uremia
Medications
Blood transfusions
Jaundice

Modified from Lawrence WT: In Cohen IK, Diegelmann RF, Lindblad WJ, editors: *Wound healing: biochemical and clinical aspects*, Philadelphia, 1992, Saunders.

Box 7-2.
Factors Contributing to Wound Infections

Trauma
Malnutrition
Immune suppression
Arterial ischemia
Venous congestion
Lymphedema
Foreign bodies
Crush injury
Necrotic tissue
Denervation
Wound maceration
Obesity
Prolonged surgery
Age

Box 7-3.
Techniques to Assess Bacterial Status of Wounds

Visual inspection
Swab culture
Quantitative wound biopsy
Rapid slide technique
Histology specimen
Allograft application
Computed tomography scan
Magnetic resonance imaging
Radioisotope scan

bacterial endotoxins and metalloproteinases contribute to changes in the inflammatory response in the wound and release enzyme collagenases that contribute to collagen turnover and tissue destruction.[111,147] Treatment of the wound should focus on decreasing the bacterial count as quickly as possible. This would include removing any devitalized tissue or foreign bodies. The wound should be dressed to avoid desiccation and to deliver topical antimicrobials to the wound bed.

WOUND HYPOXIA

Decreased oxygen in a wound is detrimental to wound healing[74,75,84,88] and results in formation of a nonhealing ulcer or impaired healing of an incision.* Although hypoxia is a stimulus for angiogenesis, the wound will not proceed through the later stages of healing without higher tissue oxygen levels.[81] Many clinical conditions affect blood vessels and can be associated with impaired healing (Box 7-4).

In the microenvironment of the skin, tissue oxygen tension levels below 35 mm Hg are associated with poor healing. At this level, wound fibroblasts are unable to replicate, and collagen production is severely impaired. Lower extremity wounds with skin oxygen tension readings below 35 to 40 mm Hg will not heal. Vascular bypass distal to the area of arterial obstruction is the standard means to improve tissue oxygenation in these patients who have poor arterial inflow. This is not effective in some patients, however, because the obstruction exists in blood vessels that are too small to be considered bypassable.

Banis et al[7] recently presented a series of patients who were not considered candidates for arterial bypass given the paucity of distal vessels seen on their arteriograms. Using microsurgical technique, they were able to anastomose the very distal vessels and achieve healing. Regardless of angiographic findings, the authors believe that a recipient distal vessel is usually present and that limb salvage is feasible in a motivated patient.

Delayed healing and chronic wounds are significant problems for patients with venous insufficiency. Although the

indicates greater than 10^5 organisms, and wound closure should not proceed.

Evidence suggests that every step in the wound healing process is altered by the presence of bacteria. Bacteria prolong the inflammatory phase and interfere with epithelialization, contraction, and collagen deposition.[111,116] The bacteria as well as the bacterial byproducts disturb normal healing. The

---

*References 73, 74, 83, 87, 144, 146.

Box 7-4.
Disorders Associated with Impaired
Blood Flow

Occlusive arterial disease
   Arteriosclerosis obliterans
   Microembolism
   Thromboangiitis obliterans (Buerger disease)
Vasospastic disease
   Cold sensitivity (Raynaud type)
   Erythromelalgia
   Livedo reticularis (severe forms)
Vasculitis
   Scleroderma
   Systemic lupus erythematosus
   Periarteritis nodosa
Hematologic disorders
   Cryoglobulinemia
   Polycythemia vera
Hypertensive ulcers

From Stadelmann WK, Digenis AG, Tobin GR: *Am J Surg* 176(suppl 2A):39S-47S, 1998.

exact mechanism is not known, evidence suggests that impaired diffusion of oxygen from the capillaries to the surrounding tissue is the cause. Proteinaceous exudate accumulates in the interstitium surrounding capillaries. This fibrin-rich fluid forms a clot, and subsequent fibrosis ensues. Over time this scar creates a barrier across which oxygen and cells must diffuse to reach the wound. Ultimately, diffusion is no longer sufficient to allow normal healing. As fibrosis occurs, leukocytes trapped in the interstitium release lysosomal enzymes and proinflammatory mediators that can exacerbate the problem and ultimately lead to tissue destruction.[128]

In the past, anemia has been considered a risk factor for impaired healing.[64,70] In a study by McGinn,[93] animals were bled to an acute anemic state and not resuscitated. These animals all demonstrated decreased wound strength. In a similar study, animals were bled but acutely resuscitated, and they did not demonstrate decreased wound strength. Any delays in resuscitation, even for 60 minutes, impair wound strength, but not to the same extent as in unresuscitated animals. The conclusion is that shock and hypovolemic hypoperfusion, more than anemia, are responsible for impaired healing.[70]

In a study of wound healing in rats made iron deficient from both chronic blood loss and dietary restrictions, breaking strength was impaired.[6] When red cell mass was reduced to 50% of that in controls, wound strength was reduced by 50% on the seventh postoperative day. Unfortunately, subsequent studies have both confirmed and refuted these results. The clinical data regarding this question are also mixed. Pure anemia without associated malnutrition or other underlying significant medical problems is uncommon.

DIABETES

Approximately 5% of the U.S. population have diabetes mellitus, characterized by hyperglycemia that results from pancreatic island cell dysfunction and decreased insulin production. An estimated 15% of diabetic patients will have a nonhealing wound some time in their life.

Diabetes is a contributing factor in more than one-half the nontraumatic lower extremity amputations performed annually. Pecoraro et al[103] found that in 81% of diabetic patients needing an amputation, abnormal wound healing was the most important contributing factor resulting in (dm4) longstanding chronic wounds. Despite multiple attempts at vascular reconstruction, ischemia progresses until limb salvage is no longer a reasonable option, and chronic wounds ensue. Although the exact mechanism is unknown, diabetes interferes with all aspects of proper wound healing and includes every stage.

The vascular end-organ damage associated with diabetes is related to the microcirculation. The capillary basement membrane thickens, blocking capillaries, causing microaneurysms, and diminishing regional blood flow. Cooley et al[18] demonstrated that a change in capillary membrane thickness is seen in both affected and nonaffected tissues. The significance of this is unclear but implies that all tissues are at risk in diabetic patients. The net result is hypoperfusion and tissue ischemia, with a decreased relative oxygen environment unable to promote wound healing.

Wound strength in diabetic wounds is greatly decreased because of altered collagen metabolism and decreased accumulation of hydroxyproline.[49,50,54] Altered granulation tissue formation results from decreases in macrophage accumulation, fibroblast ingrowth, deposition of matrix material, and alterations in angiogenesis.[94] In addition to decreases in collagen production and the net amount of collagen present in diabetic wounds, increased wound collagenase activity leads to further breakdown of the minimal collagen that has formed.[51] Functionally the collagen is less stable due to glycosylation of collagen fibers, which leads to abnormal collagen cross-linking, decreased tensile strength, and decreased wound contraction.

Epithelialization is impaired, with decreased stimulation and production of keratinocytes.[43,45] This is partially the result of decreased production of keratinocyte growth factor (KGF) by macrophages in the wound.[134] Because delays and reductions occur in the infiltration of macrophages, diabetic wounds are frequently complicated by skin infection and osteomyelitis.

Diabetic patients have difficulty fighting infection. Their wound beds may have some component of ischemia from diabetic effects on the blood supply, and their ability to handle infective pathogens is also abnormal. Immunologic complications of diabetes include alterations in the chemotaxis of granulocyte.[4] Once inside the wound environment, granulocytes have a reduced ability to phagocytize bacteria and therefore reduced bactericidal potential.[5,10] Also, adhesion of granulocytes is further reduced, decreasing their effectiveness.[3]

Separate studies by both Fowler[43] and Snip et al[127] demonstrated that superficial wounds in a rat corneal model healed without difficulty. Leukocyte infiltration into the wounds was minimal, indicating that in superficial wounds the effect of diabetes on the granulocytes is probably less important than in deeper wounds. Fortunately, the adverse effects of hyperglycemia on granulocyte function improve if serum blood glucose levels are maintained below 250 mg/dl.

Clinically, gram-positive organisms are increased in wounds of diabetic patients. Robson and Heggers[113] demonstrated that diabetic wounds tend to grow gram-positive organisms and a reduced number of gram-negative organisms. Fungal infections are also very common in diabetic patients. Any wound that does not heal despite the use of appropriate antibiotics may have a fungal infection. Fungal cultures must be obtained and the patient started on antifungal cream or oral therapy.

RADIATION

As early as 1895 the investigators who discovered radiation therapy described delayed wound healing. Becquerel noted erythema and ulceration in a chest wound he sustained after carrying 200 mg of radium in his pocket for 6 hours. The wound was red and painful and required significant time to heal.[31]

Plastic surgeons should be familiar with the different types and effects of radiation therapy. At present, high-energy megavoltage therapy has replaced low-energy orthovoltage therapy. This therapy produces a high-energy electron beam capable of sparing the skin while delivering a full dose of radiation to the deeper tissue where tumors may be located. Radiation has both acute and chronic effects on the skin. Acute effects include erythema, dry desquamation at moderate dose levels, and moist desquamation at higher dose levels. Delayed effects include increased or decreased pigmentation, thickening and fibrosis of the skin and subcutaneous tissues, telangiectasias, and alterations in sebaceous and sweat gland function. Further chronic effects can include necrosis and ultimately tumorigenesis. These effects lead to delays in wound healing as radiation therapy impacts the various components of skin and their roles in wound healing, including keratinocytes, fibroblasts, cutaneous vasculature, and adnexal structures.

Radiation damage affects the blood vessels of the skin, creating a hypoxic skin bed. Unlike in most hypoxic wound beds, however, angiogenesis is not initiated. In a radiation wound the oxygen gradient decreases from the wound edge to the center of the wound at such a gradual rate that the hypoxic stimulus for angiogenesis is not initiated. This results in wounds with poor granulation tissue. Histologic examinations of sections of skin from radiation fields have demonstrated endarteritis obliterans of the microvasculature.[90,108,121] These vascular changes contribute to the ischemia inherent in radiation wounds. Although this is an important component in radiation injury, cellular injury is considered the most significant contributor to the problem.

The keratinocytes are the critical cells in epithelialization and account for most cells in the epidermis. The keratinocytes in the basal layer divide readily and continue to cause shedding of the upper layers of the epidermis. Radiation therapy is most effective on cells in the active part of the cell cycle (i.e., G2 through M phases). Rapidly dividing cell populations are therefore most sensitive to radiation. Because of their superficial location on the skin and high replication rate, keratinocytes are very susceptible to the effects of ionizing radiation.

Activation of proteolytic enzymes is responsible for the erythema seen just after delivery of ionizing radiation. Capillary permeability is increased, which in turn causes a local inflammatory response. Cells in the basal skin layer are affected most; these cells are a major part of the immunologic system within the dermis. Injury to the basal membrane generally evokes a significant cellular response, with release of serotonin and histamines. The erythema usually develops 2 to 8 days after treatment and may persist for 2 to 3 weeks. Dry desquamation is caused by an intermediate dose of radiation that kills epidermal cells, but enough survive to repopulate the radiated area. At higher doses, insufficient epidermal cells survive to repopulate the radiated field, and moist desquamation occurs with serous oozing from the surface of the exposed dermis.[121,133] In most cases, the dose delivered to the skin is not lethal to epidermal cells but does impair their mitotic ability, causing a slow progressive desquamation.

Depending on the extent of radiation delivered to the bed, reepithelialization can continue from the adnexal structures. The rate of reepithelialization depends on not only the effect of radiation on the adnexal structures, but also the quantity of adnexal structures present. If all the adnexal structures in the dermis are injured, reepithelialization occurs from the periphery, and the long-term effect is a fragile and injury-prone epidermis. These areas are atrophic and can alternate with areas that appear thickened or hyperkeratotic. This skin is also more susceptible to the development of squamous cell tumors as a result of the atypia within the cells.

The cell most frequently injured by irradiation is the fibroblast. As in the epidermis, irradiation causes an intense inflammatory response within the dermis. This subsequently leads to edema of the collagen bundles. Coupled with a diminished ability of the dermal fibroblasts to proliferate, this causes decreased breaking strength. If the radiation injury is severe enough, full-thickness loss may ensue with necrosis and ulceration.[110]

AGING

Wound healing in the elderly patient is frequently complicated. Diabetes, peripheral vascular disease, certain medications, malnutrition, and impaired neurologic function represent known risk factors for healing in patients over age 65.[47] By 2010, it is estimated that almost one quarter of the U.S. population will be over age 65. Surgeons will be faced with an increasing group of patients considered at high risk for delayed healing because of their age, underlying medical conditions, and medications. New strategies must be developed to treat these patients and to avoid the costly postoperative wound healing complications that frequently result in limb amputation or death.

Delayed wound healing in elderly patients is the cumulative effect of all three major stages of wound healing: inflammation, proliferation, and remodeling[14] (Box 7-5). In the inflammatory stage, decreases and delays in stimulation and production of monocytes, macrophages, and B lymphocytes occur. During the proliferative phase, alterations in cell migration, proliferation, and maturation result in decreased fibroblast activity and decreased extracellular matrix formation.[63,65,66]

The role of the macrophage is critical in wound healing. Colen et al[17] demonstrated that young rats treated with a macrophage antibody heal at rates comparable to those in older rats. As a corollary, Danon et al[21] demonstrated that macrophages of young rats injected into wounds of older rats increased wound healing to rates comparable to those in younger animals. Yamura and Matsuzawa[149] demonstrated decreased rates of capillary growth in wounds of aged animals. Neovascularization is multifactorial, partly stimulated by cytokines produced by macrophages and platelets during the inflammatory stage and partly resulting from angiogenesis triggered by tissue hypoxia. In elderly patients, especially the millions affected by peripheral vascular disease, both these key mechanisms are blunted.

Carell and Ebeling[12] are credited with the earliest work recognizing delayed healing as a function of age. Based on treatment of injured World War I soldiers, they developed an index of cicatrization and found an inverse relationship between scarring and increasing age. Although this study has some limitations, it does recognize a pattern of delayed healing as persons age. Experimentally, delays in wound contractures have been identified in most animal models, including elderly rats, rabbits, and dogs. The majority of these studies examined histologic markers (e.g., collagen, elastin, extracellular matrix), in vitro growth properties, or mechanical properties. Although the conclusions are variable, evidence suggests that healing is delayed.

Studies have clearly demonstrated delayed epithelialization in shallow to intermediate partial-thickness wounds in elderly patients. Grove et al,[59] using an ammonia hydroxide blister technique, demonstrated a significant decrease in epithelialization in volunteers over age 65 compared with those under age 35. Similarly, Fatah and Ward[35] found that donor site healing in patients under age 60 was significantly faster than in those over age 60. They reported that 90% of donor sites in patients under age 60 were healed by 21 days, whereas in patients over 60, only 80% were healed in the first 3 weeks. Holt et al[67] also examined the epithelialization in elderly volunteers and found a delayed rate of epithelialization compared with controls, but unlike other studies, the ultimate thickness of the epithelium was no different than in controls.

The metabolic activity in wounds of older animals is also decreased. Heikkinen et al[63] demonstrated reduced oxygen consumption and glucose metabolism in older rats compared with those in younger animals. In the elderly animals the maximum level of glucose metabolism decreased, and the onset of glucose accumulation in the wound was delayed. Most studies agree that collagen production is decreased with advancing age, but many clinical reviews are dealing with patients who have other risk factors for delayed healing. Holt et al[67] studied normal, healthy, older volunteer patients who did not have histories of diabetes, peripheral vascular disease, or medication known to impair healing. They found marked decreases in protein accumulation, as indicated by decreased α-amino acid nitrogen content, but no differences between hydroxyproline and deoxyribonucleic acid (DNA) content. Their conclusions contradicted previously published studies.

SMOKING

Cigarette smoking has long been known to have a detrimental effect on wound healing. In 1977 Mosely and Finseth[96] reported on a patient with an underlying history of arteriosclerotic disease who continued to smoke and had delayed healing of a hand wound. Seventeen years earlier, Rottenstein demonstrated that cigarette smoking can decrease digital blood flow.[42] Although the association between cigarette smoking and delayed wound healing is accepted in clinical practice, no controlled clinical studies have proved this relationship. Much of the information in the literature is derived from animal studies that examined the individual components of cigarette smoke and tobacco, including nicotine, carbon monoxide, and hydrogen cyanide.

Nicotine has significant vasoconstrictive effects. Jensen et al[77] found that the vasoconstrictive effect, measured by subcutaneous tissue wound oxygen, lasts for up to 50 minutes after completion of smoking. This decrease in blood flow leads to a relatively ischemic environment. Nicotine also increases platelet adhesion, increasing the risk of thrombus formation in the microvasculature. Nicotine is also known to have an inhibitory effect on the proliferation of red blood cells, macrophages, and fibroblasts.

Box 7-5.
Age-related Effects on Wound Healing

Glucose metabolism
Oxygen consumption
Inflammatory cell infiltrate
Macrophage function
Fibroblast function
Capillary growth
Collagen remodeling
Incisional breakage
Contraction rate
Reepithelialization rate

Carbon monoxide serum levels are elevated in patients who smoke, causing decreased tissue oxygenation. Carbon monoxide competitively competes with oxygen for transport on the hemoglobin molecule. Because of the lower binding affinity of oxygen, carbon monoxide is selectively transported.

Hydrogen cyanide is a common byproduct of burning tobacco. It has an enzyme system that selectively inhibits oxidative metabolism in oxygen transport on the cellular level, thus interfering with normal cellular respiration.

The detrimental effect that smoking has on healing is not limited to skin. In 1993 Kyro et al[84] found a significantly longer time to clinical union and a higher incidence of delayed union in patients who smoked. They stated that smokers had 4.1-fold risk in bone fractures resulting from low-energy injuries compared with nonsmokers. A direct correlation exists between the comminution of the fracture and the number of cigarettes smoked. Silcox[126] studied the delayed effect on bone healing further by examining the rate of osteoinduction and spinal fusion.

Cigarette smoking is a significant risk factor in the formation of duodenal and oral ulcers, and the rate of healing of these ulcers is significantly delayed in patients who smoke. Fischer[39] recently indicated that smoking was one of the most significant risk factors in delayed healing of duodenal ulcers.

A variety of different techniques has been developed to ameliorate the effects of cigarette smoking on wound healing. Reus et al[17] demonstrated that if patients can stop smoking 2 weeks before a surgical intervention, the rate of healing is no different than that of nonsmokers. Upson[137] suggested that the use of topical hyperbaric oxygen could be beneficial in treating ischemic lower extremity ulcers in patients with a history of smoking. This study, however, used a patient population with multiple risk factors for nonhealing, including peripheral vascular disease and diabetes, in addition to smoking.

NUTRITION

One of the most frequently overlooked contributors to delayed healing is malnutrition. Therefore the plastic surgeon should review the patient's nutritional condition[41] (Box 7-6). Patients may be malnourished because of the primary disease or the inability to obtain adequate nutritional support. Daily calorie counts should be done to assess nutritional status. Healthy young patients who sustain a severe injury or burn can develop protein depletion within days of their injury. In an effort to decrease the morbidity associated with protein loss and other nutrients, initiation of feeding is done within hours of a patient's stabilization.[119,120]

Protein

Besides poor oral intake, the reasons for protein depletion include trauma, sepsis, nephrotic syndrome, liver disease, and burns. In starved animals a lag in the wound healing response results from impaired protein metabolism.[68] The consequences of protein depletion include decreases in angiogenesis

---

Box 7-6.
Nutritional Deficiencies Associated with Delayed Wound Healing

Decreased protein levels
Carbohydrate depletion
Decreased levels of amino acids
    Arginine
    Glutamine
Vitamins
    Decreased vitamin C
    Decreased vitamin A
    Excess vitamin E
Trace element deficiencies
    Zinc
    Iron
    Copper
    Magnesium

---

and fibroblast proliferation, resulting in decreased synthesis, accumulation, and remodeling of collagen.[9,20,46,50]

Although most studies agree that protein depletion contributes to delayed healing, the degree of depletion needed before delays are seen is not clear.[109] Albumin levels below 3.0 g/dl are associated with hypoalbuminemic tissue edema, and serious protein deficiency is seen at 2.5 g/dl.[25] Clinically, impaired wound healing is only significantly affected with severe protein losses.[22] Markers of protein stores include albumin, prealbumin, transferrin, and insulin-like growth factor I. Hypoalbuminemia as an indicator of impaired healing is controversial. Because albumin has a half-life of 3 weeks, protein malnutrition may exist long before changes in this serum marker occur. In early reports, Howe et al[68] found decreased incisional strength in animals with reduced protein stores. Felcher et al,[37] however, failed to demonstrate impaired healing in mildly albuminemic rats. Recently, Robson et al[117] demonstrated normal healing potential in clinical trials as long as serum albumin was maintained above 2.0 g/dl.

As a corollary to impaired healing in protein depletion, many studies have demonstrated improved healing in malnourished animals given supplementation.[75,86,135] These studies have shown decreased rates of muscle catabolism, increased fibroblast activity with increased collagen synthesis, and improved immune response. Chernoff et al[13] demonstrated improved healing of pressure sores in patients receiving high levels of protein supplement, regardless of whether a positive nitrogen balance could be obtained.

Vitamins

In the United States, pure protein depletion without a concomitant lack of vitamins and minerals critical for proper healing is uncommon.

VITAMIN C. Some authorities consider vitamin C deficiency to be the only true vitamin deficiency to impair wound

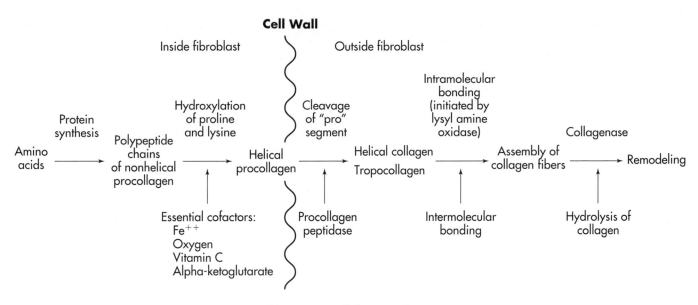

Figure 7-1. Collagen synthesis.

healing. The Vitamin C's critical role in wound healing and prevention of scurvy has been known since the early days of the British Navy. The rate and speed at which wounds heal are greatly reduced in vitamin C–deficient animals and can occur within 3 months in deprived animals.[8] Impaired healing may occur without the other symptoms of scurvy.[19,104]

In wound healing, vitamin C serves as a cofactor in the formation of hydroxyproline in procollagen (Figure 7-1). Procollagen residues are hydroxylated intracellularly to form collagen. Any deficiencies will impact both the rate and the quality of collagen production, with the net result being marked delays in healing, weaker scars, and abnormal capillary formation.[71] Severe vitamin C deficiency may even lead to the opening of previously well-healed scars.

The effects of vitamin C depletion are not limited to collagen production. Ascorbic acid increases the patient's ability to resist infection by facilitating leukocyte migration into a wound.[125] It also plays a bactericidal role by contributing to the formation of neutrophil superoxide formation.[101]

To treat vitamin C deficiencies, supplementation with 100 to 1000 g/day may be given. Supraphysiologic doses of vitamin C have been shown to improve wound healing in animal and clinical studies. Although the safety profile for vitamin C is very good, some caution must be exercised when giving large doses, since megadoses may lead to the formation of oxalate stones in the kidneys. If complicated, they can eventually lead to renal dysfunction.[54]

VITAMIN A. Vitamin A deficiencies influence most of the stages of wound healing. Weinzweig et al[141] cite monocyte and macrophage stimulation, fibronectin deposition, cellular adhesion, and tissue repair as being adversely influenced by vitamin A deficiency. Hayashi et al[60] demonstrated adverse effects on transforming growth factor beta (TGF-β) receptors in vitamin A–deficient rats. In 1968 Ehrlich and Hunt[27] demonstrated

that vitamin A supplementation could improve wound healing in steroid-impaired rats. This study prompted Freiman et al[44] to investigate whether vitamin A deficiency would impair normal wound healing. They conducted a series of experiments that showed decreased breaking strength in rat wounds as a result of decreased production of collagen, with less cross-linking.

Vitamin A deficiency is probably more common among hospitalized patients than physicians think. The detection of serum levels is costly and difficult to perform, so many cases go undetected. Isolated vitamin A deficiencies are uncommon, and most patients are considered asymptomatic.

Vitamin A also is involved with the immune response and contributes to lysosomal membrane stabilization and phagocytosis in a wound.[27] Deficiencies may be responsible for the severity of infection seen in some wounds. Vitamin A plays a role in cell-mediated cytotoxicity, cytokine production, antibody response, and epithelialization.[118] Since most malnourished patients generally have other vitamin deficiencies, supplementation usually includes vitamin A. Care must be taken when supplementing vitamin A to avoid hypervitaminosis and the effects on the liver and cornea.

OTHER VITAMINS. *Vitamin K* is vital in the normal clotting cascade. Since the initial events of the inflammatory stage of wound healing depend on blood clotting, deficiencies in vitamin K will affect the synthesis of prothrombin and factors VII, IX, and X.

Vitamin E, or α-tocopherol, is generally thought to interfere with wound healing.[28] It is a known antioxidant that possesses antiinflammatory properties. It alters prostaglandin production by inhibiting phopholipase A_2 activity. The result is decreased collagen production and decreased inflammation. Although some studies have shown improved healing in vitamin E–supplemented animals, most studies suggest that large dosages have led to healing delays.[80]

In two studies on healing tendons and skin, wound strength was impaired and collagen production decreased.[57,58] The exact role of Vitamin E is not known but appears to involve cell differentiation, epithelialization, cell-mediated immunity, the early inflammatory response, and angiogenesis.[130,131]

Trace Elements

Trace elements are critical for wounds to heal properly. Deficiencies are often overlooked. The elements most often implicated in delayed wound healing are zinc and iron.

ZINC. Zinc deficiency is uncommon but is seen in patients with large burns,[85] profuse sweating, severe surgical trauma, chronic alcoholism, cirrhosis, and gastrointestinal fistulas.[100] Zinc is an essential cofactor in normal cellular growth and replication and is involved in more than 100 different enzymatic reactions.[122] Those specifically related to wound healing include the production of DNA polymerase (essential for cellular proliferation) and superoxide dismutase. Zinc directly impacts epithelialization and fibroblast proliferation through its effects on metalloenzymes, such as ribonucleic acid (RNA) polymerase, DNA polymerase, and DNA transcriptase.[69,76,107] Zinc is also involved with many aspects of the immune response, including phagocytosis, cellular and humoral immunity, and bactericidal activity.[99,100,104]

Animal studies have demonstrated that zinc deficiency contributes to wound healing delays. Miller et al,[95] Pories et al,[104] and Weiss and Stiller[142] demonstrated decreased bursting strength in rat incisions up to 12 days postwounding in zinc-deficient animals. In Sandstead's study[122] the rate of strength gain was no different than that of the control group despite the maximum tensile strength in the study group being diminished. Subsequent studies suggest that normal wound healing is seen by 3 weeks postwounding and that zinc deficiency is responsible only for wound delays seen in the first few days to weeks after wounding.[1,2,129,139,145] Savlov et al,[124] using a radioactive zinc label, were able to demonstrate increased zinc accumulation in healing tissue, which begins gradually to disappear at day 3. Unfortunately, the same correlation has not been proved as convincingly in human trials.[36,105,106,123]

IRON. Iron is an essential cofactor in the replication of DNA. In conjunction with ribonucleotide reductase, iron is involved in producing the deoxyribonucleotides needed for DNA synthesis.[92] Ferrous iron is a cofactor needed by proline hydroxylase to convert hydroxyproline to proline. Without this, the normal collagen triple helix cannot be made.

Multiple studies have been done to examine the effects of iron deficiency anemia on wound healing.[136] Macon and Pories,[88] Waterman et al,[140] and Jurkiewicz and Garrett[79] found no significant effects of acute or chronic iron deficiency anemia on wound healing. In one of the few studies to discover a relationship among iron deficiency, anemia, and wound strength, Hugo et al[70] found tensile strength differences in the first 6 days of healing, but normalization occurred after day 9. None of these studies measured tissue oxygenation in the wound bed, and the question remains whether iron deficiencies can lead to reduced oxygen delivery, which in turn may increase the susceptibility to infection and delayed healing.

SUPPLEMENTS. Mineral supplementation is a common practice in the clinical setting. The amount of iron and zinc needed daily varies, but to date, no study has demonstrated that supraphysiologic levels of any trace element will accelerate wound healing beyond normal unless severe depletion is present.[45,67,69,95]

DRUGS

Many drugs are known to impair wound healing[16,23,40,148] (Box 7-7). Many more possess the ability to delay healing but are overlooked because the patient has more significant comorbid factors.

Chemotherapeutic Agents

Drugs used to treat cancer are by far the largest group known to delay wound healing. Wound healing and tumor growth share many physiologic and metabolic pathways. It is logical to assume that any drug that will impair tumor growth or kill cancer cells will potentially impair healing. Nine different classes of chemotherapeutic agents are used to treat cancer (Box 7-8). All of these are thought to work in a similar manner to affect wound healing.[55] These drugs tend to attenuate the inflammatory phase of healing by interfer-

---

Box 7-7.
Medications Associated with Wound Healing Delays

Anticoagulants
Antihistamines
Aspirin
Azathioprine
BAPN (β-aminoproprionitrile)
Betadine (povidone-iodine)
Chemotherapeutic agents
Chlorhexidine
Colchicine
Cyclosporine
Dakin's solution (sodium hypochlorite 0.25%)
Dilantin
Glucocorticoids
Immunosuppressive agents
Lathyrogens
Nonsteroidal antiinflammatory agents
Papaverine
Penicillamine
Phenylbutazone
Quinoline sulfate
Retinoids
Thiphenamil (Trocinate)

ing with the vascular response. Delays in the cellular infiltration in the healing wound and decreased fibrin deposition lead to poor or incomplete scaffolding for healing. These delays interfere with DNA and RNA production, protein synthesis, and cell osmosis. The primary cell affected is the fibroblast, with decreased collagen synthesis. The myofibroblast is impaired, causing delayed wound contraction in treated animals.[24,25,26,32,34]

Many of the commonly used drugs have been linked directly to delayed healing in animal studies, but the same impairment in the clinical setting is less common. Clinical studies have shown 5-fluorouracil (5-FU), methotrexate, and 6-mercaptopurine (6-MP) have to be safe, especially if treatment is not initiated until 2 weeks after surgery.[11,38] The more significant effects on healing are believed to occur if the agents are used preoperatively. This is particularly true of agents that are classified as alkylating drugs, antimetabolites, antitumor antibodies, or corticosteroids.

Tamoxifen is a synthetic nonsteroidal antiestrogen given to an increasing population of patients, particularly those with breast cancer. Unfortunately, the antitumor effects of tamoxifen are not completely known but include decreased cellular proliferation, cell cycle arrest, and interference with peptide growth factors.[98] These cellular and hormonal mechanisms are also known to play a key role in normal wound healing. Mancoll et al[89] demonstrated a dose-dependent impairment in wound tensile strength. Further cell studies also confirmed impaired fibroblast replication with tamoxifen, which was cytotoxic in concentrations greater than 16 µg. One of the proposed mechanisms is the reduction in TGF-β seen in tamoxifen-treated cells.

Steroids

Systemic glucocorticosteroids have been shown to impair wound healing by directly blunting the cellular response, which in turn impairs fibroblast proliferation and ultimately collagen synthesis. The formation of granulation tissue and extracellular matrix is also decreased in steroid-treated animals. As expected, both epithelialization and wound contraction are decreased in a dose-dependent manner. Gene transcription, particularly that associated with production of platelet-derived growth factor, is also impaired.

Box 7-8.
Classification of Chemotherapeutic Agents

Adrenocorticosteroids
Alkylating agents
Antiestrogens
Antimetabolites
Antitumor antibodies
Estrogen progestogens
Nitroureas
Plant alkaloids
Random synthetics

Erlich and Hunt[26,27] have shown the antiinflammatory effects of steroids can be reversed by the administration of vitamin A. Steroids stabilize lysosomal membranes, which are necessary to initiate part of the inflammatory response during wound healing. Vitamin A is thought to antagonize this effect and allow release of the lysosomal products.

The effect of steroids on wound strength is dose and time dependent. Low doses given for short periods will not interfere with wound healing. With chronic administration, however, Green et al[56] demonstrated impaired healing in patients receiving large doses, even up to 1 year after cessation of the drug.

Nonsteroidal Antiinflammatory Agents

Although often cited as drugs that impair wound healing, little evidence is available to suggest that NSAIDs actually delay healing. High doses of NSAIDs have been implicated in delayed healing, but not usual therapeutic doses.[91,132] Despite this, plastic surgeons should still advise patients to avoid their use preoperatively. This is more the result of concerns with bleeding than with a direct effect on wound healing.

SUMMARY

Delayed wound healing is a complication faced by all physicians regardless of their field of practice. Plastic surgeons are frequently called on to help treat patients who fail to heal properly. Therefore, plastic surgeons must be well versed in the intrinsic and extrinsic factors that can impair healing. Plastic surgeons must continue to be leaders in the search for new and innovative means by which to treat these complicated wounds.

REFERENCES

1. Agren, MS: Studies on zinc in wound healing, *Acta Derm Venereol Suppl (Stockh)* 154:1, 1990.

2. Argren MS, Franzen L: Influence of zinc deficiency on breaking strength of 3-week-old skin incisions in the rat, *Acta Chir Scand* 156:667, 1990.

3. Bagbade JD, Walters E: Impaired granulocyte adherence in mildly diabetic patients: effects of tolazamide treatment, *Diabetes* 29:309-311, 1980.

4. Bagdade JD, Root RK, Bugler RJ: Impaired leukocyte function in patients with poorly controlled diabetes, *Diabetes* 23:9-15, 1974.

5. Bagdade JD, Stewart M, Walters E: Impaired granulocyte adherence: a reversible defect in host defense with poorly controlled diabetes, *Diabetes* 27:677-681, 1978.

6. Bains JW, Crawford DT, Ketchum AS: Effect of chronic anemia on wound tensile strength: correlation with blood volume, total red cell volume, and proteins, *Ann Surg* 264:243, 1966.

7. Banis JC Jr, Richardson JD, Derr JW Jr, et al: Microsurgical adjuncts in salvage of the ischemic and diabetic lower extremity, *Clinics in Plastic Surgery,* 19(4):881-93, 1992.

8. Bobel LM: Nutritional implications for the patient with bedsores, *Clin North Am* 22:379, 1982.

9. Breslow RA, Hallfrisch J, Guy DG, et al: The importance of dietary protein in healing pressure ulcers, *J Am Geriatr Soc* 41:357-362, 1993.

10. Bybee JD, Rogers DE: The phagocytic activity of polymorphonuclear leukocytes obtained from patients with diabetes mellitus, *J Lab Clin Med* 64:1-13, 1964.

11. Calan J, Davies A: The effect of methotrexate (amethopterin) on wound healing: an experimental study, *Br J Cancer* 19:505-512, 1965.

12. Carell A, Ebeling AH: Age and multiplication of fibroblast, *J Exp Med* 34:599, 1921.

13. Chernoff RS, Milton KY, Lipschitz DA: The effect of a very high-protein liquid formula on decubitus ulcer healing in long-term tube-fed institutional patients, *J Am Diet Assoc* 90:A-130, 1990 (abstract).

14. Chvapil M, Koopmann CF: Age and other factors regulating wound healing, *Otolaryngol Clin North Am* 15:259-270, 1982.

15. Cohen BJ, Danon D, Roth GS: Wound repair in mice as influenced by age and antimacrophage serum, *J Gerontol* 42:295-301, 1987.

16. Cohen SC, Gabelnick HI, Johnson RK, et al: Effects of cyclophosphamide and Adriamycin on the healing of surgical wounds in mice, *Cancer* 36:1277-1281, 1975.

17. Reus WF 3d, Colen LB, Straker DJ: Tobacco smoking and complications in elective microsurgery, *Plast Reconstr Surg* 89(3):490, 1992.

18. Cooley BC, Hanel DP, Anderson RB, et al: The influence of diabetes on free flap transfer. I. Flap survival and microvascular healing, *Ann Plast Surg* 29(1):58-64, 1992.

19. Crandon JH, Lind CC, Dill DB: Experimental human scurvy, *N Engl J Med* 223:353, 1940.

20. Daly JM, Reynolds J, Sigal RK, et al: Effect of dietary protein and amino acids on immune function, *Crit Care Med* 18:S86, 1990.

21. Danon D, Kowatch MA, Roth GS: Promotion of wound repair in old mice by local injection of macrophages, *Proc Natl Acad Sci USA* 86:2018-2020, 1989.

22. Dempsey DT, Mulled JL, Buzby GP: The link between nutritional status and clinical outcome: can nutritional intervention modify it? *Am J Clin Nutr* 47(suppl 2):352-356, 1988.

23. Devereux DF, Thibault L, Boretos J, et al: The quantitative and qualitative impairment of wound healing by Adriamycin, *Cancer* 43:932-938, 1979.

24. Devereux DF, Triche TJ, Webber BL, et al: A study of Adriamycin-reduced wound breaking strength in rats, *Cancer* 45:2811-2815, 1980.

25. Doweiko JP, Nompleggi D: The role of albumin in human physiology and pathophysiology. Part III. Albumin and disease states, *J Parenter Enteral Nutr* 15:476, 1991.

26. Ehrlich HP, Hunt TK: The effects of cortisone and anabolic steroids on the tensile strength of healing wounds, *Ann Surg* 170:203-206, 1969.

27. Ehrlich HP, Hunt TK: Effects of cortisone and vitamin A on wound healing, *Ann Surg* 167:324, 1968.

28. Ehrlich HP, Tarver H, Hunt TK: Inhibitory effects of vitamin E on collagen synthesis and wound repair, *Ann Surg* 175:235, 1972.

29. Ehrlichman RJ, Seckel BR, Bryan DJ, et al: Common complications of wound healing: prevention and management, *Surg Clin North Am* 71:1323, 1991.

30. Elek SD: Experimental staphylococcal infections in the skin of man, *Ann NY Acad Sci* 65:85, 1956.

31. Engel D: Experiments on production of spinal deformities by radium, *Am J Roentgenol* 42:217-234, 1939.

32. Engelmann U, Grimm K, Gronniger J, et al: Influence of cis-platinum on healing of enterostomies in the rat, *Eur Urol* 9:45-49, 1983.

33. Fahrat SM, Amer NS, Weeks DS, et al: Effect of mechlorethamine hydrochloride (nitrogen mustard) on healing of abdominal wounds, *Arch Surg* 76:749-753, 1958.

34. Falcone RE, Nappi JF: Chemotherapy and wound healing, *Surg Clin North Am* 64:779-794, 1984.

35. Fatah MF, Ward CM: The morbidity of split-skin graft donor sites in the elderly: the case for mesh grafting the donor site, *Br J Plast Surg* 37:184-190, 1984.

36. Faure H, Peyrin JC, et al: Parenteral supplementation with zinc in surgical patients corrects postoperative serum-zinc drop, *Bio Trace Elem Res* 30(9):37-45, 1991.

37. Felcher A, Schwartz J, Shechter C, et al: Wound healing in normal and albuminemic (NAR) rats, *J Surg Res* 43:546-549, 1987.

38. Ferguson MK: The effect of antineoplastic agents on wound healing, *Surg Gynecol Obstet* 154:421-429, 1982.

39. Fischer BH: Topical hyperbaric oxygen treatment of pressure sores and skin ulcers, *Lancet* 23;2(7617):405-9, 1969.

40. Fitzpatrick DW, Fisher H: Carnosine, histidine, and wound healing, *Surgery* 91:56-60, 1982.

41. Flanigan KH: Nutritional aspects of wound healing, *Adv Wound Care* 10(3):48-52, 1997.

42. Forrest CR, Pang CY, Lindsay WK: Dose and time effects of nicotine treatment on the capillary blood flow and viability of random-pattern skin flaps in the rat, *Br J Plast Surg* 40:295-299, 1987.

43. Fowler SA: Wound healing in the corneal epithelium in diabetic and normal rats, *Exp Eye Res* 31:167-179, 1980.

44. Freiman ME, Seifter E, et al: Vitamin A deficiency and surgical stress, *Surg Forum* 21:81, 1970.

45. Frosch PJ, Czarnetzki BM: Effect of retinoids on wound healing in diabetic rats, *Arch Dermatol Res* 282:424, 1989.

46. Garrow JS: Protein nutrition and wound healing, *Proc Nutr Soc* 28:242-248, 1969.

47. Geriatric Panel Discussions: Practical nutritional advice for the elderly. Part I. Evaluations, supplements, RDAs, *Geriatrics* 45:28, 1990.

48. Goodson WH, III, Hunt TK: Studies of wound healing in experimental diabetes mellitus, *J Surg Res* 22:221-227, 1977.

49. Goodson WH III, Hunt TK: Wound healing in experimental diabetes mellitus: importance of early insulin therapy, *Surg Forum* 29:95-98, 1978.

50. Goodson WH III, Hunt TK: Deficient collagen formation by obese mice in a standard wound model, *Am J Surg* 138:692-694, 1979.

51. Goodson WH III, Hunt TK: Wound healing and the diabetic patient, *Surg Gynecol Obstet* 149:600-608, 1979.

53. Gottrup F, Andreassen TT: Healing of incisional wounds in stomach and duodenum: the influence of experimental diabetes, *J Surg Res* 31:61-68, 1981.

54. Gottschlich MM, Warden GD: Vitamin supplementation in the patient with burns, *J Burn Care Rehabil* 11(3):275-9, 1990.

55. Graf WS, Weiber S, et al: The roles of nutritional depletion and drug concentration in 5-fluorouracil–induced inhibition of colonic healing, *J Surg Res* 56:452-456, 1994.

56. Lee PW, Green MA, Long WB 3d, et al: Zinc and wound healing, *Surg Gynecol Obstet* 143(4):549-554, 1976.

57. Greenwald DP, Sharzer LA, Padawer J, et al: Zone II flexor tendon repair: effects of vitamins A, E, beta-carotene, *J Surg Res* 49(1):98-102, 1990.

58. Greenwald D, Mass D, Gottlieb L, et al: Biomechanical analysis of intrinsic tendon healing in vitro and the effects of vitamins A and E, *Plast Reconstr Surg* 87(5):925-930; discussion 931-932, 1991.

59. Grove GL: Age-related differences in healing of superficial skin wounds in humans, *Arch Dermatol Res* 272(3-4):381-385, 1982.

60. Hayashi K, Frangieh G, Wolf G, et al: Expression of transforming growth factor-beta in wound healing of vitamin A–deficient rat corneas, *Invest Ophthalmol Vis Sci* 30:239, 1989.

61. Heggers JP, Robson MC: *Quantitative bacteriology: its role in the armamentarium of a surgeon,* Boca Raton, Fla, 1991, CRC Press.

62. Heggers JP, Robson MC, Doran ET: Quantitative assessment of bacterial contamination of open wounds by a slide technique, *Trans R Soc Trop Med Hyg* 63:632-634, 1969.

63. Heikkinen E, Aalto M, et al: Age factor in the formulation and metabolism of experimental granulation tissue, *Gerontology* 26:294-298, 1971.

64. Heughan C, Grislis G, Hunt TK: The effects of anemia on wound healing, *Ann Surg* 179:163, 1974.

65. Holm-Petersen P, Zenderfeldt B: Granulation tissue formation in subcutaneously implanted cellulose sponges in young and old rats, *Scand J Plast Reconstr Surg* 5:13-16, 1971.

66. Holm-Petersen P, Zenderfeldt B: Strength development of skin incisions in young and old rats, *Scand J Plast Reconstr Surg* 5:7-12, 1971.

67. Holt DR, Kirk SJ, et al: Effect of age on wound healing in healthy human beings, *Surgery* 112:293-298, 1992.

68. Howes EL: Strength of wounds sutured with cat gut and silk, *Surg Gynecol Obstet* 57:309-317, 1933.

69. Hsu THS, Hsu JM: Zinc deficiency and epithelial wound repair: an autoradiographic study of H-thymidine incorporation, *Proc Soc Exp Biol Med* 140:157, 1972.

70. Hugo NE, Thompson LW, Zook EG, et al: Effect of chronic anemia on the tensile strength of healing wounds, *Surgery* 66:741, 1969.

71. Hunt AH: The role of vitamin C in wound healing, *Br J Surg* 28:436, 1940.

72. Hunt TK: Disorders of wound healing, *World J Surg* 4:271-277, 1980.

73. Hunt TK: Distribution of oxygen and its significance in healing tissue. In Longacre JJ, editor: *The ultrastructure of collagen,* Springfield, Ill, 1976, Thomas.

74. Hunt TK, Zederfeldt B, et al: Oxygen and healing, *Am J Surg* 118:521-525, 1969.

75. Irvin TT: Effects of malnutrition and hyperalimentation on wound healing, *Surg Gynecol Obstet* 146:33-37, 1978.

76. Jeejeebhoy KN: Rhoads lecture—1988. Bulk or bounce—the object of nutritional support, *JPEN J Parenter Enteral Nutr* 12(6):539-549, 1988.

77. Jensen JA, Goodson WH, Hopf HW, et al: Cigarette smoking decreases tissue oxygen, *Arch Surg* 126(9):1131-1134, 1991.

78. Jonsson K, Jensen JA, et al: Tissue oxygenation, anemia, and perfusion in relation to wound healing in surgical patients, *Ann Surg* 214:605-613, 1991.

79. Jurkiewicz MJ, Garrett LP: Studies on the influence of anemia on wound healing, *Am Surg* 30:23, 1964.

80. Kim JE, Shklar G: The effect of vitamin E on the healing of gingival wounds in rats, *J Periodontol* 54:305, 1983.

81. Knighton DR, Hunt TK, et al: Oxygen tension regulates the expression of angiogenesis factor by macrophages, *Science* 221:1283-1285, 1983.

82. Krizak TJ, Robson MC, Kho E: Bacterial growth and skin graft survival, *Surg Forum* 18:518, 1967.

83. Kulonen E, Niinikoski J, et al: Effect of the supply of oxygen on the tensile strength of healing skin wound and granulation tissue, *Acta Physiol Scand* 70:112-115, 1967.

84. Kyro A, Usenius JP, Aarnio M, et al: Are smokers a risk group for delayed healing of tibial shaft fractures? *Ann Chir Gynaecol* 82(4):254-262, 1993.

85. Larson DL, Maxwell R, Abston S, Dobrksovsky M: Zinc deficiency in burned children, *Plast Reconstr Surg* 46:13, 1970.

86. Law NW, Ellis H: The effect of parenteral nutrition on the healing of abdominal wall wounds and colonic anastomoses in protein-malnourished rats, *Surgery* 107:449-454, 1990.

87. Lundgren CE, Zederfeldt BH: Influence of low oxygen pressure on wound healing, *Acta Chir Scand* 135:555-558, 1969.

88. Macon WL, Pories WJ: The effect of iron deficiency anemia on wound healing, *Surgery* 69:792-796, 1971.

89. Mancoll JS, Zhao J, Phillips L: Inhibitory effects of tamoxifen on wound tensile strength (submitted, 1999).

90. Marino H: Biologic excision: its value in treatment of radionecrotic lesions, *Plast Reconstr Surg* 40:180, 1967.

91. Mastboom WJB, Hendriks T, van Elteren P, et al: The influence of NSAIDs on experimental intestinal anastomoses, *Dis Colon Rectum* 34:236, 1991.

92. Mazzotta MY: Nutrition and wound healing, *J Am Podiatr Med Assoc* 84:456-462, 1994.

93. McGinn FP: Proceedings: Effect of haemorrhage on wound healing in the rat, *Br J Surg* 63(2):163, 1976.

94. McMurry JF: Wound healing with diabetes mellitus, *Surg Clin North Am* 64:769-778, 1984.

95. Miller WJ, Morton JD, Pitts WJ, Clifton CM: Effect of zinc deficiency and restricted feeding on wound healing in bovine, *Proc Soc Exp Biol Med* 118:427, 1965.

96. Mosely LH, Finseth F: Cigarette smoking: impairment of digital blood flow and wound healing in the hand, *Hand* 9(2):97-101, 1977.

97. Mowat AG, Baum J: Chemotaxis of polymorphonuclear leukocytes from patients with diabetes mellitus, *N Engl J Med* 284:621-627, 1971.

98. Nayfield SG, Karp JE, Ford LG, et al: Potential role of tamoxifen in prevention of breast cancer, *J Nat Cancer Inst* 83(20):1450-1459, 1991.

99. Norman JN, Rahmat A, Smith G: Effect of supplements of zinc salts on the healing of granulating wounds in the rat and guinea pig, *J Nutr* 105:815-821, 1975.

100. Orberleas D, Seymour JK: Effect of zinc deficiency on wound-healing in rats, *Am J Surg* 121:566-568, 1971.

101. Orgill D, Demling RH: Current concepts and approaches to wound healing, *Crit Care Med* 16(9):899-908, 1988.

103. Pecoraro RE: The nonhealing diabetic ulcer—a major cause for limb loss, *Prog Clin Biol RES* 365:27-43, 1991.

104. Pories WJ, Henzel JH, Rob CG, Strain WH: Acceleration of wound healing in man with zinc sulfate given by mouth, *Lancet* 1:121, 1967.

105. Prasad AS: Clinical manifestations of zinc deficiency, *Ann Rev Nutr* 5:341-363, 1985.

106. Prasad AS: Zinc and growth in development and the spectrum of human zinc deficiency, *J Am Coll Nutr* 7:377, 1988.

107. Prasad AS, Oberleas D: Changes in activities of zinc-dependent enzymes in zinc deficient tissues of rats, *J Appl Physiol* 31:842, 1971.

108. Reinisch JF, Puckett CL: Management of radiation wounds, *Surg Clin North Am* 64:795-802, 1984.

109. Rhoads JE, Fliegelman MT, Panzer LM: The mechanism of delayed wound healing in the presence of hypoproteinemia, *JAMA* 118:21, 1942.

110. Robinson DW: Surgical problems in the excision and repair of radiated tissue, *Plast Reconstr Surg* 55:41, 1975.

111. Robson MC: Wound infection, *Surg Clin North Am* 77:637-650, 1997.

112. Robson MC, Heggers JP: Bacterial quantification of open wounds, *Milit Med* 134:19, 1969.

113. Robson MC, Heggers JP: Effect of hyperglycemia on survival of bacteria, *Surg Forum* 20:56-57, 1969.

114. Robson MC, Heggers JP: Surgical infection. II. The "B" hemolytic streptococcus, *J Surg Res* 9:289-292, 1969.

115. Robson MC, Lea CE, Dalton JB, Heggers JP: Quantitative bacteriology and delayed wound closure, *Surg Forum* 19:501-502, 1968.

116. Robson MC, Stenberg BD, Heggers JP: Wound healing alterations caused by bacteria, *Clin Plast Surg* 3:485-492, 1990.

118. Ross AC: Vitamin A and protective immunity, *Nutr Today* 27:18, 1992.

119. Ruberg RL: Role of nutrition in wound healing, *Surg Clin North Am* 64:705-714, 1984.

120. Ruberg RL: The role of nutrition in plastic surgical practice: a review, *Plast Reconstr Surg* 65:363, 1980.

121. Rudolph R, Utley J, Woodard N, et al: The ultrastructure of chronic radiation damage in rat skin, *Surg Gynecol Obstet* 152:171, 1981.

122. Sandstead HH, Shepard GH: The effect of zinc deficiency on the tensile strength of healing surgical incisions in the integument of the rat, *Proc Soc Exp Biol Med* 128:687-689, 1968.

123. Sandstead HH, Lanier VC Jr, Shephard GH, Gillespie DD: Zinc and wound healing: effects of zinc deficiency and zinc supplementation, *Am J Clin Nutr* 23:514, 1970.

124. Savlov ED, Strain WH, Huegin F: Radiozinc studies in experimental wound healing, *J Surg Res* 2:209-212, 1962.

125. Schwartz PL: Ascorbic acid in wound healing—a review, *J Am Diet Assoc* 56:497-503, 1970.

126. Silcox DH 3rd, Daftari T, Boden SD, et al: The effect of nicotine on spinal fusion, *Spine* 20(14):1549-1553, 1995.

127. Snip RC, Thoft RA, Tolentino FE: Similar epithelial healing rates of the corneas of diabetic and nondiabetic patients, *Am J Ophthalmol* 90:463-468, 1980.

128. Stadelmann WK, Digenis AG, Tobin GR: Impediments to wound healing, *Am J Surg* 176(suppl 2A):39S-47S, 1998.

129. Stephan JK, Hsu JM: Effect of zinc deficiency and wound on DNA synthesis in rat skin, *J Nutr* 103:548, 1973.

130. Tanka TH, Fujiwara H, Torisu M: Vitamin E and the immune response, *Immunology* 38:727, 1979.

131. Taren DL, Chavpil M, Weber CW: Increasing the breaking strength of wounds exposed to preoperative irradiation using vitamin E supplements, *Int J Vit Nutr Res* 57:133, 1987.

132. Telfer NR, Moy RL: Drug and nutrient aspects of wound healing, *Dermatol Clin* 11:729-737, 1993.

133. Telok HA, Mason ML, Wheelock MD: Histopathologic study of radiation injuries in the skin, *Surg Gynecol Obstet* 90:335, 1950.

134. Thakral KK, Goodson WH III, Hunt TK: Stimulation of wound blood vessel growth by wound macrophages, *J Surg Res* 26:430, 1979.

135. Thomas DR: Specific nutritional factors in wound healing, *Adv Wound Care* 10(4):40-43, 1997.

136. Trueblood HW, Nelsen TS, Oberhelman HA: The effect of acute anemia and iron deficiency on wound healing, *Arch Surg* 99:113, 1969.

137. Upson AV: Topical hyperbaric oxygenation in the treatment of recalcitrant open wounds: a clinical report, *Phys Ther* 66(9):1408-1412, 1986.

138. Van Winkle W: The tensile strength of wounds and factors that influence it, *Surg Gynecol Obstet* 129:819, 1969.

139. Watanabe T, Arakawa T, Fukuda T, et al: Zinc deficiency delays gastric ulcer healing in rats, *Dig Dis Sci* 40:1340-1344, 1995.

140. Waterman DF, Birkhill FR, Pirani CL, Levenson SM: The healing of wounds in the presence of anemia, *Surgery* 31:821, 1952.

141. Weinzweig J, Levenson SM, Rettura G, et al: Supplemental vitamin A prevents the tumor-induced defect in wound healing, *Ann Surg* 211:269, 1990.

142. Roth RN, Weiss LD: Hyperbaric oxygen and wound healing, *Clin Dermatol* 12(1):141-156, 1994.

143. Weissman G, Simolen JE, Korchak HM: Release of inflammatory mediators from stimulated neutrophils, *N Engl J Med* 303:27, 1980.

144. Whitney JD: Physiologic effects of tissue oxygenation on wound healing, *Heart Lung* 18:466-474, 1989.

145. Williams RB, Chesters JK: The effects of early zinc deficiency on DNA and protein synthesis in the rat, *Br J Nutr* 24:1053, 1970.

146. Winter GD: Oxygen and epidermal wound healing, *Adv Exp Med Biol* 94:673-678, 1977.

147. Witte MB, Barbul A: General principles of wound healing, *Surg Clin North Am* 77:509-527, 1997.

148. Wiznitzer T, Orda R, Bawnik JB, et al: Mitomycin and the healing of intestinal anastomosis, *Arch Surg* 106:314-319, 1973.

149. Yamura H, Matsuzawa T: Decrease in capillary growth during aging, *Exp Gerontol* 15:145-150, 1980.

CHAPTER 8

Healing of Nerves, Blood Vessels, Muscle, Tendon, Cartilage, and Bone

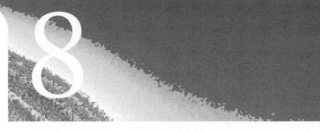

W. Thomas Lawrence

Ajaya Kashyap

The body's response to injury has many common themes that pertain to virtually all types of tissue. Soon after injury an inflammatory response occurs in which damaged cells and tissue are phagocytized and cytokines are released. The next phase is characterized by significant migratory and proliferative cellular activity, followed by a phase of synthetic activities. The final phase of healing is characterized by maturation of the healed tissues.

Despite these common themes, tissues differ in terms of the specific activities that occur in response to injury. Many tissues in the body have very specialized functions, and some have almost unique structures. Although humans cannot regenerate any damaged part completely, the response to injury must reproduce a structure that can continue the tissue's original function to some degree. The healing process therefore generally involves a component of regeneration, combined with a component of repair.

Unique and individualized nuances of the response to injury are seen in peripheral nerves, blood vessels, muscle, tendon, cartilage, and bone. In each a different balance of regeneration and repair generates the clinical results seen after injury.

PERIPHERAL NERVES

Anatomy

Because of their unique morphology and function, the healing of peripheral nerves involves many special considerations. The cell bodies of motor nerves are found in the anterior horn of the spinal cord, whereas the cell bodies of sensory nerves reside adjacent to the spinal cord in the dorsal root ganglia. The axons extend from the cell bodies and course along the length of the peripheral nerves. Motor nerves terminate at motor end plates in muscle, and sensory nerves terminate in sensory receptors in skin or other structures. Individual neurons are therefore extremely long, which allows injury to occur to a limited part of the cell (Fig. 8-1).

When a neuronal cell body is damaged, the entire cell dies; the body's response is similar to that in other tissues. Cells migrate into the damaged area from the periphery, and a scar is produced, leading to the complete loss of nerve function. This type of injury occurs infrequently because the spinal cord and adjacent dorsal root ganglia are relatively well protected by the vertebrae and adjacent musculature. Peripheral nerves are injured more often at a more distal level, where the axon is the primary cellular structure damaged. Such injuries do not result in cell death. Instead, the damaged neurons respond by regenerating new distal axonal segments.

Peripheral nerves are made up of axons that have many neurons running together. Most axons are surrounded by myelin sheaths, which in turn are encompassed by Schwann cells. These structures are surrounded by an *endoneurium,* which also serves as a basement membrane for the adjacent Schwann cells. Groups of these endoneurially surrounded axons are bounded by a *perineurium* and make up nerve fascicles. Groups of perineurially bounded bundles are surrounded by an *epineurium.* An inner epineurium often surrounds one or more fascicular bundles within larger peripheral nerves, with the outer epineurium surrounding the entire peripheral nerve. The outer epineurium is the nerve sheath that incorporates peripheral nerves when they are intact.

At each level of organization within the nerve, connective tissue elements are interspersed between the nerve structures within the surrounding sheaths. Also at all levels, blood vessels provide a vascular supply to the neural elements (Fig. 8-2).

The cell nucleus and many other, more metabolically active cellular subunits reside within the neuronal cell body centrally. Proteins and other substances required for maintenance of cellular homeostasis and for signal transmission are synthesized primarily within the cell body. These compounds are then transmitted down the axon through a microtubular system to the site where they are needed.

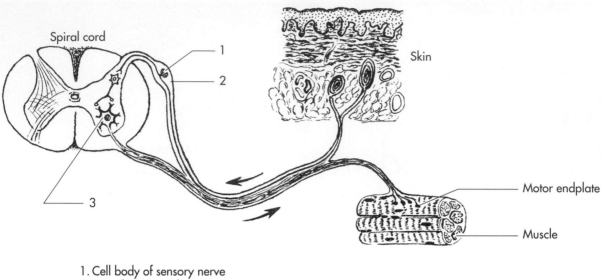

1. Cell body of sensory nerve
2. Dorsal root ganglion
3. Cell body of motor nerve

Figure 8-1. Peripheral nerve anatomy.

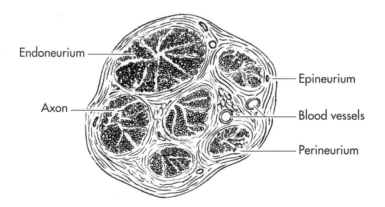

Figure 8-2. Cross section of peripheral nerve.

Nerve Injury

When the axon of a peripheral nerve axon is injured, different processes occur proximal and distal to the site of injury. *Wallerian degeneration* occurs distally; because the cellular elements distal to the injury do not include a nucleus or other essential synthetic subunits, they degenerate along with the surrounding myelin. The injury causes the release of calcium ions, which mediate the activation of various proteases and contribute to the formation of free radicals. Both the proteases and the free radicals participate in tissue breakdown.

As tissue degeneration proceeds, the adjacent Schwann cells proliferate and become phagocytic. They phagocytize degenerating axonal elements and myelin, contributing to the clearing of the distal neuronal elements. Macrophages are also recruited to the distal axonal segment and also contribute to the phagocytic process.

As neural elements are broken down, residual clumps of neurofilaments and microtubules are initially seen within distal axonal segments. Over time these segments swell and break into smaller segments before eventually being eliminated completely. The combined effect of this chemical and cellular debridement is a hollow endoneural sheath, which then collapses. It can take weeks to completely eliminate residual neuronal material and myelin from the distal nerve segment. What remains is empty endoneural tubes with their adjacent Schwann cells.

Immediately proximal to the site of injury, limited degeneration occurs in a similar manner. The distance that the axons degenerate proximally depends on the severity of the injury but also is usually limited.

In addition to contributing to phagocytosis, Schwann cells secrete cytokines, such as nerve growth factor (NGF), that promote axonal extension.[23,44] Macrophages contribute NGF, insulin-like growth factor (IGF), platelet-derived growth factor (PDGF), and apolipoprotein E (apo E). IGF, as with NGF, is a known stimulant of axonal elongation. Apo E contributes to axonal elongation and remyelination.

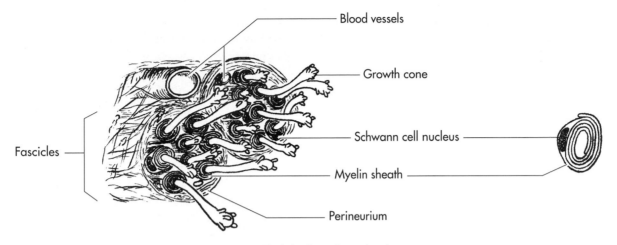

Figure 8-3. Early healing of peripheral nerves.

Changes also occur in the cell body. The cell nucleus swells and migrates closer to the cell membrane from a more central location, and the entire cell body becomes rounder. The number of ribosomes increases, and the rough endoplasmic reticulum breaks apart and moves to the cell periphery. The marginated endoplasmic reticulum fragments are referred to as *Nissl's substance,* or *Nissl bodies.*

These histologic changes have been termed *chromatolysis.* As these histologic changes occur, the synthesis of neurotransmitter substances diminishes dramatically, whereas the synthesis of lipids and structural proteins (e.g., tubulin) increases. These are then transported down the axon to the site of injury.

At the site of injury, axons sprout from the proximal nerve segment within 24 hours after injury (Fig. 8-3). They derive from both the cut axonal end and from nodes of Ranvier several segments proximal to the axon tip. They are initially unmyelinated, and individual axons may produce more than one sprout.

A region of axoplasmic enlargement known as a *growth cone* develops at the tip of the sprouts. The growth cone includes many intracellular structures, including smooth endoplasmic reticulum, microtubules, microfilaments, large mitochondria, and lysosomes. They also include Schwann cells at their periphery.

Actin-rich *filopodia* extend out and then retract from the most distal part of the growth cones in an ameboid fashion. These fibropodia reach out from the injured nerve and move in different directions until they come in contact with a favorable physical substrate.[34] Favorable substrates include those with Schwann cells and attachment factors such as fibronectin and laminin, substances found within the endoneural sheaths. The fibropodia will not grow into solid structures even if they contain the desired attachment factors.

Once a sheath containing attachment factor is found, the axon will grow into it. This usually occurs within several days after injury. Although multiple sprouts may have initially been generated from an injured nerve, the auxiliary sprouts degenerate once one finds a desirable milieu and begins to grow.

In order for the axon to grow, new cytoskeletal components are required. As mentioned, these are synthesized in the cell body and are transported down the axon to the site of injury. Some compounds can be transported down the axons relatively quickly (400 mm/day), but the actin, tubulin, and neurofilaments required for axonal regeneration are transported by slow axonal transport mechanisms (less than 30 mm/day). The rate of slow axonal transport is the rate-limiting component of nerve regeneration. Whether myelin is produced or not to surround the regenerating sprout is determined by the nature of the neuron, not by the distal site into which it grows.

Neurotrophic factors released by the denervated structure probably contribute to the growth of the axon toward it. In both rat and primate models, axons regenerate toward appropriate nerve end organs.[26] Additional studies have demonstrated that this directed regeneration applies to both motor and sensory nerves. NGF is one of the factors that contribute to accelerated and directed growth of axons; IGF may also have a role. Both fibroblast growth factor (FGF)[40] and interleukin-1 (IL-1) stimulate Schwann cell proliferation and may be involved, along with ciliary neurotrophic factor.

Beginning approximately 1 month after injury, additional endoneural collagen is noted within the axon sheaths in the distal nerve segments. If no axon grows into the endoneural sheaths, they shrink over time to only 1% of their original size 1 year after injury. The blood supply contracts concurrently. Although a sheath can reexpand if an axon grows into it later, the blood supply never returns completely to its premorbid state, and the regenerating axon will be smaller than its original size.

The loss of axonal continuity leads to the loss of synaptic transmission of neural signals. At the nerve terminal the normal whorls of neurofilaments that surround mitochondria become disrupted and swollen. If a nerve ending is at some distance from the site of injury, substrate in the distal cellular structures may be adequate to maintain synaptic transmission for several days after injury. The signal cannot be transmitted centrally, but evidence suggests positive nerve excitability distally.

If the injury is closer to the nerve ending, synaptic activity diminishes much more quickly. Motor end plates in the most distal portion of motor nerves atrophy after injury, although recovery can occur if they become reinnervated up to 12 to 24 months after injury. Sensory end organs can regain function if reinnervated years after injury, but the quality of renewed sensation may diminish if a long time has elapsed between injury and repair. Despite neurotrophic factors contributing to the regeneration of axons to appropriate end organs, the ultimate number of axons reaching an appropriate end organ is generally less than the preinjury number. Often, central compensation and reeducation must occur to maximize the final functional result.

Injury Classification

The severity of injury to the axon can vary and affects the healing response. Seddon[36] provided one of the earliest classifications of nerve injury in 1943, which Sunderland[38] expanded in 1951 (Table 8-1).

Table 8-1.
Classification of Nerve Injuries

SEDDON	SUNDERLAND
Neuropraxia (first degree)	Level I: interruption of conduction within axons with preservation of anatomic continuity
Axonotmesis (second degree)	Level II: loss of axonal continuity without loss of endoneurial continuity
	Level III: loss of nerve fiber continuity, including axon, myelin sheath, and Schwann cells
	Level IV: loss of fascicular continuity, including perineurium
Neurotmesis (third degree)	Level V: loss of nerve trunk continuity

Seddon's *neuropraxia,* which corresponds to Sunderland's *level I injury,* involves a conduction block but no actual structural damage to the cell. Axonal regeneration is not required after this type of injury, which is generally produced by transient nerve compression.

Seddon's intermediate grade of injury is termed *axonotmesis* and involves damage to internal nerve structures, whereas the outermost epineurium remains intact. Sunderland subclassifies this group according to which of the nerve structures is actually damaged. A *level II injury* involves an injury to the axon alone, whereas a *level III injury* also involves the endoneurium surrounding it. A *level IV injury* includes the perineurium in addition to the axon and endoneurium.

As the severity of injury increases, the likelihood of improper axonal regeneration increases. With any such injury, however, at least some structural elements remain intact to provide guidance to the growing axons. Seddon's *neurotmesis* corresponds to Sunderland's *level V injury* and consists of an injury that involves all peripheral nerve structures, such as laceration of a peripheral nerve. Level V injuries are the most common types leading to surgical intervention.

Repair Process

A number of factors influence the results of nerve repair after injury (Box 8-1).

Lacerations at multiple levels and more severe injuries create defects with significant scarring between proximal and distal segments of the sheath. This is especially true with a severe ischemic insult. Regenerating axons have limited ability to generate the proteases required for scar penetration and frequently branch in response to it. Whereas growth through a nerve graft is generally 2 to 3 mm/day, growth through a scarred sheath may occur at a rate of only 0.25 mm/day. As the severity of injury increases, the likelihood of any injured nerve not finding its appropriate distal sheath increases, and the quality of the functional result decreases.

If a long time passes between injury and repair, the sheaths diminish in size, limiting axonal size, myelin thickness, and the functional result. The deleterious effect of a long interval between injury and repair is particularly evident in motor nerves, where, as mentioned, the motor end plates atrophy and become less functional with time.

Age is a significant variable affecting results, with individuals over 40 achieving much poorer results than those under 40. This may involve cortical plasticity more than the axon's ability to regenerate.

Box 8-1.
Adverse Factors in Nerve Repairs

Injury at multiple levels
Injury to proximal nerve
Concomitant injuries
Devascularization
Delayed repair
Patient over age 40

Repairs of injuries more proximal to involved muscles and sensory end organs achieve much better results than when structures must regenerate over longer distances. This is partly the result of target organ degeneration and the increasing homogeneity of distal nerves, which leads to less cross-innervation. In addition, more proximal muscles tend to require less precise function than some more distal muscles, such as those of the hand.

Efforts have been made to improve healing of nerves by more precisely aligning neural elements during surgical repairs. This has involved approximating individual fasciculi within nerves. Biologically, improved alignment of proximal and distal segments should result in improved function, but clinical results generally have not been significantly better when fascicular repairs are compared with those that approximate only the epineurium. This most likely results from the increased scarring generated by the intraneural stitches.

Fibrin glue and lasers have been used to repair nerve ends, but at this time, neither has been shown to produce better results than those obtained with sutures.

The following basic principles are the most reliable and beneficial:

1. Careful handling of tissues
2. Limited devascularization of proximal and distal nerves
3. Tension-free closures
4. Careful coaptation of nerve ends

Supplements, including hormones and gangliosides, have been used to improve the results of healing, with some success reported.[44] Early results with electrical stimulation have also been encouraging. No supplement or mechanical stimulant, however, has definitively been shown to be of clinical benefit at this time.

Conclusion

Nerves are particularly dependent on regeneration to maintain function. Proximal injuries to the cell body and severe distal injuries that limit regeneration result in scarring and a loss of neural function. Regeneration is often possible, however, in less severe, well-managed peripheral nerve injuries. Therefore, when managing nerve injuries, it is especially important to create a healing environment where regeneration is optimized.

BLOOD VESSELS

The healing of blood vessels is unique because of their critical function as blood conduits. Maintenance of a blood supply is essential to sustain tissue viability. When larger, more essential vessels are either surgically reconstructed or repaired after injury, maintenance of blood flow is a primary consideration, and healing in a manner that reconstructs the vessel's function as a conduit is essential.

At the same time, mechanisms must plug smaller lacerated vessels to prevent exsanguinating hemorrhage after minor injuries. When a small vessel is traumatically damaged, optimal healing generally involves occlusion of the vessel with scarring.

Anatomy

Blood vessels vary significantly in different parts of the body. Vessels in the lower extremity generally are thicker than those in the head and neck. Arteries and veins differ in wall thickness and structure, and capillaries differ from these larger vessels.

The innermost layer of essentially all blood vessels includes endothelial cells, which rest on a basement membrane. In arteries an additional connective tissue layer contains elastin, microfibrils, and myointimal cells adjacent to the basement membrane. These structures make up the *intima*. Peripheral to the intima is the *media*, which includes collagen, smooth muscle, and elastic fibers.

The outermost layer of a blood vessel is the *adventitia*, which includes connective tissue, and the *vasa vasorum*, which provide the vessels with a blood supply. Most arteries have an additional inner elastic lamina between the intima and media, and larger arteries have an external elastic lamina peripheral to the media as well (Fig. 8-4).

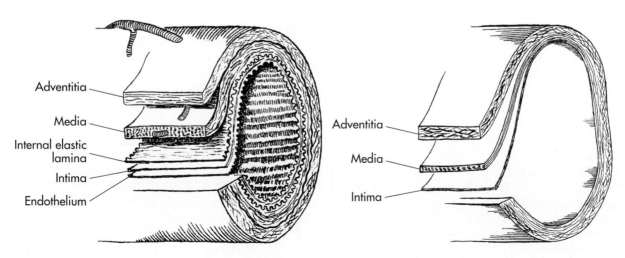

Figure 8-4. Cross section of blood vessels.

Vessel Injury

Injuries limited to the endothelium can be produced by minor trauma. Surgical dissection of a blood vessel, desiccation of the vessel, prolonged spasm, or the application of a microvascular clamp can cause endothelial loss. When such an injury occurs, the endothelium is reconstituted by endothelial cells that migrate from the edges of the denuded area. A 1-cm to 1.5-cm area of denudement is generally completely covered in 7 to 10 days (Box 8-2).

Healing at an anastomosis requires the healing of all tissue layers. This usually is supplemented by the sutures used to approximate the vessels. In an anastomotic portion of an artery, endothelium is lost as well as internal elastic lamina, exposing the connective tissue elements of the deeper layers. Endothelial damage from surgical manipulation extends over a wider area.

Platelets aggregate where subendothelial collagen is exposed. Subendothelial microfibrils and basement membrane stimulate platelet aggregation to a lesser degree, as do sutures. Despite these factors that contribute to platelet aggregation, however, only a thin layer of platelets will adhere in the region of a well-formed anastomosis.

This carpet of platelets begins to form immediately after blood flow returns to an anastomosis.[35] Platelet deposition peaks several hours after blood flow is restored to the anastomotic site. Although some fibrin and red blood cells (RBCs) are included in the platelet thrombus, significant amounts of fibrin are not produced unless there is significant constriction of the vessel or extensive exposure of the media. The layer of platelets and thrombus is thickest in the anastomotic area with veins, which generally create thicker layers than arteries.

The thickness of the platelet carpet increases for the first 4 hours postoperatively and then gradually diminishes in size. The platelets slowly disappear over 3 to 7 days, as endothelial proliferation becomes increasingly apparent. Fibrinolysis also occurs during this period.

Studies have not been able to delineate whether endothelial cells migrate under or over the platelet thrombus. The migrating endothelial cells derive both from the periphery of the injured area and from myointimal cells that migrate into the injured area from below.

Neutrophils are seen at the anastomotic site within an hour of a vascular repair and begin to replace the RBCs initially seen. Macrophages are seen in large numbers approximately 3 days after a vascular repair. These phagocytic cells contribute to the gradual decrease in the size of the thrombus over the first week.

When examined sequentially over time, sutures at an anastomotic site are gradually covered by tissue.[15] At 5 days they are covered by a pseudointima consisting of thrombus, fibrin, and leukocytes. Endothelial cell migration across the anastomotic site begins several days after the procedure, and by 14 days the sutures are completely covered by endothelial cells.[15,43] At this point, however, the endothelial layer at the anastomotic site has significant irregularities. Up to 8 weeks may pass before the endothelial surface is flat and smooth (Table 8-2).

Repair Process

The endothelial repair process is modulated both by the matrix on which the cells migrate and by cytokines that stimulate endothelial cell activities. Endothelial cell migration involves the following[21]:

1. Regulated attachment and detachment of cells
2. Contraction of cytoplasmic filaments
3. Changes in the plasticity of the cytoskeleton
4. Regulated cell-to-cell communications

The dissolution of existing cell-substrate binding involves collagenases and other proteolytic enzymes. Adhesion of the cells to new areas is largely regulated by components of the underlying matrix. Laminin and collagen types I, III, and IV induce cytoskeletal changes associated with migration, whereas fibronectin does not.[27] Some matrix binding depends on integrin.

Several cytokines influence endothelial cell activity, including basic fibroblast growth factor (bFGF), acidic fibroblast growth factor (aFGF), epidermal growth factor (EGF), transforming growth factor alpha (TGF-α), insulin-like growth factor I (IGF-I), endothelial cell PDGF, and vascular endothelial growth factor.[4] Cytokines such as IL-1 and tumor necrosis factor alpha (TNF-α) may help stimulate vascular smooth muscle cells to synthesize the collagenase involved in degradation of damaged matrix.[10] Endothelial cells synthesize some of these cytokines, including bFGF, PDGF, TGF, and IGF-I, although other cells also contribute cytokines to the repair process. Vascular smooth muscle cells, for example, are a source of both aFGF and bFGF.

Healing in the deeper vessel layers continues for months at an anastomotic site. Some medial necrosis is produced by the sutures, and smooth muscle cells and fibroblasts migrate into the area from adjacent areas. They produce collagen and other connective tissue elements, which seal the deeper vessel layers.

Box 8-2.
Causes of Endothelial Loss

Surgical desiccation
Dessication
Prolonged spasm
Clamp application

Table 8-2.
Healing of Vascular Anastomosis

TIME	SITE COVERAGE
Day 5	Pseudointima
Day 14	Endothelium
8 weeks	Flat endothelial surface

At times, excessive collagen production can lead to intimal thickening or hyperplasia. Myointimal thickening may occur as early as 10 days after an anastomosis, and at 3 months, vessel wall thickness in arteries may be doubled.[24]

This process is much more active in arteries than veins, where the degree of thickening is much less extreme and is primarily mediated by smooth muscle cells, which migrate into the area and proliferate. The release of PDGF and transforming growth factor beta$_1$ (TGF-β_1) by aggregating platelets may contribute to this. PDGF and TGF-β_1 stimulate both smooth muscle cell proliferation and migration.

As with endothelial cells, migration of mesenchymal cells involves proteolytic dissolution of cell-matrix bonds and upregulation of binding proteins (e.g., integrins), as well as cytoskeletal reorganization and synthesis of additional proteins (e.g., fibronectin) that can provide a suitable migratory matrix.[27] Interestingly, fibronectin and TGF-β_1 stimulate smooth muscle cell migration while limiting endothelial cell migration.

With scar remodeling, blood vessels gradually decrease in thickness for up to a year after vascular repair.

When vein grafts are used in arteries, the endothelium initially sloughs from a large portion of the vessel.[32] This begins very early after the anastomosis, with neutrophils playing a major role in the process. At the anastomotic site, all endothelium is lost, whereas farther from the anastomosis, only partial endothelial loss may occur. By 4 hours after an anastomosis, up to 50% of the endothelium is sloughed. Areas of endothelial loss are covered with a platelet thrombus, and mural edema and cellular degeneration occur in the media and adventitia. The endothelium is regenerated, at least in small grafts, by 14 days.

The normal media and intima are replaced by a fibromuscular neointima with long smooth muscle cells, fibroblasts, and collagen. The smooth muscle cells have fewer contractile elements and more synthetic elements than usually seen, and these cells contribute significantly to the synthesis of matrix components. The cellular elements most likely originate from the native vessel and migrate into the graft.

Myointimal thickening is most apparent at 14 days and gradually improves with scar remodeling. At 6 months, many macrophages still contain lipid in the walls of a vein graft, although the numbers of lipid-laden cells diminishes by 12 months. Even at 6 months, necrotic areas within the graft remain. Vein grafts in the venous position are not subjected to the additional trauma created by pulsatile blood flow and maintain a more normal appearance.

Conclusion

To optimize the healing of vascular anastomoses clinically, careful surgical technique is critical. Important technical points include the following:

1. Ensuring accurate apposition of vessel walls
2. Minimizing number of sutures used
3. Avoiding excessive tension on sutures to limit medial necrosis

These technical requirements are essentially the same as those required in nerve repairs. Attention to these details will facilitate the regeneration required for the endothelial layer while minimizing the scarring produced in the vessel's deeper layers.

MUSCLE

In response to injury, muscle can either regenerate itself or form a scar in a manner similar to skin and many other tissues. Multiple factors determine which response is generated.

A key factor is whether the muscle involved is smooth muscle, skeletal muscle, or cardiac muscle. Skeletal muscle more often responds to injury through regeneration of functional muscle, whereas smooth muscle and cardiac muscle more frequently heal through collagen production and scar formation. Regeneration of cardiac muscle may occur, however, when individual fibers have been damaged with preservation of endomysium.

Since mechanism of healing of cardiac and smooth muscle does not differ significantly from the mechanism seen in skin, this discussion focuses primarily on skeletal muscle.

Another key factor determining the response to injury is the nature of the insult. Limited injuries to skeletal muscle, such as muscular contusions from a direct blow to a muscle belly, minor muscular tears, mild thermal injuries, and most lacerations induced by trauma or surgery, heal primarily by muscle regeneration. For regeneration to occur, the muscle components must remain in reasonable approximation. When skeletal muscle damage is extreme, particularly if accompanied by ischemia and infarction, healing is mainly by scar tissue, as in Volkmann's ischemic contracture.

Anatomy

Skeletal muscles consist of multiple elongated cells packed into fiber bundles (Fig. 8-5). These cells have multiple nuclei and a large amount of cytoplasm containing myofibrils. Each cell is circumscribed by its *sarcolemma,* which includes the cellular membrane, a basement membrane, and an *endomysium* consisting of connective tissue elements. Bundles of muscle fibers, known as *fascicles,* are circumscribed by a *perimysium.* The muscle as a whole is surrounded by an *epimysium.*

The vascular and neural supply to the muscle courses within the sarcolemma. With any injury, therefore, local muscle degeneration results from damage to these small nerve fibers, even if the primary neural supply to the muscle remains intact. The surgeon must consider regeneration of neural function as well as restoration of muscle continuity in order for the muscle to function normally.

Muscle Injury

When a muscle is lacerated, the cellular elements retract, leaving the sarcolemma gaping and empty for a short distance. At this point, three distinct areas can be identified in the zone of injury, as follows[18] (Fig. 8-6):

1. Uninjured zone proximal to injury
2. Central area of wound, including clot
3. Intermediate "surviving zone," including sarcolemmal membranes.[18]

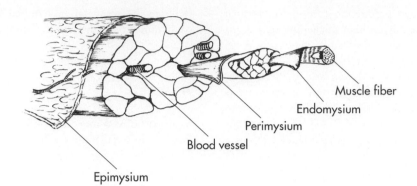

Figure 8-5. Cross section of skeletal muscle.

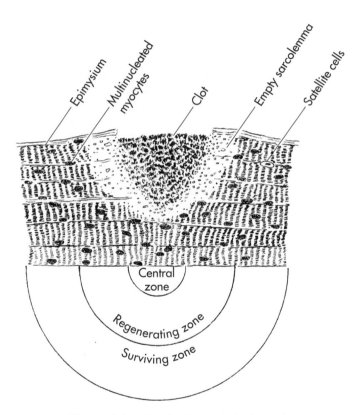

Figure 8-6. Early healing in skeletal muscle.

The dense clot at the end of the retracted portion of muscle fibers appears as a cap over the injured muscle. This includes fibrin, generated by the coagulation cascade, and fibronectin, probably initially released by cellular elements from the plasma. This matrix facilitates the migration of inflammatory cells and then fibroblasts into the injured areas.

During the first 2 days the injured myocyte seals with the formation of a new membrane,[18] and neutrophils and macrophages migrate into the injured muscle. By the third day the basal laminae of the empty sarcolemmal sheaths are lined by macrophages, which are actively phagocytizing degenerating cellular elements and debris. The hematoma remains in the central portion of the sheath. During this period, revascularization of the injured area is also occurring under the influence of bFGF and TGF-β.[20]

Inflammatory cells persist in the injured area for several days, but their numbers begin to diminish by day 5 after injury, and by day 10 they are rarely seen.[19] Also, extensive fibroplastic proliferation occurs in the endomysium. Increased amounts of collagen are noted beginning several days after injury. Initially, type III collagen is mainly seen, but within days, more type I collagen develops.[22] The collagen is located in the granulation tissue and clot at the injury site, as well as in the endomysium.

Regeneration Process

At the same time, muscle cells are beginning to regenerate. The source of regenerating muscular elements are small cells that adhere to the basal lamina of the sarcolemma and lie adjacent to the larger muscle cells.[2] Unlike the elongated, multinucleated muscle cells, which have a prominent cytoplasm containing myofibrils, these *satellite cells* have large nuclei and scant cytoplasm.

Satellite cells are found only in skeletal muscle, not in smooth or cardiac muscle, which explains why skeletal muscle is the only muscle type with significant capacity for regeneration. Satellite cells provide approximately 5% of the nuclei found in a muscle fiber, although more are present during fetal development and after repeated injury. Satellite cells are the only cells in muscle with the capacity for mitosis. Mature, multinucleated muscle cells do not have this capability.

After injury, these satellite cells become myoblasts and, through repeated mitosis, repopulate the injured area with muscular elements. This process is stimulated by bFGF, IGF-I, and TGF-β.[13] After many cells are generated, they fuse to produce larger multinucleated cells, which then produce contractile proteins. Only the multinucleated, muscle cells can synthesize these proteins, so fusion is necessary before synthesis can occur. Fibronectin blocks myoblast fusion and therefore potentiates further cell division, whereas a decrease in fibronectin facilitates fusion. Fibronectin appears to be at least one key mediator of the regeneration process.

The earliest regenerative phase, when myoblasts are predominantly dividing, is the *myoblastic phase,* which reaches its peak 48 to 72 hours after injury.[6] By days 4 to 6 after injury the sarcolemmal tubes are lined by myoblasts.[1]

The *myotubular phase* occurs when fibronectin concentrations diminish and myoblasts fuse and become synthetic.[31] During this phase the intracellular myofibrils gradually become longer and longer as more actin and myosin are synthesized. Grossly, muscle cells begin to extend from the sarcolemmal tube. This process is evident 4 to 7 days after injury.

By day 7, myofibrils begin to demonstrate a cross-striated appearance. By day 14, at least in experimental systems, they have been observed to bridge the gap created by the injury. At this stage the muscle fibers still are somewhat attenuated and have a disorgainzed appearance. By day 21, myofibrils are deeply staining with abundant cross-striations, and a clear sarcolemma has formed.

During the *maturational stage,* final architecture is restored, cross-striations become more prominent in the myofibrils, and the myofibers gradually increase in thickness. Tension across the muscle appears to be necessary in order for the myofibrillar orientation to regenerate in a near-natural manner.

Reinnervation takes place during this final stage of healing. Five days after injury, fibrillation is evident in the injured area, as is characteristic of areas of denervation.[18] By days 7 to 10 after injury, fibrillation potentials and positive sharp waves are seen proximal and distal to the site of injury. These findings are consistent with those in nerve injury alone. These potentials and waves disappear in the proximal muscle by day 14 and in the distal muscle by day 21, as reinnervation of the damaged portion of muscle occurs.

Ideally, fibroblasts generate a framework through which the muscle cells regenerate, yielding a functional muscle. If this process becomes imbalanced and excessive scar tissue is produced, a mechanical barrier to muscle regeneration develops across the traumatic gap, and a less functional result is achieved. This process may occur to a greater or lesser degree depending on the injury.

In severe injuries resulting in *muscle ischemia,* muscle fibers in the ischemic areas rapidly die. Although sarcolemmal and endomysial membranes may initially remain intact, the satellite cells required for the regenerative process do not survive. Endomysial edema soon occurs, followed by inflammatory cells invading the area.

As phagocytosis occurs, fibroblasts grow around the endomysial tubes. Growing sprouts may develop from intact muscle at the periphery of the injured area, but the extent of injury is too severe to allow complete regeneration of a normal muscle. Collagenous scar is interposed between the muscular elements in the surrounding healthy tissue. A similar reaction occurs with extensive thermal injury.

Complete muscle regeneration is also impossible when the muscle elements remain widely separated.

The other extreme in terms of muscular injury is a *mild strain.* In this type of injury, cellular damage is limited. During a transient period of inflammation, macrophages appear within 48 hours and phagocytose any damaged tissue. Cellular damage is repaired through regeneration of muscle elements (Box 8-3).

Management and Mobilization

The management of muscle injuries is difficult to optimize. Mobilization accelerates revascularization and allows for more rapid regeneration of normal architecture and function in the muscle. Mobilization can also lead to further muscle disruption resulting in increased granulation tissue formation and fibrosis.

Optimal management of injured muscle was addressed in a rat model.[18] After 5 days of initial immobilization, sufficient tensile strength was regained to prevent rerupture of injured muscle when mobilization was subsequently started. Mobilization allowed for better regeneration of functional muscle and resorption of remaining connective tissue synthesized in the injured area after the injury. Earlier mobilization resulted in disruption of the muscle fibers and more fibrosis between the healing muscle segments.

Therefore, although typically thought to limit the quality of the ultimate result, collagen synthesis is required to facilitate optimal muscle regeneration. Prolonged immobilization results in increased amounts of collagen and less organized muscle regeneration.

Box 8-3.
Impediments to Muscle Regeneration

Severe tissue damage
Extensive devascularization
Large gap between muscle ends

Conclusion

Healing in skeletal muscle is optimized when regeneration predominates and scar formation is limited. Careful handling of tissues, approximation of disrupted muscle segments, and the postoperative protocols just discussed can help promote regeneration.

TENDONS

Tendons transmit the force from a contracting muscle to the joints between the muscle's origin and the tendon's insertion. Functioning tendon must be able to glide through surrounding tissue. For this to occur after injury, scarring to adjacent tissues must be limited.

Anatomy

Tendon is a relatively inelastic tissue that consists of fibrils composed of predominantly type I collagen in a ground substance with a high proportion of dermatan sulfate. The fibrils are bundled together into fibers that have a characteristic crimp at rest. This slack is removed when stress is applied to the tendon. Fibroblasts are the primary cell type within tendon.

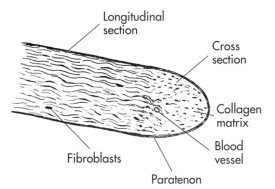

Figure 8-7. Cross section of tendon.

Tendons are encased in a *paratenon* consisting of loose areolar vascular tissue. Fine connective tissue layers known as *endotenon* extend from the paratenon to the more central portions of the tendon. Blood vessels enter the paratenon from the muscular tissue at one end of the tendon and from the bone at the other end. Smaller blood vessels and lymphatics branch from the vessels in the paratenon and course through the endotenon to provide a blood supply to the tendon's more central portions (Fig. 8-7).

In the fingers, vincula run within the tendon sheaths and provide additional blood supply to the flexor tendons in the hand. Flexor tendons do not depend on the vincular blood supply for survival, but better clinical results are obtained after tendon injuries when the vincular system is intact.[3]

Blood flow to tendons is low, usually less than 10 ml/100 g/min. The blood supply varies from one part of the tendon to another depending on the distance from the source of blood and possibly the degree of compression.

In the hand, flexor tendons are encased in a bilayered tendon sheath. The outer wall of the sheath is more ligamentous and includes the pulley system. The internal layer, known as the *epitenon,* directly surrounds the tendon and is more synovial. Synovial fluid fills the space between these two layers of the tendon sheath (Fig. 8-8). Tendons within tendon sheaths derive additional nutrition from the synovial fluid and are not totally dependent on their blood supply. Poorly vascularized areas within the tendon may be more dependent on the synovial nutritional supply. Tendons can survive on nutrients provided by synovial fluid alone in the absence of a blood supply.[28]

Tendons in locations where they are compressed differ physiologically and pathologically from tendons under tension. Tendons under tension have higher proteoglycan levels, are more vascular, and have larger fibrils than tendons under compression. The fibril orientation of tendons under tension is parallel to lines of tension, unlike tendons under compression.

Tendon Injury

Under normal circumstances, tendons are not particularly metabolically active. This observation encouraged Peacock[30]

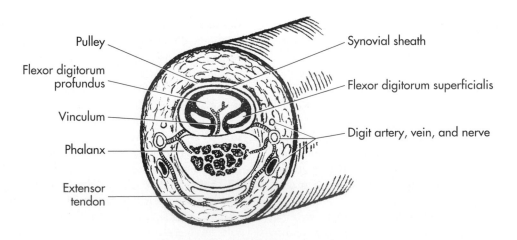

Figure 8-8. Cross section of finger.

and others to claim that after a laceration, tendon healing required the formation of adhesions to surrounding tissues to provide a route of ingrowth for cells and vessels. This finding was contradicted by the classic studies of Lundborg and Rank,[25] who demonstrated that lacerated rabbit tendons were capable of healing when separated from adhesions within a knee joint or in subcutaneous tissue. Subsequent work has demonstrated that tendons totally separated from biologic input can also mount a healing response in tissue culture systems.

The healing process in tendon therefore has two potential contributors: (1) adhesions from the surrounding tissues and (2) intrinsic healing driven by the fibroblasts within the tendon (Fig. 8-9). Under most circumstances, both mechanisms probably contribute to healing.

Healing through *adhesion formation* is maximized by tendon immobilization after injury. The healing response through ingrowth of adhesions is relatively similar to that in skin and other tissues. Erythrocytes, platelets, and fibrin are seen shortly after injury. A bridge of fibrin and platelets initially forms between the tendon and the surrounding tissues, and inflammatory cells migrate over the bridge, followed by mesenchymal cells.

Neutrophils and macrophages are seen in the adhesive bridge and the adjacent tendon early after injury. Granulation tissue, including fibroblasts, collagen, and neovascular elements, is generated within the adhesive bridge in the first few days after wounding. Fibroblasts and neovascular elements are also noted in the tendon during this phase of healing.

In the hand the bridge develops between the surrounding synovial sheath and the tendon. The surrounding tissue and fibroblasts from the tendon contribute to adhesion formation. Significant amounts of collagen are synthesized within the tendon by day 7 after injury, creating strength in the damaged tendon.

In the final phase of healing, tendon remodeling occurs at the repair site. Mechanical forces govern the nature of the remodeling, which is essential to restore functional glide to the damaged tendon. During this remodeling the adhesive bridges become thin and more flexible to facilitate tendon movement. Many functional problems after tendon repair result from the persistence of adhesive, tendinous bands between healed tendon and surrounding tissue.

Intrinsic healing appears to depend much less on an inflammatory response. Early controlled motion of the tendon tends to generate more intrinsic healing. It is unclear whether the motion actively promotes intrinsic healing mechanisms or simply limits the participation of adhesions, which otherwise would overwhelm the intrinsic response.

In this setting, fibroblasts migrate primarily from the epitenon into the damaged area in a process facilitated by fibronectin.[8] EGF and PDGF are upregulated in response to tendon injury, and increased concentrations of these cytokines may be involved in stimulating this migratory response.[12] Damaged tissue is phagocytosed by cells derived from the epitenon.

Neovascularization also occurs in the early postwounding period, with increased numbers of longitudinally oriented vessels across the site of injury. Basic FGF is present in tendons and most likely participates in neovascularization.[8] Collagen is synthesized primarily by fibroblasts from the epitenon, although fibroblasts from the endotenon may contribute 2 to 3 weeks after injury.[11] PDGF and EGF may also be involved in the stimulation of synthetic activity.

Early tendon motion encourages significant participation of the intrinsic component of the healing response. This results in a quicker gain in tensile strength than when tendons are immobilized and heal more through adhesion formation.[17]

Several injury factors influence tendon healing (Box 8-4). These include extent of initial injury, amount of associated crush, degree of bacterial contamination, degree of tendon end separation, and degree of vascularity. Healing involving adhesions is more likely to predominate with extensive injuries

---

Box 8-4.
Tendon Injuries with Adhesion Formation

Severe crush injuries
Damage to surrounding structures
Devascularizing injuries
Damage to large segment of tendon
Injuries with poor apposition of tendon ends
Injuries with significant bacterial contamination

Tendon Healing

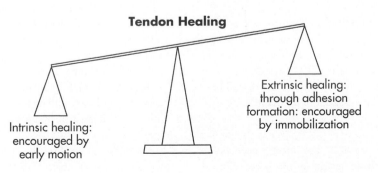

Intrinsic healing:
encouraged by
early motion

Extrinsic healing:
through adhesion
formation: encouraged
by immobilization

Figure 8-9. Wound healing in tendons: a dynamic balance.

Box 8-5.
Technical Considerations in Tendon Repairs

Careful handling of tissues
Accurate apposition of tendon ends
Limited dissection and devascularization
Repair within several days of injury
Preservation of tendon sheath
Postoperative controlled mobilization

Table 8-3.
Types of Cartilage

TYPE	FUNCTION	LOCATION
Hyaline	Dissipates loads on bone in joints	Joints, rib cage, trachea
Elastic	Provides semirigid support	Ear, larynx
Fibrocartilage	Transfers loads between tendon and bones	Intervertebral disks

that devascularize or damage large segments of tendon and when surrounding tissues are also damaged. Intrinsic healing is limited when a substantial gap exists between the tendon ends. Bacterial contamination slows the healing process in any wound and stimulates an inflammatory response, which is more likely to favor adhesion formation.

Repair Techniques

Surgical techniques used for tendon repair can have a major influence on the quality of the clinical result (Box 8-5). Gentle technique and accurate apposition of tendon ends are essential. Primary repair within the first few days after injury also contributes to improved clinical results, although primary repair may still be possible later.

Resection of tendon sheaths can lead to adhesions, and the sheaths should be preserved as much as possible. Some believe that reconstruction of tendon sheaths limits tissue adhesion formation and promotes intrinsic healing,[29] but this concept has not been validated. Autogenous sheath grafts have been used to limit adhesion formation and improve functional results with only limited success.[39]

Synthetic materials have also been placed between injured tendons and surrounding tissues to limit adhesion formation and promote intrinsic healing. No material has been demonstrated to eliminate adhesion formation completely or to improve clinical results.

Some particularly favor reconstructing tendon sheaths when there is concomitant bony injury and significant adhesion formation is likely as suggested by the one wound–one scar theory of Peacock,[30] despite the lack of supporting evidence for these protocols. Hyaluronic acid and other agents have been considered as supplements to accelerate intrinsic healing and reduce adhesion formation, although their efficacy also has not been proved.

Postoperative controlled mobilization has also been used to limit adhesion formation and promote intrinsic healing. These methods of rehabilitation involve active or passive range of motion or continuous passive motion (CPM) machines, which take the injured part through passive range of motion. These protocols are being actively investigated in the hand.

Conclusion

In tendon, methods that promote the more regenerative intrinsic component of healing result in improved clinical results.

CARTILAGE

Cartilage is a specialized connective tissue consisting of chondrocytes in an extracellular matrix composed of proteoglycans, collagen, and water. Cartilage can be classified as *hyaline* (joints, rib cage, tracheobronchial tree), *elastic* (external ear, larynx), and *fibrocartilage* (intervertebral disks, tendon attachments).

Each cartilage has a different function. Hyaline cartilage dissipates loads on bones in joints, and elastic cartilage provides flexible, semirigid support to anatomic structures. Fibrocartilage participates in the transfer of loads between tendon and bones. The structure of each type of cartilage is slightly different to provide specific functional characteristics (Table 8-3). Many of these specialized functions could be restored after injury only by a regenerative response.

Anatomy

All types of cartilage are composed of smaller units called *chondrons,* which include chondrocytes surrounded by a multilaminated, capsulelike structure[37] (Fig. 8-10). The inner layer adjacent to the cell membrane is enriched with hyaluronic acid and proteoglycans. This layer is surrounded by an additional layer enriched with type II collagen.

Outside this unit is additional interterritorial matrix consisting of more collagen and proteoglycans. This matrix between the chondrons includes collagen fibers that have thinner fibrils and are more loosely packed than in the collagenous layer closer to the chondrocytes.

Type II is the predominant collagen in hyaline and elastic cartilage, with small quantities of type IX, type XI, and other types. The primary collagen in fibrocartilage is type I (90%), with lesser quantities of type III (about 10%), type II, and type V.[37]

Proteoglycans consist of a protein core and one or more glycoaminoglycan chains. Within cartilage, large aggregating proteoglycan monomers known as *aggrecans* are rich in

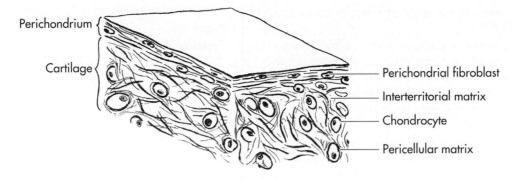

Figure 8-10. Cross section of cartilage.

Table 8-4. **Response of Cartilage to Injury**	
TYPE	**RESPONSE**
Elastic	Limited intrinsic healing
	Cell migration from surrounding tissue
	Scar formation
Hyaline	Limited intrinsic healing
	Regeneration only with adjacent bone injury
Fibrocartilage	Regeneration

chondroitin sulfate and keratin sulfate.[5] Smaller nonaggregating proteoglycans include *fibromodulin* and two forms of dermatan sulfate, *biglycan* and *decorin.* The proteoglycans and collagen of the cartilaginous matrix are generally organized around threads of hyaluronic acid.

Noncollagenous proteins also exist in the matrix within cartilage. *Elastin* is present in large amounts within the matrix of elastic cartilage. *Anchorin CII* helps attach chondrocytes to the surrounding matrix elements.

Cartilage has no blood supply or lymphatic vessels. It obtains nutrition primarily by diffusion of nutrients in water found in the matrix. Because of this limited supply of nutrients, chondrocytes normally are not very metabolically active and divide very slowly in adults.

Cartilaginous Injury

The response of cartilage to injury varies depending on the injury and type of cartilage, although cartilage cells generally have a limited response (Table 8-4). In most injuries to elastic cartilage, surrounding vascularized soft tissues are also injured, resulting in bleeding, platelet aggregation, inflammation, cytokine release, mesenchymal cell migration and proliferation, and eventually collagenous scarring.

SUPERFICIAL. With a superficial injury to hyaline cartilage, the healing response is more limited. Hyaline cartilage typically abuts synovium-lined spaces in joints, and an isolated injury in this location does not necessarily lead to bleeding. Therefore no platelets or inflammatory cells are available to release cytokines and stimulate a healing response. If the wound is less than 3 mm, the edges of the cartilage become rounded, and a new layer of cartilage is generated. This new cartilage is often worn off over time.

DePalma et al[7] showed that partial-thickness cartilage defects in deeper tissue do not show significant reparative changes even after 66 weeks. Fuller and Ghadially[9] confirmed that even though a superficial injury to cartilage may result in a brief metabolic and enzymatic response, chondrocyte proliferation or matrix synthesis is insufficient to fill a wound defect. Some proliferation and reconstitution may occur, but the response to any injury confined to the cartilage is minimal.

DEEP. With a slightly deeper injury to hyaline cartilage that damages surrounding tissue and generates bleeding, the healing response is greater. As with skin and cartilage in more vascular locations, injury initiates the clotting mechanism and an inflammatory response. Fibroblasts are attracted to the area, and fibrous scar tissue is eventually synthesized. These deeper wounds are primarily filled with fibrous scar.

When an injury to hyaline cartilage extends into adjacent bone, the response to injury is different.[41] As with injuries not involving bone, bleeding is associated with platelet aggregation, and an inflammatory response results in cytokine release. Mesenchymal cells are attracted to the area, proliferate, and synthesize fibrous tissue.

This type of injury differs from more superficial injuries, since it allows bone cells to migrate into the area and participate in the healing process as well. Initially the wound base is filled with new cancellous bone, whereas connective tissue and scarring are seen more superficially. By 4 weeks after injury the wound is completely filled with various types of mesenchymal tissue, and by 12 weeks, subchondral bone forms at the base of the defect. A cover layer of fibrous cartilage thinner than the surrounding cartilage is regenerated as well.

By 24 weeks after wounding the regenerating cartilage layer is thicker but remains attenuated and is more like fibrocartilage. This fibrocartilage intermediate is eventually replaced by hyaline cartilage.

The primary mediator of this regeneration of hyaline cartilage is the mesenchymal cells of the marrow, not chondrocytes from residual articular cartilage. This response appears to be a result of the proliferation and differentiation of primordial mesenchymal cells in the bone marrow, which may require 12 months to reach maturity.

Fibrocartilage and immature cartilage appear to have more intrinsic ability to regenerate in response to injury.[33] Fibrocartilage resides in areas where blood will be shed from surrounding vessels when an injury occurs, so there will be cytokine exposure. In addition to fibroblast invasion and proliferation followed by scar production, cartilage cells appear to be directly stimulated to proliferate and synthesize new matrix.

Multiple interleukins and growth factors are activated by cartilaginous injury. The major family of growth factors that affect cartilage growth and regeneration as well as synthesis of matrix components are the IGFs, or somatomedins.[37] Other factors (e.g., FGF, TGF-β, PDGF), as well as cartilage-derived and epidermal growth factors, may also be involved.

Conclusion

A regenerative response to injury recreates functional cartilage, but this does not always occur, especially in elastic cartilage and hyaline cartilage. Cartilage's lack of blood supply and decreased metabolic activity limit its ability to respond to injury in this manner. If injury to surrounding structures results in blood loss, scar formation is stimulated.

True cartilage re-formation can occur in hyaline cartilage only if bone is injured concurrently. Bone supplies primordial mesenchymal cells to participate in the healing process and produce cartilage. Fibrocartilage has greater regenerative capacity than hyaline or elastic cartilage.

BONE

The special structure and function of bone require a unique response to injury. Bones provide rigid structure and support to the skeleton, and these features must be reconstituted after injury. Collagenous scar tissue alone cannot provide the strength and rigidity required to support the body, and therefore a more regenerative response to injury is necessary to maintain function.

Anatomy

Bones are embryologically derived from mesenchymal tissue. They may be classified as endochondral or membranous depending on the manner in which they ossify (Table 8-5).

Endochondral bone is initially laid down as cartilage at the bony epiphysis and subsequently ossifies. In *membranous bone*, preexisting mesenchymal cells differentiate into osteoblasts, which lay down osteoid directly without cartilaginous interme-

Table 8-5.
Types of Bone

TYPE	METHOD OF OSSIFICATION	EXAMPLES
Endochondral	Cartilaginous precursors subsequently ossify	Long bones
Membranous	Osteoblasts lay down bone primarily	Facial bones

diates. The long bones of the axial skeleton are endochondral bones, whereas membranous bones include the bones of the skull and most of the facial skeleton. Bones may also be classified as cortical (compact) or cancellous based on their morphology.

During development, bone is generated by *osteoblasts,* which manufacture the collagen fibers and proteoglycans that make up the bony matrix. The osteoblasts become completely surrounded by the matrix they produce. After the matrix ossifies, the cells are trapped in this lacunar space. Once entrapped in bone, these cells become smaller and are called *osteocytes.*

In *cortical bone,* osteocytes with the surrounding matrix are primarily arranged in concentric lamellae around haversian canals, which contain blood vessels. The osteocytes intercommunicate with the haversian system by fine canaliculi that persist in the bony matrix. Additional lamellae are circumferentially around the periphery of long bones, underlying the periosteal blood supply. Each osteocyte must have at least one component no farther than 0.1 mm from a capillary (Fig. 8-11).

Cancellous bone is structured differently, with both large and small units of mineralized bone known as *trabeculae* and *spicules,* respectively. The axis of trabeculae and spicules is generally perpendicular to muscular and gravitational forces. These units also consist of osteocytes surrounded by osseous matrix, although the bone is not as compact and organized as cortical bone. Osteoblasts are present on the surface of the trabeculae as well.

Bones are hard because they are 92% solid material and only 8% water.[16] The bone matrix itself is 98% collagen and 2% glycosaminoglycans and proteoglycans. Type I is the primary collagen in bone. Bone crystals within the collagen fibrils consist primarily of hydroxyapatite.

Bone healing involves both osteoinduction and osteoconduction. *Osteoinduction* involves transformation of pluripotent mesenchymal cells into bone cells by means of chemical, humeral, and physical signals. *Osteoconduction* is the ingrowth of capillaries and osteoprogenitor cells into the fracture from surrounding bone and soft tissue.

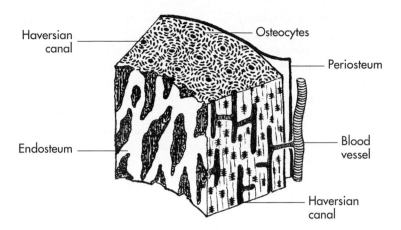

Figure 8-11. Cross section of long bone.

Table 8-6. Bone Healing	
METHOD	**BONE STATUS**
Callus formation	Reasonable approximation
	Relatively immobile
Primary healing	Rigidly fixed
	Anatomic approximation
Fibrous union	Poorly approximated
	Mobile

Bone Injury

After bone is injured, healing can occur in one of several ways (Table 8-6). The nature of the healing response depends on many factors, including proximity of the fractured fragments, vascularity of the injured bone, and immobilization of the bone ends.

If fracture fragments are widely displaced and poorly immobilized or vascularized, collagenous scar tissue is produced in response to injury. When this occurs, bone loses its structural rigidity, and function is frequently lost. Bones are immobilized after injury to prevent such fibrous unions.

When endochondral bones are held in reasonable proximity and are immobilized, the healing process results in new bone formation. This process includes intermediate stages in which cartilage is synthesized and callus is formed[45] (Fig. 8-12).

INFLAMMATION. Bone injury results in direct damage to the *osteons* (basic compact bone units) in the area of injury. Devitalization and necrosis affect a larger area as a result of damage to the blood supply. Immediately after injury, bleeding ensues and a hematoma forms.

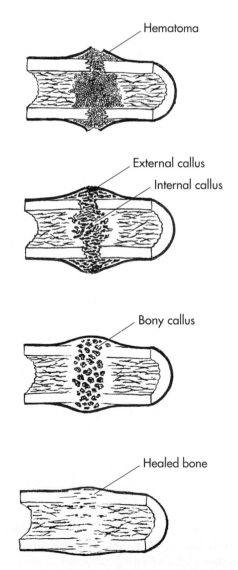

Figure 8-12. Stages in healing of endochondral bones.

This tissue damage incites a rapid inflammatory response, with increased blood flow, exudate formation, and edema, as occurs with inflammation elsewhere in the body. The fibrin trellis within the clot facilitates the migration of neutrophils, macrophages, and mast cells into the injured area. These inflammatory cells participate in the phagocytosis of damaged cells and matrix in the area of injury.

As in most injuries, platelets and macrophages provide cytokines that participate in the healing process. Osteoclasts aid macrophages and other inflammatory cells in removing debris and resorbing hematoma. Osteoclasts are derived from cells of the macrophage series and are generated through the fusion of multiple cells. They resorb and remove dead bone at fracture surfaces.

Clinically, this initial phase of healing is associated with inflammation and pain. Radiologically, decreased density is seen in the injured area.

SOFT CALLUS. The second stage of bone healing involves formation of soft callus. It begins 3 to 4 days after injury and continues for several weeks. Endothelial and smooth muscle cells migrate into the damaged area and contribute to neovascularization. The periosteum is the primary source of these neovascular elements, especially initially, although adjacent muscle, marrow, and endosteum also contribute. Precursor mesenchymal cells and osteoprogenitor cells migrate into the injured area as well.

After migrating into the injured area, these precursor cells differentiate into fibroblasts, chondroblasts, and osteoblasts. They subsequently proliferate and synthesize the collagen, cartilage, and osteoid that make up the immature woven bone, or soft callus, that characterizes this phase of healing.

Callus forms externally along the bone shaft and internally along the marrow cavity and produces a sheath of soft tissue around the fracture site. The primary component of soft callus is generally unmineralized cartilage, but the relative proportions of cartilage, fibrous tissue, and bone vary with the degree of bone displacement, vascularity, soft tissue injury, and fracture comminution.

Type II collagen makes up 40% to 60% of the collagen found in this immature healing bone. This fibrocartilaginous union limits motion at the fracture site; clinically, this is the end of inflammation and pain.

HARD CALLUS. The third stage of healing involves mineralization of the soft callus, resulting in a hard callus. This begins approximately 3 to 4 weeks after injury and continues until a firm union is created. This may require 3 to 4 months in major long bones.

During this phase of healing, osteoclasts complete their task of removing damaged bone. Enchondral ossification takes place as cartilaginous intermediates, primarily type II collagen, are gradually replaced by type I collagen. Calcium hydroxyapatite crystals are deposited in the collagenous matrix, generating a calcified lattice.

The vascularity of the area improves as a result of both periosteal and endosteal contributions. The new blood vessels run through the interstices of the new bone being formed. Additional osteogenic cells migrate into the area along the new vascular strands. These osteogenic cells differentiate into osteoblasts and lay down additional immature woven bone. The woven bone forms a network of fine trabeculae, which contribute to hard callus formation and bony union.

Hard callus histologically consists of woven bone following lines of capillary ingrowth. Clinically this is seen as stabilization of the fracture and radiographically as healing. Although the fracture site has stability, excess bone is present both externally and internally within the marrow.

The electronegativity or electropositivity at the fracture site can influence healing. Concave surfaces tend to be electronegative and convex surfaces electropositive. Bone develops a more significant callus on an electronegative concave surface than on electropositive convex surfaces, which tend to be osteoclastic.

RESHAPING. The fourth stage consists of modeling and remodeling the callus into dense compact bone. *Modeling* refers to cellular interactions that result in normalization of bony macrostructure such that its orientation reflects lines of stress. This ability of bone to reorient its fibers along lines of biomechanical stress is known as *Wolff's law.*

Remodeling refers to cell-mediated breakdown and formation of bone, leading to a stable orientation of bony infrastructure. The woven fibrous bone in hard callus is replaced by successive layers of mature lamellar bone under the influence of functional stress. The cortical callus seen as a bump on the healing bone is replaced by dense compact bone.

Mineralization occurs with restoration of the normal structure of mature bone and reestablishment of a marrow cavity and the haversian system. Some thickening may be seen radiologically, but otherwise a well-healed fracture is indistinguishable from normal bone.

This process of bone reshaping and bone marrow restoration may take years. The pediatric population is better able to remodel fracture sites.

Primary Bone Healing

The third type of response to bony injury involves healing without cartilaginous intermediates and callus formation and is called primary bone healing. This is the principal mode of bone healing for membranous bone. It also occurs in endochondral bone when the fracture fragments are well vascularized and held in close approximation by rigid fixation. When this occurs, the stages described earlier are not followed.

New bone bridges the fracture site during the early phases of healing, and modeling and remodeling begin immediately. There is no evidence of external soft or hard callus. Osteoclasts form spearheads at the end of haversian canals and advance across the fracture site, creating new haversian-like canals in the damaged space between the immobilized bone segments. Osteoblasts follow the osteoclasts and generate new osteons, with lamellae of bone surrounding the new haversian canals. It takes approximately 6 weeks for new osteons to form.

No intermediate phase occurs in which type II collagen predominates. Instead, type I collagen is seen from the beginning.

Repair Techniques

Clinically, efforts are frequently made to align fractured bones precisely with rigid fixation to encourage more primary bone healing whenever possible. Bone healing through callus formation can produce satisfactory results, however, and is relied on in many clinical circumstances.

Several cytokines have been demonstrated to contribute to the process of bone healing.[45] PDGF, TGF-β, and EGF are all mitogenic for bone cells and fibroblasts. EGF, FGF, IGF, and cartilage-derived growth factors 1 and 2 can stimulate cartilage cell proliferation. Bone matrix synthesis is stimulated by TGF-β and cartilage matrix synthesis by PDGF and IGF.

Other inductive factors are involved in bone healing and have been isolated from demineralized bone.[42] These have been collectively called *osteogenins*. *Bone morphogenic protein* (BMP) is the best known factor. Eight distinct BMPs have been identified in human bone, and they constitute a subfamily of the TGF-β and inhibin family of proteins. They may be released from damaged bone as the osteoclasts remove this bone after injury.

BMP induces perivascular connective tissue cells to transform into chondroblasts and osteoprogenitor cells, which generate new bone. BMP also probably stimulates proliferation of these cells and production of new bone elements. Bone defects treated with BMP regenerate more completely than untreated defects.

A new clinical method of modulating bone healing and regenerating new bone was pioneered by Ilizarov for long bones and subsequently in craniofacial surgery by McCarthy.[14] A corticotomy is created in the bone, and pins are placed in each of the bone fragments. Gradual distraction is applied to the bone with a distraction device. If the rate of distraction is limited, new bone is regenerated as the bones are distracted; a rate of 1 mm/day appears to be functional. Distraction at too fast a rate results in nonunion, whereas slower distraction can result in union, preventing further bone regeneration.

In long bones, endosteum seems to provide the cellular elements that generate the new bone. In the facial skeleton, however, periosteal contributions appear critical.

This method of manipulating the healing process has great potential as a technique for reconstructing a variety of bone defects.

Conclusion

Bone probably has the most regenerative potential of any of the tissues discussed in this chapter. Scar formation and fibrous unions can occur, but proper clinical management in terms of immobilization can generally shift the healing response to a regenerative one.

SUMMARY

Nerves, blood vessels, muscle, tendon, cartilage, and bone have unique structural characteristics that allow them to provide specialized functions. To maintain function after injury, these structural elements must be restored. In all these tissue types, a response to injury blends the production of dysfunctional scar tissue with the regeneration of specialized tissues. The mix of regeneration versus healing by scar formation varies in different tissues, but this blend of responses is the common bond among these specialized tissues in terms of their response to injury.

REFERENCES

1. Allbrook D: Skeletal muscle regeneration, *Muscle Nerve* 4:234-245, 1981.

2. Allbrook D, Baker WD, Kirkaldy-Willis WH: Muscle regeneration in experimental animals and man: the cycle of tissue changes that follow trauma in the injured limb syndrome, *J Bone Joint Surg* 48B:153-169, 1966.

3. Amadio PC, Hunter JM, Jaeger SH, et al: The effect of vincular injury on the results of flexor tendon surgery in zone 2, *J Hand Surg* 10A:626-632, 1985.

4. Bio S, Yu Y-M, Smale G, et al: Expression and subcellular distribution of basic fibroblast growth factor are regulated during migration of endothelial cells, *Circ Res* 74:485-494, 1994.

5. Buckwalter JA, Mankin HJ: Articular cartilage. Part I. Tissue design and chondrocyte-matrix interactions, *J Bone Joint Surg* 79A:600-611, 1997.

6. Carlson BM: The regeneration of skeletal muscle: a review, *Am J Anat* 137:119-150, 1973.

7. DePalma AF, McKeever CD, Subin DK: Process of repair of articular cartilage demonstrated by histology and autoradiography with titrated thymidine, *Clin Orthop* 48:229-242, 1966.

8. Duffy FJ, Seiler JG, Gelberman RH, Hergreuter CA: Growth factors and canine flexor tendon healing: initial studies in uninjured and repair models, *J Hand Surg* 20A:645-649, 1995.

9. Fuller JA, Ghadially FN: Ultrastructural observations on surgically produced partial thickness defects in articular cartilage, *Clin Orthop* 86:193-205, 1972.

10. Galis ZS, Muszynski M, Sukhova GK, et al: Cytokine-stimulated human vascular smooth-muscle cells synthesize complement of enzymes required for extracellular matrix digestion, *Circ Res* 75:181-189, 1994.

11. Garner WL, McDonald JA, Kuhn C, Weeks PM: Autonomous healing of chicken flexor tendons in vitro, *J Hand Surg* 13A:697-700, 1988.

12. Gelberman RH, Vanderberg JS, Manske PR, Akeson WH: The early stages of flexor tendon healing: a morphologic study of the first fourteen days, *J Hand Surg* 10A:776-784, 1985.

13. Grounds MD: Towards understanding muscle regeneration, *Path Res Pract* 187:1-22, 1991.

14. Habal MB: Bone repair by regeneration, *Clin Plast Surg* 23:93-101, 1996.

15. Harashina T, Fujino T, Watanabe S: The intimal healing of microvascular anastomoses, *Plast Reconstr Surg* 58:608-613, 1976.

16. Heppenstall RB: Fracture healing. In Hunt TK, Heppenstall RB, Pines E, Rovee D, editors: *Soft and hard tissue repair,* New York, 1984, Praeger.

17. Hitchcock TF, Light TR, Bunch WH, et al: The effect of immediate constrained digital motion on the strength of flexor tendon repairs in chickens, *J Hand Surg* 12A:590-595, 1987.

18. Hurme T, Lehto M, Falck B, et al: Electromyography and morphology during regeneration of muscle injury in rats, *Acta Physiol Scand* 142:443-456, 1991.

19. Jarvinien M, Aho AJ, Toivonen H: Age dependent repair of muscle rupture: a histological and microangiographical study in rats, *Acta Orthop Scand* 54:64-74, 1983.

20. Lafaucheur JP, Gjata B, Lafont H, Sebille A: Angiogenic and inflammatory responses following skeletal muscle injury are altered by immune neutralization of endogenous basic fibroblast growth factor, insulin-like growth factor-1 and transforming growth factor-β 1, *J Neuroimmunol* 70:37-44, 1996.

21. Larson DM, Haudenschild CC: Junctional transfer in wounded cultures of bovine aortic endothelial cells, *Lab Invest* 59:373-379, 1988.

22. Lehto M, Duance VC, Restall D: Collagen and fibronectin in a healing skeletal muscle injury: an immunohistological study of the effects of physical activity on the repair of injured gastrocnemius muscle in the rat, *J Bone Joint Surg* 67B:820-828, 1985.

23. Levi-Montalcini R: The nerve growth factor thirty five years later, *In Vitro Cell Dev Biol* 23:227-238, 1987.

24. Lidman D, Lyczakowski T, Daniel RK: The morphology and patency of arterial and venous anastomoses throughout the first post-operative year, *Scand J Plast Reconstr Surg* 15:103-110, 1984.

25. Lundborg G, Rank F: Experimental intrinsic healing of flexor tendons based upon synovial fluid nutrition, *J Hand Surg* 3:21-31, 1978.

26. MacKinnon SE, Dellon AL, Lundborg G, et al: A study of neurotropism in a primate model, *J Hand Surg* 11A:888-894, 1986.

27. Madri JA, Bell L, Marx M, et al: Effects of soluble factors and extracellular matrix components on vascular cell behavior in vitro and in vivo: models of de-endothelialization and repair, *J Cell Biochem* 45:123-130, 1991.

28. Manske PR, Lesker PA: Flexor tendon nutrition, *Hand Clin* 1:13-24, 1985.

29. Oei TS, Klopper PJ, Spaas JA, Buma P: Reconstruction of the flexor tendon sheath: an experimental study in rabbits, *J Hand Surg* 21B:72-83, 1996.

30. Peacock EE: Biology of tendon repair, *N Engl J Med* 276:680-683, 1967.

31. Podleski TR, Greenberg I, Schersinger J, Yamada KM: Fibronectin delays the fusion of L6 myoblasts, *Exp Cell Res* 122:317-326, 1979.

32. Rao VK, Nightingale G, O'Brien BM: Scanning electron microscopic study of microvenous grafts to artery, *Plast Reconstr Surg* 71:98-106, 1983.

33. Robinson PD: Articular cartilage of the temporomandibular joint: can it regenerate? *Ann R Coll Surg Engl* 75:231-236, 1993.

34. Rogers SL, Letorneau PC, Palm SL, et al: Neurite extension by peripheral and central nervous system neurons in response to substratum-bound fibronectin and laminin, *Dev Biol* 95:212-220, 1983.

35. Rosenbaum TJ, Sundt TM: Thrombus formation and endothelial alterations in microarterial anastomoses, *J Neurosurg* 47:430-441, 1977.

36. Seddon HJ: Three types of nerve injury, *Brain* 66:237-288, 1943.

37. Silver FH, Glasgold AI: Cartilage wound healing: an overview, *Otolaryngol Clin North Am* 28:847-864, 1995.

38. Sunderland S: *Nerves and nerve injuries,* ed 2, Edinburgh, 1978, Churchill Livingstone.

39. Tang JB, Ishii S, Usui M, Aoki M: Dorsal and circumferential sheath reconstructions for flexor sheath defect with concomitant bony injury, *J Hand Surg* 19A:61-69, 1994.

40. Unsicker K, Grothe C, Otto D, Westermann R: Basic fibroblast growth factor in neurons and its putative functions, *Ann NY Acad Sci* 638:300-305, 1991.

41. Vachon A, Bramlage LR, Gabell AA, Weistrode S: Evaluation of the repair process of cartilage defects of the equine third carpal bone with and without subchondral bone perforation, *Am J Vet Res* 47:2637-2645, 1986.

42. Wang EA: Bone morphogenetic proteins (BMPs): therapeutic potential in healing bone defects, *Trends Biotechnol* 11:379-383, 1993.

43. Wieslander JB, Mecklenberg CV, Aberg M: Endothelialization following end-to-end and end-in-end microarterial anastomoses: a scanning electron microscopic study, *Scand J Plast Reconstr Surg* 18:193-199, 1984.

44. Wong BJF, Crumley RL: Nerve wound healing: an overview, *Otolaryngol Clin North Am* 28:881-895, 1995.

45. Wornom IL, Buchman SR: Bone and cartilaginous tissue. In Cohen IK, Diegelmann RF, Lindblad WJ, editors: *Wound healing: biochemical and clinical aspects,* Philadelphia, 1992, Saunders.

CHAPTER 9

Fetal Healing

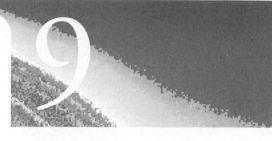

Vivian Ting
George K. Gittes
Michael T. Longaker

Cutaneous scarring can be defined as a macroscopic functional and structural disturbance in the normal skin architecture created during the process of wound repair. This can result in changes in texture, color, vascularity, innervation, and mechanical characteristics. Histologically this is characterized by collagen organization that is abnormal compared with the surrounding uninvolved tissue.[21] The discovery that fetal skin wounds in certain animal models heal with minimal or no scarring (seen macroscopically) has created a rapidly growing field of surgical research devoted to the biology of fetal healing and the manipulation of scar formation in adult models.

Advances in prenatal diagnosis have led to the development of fetal therapy as an exciting new technology in the correction of highly selected congenital anomalies. The ability to repair craniofacial malformations such as cleft lip in utero with scarless healing of dermal and skeletal components could revolutionize the field of reconstructive plastic surgery. Fetal surgery has been performed successfully for more than a decade to treat a variety of life-threatening conditions, including congenital diaphragmatic hernia, sacrococcygeal teratoma, and obstructive uropathies.[1] Currently the risks to mother and fetus cannot be justified in the correction of a nonlethal condition. This chapter discusses this issue further in light of the potential future applications for plastic surgery.

NORMAL ADULT WOUND HEALING

In the adult, wound healing is traditionally divided into three stages: inflammation, fibroplasia, and maturation (see Chapter 5). The acute inflammatory phase involves a series of events initiated by a hemostatic response involving vasoconstriction of arterioles, platelet activation, histamine release with increase in vascular permeability, and edema formation. This extravasation perpetuates the inflammatory response by activating inflammatory cells, such as neutrophils, monocytes, and lymphocytes; initiating coagulation, kinin, and complement cascades; and stimulating the elaboration of growth factors, cytokines, and extracellular matrix (ECM) components.

Neutrophils serve important phagocytic and microbicidal roles, but the inflammatory cell essential for wound healing in the adult is the *macrophage,* which orchestrates the proliferative phases of wound healing. Macrophage products influencing repair include neutral proteases, complement factors, oxygen metabolites, fibroblast and angiogenic growth factors, arachidonic acid metabolites, fibronectin, and interleukin-1 (IL-1). Macrophages are involved in debridement (removal of microorganisms and debris), degradation of the ECM (enzyme secretion and phagocytosis), and matrix remodeling through cytokine secretion.[48]

Macrophage cytokines include platelet-derived growth factor (PDGF), transforming growth factors alpha (TGF-α) and beta (TGF-β), IL-1, IL-6, and tumor necrosis factor (TNF). TGF-β, which is released by platelets, activated lymphocytes, and macrophages, is a potent chemoattractant for macrophages and fibroblasts, stimulates angiogenesis, and blocks plasminogen inhibitor. TGF-β stimulates collagen synthesis, inhibits collagenase, and induces inhibitors of metalloproteinases, all of which lead to the accumulation of matrix components. TGF-β also induces expression of alpha smooth muscle actin in fibroblasts, which may implicate it in wound contraction. Expression of TGF-β is correlated with pathologic scar conditions, such as cirrhosis, abdominal adhesions, proliferative vitreoretinopathy, scleroderma, and interstitial pulmonary fibrosis. Antiserum to TGF-β1 suppresses pathologic matrix deposition in glomerulonephritis.[54]

PDGF is secreted by platelets, endothelial cells, macrophages, and neoplastic cells. It is mitogenic and chemotactic for a variety of mesenchymal cells, including endothelial cells, fibroblasts, chondroblasts, osteoblasts, smooth muscle cells, and glial cells. PDGF initiates deoxyribonucleic acid (DNA) synthesis, activates expression of interferon-β and proto-oncogenes c-*myc* and c-*fos,* reorganizes intracellular actin needed in cell division and migration, and stimulates elaboration of ECM and collagen in the healing wound. TNF-α, secreted by activated macrophages, is angiogenic and may play a role in angiogenesis in the healing wound.[16]

Fibroplasia, the second phase of adult wound healing, is established by the fifth day after wounding and can last up to 2 weeks. This stage entails, in order, fibroblast migration and proliferation, ECM formation, contraction, angiogenesis, and epithelialization. The early ECM is rich in hyaluronic acid and fibronectin, which facilitate cellular migration. High levels of hyaluronic acid are required for cellular migration in both wound healing and embryogenesis. Fibronectin binds to both matrix and fibroblast, serving as a skeleton along which the fibroblast can migrate.[48]

Fibroblast chemotaxis and proliferation are stimulated by PDGF, whereas fibroblast proliferation and production of collagen and fibronectin are stimulated by TGF-β. As fibroblasts invade the wound, they produce matrix components, including proteoglycans and structural proteins such as collagen types I and III and elastin. The macrophage is important to regulation of fibroblast activity and collagen production. Studies using transparent wound chambers show macrophages at the leading edge of cells migrating into the wound, followed by fibroblasts, which multiply to surround new endothelial buds.[28]

After fibroblast migration and proliferation, the wound undergoes *contraction,* a process that is not well understood. The *myofibroblast,* a cell found in granulation tissue, is morphologically intermediate between smooth muscle and fibroblasts, and has been implicated in the process of contraction. It appears at the onset of wound contraction and disappears by the completion of this phase. Whether this cell is critical to wound contracture is controversial, since studies involving in vitro collagen lattices have demonstrated contraction in the absence of these cells. Understanding the mechanisms underlying contraction would be crucial to managing patients with unwanted contractures (e.g., burn victims).[16]

Angiogenesis is stimulated by a number of angiogenic factors, including acidic and basic fibroblast growth factor (FGF), angiogenin, TGF, prostaglandins, and ground substances such as heparin and heparan sulfate.[22] The process of angiogenesis during repair involves migration and proliferation of endothelial cells with formation of neovasculature. Angiogenesis may be subsequently inhibited by factors such as TGF-β and higher oxygen tension.[16]

Epithelialization of the wound, which begins 12 hours after epithelial wounding, involves migration of epithelial cells over the exposed collagen-fibronectin surface in a sheetlike progression from the wound edges. Successive parabasal cells roll over attached basal cells and become attached to the basal lamina. Proliferation occurs behind the wound edge, where stem cells in contact with the basal lamina divide. The epithelial cells secrete their own matrix, and the process of epithelialization is complete when the appropriate epidermal thickness is achieved.[16]

The final stage of wound healing, *maturation* or *remodeling,* commences during the second week of repair and continues indefinitely. The process represents a balance among synthesis, deposition, and degradation, with increasing wound strength in the absence of further collagen deposition. In early remodeling, hyaluronidase, plasminogen activators, collagenases, and elastases are active in matrix degradation; late remodeling involves primarily collagenase activity. Hyaluronic acid is replaced by sulfated proteoglycans, with resultant loss of water from the wound. Collagen fibers increase in strength and resistance to proteolysis, becoming organized over stress lines and undergoing increased fibril cross-linking to form a mature scar.[48]

BIOLOGY OF FETAL REPAIR

The observation that the human fetus appears to heal without scarring was made by Rowlatt in 1979, who stated that the midgestational fetus heals by mesenchymal proliferation and without the formation of normal adult scar tissue[32] (Table 9-1). Over the past 15 years, evolving fetal surgery for highly selected life-threatening conditions, performed primarily at the Fetal Treatment Program at the University of California at San Francisco (UCSF) under Michael R. Harrison, has confirmed this finding. Subsequent studies have used different animal models, including chick, guinea pig, mouse, rat, opossum, rabbit, sheep, and monkey.[2]

Table 9-1.
Comparison of Adult and Fetal Wound Healing Characteristics

CHARACTERISTIC	ADULT	FETUS
Scar	Present	Absent
Cell proliferation	Slower	Faster
Speed to closure	Slower	Faster
Scab	Present	Absent
Oxygen tension	Greater	Lesser
Fluid environment	Absent	Present
Sterile environment	Absent	Present
Skin temperature	Cooler	Warmer
Acute inflammation	Greater	Lesser
Matrix deposition	Slower, disorganized	Faster, organized
TGF-β, bFGF	Greater	Lesser
Angiogenesis	Greater	Lesser
Epithelialization	Slower	Faster
Keratinization	Present	Immature

From Adzick NS, Lorenz HP: *Ann Surg* 220:10-18, 1994.
TGF-β, Transforming growth factor beta; *bFGF,* basic fibroblast growth factor.

Differences in wounding techniques employed and variations with respect to gestational age, time of wounding, and other species-specific variations make comparison of any one animal model to human repair difficult. Despite this, all models are aimed at elucidating the differences between fetal and adult healing and at determining whether scarless healing is a result of the fetal environment, fetal tissue itself, or a combination of both. A broad understanding of fetal healing biology with applications for the human fetus is slowly emerging and will have a profound impact in developing future interventions in fetal surgery and wound healing.

The Fetal Environment

The following differences between fetal and adult wound environments may or may not affect healing:

1. The fetal wound is bathed in amniotic fluid, which provides a warm, moist environment containing a rich source of ECM components, including hyaluronic acid and fibronectin, as well as growth factors critical to fetal development.[34] Amniotic fluid may contain a wound contraction inhibitor in some animal models, whereas in others it stimulates fetal wound contraction. Either the stimulatory or the inhibitory activity of amniotic fluid may influence excisional fetal wound repair.[55]

2. Fetal tissue is hypoxemic relative to adult tissue. Using a miniature oximeter probe, Adzick and Lorenz[3] showed that the tissue oxygen pressure in midgestational fetal lambs is 16 mm Hg, compared with 45 to 60 mm Hg in the adult. The human fetus has an arterial oxygen tension of 20 mm Hg. Fetal hemoglobin, with its greater affinity for oxygen, may partially compensate for this. Contrary to findings in adult wounds that poor tissue oxygenation results in delayed healing, impaired leukocyte function, and higher infection rates, fetal wounds appear to heal rapidly in such an environment.

3. Fetal serum contains a different growth factor composition, with much higher levels of insulin-like growth factor II and hyaluronic acid–stimulating factor, the relative balance of which may be crucial to the unique properties of fetal repair.[18,36]

The importance of these factors to scarless healing is debatable. To test the effects of environment on wound healing, it is necessary either to transplant the fetal wound into the adult environment or to bring adult skin into the fetal environment. Studies during the early gestation of *Monodelphis domestica* (a marsupial opossum), which undergoes a fetal stage of development outside of the womb, demonstrate scar-free healing after birth and migration of the fetus into its mother's pouch, suggesting that the amniotic environment is not necessary to scarless healing.[5]

Longaker et al[42] examined the effect of transplanting adult sheep skin onto fetal lambs at 60 days' gestation (term gestation 145 days). The adult skin, bathed by amniotic fluid and perfused with fetal blood, continued to heal with adult-pattern scar formation after wounding was performed 40 days later (at 100 days' gestation). This study suggests that fetal skin repair is regulated by properties intrinsic to fetal skin

and not the environment. Similarly, in vitro studies of rat fetal skin placed in organ culture show that scarless healing of wounds is retained even in the absence of the in utero environment while in the presence of culture media.[29]

In support of these observations, studies involving human fetal skin grafts placed onto adult athymic mice and subsequently wounded showed that fetal skin grafted onto the mouse in a cutaneous position healed with scar formation. In contrast, fetal skin implanted subcutaneously showed scarless healing. Microscopic examination revealed that the scarred cutaneous grafts showed infiltration by adult murine fibroblasts, whereas the subcutaneous grafts showed only the presence of human fetal fibroblasts, which continued to deposit collagen in a scarless fetal pattern.[45] Thus, in broad terms, scar-free fetal skin repair appears to be dictated by characteristics of fetal cells that are distinct from their adult phenotype, rather than by environment.

Intrinsic Factors Influencing Fetal Repair

GESTATIONAL AGE. Studies in the sheep, mouse, and rat demonstrate a clear transition from scarless healing to scar formation as a function of gestational age.[21] In the lamb, for incisional skin wounds, this transition occurs between the second and third trimesters. The histologic changes that occur with gradual loss of scar-free healing ability have also been described in primates (Figure 9-1). Initially, wounds lose the ability to regenerate dermal elements such as hair follicles but retain the ability to heal the dermis without scar. Wounds formed later in gestation are characterized by disorganized dermis resulting in a thin scar, with full adult-type scar formation and densely packed collagen deposition in early third-trimester wounding.[46]

Transition of wounds from scar-free to scar-forming repair is correlated with an increasing ability to generate an inflammatory response at the wound site, with subsequent cytokine alterations and increasing complexity of dermal and subcutaneous architecture.[5] Scarless healing occurs only before a certain gestational age (probably before middle second trimester in humans), and open fetal surgery can be performed safely only within a period of time distinct for each species because of the risk of premature labor and fetal demise. At present, fetal surgery is only performed in humans between 18 and 28 weeks of gestation.[37]

SPECIES AND STRAIN DIFFERENCES. Knowledge of species-specific differences in fetal healing is critical when reviewing studies in fetal wound healing. These can include differences in gestational length, manner of placentation, and intrinsic wound healing characteristics. This is most clearly demonstrated in comparisons of wound contraction. Fetal rabbit wounds, for example, do not contract in the presence of amniotic fluid but do contract when excluded from amniotic fluid. This results from a characteristic of rabbit amniotic fluid that inhibits fibroblast contraction, which has been confirmed in vitro using a fibroblast-populated collagen lattice model.[32] Rabbit amniotic fluid is known to contain large numbers of high-molecular-weight proteins such as immunoglobulins that

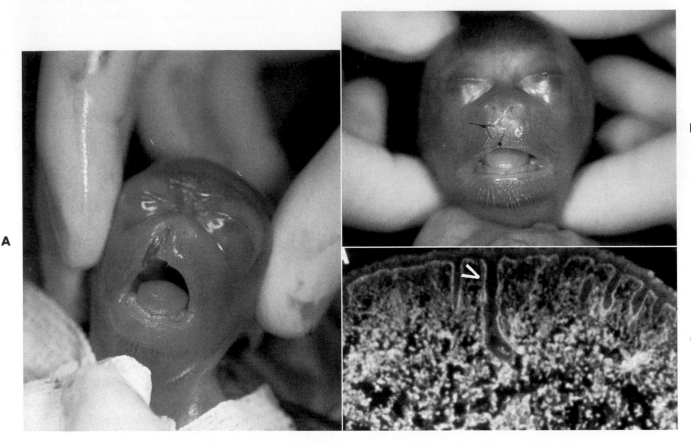

Figure 9-1. **A,** Intraoperative photograph of fetal rhesus monkey at 75 days' gestation (term 165 days) with 2-mm excisional wound in upper lip. **B,** Wound approximation with sutures demonstrates scarless repair. Wound is not visible except for suture placement. **C,** Immunohistochemical staining for collagen type III demonstrates scarless fetal wound repair in different monkey lip, also at 75 days' gestation. Reticular collagen pattern is indistinguishable from unwounded dermis. Sebaceous gland and hair follicle patterns are unchanged. Arrow indicates site of wound. (Magnification 50×.) (From Lorenz HP, Whitby DJ, Longaker MT, et al: *Ann Surg* 217:391-396, 1993.)

may be responsible for this phenomenon.[3] In contrast, amniotic fluid in sheep can stimulate sheep fibroblast contraction of in vitro collagen lattices in a dose-dependent manner. A 40-kD protein isolated from sheep amniotic fluid stimulates human fibroblast contraction in vitro.[55] Wounds in embryonic mice contract by undergoing purse-string closure through polymerization of actin cables, demonstrating yet another means of closure.[47]

When applying animal models toward human wound healing, differences in breeding technique may affect individual variation in healing. Most laboratory animals used in wound healing research (mice, rats) are inbred to eliminate variation. Laboratory sheep, pigs, and monkeys are more outbred but still show less individual variation than humans.[2] The fetal opossum *Monodelphis domestica,* a relatively outbred animal, shows individual variation in transition time from scarless to scar-forming healing, as well as in extent of scarring.[5] Further study in humans is needed to determine the gestational range of individual variations in scarless repair for application toward future in utero interventions.

HISTOLOGY AND ORGAN SPECIFICITY. The histologic development of fetal skin is distinct from that of adult wounds.

The human fetal epidermis is a stratified epithelium at 9 to 14 weeks' gestation that undergoes follicular keratinization at 14 to 24 weeks and subsequent interfollicular keratinization thereafter. Superficial to the epidermis is the periderm, which is present between 4 and 24 weeks. This layer has multiple microvilli projecting off its surface, which may have an absorptive function in the amniotic environment.[32]

Different fetal tissues may possess different regenerative patterns. Human fetal surgery revealed that extensive intraabdominal adhesions occur after diaphragmatic hernia repair, but the thoracic skin incision showed no evidence of scar formation. Studies in early-gestation fetal lambs show that diaphragm and gastric wounds heal with scar, whereas concurrent skin wounds heal without scar.[50] It is possible that some organ systems cannot heal without scarring; however, this is unlikely given that early embryos heal perfectly.[21] These findings suggest that differences exist in the timing or mechanism of repair in wounds from different tissues of embryonic origin. In contrast to other tissues of mesodermal origin, midgestational fetal lamb bone healing mirrors fetal skin healing. Fetal long bones heal with minimal callus and demonstrate both intramembranous and enchondral ossification. More strikingly, fetal bones can heal defects that would be of critical size in postnatal situations (i.e., defects three times the bony width, including periosteum) with generation of new overlying periosteum.[38] Understanding the timing of repair in various organ systems may be crucial in planning any human fetal surgery.

FETAL FIBROBLAST. Fetal fibroblasts possess the ability to deposit collagen and matrix in the organized pattern seen in normal skin and retain this ability even when placed in an adult host environment. Differences in gene regulation distinguish the fetal fibroblast from its adult phenotype. Expression of *prolyl hydroxylase,* an enzyme controlling a rate-limiting step in collagen production, is much greater in fetal fibroblasts until 20 weeks' gestation, after which levels decrease to those seen in adult cells. In the fetal fibroblast, expression of this enzyme is controlled by poly–adenosine diphosphate–ribose synthetase, an enzyme important in cell repair and tumor development.[3]

Fibroblast phenotypic expression in the fetal lamb demonstrates that the onset of expression of alpha smooth muscle actin (ASMA) coincides with the onset of scar formation. In adult wound healing the myofibroblast is thought to play a role in wound contraction and scar formation and is characterized by ASMA expression. Immunohistochemical techniques show that excisional wounds in fetal lamb made at day 75 of gestation heal without scar or contraction in the absence of ASMA expression. At 100 days' gestation, fibroblasts expressing ASMA first appear at the same time that scar formation begins to occur. Electron microscopy demonstrates increasing organization of microfilament bundles over time with gradual formation of a tight, parallel organization of matrix associated with myofibroblast contraction. In both the adult wound and the late-gestation fetal wound, contractile forces generated by myofibroblast phenotypic expression alter the orientation of collagen fibrils with formation of scar.[19]

EXTRACELLULAR MATRIX COMPONENTS. The ECM is a cross-linked network of structural proteins, polysaccharides, and adhesion molecules. The fetal wound synthesizes many of the same matrix components seen in adult wounds, but the timing and relative concentration of these various compounds in fetal wounds differ from adult deposition and contribute to the generation of organized healing with the pattern of native intact skin.

Collagen, the most abundant protein in adult ECM, is of particular interest in fetal healing because the quantity and pattern of collagen deposition dictate scar formation. Fetal animal wounds demonstrate more orderly and rapid collagen deposition than adult wounds, with a reticular pattern indistinguishable from surrounding intact skin. Postnatal and adult wounds demonstrate excessive, disorganized collagen bundles aligned perpendicularly to the plane of injury. Immunohistochemistry using antibodies to collagen types I, III, IV, and VI shows rapid deposition in fetal incisional wounds of lambs at 75, 100, and 120 days' gestation. Two weeks after wounding the pattern of collagen deposition in the 75-day and 100-day groups is indistinguishable from normal fetal skin. Incisional wounds created on 120-day fetuses show

transition to adult-pattern healing with formation of a dense collagen scar.[41]

Collagen gene expression in fetal cells is upregulated compared with adult cells. Hydroxy-L-proline, a marker of collagen synthesis, is detected earlier in fetal rabbit than in similar adult rabbit wounds. In vitro studies of fetal dermal fibroblasts show greater capacity for collagen synthesis than their adult counterparts. First-passage fetal rabbit fibroblasts in culture produce significantly higher levels of collagen synthesis with more type III and V collagen than in adult fibroblasts.[54]

The type of collagen synthesized in fetal wounds is also thought to contribute to differences in dermal healing. Both adult and fetal wounds synthesize types I, III, V, and VI collagen. Although type I collagen is the predominant form, fetal dermis contains more type III collagen than the adult.[49] As the fetus matures, the ratio of type III to type I collagen decreases, approaching adult levels. This may have implications for the role of collagen fibril size in healing, since small-diameter collagen I fibrils with a configuration similar to fetal-type collagen (type III in association with type I aminopropeptides) are seen near the epidermal-dermal junction in adult skin, where minimal scarring occurs.[3] Such ultrastructural differences may have great impact in modulating repair.

Proteoglycans, macromolecules consisting of a protein core to which sulfated glycosaminoglycans (GAGs) are covalently bound, are important factors in wound healing. They modulate cell migration and proliferation, collagen synthesis, collagen and fibril organization, and the rate of collagen degradation. Fetal wound matrix is rich in GAGs. Fetal rabbit wounds, for example, demonstrate three times the GAG level seen in adult wounds and 10 times the level of unwounded fetal skin.[14] Hyaluronic acid (HA) is a large molecule composed of alternating units of glucuronic acid and *N*-acetylglucosamine. It is the most abundant GAG in the fetal ECM. In both fetal and adult wounds, HA precedes the appearance of sulfated GAGs, and the replacement of HA levels by sulfated GAGs is thought to stimulate cell differentiation in several fetal models.[3]

The extended presence of HA in fetal wounds may provide the matrix signal needed for scarless repair. Degradation of HA by hyaluronidase added to polyvinyl alcohol (PVA) sponges in fetal wounds leads to greater inflammation and fibrosis. Conversely, the addition of HA degradation products to PVA sponges in fetal wounds also increases fibrosis and neovascularization. The presence of HA seems to favor scarless healing, whereas HA degradation products favor scar formation.[54]

Amniotic fluid, fetal wound fluid, and fetal urine all possess *hyaluronic acid–stimulating activity* (HASA) because of a 55-kD glycoprotein that peaks in midgestational fetal lambs and calves and is low in postnatal sera.[34,36] Longaker et al[36] showed that Hunt-Schilling chambers implanted into midgestational fetal lambs for 1 to 14 days yielded greatly elevated HASA levels, whereas adult wounds did not demonstrate this. HASA levels showed a bimodal distribution, with the first peak (days 1 to 4) thought to represent fetal serum HASA and the second peak (days 8 to 14) caused by local wound fibroblast HASA production. In amniotic fluid, HASA levels peak at term gestational age. This reflects the contribution of fetal urine to amniotic fluid because fetal urine is rich in HASA.[34] The presence of HASA and HA in amniotic fluid bathing the fetal skin provides an additional route for fetal exposure to these factors. Levels of both HA and HASA in fetal lamb wound fluid decrease significantly at 120 days' gestation, marking the transition from fetal to adult-type healing. Total GAG and HA content decrease with gestational age, and replacement of HA by sulfated GAGs (e.g., decorin, heparan sulfate) coincides with the development of scar-forming ability in late gestation.[32]

In contrast to fetal wounds, adult wounds demonstrate HA only in the earliest stages of wound healing, after which hyaluronidase production removes HA and the wound ECM is filled with collagen. HA deposition in adult wounds is mediated by platelet plug and fibrin clot formation rather than by HASA stimulation. The presence of HASA is seen only in the fetal wound, resulting in the prolonged presence of HA, which does not occur in adults.[32] HA stimulates cell motility and proliferation. Migration of fetal fibroblasts into a loose ECM rich in HA may be responsible for the unique reticular array of collagen deposition in the fetus, in contrast to the dense collagen arrangement seen in adult wounds. The response to HA may be mediated by the fetal fibroblast, since fetal rabbit fibroblasts have been shown to possess more CD44 receptors than adult rabbit fibroblasts. The *CD44 receptor* is a member of the immunoglobulin superfamily and one of the two major HA receptors. Binding of fibroblast CD44 receptors may alter fibroblast gene expression.[54]

Adhesion molecules, known as *integrins,* also play a key role in fetal healing and embryogenesis. The ECM acts as a scaffold for cell attachment and migration. Adhesion glycoproteins found in the ECM (e.g., tenascin, fibronectin, thrombospondin) may be responsible for cell-ECM interactions. *Fibronectin* is normally expressed in large quantities in adult wounds and is seen in association with fibrin clot formation and platelet granules. Application of fibronectin to rat wounds accelerates healing. Fibronectin is more abundant in fetal than in neonatal or adult skin, which may create a more favorable environment for cell migration and proliferation in fetal wounds. Expression of fibronectin occurs earlier in fetal than in adult rabbit skin wounds, and amniotic fluid, which also contains fibronectin, may provide an additional source. *Tenascin* is thought to play a role in fetal epithelial-mesenchymal interactions. Its deposition antagonizes the adhesive effect of fibronectin, permitting cells to migrate from the ECM. This counteraction of tenascin and fibronectin in the ECM may help to promote rapid epithelialization of fetal wounds.[32]

INFLAMMATORY RESPONSE AND CYTOKINE EXPRESSION. The fetal immune system is characterized by a lack of self-nonself immunologic identity, at least until midgestation, and also lacks the typical inflammatory response generated in adult wounds. Fetal wounds are relatively neutropenic, and fetal polymorphonuclear neutrophils (PMNs) may not possess the chemotactic abilities of their adult counterparts. In addition, minimal scarring in some fetal wounds has also been

associated with a greatly reduced mononuclear infiltrate and absence of endogenous immunoglobulin expression.[3] The level of inflammation correlates with gestational age; studies in fetal rabbits and monkeys demonstrate increasing degrees of cellular inflammatory response to foreign stimuli with increasing gestational age.[32]

Do fetal immune system components respond differently to normal stimuli of inflammation in wounding? In fetal lambs, neutrophil function has been shown to have limited ability to phagocytose adequately opsonized *Staphylococcus aureus,* a defect that is resolved by the third trimester. The ability of fetal lamb plasma to opsonize bacteria, however, remains ineffective until after birth, indicating variability in function among different components of the fetal immune system based on gestational age.[30] Fetal rabbit neutrophils are capable of responding to standard neutrophil chemoattractants, such as *N*-formyl-methionyl-leucyl-phenylalanine (FMLP). Fetal PMNs have been shown to migrate into FMLP-treated PVA sponges implanted into rabbit fetuses on gestational day 24 (term 31 days), along with fibroblast infiltration and collagen deposition. If the same PVA sponges are first implanted in adult pregnant rabbits, then transplanted to the fetus, PMNs are seen in greater numbers in the transplanted sponges than in control adults. Despite this influx of PMNs, the normal fibrotic reaction seen in adult controls is absent in those sponges transplanted into fetuses. This suggests differences in the recruitment of fetal versus adult fibroblasts and inflammatory cells as well as differences in mediators affecting cellular expression.[52] Other inflammatory cells (e.g., macrophages, lymphocytes) have also been shown to be functional in the fetus when adequately stimulated. Fetal wound macrophages may orchestrate healing through growth factor secretion and through rapid matrix remodeling with proteinase and proteinase inhibitor production.[32]

Differences in cytokine expression may be responsible for the absence of inflammation in fetal wounds and may contribute significantly to fetal repair. This has led to intense interest in fetal cytokine expression and an avid search for the "key ingredient" in scarless wound healing. No one factor is probably responsible for scarless repair, and the balance of various cytokines may provide the answer. Factors examined to date include epidermal growth factor (EGF), TGF-α, TGF-β, basic fibroblast growth factor (bFGF), and PDGF. EGF is a mitogen that causes epithelialization in adult wounds. When placed on excisional fetal rabbit wounds, epithelialization occurs at a significantly greater rate, suggesting that EGF can accelerate fetal wound healing.[13] In contrast to EGF, fetal excisional wounds treated with TGF-α, a factor structurally similar to EGF, show mesenchymal cell infiltrates without reepithelialization, indicating that the mechanism of action of these growth factors needs to be examined with greater detail using the same model.[32]

TGF-β is probably the most studied of all the growth factors in wound healing. It is produced by a variety of cell types, and its activities vary depending on the local environment and target cell. The effects of the various types of TGF-β on fetal wound healing are controversial. Application of

TGF-β to adult rat wounds increases wound strength and the rate of healing with scar formation.[56] Addition of TGF-β to PVA sponges placed into fetal rabbits on day 24 of gestation similarly produces inflammation and fibrosis, and when added to human fetal skin wounds in vitro as a slow-release disk, scar is formed.[54] TGF-β upregulates collagen expression in cultured fetal dermal fibroblasts, indicating the response of fetal fibroblasts is similar to the adult response.[44] Fetal fibroblasts respond to TGF-β by collagen synthesis and cell proliferation. Expression of the TGF-β gene by fetal fibroblasts may be blunted under hypoxic conditions, which has led some to suggest that the uterine environment results in lower production of this factor. Immunolocalization studies in fetal mouse and rabbit skin, as well as in human fetal skin wounds transplanted subcutaneously into nude mice, reveal a relative deficiency of TGF-β compared with that in adult skin. TGF-β may be significant in fetal wound healing because fetal cells are exposed to diminished levels of TGF-β or to different relative concentrations of its various types (β1, β2, β3).[54]

More recent observations question these findings. After immunohistochemical localization of TGF-β isoforms in fetal mouse lip wounds at 16 days' gestation (term 19 days), fetal unwounded skin showed strong staining for all three isoforms, with relatively little staining in adult unwounded skin. After wounding, fetal wounds showed only minimally increased staining at the wound margins, and by 48 hours postwounding, when the wound has completely reepithelialized, dermal staining was the same as in normal fetal tissue. In the adult wound, however, staining remained strongly positive for all three isoforms through day 7 after wounding. This suggests that differences in fetal and adult healing are not caused by simply an absence of TGF-β in the fetal wound, and differential regulation of the biologic activity of TGF-β in adult and fetal wounds may be important in explaining differences in repair.[62]

Wound fluid analysis studies also demonstrate greater presence of TGF-β in fetal sheep wounds compared with adult wounds.[35] In cell growth inhibition assays, TGF-β increased in adult, 100-day fetal, and 120-day fetal sheep wound fluids, with significantly more TGF-β in the fetal groups. When the fluid was analyzed for specific isoform concentrations using the sandwich enzyme-linked immunosorbent assay technique, the highest amount and concentration of total TGF-β1 and TGF-β2 were found in 100-day fetal wound fluid, followed by 120-day fetal wounds, with the least amount detected in adult wounds. Such wound fluid data suggest that the concentration of TGF-β isoforms in wound fluid may determine biologic activity and scarring, contrary to earlier findings.

It has also been hypothesized that the relative concentrations of TGF-β isoforms may explain differences in healing. Adult rat wounds treated with a polyclonal antibody to TGF-β showed extremely diminished scarring, normal tensile strength, and normal dermal architecture. Antibody application only at the time of wounding was necessary to prevent induction of TGF-β messenger ribonucleic acid (mRNA) and limit macrophage infiltration and TGF-β release. Shah et al[56] showed that application of antibodies to both TGF-β1 and

TGF-β2 had a synergistic antiscarring result greater than that achieved by blocking either isoform alone. TGF-β3, which downregulates β1 and β2 production, achieved the same antiscarring effect.

In contrast, another study examined the relative effects of TGF-β isoforms injected subcutaneously into newborn mice. Injections of β1, β2, and β3 showed similar results, with extensive subcutaneous fibrin deposition, edema, inflammation, fibroblast recruitment, and vascular endothelial activation. No differences were noted in comparing mice injected with a combination of the isoforms in the ratios typical for fetal wound concentrations (50% β1 : 50% β2) with those injected with adult wound concentrations (90% β1 : 10% β2) and with equal concentrations of all three (33% each of β1, β2, and β3).[7] This suggests that greater understanding of the relative importance of these various isoforms is needed in both adult and fetal wound studies before conclusions can be drawn regarding their relative significance in scarless repair.

As with TGF-β, bFGF is found in large amounts in postnatal mouse lip wounds but is not detected in fetal wounds. It is strongly angiogenic, and therefore the increased rate of neovascularization seen in adult wounds may partly result from bFGF. Rapid angiogenesis results in earlier arrival of inflammatory cells and scar development.[3]

PDGF is chemotactic for smooth muscle cells and fibroblasts. Fetal mouse limbs wounded late in gestation and treated with antibodies to PDGF show reduced scarring, suggesting that PDGF also exerts a fibrotic response similar to that of TGF-β.[27] PDGF-treated PVA sponges placed in fetal rabbit wounds induce fibrosis and neovascularization. Along with TGF-β1 and TGF-β2, the expression of PDGF in fetal porcine sera is lower than in the adult. PDGF thus appears to share not only paracrine effects in fetal and adult wound healing similar to TGF-β, but also profiles of expression in fetal and adult wounds.[54]

The *relative* expression of multiple cytokines, including TGF-β, bFGF, and PDGF, may be important to adult scar formation. Unique expression of these cytokines in fetal wounds may be an important component in the regulation of scarless repair.

PREOPERATIVE CONSIDERATIONS IN HUMAN FETAL SURGERY

Prenatal Diagnosis
Current techniques available for prenatal diagnosis include fetal ultrasound (US), amniocentesis, percutaneous umbilical blood sampling (PUBS), and chorionic villus sampling (CVS).[10] Ultrasound remains a highly reliable means of initial diagnosis; fetal cleft lip and palate, for example, can be accurately diagnosed as early as 15 to 20 weeks' gestation.[8] Fast-scan magnetic resonance imaging (MRI) is becoming a useful tool in fetal evaluation, allowing clear imaging in high-risk situations such as maternal obesity and oligohydramnios. It provides superior soft tissue resolution and has been used to image the brain, spinal cord, skeleton, lungs, liver,

heart, limbs, subcutaneous tissue, and placenta in fetuses between 28 and 40 weeks' gestation, with less consistent visualization of intracranial anatomy. If it can be adapted to younger gestational ages, MRI may be used as a noninvasive diagnostic tool in preoperative selection.[23]

After initial screening, more focused testing can include specialized tests such as fetal echocardiograms, fetal urinary electrolyte analysis, fetal tissue biopsy, thoracentesis, immunoglobulin G (IgG) analysis, and polymerase chain reaction (PCR) analysis.[10] A thorough review of all organ systems is required before any fetal surgical intervention, with an in-depth anatomic and functional assessment of the particular organ of surgical interest. Functional assessment of in utero intracranial disease may be possible in the future, as visual-evoked potential in fetal lambs correlates with hypoxia, intracranial pressure, and hydrocephaly.[6]

Using this technology, a wide variety of anomalies involving genitourinary, thoracic, abdominal, neurologic, skeletal, and head and neck defects can be detected, as well as a variety of prenatal tumors (Table 9-2). A review of prenatal diagnosis on

Table 9-2.
Fetal Anomalies Prompting Prenatal Pediatric Surgical Consultation

SITE/OTHER	DIAGNOSIS	NUMBER	ALTERED DELIVERY PLAN			TOP	AVOID TOP	FETAL THERAPY
			SITE	MODE	TIMING			
Head and neck (n = 6)	Cervical teratoma	1	1	1			1	
	Lymphangioma	2	1	1		1		
	Cleft lip/palate	2						
	Laryngeal atresia	1						
Thoracic (n = 38)	Congenital diaphragmatic hernia	8	6	1	1	2	1	
	Bronchopulmonary sequestration	3				3		
	Congenital cystic adenomatoid malformation	2	1					
	Fetal hydrothorax	9	2			1		3
	Esophageal atresia	10	7					
	Complete heart block	2	2					
	Lymphangioma	1	1	1	1			1
	Teratoma	1				1		
	Ectopia cordis	2	2					
Abdominal wall (n = 25)	Omphalocele	13	11	3		3		
	Gastroschisis	8	8		2	1		
	Pentalogy of Cantrell	2	2					
	Cloacal exstrophy	2				2		
Intraabdominal (n = 34)	Meconium peritonitis	9	4					
	Choledochal cyst	1	1					
	Ovarian cyst	2	2					
	Duodenal atresia	3	3					
	Liver calcifications	2						
	Echogenic bowel	1						
	Heterotaxy	3	3				1	
	Bowel dilation	6						
	Gallstones	1						
	Abdominal mass	2						
	Splenic cyst	4						

From Crombleholme TM, D'Alton M, Cendron M, et al: J Pediatr Surg 31:156-163, 1996.
SITE, Change to tertiary care facility for site of delivery; MODE, mode of delivery; changed in 6.8% if cesarean section was recommended for fetal indications or to vaginal delivery without monitoring in cases with dismal prognosis; TIMING, time of delivery; changed to early delivery in 4.5% of cases (between 32-36 weeks gestation to ensure long maturity) due to concern over ongoing fetal organ damage or to coordinate care during delivery for complex cases; TOP, termination of pregnancy; UPJ, ureteropelvic junction; MCDK, multicystic dysplastic kidney.

perinatal management shows an algorithm that is used in prenatal evaluation and diagnosis (Figure 9-2). Prenatal diagnosis can have a significant impact on the management of a fetus, including decision to terminate the pregnancy; changes in site, timing, and mode of delivery; and decision to pursue in utero correction of congenital abnormalities. With careful screening and selection for correctable, life-threatening congenital disorders, the number of patients selected as appropriate for human fetal surgery was only 5% in one study at the New England Medical Center. Similar numbers were obtained at UCSF, with 27 fetuses undergoing surgery over 10 years after evaluation of 300 candidates.[10,37]

Several issues arise when considering application of prenatal diagnosis in performing fetal interventions for nonlethal conditions, such as craniofacial anomalies. Because of the nonlethal nature of these lesions, careful risk-benefit analysis is necessary before clinical applications. Another issue involves the accuracy of prenatal US in correctly diagnosing the disorder and the extent of any associated syndrome of anomalies. Even at major referral centers with experienced ultrasonographers, false-positive diagnoses of cleft lip and palate can occur. The accuracy of US and other modalities must reach 100% before fetal surgery for nonlethal diagnoses can be attempted on a large scale.[25]

Among children born with cleft lip and palate, 2% to 13% demonstrate associated syndromes; other studies suggest percentages as high as 60%. Facial clefts can be associated with derangements in any chromosome, many of which are incompatible with life. Fetuses with clefting diagnosed in utero may have other lethal syndromes not detected by US and may therefore have a higher mortality rate compared with infants who survive to term and are incidentally born with clefts. This hidden mortality has also been seen with fetuses diagnosed with cystic hygroma.[40] A more recent review of 32 fetuses with US-diagnosed cleft lip and palate at two major institutions illustrates this finding. Of 24 fetuses with complete records, eight were therapeutically aborted, seven of whom demonstrated significant associated anomalies. Three other fetuses died in utero, and four others died postnatally, all with associated anomalies. Of the 24 fetuses,

Table 9-2.
Fetal Anomalies Prompting Prenatal Pediatric Surgical Consultation—cont'd

| SITE/OTHER | DIAGNOSIS | NUMBER | ALTERED DELIVERY PLAN | | | TOP | AVOID TOP | FETAL THERAPY |
			SITE	MODE	TIMING			
Tumors (n = 6)	Neuroblastoma	2	2					
	Sacrococcygeal teratoma	2	1	1	1			
	Cervical teratoma	1	1	1	1			
	Teratoma (other)	1				1		
Urologic (n = 84)	UPJ obstruction	57	1	2				
	Posterior urethral valves	6	2	1	2	4		5
	Ectopic ureterocele	4	1					
	Renal agenesis	6	1	2			1	
	MCDK	4	3		1			
	Polycystic kidneys	3	2					
	Megaureter	2	1					
	Ambiguous genitalia	2	1			1		
Neurologic (n = 21)	Neural tube defects	7					1	
	Hydrocephalus	9	1	1	1	1		
	Dandy-Walker variants	3	3				1	
	Partial agenesis of corpus callosum	1					1	
	Craniosynotosis	1						
Musculoskeletal (n = 14)	Skeletal dysplasia	8						
	Clubfoot	5						
	Persistent tail bone	1					1	
Twins (6 sets)	Twin-twin transfusion syndrome	5	5					5
	Discordant anomaly, monozygous twins	1	1					1

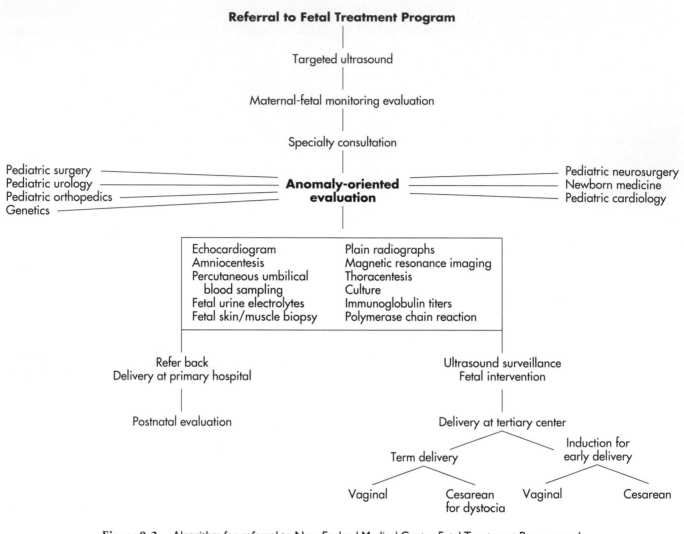

Figure 9-2. Algorithm for referral to New England Medical Center Fetal Treatment Program and subsequent evaluation. (Modified from Crombleholme TM, D'Alton M, Cendron M, et al: *J Pediatr Surg* 31:156-163, 1996.)

only nine survived, three of whom had significant other anomalies.[25]

Further studies in fetal craniofacial diagnosis need to be performed so that only patients with isolated, simple anatomic defects that are potentially correctable in utero and have good probability for survival are selected for future applications in fetal plastic surgery.

Maternal Risk

The experience of the UCSF Fetal Treatment Program over the past decade suggests that in utero surgery can be performed without maternal mortality. The mother still is placed at certain risk, which must be taken into serious consideration, especially when efforts are directed toward correcting nonlethal defects. The most obvious concern is the risk involved in undergoing two major surgeries over a short time, that is, general anesthesia and cesarean birth both during fetal surgery and at delivery.

Another factor is preterm labor and its prophylaxis. Tocolytics themselves carry risks to both mother and fetus.

Maternal pulmonary edema is a side effect of magnesium sulfate and β-mimetics, and fluid restriction only serves to jeopardize maternal-fetal circulation and result in preterm labor. Halothane anesthesia can lead to maternal and fetal myocardial depression and decreased placental perfusion. Indomethacin can cause constriction of the fetal ductus arteriosus, with tricuspid regurgitation and right-sided heart failure.[1]

Risks related to the hysterotomy performed for in utero surgery include subsequent amniotic fluid leakage, chorioamnionitis, premature rupture of membranes, and uterine rupture, either during the current pregnancy or with future pregnancies.[9] Still another issue is the effect of hysterotomy and fetal surgery on future maternal fertility. It is promising, however, that eight of 17 maternal patients reviewed who received fetal surgery underwent subsequent pregnancies, all with cesarean deliveries and good outcomes.[37]

A review of the 47 cases of fetal surgery performed at UCSF between 1981 and 1994 revealed the following maternal complications. Amniotic leaks occurred in five patients: two through the hysterotomy, necessitating repeat surgery and closure, and three vaginal leaks through internal fluid dissection from the hysterotomy to the cervix. Five patients required blood transfusions. One mother developed pulmonary edema from tocolytic therapy and was treated. Two cases of infection were reported: one superficial wound infection and one case of pseudomembranous colitis treated with vancomycin. Two mothers had mirror syndrome, requiring early fetal removal. No cases of maternal mortality have occurred.[1]

Fetal Risk

The risks to the fetus are primarily the same as for the mother, with the additional risks of preterm labor and delivery of a premature, nonsalvageable fetus, as well as postoperative intrauterine fetal demise. Despite oral or subcutaneous tocolytic therapy, all human subjects studied so far have delivered prematurely between 25 to 36 weeks of gestation. For example, in the review of the first seven human fetal procedures performed for bilateral hydronephrosis at UCSF, fetal complications included two neonates born prematurely with complications of pulmonary hypoplasia, one case of septicemia, and one premature delivery due to noncompliance with tocolytic therapy.[40] Preterm labor also carries the risk of uterine disruption and fetal demise if not detected in time for the standard cesarean procedure. Future advances in tocolytic therapy and in minimizing fetal exposure and manipulation (e.g., fetal endoscopy) may circumvent the problem of preterm labor.

The demands of in utero surgery and preterm labor can pose significant physiologic challenges to the premature infant, whose immature brain is particularly susceptible to anoxic injury and hemorrhage. In 33 fetuses followed for neurologic outcome after in utero surgery, seven sustained neurologic injury consisting of periventricular hemorrhage, intraventricular hemorrhage with and without hydrocephalus, and periventricular leukomalacia. Four had documented fetal bradycardia or neonatal hypotension, indicating asphyxia as an etiologic factor. Sudden changes in cerebral perfusion due to maternal hypoxia and tocolytic drugs (e.g., indomethacin, terbutaline) may have devastating results.[6]

Fetal demise can result from any number of potential factors, including chorioamnionitis and fetal sepsis, dehydration from prolonged exposure times, fetal hypoxia due to maternal hypoxia or disruption of placental perfusion from tocolytic agents, umbilical kinking or placental-uterine separation during in utero procedures. A review of surgeries performed on fetuses between 18 and 28 weeks' gestation revealed a relatively low rate of miscarriage with procedures performed before 22 weeks. The precise range of early gestational ages during which fetal surgery can be performed for scarless healing has yet to be determined.[40]

Occasionally, maternal complications may affect fetal outcome. *Mirror syndrome,* a poorly understood condition in which the mother develops the physiologic manifestations of the fetus (e.g., hydrops, high-output cardiac failure) is thought to result from release of placental hormones or vasoactive compounds. Two patients with this syndrome, one carrying a

fetus with sacrococcygeal teratoma and one with a congenital cystic adenomatoid malformation, have been reported. In both cases, fetal surgery did not resolve the maternal condition, and both fetuses had to be sacrificed soon after fetal surgery to resolve the maternal symptoms.[37]

Fetal Surgical Techniques

Fetal surgical techniques have been developed and refined over the past 15 years by performing more than 1600 procedures in fetal lambs and 400 in fetal rhesus monkeys at UCSF.[1] In an extensive study in primates involving 94 gravid monkeys at 94 to 152 days' gestation, 102 fetal surgical procedures were performed, ranging from urinary tract obstruction to drainage of hydrocephalus. A classic cesarean-type hysterotomy was performed in the upper segment of the uterine corpus using (1) electrocautery with layered closure using polyglycolic or polyglactin suture, (2) a metal gastrointestinal anastomosis (GIA) stapling device with subsequent TA-90 closure*, or (3) a prototypic GIA or TA device using a double layer of staggered absorbable polyglycolic staples.

Three maternal deaths were reported: one from anesthetic mismanagement, one from eclampsia and subsequent convulsions, and the third from uterine rupture and peritonitis during preterm labor. Lesser complications included two patients with wound dehiscence and three with wound infections; all recovered uneventfully. More significantly, of 67 mothers undergoing subsequent vaginal delivery after fetal surgery, five sustained uterine rupture during delivery. One occurred during preterm labor, two from technical failure of the prototypic absorbable staple device, and two at term labor. Despite this, no cases of rupture occurred during subsequent pregnancies, even with vaginal delivery. The use of metal staple closure was associated with a significantly decreased fertility rate ($p < 0.01$) compared with use of absorbable suture, with migration of staples through the uterine wall into the endometrial cavity.[4]

The following conclusions were drawn from this study:
1. Fetal surgery can be performed safely, with survival of both mother and fetus and minimal morbidity in most patients.
2. Cesarean delivery should be mandatory after fetal surgery to prevent the risk of uterine rupture during labor through a relatively fresh uterine wound.
3. Fetal surgery does not preclude safe vaginal delivery in subsequent pregnancies.
4. Closure with absorbable suture is important for maintaining fertility.
5. After refinement, the absorbable stapling device can be used safely, minimizing blood loss and preventing separation of fetal membranes from the uterine wall.[4]

A number of techniques can be used to minimize maternal and fetal risk and provide adequate monitoring during fetal surgery. These were developed over 8 years at UCSF, from 1981 to 1989. The mother is admitted the night before surgery

---

*TA-90 is a trademark for a stapler originally marketed by United States Surgical Corporation.

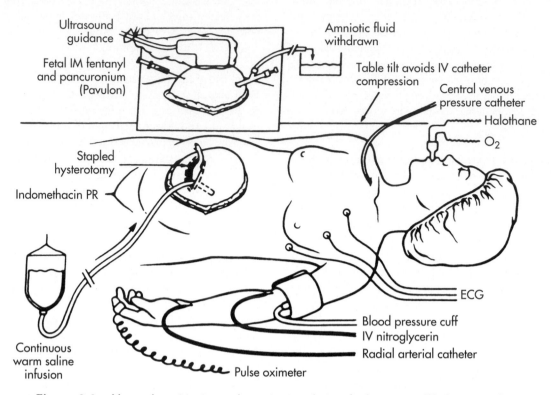

Figure 9-3. Maternal positioning and monitoring during fetal surgery. *IM,* Intramuscular; *IV,* intravenous; *PR,* per rectum. (From Longaker MT, Golbus MS, Filly RA, et al: *JAMA* 265: 737-741, 1991.)

and is begun on tocolytic therapy with indomethacin, 50 mg at bedtime and on call to the operating room. Heparin prophylaxis for thrombosis is generally not used. In the OR, mother and fetus are anesthetized with halothane, which also provides maximal uterine relaxation.[37] The mother is positioned supine with her right side elevated slightly to prevent aortocaval compression by the gravid uterus. A maternal central venous pressure catheter and radial arterial line are placed in addition to blood pressure cuff, bladder catheter, electrocardiogram (ECG) leads and pulse oximeter (Figure 9-3).

For fetal monitoring, a miniature pulse oximetry probe is wrapped around the fetal hand, and a radiotelemetric device is implanted to measure the fetal ECG and core temperature both intraoperatively and postoperatively. It is removed with local anesthesia in the postoperative period (Figure 9-4). An intrauterine pressure monitor is also placed. Blood pressure, oxygen saturation, and heart rate are continuously monitored. Intravenous (IV) tocolytics are administered, including magnesium sulfate, calcium channel blockers, and more recently, nitroglycerin, as a means of delivering nitric oxide, a smooth muscle relaxant.[43]

Postoperatively the mother and fetus are monitored in the maternal-fetal intensive care unit, and the mother is kept on bedrest for 3 days. Epidural morphine can be used for analgesia. An IV first-generation cephalosporin is administered for 48 hours postoperatively. The fetal heart rate is monitored

continuously for the first 24 hours, then as needed. Fetal US is performed daily for the first postoperative week, then weekly to monitor fetal growth and amniotic fluid volume. IV tocolytics are administered until uterine contractions cease. The mother is then switched to oral or subcutaneous tocolytics for the remainder of the pregnancy. Bedrest after the initial postoperative period is unnecessary unless warranted by preterm labor. Hospitalization usually lasts 1 week.[37]

OPEN FETAL SURGERY. The following techniques have proved helpful in open fetal surgery. A low transverse skin incision is made to expose the uterus. The site of hysterotomy is determined using intraoperative US to localize and avoid the placenta. Rather than a low transverse approach, a classic cesarean hysterotomy is used in fetal surgery and therefore carries an increased potential for uterine rupture with labor. The hysterotomy is made at least 6 cm away from the placenta. If necessary, a posterior hysterotomy can be made by tipping the uterus forward. Strategies to minimize blood loss during hysterotomy include a combination of (1) electrocautery to make a 1-cm full-thickness incision through the uterine wall, (2) trocar decompression of amniotic fluid, (3) reverse-biting atraumatic uterine clamps that compress the edges of the hysterotomy (Figure 9-5), and (4) manual compression of the uterus to decrease venous bleeding.

The repair is carried out with the least fetal exposure as necessary; exposure time has been as long as 95 minutes.

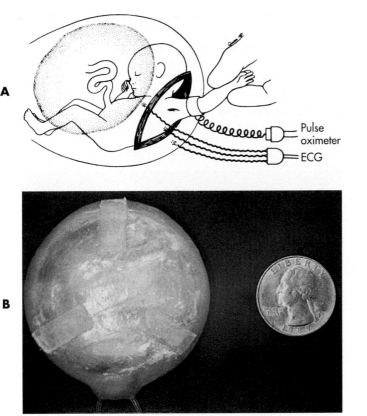

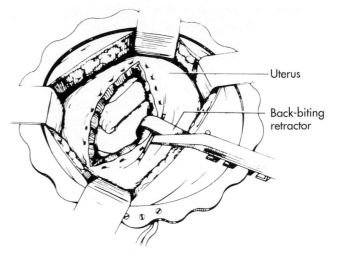

Figure 9-5. Hysterotomy is extended from trocar site with uterine stapling device. Back-biting (reverse-biting) uterine retractors gently compress uterine edges and are attached to abdominal ring retractor to facilitate exposure. (From Longaker MT, et al: *JAMA* 265(6):737-741, 1991.)

Figure 9-4. A, Fetal left arm and chest exteriorized, with monitors placed through subcostal incision. Miniaturized radiotelemetry device can be placed subcutaneously for perioperative fetal electrocardiogram *(ECG)*, temperature, and activity monitoring. **B,** Fetal radiotelemeter weighs 32 g and can transmit temperature and ECG data continuously for 4 months. Transmission range is about 2 m (6½ feet) from maternal abdomen. (**A** from Harrison MR, Adzick NS, Flake AW, et al: *Ann Surg* 213:279-291, 1991; **B** from Jennings RW, Adzick NS, Longaker MT, et al: *J Pediatr Surg* 27:1329-1333, 1992.)

Problems with fetal hypothermia can decrease placental blood flow. To minimize this, the OR must be kept warm, and the fetus is irrigated frequently with warm saline. No excessive problems with bleeding or dehydration have been reported. After the fetal repair is complete, the amniotic fluid is restored with normal saline or lactated Ringer's solution containing 1 g of nafcillin.

A two-layer or three-layer uterine closure is performed at the end of surgery using absorbable monofilament suture, with care taken to close the amniotic membranes and myometrium with an inner running layer to prevent amniotic fluid leakage. Fibrin glue can be used between the layers to seal the membranes and minimize amniotic fluid leakage. A thin, transparent dressing is placed on the laparotomy wound to avoid interference with US monitoring.[37]

FETAL ENDOSCOPY. Open fetal surgery carries a significant risk of preterm labor. Other techniques developed to circumvent this include percutaneous techniques to allow fluid drainage or catheter placement for conditions such as fetal hydrothorax or urinary outlet obstruction. Recent advances have led to the development of fetal endoscopy as a potentially less invasive technique for in utero surgery.

Estes et al[17] examined the use of endoscopic fetal surgery in lambs for correction of an experimental model of obstructive uropathy. Standard endoscopic techniques and instruments were used. A midline laparotomy was performed in two pregnant ewes, and the uterus was delivered into the wound. A camera port site was chosen, and a silk purse string incorporating all layers of the uterus and membranes was placed. A Veress needle was inserted perpendicularly through all layers and into the amniotic fluid, producing a single, characteristic pop. Placement was confirmed by amniotic fluid aspiration. Carbon dioxide insufflation was performed, since preliminary studies revealed that the electrolyte-rich environment of the amniotic fluid made cautery ineffective, and particulate debris produced excessive light scatter. Insufflation was performed at a slow rate and maintained at no higher than 3 to 5 cm H_2O (earlier studies resulted in fetal deaths from excessive insufflation, most likely due to separation of the placenta from the uterus). The Veress needle was replaced by a 5-mm trocar, and a 5-mm zero-degree telescopic lens was placed through this and connected to a xenon light source. An accessory port was subsequently placed under endoscopic visualization. The fetus was positioned by external manipulation.

Estes et al[17] were able to place a wire bladder stent successfully in this manner with no fetal or maternal morbidity. The uterus was subsequently deflated, and lactated Ringer's solution with penicillin was introduced into the uterine cavity. The purse-string sutures were tied and the port site closures reinforced with interrupted 2.0 silk suture.

If preterm labor can be avoided and maternal surgical risk decreased, this technique may prove to be particularly useful in procedures for nonlethal conditions. The magnification provided by endoscopy permits fetal procedures earlier in gestation, which is especially important if a scarless result is desired. An endoscopic model of congenital cleft lip has been created and repaired successfully in midgestational fetal lambs.[20] Future applications in human fetal surgery could include repairing cleft lip and palate, neural tube defects, and amniotic bands, as well as providing a simple means to perform lesser procedures, such as catheter or IV access placement (Tables 9-3 and 9-4).

Fetal endoscopic surgery is still in its infancy. Further study is needed to assess potential side effects, such as fetal eye injury from xenon light exposure and the impact of carbon dioxide and nitrous oxide insufflation on fetal hemodynamics and acid-base balance. More recent studies manipulating amniotic pressures in pregnant ewes suggest that amniotic pressure

Table 9-3.
Fetal Malformations Treatable by Fetoscopic Techniques

FETAL MALFORMATION	FETAL PRESENTATION	FETAL/NEONATAL EFFECTS
Posterior urethral valves	Hydronephrosis	Renal dysplasia Renal insufficiency
	Oligohydramnios	Pulmonary hypoplasia Respiratory insufficiency

Twin-twin transfusion syndrome
  Fetoscopic cord ligation
  Fetoscopic laser ablation
  Fetoscopic cord injection
	Acephalic-acardiac twin	Intrauterine fetal demise
		Multifocal leukoencephalomalacia

Potential applications
  Myelomeningocele
  Amniotic band syndrome
  Prenatal tracheal occlusion
  Fetal tracheoscopy		

From Crombleholme TM: *Semin Perinatol* 18:385-397, 1994.

Table 9-4.
Fetal Malformations Treatable by Shunting Procedures and Needle Decompression

FETAL MALFORMATION	FETAL PRESENTATION	FETAL/NEONATAL EFFECTS
Posterior urethral valves	Hydronephrosis	Renal dysplasia Renal insufficiency
	Oligohydramnios	Pulmonary hypoplasia Respiratory insufficiency
Cystic adenomatoid malformations of lung, Stocker type I (cyst)	Mediastinal shift Hydrops	Pulmonary hypoplasia
Aqueductal stenosis	Hydrocephalus	Neurologic damage
Fetal hydrothorax	Mediastinal shift Hydrops Polyhydramnios	Pulmonary hypoplasia
Ovarian cyst	Wandering cystic abdominal mass Polyhydramnios	Ovarian torsion

From Crombleholme TM: *Semin Perinatol* 18:385-397, 1994.

above 20 mm Hg results in a significant decrease in placental blood flow as determined by ultrasonic probes, producing fetal hypoxia. Pressures below 20 mm Hg result in maintenance of placental perfusion. Technical advances, such as the development of percutaneous methods for port placement to avoid maternal laparotomy, would minimize maternal surgical morbidity significantly.[57]

FETAL SURGICAL INTERVENTIONS

As stated earlier, the current indications for in utero surgery "consist of simple anatomic defects that have progressive, deleterious physiologic effects during pregnancy and life-threatening consequences after birth."[37] Fetal surgeries that have been performed over the past 15 years include procedures for the treatment of congenital diaphragmatic hernia (CDH), congenital cystic adenomatoid malformation, obstructive ur-

opathy, pleural effusion, sacrococcygeal teratoma, twin-twin transfusion syndrome, complete heart block, aqueductal stenosis with hydrocephalus, and aortic valve obstruction (Table 9-5).[1]

A review of the fetal therapeutic trials for CDH illustrates the evolution of fetal surgery with increasing experience. The frequency of CDH is 1 in 2400 births. Most infants die postnatally from pulmonary hypoplasia secondary to lung compression caused by herniated viscera during fetal development. Postnatal surgical repair of the diaphragm does not reverse severe pulmonary hypoplasia. One prospective study of 83 fetuses with CDH demonstrated a 58% mortality rate despite optimal care, and of the 35 survivors, nine had chronic illness from extracorporeal membrane oxygenation therapy. Given these odds, open fetal surgery was attempted in a series of 14 fetuses with CDH.[24] Repair was successful in nine fetuses, but only four survived, the others succumbing to in utero demise from impaired umbilical blood flow due to

---

Table 9-5.
Fetal Malformations that Interfere with Development and Surgical Options

DEFECT	EFFECT ON DEVELOPMENT (RATIONALE FOR TREATMENT)	TREATMENT
Urinary obstruction (urethral valves)	Hydronephrosis (renal failure) Lung hypoplasia (pulmonary failure)	Vesicoamniotic shunt Videofetoscopic vesicostomy Open vesicostomy
Cystic adenomatoid malformation	Lung hypoplasia, hydrops (fetal hydrops, death)	Open pulmonary lobectomy
Chylothorax	Lung hypoplasia, hydrops (fetal hydrops, death)	Thoracoamniotic shunt
Diaphragmatic hernia	Lung hypoplasia (pulmonary failure)	Open repair Temporary tracheal occlusion
Sacrococcygeal teratoma	High-output failure (fetal hydrops, death)	Resect tumor Videofetoscopic vascular occlusion*
Twin-twin transfusion syndrome	Vascular steal through placenta (fetal hydrops, death)	Open fetectomy Videofetoscopic division of placenta
Complete heart block	Low output failure (fetal hydrops, death)	Percutaneous pacemaker Open pacemaker
Aqueductal stenosis	Hydrocephalus (brain damage)	Ventriculoamniotic shunt Open ventriculoperitoneal shunt*
Pulmonary and aortic valve obstruction	Ventricular maldevelopment (heart failure)	Percutaneous valvuloplasty Open valvuloplasty*
Laryngeal atresia and stenosis	Overdistention by lung fluid (hydrops, death)	Videofetoscopic tracheostomy* Open tracheostomy*

From Adzick NS, Harrison MR: *Lancet* 343:897-902, 1994.
*Not yet attempted in human fetuses.

reduction of the liver into the abdomen ($n = 3$) and premature delivery ($n = 2$).

This has led to more careful US evaluation of the umbilical vein and ductus venosus, and fetuses with liver herniation and vessels above the diaphragm no longer undergo complete in utero repair. A less invasive approach has been developed to enhance lung growth in these patients. In fetal lambs with surgical models of CDH, obstruction of the normal outflow of lung fluid leads to accumulation of lung fluid with distention of the hypoplastic lungs and reduction of the viscera into the abdomen. This technique of *prenatal tracheal occlusion* (PLUG: "plug the lung until it grows") has now been applied to human fetuses with large liver herniations. Comparison of the safety, efficacy, and cost-effectiveness of these procedures with that of postnatal therapy is underway.[1]

Related areas of fetal surgical research include the development of *transplantation of cells* to and from the fetus. Transplantation of fetal islet cells in rodent models in the study of diabetes and transplantation of fetal dopaminergic neurons for the treatment of Parkinson's disease have been well publicized. The concept of fetal hematopoietic stem cell transplantation developed because of the multiple potential complications with postnatal allogeneic bone marrow stem cell transplantation used to treat congenital hematologic diseases such as β-thalassemia and severe combined immunodeficiency syndrome. Successful transplantation of fetal hematopoietic cells into a preimmunocompetent fetus may avoid problems of graft-versus-host disease (GVHD), rejection, and infection risks seen with marrow ablation.

Even more fascinating is the possibility of using fetal hematopoietic stem cells as a vehicle for gene transfer. This has been performed successfully in the fetal lamb, using cells transfected with a vector carrying the neomycin resistance gene. Hematopoietic stem cell transplantation has also been performed successfully in rhesus monkeys, with formation of stable hematopoietic chimeras and no evidence of GVHD. Xenogeneic hematopoietic chimeras have even been made, using human stem cells injected into fetal sheep, raising the possibilities of cross-species transplantation as a source of organs and other donor tissues.[12] It is intriguing to contemplate the future possibilities of using a similar mode of genetically engineered fetal cell delivery to treat congenital craniofacial syndromes or malformations caused by a single genetic mutation.

FUTURE INDICATIONS AND APPLICATIONS IN PLASTIC SURGERY

At present, **no** fetal procedures are indicated in plastic surgery. The risks to mother and fetus make surgery for nonlethal conditions unjustifiable under the conditions of current fetal surgical technology. With rapid advances being made in surgery for life-threatening fetal malformations, however, fetal plastic surgery may become a reality.

The following sections discuss some of the experimental animal models for fetal repair of conditions that are potential

---

Box 9-1.
Potential Indications for Fetal Plastic Surgery

CRANIOFACIAL APPLICATIONS
Cleft lip
Cleft palate
Craniofacial clefts
Severe craniosynostoses

OTHER RECONSTRUCTIVE/APPLICATIONS
Flap procedures for soft tissue coverage
  (e.g., myelomeningocele)
Syndactyly
Amniotic band syndrome

---

indications for fetal reconstructive plastic surgery (Box 9-1). Even more significantly, understanding the biology of fetal repair and scarless healing will lead to wide-ranging applications in manipulating adult wound repair to become more fetal in nature.

Cleft Lip and Palate

Cleft lip and cleft palate are the most common congenital craniofacial anomalies. Excellent aesthetic and functional results can be achieved with routine surgery, but cases requiring repeated surgical procedures can lead to scar formation and midface growth retardation in a number of patients. Secondary growth anomalies can include nasal asymmetry, septal deviation, and maxillary hypoplasia, frequently resulting in class III malocclusion.

In utero repair of lip or palate clefting may allow healing without inflammatory response or scarring, resulting in a perfect aesthetic result free of secondary midface growth pathology. Of the craniofacial anomalies being considered for fetal application, repair of cleft lip and palate may be the simplest to perform technically, making it the most likely initial reconstructive procedure to be attempted in humans.

The biology of lip wounds has been extensively studied in the mouse and rat. Whitby and Ferguson[61] demonstrated that fetal mouse lip wounds showed restoration of normal collagen pattern with rapid closure and scarless repair, with distinct patterns of collagen, tenascin, and chondroitin sulfate expression. Hallock described the first animal model for cleft lip, created by maternal exposure to diphenylhydantoin, with successful in utero repair on day 17 of the normal 19 days' gestation. He later repeated this in a primate model using a surgically created cleft lip.[4] Studies of orofacial wounds in fetal rats also show complete epithelialization of oral and skin wounds, with no evidence of inflammation or scar. Nasal cartilage wounds healed with intact perichondrium and without callus formation.[4]

A surgical model for cleft lip has been created in fetal rabbits with excision of a paramedian section of the fetal lip and anterior maxillary alveolus to form a full-thickness nasal fistula. The cleft was immediately repaired in linear fashion using two

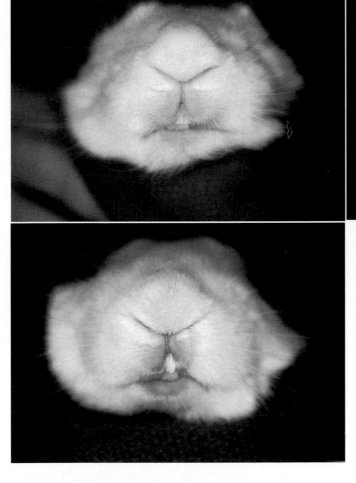

Figure 9-6. Fetal rabbit model for cleft lip repair, 12 days after birth. **A,** Normal control animal. **B,** Unrepaired study animal has slight flattening and asymmetry of nose. Cleft remains open, with epithelialization at edge but no continuity across defect. **C,** Repaired animal has symmetric nose and full lip on cleft side. Linear depression in area of cleft is covered with epithelium, with no scar grossly. Distance from midline to commissure is decreased on cleft side, a reflection of resected tissue. (From Longaker MT, Dodson TB, Kaban LB: *J Oral Maxillofac Surg* 48:714-719, 1990.)

full-thickness 10.0 chromic gut sutures. Fetuses that underwent in utero repair showed epithelialization across the defect and scarless healing, with less facial asymmetry than unrepaired controls after birth (Figure 9-6).[33] The model was then used to determine the effects of in utero cleft lip repair on postnatal facial growth. Compared with normal controls, the rabbits that received repair showed no difference in anterior maxillary length or in anterior, posterior, or premaxillary width when followed postnatally for 26 weeks. These data suggest that in utero cleft lip repair can result in normal postnatal midface growth.[31]

The fetal lamb has proved to be a particularly useful model in the study of cleft lip repair. Longaker et al[39] created a similar model of cleft lip in midgestational fetal lambs (day 73 of 145) by excising a 3-mm–wide left paramedian section of fetal lip and premaxilla. These were closed in experimental animals using 7.0 chromic sutures to make a linear repair of mucosa, muscle, and skin, taking care to approximate the vermilion border and nasal sill. The fetuses were harvested 7, 14, 21, and 70 days (term gestation) postoperatively. The wounds on the repaired fetuses were not visible at any of these time points, with no distortion of the fetal nares or lip (Figure 9-7). Despite an intraoral indentation at the site of the alveolar cleft, the maxilla remained symmetric in all groups, with no evidence of midfacial growth inhibition (Figure 9-8). Histologically, all

wounds showed reepithelialization without inflammation. Collagen staining revealed that the pattern of collagen deposition was indistinguishable from uninjured fetal skin. Hair follicles regenerated, and muscle regeneration was seen as growing bundles across the defect, which may be significant in allowing normal midface growth.[39]

A similar model created incisional or excisional clefts in fetal lambs at 58 to 62 days of gestation. These were later repaired in utero after a delay of 2 weeks to mimic true human cleft lip conditions that involve epithelialized lip margins. Both the incisional and the excisional defects completely healed without scar, but the excisional wounds showed loss of skin appendages (hair follicles, glands) and lack of regeneration of lip muscle in the deeper dermis. The latter finding may indicate formation of a transition wound, representing the transition from scarless to adult-type healing related to gestational age.[26]

The first endoscopic repair of fetal cleft lip was performed using the lamb model. Standard endoscopic instruments were used, as described earlier, along with 5-mm trocars and a zero-degree telescopic lens. A Veress needle was used to insufflate the uterus with carbon dioxide to a pressure of no more than 3 to 5 cm H_2O. Miniaturized endoscopic graspers and needle holders capable of performing microsurgical functions were developed. A full-thickness lip incision was

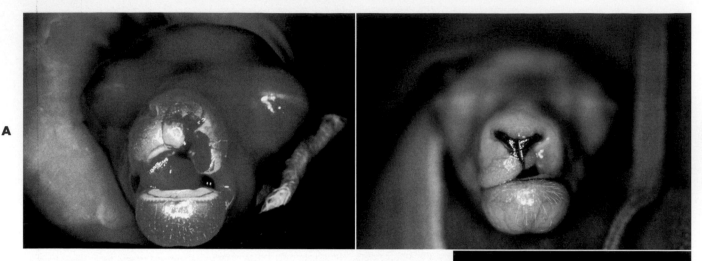

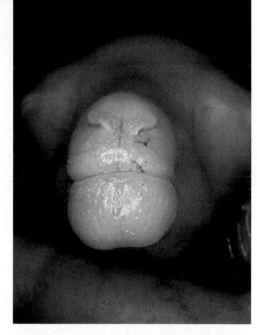

Figure 9-7. Fetal lamb model for cleft lip repair. **A,** Cleft lip created by excising 3-mm segment of upper lip and maxillary alveolus. **B,** Unrepaired fetus, frontal view, 14 days postoperatively. Defect is reepithelialized at edges but has not completely closed. Face is asymmetric. Naris on left (cleft) side is depressed, and distance from labial commissure to midline is decreased, indicating retraction of soft tissue into cleft and maxillary asymmetry. **C,** Repaired fetus, frontal view, 14 days postoperatively. Wound is not visible and is marked only by two sutures. Midface and nose are symmetric. (From Longaker MT, Stern M, Lorenz HP, et al: *Plast Reconstr Surg* 90:750-756, 1992.)

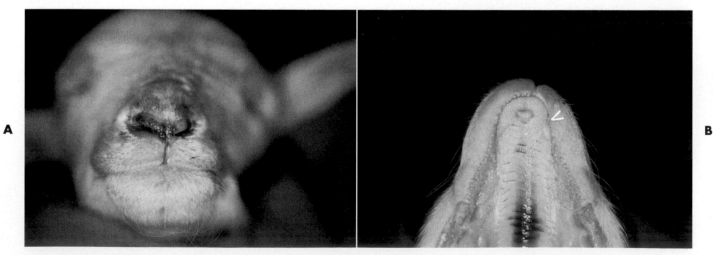

Figure 9-8. Fetal lamb cleft lip repair model, at term. **A,** Repaired fetus, frontal view. Wound (left side) is not visible, and face and nose are symmetric. **B,** Repaired fetus, palatal view. Alveolar cleft has completely healed and is visible as faint indentation *(arrow)*. (From Longaker MT, Stern M, Lorenz HP, et al: *Plast Reconstr Surg* 90:750-756, 1992.)

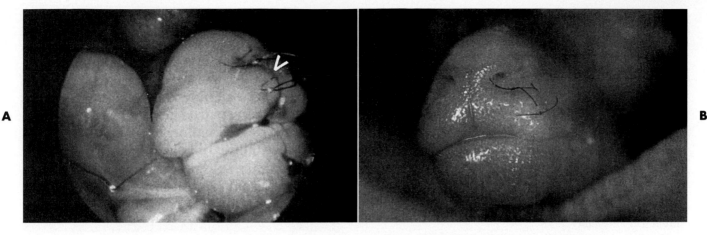

Figure 9-9. Endoscopic repair of incisional cleft lip in fetal lamb. **A,** Lip wound *(arrow)* immediately after repair, seen through endoscope. **B,** Lip wound 14 days after endoscopic repair. Fetus has been removed from uterus. (From Estes JM, Whitby DJ, Lorenz HP, et al: *Plast Reconstr Surg* 90:743-749, 1992.)

created. The wound was closed immediately with two or three interrupted 6.0 nylon sutures using intracorporeal technique (Figure 9-9). The fetuses were harvested 2 weeks later and demonstrated complete healing without scar formation.[20]

Further endoscopic techniques to limit wound tension and facilitate approximation need to be developed before this can become a viable method for repair in humans. At present, fetal cleft lip and palate repair may be justified only in the patient undergoing simultaneous correction of a life-threatening condition with open uterine exposure.

Craniosynostosis

In utero experiments provide an excellent means to study the pathophysiology of craniosynostosis and other congenital craniofacial anomalies. In 1992 Duncan et al[15] reported an in utero model of craniosynostosis. They performed coronal suture strip craniectomies in 36 fetal rabbits at 25 days of gestation (term 31 days). In each fetus the head was exposed through a limited hysterotomy. Through a coronal incision, anterior and posterior scalp flaps were elevated, and a bilateral strip craniectomy was carried out to excise the coronal suture. In experimental animals (craniosynostosis model), demineralized bone matrix (DBM) was placed within the craniectomy. Of the surviving fetuses, those that received DBM within the craniectomy showed bone formation filling the craniectomy defect with ablation of the coronal suture, providing a true bony fusion. Controls that underwent craniectomy but no DBM showed persistent defects in the area of the excised coronal suture. Computed tomography (CT) scans showed that the experimental animals developed significantly wider and taller cranial vaults than littermate controls.[15]

Since the rabbit model involved high prenatal mortality because of short gestation, Stelnicki et al[60] repeated this method for creating craniosynostosis in a lamb model. Sheep DBM with bone morphogenetic protein-2 and poly–TGF-β was placed in a right coronal strip craniectomy made in 10 fetuses at 70 days' gestation. Two of the animals died

postoperatively from preterm labor and intrauterine fetal demise. Four of the remaining eight fetuses were examined at 90 days' gestation. Complete fusion was noted by 90 days, with right-sided frontal bone flattening and supraorbital rim elevation. The remaining four fetuses were examined at 140 days' gestation (near term) and found to have even more pronounced deformities, including increased right forehead flattening, posterior and superior orbital displacement, flattening of the cranial base, and deviation of the nasal tip away from the side of the defect. Two animals formed a bony ridge at the fusion site. Such findings are consistent with those seen in clinical unilateral coronal synostosis.[60]

Using this model, correction of the right coronal craniosynostosis was then performed. After creating unilateral right craniosynostosis in eight lamb fetuses at 70 days' gestation, repair was performed in four lambs at 91 days' gestation by excising the area of fusion with a 4 × 12–mm strip craniectomy to open the entire fused right coronal suture. The excisional margins were wrapped with Goretex to prevent refusion. At term (140 days), all treated lambs had a widely open craniectomy site without evidence of bone refusion or regeneration. This produced improvements in craniofacial morphology with respect to orbital position, skull length, and frontal bone shape in three of the four animals.[59]

The fetal lamb model, although the best available for the study of surgically created craniosynostosis, may be somewhat limited compared with naturally occurring craniosynostosis. The clinical disorder may be caused by a genetic defect that may have adverse effects on central nervous system growth and subsequent overlying bone growth centers. Nevertheless, these promising results increase the possibility of fetal correction of such conditions as Apert's syndrome if studies can demonstrate that secondary growth of the midface and cranial base can be successfully restored by early intervention in utero. It is hoped that similar models for other forms of craniofacial anomalies, such as hemifacial microsomia or facial clefts in Treacher Collins syndrome, will show equal success in manipulating the plasticity of fetal bone growth, sparing future infants the sequence of postnatal surgeries traditionally performed for these conditions, with all their psychologic and physical morbidity.

Amniotic Band Syndrome

Amniotic band syndrome (ABS), also known as the *amnion rupture sequence,* is a fetal condition consisting of constrictive amniotic bands that result in limb, craniofacial, and trunk deformities. It occurs in 1 in 1200 to 15,000 live births. Consequences can range from minor (e.g., syndactyly) to the extreme (elephantiasis requiring amputation). Because the pathophysiologic mechanism for this condition is simple mechanical obstruction, release of the band should resolve or prevent fetal morbidity.[11]

Crombleholme et al[11] designed a model of ABS using 24 limbs from six fetal lambs at 100 days' gestation. In the first group of limbs studied, 15 limbs were banded with umbilical tape as tightly as possible without affecting blood flow. Of these limbs, six were fetoscopically released at 125 days' gestation. In the second group, four limbs were banded to produce a 10% to 25% reduction in blood flow, as determined by laser Doppler studies. These were not released and progressed to term. The remaining five limbs were not banded, serving as a sham surgical group. Sonographic evaluation of the fetuses after banding demonstrated hydropic limbs similar in appearance to those of human fetuses with ABS. All the surviving fetuses were allowed to progress to term, then sacrificed. All banded limbs demonstrated brawny edema and absence of wool formation below the band, as well as shorter limb length, increased hoof circumference, and decreased range of motion.

Histologically, the banded limbs revealed edema, lymphatic and venous congestion, and fibrosis, with more severe findings in limbs with diminished blood flow. The limbs that were released fetoscopically, however, were identical to normal control limbs in gross appearance and function, indicating that fetoscopic release successfully halted the progression of obstructive complications (Figure 9-10). Histology of the released limbs, however, revealed mild venous and lymphatic congestion with increased fibrosis, confirming the adequacy of the banding method.

This may be a useful model for further study of ABS and its role in the pathogenesis of craniofacial and skeletal deformities. Endoscopic release may become a simple method for correction of this disorder.[11]

Myelomeningocele

Myelomeningocele, a frequent congenital disorder resulting in paraplegia, incontinence, sexual dysfunction, hydrocephalus, and skeletal abnormalities, is thought to be caused by a defect in neural tube formation during early embyogenesis. Recent in utero studies, however, suggest that the condition may be caused by a failure of mesodermal migration, resulting in malformation of the posterior spine, meninges, and soft tissues. This leads to spina bifida with open dura and pia mater and subsequent mechanical and chemical damage to the exposed spinal cord.

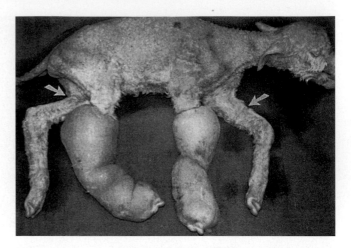

Figure 9-10. Newborn lamb that underwent banding of all four limbs at 100 days' gestation, with fetoscopic release of bands around left limbs *(arrows)* at 125 days' gestation. (From Crombleholme TM, Dirkes K, Whitney TM, et al: *J Pediatr Surg* 30:974-978, 1995.)

Meuli et al[51] created a model of myelomeningocele in fetal lambs to test this hypothesis. In 75-day and 60-day gestational lambs, the lumbar spinal cord was exposed by laminectomy with excision of skin and paraspinal soft tissues. At 100 days the 75-day group demonstrated pathology consistent with myelomeningocele formation, including herniation of the spinal cord into a cystic sac, flattening of the neural tissue, and loss of cytoarchitecture (Figure 9-11, *A*). In contrast, the 60-day group showed healed skin wounds with almost normal spinal cord histology. Fetuses allowed to progress to term were paraplegic in the 75-day group, but the 60-day group showed only a mild paraparesis.[51]

To test this hypothesis further, Meuli et al[52] repeated the experiment using 12 lamb fetuses at 75 days' gestation and subsequently performed delayed in utero repair at 100 days' gestation. This involved creation of a latissimus dorsi flap by dissection of the muscle through a flank incision between the scapula and iliac crest. The muscle was transected at the humeral origin, proximal vascular pedicle, and paraspinal insertions, leaving the muscle attached to the posterior iliac crest and distal vascular pedicle. A subcutaneous tract was created between the flank incision and the area around the lesion, through which the flap was guided to allow placement over the cord. The flap was sutured to the surrounding soft tissues (Figure 9-11, *B*). After cesarean delivery at 145 days, the lambs were found to have healed skin wounds and almost normal neurologic function, with retention of sensory and motor function despite a mild paraparesis, and preservation of continence. No significant donor site defect was noted. Histologic findings showed cord deformation but gross preservation of cord anatomy and cytoarchitecture (Figure 9-11, *C*).

Although fetal mortality was high in this study, with 42% of fetuses with created myelomeningocele and 57% of repaired fetuses dying before term, this was attributed to the ovine model used rather than the procedures involved.[52] A large flap from a remote area is thought to be important to the repair,

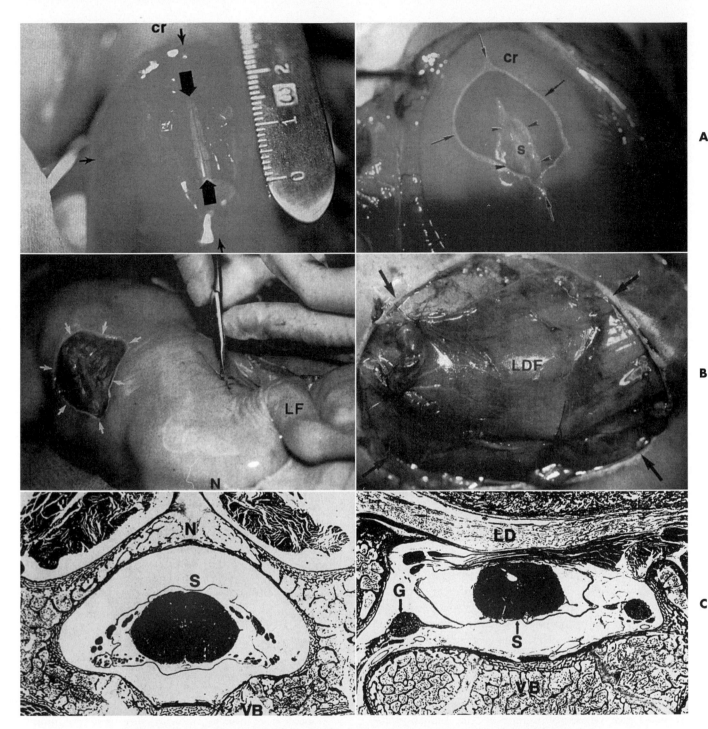

Figure 9-11. **A,** *Left,* Spina bifida type of defect created at 75 days' gestation. Normal and undamaged spinal cord is openly exposed for 2 cm between lumbar levels 1 and 4 *(thick arrows)*. *Thin arrows,* skin defect; *cr,* cranial end of defect. *Right,* Developing myelomeningocele lesion at 100 days' gestation before repair shows large skin defect *(arrows)* and bony spina bifida defect *(arrowheads)*. Note slight herniation of spinal cord *(S)* out of spinal canal. **B,** *Left,* Exteriorized sheep fetus at 100 days' gestation. Myelomeningocele type of lesion measures 4 cm² *(arrows)*. Left-sided thoracodorsal incision for latissimus dorsi flap harvest is placed. *LF,* Left forelimb; *N,* neck. *Right,* Latissimus dorsi flap *(LDF)* is sutured over myelomeningocele lesion *(arrows)*. **C,** *Left,* Photomicrograph of cross section through normal lumbar spine of neonatal lamb. *VB,* Vertebral body; *N,* neural arches; *S,* spinal cord. *Right,* Cross section of myelomeningocele model after repair. Spinal cord *(S)* is moderately deformed, but anatomic hallmarks of cord, as well as spinal ganglia *(G),* are preserved. Skin is healed, and viable muscle flap *(LD)* covers entire defect. *VB,* Vertebral body. (Gomori trichrome stain; magnification 10×.) (**A** and **C** from Meuli M, Meuli-Simmen C, Yingling CD, et al: *J Pediatr Surg* 31:397-402, 1996; **B** from Meuli-Simmen C, Meuli M, Hutchins GM, et al: *Plast Reconstr Surg* 96:1007-1011, 1995.)

since it provides adequate tension-free coverage and leaves the potentially functional erector spinae muscles intact. The latissimus dorsi flap is especially useful because it can be based proximally or distally and used as a transpositional or reversed flap. Anatomic dissections in stillborn fetuses at 25 and 29 weeks' gestation have been performed to confirm the versatility of this flap. In this manner, every level of spinal defect could potentially be covered by a latissimus flap.[53]

These studies are highly encouraging in their possible future application toward human fetuses in preventing this debilitating and otherwise irreversible neurologic condition.

Cost-effectiveness of Fetal Plastic Surgery

A review of the cost of fetal surgery at UCSF indicates that fetal surgery may be a cost-effective alternative to traditional care. The average cost of fetal surgery at UCSF in 1989 was $10,425.82 for all surgeries performed, with a range of $5593.88 to $22,315.24.[37] Considering the tremendous costs that can accumulate in supporting an infant with severe craniofacial and associated syndromal anomalies, including neonatal intensive care, airway management problems in the hospital or at home (particularly with tracheostomy patients), a succession of postnatal surgeries, orthodontic treatment, and therapy for speech and eating disorders, fetal surgery may be a highly cost-beneficial alternative to postnatal treatment.

Application Toward Adult Wound Healing

The future application of fetal wound healing biology toward improving adult wound healing and preventing scar formation after surgery or trauma is an intriguing possibility. In experimental models, alteration of the growth factor profile in the early stages of wound healing has resulted in modulation of scar formation.

Much of the work has been done on TGF-β, as mentioned earlier. A single application of neutralizing antibody to TGF-β1 and TGF-β2 at wounding was sufficient in virtually eliminating scar formation. This finding would have great significance in adaptation for clinical use because it would eliminate problems of delivery or patient compliance.[56] Histologically the neutralizing antibodies resulted in decreased deposition of fibronectin and collagen, a lesser degree of angiogenesis in the first 14 days of healing, and a smaller monocytic infiltrate. The organization of the wound ECM resembled that of normal uninjured skin, similar to the findings in fetal wound healing. Wound strength was found to be equal or stronger than control wounds, improved by the more normal dermal architecture achieved.

Other studies reducing the activity of TGF-β1 and TGF-β2 in wounds, such as addition of antisense oligonucleotides to TGF or competitive inhibitors of TGF activation (e.g., mannose-6-phosphate), have demonstrated similar antiscarring responses.[21]

The relative balance of TGF-β1 and TGF-β2 with TGF-β3 may be crucial in scar formation. Addition of TGF-β3 to wounds also reduces scarring. When all three TGF-β forms are blocked with neutralizing antibodies, however, no improvement in scar formation is seen. Similarly, complete reduction of several growth factors by the agent suramin produces no antiscarring ability. This suggests that drugs merely serving as indiscriminate antiinflammatory agents (e.g., corticosteroids) will have limited use in scar reduction. Cytokine strategies to improve healing may require modulating the balance among the various TGF-β isoforms and the factors that influence their expression, such as PDGF.[21]

Therapeutic interventions to reduce or eliminate scarring will have wide-reaching applications in all fields of medicine and surgery. In plastic surgery, it is hoped that such therapy will have tremendous impact on functional as well as cosmetic outcome and reduce the need for secondary surgeries to resolve complications of scarring. In microsurgery, for example, neuroma formation and neointimal hyperplasia may be circumvented, resulting in preservation of function of nerve and vascular anastomoses. In general surgery, applications may include prevention of postlaparotomy abdominal adhesions and cardiac, vascular, biliary, intestinal, tracheal, urinary, and transplant anastomotic obstructions.

Because scar processes in different organ systems seem to share similar characteristics, the application of fetal healing biology toward correction of a vast array of fibroproliferative diseases, such as cirrhosis and pulmonary fibrosis, may become a reality.

REFERENCES

1. Adzick NS, Harrison MR: Fetal surgical therapy, *Lancet* 343:897-902, 1994.

2. Adzick NS, Longaker MT: Animal models for the study of fetal tissue repair, *J Surg Res* 51:216-222, 1991.

3. Adzick NS, Lorenz HP: Cells, matrix, growth factors, and the surgeon: the biology of scarless fetal wound repair, *Ann Surg* 220:10-18, 1994.

4. Adzick NS, Harrison MR, Glick PL, et al: Fetal surgery in the primate. III. Maternal outcome after fetal surgery, *J Pediatr Surg* 21:477-480, 1986.

5. Armstrong JR, Ferguson MWJ: Ontogeny of the skin and transition from scar-free to scarring phenotype during wound healing in the pouch young of a marsupial, *Monodelphis domestica*, *Dev Biol* 169:242-260, 1995.

6. Bealer JF, Raisanen J, Skarsgard ED, et al: The incidence and spectrum of neurological injury after open fetal surgery, *J Pediatr Surg* 1:1150-1154, 1995.

7. Bouhana KS, Longaker MT, Banda MJ, et al: In vivo analysis of TGF-β isoforms injected individually and in combinations, *Surg Forum* 46:751-752, 1995.

8. Christ JE, Meininger ME: Ultrasound diagnosis of cleft lip and palate before birth, *Plast Reconstr Surg* 68:854-859, 1981.

9. Crombleholme TM: Invasive fetal therapy: current status and future directions, *Semin Perinatol* 18:385-397, 1994.

10. Crombleholme TM, D'Alton M, Cendron M, et al: Prenatal diagnosis and the pediatric surgeon: the impact of prenatal consultation on perinatal management, *J Pediatr Surg* 31:156-163, 1996.

11. Crombleholme TM, Dirkes K, Whitney TM, et al: Amniotic band syndrome in fetal lambs. I. Fetoscopic release and morphometric outcome, *J Pediatr Surg* 30:974-978, 1995.

12. Crombleholme TM, Langer JC, Harrison MR, et al: Transplantation of fetal cells, *Am J Obstet Gynecol* 164:218-230, 1991.

13. DeLozier J, Nanney LB, Hago K, et al: Epidermal growth factor enhances fetal reepithelialization, *Surg Forum* 38:623-626, 1987.

14. DePalma RL, Krummel TM, Durham LA, et al: Characterization and quantitation of wound matrix in the fetal rabbit, *Matrix* 9:224-231, 1989.

15. Duncan BW, Adzick NS, Moelleken BRW, et al: An in utero model of craniosynostosis, *J Craniofac Surg* 3:70-79, 1992.

16. Edington HD: Wound healing. In *Basic science review for surgeons,* Philadelphia, 1992, Saunders.

17. Estes JM, MacGillivray TE, Hedrick MH, et al: Fetoscopic surgery for the treatment of congenital anomalies, *J Pediatr Surg* 27:950-954, 1992.

18. Estes JM, Spencer EM, Longaker MT, et al: Insulin-like growth factor-II in ovine wound fluid: evidence for developmental regulation, *Surg Forum* 42:659-661, 1991.

19. Estes JM, Vandeberg JS, Adzick NS, et al: Phenotypic and functional features of myofibroblast in sheep fetal wounds, *Differentiation* 56:173-181, 1994.

20. Estes JM, Whitby DJ, Lorenz HP, et al: Endoscopic creation and repair of fetal cleft lip, *Plast Reconstr Surg* 90:743-749, 1992.

21. Ferguson MWJ, Whitby DJ, Shah M, et al: Scar formation: the spectral nature of fetal and adult wound repair, *Plast Reconstr Surg* 97:854-860, 1996.

22. Folkman MJ et al: Angiogenic factors, *Science* 235:442-447, 1987.

23. Garden AS, Griffiths RD, Weindling AM, et al: Fast-scan magnetic resonance imaging in fetal visualization, *Am J Obstet Gynecol* 164:1190-1196, 1991.

24. Harrison MR, Adzick NS, Flake AW, et al: Correction of congenital diaphragmatic hernia in utero. VI. Hard-earned lessons, *J Pediatr Surg* 28:1411-1418, 1993.

25. Hedrick MH, Montgomery L, Hoffman WY, et al: Natural history of fetuses with cleft lip and palate, *Plast Reconstr Surg* 103:34, 1999.

26. Hedrick MH, Rice HE, Vanderwall KJ, et al: Delayed in utero repair of surgically created fetal cleft lip and palate, *Plast Reconstr Surg* 97:900-907, 1996.

27. Houghton PE, Keefer KA, Krummel TM: Scar formation in wounded fetal mouse limbs is reduced by platelet derived growth factor neutralizing antibody, *Wound Rep Reg* 2:80, 1994.

28. Hunt TK et al: Studies on inflammation and wound healing: angiogenesis and collagen synthesis stimulated in vivo by resident and activated wound macrophages, *Surgery* 96:48-54, 1984.

29. Ihara I, Motobayashi Y: Wound closure in foetal rat skin, *Development* 114:573-582, 1992.

30. Jennings RW, Adzick NS, Longaker MT, et al: Ontogeny of fetal sheep polymorphonuclear leukocyte phagocytosis, *J Pediatr Surg* 26:853-855, 1991.

31. Kaban LB, Dodson TB, Longaker MT, et al: Fetal cleft lip repair in rabbits: long term clinical and cephalometric results, *Cleft Palate Craniofac J* 30:13-21, 1993.

32. Longaker MT, Adzick NS: The biology of fetal wound healing: a review, *Plast Reconstr Surg* 87:788-798, 1991.

33. Longaker MT, Dodson TB, Kaban LB: A rabbit model for fetal cleft lip repair, *J Oral Maxillofac Surg* 48:714-719, 1990.

34. Longaker MT, Adzick NS, Hall JL, et al: Studies in fetal wound healing. VII. Fetal wound healing may be modulated by elevated hyaluronic acid stimulating activity in amniotic fluid, *J Pediatr Surg* 25:430-433, 1990.

35. Longaker MT, Bouhana KS, Harrison MR, et al: Wound healing in the fetus: possible role for macrophages and transforming growth factor-β isoforms, *Wound Rep Reg* 2:104-112, 1994.

36. Longaker MT, Chiu ES, Harrison MR, et al: Studies in fetal wound healing. IV. Hyaluronic acid stimulating activity distinguishes fetal from adult wound fluid, *Ann Surg* 210:667-672, 1989.

37. Longaker MT, Golbus MS, Filly RA, et al: Maternal outcome after open fetal surgery: a review of the first 17 human cases, *JAMA* 265:737-741, 1991.

38. Longaker MT, Moelleken BRW, Cheng JC, et al: Fetal fracture healing in a lamb model, *Plast Reconstr Surg* 90:161-171, 1992.

39. Longaker MT, Stern M, Lorenz HP, et al: A model for fetal cleft lip repair in lambs, *Plast Reconstr Surg* 90:750-756, 1992.

40. Longaker MT, Whitby DJ, Adzick NS, et al: Fetal surgery for cleft lip: a plea for caution, *Plast Reconstr Surg* 88:1087-1092, 1991.

41. Longaker MT, Whitby DJ, Adzick NS, et al: Studies in fetal wound healing. VI. Second and early third trimester fetal wounds demonstrate rapid collagen deposition without scar formation, *J Pediatr Surg* 25:63-69, 1990.

42. Longaker MT, Whitby DJ, Ferguson MWJ, et al: Adult skin wounds in the fetal environment heal with scar formation, *Ann Surg* 219:65-72, 1994.

43. Lorenz HP, Adzick NS, Harrison MR: Fetal surgical techniques, *Semin Pediatr Surg* 2:136-142, 1993.

44. Lorenz HP, Chang J, Longaker MT, et al: Transforming growth factors beta-1 and beta-2 synergistically increase gene expression of collagen types I and III in fetal but not adult fibroblasts, *Surg Forum* 44:723-725, 1993.

45. Lorenz HP, Longaker MT, Perkocha LA, et al: Scarless wound repair: a human fetal skin model, *Development* 114:253-259, 1992.

46. Lorenz HP, Whitby DJ, Longaker MT, et al: Fetal wound healing: the ontogeny of scar formation in the non-human primate, *Ann Surg* 217:391-396, 1993.

47. Martin P, Lewis J: Actin cables and epidermal movement in embryonic wound healing, *Nature* 360:179, 1992.

48. Mathes SJ, Abouljord M: Wound healing. In Davis JH, editor: *Clinical surgery,* St Louis, 1987, Mosby.

49. Merkel JR, DiPaolo BR, Hallock GG, et al: Type I and type III collagen content of healing wounds in fetal and adult rats, *Proc Soc Exp Biol Med* 187:493-497, 1988.

50. Meuli M, Lorenz HP, Hedrick MM, et al: Scar formation in the fetal alimentary tract, *J Pediatr Surg* 30:392-395, 1995.

51. Meuli M, Meuli-Simmen C, Yingling CD, et al: Creation of myelomeningocele in utero: a model of functional damage from spinal cord exposure in fetal sheep, *J Pediatr Surg* 30:1028-1033, 1995.

52. Meuli M, Meuli-Simmen C, Yingling CD, et al: In utero repair of experimental myelomeningocele saves neurological function at birth, *J Pediatr Surg* 31:397-402, 1996.

53. Meuli-Simmen C, Meuli M, Hutchins GM, et al: Fetal reconstructive surgery: experimental use of the latissimus dorsi flap to correct myelomeningocele in utero, *Plast Reconstr Surg* 96:1007-1011, 1995.

54. Olutoye OO, Cohen IK: Fetal wound healing: an overview, *Wound Rep Reg* 4:66-74, 1996.

55. Rittenberg T, Longaker MT, Adzick NS, et al: Sheep amniotic fluid has a protein factor which stimulates human fibroblast populated collagen lattice contraction, *J Cell Physiol* 149:444-450, 1991.

56. Shah M, Foreman DM, Ferguson MWJ: Neutralization of TGF-beta 1 and TGF-beta 2 or exogenous addition of TGF-beta 3 to cutaneous rat wounds reduces scarring, *J Cell Sci* 108:985-1002, 1995.

57. Skarsgard ED, Bealer JF, Meuli M, et al: Fetal endoscopic ("Fetendo") surgery: the relationship between insufflating pressure and the fetoplacental circulation, *J Pediatr Surg* 30:1165-1168, 1995.

58. Somasundaram K, Prathap K: The effect of exclusion of amniotic fluid on intra-uterine healing of skin wounds in rabbit foetuses, *J Pathol* 107:127-130, 1972.

59. Stelnicki EJ, Vanderwall K, Harrison MR, et al: The in utero correction of unilateral coronal craniosynostosis, *Plast Reconstr Surg,* 101:287-296, 1998.

60. Stelnicki EJ, Vanderwall K, Hoffman WY, et al: A new in utero sheep model for coronal craniosynostosis, *Plast Reconstr Surg,* 101:278-286, 1998.

61. Whitby DJ, Ferguson MWJ: The extracellular matrix of lip wounds in fetal, neonatal and adult mice, *Development* 112:651-668, 1991.

62. Whitby DJ, McMullen HF, Sung JJ, et al: Localization of TGF-β isoforms in adult and fetal mouse lip wounds, *Surg Forum* 46:651-652, 1995.

Practice Management

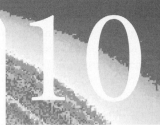

Brian M. Kinney

THE CHANGING HEALTH CARE LANDSCAPE

For many years a physician simply finished a residency, chose almost any location, and opened an office, whether in private practice or a university setting. Options abounded; not much research was needed. The surgeon joined the medical staff of several hospitals and introduced himself or herself to the community and colleagues. He or she busily began practicing plastic surgery, sat for the written and oral American Board of Plastic Surgery examinations,[2] and went on to decades of a successful and rewarding practice of plastic surgery. A good knowledge of the principles of plastic surgery, moderate experience with various procedures, and suture, scalpel, forceps, basic office staff, and a presence in the community were the essentials. The "three A's" of availability, ability, and affability served well. The plastic surgeon's individual talent, drive, and characteristics were the dominant variables in the prosperity, style, and case mix of the practice.

Personal choices were unencumbered by the outside influences of today, such as an insurance company's preauthorization rules and credentialing requirements or the denial and micromanagement of care by innumerable third-party agencies. A physician simply engaged in the practice of medicine, and the physician-patient relationship reigned supreme.

The stability of this traditional paradigm of health care is gone. Plastic surgery is becoming technology intensive and moving at a faster and faster pace as medical knowledge increases more rapidly. Surgery is now a technology-based discipline, and surgeons practice in conjunction with computers, endoscopes, lasers, microsurgical techniques, ultrasonic equipment, the Internet, and a newly touted and "revolutionary" procedure several times a year. Their practice armamentarium experiences a complete turnover in just a few years, and they must reinvent themselves repeatedly to stay current. Change is accelerating and inevitable.

Plastic surgeons must also engage in the "business" of running a medical practice instead of the "practice" of medicine and deal with other businesses, insurance companies, the government, legal mandates, malpractice litigation, political lobbies, patient advocacy groups, and much more. It can be overwhelming. New thought processes and technologies, organizational and management skills, information processing, computer training, surgical techniques, flexibility, insight, perseverance, and patient care methods are necessary to survive and prosper.

In the 1950s, patients paid the physician directly for their health care at the time of service. Physicians treated underprivileged patients without compensation, or charitable organizations and hospitals cared for patients without regard for their ability to pay. Large national businesses began to offer private health care through private insurance carriers 30 to 40 years ago.[22] These benefits proved to be very popular with employees, who saw them as a basic part of having a job in many industries. Insurance companies, however, were silent partners in the physician-patient relationship and simply "paid the bills." In addition, starting with the formation of Medicare in the Social Security Act of 1965,[1] the federal government, as well as state governments through the Medicaid programs, became increasingly involved in health care. The Health Care Finance Administration (HCFA) grew out of this legislation and pays for Medicare.[24]

The depth and breadth of this health insurance coverage increased over the years until the cost of these benefits began to be a major part of a business' and the government's expense. Businesses, through their partnerships with insurance companies, the federal government, and not patients themselves, have largely paid for health care in the United States in recent years. People were living longer, and use of health services dramatically increased. With enormous investment in expensive new technologies and with patients disconnected from the financial impact of the health care bill, utilization of resources increased dramatically. Costs began to go out of control. Health care rose to about 17% of the nation's gross domestic product (GDP) by the early 1990s. To control these costs, businesses, insurance carriers, and the government began to impose restrictions on the practice of medicine, various procedures, and the care that patients saw as a basic covered service.[17] All this began to affect the ability of physicians to manage their practices.

Finally, in 1992 and 1993, after several decades of setting policy and influencing the private sector, the federal government considered, but did not implement, a national health care initiative.[21] Although this effort failed, a new mindset took hold. A relentless pressure has remained to make medicine more accountable, efficient, accessible, and inexpensive, and change continues to impact the medical profession.[23]

Health maintenance organizations (HMOs), organized by the large insurance companies to serve businesses' desire to keep costs down, have become the primary third-party insurers in many regions of the United States and continue to grow rapidly. Large, multinational hospital corporations have spread state by state and begun buying hospitals, surgicenters, and physicians' practices. Some of them now own hundreds of hospitals and have great influence over the marketing of health care. Many more physicians now are employees of, or have formal contracts with, hospitals, universities, HMOs, independent practice associations (IPAs), preferred provider organizations (PPOs), and an array of new legal entities with assorted acronyms. An understanding of contract law and how one coexists with large organizations is now required.

Recently, in response to cost pressures from business, patients, and the government, third-party insurers have restricted or eliminated reimbursement for many physicians' services. In many cases, these "financial" restrictions on various procedures have affected physicians' ability to provide their patients with the standard of care or the latest innovations. In many states the insurers have deemed such important procedures as postmastectomy reconstruction and craniofacial surgery as "cosmetic" and do not cover them.

Now the companies are marketing cosmetic surgery for pay to their insured population and contracting with "providers," often any physician, board certified or not, who is willing to provide "plastic surgery" services. Other medical specialties have found their reimbursement from carriers decreasing, and their members, armed with the latest information from short seminars, have begun to perform procedures traditionally the sole domain of plastic surgery. Competition is intense, and the dividing lines among various specialties are blurred.

Projections show a severe oversupply of all types of physicians, including plastic surgeons. Advertising has created the potential for conflicts of interest. Office surgery centers have become commonplace and have led to loss of hospital-based peer review. The time-honored process of peer review, the morbidity and mortality conference, is not required in this setting. In response to this problem, many states have passed legislation requiring certification by an appropriate agency. Regional, state, and national certification programs also have become commonplace, but they are not the law in all states.

When opening a new practice or managing an ongoing practice, the plastic surgeon must face many important decisions.[12,18] Each decision will critically impact the profitability of the practice, the type of surgery performed, and the practitioner's professional and personal satisfaction. The list includes practice location, case mix (cosmetic versus reconstructive), business form of the practice (solo, group, multispecialty group, university, insurance company, HMO), contracts with third-party payers, financial issues, personnel issues, planning and construction of the physical space, continuing education, innovations, and advances in technology.

INFORMATION AND BUSINESS

The rationale for practice management is simple: one must have access to high-quality information to be able to make good decisions. Information is the lifeline of successful practice management, and access to information is neither free nor easy. Tim Berners-Lee, the developer of the World Wide Web, has stated that "machines must be able to verify the authenticity of assertions found over the Web."[7] Access to good information comes from hard work, and maintenance of reliable information systems is a continual effort. In recent years, insurance carriers, the government, and patients themselves have spent enormous resources on building information infrastructure. They now have excellent access to not only medical information, but also information about physicians, their practices, and even their malpractice record through the National Practitioner's Data Bank in Washington, D.C. This information is found on the Internet at http://www.npdb.com and is available to anyone.

The environment in medicine is more competitive than ever before, and good information has never been more critical. Population demographics, the setting (urban versus rural), the type of insurance carriers dominating the region, the number of surgeons in the area, state and county taxes and regulations, services provided by the hospitals, the weather, economic environment, and many other external factors influence the practice. All this information, and more, is available from the local library or by using a computer and the Internet.[13,14,25,26]

Plastic surgeons must make time for the business side of the practice no matter how undesirable it may seem or how busy they become with patient care. Although surgery and patient care must remain the central endeavor of any surgeon's practice, unless surgeons take care of the business, they will be unable to take care of their patients.[5] Surgeons must build a team of good advisors and resources. Frequent contact with an accountant, attorney, or business advisor helps surgeons to define goals and implement plans. The physician should be aware of these advisors' fee schedule (monthly retainer, hourly rate, fee for service) in advance to avoid surprises.

Once the practice becomes well managed, less time is consumed reacting to immediate concerns. The surgeon can anticipate changes and plan for the future. Knowing what surgical or business methods to keep, improve, discard, or develop is one of the keys to efficient practice management. Ineffective practice management risks loss of patients, a compromise of patient care, a degradation of surgical skills, a lack of productivity, poor employee morale, financial difficulties, and other problems.

One prominent method of good practice management is achieved by implementing an ongoing program of *total quality management,* a concept developed by Edward Deming[10] and Joseph M. Juran,[20] two American scientists who helped the Japanese rebuild their economy after World War II. Total quality management enhances the practice by improving its efficiency, focusing on patient satisfaction, and empowering employees to serve the patients. The practice is continuously monitored, measured, and revamped. Knowing which features of a practice to keep and which to discard can be determined by listening to patients and reflecting on their needs. The seven broad categories of this system are as follows[11]:

1. Vision and values
2. Commitment and participation
3. Quality measurement
4. Continuous improvement
5. Human resource development
6. Rewards
7. Technology and systems

These values are applicable to the individual practice as well as to the design of the entire health care system of a company or a country.[19]

MODELS OF MANAGEMENT

In the past a physician could practice medicine and not have to run a business. The business would "run itself." The clinical part of the practice was essentially the practice. The rent, employees, medical suppliers, and insurance had to be paid, but otherwise management was not a major obligation. Paperwork, other than the traditional patient chart and professional correspondence, was minimal.

Today a physician confronts federal and state regulations for blood-borne pathogens, legal issues of informed consent, the American with Disabilities Act, the Occupational Safety and Health Administration (OSHA), state regulations, HMO and insurance company legal documents, federally and state mandated employee obligations, marketing campaigns, competition from other specialties, and many other considerations. Effectively managing each of these requires time, effort, and planning with careful implementation of policy. The physician who does not confront these factors loses the ability to manage the practice and therefore to practice medicine.

Several models are available for implementing an effective strategy to manage all these factors. The first, employment in an academic setting, alleviates these management obligations from everyone except the department chairman. Working in the military, a large managed care organization, or prepaid health plan also means the surgeon is the employee. Professionally trained administrators manage the practice, and the physician practices medicine relatively unimpeded. Many plastic surgeons enjoy this relief from the hassles of business. Unfortunately, most are not in this situation.

Other plastic surgeons find that the loss of autonomy is frustrating. They may choose to work in a *group practice,* where some autonomy may be found. Multispecialty practices may have dozens of physicians, whereas plastic surgery groups rarely include more than a half-dozen surgeons. Both require practice meetings, election or appointment of a board of directors, discussions, and revenue and expense sharing agreements. Legal documents must be created and accounting methods developed. Cross-coverage for after-hours call is built in to the practice but must be negotiated. Consultation with colleagues is readily available. Expense sharing reduces overhead. Everyday contact enhances the educational interchange among surgeons.

A *solo practice* offers the most autonomy but places full responsibility on the physician to manage all aspects of the practice. Economies of scale are lost, with less efficient use of equipment, supplies, and employees' hours. An in-office operating room (OR) and equipment often sit idle, and employees are not always involved in patient care. When the sole physician is not working, the expenses accumulate without production of income. Fixed costs are a higher percentage of the practice. Excellent planning and budgeting are necessary.

Finally, other models of practicing medicine include nonclinical positions. Medical-legal work, insurance company position, full-time research, medical broadcasting, and journalism are some possibilities. This discussion, however, addresses the clinical fields only.

Outside Services

Each of these forms of practice may retain or consult several outside professionals to provide various business services. The consultant usually charges a fee for service but may charge a percentage of revenue or a standard monthly retainer. Charges may run several thousand dollars a month or higher.

Outside expertise is crucial, and the surgeon must choose those services carefully. Paying too little for poor advice wastes money and eventually may lead to unanticipated crises. Overpaying for inflated services that are not effective is another danger. Many "experts" are willing to charge large amounts of money to give unnecessary advice. Simple services may consist of internal marketing, computer training, or a referral arrangement with outside parties. Advanced services include orchestration of an advertising campaign, computer graphic design of patient education materials, logos and stationery, installation of computer hardware, and networking. Architectural design of the office, the OR suite, and consultation services for certification of a surgicenter are other examples.

Some services are essential and must be procured for the office to run. Every practice requires an accountant or CPA to evaluate tax matters, establish appropriate record keeping, and give counsel on the office's financial growth and development. Legal advice on advanced financial matters also may be necessary. Many accountants work closely with tax attorneys and can give a referral for a legal adviser in tax matters. Employment agreements, contracts with insurance companies, office leases, and other office items usually require legal attention from an attorney experienced in general law as well as medical contracts. Because many attorneys specialize as physicians do, this may be a different lawyer than the tax attorney.

A banker will lend money, offer financial advice on investments, savings, and retirements. Broad financial services are needed to run an office. Insurance needs are available through a personal broker or the county, state, or national medical society. Malpractice, disability, office overhead, life, property and casualty, auto, and other types of insurance are essential to protect the practice. Workers' compensation insurance for employees is required by state law. Unemployment and disability insurance taxes are withheld from employees' paychecks to protect them in case of a layoff, accident, or illness. If the practice is large, a pension fund manager may be required to manage the staff's retirement plan. Real estate brokers may assist in the purchase of office space or negotiate a business lease.

Management consultants or business managers oversee all aspects of the office, but they are expensive. Some accounting firms provide this type of service. A public relations manager oversees marketing and advertising campaigns, pursues new patient markets and hospital affiliations, interacts with the public in educational forums, and may help design themes or the general style of the office. Outside consultants may also provide computer training and maintenance, continuing medical education (e.g., CPR, laser training), and advice on permanent makeup, massage, cosmetics, skin care, occupational therapy, or other allied health care.

Each of these outside experts adds value to a practice, but not all practices require each one. Before starting a new business relationship, the surgeon must ask whether the practice needs this type of service. If it is not essential, the costs in money, time, and loss of autonomy in procuring the outside services must be balanced against the gains in expertise, improved quality of patient care, and potential increased income.

Risks and Benefits

In the academic, military, or employee model the surgeon is at risk from decisions by management, outside market forces, and government policies. A university professor must actively engage in and publish original research. Inadequate self-generated funding or publication of original research may prevent attainment of tenure at the university. A new department chairman may choose to take the faculty in a new direction or remove members from the department for reasons other than performance. The military may close a facility, the commanding officer or the government may force the physician to transfer to another location, or the practice may be downsized.

The plastic surgeon in private practice should have a marketing plan, outside consultants for specialized tasks, and adequate space in a modern facility. Surgeons must choose carefully whether to run their own surgicenter, which is convenient, private, and more comfortable for the patient. The patient may only have to see four or five people, without the elaborate protocol of the hospital setting. Cleanliness is easier to maintain in the small OR, and scheduling certain procedures in the hospital keeps the infection rate low. Managing an OR, however, requires a much higher administrative overhead, paperwork, inspections by local and national organizations, certification and recertification, and liability. Liability issues also arise if another surgeon is using the OR when problems occur. In short, surgicenters are very expensive to maintain and require constant attention.

EMPLOYEES AND RISK MANAGEMENT

Personnel are the most important resource in surgical practice other than the surgeon. They should be well trained, professional, and extremely patient oriented. Each must have well-defined responsibilities. Their job descriptions and duties must be prepared in detail in writing. Recruitment of employees may come from newspaper and classified advertisements, employment agencies, local schools and colleges, medical societies, or word of mouth. Many state and federal guidelines involve employees, employment, and applications. A comprehensive employee manual is required, covering work hours, duties, time off, pay rates, appearance, evaluations, retirement plan benefits, conduct, and other details.

Aided by outside services (e.g., transcription service, per diem registered nurses), a streamlined and efficient practice may only require three or four cross-trained employees, even if the surgeon is performing more than 20 major surgeries per month. When the practice is small, each employee must be able to perform many types of duties for efficiency and economy. Each employee must be flexible and able to work in the front and back office. As the practice grows, more employees will be required.

Up to 10 different types of employees may be needed if the practice is large and diverse. A practice manager supervises financial affairs, patient care, personnel, advertising, and marketing and coordinates all physician activities. Registered nurses may perform preoperative and postoperative clinical duties with minimal physician supervision, oversee the work of physician's assistants, assist in surgery, and run specialty services such as skin care. A physician's assistant or surgical technician may serve as a part-time receptionist and carry out duties similar to a registered nurse, but in a supervised setting. A medical assistant, with less formal training, should handle routine chart work and procedures, examine patients with the physician, and prepare patients and the OR for surgery. A receptionist greets patients and oversees the front desk, telephones, appointments, and general office communications. The duties of a trained medical assistant may overlap those of a receptionist, but also include bookkeeping, billing, accounting, and insurance filing. In the large office a special insurance secretary may devote all work hours to claims, reports, collections, and patient education in insurance matters. Medical transcription services are inexpensive and efficient and usually have a turnaround time of 1 day on dictated reports. In the large group, this job may be performed in house. A patient coordinator serves as the liaison between the physician and the patients and is responsible for patient education, discussion of surgical routines, insurance coverage, follow-up, and general patient services.

Risk management techniques should be used daily in the practice, along with high-quality patient care. The costs of malpractice insurance have soared in recent years. In an era with unprecedented personal options, the public feels less responsible for the choices they make. If an adverse event occurs, the attitude may be "someone must pay for what happened to me," even if no "fault" is attributable to anyone.

The vast dissemination of medical knowledge, fantastic media coverage of "medical miracles," exaggerated advertising claims, and publicity of multimillion-dollar malpractice awards heighten the tendency for the public to sue. Expectations have never been higher. Loyalty to and respect for the physician is at a historic low. Risk management training reduces legal problems with the unhappy patient and leads to improved patient care.

The office manager must have an excellent knowledge of the intricacies of Medicare and Medicaid, workers' compensation insurance, indemnity insurance billing, and managed care plans. Literally thousands of insurance plans are available. Group insurance plans are much more common than individual plans, but they are similar in practice. An employer or association purchases them on behalf of the individual and usually has an annual deductible that the beneficiary must pay. An additional co-payment requirement may range from 10% to 40% of the bill.

Managed care plans include HMOs, PPOs, and a variety of other structures.[22] Generally, the employer or association makes fixed payments in advance on behalf of the beneficiary. The HMO plan capitates the physician and pays a fixed amount regardless of the services provided. A PPO plan may operate as an indemnity insurance plan, but simply refer its enrollees to a practice for a fixed reduction in fee. Medicare, Medicaid, and workers' compensation each pay a fixed amount for each item, subject to severe restrictions by state and federal law. The workers' compensation laws require a variety of reports, protocols, evaluations, and procedures and vary state by state.

Management of the surgical practice's finances is an intricate task in the face of this large body of rules and regulations. Information on HCFA may be obtained from the World Wide Web.[16]

A daily record must be kept of accounts payable and receivable, receipts of deposits, and each patient's charges and payments. A system of checks and balances with a division of responsibilities among employees decreases the chance of embezzlement. Even with complete payment at the time of service in a cosmetic practice, managing without computers risks financial mismanagement from lack of information. Many reports are helpful if not essential. Accounts receivable may run two to four times the monthly gross income of a reconstructive practice and much less in a largely cosmetic practice. Some insurance carriers may pay slowly or much less than others. Patients slow to pay a bill should be contacted monthly. It is important to write off nonperforming accounts receivable. A good insurance-billing program and staff computer training are essential parts of a modern, well-designed practice, as are knowledge about the myriad of forms and maintenance of medical records.

A working familiarity with employment laws and contracts, employee oversight and relations, financial management, and local, state, and federal tax laws and regulations is necessary for efficiency. Usually an in-house employee manages these issues within the practice, but a larger group may require an outside consultant.

STRUCTURAL PROBLEMS

Many structural problems can occur in a surgical practice. Perhaps the most obvious are not keeping up with the latest techniques and not actively engaging in continuing education. The advent of microsurgery in the late 1980s and early 1990s led to a dramatic change in breast surgery, facial and extremity reconstruction, and hand surgery. Failure to learn current techniques would have a dramatic effect on patient care and physician satisfaction. Being incapable of endoscopic surgery and laser techniques would place the surgeon years behind more current surgeons. If the local hospital did not obtain a new operating microscope, endoscope, or laser, problems would arise even if the surgeon was trained.

With an excess of physicians, the light workload may lead to physician dissatisfaction or a diminution of surgical skills. Some practices have too few physicians in an area with a great workload, and physicians may be overworked. Performing a variety of difficult procedures (e.g., replantation, microsurgery) without an assistant surgeon can be taxing. This is more common in a rural setting than in the city, where many specialists are available.

Heavy dependence on a particular HMO, type of surgery, legal work, or workers' compensation can lead to disaster when the environment suddenly changes. HMOs have released excellent physicians for financial reasons or because they have too many physicians on their roster. A practice that relied highly on breast implant surgery in the early 1990s would have suffered severely for several years during the Food and Drug Administration (FDA) silicone implant ban. Some practices were geared heavily toward explanation and reconstructive surgery during the breast implant crisis. To expect reimbursements based on the national class action lawsuit was to invite financial trouble. The global settlement went through many changes before final resolution and court ordered reimbursement to physicians for surgery is based on the global settlement.

Structural problems with staff are a critical issue in managing a practice. Overemployment will lead to financial problems of excessive financial overhead. Idle time during work hours will affect staff-patient interactions. With just a few overworked staff members, burnout and poor morale are likely. A spouse may work in the office or may be the office manager, which inevitably alters the workplace. Some offices can work well under these conditions; others cannot. Employees always know that one worker is "special" despite all attempts at fairness. Relatives or close friends who work in the office may be excellent but are difficult to hire and fire. The relationships outside of the office may be affected as well.

A good office in a poor location may not work well. Changing demographics are important to monitor. An urban area may experience growth in a direction away from the surgeon's present location. The area may undergo a transition from a residential to an industrial neighborhood, adversely affecting admissions. The management of a leased building may not choose to update the premises, which may compromise the ability to attract patients or deliver services. Lack of fresh carpet, clean exterior, or gardens may only be cosmetic. Lack of a good electrical or plumbing system, however, limits the use of 240-volt outlets for lasers, improved water systems for the OR, or the heating and air conditioning.

Marketing issues affect the structure of a practice.[4] Too little or no marketing results in physicians or patients being unaware of the surgeon's skills or specialties. Overreliance on marketing and advertising may require excessive consultation to book patients for surgery. A high volume of surgery may be necessary to cover the high expenses and may lead to burnout, excessive complications, or poor patient care.

Documentation, accounting, and record keeping are vital, and any imbalance or compromise quickly leads to severe problems. Every practice must have excellent access to information, good financial accounting, and a system of charts, files, and records that is powerful and easy to use. It is becoming increasingly difficult and unreasonable to do this without a computer. The demand for information is simply too great to handle it well without automation. Modern information technology is essential to a surgical practice, and every employee should be comfortable with computer basics.

Medical records are closely associated with good patient care and medical-legal affairs. All medical records must be accurate, legible, and well organized. Access must be fast and efficient. Paper copies and records should be clear, clean, and easily available. Word processing, spreadsheets, accounting and bill-paying software, and insurance and patient database programs are the basic tools necessary. Digital photography, Internet access, multimedia capabilities, electronic insurance claim submission, remote-access software, desktop publishing, and digital presentation software are increasingly used in surgical practice. Telemedicine, surgical simulation, virtual reality, and remote robotic surgery will be used in the near future.

CLINICAL PROBLEMS

The surgical outcome for a patient may be substandard or inadequate when the most modern, proven techniques are not used. Traditional operations gradually become outmoded when a new technique withstands peer review scrutiny and surgeons overcome the initial learning curve. Complication rates rise when a surgeon does not keep up with improved techniques and equipment. When a surgeon depends heavily on a few procedures and the demographics of the marketplace change, the surgeon will become outdated and need retraining. Patients will sense this and go to other physicians. Examples would be to rely on a pedicle flap for lower extremity reconstruction, on dermabrasion for facial resurfacing, or on tissue expanders for breast reconstruction.

Disgruntled employees or an unqualified relative with too much authority in the office can cause problems with patient care and employee relations. Extravagances in office decor, overspending on expensive OR equipment or computers, excessive time off or employee benefits, or too many vacations for the surgeon will lead to overhead problems. Demographics,

location, and a changing medical environment must always be considered to prevent compromise of the practice. Avoiding managed care in an area with few traditional indemnity carriers will lead to financial stress. Attempting to practice cosmetic surgery alone in a rural area is likely to fail. Poorly educated or trained employees will always threaten quality patient care. Continuing education is required for nurses, surgical technicians, receptionists, and office managers; national organizations with excellent programs are available. Financial and medical-legal problems always closely follow poor record keeping and substandard patient care.

OPTIMIZING FUNCTION

A smoothly functioning practice is not only more satisfying, but also more efficient, safer, and better for the quality of patient care. After infrastructure is built and protocols are well developed, management becomes easier. When an office is well organized, it will attract many patients. If the patients enjoy good clinical outcomes, the surgeon will be compensated. Besides detrimental to the patient, complications are expensive. When the surgeon is busy, well-trained employees find a stimulating and challenging workday. Physicians and the staff derive great satisfaction from providing excellent care and seeing grateful patients recover from surgery. Once learned by the surgeon, offering state-of-the-art procedures is in the patient's best interest. Incorporating the latest techniques without a thorough period of training, however, can be disastrous in regard to complications, staff frustration with new methods, and extra time taken from routine patient care.

Short-term success in a practice is possible with structural problems present, but long-term success and financial security can only be achieved when excellence in patient care comes first.

EVOLUTION OF SOLUTIONS

The practice of medicine had been stable for many years until the 1990s. Recently, medicine has been in accelerated evolution, with no end in sight to the upcoming changes. The federal government has drastically cut back its financial support for residency training programs. Large multinational hospital chains and insurance companies have engaged in mergers, buyouts, and acquisitions. HMOs, PPOs, IPAs, medical service organizations (MSOs), and a myriad of other groups have been formed. As fast as one entity is created, another replaces it. Even physicians have formed their own managed care plans to compete with the commercial carriers of insurance.

In the Balanced Budget Bill of 1997 a regulation established that telemedicine consultation (roughly equivalent to regular face-to-face consultation) is reimbursable through HCFA, the government agency that administers Medicare. This is a little-known but fundamentally important portent of the future. Remote consultation without the opportunity to palpate, auscultate, or percuss will become a more prominent part of the practice of medicine. Inevitably, this will bring about major changes.

University departments have begun to compete with private practitioners, reach out to the surrounding communities, and market themselves as the "gold standard" of care. Many have established satellite clinics at distant outposts to increase their outreach. Some university medical centers are merging with each other, a possibility almost unheard of just a few years ago. Economies of scale may provide them with lower overhead, greater marketing power, and improved negotiations with managed care and hospital chains. HMOs and group practices have aggressively looked for more patients to include in their plans. Concurrently, many "caregivers" experience restrictions on what procedures they may perform. Formation of small groups (some multispecialty, many single specialty) among private practitioners has accelerated in recent years.

Fewer and fewer surgeons are in solo practice. Physicians have formed publicly held corporations that own medical practices. Buyers and sellers trade shares openly in the stock market. Many of these companies own medical practices in dozens of states, and many physicians are prominent stockholders in these corporations that own their practices. The corporation pays them a salary and stock options based on their profitability. The for-profit motive and the shareholder's interests represent a fundamental conflict that must be resolved with the patient's best interest and quality of care in mind.

Formerly, physicians could refer patients to entities in which they had part ownership. The U.S. Congress passed the Stark law to prevent a physician from referring a patient to a medical laboratory, supply house, or other entity in which the physician has a financial interest, except in unusual circumstances and with prior disclosure to the patients. Although no widely publicized problems occurred with "self-referral," the drive to eliminate potential conflicts of interest led to this effort.

Solutions are still in evolution. In late 1997 plans circulated in Congress to lower the Medicare coverage age to 55 years. A "Medicare" program for children up to age 18 has also been discussed. The practice of medicine will continue to change as physicians and others strive to meet increasing health care demands more efficiently.

Surgical practices experience more educational, competitive, and financial demands. The acceleration of technology has increased the effort required to stay current and has pressured surgeons to abandon the practice of "general" plastic surgery. Many physicians promote themselves as specialists in one small area to achieve a competitive advantage in the public's eye. Many HMOs, insurance companies, and corporate entities promote their special expertise in a certain area to gain "market share." Meanwhile, for greater efficiency, some of the same insurers are forcing physicians in the opposite direction, to care for all patients in the insurer's plan, regardless of the physician's skills. Surgeons must perform procedures that they do not perform regularly.

AUTHOR'S PREFERRED PRACTICE MANAGEMENT

A streamlined solo practice still represents one of the most desirable models, but it is becoming increasingly rare. It is simply too inefficient to run an office easily in this manner. The margin for error in management is very narrow. Agreements for overhead and expense sharing among several solo practitioners in the same office suite are now the most popular choice for new graduates because of the high costs of setting up an office. Many experienced surgeons are also joining in overhead-sharing arrangements for the same reasons.

I have been in both a solo practice and a group arrangement with shared overhead as a junior and senior member. My preference is group sharing of expenses because it allows for maximum individual freedom and has the advantages of reduced overhead. Clinical duties are shared on a reliable but informal basis, with few meetings and administrative duties.

Group practices of plastic surgeons who pool and share revenue and clinical duties are growing, and some have as many as 10 surgeons. Except in the university settings, these were extremely rare until recent years. Academic surgeons generally share funds as a group and negotiate arrangements with the university, often with a fixed base income and a graduated tax on increased productivity. The university medical center usually mixes the revenue in a pool with physicians in other disciplines. Fee-for-service multispecialty practices have been modeled after the Mayo Clinic for decades, but only a small percentage of plastic surgeons have been members. The Kaiser Permanente model, in effect since World War II, is similar but is generally a salaried plan for physicians.

Some physicians sell their practice to a private corporation in the form of an MSO. The physician becomes an employee of the corporation that owns the practice, and the corporation pays a salary and possibly bonuses to the physicians. Some of these publicly held companies will pay bonuses through stocks or stock options. Most physicians belong to at least a few insurance carriers (e.g., HMOs), and in a few states they have formed their own organizations. Until recently, no program included a medically oriented MBA, and now a few U.S. universities offer just such a degree. The number of physicians who are law school graduates continues to rise.

Advantages and Disadvantages

The chief advantage of solo practice is great individual freedom, and its greatest drawback is the financial burden. The practice remains small, efficient, and streamlined. The group model, whether in private practice or the university setting, possesses increased efficiency and sharing of fixed financial costs, but some administrative obligation is involved. Professional interchange among colleagues offers distinct advantages. As the group becomes larger, the administrative duties grow. Entities such as the MSO and publicly held stock company offer even more relief from administrative duties and fixed overhead, but the arrangement increasingly resembles an employee-employer relationship. The larger and more complicated the group, the more the surgeon's duties become those of an employee.

Strategies and Structure

Regardless of the form of the practice, a strategy must be built according to the types of surgery performed and the population of patients served. Surgeons have a few favorite procedures or those they are particularly adept at performing. These may or may not be lucrative. Surgical procedures fall into seven broad categories: (1) congenital anomalies, (2) hand surgery, (3) aesthetic surgery, (4) trauma, (5) breast surgery, (6) cancer, and (7) burns. No surgeon is an expert in all these areas.

Early in the practice, before a strategy is fully realized, circumstances may dictate that the surgeon work on a broad range of patient problems. Extensive clinical experience is essential for the maturation of surgical judgment and patient management. Satisfied patients are a practice's best promotion. Attaining a "critical mass" of postresidency experience and postoperative expertise is important. In time, however, this will begin to change as some specialization occurs. Few surgeons are busy in more than three of the seven categories. It is difficult to maintain state-of-the-art skills in many areas. Surgeons develop a few areas of expertise that they become known for and enjoy. It may take 5 to 7 years for the surgeon to narrow the choices and for the practice to mature in such a way. Occasionally the surgeon still may perform all types of surgery.

Surgeons should also divide their practice into broad categories based on financial issues and personal interest. The ideal situation is a financially positive procedure that the surgeon truly enjoys. The least desirable situation is a very expensive or poorly reimbursed procedure that the surgeon is not adept at performing or does not enjoy. The other two combinations lie between these extremes. Income from the lucrative procedures will compensate or subsidize the other procedures.

Surgeons should not abandon favorite procedures only because they are not lucrative. The contributions to society by generous surgeons are enormous and often unrecognized by those outside the field. Many plastic surgeons have participated in charitable organizations, such as Interplast, Operation Smile, and Operation Rainbow. Some specialize in techniques such as cleft lip and craniofacial reconstruction; others perform operations without compensation on inner-city youths, the poor, refugees, war casualties, crime victims, and burn patients. Maintaining the surgical skills required to perform these procedures improves results in other areas. These efforts also create immeasurable good will and personal satisfaction. This remains a fundamental part of the higher calling in the practice of plastic surgery.

TECHNOLOGY

The advances of information technology in the last decade have dramatically impacted the practice of medicine. Although an information system requires major expenditure of capital for the hardware, software, and employee training, the benefits are substantial when the office properly implements the program. Information is power, but it is the knowledge from this information that is so vital. The effective use of data leads to optimization of patient and financial outcomes for the practice.

Medicine as a business is much more complex now. Insurance and government regulations are so overwhelming that a reliable means of handling large amounts of data is required. Patient demands for access to medical information is at an all-time high. Rapid communications and the automation of repetitive tasks are what computers do best.

Information technology is useful in many areas. Word processing improves office correspondence and writing of papers, with formatting, spell checking, and grammar checking for documents. The computer novice usually tries this type of software first. The improvements in productivity and ease of use are often enough to convince the most reluctant users that they must incorporate computers into the practice. The preparation of slides for lectures is another area that has immediate benefits. Over time the surgeon may choose to use a laptop computer to present lectures directly without the intermediate and expensive step of preparing slides for a projector. Full multimedia presentations with movies, animations, dynamic graphic transitions, morphs, and many other improvements are possible.

Spreadsheet programs provide data analysis and solve common office problems. A contact manager provides a database of people important to the practice. Integrated office suites contain word-processing software, spreadsheets, presentation packages, and a database program, as well as many ancillary utilities. Preparation of marketing brochures, newsletters, and mailing lists with desktop-publishing software helps to educate patients, colleagues, and third-party payers.

Most offices have now converted to computer billing programs, a repetitive task ideal for the personal computer. Submission of bills to third-party payers is now possible by electronic means. Unfortunately, hundreds of closed-architecture, proprietary systems use expensive programs. These programs may cost 10 to 100 times as much as the other programs. The medical marketplace still awaits the arrival of inexpensive, interchangeable systems for insurance billing. Fortunately, financial management and accounting programs for general use abound in the inexpensive price range. They are easy to use, are extremely powerful, and significantly improve efficiency in paying bills, tracking expenses, and collecting information for tax matters. Many of these cost less than $100.

Digital photography is still an emerging field and does not offer the quality, reliability, and simplicity of traditional film photography. Within the next 5 years, however, digital imaging will probably become the standard method for clinical imaging. This will have a profound effect on the use of photography in plastic surgery. Professional standards must be devised for the protection of the digital image from improper computer manipulation. Legal standards will develop as imaging issues arise in malpractice, workers' compensation, and personal injury cases.

Computer modems in the 1970s transmitted bits at less than 100 baud (bit audio density). Currently, inexpensive modems transmit at 56,000 baud (56k), and businesses typically transmit information at more than 1 megabit per second (Mbs). This bandwidth allows for the transmission of streaming audio and video information rapidly and easily over the Internet. This capability, along with the exponential growth of the Internet, has fundamentally changed the world and the world of medicine.[7] Worldwide more than 100 million users joined the Internet in the 1990s. This unprecedented increase in people's ability to communicate transcends all national borders, cultures, and professions.

The physician must make the commitment to change. The relentless innovation of the information age yields greater power at a lower purchase price each year. The total cost of ownership, however, involves many other issues. Ongoing staff training may be the greatest expense in computerization of the office. Hardware upgrades are required every 2 to 3 years. Although the old equipment is still functional, it may not serve the office well and may cost more to maintain. Software upgrades are less problematic, but they occur as often as twice a year. Newly upgraded software often contains imperfect computer codes, or bugs, which may lead to inefficiency in employee production.

Moving forward too fast, however, involves many perils. Employees should not take on too many new software programs at once because it will interrupt normal office flow and frustrate them. A new computer will not eliminate the need for an employee, but it will enable the worker to be more productive. For the physician, telemedicine for consultation is in the immediate future, and telesurgery (or remote surgery) may arrive within 10 to 20 years.

The practice manager must start with specific goals for information management, purchasing equipment or software to solve specific problems in the office, not because of their potential or their ability to perform many other tasks. Not spending enough on computer equipment is just as harmful as overspending. Both can lead to poor productivity. The amount of time each employee will spend with computer equipment and the employee's specific role should be considered. Employees should take instructional courses at regular intervals. The manager must understand how employees can best learn new computer software. Many methods, such as video instruction or sitting in a classroom listening to lectures, may be ineffective.[15] Computer literacy should be a prerequisite for new employees.

STAFF EDUCATION

Continuing education has been a professional requirement for physicians for many years and should include management issues. Registered nurses have similar professional guidelines, and other employees should have continuing education as well. Seminars cover insurance billing, anatomy for office personnel, office management, employee relations, word processing, Windows or Macintosh operating systems, spreadsheets,

billing, marketing, and advertising. On-the-job employee training is cost-effective over time and should be included in the office budget.

The effective manager must manage the office's most valuable resource, the employees. In the service "business" of medicine, what ultimately counts is the human factor. In the practice of medicine, excellent training and high-quality patient care are paramount.

TOTAL QUALITY MANAGEMENT

Preoperative and postoperative management should embody the principles of total quality management (TQM), a well-known Japanese business principle applied in America in recent years. TQM is the global focus on the continuous improvement of quality. The office can achieve success in TQM by improving the efficiency of the process, focusing on satisfying the patient, and empowering the employees to deliver quality and excellence in patient care.[9] It is similar to the iterative process in computer programming. Continuous monitoring and measurement of quality and effectiveness is the central task in TQM. Deciding which features to keep and which to discard can be determined by focusing on the patients, evaluating the outcome of surgery, and receiving feedback on their needs and satisfaction.

Deming, one of the fathers of TQM, proposed 14 points that fall into seven categories as the core of the process.[8] These ideas can be applied to the plastic surgery practice as follows:

1. The practice must have a particular vision and a core set of values, including an understanding of what type of surgery will be performed and how the medical staff will carry out their mission.
2. Each employee must have a sense of commitment and be eager to participate in a culture of quality patient care, with a true desire to serve the patient's needs.
3. A mechanism must exist for evaluating results, both surgical and with regard to patient satisfaction. Reproducible standards must be met.
4. The process of improvement must be an integral part of patient care from the first consultation and evaluation until final discharge.
5. The employees are the most important resource of the practice. Openness, creativity, communication, and continuous discourse are essential to the process and to the new culture of the practice. The employees must focus not on profits, vacation time, or number of procedures performed, but on continuous change, quality, and improvement. This is the most difficult part of the process. It requires a fundamental change in the culture and mindset of the employees.
6. The physician must emphasize the human aspects of recognition, rewards, and the work environment. These are as important to employee satisfaction as monetary factors. Personal involvement in the employees' performance by showing appreciation for a job well done demonstrates great care for them.

7. If the entire step-by-step process is high quality, the final result will be high quality. High quality cannot be achieved efficiently without accurate information and good technology. The patient is central to the process. Continuous quality improvement is required. Prevention of mistakes and a well-designed patient care plan are crucial. Every member of the team is responsible for the results.

SECONDARY MANAGEMENT PROCEDURES

Many agencies inspect, evaluate, or regulate the practice of medicine. First, periodic self-assessment should take place. This is done on the clinical side of the practice through take-home examinations, recertification by the American Board of Plastic Surgery (ABPS), and biannual continuing medical education requirements. Each plastic surgeon must fulfill the requirements of the particular state. Most require about 150 total hours every 2 years. About 90 hours must be in the field of plastic surgery and the remaining 60 hours in a field related to the practice of plastic surgery or office management.

Accounting or business consultants can review the surgeon's image, marketing, advertising, workplace, flow of patient care, and other office matters. Some of these factors may be very valuable in improving the work environment. Organizations such as the American Association for Accreditation of Ambulatory Surgical Facilities (AAAASF), American Association for Accreditation of Ambulatory Health Centers (AAAHC), and Medicare inspect and certify outpatient surgicenters and in-office OR facilities. They usually have a 2-year or 3-year cycle for reinspection and recertification. Extensive record-keeping methods are required. The quality of these centers has greatly improved with these programs.

OSHA and its state counterparts may engage in surprise inspection of the work environment. Many regulations apply to the handling of hazardous materials, and an ongoing program of biologic waste disposal is mandatory in most states. All these agencies oversee processes that should be an essential part of a healthy medical practice.

ROLE OF STATISTICS

Interesting and valuable statistical and quantitative data are available as a qualitative guide to overall office management and choices in practice mix, but actual clinical outcome data are just beginning to emerge in plastic surgery.[3] Without forceful economic pressure and a large information infrastructure, no significant effort had been made until recent years to accumulate this type of information. The immediate practical application of these data is not clear, but groups of surgeons can show large insurance carriers their results with a particular procedure to justify expenditures by the company to treat a condition surgically. Cost information on endoscopic versus open carpal tunnel release and autologous tissue versus breast implant reconstruction are two examples, but they show

conflicting data. Much of this depends on the technique and the physician, and studies support each of the methods. A formal program in breast reduction is underway. Clinical outcome data in many other areas should be available in a few years.

The American Society of Plastic and Reconstructive Surgeons (ASPRS) Department of Communications accumulates data on reconstructive and cosmetic procedures every year.[3] The process is improving with the computerization of data collection at each physician's office. The top reconstructive procedure in 1996, for example, was tumor removal (including skin lesions), with 542,063 cases, followed by 153,581 hand surgery cases, 146,470 "other reconstructive" procedures, and 115,998 laceration repairs. Data are also available for the prices of cosmetic and reconstructive procedures by various categories, including region, state, race, and type of OR setting.

Although knowing these data may prove interesting, it is more useful to know the demographic information of the population near the office. Many commercial sources of data are available on income, race, types of occupations, taxes, and other items. The U.S. Census Bureau is the original source of much of this information, however, and has a large searchable database.[26] Any large public or university library contains a wealth of information. Polling companies and marketing companies have carefully studied the public's interest in cosmetic surgery. One firm, Markets Facts of Chicago, sponsored a large study of general interest in cosmetic surgery. The physician also may purchase many popular books with statistics on hospitals, medical schools, business regulation, tax rates, climate, recreational activities, income, lifestyle, and other factors that impact the choice of a practice location.

Surveys on computer software and learning counter the most popularly held ideas about mastering hardware and software training.[15] The twenty-third most useful method of learning new software is attending a formal training seminar on the software, whereas the seventh is asking an instructor a question after a training course. Number one is experimenting with the program, number two is relying on program consistency, number three is asking co-workers for help, and number four is searching program menus. Number 29 of 30 is watching videotaped lectures and demonstrations.

Understanding how to learn new technology is essential to appropriate utilization of human resources. This applies to computer software, office staff training, patient relations, and new surgical techniques.

The choice of location, management style, and partnership arrangement dramatically affects the finances and development of the practice,[6] as discussed earlier. The model should be consistent with the surgeon's practice and lifestyle. A busy practice may result in higher income but much longer work hours and fewer opportunities to pursue other interests, such as family, sports, the arts, or hobbies. A more complicated practice requires greater financial and "personal" overhead to maintain. No formal data exist for this area in practice management. In the future, widespread surveys in plastic surgery may characterize these issues.

ECONOMIC ISSUES

To maximize revenues, the surgeon must examine each of the practice's payers. Working with insurance companies is often very difficult, and each has its own set of rules. If difficulties arise in keeping up with too many companies, concentrating on a few payers may help. The surgeon should establish close relationships with as many claims adjusters as possible, know them by their first name, and have the staff keep in close contact with them. Such efforts should be cooperative and consultative in achieving a common goal, "enlisting" adjusters as team members in the common effort to complete claims processing. The surgeon should learn how to preauthorize quickly and appeal denials or poor reimbursement when necessary but must not lower quality of care, agree to operate without an assistant surgeon, or compromise the practice for any insurance company or patient.

A busy practice needs patients. Telephones should be available all day, if possible, and answered quickly. Telephones on an answering service means the surgeon is unavailable to patients; no more than 1 hour a day is reasonable. An understanding of patient mix and a streamlined practice are essential to provide services. A rigorous financial analysis of each office activity shows the costs to manage each activity and the resulting revenue. Knowing fixed costs (e.g., rent, electricity, malpractice insurance, loan payments) helps determine how to restructure or renegotiate them. Identifying variable costs (e.g., OR supplies, advertising, marketing) and part-time employees' salaries helps determine how to share, reduce, or change them.

Controlling overhead expenses is one of the most important factors in maintaining the financial health of the practice. Physician salaries, taxes, disability insurance premiums, auto expenses, and health benefits are generally excluded from the overhead numbers, as are physicans' continuing education, travel, and entertainment expenses. Personnel costs are often the largest item in the overhead. A bonus, incentive, or productivity plan with a lower base salary for employees will save regular payroll dollars, but reward efforts that promote the practice. Efficient organization minimizes overtime costs. The manager should maintain accurate and up-to-date job descriptions for each employee, evaluate productivity standards at least yearly, and nurture employee morale. Contented employees are much more likely to stay. Training new employees takes several months, disrupting the office flow. The surgeon should consider merging with other surgeons to share overhead, while still maintaining independence.

A major economic issue is the complication rate in surgery. Higher rates lead to higher returns to the OR for repeat surgery. Many times a third party and the patient do not cover these costs. The physician must pay for the expenses associated with the secondary surgery. The costs of secondary surgery, high complication rates, and isolated cases of spectacular complications may bring a practice to financial ruin. The simplest way to avoid this is to practice the highest patient care standards and keep up with current knowledge. Large practices with a high volume of surgery spend less time with each patient. Less development of the physician-patient relationship could lead to more problems in the risk management issues.

AESTHETIC AND LIFESTYLE ISSUES

Significant lifestyle issues are associated with the various practice choices. Individual choices should be based on a careful set of compromises and personal preferences. A rural setting has many advantages of a quieter, less expensive, cleaner, less crowded environment with fewer hassles. On the other hand, it is often stressful to practice in relative isolation and manage difficult cases without assistance. The academic setting contains the rigors of "publish or perish," the emphasis on generating outside research funding, and the duties of teaching students that compete with the surgical caseload. However, the stimulation of interaction with colleagues, a built-in referral base, and the challenging nature of the patient care may be more important as a career consideration.

The urban setting in private practice has too many specialists, stiff competition from well-trained physicians, higher costs, more taxes and regulations, and access difficulties for patients. These practices place the physician close to all the cultural advantages of a lively and active urban area. A checklist of the top 10 advantages and drawbacks of each choice can help in making this decision.

DEMOGRAPHIC CONSIDERATIONS

More than 30% of the board-certified plastic surgeons in the United States live in one of four states: California, New York, Florida, and Texas.[3] Not surprisingly, all these states have large populations, as well as a higher percentage of the population interested in cosmetic surgery. The ratio of board-certified plastic surgeons to the population significantly affects a surgical practice. Some areas, such as Washington, D.C., Nevada, Hawaii, and Utah, have small populations but many plastic surgeons and stiffer competition. Other states, such as Florida, Maryland, and New York, have a large population and a large number of plastic surgeons. In a smaller, rural state a plastic surgeon cannot perform many cosmetic procedures, although fewer plastic surgeons means less competition. It is also unlikely that a surgeon would perform a large number of reconstructive procedures in the shadow of a major university medical center.

Many physicians perform the more lucrative cosmetic procedures in urban areas, and the community standard may be extremely high. The presence of an internationally known, prominent surgeon in the community nearby affects other physicians' ability to draw patients to their office. Cultural considerations are also extremely important. Cultural groups appear to vary in their likelihood to undergo certain surgical procedures, but data are not available. The ability to speak several foreign languages can improve the quality of care to patients not fluent in English and may attract more patients than if translators are required for communication.

PATIENT SATISFACTION

High patient satisfaction directly follows high-quality patient care. Nonmedical factors, such as parking, ambience, decor, music, free samples of supplies, and brochures, amplify the patient's experience in your office but are built on the foundation of practicing medicine well. Without a consistent pattern of good clinical outcome, the benefits of these diminish dramatically. Basic medical principles must come first, and surgeons must never forget this. Patient satisfaction depends on a well-managed treatment plan and precise surgery that result in a good outcome.

Some patients with more unusual medical conditions enjoy the atmosphere of higher learning and the cutting edge of university research. Others, however, dislike the parade of specialists, students, and residents who visit them for a routine procedure in a teaching hospital. Many industrial workers who undergo a reconstructive procedure value simple surroundings, quick and easy access to the office, inexpensive parking, and small clinics or hospitals. A lower-priced area with simple but efficient facilities would be preferable under those circumstances. Many patients prefer more privacy than the university setting allows but also want fancy spalike environments. The private practice offers the personal service, privacy, streamlining, and lack of bureaucracy that many busy, higher-income patients may prefer. Surgeons should tailor the practice to the type of patients they expect to treat.

Regardless of the type of practice or the type of patients that predominate, quality of patient care is the most important consideration. The same principles of medical practice apply, the same diagnoses and indications must be formulated, the same indications are used, the same surgeries are performed, the same preoperative and postoperative management is implemented, and the outcomes should be the same.

REFERENCES

1. Altmeyer A: *Formative years of Social Security,* Madison, Wis, 1966, University of Wisconsin Press.
2. American Board of Plastic Surgery: *ABPS booklet of information,* Philadelphia, 1999, ABPS Publishing, published annually.
3. American Society of Plastic and Reconstructive Surgeons: Plastic Surgery Information Service: http://www.plasticsurgery.org/mediactr.
4. American Society of Plastic and Reconstructive Surgeons: *Marketing your cosmetic practice,* Arlington Heights, Ill, 1995, ASPRS Publishing.
5. American Society of Plastic and Reconstructive Surgeons: *Practice management guide,* Arlington Heights, Ill, 1992, ASPRS Publishing.
6. American Society of Plastic and Reconstructive Surgeons: *Increasing your practice profitability,* Arlington Heights, Ill, 1997, ASPRS Publishing.
7. Berners-Lee T: WWW: past, present, and future, *IEEE Comput* 29:76, 1996.
8. Bidgoli H: *Modern information systems for managers,* San Diego, 1997, Academic Press.
9. Blumenthal D, Scheck A, editors: *Improving clinical practice: total quality management and the physician,* San Francisco, 1995, Jossey-Bass.
10. Deming WE: *Out of the crisis,* Cambridge, Mass, 1986, MIT Press.
11. Esichaikal V, Medey GR, Smith RD: Problem-solving support for TQM, *Information Systems Management,* Winter 1994, p 47.
12. Fox Y, Levine BA: *How to join, buy or merge a physician's practice,* St Louis, 1998, Mosby.
13. Garoogian R, editor: *America's top rated cities: a statistical handbook,* Boca Raton, Fla, 1997, Universal Reference Publications.
14. Garoogian R, editor: *America's top rated smaller cities 1996-97: a statistical handbook,* Boca Raton, Fla, 1997, Universal Reference Publications.
15. Harp C: Winging it, *Computerworld* 30:107-109, 1996.
16. Health Care Finance Administration: http://www.hcfa.gov.
17. Helms R: *American health care policy: critical issues for reform,* Washington, DC, 1993, American Enterprise Institute.
18. Holliman CJ: *Resident's guide to starting in medical practice,* Baltimore, 1995, Williams & Wilkins.
19. Joss R, Kogan M: *Advancing quality: TQM in the National Health Service,* Buckingham, UK, 1995, Open University Press.
20. Juran JM: *Managerial breakthrough: the classic book on improving management performance,* New York, 1995, McGraw-Hill.
21. Laham N: *A lost cause: Bill Clinton's campaign for national health insurance,* New York, 1996, Praeger.
22. Miller I: *American health care blues: Blue Cross, HMO's and pragmatic reform since 1960,* New Brunswick, NJ, 1996, Transaction.
23. Morreim EH: *Balancing act: the new medical ethics of medicine's new economics,* Washington, DC, 1997, Georgetown University Press.
24. Robinson C: *The bureaucracy and the legislative process: a case study of the HCFA,* Washington, DC, 1991, University Press of America.
25. Savageau D, Loftus G: *Places rated almanac,* ed 5, Indianapolis, 1997, MacMillan.
26. US Census Bureau: http://www.census.gov.

CHAPTER 11

Photography

John Di Saia

Plastic surgeons have a definite need for a system of reliable image generation within their specialty. Images are necessary not only to teach techniques and outcomes to other surgeons, but also to document the following:

1. Preoperative status and postoperative results
2. Any case involving extensive trauma
3. Any case with a high probability of a poor outcome
4. Unsuspected findings in the operating room
5. Interesting or new surgical cases and techniques

Since few surgeons really understand the process of photography, this chapter briefly reviews the basic elements and provides case examples and standardized views used in plastic surgery.

THE BASICS

A camera is a light-gathering device (the lens) closely juxtaposed to a photographically sensitive medium (in the photographic example here, this is the film). The *lens* is a special device that allows objects to be focused and framed by the operator. An *aperture* varies the amount of light that is allowed to reach the film, which results in an exposure. Apertures are commonly referred to as "f stops." The confusing issue with f stops is that a larger amount of light is designated by a smaller number (e.g., an aperture of 1.7 allows twice as much light to reach the film as one of 3.5). Smaller apertures allow for a greater range of objects to be in focus, a concept called *depth of field.* Shutter speed determines the length of time that the light is allowed to pass through the aperture to expose the film.

Photographic film has a varied light sensitivity designated by an ASA number. A higher ASA represents more light sensitivity (e.g., an ASA 200 film is twice as light sensitive, or twice as "fast," as ASA 100 film). Film is also balanced for a particular light source. Light has an associated color temperature. Most film commercially available is balanced for daylight, or white light. This form of light has all wavelengths included. This "dedication" is significant because daylight film exposed under common light bulbs (tungsten light) will result in a yellow hue. Similarly, the same film exposed under fluorescent light will appear green. Fortunately, the light from common flash units is white light, which should be used to expose daylight film indoors for a proper tonal result.

A final issue with film is the choice of slide film versus negative film. Professional photographers prefer slide films because these have a much greater tonal range than print films. Slides also have a much smaller margin for error in relation to the actual exposure *(exposure latitude).* Contrast is much higher in slide film, but black appears as black, which cannot always be assumed with negative films. This fact also readily allows for harsh shadows. The camera operator should attempt to cast these distracting shadows out of the frame.

GENERAL EQUIPMENT

The best general-purpose camera at present is the 35-mm single lens reflex (SLR). This format provides high-quality images at a moderate price. A good general-purpose lens (portraiture) is between 80 and 105 mm. Consideration of a macro lens (designed for close-up photography) purchase is also warranted depending on the surgeon's exact needs. The use of diopters (simple magnifiers) attached to an existing lens usually results in poor-quality images with exceptionally poor depth of field.

The zoom lens, a lens with multiple focal lengths, is becoming a more reasonable alternative to carrying several fixed–focal length lenses. The loss in resolution was once much higher than it is at present. In using such a lens, a single 35-mm to 105-mm unit can replace three popular focal lengths, allowing for a moderate-wide-angle (35 mm), general-purpose (50 mm), and portraiture-length (105 mm) lens all in one.

A flash unit is essential, especially for operative photography. The purist will choose a *ring light,* a donut-shaped unit that fits around the lens. The advantage is that such a unit provides multidirectional light that virtually eliminates shadows. A simple top-mounted flash unit can be used, but care must be taken to avoid harsh shadows and reflections.

In the office a small studio is optimal. The walls should be painted a soft-white color. Strong-colored wall paint should be avoided because this can easily result in a color bias in the pictures. A background of a similar neutral color should be selected for similar reasons. At least two flash units should be available. The simplest arrangement involves the placement of one unit on each side of the camera in front of the subject (Figure 11-1). Each source strikes the subject obliquely, thereby eliminating shadow. The light can also be softened by using a flash umbrella; the light is bounced from the umbrella onto the subject.

My preferred film is ASA 100 E6 slide film. This film is readily developed by many laboratories in 1 or 2 hours. "Faster" films (with higher ASA ratings) are available, but at the cost of increased "graininess" in the final product. Although not obvious at ASA 200, graininess increases above this rating. The advantage of faster and therefore more light-sensitive films is that a smaller aperture can be used, resulting in a greater depth of field. With close-up work, occasionally this increase in depth of field may warrant the use of faster films.

A professional laboratory should be used for film developing. Although these are more costly than the many "economy" film-developing services available, the professional laboratory offers development to more exacting specifications with more frequently changed chemicals. Nothing may mar surgical results more than lost or poorly developed images.

Since the average surgeon will produce thousands of slides annually, film storage becomes a concern. Fortunately, many filing systems are commercially available. The key elements to storage are the temperature, brightness, and humidity to which the slides are exposed. Slides films are sensitive to warm, bright, humid conditions, which accelerate their degradation. Photographic dyes in the slide change over time, but this occurs less rapidly in a cool, dark, dry environment.

INFORMED CONSENT

The special physician-patient relationship has implications for photography. Patients are often curious about the use of photographs taken by the surgeon. Few know who specifically may see these images or precisely what they reveal. A medical-ethical issue results if a patient is done harm because of the inappropriate use of a photograph. The issue of informed consent therefore becomes important.

A person should be informed of the purpose and potential uses of the images at the time of photography. Emphasizing that the images are the physician's property may avert problems later should the patient ask for the originals. Any recognizable person in a photograph taken by or for the physician may require a release, which is certainly needed if the intent is publication. Even if the person is not recognizable, a release may still be helpful because it documents the informed consent. Be advised that a release does not prevent a lawsuit; it merely helps to protect the physician if one is filed.

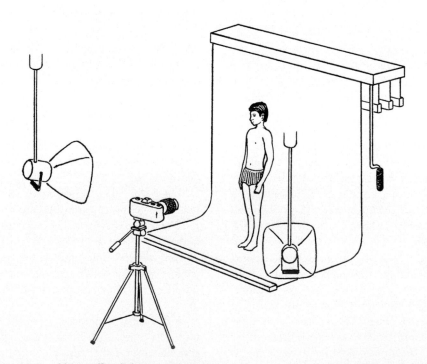

Figure 11-1. Most office-lighting arrangements use two frontal light units and a simple background.

The original photographs should remain in the surgeon's possession. If an attorney requests photographs, copies can be provided after the appropriate release from the patient has been obtained.

A related medical-legal issue involves photography and acute complications. The appropriate procedure for photographing the patient with complications is controversial. The degree to which complications are an issue relates to the preoperative discussion between the physician and patient. The proper time for documentation of a complication is the time when it is observed. An upset patient, however, may not react favorably when abruptly thrust into a photographic session. Although documentation of the complication is important, under these circumstances it may be better to postpone the photograph.

TECHNIQUES

Composition
Since photography represents a three-dimensional object in two dimensions, the need for multiple views is readily apparent. Standardization of these views, however, is equally important for later comparisons among the same and different subjects. The literature has addressed the importance of standardization.[1,3,5] The quality of images used in presentations and even in the literature, however, have been variable.

Standardization includes many elements that should be the same as much as possible for all images of a subject. These elements include viewpoint, light source, lens, background, and the size of the subject in the frame. The purist would photograph the subject with the same camera and lens using the same lighting and background at the same aperture and distance every time.

BASIC VIEWPOINTS. Basic viewpoints include frontal (anterior), profile (lateral), and oblique. A frontal view should be exactly that: a direct anterior view. Symmetry can be judged well from this perspective if the illumination by the flash is symmetric. When seen along with a frontal view, a lateral view allows one to imply three-dimensional character to the subject. This should be a direct profile. An oblique view would result from a poorly shot lateral. The oblique viewpoint, however, has the advantage of implying a three-dimensional character better than either of the other views. As a single view, it is of little value.

Emphasizing the Subject
An early adjustment for the photographer is to begin visualizing how the camera will render a subject. Beginners often fail to realize that a subject that takes up little of the camera frame will not appear well in a photograph. Because surgeons are seeking to document their subjects, they must fill the frame with them. Once they have accomplished this, the goal becomes orientation of the subject so that its exact nature is clearly apparent. Extraneous objects should be removed from view so that only the subject is available for examination.

SPECIAL CASES

Operative Photography
When shooting in the operating room (OR), it is prudent once again to develop a consistent technique. This avoids wasting time and thus delaying the cases that follow. Shooting in the OR is akin to the professional photographer shooting "on location." Many of the controls set up in the office studio are not available, so obtaining quality results requires extra thought.

OR lighting is not white light; it has a yellow tint when used to expose daylight film. These lights should be turned away and a flash used. Similarly, fluorescent light has its own color temperature (green); the photographer should not rely on it to expose the film. The flash is the lighting of choice in the OR. Problems with flash lighting (except for the ring) include harsh shadows. These can be adeptly cast away from the background by the photographer and not included in the image.

The subject should be cleaned before shooting, with blood and debris removed and the object framed with clean blue towels. The photographer should remember to orient such that the viewer will be able to recognize the subject easily. If the object's size is a key aspect, placing a paper or plastic ruler in the field helps to indicate the relative scale. A metal ruler tends to reflect flash light and is generally a poor choice for this purpose. A series of pictures in a complicated case will clarify not only what the subject is, but also what the procedure has accomplished.

Another special case in the OR involves photographing radiographs. It is useful in record keeping to shoot the occasional computed tomography (CT) image to complement the clinical photograph, especially for presentations. The OR situation is suboptimal because viewing-box fluorescent light is mixed with the tungsten of the overhead lights. Surprisingly, the images obtained when photographing under these conditions can be adequate, if not perfect. My technique involves shooting under ambient light (no flash) at a slow shutter speed (about $\frac{1}{30}$ second) at a midrange aperture (f 8). Focusing on one slice from a CT scan or on a small plain radiograph results in a readable image when projected (slide film). The photographer must accept the color shift (generally light yellow) and a slight loss of contrast. When these CT images or radiographs need to be perfect, it is still best to have them produced as slides by a professional audiovisual department.

Digital Photography
With the rapid improvements in the personal computer and digital image generation, it is apparent that the future of medical photography is digital. Presently, however, the issue of electronic manipulation is paramount.[4] Using widely available

software and the home computer, any photograph can be substantially retouched. The image is scanned into the computer and manipulated with one of several software packages. The resulting image is then converted to a hard copy (slide or photograph) with a film recorder.

After considering this process and its widespread availability, the American Board of Plastic and Reconstructive Surgery began accepting digital photographs for board-related cases in September 1999.

CASE EXAMPLES

Plastic surgeons can become as critical of their photography as they are of their surgery. There is, literally, always room for improvement. All the following photographs were taken using a 35-mm camera with a top-mounted flash unit. Because operative photography seems the most difficult to master, this is the focus here.

Figure 11-2 demonstrates a burn contracture of the axilla. The subject is isolated to an extent by the application of a blue towel laterally. Although the patient's humerus and forearm lead the viewer to the contracture, the frame is not placed widely enough. Without the previous description, the contracture and its anatomic location are not readily apparent.

Figure 11-3 illustrates a simple skin graft case before and after application of the graft. The position of the hand is quite similar between the images. The hand is included in the frame to identify the limb, and the arm is isolated from debris with blue towels.

Placing an object in the field beside the subject allows the viewer to infer relative scale. In Figure 11-4 a venous malformation of the long finger is centered for emphasis. The restraining fingers of an assistant provide optimum positioning as well as this relative scale.

Figures 11-5 to 11-8 illustrate the standardized views used for photographic documentation in burn patients.

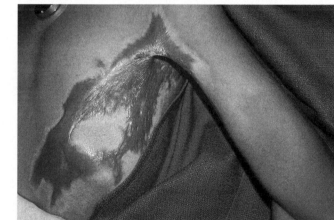

Figure 11-2. Burn contracture of axilla. Image is composed without providing enough anatomic information to allow easy identification.

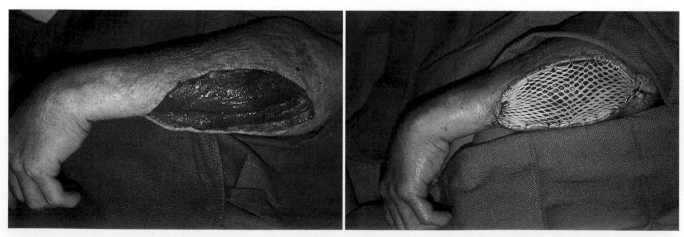

A

B

Figure 11-3. **(A)** Preoperative and postoperative **(B)** photographs of skin graft case. Each image is similarly constructed, including position of arm and isolation with towels.

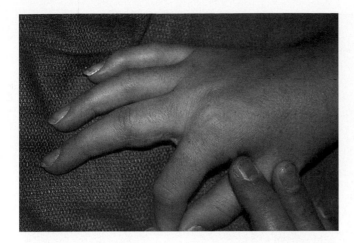

Figure 11-4. Venous malformation of long finger. Image is centered for emphasis. Scale is added (and position held) with help of an assistant's fingers.

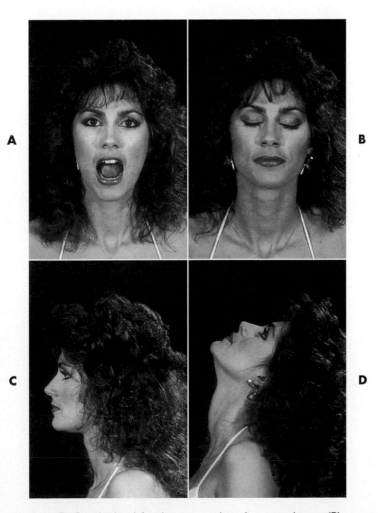

Figure 11-5. **A** to **D,** Standardized facial views used to document burns. (Photographs by Jeff Higgs, Scientific Photographer, Division of Plastic Surgery, SIU School of Medicine; and Elof Eriksson.)

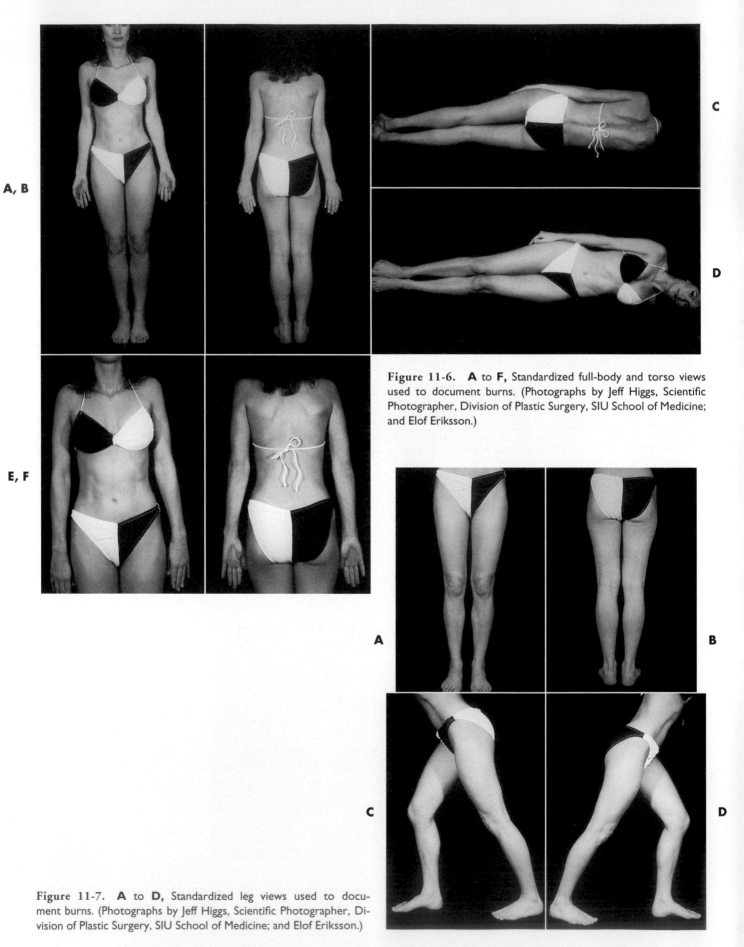

A, B

E, F

C

D

Figure 11-6. **A** to **F,** Standardized full-body and torso views used to document burns. (Photographs by Jeff Higgs, Scientific Photographer, Division of Plastic Surgery, SIU School of Medicine; and Elof Eriksson.)

A

B

C

D

Figure 11-7. **A** to **D,** Standardized leg views used to document burns. (Photographs by Jeff Higgs, Scientific Photographer, Division of Plastic Surgery, SIU School of Medicine; and Elof Eriksson.)

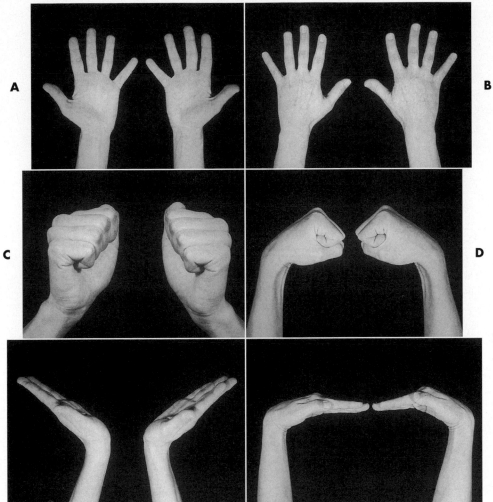

Figure 11-8. **A** to **F,** Standardized hand views used to document burns. (Photographs by Jeff Higgs, Scientific Photographer, Division of Plastic Surgery, SIU School of Medicine; and Elof Eriksson.)

REFERENCES

1. Clinical Photography Committee: *Photographic standards in plastic surgery,* Philadelphia, 1991, Plastic Surgery Educational Foundation.

2. Gilson CC: Ethical and legal aspects of illustrative clinical recording, *Br J Hosp Med* 52:225-229, 1994.

3. Jemec BIE, Jemec GBE: Photographic surgery: standards in clinical photography, *Aesthetic Plast Surg* 10:177-180, 1986.

4. Perniciaro C: Electronic manipulation to enhance medical photographs, *Mayo Clin Proc* 68:1220-1221, 1993.

5. Sherr D: Clinical photography: an important documentation of the plastic surgeon's practice, *Plast Surg News* 9b(2):5, 1997.

CHAPTER

Patient Selection and Risk Factors

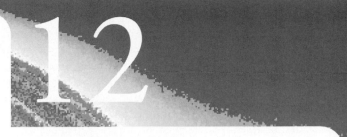

Lawrence J. Gottlieb
Judith M. Gurley
Robert W. Parsons

Proper selection of patients for plastic surgery will optimize surgical outcomes, increase patient satisfaction, and perhaps lead to appropriate referral for those patients whose problems should not be surgically treated. This chapter describes the evaluation of patients using the familiar medical workup format, discusses risk factors that may lead to an unfavorable outcome, and considers the nature and role of informed consent in the process.

PRELIMINARY CONSIDERATIONS

Patient selection is too often regarded as simply the process of "selecting out" those patients who represent undue risk for litigation. Although this is certainly a consideration, the selection process should involve much more. The patient sometimes may see the consultation as placing an order, as if buying a commodity.[12] The surgeon, on the other hand, needs to recognize that diagnosis precedes treatment. The nature of the problem needs to be identified and evaluated to ensure that the procedure requested is appropriate.[13] It is also clearly essential to ascertain that the patient is in good health, can and will comply with the essential preoperative and postoperative care, and has realistic expectations of the surgical results.[18]

Edgerton et al[6] have pointed out that the only good reason for aesthetic surgery is to improve the patient's emotional health. This would apply to any surgery to improve appearance, whether the intent is cosmetic improvement of a normal feature or correction of deformity. It does not imply that everyone who requests surgery for aesthetic improvement has a psychiatric problem. It does emphasize the psychologic response to plastic surgery, which enhances the quality of life of patients by facilitating improvements in the body image.[8]

Body image has been defined as the mental picture that persons have of their own physical appearance, and it is rarely the same as the image a photograph would portray.[23,27] It has been compared with the homunculus often depicted on the sylvian fissure in drawings of the cerebral cortex, in that it often greatly exaggerates what persons see as their best and worst

features. Disparity between the body image and what the patient perceives as normal leads to the emotional discomfort or distress that motivates the request for surgery. When injury causes an abrupt change in the body, acute distress may be caused by the incongruity of the deformity with the established body image. This distress may persist for a lifetime.

Patient satisfaction is conditioned by the type of surgery.[28] Restorative operations, which return the appearance toward the previous body image, such as a facelift or mammary reconstruction after mastectomy, more readily result in a satisfied patient than operations that alter an appearance that is an integral part of the body image. Procedures such as a rhinoplasty or mammary augmentation produce a new appearance that contrasts with the established self-perception and may cause anxiety until the changes are incorporated into the body image.[8,10] Adolescents tend to accept surgical changes more readily than older individuals, probably because their body images are already undergoing continuing change.

Initially, patient selection may seem to focus on the cosmetic surgery patient. Careful evaluation is equally important in all elective surgery, however, especially when considering correction of longstanding disabilities or deformities. The risks involved with compliance issues and unrealistic expectations extend even to urgent surgery for cancer and emergency procedures for trauma. Although these latter patients are rarely selected out or referred to another physician, it is important to recognize that these issues require consideration.

INITIAL EVALUATION

The traditional medical workup format is still effective for eliciting and recording the important data in patient selection. With medical practice now forced into a more businesslike mold, the workup also reminds plastic surgeons that they are still physicians dealing with patients.

Both the patient and the surgeon approach the initial interview with preconceptions, and it is important to understand these as clearly as possible. The patient's understanding of what the surgeon says will be conditioned by what the patient has been told by referring physicians or previous patients or has gleaned from the media. Too often a referring colleague may have said surgery can eliminate a scar or make someone "as good as new" and thereby exaggerate and distort plastic surgeons' skills. Some patients, especially those who have "shopped around" for a plastic surgeon, may try to give the "correct" answers to questions, as if the object were to pass a test in order to be accepted for surgery. Perhaps more often, significant factors in the history, such as illnesses, previous operations, and drug or alcohol abuse, are forgotten or omitted unless specific questions are asked.[18]

The surgeon, on the other hand, tends to assume that any patient with an appointment is expecting an operation. In fact, some are seeking a second opinion in the hope of avoiding an operation, and many others have not yet decided whether to have surgery. The surgeon must be sensitive and willing to listen to the patient in order to uncover the reason for the consultation. Open-ended questions facilitate gathering information to formulate a diagnosis and design a treatment plan.

It is essential to begin by eliciting the chief complaint. It is surprising how often the first steps in interviewing a patient are either ignored or glossed over. The receptionist may have the patient fill out a form that asks, "What did you come to see the doctor about today?" The answer, such as "a facelift" or "my scar," is taken as sufficient for both the chief complaint and the history. Open-ended questions in the face-to-face interview may result in a straightforward discussion about wrinkles and jowls. It is not unusual, however, to discover that the patient has been feeling depressed since her husband died, for example, and thinks that an operation would reawaken her interest in life. Perhaps the patient has recently been divorced, needs to reenter the job market, has lost a job, or has been passed over for promotion. It is crucial to identify patients using surgery for a secondary, unrealistic gain.[8]

The important thing is to determine the patient's real concern. As a rule of thumb, no patient seeks surgery simply because a perceived defect is present. The *effect* of this perceived defect on the patient's quality of life results in the consultation. The emotional distress is a combination of negative emotions, defensive behavior, and self-defeating thinking patterns.[23] These patients always have the desire for correction to relieve this emotional distress. Patient selection chooses those for whom surgery can be expected to produce this relief.

Thus it is important to ask about the history of the presenting complaint to answer the following:

- How long has the problem or deformity been present?
- How long has it been a concern?
- Under what circumstances is the patient self-conscious about the problem?
- How has the patient dealt with it in the past?
- What has changed to cause consideration of surgery at this time?
- Has the patient had previous operations for this or other problems, and was that surgery successful?
- Why is correction important?

- Why is the patient willing to consider spending the time and money and enduring the discomfort and inconvenience of surgery?
- Have friends had similar surgery, and were they pleased with the results?
- How will life be better after successful surgery?

All these considerations are important in assessing whether the patient's goals are realistic.

Many patients are somewhat frightened or intimidated on the initial visit. It helps to ease their minds if they are told, after a brief discussion of their primary concerns, that probably no final decision about surgery will be made on the first visit. The surgeon explains that this visit is to evaluate the problem; do a careful examination; explain the options for management, including the potential risks and benefits; and give the patient an opportunity to ask questions. We encourage as many preoperative visits as necessary to achieve a mutual understanding between surgeon and patient.

A useful technique is to tell the patient that you will summarize the points discussed in a letter, which they can refer to while considering surgery. This is also an excellent opportunity to document the points of informed consent in writing and to add any important information that may have been omitted in the interview.[14] Standard letters can be devised and personalized for each patient.

The initial interview must include a brief but careful medical history. Even if the patient's form covers the past medical history, specific inquiry is essential regarding major illnesses (e.g., hepatitis, HIV infection),[7] current and past medications, allergies, and past surgeries and complications. Chronic problems such as asthma, migraine, or depression may be currently asymptomatic and therefore not mentioned; alcohol and substance abuse are infrequently volunteered.[8,10,18]

Elements of the family and social history may be covered conversationally throughout the interview but are no less important. The patient's job or profession, employment history, recreational pursuits, marital status, and sexual orientation may provide useful insights regarding motivation. For example, the chronically unemployed actor who thinks a rhinoplasty is the key to successful auditions is unlikely to have a dramatic career upswing after surgery. The same is true of the middle-aged woman who believes a facelift will bring back the husband who left her.

It is not unusual for a patient to have had one or more previous plastic surgical procedures. The perception of the success or failure of that surgery and the attitude toward the previous surgeon can be helpful in this evaluation. Patients who have been pleased with the results of previous operations are likely to be pleased with the results of a further procedure. If the earlier surgery was not successful, it is helpful to know the patient's understanding of what went wrong. When a complication has occurred, it may help to contact the surgeon to learn what happened, especially if the previous surgery was for the same problem. It is both arrogant and foolhardy to assume that the outcome of a new operation will be better unless the reason for the disappointing result can be identified. When the patient is unwilling to reveal the name of the first surgeon or to permit inquiry, the physician should proceed with greatest caution. The reason for the unfavorable result may not be a poorly executed operation, but a noncompliant patient.[19]

When the patient is hostile and angry toward the original surgeon, it is important to ask whether a lawsuit is contemplated or in progress.[18] Surgeons are often surprised to discover that the patient they are evaluating for possible surgery is really looking for a witness who disagrees with the previous surgeon. Patients and attorneys often fail to appreciate that a potential expert witness will need to focus on different information than a surgeon planning a new operation, and they may wait until after the appointment to bring up the subject.

The examination really begins when the surgeon first meets the patient. Personality characteristics, attitude and affect, and manner of speaking are noted. Does the patient's physical appearance match the kind of change being requested?

At the initial visit the physical examination focuses on the defect or deformity that is the subject of the chief complaint. The general physical examination, although important before scheduling surgery, usually can be deferred until a later visit. Does the patient's complaint correspond with what the surgeon sees? A relatively inapparent scar, for example, may seem grossly deforming to the patient because of the emotions associated with the injury that caused it. Evaluation includes determining whether surgery can relieve the patient's concern. The focus of the initial examination is on the anatomy of the problem and the technical aspects of fashioning the desired changes.[10]

RISK FACTORS

Plastic surgery enhances the quality of life by facilitating improvements in the body image. Anatomic improvements, however, are not always directly reflected in body image changes. Many important risk factors are related to this fact.

Unrealistic Expectations

Persistent unrealistic expectations, when recognized, constitute an absolute contraindication to surgery. Often they are unrecognized, however, or not even sought. The patient may want a result that is technically unrealistic; stating this does not necessarily mean that the patient has understood. It may require several preoperative visits to be sure that unrealistic expectations have been abandoned.[18]

It is essential to reemphasize that patients do not request surgery simply because a feature has a particular shape or deformity. Motivation for surgery may be internal or external.[5,9,27,29] That is, the patient may seek to feel more comfortable about the normality of their appearance, or the desire for change may come from a desire to change the actions or reactions of others. Patients experience distress because of their perception that the appearance does not match their mental picture of normal.[23] When surgical success depends on changing others' behavior, a good outcome is impossible. If success means getting a job, for example, the money would usually be better spent in acquiring needed skills.

Compliance

The patient must comply with preoperative and postoperative instructions for surgery to succeed. Therefore the surgeon should determine if the patient can cooperate. At the simplest level this means keeping appointments and being on time. If patients have difficulty fitting preoperative routines into their schedules, they probably will be unable to comply with postoperative appointments and care.

The patient who repeatedly defers surgery or cancels scheduled dates may also have difficulty with compliance. Those who travel extensively, are from a distant city, or simply have transportation problems should not be considered for surgery until it is clear they can return as necessary for postoperative appointments. Patients view this as the surgeon's fault when postoperative care is compromised.

A special category of the noncompliant patient is the chronic alcoholic or drug abuser. Such individuals are often truly unable to cooperate with instructions for appointments, dressings, care, and surgical wound protection. Lewis et al[18] discuss how to identify patients with alcohol and potential compliance problems.

It is essential to ask patients with previous unfavorable surgery about their postoperative management and to talk with the surgeon. Patients unable or unwilling to discuss problems with postoperative management should not be accepted for surgery.

Poor Communication

Inability to communicate clearly during the initial interview may simply be a sign that further discussion is needed. Patients may need time to gain the trust to discuss their real concerns with the surgeon, and complaints may seem vague at first. Some patients, however, are never able to describe their concern clearly. Some attempt flattery, saying they trust the surgeon's professional judgment. Others cannot focus on a single problem, talking about the nose, the breasts, and then liposuction, unable to say exactly what anatomic change they desire.

Communication involves not only patients' ability to express themselves but also their ability to hear and understand the surgeon. Two or more preoperative visits may be required. Ultimately, surgery may be contraindicated because no surgical solution can be matched to the patient's complaints. Patients who repeatedly defer surgery also may fall into this category, sensing that they have not really identified their concerns to themselves or to the surgeon.[10]

Minimal Deformity

Although not always a risk factor, minimal deformity should alert the surgeon to proceed carefully. If the patient is consistent, specific, and not looking for an unlikely secondary gain, surgery may be very successful. Problems arise if the surgeon does not see the deformity the patient sees or does not clearly understand the specific change requested. Pruzinsky[23] notes that the minimal deformity patient may be narcissistic and that such patients often have a "sense of entitlement," which makes relating to them difficult, both before and after surgery.

Repeat Surgery

When the patient requests surgery again for the same complaints, as noted earlier, the surgeon must decide whether the unfavorable outcome was technical or whether unrealistic expectations, poor communication, or noncompliance was responsible. A second operation is *never* indicated if the reason for the unfavorable result cannot be reasonably identified. Sometimes the wrong operation was performed, or a procedure was done for the wrong reason. The surgeon should resist the temptation to assume too quickly that the previous surgeon was incompetent or technically inept. These patients may use "catch words" or phrases in an attempt to influence the surgeon's judgment.

Children

When dealing with children, patient selection and risk factors are often overlooked. With young children, surgeons must address the parents' distress and guilt feelings about the body image–deformity disparity. The key risk factors of unrealistic expectations and compliance require special consideration in acute trauma, posttrauma scarring, and congenital deformities. These situations often involve parental guilt and the desire to erase the problem surgically. When the inevitable scar is evident, parents become anxious or even angry.

Even in acute trauma, informed consent is essential. The surgeon should always explain *before repair* that (1) a scar will form; (2) its quality depends more on the injury than the suturing; (3) scar maturation requires time; (4) the final result will not be evident for a year or more; and (5) the parents' cooperation is essential in the postoperative period.

Parents are often rightly concerned about the psychologic consequences of deformities in children. In general, the child accepts congenital deformity better than acquired problems incurred in the school years or later.[24] Preschool children often notice and talk about individual differences in a completely neutral way. Beginning at 5 to 6 years, however, school-age children learn to tease and may cause considerable emotional distress. Therefore, in general, children should have surgery before they begin school, even though they may have more internal motivation later. Such emotional considerations should not confuse good surgical judgment regarding other contraindications.

Compliance in pediatric patients is related to the balance between their concern about the problem and their fear of surgery. Cooperation can often be enlisted by directly addressing the child's fears and questions in a nonthreatening setting. The child should be told in simple terms what is going to happen and why.[15] The patient must see the defect as important to understand the hardships during the recovery period and to have the motivation to follow instructions regarding activity and protection of the surgical site. Although parental concerns are important and their postoperative compliance is crucial, too often all discussion is with the parents, which isolates the child.

The timing of elective surgery in children depends on special compliance risks at various ages. At age 1 year the release of a palmar contracture may be thwarted because immobilization with a plaster splint cannot be maintained. A facial scar revision in a school-age boy who has frequent fights with his older brother, or a cosmetic rhinoplasty in a budding rugby player, can be an exercise in futility.

Male Aesthetic Patients

For many years the plastic surgery literature cautioned about special risks with male patients who requested aesthetic surgery.[3] According to reports, men exhibited more psychopathology and were less satisfied after surgery than their female counterparts.[26,27] At the same time there seemed to be a societal bias against the idea that men would want cosmetic improvement.

More men have been requesting aesthetic procedures over the years, and any social stigma seems to be decreasing.[1,10,16] As the emphasis on youth, fitness, and physical attractiveness has permeated our culture, it has become more acceptable and perhaps more important for men to try to maintain these qualities through lifestyle changes, physical activity, and even surgery. If the earlier observations about special risks in male cosmetic patients had empiric validity, the risk has been significantly diluted by the broader spectrum of individuals now requesting aesthetic surgery.[29]

Historically, the cautionary comments have focused on the male rhinoplasty patient. In both men and women, as previously noted, psychologic differences exist between *changing* the appearance and *restoring* a more youthful appearance. In some men, important questions of motivation should be explored, just as in women. Again, the question is whether expectations are realistic. At present the surgeon should evaluate men by the same criteria as other patients, by exploring their expectations and compliance issues.

One group of patients, often young men, has been called "insatiable" surgical patients. They often acknowledge each procedure as an improvement but always want slightly more. These patients often fit the diagnostic criteria for body dysmorphic disorder.[23]

Traumatic Deformity

Traumatic deformity frequently is accompanied by a heavy emotional burden related to the circumstances of the injury. Pruzinsky has developed a way of measuring quality of life by using the cognitive behavioral theory (CBT) perspective and found that "acquired disfigurement is more disruptive than congenital disfigurement."[23,24] Traumatized patients may have current or past alcohol or drug problems and serious compliance problems. The plastic surgeon must carefully explore how the patient has attempted to cope with the deformity and its associated emotional problems.

When a longstanding deformity is present, the surgeon should know why the patient is requesting surgery now and has a need to replace previous coping strategies. Often the patient has new emotional stresses, and surgery may or may not offer the means to deal with them. Using the CBT, the surgeon can better estimate the effects of plastic surgery on the patient's quality of living.

Surgeon's Viewpoint

The concept of the surgeon's *comfort zone* should receive more consideration in patient selection. At the first level the surgeon may simply be uncomfortable with performing a particular operation. More often, however, the surgeon is not comfortable performing surgery on a particular patient. Although the nature of the problem may be the reason, more likely the surgeon has an emotional reaction to some aspect of the patient's personality. The surgeon should recognize this and not accept the patient for surgery until this uneasiness is resolved. Just as all people do not get along, some surgeons will not be comfortable with every patient. It can be difficult caring for and about such patients, especially when postoperative problems occur.

At times the surgeon's discomfort results from the sense that the patient is approaching the evaluation and surgery with a hostile attitude. This may be masked in the surgeon's presence but more apparent to the office personnel. Such an attitude may be simply a manifestation of apprehension. If it persists throughout the interview, however, or is still noted on the second visit, the patient will be difficult to satisfy, even with a good anatomic result.

Coexisting Psychopathology

Pruzinsky has emphasized that "the ultimate success of plastic surgery is determined as much by the psychology of the patient as it is by the outcome of surgery."[23] During the standard medical interview the surgeon will gain a sense of the patient's behavior, personality, and ability to think rationally, as well as uncover any history of psychiatric treatment. The diagnosis or suspicion of a coexisting psychiatric problem may prompt referral to the patient's own therapist or an appropriate mental health consultant for evaluation, diagnosis, and recommendations regarding surgery.

The surgeon may be uncomfortable explaining to the patient the importance of psychiatric evaluation and the need to delay decisions about surgery until consultation is obtained. Goin and Goin[8] recommend telling the patient openly and directly, by equating the seriousness of a mental disorder with a physical one. For example, a surgeon would not accept a patient for a facelift without consultation for suspected or known heart disease. The authors also emphasize the importance of consultation with a psychiatrist knowledgeable about patients seeking elective plastic surgery.

In the past, surgeons have been warned to avoid surgery for patients with psychiatric disorders because of the risks of precipitating problems and inviting a negative outcome. Over the past 40 years, however, Edgerton et al[4-6] and others[25,28] have provided substantial data to show that a psychiatric diagnosis itself is not a contraindication to surgery. Some patients with mental or personality disorders gain significant benefits from plastic surgery.

Once the diagnosis of a psychiatric disorder is made, the plastic surgeon still must decide whether surgery is indicated or perhaps is contraindicated. As in all other patients, this means assessing the individual's motivation, expectations, ability to communicate, and compliance. The surgeon must also remember that surgical changes in the body's size and shape can have disturbing effects on the body image, even in psychiatrically normal patients. Those whose overall evaluation is compatible with a positive surgical result can be expected to do well. Although patients with psychiatric diagnoses may require more reassurance and attention, they may also be more appreciative than their more normal counterparts.

OTHER CONSIDERATIONS

Refusing Surgery

Too often surgeons hear colleagues say, "I didn't want to operate on him, but he kept insisting, so I finally did." This is simply a statement that the surgeon has lost control of the situation and abdicated the role of medical decision maker to the patient. It is often difficult, however, to tell an eager patient that the requested surgery should not be done.[5,12] A common reaction of patients is that they have somehow failed a test or not measured up to the surgeon's requirements.

The first rule is to present the case for treatment refusal in unequivocal terms, not as if the decision is still open to further discussion. The surgeon might say, "I have carefully evaluated what you have told me, along with my findings, and I have concluded that an operation will not give you the result you want." The surgeon can explain factors that went into the decision, such as inability to obtain an accurate picture of what the patient wants or needs, but again should avoid any indication that this is a subject for debate. Surgeons must forget ego when they need to say, "I don't know how to do an operation that will give you the result you want."

If the surgeon has concluded that surgery is not appropriate for the patient, it is inconsistent then to make a referral to another plastic surgeon. Such a referral may be appropriate only when the reason for deciding against surgery is the surgeon's comfort level, and discussion has not revealed other contraindications. The surgeon should not succumb to the inappropriate thought process, "The patient will shop around and finally find a plastic surgeon to operate, so I might as well do it," if the surgery is not indicated.

Managing Risks

Medical-legal risk management begins with the first patient contact, and all the factors considered in this chapter are important. Patients who sue are not always identifiably litigious during the preoperative evaluation. However, they are always dissatisfied and unhappy with the surgical result, especially if it comes as a surprise. The selection process discussed earlier is crucial to risk management. The patient's problem must be clearly understood by both the patient and the surgeon, as must the expected surgical result.[18]

In arriving at the level of understanding needed before surgery, informed consent plays a crucial role.[9] It is not a paper that the patient signs, and it does not preclude a lawsuit. *Informed consent* is the process by which the surgeon provides enough information so that the patient can make a reasonable decision for or against surgery.[2,21] This includes information about the procedure, the expected postoperative course, final result, and possible risks and complications. Patients must be aware of their surgical and nonsurgical options to be fully informed.[17,24]

Accurate documentation is essential in all aspects of patient care. In a court of law, what is believed to be true is not necessarily what happened, or what the physician or patient says happened. It is most often what was contemporaneously documented in the chart.[20] A medically adequate, accurate record of all interactions with the patient, whether in the office or on the phone, needs to be filed in the chart. This may include the letter suggested earlier as a follow-up to the initial visit, as well as any other letters.

Controlling Anger

Angry, unhappy patients believe they somehow have been betrayed. It is essential to determine the reason and seek to clarify the problem. Even if the patient is completely wrong in being angry, the surgeon must never show anger in return. It is always tempting to avoid the angry patient, and often the office personnel try to shield the surgeon from disturbing phone calls. It is imperative that the surgeon be available, however, and that the disappointed patient not feel isolated or abandoned, especially when surgical complications have occurred.[8,10,11,19]

REFERENCES

1. Baker DC, Aston SJ, Guy CL, Rees TD: The male rhytidectomy, *Plast Reconstr Surg* 604:514, 1977.
2. Cassileth BR, Zupkis RV, Sutton-Smith K, March V: Informed consent: why are its goals imperfectly realized? *N Engl J Med* 302:896, 1980.
3. Dillerud E: Suction lipoplasty: a report on complications, undesired results, and patient satisfaction based on 3511 procedures, *Plast Reconstr Surg* 88:239, 1991.
4. Edgerton MT: Plastic surgery: the rainbow profession, *Ann Plast Surg* 38:197, 1997.
5. Edgerton MT, Knorr NJ: Motivational patterns of patients seeking cosmetic (esthetic) surgery, *Plast Reconstr Surg* 48:551, 1971.
6. Edgerton MT, Langman MW, Pruzinsky T: Plastic surgery and psychotherapy in the treatment of 100 psychologically disturbed patients, *Plast Reconstr Surg* 88:594, 1991.
7. Fisher JC, Gorney M: AIDS, wound healing, and the surgeon's well-being, *Ann Plast Surg* 21:297, 1991.
8. Goin JM, Goin MK: *Changing the body: psychological effects of plastic surgery,* Baltimore, 1981, Williams & Wilkins.
9. Goin MK, Burgoyne RW, Goin JM: Face-lift operation: the patient's secret motivations and reactions to "informed consent," *Plast Reconstr Surg* 58:273, 1976.
10. Goldwyn RM: *The patient and the plastic surgeon,* ed 2, Boston, 1991, Little, Brown.
11. Goldwyn RM: *Beyond appearance: reflections of a plastic surgeon,* New York, 1986, Dodd, Mead.
12. Gorney M: Choosing patients for aesthetic surgery, *Plast Reconstr Surg* 88:917, 1991.
13. Gorney M: Plastic surgery is not a casual thing, *Ann Plast Surg* 1:531, 1978.
14. Krizek TJ: Personal communication, 1984.
15. Lantos JD: Should we always tell children the truth? *Perspect Biol Med* 40:78, 1996.
16. Lawson W, Naidu RK: The male facelift, *Arch Otolaryngol Head Neck Surg* 119:535, 1993.
17. Leeb D, Bowers DG, Lynch JB: Observations on the myth of "informed consent," *Plast Reconstr Surg* 58:280, 1976.
18. Lewis CM, Lavell Sharie, Simpson MF: Patient selection and patient satisfaction, *Clin Plast Surg* 10:321, 1983.
19. Moyer P: Dissatisfied patients should be handled with care, *Cosmet Surg Times,* p. 26, 1997.
20. Nisonson I: Proper documentation: the medical record. In Nora PF, editor: *Professional liability/risk management: a manual for surgeons,* Chicago, 1991, American College of Surgeons.
21. Palmisano DJ: Consent and the process of informed consent. In Nora PF, editor: *Professional liability/risk management: a manual for surgeons,* Chicago, 1991, American College of Surgeons.
22. Pruzinsky T: The psychology of plastic surgery: advances in evaluating body image, quality of life, and psychopathology. In Habal MB, Lineaweaver WC, Parsons RW, Woods JE, editors: *Advances in plastic and reconstructive surgery,* vol 12, St Louis, 1996, Mosby.
23. Pruzinsky T: Social and psychological effects of major craniofacial deformity, *Cleft Palate Craniofac J* 29:578, 1992.
24. Robinson G, Merav A: Informed consent: recall by patients tested postoperatively, *Ann Thorac Surg* 22:209, 1976.
25. Slator R, Harris DL: Are rhinoplasty patients potentially mad? *Br J Plast Surg* 45:307, 1992.
26. Thomson JA Jr, Knorr NJ, Edgerton MT Jr: Cosmetic surgery: the psychiatric perspective, *Psychosomatics* 7, 19(1): 7-15, 1978.
27. Webb WL, Slaughter R, Meyer E, Edgerton M: Mechanisms of psychosocial adjustment in patients seeking "face lift" operation, *Psychosom Med* 27:183, 1965.
28. Wengle HP: The psychology of cosmetic surgery: old problems in patient selection seen in a new way. Part II, *Ann Plast Surg* 16:487, 1986.

CHAPTER 13

Plastic Surgery Techniques

Stefan Preuss
Karl H. Breuing
Elof Eriksson

The specialty of plastic surgery received its name in 1838 in a publication by Zeiss.[24] Plastic surgery means formative surgery (from physics, plastic versus elastic deformation). The art and science of plastic surgery have always been at the forefront in the development of surgical principles and techniques. The foundation for these principles is the biology of wound healing, as well as philosophic and ethical tenets (e.g., "do no harm"). The diverse principles and techniques described in this chapter are the basis for analysis and discussion of diagnoses, treatments, complications, and outcomes in plastic surgery.

A principle is "a general or fundamental doctrine or tenet." A technique is "the manner of performance, or the details, of any surgical operation, experiment, or mechanical act."[20] A plastic surgeon must know the principles and be able to master the various techniques better than most surgeons. Pathophysiologic factors (e.g., tissue ischemia) and aesthetic demands (e.g., eyelid, nose, or lip procedures) greatly reduce the tolerances for technical error in plastic surgery.

The goal is to learn, comprehend, and master the principles of surgery and to exercise all useful techniques. Plastic surgeons must know several of the best techniques for optimum treatment of patients. Therefore titles such as "microsurgeon" and "laparoscopic surgeon" are paradoxic. For example, a microsurgeon not only must master the techniques in microsurgery, but also must be equally proficient in the use of nonmicrosurgical techniques when treating patients.

TRAUMA OF WOUNDING

A patient becomes much more ill from a large injury than a small one. The patient with a full-thickness burn to 50% of the body surface area becomes much sicker than the patient with a 1% surface burn. The same is true with trauma to a limited part of the body. For example, the patient with a linear fracture of the midtibia from a skiing accident has much less of a problem than the patient who receives a tibial fracture from being pinned between the bumpers of two cars and also has significant soft tissue injury.

The same observations apply to surgical trauma. For example, the surgical removal of a small skin lesion on the face makes the patient less ill than the patient who has a colectomy. It is therefore logical always to minimize the trauma from surgery. Most surgeons would agree with this principle, but many, including plastic surgeons, do not apply it to their technical execution. Use of crushing instruments, desiccation of tissues, injudicious use of cautery, and application of cytotoxic substances (e.g., peroxide, chlorine) to wounds are examples of the disconnection between knowledge of principle and execution of technique.

The two main determinants of postsurgical wound complications are the type of surgical procedure and the surgeon. Some surgeons have complication rates up to one order of magnitude greater than the complication rates of the best surgeons, probably because they do not use optimal surgical technique. All surgical procedures are traumatic, and every surgeon must continually strive to minimize surgical trauma.

DEBRIDEMENT AND IRRIGATION

Debridement primarily involves removal of devitalized and highly contaminated tissues with maximal preservation of critical anatomic structures, such as nerves, blood vessels, tendons, and bone. More reconstructions after trauma and infections fail because of inadequate debridement than because of failed reconstructive technique.[5] Immediately after trauma, the surgeon is faced with the dilemma of not being able to determine precisely the border between irreversibly damaged tissue and tissue that is salvageable with proper management. Also, most methods of delayed debridement cause progression of necrosis resulting from (1) desiccation of the surface of the traumatized wound and (2) gradual multiplication of the contaminating bacteria at the interface between viable and nonviable tissue. This has been well documented in burn injuries and also occurs in many cases of nonthermal trauma.[18,23] In particular, traumatized and exposed nerves, tendons, joints, and bone show progressive necrosis, most likely from desiccation of the structure's surface.

A practical strategy for debridement was developed during the Vietnam War.[17] Traumatic wounds were debrided on admission to the surgical unit, packed with saline gauze, and then debrided again at intervals of 48 hours until deemed sufficiently free of devitalized tissue and contamination to be closed. This has become a useful practical strategy when, for example, treating victims of high-speed automobile accidents and gunshot wounds. It does not solve the problem of desiccation, however, because the water in the saline gauze soon evaporates and transforms the dressing into a dry one. This technique of debridement is also labor intensive and consumes significant resources.

Surgeons clearly need better methods to evaluate sustainable viability of various tissues immediately after trauma, as well as better methods to treat early traumatic wounds and thus prevent progression of injury.

In 1964 Ferguson's group in Chicago contaminated incisional wounds in guinea pigs with bacterial cultures, saliva, feces, urine, soil, and pus. After 24 hours of inoculation the wounds were copiously irrigated and closed. The group concluded that all these contaminants except pus could be successfully removed from the wound and that healing would occur without a significantly increased rate of wound infections.[4] Since that time, irrigation, preferably with a pulsatile jet lavage system, has become a cornerstone in the treatment of traumatic wounds.[3]

Technically, debridement can be labeled as mechanical, autolytic, and chemical. *Mechanical debridement* is done in the emergency room (ER) or operating room (OR) with scalpel, scissors, curets, or other instruments in combination with copious irrigation employing pulsatile jet lavage. *Gauze debridement* is usually done by applying saline-moistened gauze to the wound, letting it desiccate, and then removing the gauze at frequent intervals, usually two or three times per day. It is a useful complement to surgical debridement when most of the devitalized or contaminated tissue has been removed but necrotic tissue or significant contamination remains. This saline gauze treatment of wounds is a debridement technique, not a technique to heal wounds. Some wounds will heal when treated with repeated saline gauze changes, but other techniques, particularly employing a controlled hydration dressing, will heal these wounds much faster, with less nursing or patient effort and less pain.

Autolytic debridement, as defined by the National Pressure Ulcer Advisory Panel on pressure sore treatment, is a process of debridement that uses the body's digestive enzymes to break down necrotic tissue.[16,21] It is useful in the treatment of pressure sores and extremity ulcers but is less helpful with other acute traumatic wounds.

Chemical debridement has been particularly used when removing burn eschar. The debriding agent is usually an enzyme, but other molecules have been suggested. The first widely used agent was the enzyme of the *soutilens* bacteria (Travase).[22] When applied in liquid form to the burn eschar, it would turn some of the eschar into a gel that could be mechanically removed. The main disadvantages were the absence of a practi-

cal delivery method, severe pain on application, and the promotion of sepsis in certain patients.

The combination of the enzymes *streptokinase* and *streptodornase* (SKSD) and, more recently, *collagenase* (Santyl) have been studied and widely used.[10] Manufacturers claim all the enzymes only attack devitalized tissue and are not harmful to live tissue. These drugs' therapeutic range (between level of effectiveness and level of toxicity), however, is relatively narrow. The ideal chemical agent would have a practical application method, wide therapeutic range, minimal pain, and no infection or other complications.

WOUND CLOSURE

Traumatic wounds illustrate the spectrum of problems and possible solutions when attempting wound closure. When dealing with a wound, the first major consideration is the *diagnosis.* Anatomic, radiologic, and microbial diagnoses are probably most important in the diagnosis of an acute wound. The diagnosis of a chronic wound is much more complex. For many chronic wounds, a precise diagnosis cannot be established despite optimal effort (Table 13-1).[12]

Once a diagnosis has been established, the next step is to determine the expertise and the resources needed to treat the wound. These factors have been well defined for burn wounds but have not been as well established for other traumatic wounds. Most plastic surgeons are experts at treating traumatic wounds, and suboptimal treatment often results from the ER triage person failing to recognize the wound's severity and the difficulty of treatment.

Timing

The principle governing the timing of wound closure is that any traumatic wound should be closed as soon as possible with minimal complications. Traditional teaching was that a laceration should be closed within 6 hours or, if this was not possible, left open to healing by so-called secondary intention.[7] Gradually the 6 hours became 8 hours and 12 hours in some cases. Biology and pathophysiology represent a continuum, however, outside the arbitrary time limits set by physicians. In many patients, therefore, particularly those with facial lacerations, the surgeon might elect to close the wound after as long as 24 or 48 hours after adequate debridement, irrigation, and antibacterial treatment.[13]

When expanding the time from laceration to closure, which can be equated with a longer inoculation phase for bacteria in the wound, the rate of wound complications is higher. Therefore this must be stressed to the patient when providing the informed consent before wound treatment. The general rule is still that a laceration should be closed within approximately 12 hours and preferably shorter, although a plastic surgeon can often achieve uncomplicated closure later than that.

Methods

The goal is to achieve wound closure as soon as safely possible with the fewest complications using the technique that is the most advantageous to the patient in regard to complexity,

Table 13-1.
Algorithm for Treatment of Chronic Wounds

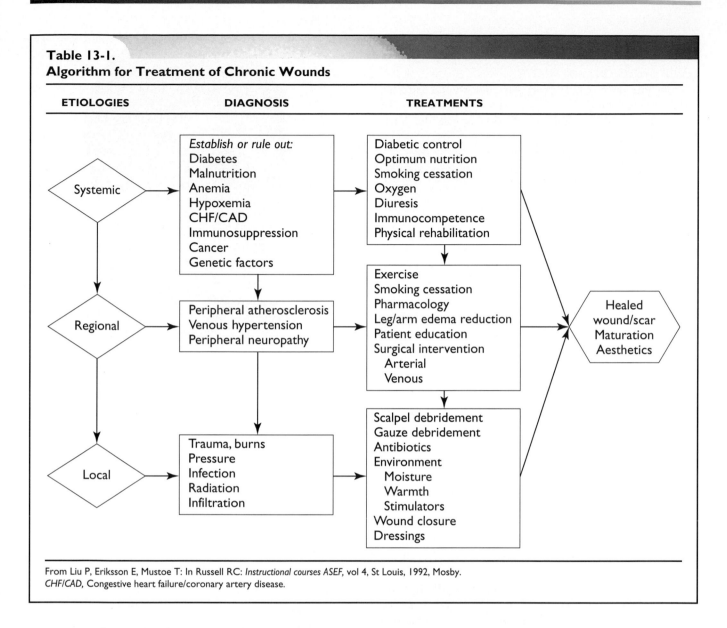

ETIOLOGIES	DIAGNOSIS	TREATMENTS
Systemic	*Establish or rule out:* Diabetes, Malnutrition, Anemia, Hypoxemia, CHF/CAD, Immunosuppression, Cancer, Genetic factors	Diabetic control, Optimum nutrition, Smoking cessation, Oxygen, Diuresis, Immunocompetence, Physical rehabilitation
Regional	Peripheral atherosclerosis, Venous hypertension, Peripheral neuropathy	Exercise, Smoking cessation, Pharmacology, Leg/arm edema reduction, Patient education, Surgical intervention — Arterial, Venous
Local	Trauma, burns, Pressure, Infection, Radiation, Infiltration	Scalpel debridement, Gauze debridement, Antibiotics, Environment — Moisture, Warmth, Stimulators, Wound closure, Dressings

Healed wound/scar, Maturation, Aesthetics

From Liu P, Eriksson E, Mustoe T: In Russell RC: *Instructional courses ASEF,* vol 4, St Louis, 1992, Mosby.
CHF/CAD, Congestive heart failure/coronary artery disease.

pain, time of recovery, functional and aesthetic recovery, and cost. The techniques in the reconstructive ladder are as follows:

1. Linear closure
2. Skin graft
3. Skin flap
4. Muscle flap
5. Skin-muscle flap
6. Bone-tendon-nerve flap
7. Skin-muscle-bone flap
8. Skin-muscle free flap

The first choice is always a linear closure with or without undermining the adjacent skin, provided that the closure can be achieved without unacceptable tension. (The proper term is *linear closure;* "primary closure" describes only the timing of the closure in relation to elective incisions or wounding.) Exceptions to this rule include most notably pressure sores, where the first choice usually is a flap procedure. If linear closure is attempted for the common pressure sore, the closure is placed under tension immediately over the bony prominence. It is therefore preferable to use a flap that allows a tension-free closure away from the bony prominence. A similar principle applies to closures in the plantar surface of the foot, where flaps are sometimes used to move the suture line away from a pressure point, particularly over the metatarsal heads.

In certain situations, reconstruction can be achieved with either a skin flap or a skin (or composite) graft. A *skin flap* can generally provide better color, texture, and thickness for the reconstruction. The main drawback is that it creates additional scarring in the area of the reconstruction from the flap donor site. A *skin graft,* particularly if the recipient site has sufficient vascularity to accept a composite graft with full thickness of skin and additional fat, allows the surgeon to create an even contour. Skin and composite grafts can be made quite thick if they have a "pie crust" to permit drainage.

ANTIBIOTIC PROPHYLAXIS

Antibiotic prophylaxis is considered mandatory in patients who have prosthetic heart valves, as well as in patients who are immune depressed or otherwise at high risk for infection. It is also indicated for patients with contaminated or infected wounds. Many surgeons provide antibiotic prophylaxis in "clean" operations as well.

Principles of antibiotic prophylaxis for wound infection include the following:[15]

1. Select antibiotic that is effective against the likely pathogen.
2. Single-agent prophylaxis is almost always effective.
3. Half-life must be long enough to maintain adequate tissue levels throughout the operation.
4. Give single dose equal to full therapeutic dose intravenously immediately before skin incision.

An area that has been studied extensively is the treatment of dog bites, for which copious irrigation and debridement are recommended, but not antibiotic prophylaxis.

SKIN INCISIONS

The following principles apply to the placement of skin incisions:

1. Place incisions inconspicuously, ideally so that neither the patient nor others can see them. An example is the facelift incision, a significant portion of which is placed in the hair or hairline.
2. Place the incisions in the relaxed skin tension lines (Figure 13-1).[11]
3. Make the incision as short as possible.
4. If an excision is made, make certain that the incision is placed so that an adequate amount of skin can be mobilized to allow a closure with acceptable tension. This is particularly true in the extremities, where a longitudinal incision usually allows for more mobilization of the skin than a transverse incision.
5. Ensure that the operation can be made through the incision used. In particularly traumatic cases, this also means that the surgeon can lengthen the incision, if necessary.
6. If the patient may need a local or regional flap, place the incision so that it does not limit flap design.
7. Be compulsive about minimizing scarring. In particular, avoid making a scar in the triangle over the anterior chest, which is created by connecting lines between the tips of each shoulder and the xiphoid process. Incisions in this area heal with a conspicuous scar, which is often hypertrophic or keloidal (Figure 13-2, A).
8. If possible, avoid incisions in the plantar area of the foot because temporary or permanent pain in the area of the scar is common (Figure 13-2, B).

Healing skin wounds predictably contract in three dimensions. In a *longitudinal* direction, skin wounds contract between 1% and 10%, depending on the skin tension opposing the contraction. The contraction in a longitudinal direction is usually obvious and can be functionally incapacitating if it occurs, for instance, across the flexor surface of a joint. Contraction in a plane *perpendicular* to the skin usually does not have functional implications. If it results in a depression, however, this contraction can make the scar conspicuous and unsightly.

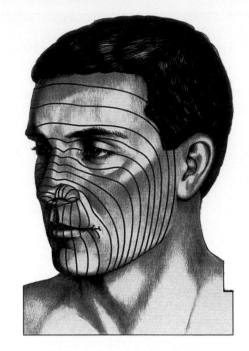

Figure 13-1. Relaxed skin tension lines. (From Larrabee WF: *Principles of facial reconstruction,* Philadelphia, 1995, Lippincott-Raven.)

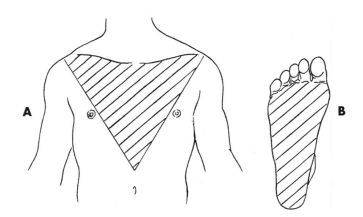

Figure 13-2. Danger areas. **A,** High risk of keloids and hypertrophic scarring. **B,** Risk of long-term postoperative pain.

Contraction in a *transverse* plane parallel to the skin is usually of no significance.

The impact of the contraction in the longitudinal direction of an incision can be minimized (1) by placing the incisions in the relaxed skin tension lines and (2) by placing them away from extensor and flexion surfaces, such as midaxial in the extremities. Traditionally, using everting sutures has been advocated to reduce contraction in the plane perpendicular to the skin. This is important, and everting sutures should always be used, for example, in the nose and the ear. It is equally important to cause eversion by design when performing a tissue excision (Figure 13-3). If both of these measures are taken, depressed scars can usually be avoided.

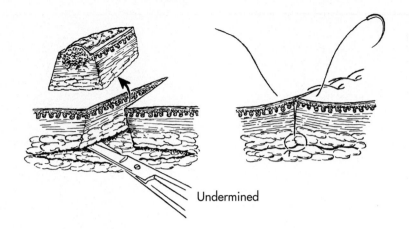

Figure 13-3. Wound eversion by design of excision. Predictably, skin wounds will contract in all three dimensions. Eversion by design reduces risk of depressed scar.

TECHNIQUES FOR WOUND CLOSURE

The principle is to achieve anatomic realignment of the wound edges and provide adequate strength while the wound is healing. At the same time, surgeons attempt to minimize functional and aesthetic complications. Frequently used techniques employ sutures, needles, knots, staples, tape, and glue.[8]

Sutures

Sutures can generally be divided into absorbable and non-absorbable types (Tables 13-2 to 13-4). Of the absorbable sutures, catgut is harvested from the submucosa of ovine gut or the serosa of bovine gut. Untreated catgut is broken down in the tissue within a few days, whereas catgut that has been tanned in chromic acid lasts two to four times longer.

Other absorbable sutures are synthesized with chemical methods and then modified physically to be maximally functional for the intended purpose. In general, fast-absorbing sutures are used for approximation of mucosa, whereas slow-absorbing sutures are preferred when used for approximation of the dermis. Nonabsorbable sutures can consist of multiple natural fibers, such as linen, cotton, or silk, that are twisted or braided. Synthetic fibers such as nylon also can be braided. Generally, smooth monofilament synthetic sutures are preferred because they cause less tissue reaction. The most common sutures are made of polypropylene or polyethylene (nylon).

Stainless steel sutures can be used either as a monofilament or as a multifilament twisted suture. Stainless steel has excellent breaking strength but is often difficult to handle.

Needles

Needles are usually attached to the suture and can be straight or curved. The curve of a needle can be anywhere from one quarter to five eighths of a circle. We generally prefer needles that are three eighths of a circle. The needle tip can be either tapered or cutting.

The cutting needle can have either a conventional or a reverse cutting design. We also generally prefer a reversed cutting needle, except for vascular sutures, when we use a tapered needle. Straight needles are not often used for routine surgical procedures but are sometimes found in emergency suture kits. They do not require a needle holder, and the suture can be cut with a needle, eliminating the need for scissors.

Suturing Techniques

Figure 13-4 to 13-8 illustrate various skin suturing techniques. In general the authors prefer deep dermal interrupted sutures with a buried knot. The superficial dermis and epidermis are then approximated with an intradermal running suture (Figure 13-6). The preferred suture for this closure in the skin is a slowly absorbable suture such as Polydioxanone or Poliglecaprone (see Table 13-3). The closure is then reinforced with surgical tape (Figure 13-9).

Tape and Adhesives

Surgical tape can be used alone or with sutures and glue. The surgeon must be careful not to place too much tension on the tape because this can result in blistering of the skin. In the face the surgical tape is often placed longitudinally. In addition to supporting the wound closure, tape also acts as a dressing that protects and conceals the wound during healing. Surgical tape is usually left on the wound as long as it stays there.

A number of biologic or synthetic wound adhesives are being tested for use in wound closure. The fibrin-type adhesives are not as strong as the synthetic adhesives but seem to be better tolerated by the tissue. They can be used alone or with sutures.

Synthetic adhesives such as acrylic glues are used on top of the wound. The wound glues are useful because they often eliminate the need for local anesthetics when closing a wound. Their precise role in elective and nonelective surgical procedures has yet to be determined (Figure 13-10).

Staples

Various stapling devices are sometimes useful in skin closure. We frequently use them for temporary closure during a surgical procedure, then replace them with sutures. We also prefer staples when securing large areas of skin grafts in burn or other major reconstructive procedures.

Text continued on p. 156

Table 13-2.
Natural Fibers for Absorbable and Nonabsorbable Sutures

NAME	SOURCE	SPECIAL PROCESSING	FILAMENT	RELATIVE TENSILE STRENGTH*	TENSILE STRENGTH PROFILE†	ABSORPTION PROFILE	TISSUE REACTION‡	EASE OF USE§
ABSORBABLE								
Plain gut	Highly purified (nearly 100%) collagen derived from submucosa of sheep intestines or serosa of beef intestine	None	Twisted	2	75% at 7 days	70 days proteolysis		
Chromic gut		Chromium salt treatment resists breakdown	"virtual" monofilament	2	75% at 14 days	90 days proteolysis	5	4
Fast-absorbing gut		Heat treated to speed up degradation	monofilament	2	75% at 5 days	60–70 days proteolysis		
Plain collagen	Beef Achilles tendon	Chromium salt treatment	Twisted "virtual" monofilament		75% at 7 days	70 days proteolysis		
Chromic collagen		Chromium salt treatment	monofilament		35% at 14 days	90 days proteolysis	4	3
NONABSORBABLE								
Silk	Silkworm	Coating with beeswax or silicone; dyed	Braided	1	Progressive loss over 1 year	Significant at 2 years proteolysis	4	1 (gold standard)
Cotton	Cotton seed		Twisted	1				2
Linen	Flax seed		Twisted	2				2
Surgical steel			Braided or monofilament	5	Significant loss only if kinked		1	5

From Sykes JM, Byorth PJ: In Baker SR, Swanson NA: *Local flaps in facial reconstruction,* St Louis, 1995, Mosby.
*Scale: *1,* least; *5,* greatest. Parentheses indicate relative rank within a relative strength class: (*1*), greatest; (*5*), least.
†Percentage of original, dry tensile strength.
‡Scale: *1,* least; *5,* greatest.
§Scale: *1,* easiest; *5,* most difficult.

Table 13-3.
Absorbable Synthetic Sutures

NAME	SOURCE	SPECIAL PROCESSING	FILAMENT	RELATIVE TENSILE STRENGTH*	TENSILE STRENGTH PROFILE†	ABSORPTION PROFILE	TISSUE REACTION‡	EASE OF USE§
Poliglecaprone 25 (Monocryl, Ethicon)	Synthetic copolymer glycolide and caprolate	Undyed	Monofilament	4 (1)	50-60% at 1 wk 20-30% at 2 wk 20% at 3 wk	90-120 days hydrolysis	2	1—very pliable elastic
Polydioxanone (PDSII, Ethicon)	Synthetic polymer polydioxanone	Undyed	Monofilament	4 (4)	70% at 3 wk 50% at 4 wk 25% at 6 wk	180-210 days hydrolysis	2	3
Polygalactin 910 (Vicryl, Ethicon)	Synthetic copolymer glycolide lactide	Dyed violet or undyed, coated galactin 370	Braid	4 (2)	65% at 2 wk 40% at 3 wk 8% at 4 wk	56-70 days hydrolysis	3	2
Polyglycolic acid (Dexon II Dexon"s," Davis & Geck)	Synthetic polymer	Dyed or undyed, coated polycaprolate	Braid	4 (3)	65% at 1 wk 35% at 2 wk 5% at 4 wk	90-120 days hydrolysis	3	2
Polyglyconate (Maxon, Davis & Geck)	Synthetic polymer polytrimethylene carbonate	Dyed	Monofilament	4 (1)	75% at 2 wk 50% at 4 wk 25% at 6 wk	180-210 days hydrolysis	2	2

From Sykes JM, Byorth PJ: In Baker SR, Swanson NA: *Local flaps in facial reconstruction*, St Louis, 1995, Mosby. See Table 13-2 footnotes.

Table 13-4.
Nonabsorbable Synthetic Sutures

NAME	SOURCE	SPECIAL PROCESSING	FILAMENT	RELATIVE TENSILE STRENGTH*	TENSILE STRENGTH PROFILE†	ABSORPTION PROFILE	TISSUE REACTION‡	EASE OF USE§
Nylon Dermalon (Davis & Geck) Ethilon (Ethicon)	Synthetic polyamide	Clear or dyed	Monofilament	3	81% at 1 yr 72% at 2 yr 66% at 11 yr	Slow hydrolysis stable at 2 yr	2	2—low coefficient of friction
Nurolon (Ethicon) Surgilon (Davis & Geck)		Dyed, silicone coated	Braided	2	Same as above	Same as above	2+	1
Polybutester Novafil (Davis & Geck)	Synthetic copolymer polyglycol terephthate polytrithylene terephthate	Dyed blue	Monofilament	3	—	None	1	2—very elastic, very low coefficient of friction
Polyester Ticron (Davis & Geck) Ethibond extra (Ethicon)	Synthetic Dacron polyester	Dyed, silicone coated	Braided	3	—	None	2	2
Dacron (Davis & Geck) Mersilene (Ethicon)	Synthetic Dacron polyester	Dyed, uncoated	Braided	2	—	None	2	3
Polypropylene prolene (Ethicon) Surgilene (Davis & Geck)	Synthetic polymer propylene	Dyed blue	Monofilament	2		None	1	3—very low coefficient of friction

From Sykes JM, Byorth PJ: In Baker SR, Swanson NA: *Local flaps in facial reconstruction*, St Louis, 1995, Mosby.
See Table 13-2 footnotes.

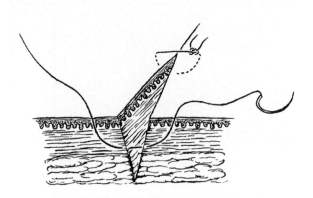

Figure 13-4. Simple interrupted suture.

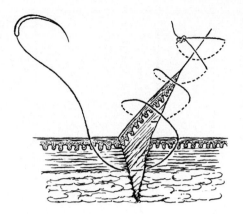

Figure 13-5. Continuous running suture.

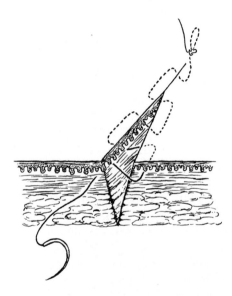

Figure 13-6. Running intradermal suture.

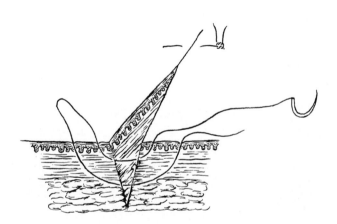

Figure 13-7. Vertical mattress suture.

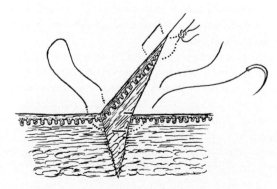

Figure 13-8. Horizontal mattress suture.

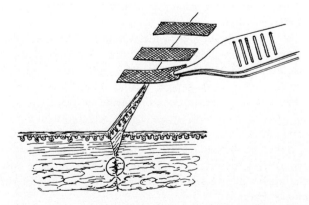

Figure 13-9. Skin closure with deep dermal sutures and surgical tape.

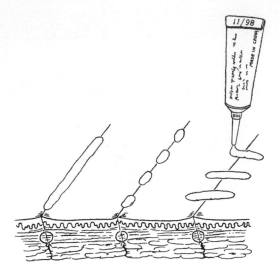

Figure 13-10. Skin closure with deep dermal sutures and surgical glue.

The two major drawbacks with staples follow:
1. With staples it is difficult to achieve the precision and approximation of the skin edges possible with sutures.
2. It is almost always more painful to remove staples than sutures.

The stapling device that eliminated these two disadvantages would be of great practical use.

Removal of Sutures, Staples, and Tape

The principle is to remove sutures and staples as soon as the wound's breaking strength is sufficient to avoid wound dehiscence. The breaking strength never returns to normal completely, and several weeks are required before the wound is strong enough to withstand trauma from, for instance, a hit by an elbow in contact sports (Figure 13-11).[11]

The earlier that sutures that penetrate the epidermis can be removed, however, the less likely that suture marks are seen when the wound is healed. This is also true for staples. Surgical tape rarely leaves any permanent marks, and it is therefore advisable to keep the wound taped together as long as possible. It is also advisable to tape the wound after removal of sutures or staples if there is a significant risk of wound separation.

The time of healing until the wound can withstand the skin tension varies greatly from one area of the body to the other. Although the suture in the eyelid can usually be removed after 3 to 5 days, a wound in the lower leg or lumbar back may need to have the sutures in place for more than 2 weeks. If a strong closure can be achieved with buried dermal sutures, this period is shortened, sometimes to the point that no transepidermal sutures are needed. In some older patients, however, it may be impossible to place adequate buried dermal sutures because of the thinness of the atrophic dermis.

Table 13-5 lists the average interval between the operation and suture removal.

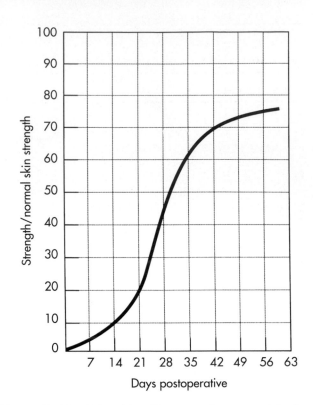

Figure 13-11. Wound breaking strength, measured by force necessary to separate wound edges. (From Larrabee WF: *Principles of facial reconstruction,* Philadelphia, 1995, Lippincott-Raven.)

POSTOPERATIVE WOUND MANAGEMENT

A dressing that covers a closed wound has the following purposes:
1. Protection
2. Absorption
3. Compression
4. Immobilization
5. Aesthetics

All these functions are not important in every wound, but one or more are usually to healing. The current surgical teaching is that a wound will be "sealed" within 8 hours postoperatively. Studies have shown that a closed wound is unlikely to be contaminated from the outside after this period. It takes at least 4 days, however, until the epidermal barrier has reduced protein leakage to normal.[12]

Many weeks must pass before water vapor permeability begins to approach normal.[9] Therefore a controlled hydration dressing should be used over a wound several weeks after the operation to minimize wound desiccation and scarring. Once the dressing has been removed, an ointment or water-retaining cream can be used.

Several modalities of treatment have been suggested to reduce scarring. Compression[6] and treatment with silicone sheets[1] appear to be the best-documented approaches. Compression is particularly important in the extremities, where it also has a major function in reducing limb edema.

Table 13-5.
Recommended Suture Types and Intervals for Suture Removal*

BODY REGION	PERCUTANEOUS	DEEP (DERMAL)	REMOVAL (DAYS)
Scalp	4-0/5-0 Monofilament	3-0/4-0 Polydioxanone, Poliglecaprone	6-8
Ear	6-0 Monofilament	5-0	10-14
Eyelid	6-0/7-0 Monofilament	—	3-4
Eyebrow	5-0/6-0 Monofilament	5-0 Absorbable	3-5
Nose	6-0 Monofilament	5-0 Absorbable	3-5
Lip	6-0/7-0 Monofilament	5-0 Absorbable	3-4
Oral mucosa, other facial areas	6-0/7-0 Monofilament	5-0 Absorbable	3-4
Breast and trunk	4-0/5-0 Monofilament	3-0 Absorbable 3-0/4-0 Polydioxanone	NA
Extremities	4-0/5-0 Monofilament	4-0 Absorbable	8-10
Hand	5-0 Monofilament	5-0 Absorbable	8-10
Foot/sole	3-0/4-0 Monofilament	4-0 Absorbable	12-14
Penis	5-0/6-0 Monofilament	—	8-10

*Surgical tape is added for reinforcement whenever possible.

Surgical Treatment of Scars

Every surgical or traumatic wound heals with a scar (see Chapters 5 and 7). Scarring can be reduced by (1) optimal placement of incisions, (2) minimization of trauma during the operation, and (3) use of proper suturing and dressing techniques. Scarring usually is worse in very young patients and in African and Asian populations. Also, some patients of any skin type seem to scar more than other individuals.

During the first year after trauma or an elective operation, the scar usually becomes more conspicuous for approximately 3 months, then regresses over the ensuing months. In general the scar has attained its final appearance by 1 year, but some scars continue to improve or worsen for 2 or more years. After removal of the initial dressing and the sutures, scarring can be reduced by prolonged treatment with controlled hydration dressings, treatment with silicone sheets, pressure treatment, and topical therapy with steroids and bleaching agents.

Surgical correction of scars is usually delayed until the scar has matured for 1 year, except for patients in whom earlier scar revision becomes clinically necessary to maintain joint mobility or prevent corneal desiccation in an ectropion. Posttraumatic scars involving a significant area of skin may require resurfacing with either a skin graft or a skin flap. Depressed scars may require a flap to replace a tissue deficit. Tissue expansion may be useful in many of these situations. The most common scars are either linear or close to linear, and these scars are usually treated with excision alone or in conjunction with a Z-plasty or W-plasty.

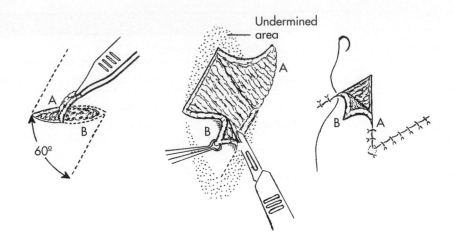

Figure 13-12. Z-plasty involves transposition of two interdigitating equal triangular flaps. Z-plasty at 60-degree angle shows a gain in length along direction of common limb. Direction of common limb of Z is changed.

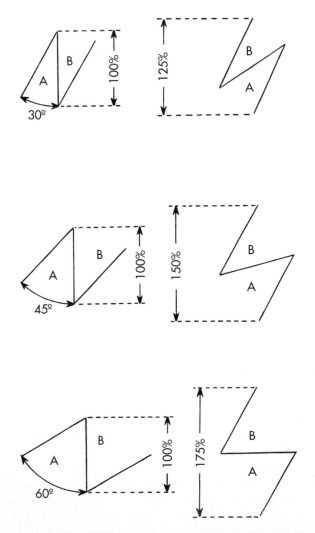

Figure 13-13. Different angles change percentage increase of length. Larger angles provide greater lengthening. Contracted scar lengthens at expense of lateral skin, so that with increasing angle size, lateral wall tension increases and becomes key limiting factor.

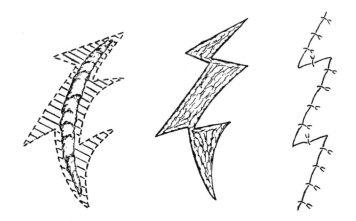

Figure 13-14. Asymmetric Z-plasty.

Z-PLASTY. The Z-plasty was first described by William E. Horner of Philadelphia in 1837. He used the procedure for correction of an ectropion of the lower eyelid. Many surgeons later described various uses for the Z-plasty, most comprehensively by Borges[2] and the McGregor.[14]

In principle the Z-plasty lengthens a scar by mobilizing skin on both sides of the scar (Figure 13-12). It is therefore best used when the scar itself is contracted and when there is significant laxity of the surrounding skin. A Z-plasty can be designed in many ways (Figure 13-13). We prefer to determine the desired main oblique axis of the Z-plasty first, then design the individual limbs accordingly. Z-plasties can be single, multiple, asymmetric, and opposing (Figure 13-14).

If multiple Z-plasties are designed, it is usually advantageous to make the flaps of a Z-plasty at the end of a scar smaller than the flaps in the center. Each Z-plasty flap can become necrotic at the tip, so generally the flap should be given a pyramid shape to increase the blood supply by broadening its base. Multiple Z-plasties may benefit from use of the Y-to-V advancement principle. Specialized applications for Z-plasties

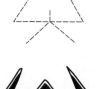
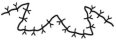

Figure 13-15. Classic double-opposing Z-plasty and flap transfers after mobilization. Used for contractures of web spaces or epicanthal folds.

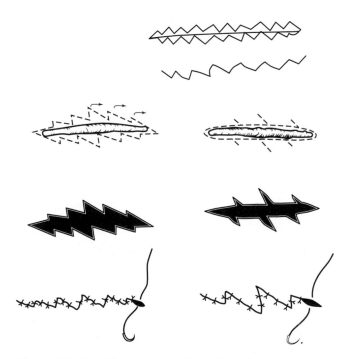

Figure 13-16. W-plasty is useful method for correction of contracted facial scars, especially on forehead and cheeks. Procedure consists of conversion of contracted scar to multiple small scars, which in turn are able to change direction of contracture itself, resulting in overall scar improvement.

include the four-flap and five-flap Z procedures used for contractures of the thumb and digital web spaces. Opposing Z-plasties can also be used for small contractures of web spaces or epicanthal folds (Figure 13-15).

Overall the Z-plasty procedure is very useful, and even if its principle and basic technique seem simple, optimal results require careful planning. In the face, Z-plasties are usually placed in periorbital and perioral areas with skin creases. It is

important to label the Z-plasty flaps before elevation and transposition to prevent flaps from being elevated and then accidentally put back down in their original position. If Z-plasty flaps have been transposed correctly, the original orientation of the scar should have been changed.

W-PLASTY. A W-plasty changes the appearance of a scar by turning the scar into a zigzag line. No transposition of local flaps occurs (Figure 13-16).

To reduce the conspicuousness of a W-plasty, its limbs should usually not exceed 6 mm in length.[2] The W-plasty flaps (and often Z-plasty flaps) are best made with the no. 11 scalpel used in a sawing motion. When a contracted scar has formed a skin web, such as in a longstanding contracture in the axilla, a W-plasty used with the Y-to-V advancement technique is often beneficial.

In the face the W-plasties are usually preferred in the forehead, zygomatic region, nose, and chin. In these locations it is important to undermine the skin widely to allow advancement without tension.

SKIN GRAFTING

Skin can successfully be transplanted as a split-thickness skin graft (STSG), a full-thickness skin graft (FTSG), or a composite graft (Figure 13-17).[14] No clear boundaries exist among these different grafts, since the design of the graft's thickness usually is determined by the defect that is reconstructed.

Split-thickness Grafts

STSGs consist of epidermis and a portion of the underlying dermis. They are measured in thousandths of an inch, with the thickness of the space set in the dermatome being measured, not the graft's thickness. The thickness should therefore be considered relative. A thin graft is usually 0.005 to 0.012 inch thick, intermediate graft 0.012 to 0.018 inch thick, and a thick graft 0.018 to 0.028 inch thick. The grafts are generally harvested with a dermatome from an available donor site.

In children, when concealment of the donor site is important, a typical donor site for an STSG is the buttock. In the older person the anterior or lateral thigh constitutes an excellent donor site. If only a small graft is needed, split-thickness skin can be harvested from the groin, after which the wound can be closed in a linear fashion.

Once harvested, grafts can be either used as they are or meshed with or without expansion. We believe that skin grafts to the face, hand, and forearm should not be meshed unless absolutely necessary. In other areas, meshing is an option, particularly if large surface areas need to be covered. Meshing gives the graft a waffled appearance and allows expansion up to approximately six times. A meshed graft conforms better to an uneven surface and allows drainage from the recipient site through its openings.

We prefer the compressed air–powered dermatome made by Zimmer because it allows for good control of the speed of the oscillating blade. For soft donor site surfaces, such as the

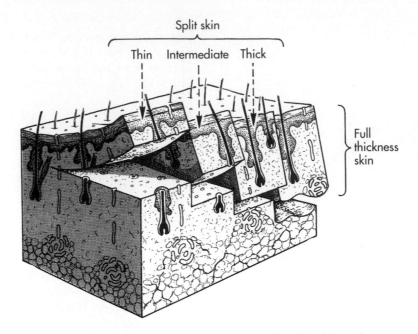

Figure 13-17. Various types of skin grafts in relation to epidermal and dermal anatomy.

abdominal wall, we prefer the drum-type dermatome made by Padgett. It uses an adhesive interface between the skin surface and dermatome drum. Therefore the graft can be harvested without depending on counterpressure from the underlying tissues.

After the recipient site has been cleared of necrotic tissue and hemostasis established, an STSG is secured in place with sutures (we prefer 5-0 chromic sutures). When skin grafting very large areas, such as in burns, staples can be used to save time. A tie-over dressing is useful to stabilize the STSG to the underlying recipient tissue, except over bony prominences, where it could cause necrosis. In the scalp, we cautiously use a tie-over dressing to avoid pressure necrosis of the galea or periosteum.

If the recipient site is clean and uncontaminated, the dressing is left in place for 1 week, whereas in contaminated wounds it is usually changed after 48 to 72 hours. To prevent relative motion between the graft and the underlying recipient tissues, a plaster splint can be used to immobilize the body part being grafted. An elastic wrap is used for compression, and the grafted site usually is elevated for at least 1 week.

The donor site should be protected from desiccation and contamination and therefore preferably covered with a controlled hydration dressing. Compared with any dry dressing technique, such as Xeroform gauze treatment, a controlled hydration dressing allows faster healing (on average by about 50%) and greatly reduces pain. If the grafted area is small, the procedure can usually be done without hospitalization.

Full-Thickness and Composite Grafts

FTSGs contain both dermis and epidermis, and composite grafts may contain fat, cartilage, or muscle as well. In principle the graft should be of approximately the thickness required to fill the defect. A thick composite graft will only survive in a well-vascularized bed and if it has a "pie crust" to allow drainage.

FTSGs usually heal with a better match in color and texture compared with STSGs. FTSGs, however, tend to undergo "biscuiting," or elevation of the graft's center and depression of its periphery. FTSGs also benefit from tie-over dressings.

Few skin grafts fail unless the recipient site provides poor vascularity or is heavily contaminated or some technical error has occurred.

Composite grafts from the ear are sometimes used to reconstruct the ala of the nose. In these grafts the upper limit in size is 1 cm^2.

Once healed, the donor site and the grafted site frequently need to be treated with compression, silicone sheets, topical steroids, and bleaching creams.

REFERENCES

1. Ahn S, Monafo WW, Mustoe T: Topical silicone gel for the prevention and treatment of hypertrophic scar, *Arch Surg* 126:499-504, 1991.

2. Borges AF: *Elective incisions and scar revision,* Boston, 1973, Little, Brown.

3. Brown LL, Shelton HT, Bornside GH, et al: Evaluation of wound irrigation by pulsatile jet and conventional methods, *Ann Surg* 187:170-173, 1978.

4. Candie JP, Ferguson DJ: Irrigation of copious amounts of Ringer lactate by pulsatile jet, *Surgery* 50:367, 1961.

5. Godina M: Early microsurgical reconstruction of complex trauma of the extremities, *Plast Reconstr Surg* 78:285-292, 1986.

6. Heimbach DM, Engrav LH: *Surgical management of the burn wound,* New York, 1984, Raven.

7. Hollander JE, Singer AJ, Valentine S, et al: Wound registry: development and validation, *Ann Emerg Med* 25:675-685, 1995.

8. Holmlund D, Tera H, Wiberg Y, et al: *Sutur när var hur,* Uppsala, Sweden, 1976, Andra Upplagan Universtetsförlaget Uppsala.

9. Jonkman MF: Epidermal wound healing between moist and dry, Groningen, Belgium, Cip-Gegevens Koninklijke Bibliotheek, den Haag; 5:59-65, 1989.

10. Kennedy KL, Tritch DL: Debridement. In Krasner D, Dean K, editors: *Chronic wound care: a clinical source book for healthcare professionals,* ed 2, Wayne, Pa, 1997, Health Management.

11. Larrabee WF: *Principles of facial reconstruction,* Philadelphia, 1995, Lippincott-Raven.

12. Liu P, Eriksson E, Mustoe T: Wound healing: practical aspects. In Russell RC: *Instructional courses ASEF,* vol 4, St Louis, 1992, Mosby.

13. Losken HW, Auchinloss JA: Human bites of the lip, *Clin Plast Surg* 11:159-161, 1984.

14. McGregor IA, McGregor AD: *Fundamental techniques of plastic surgery,* ed 9, Edinburgh, 1995, Churchill-Livingstone.

15. Meakins JL: Prophylactic antibiotics. In Taylor EW: *Infection in surgical practice,* Oxford, UK, 1992, Oxford University Press.

16. National Pressure Ulcer Advisory Panel: Pressure ulcer healing: controversy to consensus assessment methods and outcomes, Washington, DC, 1995, Consensus Conference.

17. Norman R, Wind G, editor: *Principles of surgical technique: the art of surgery,* ed 2, Baltimore, 1987, Urban & Schwarzenberg.

18. Robson MC: Burn wound microbiology, *Am J Clin Pathol* 76:246-247, 1981.

19. Sykes JM, Byorth PJ: Sutures, needles and techniques for wound closure. In Baker SR, Swanson NA: *Local flaps in facial reconstruction,* St Louis, 1995, Mosby.

20. *Stedman's Medical dictionary,* ed 26, Baltimore, 1995, Wilkins & Wilkins.

21. Treatment of pressure sore ulcers, Clinical Practice Guideline, no 15, Washington, DC, 1994, US Dept. of Health and Human Services, Public Health Service, Agency for Health Care Policy and Research.

22. Zawacki BE: The effect of Travase on heat injured skin, *Surgery* 77:132-136, 1975.

23. Zawacki BE: The natural history of reversible burn injury, *Surg Gynecol Obstet* 139:867-872, 1974.

24. Zeiss E: *Handbuch der Plastischen Chirurgie,* Reimer. Berlin, 1838.

Microsurgery

Denton D. Weiss

Julian J. Pribaz

Microsurgery is that surgical specialty requiring magnification for its completion. This area of surgery embraces numerous specialties, including plastic surgery, ophthalmology, neurosurgery, orthopedic surgery, urology, otolaryngology, and gynecology. Although the compound word "micro-surgery" would suggest a particular scale of 10^{-6}, actually the scale is limited by the power ($\times$) of the magnification and the steadiness of the instruments in the human hand. Conceivably, therefore, in the years ahead the scale will continue to shrink, especially as the emerging area of surgery on the unborn child develops. As a result, plastic surgeons can expect new technical and ethical challenges.

HISTORY

The developments of vascular surgery and microsurgery have had a long and paralleled history, but not until the twentieth century did the two merge into a single field. Vascular surgical techniques were first described by the rustic barber's apprentice and later army surgeon Ambroise Paré in 1552. Zacharias Janssen invented the compound microscope in 1590. Athanasius Kircher, a Jesuit priest, is considered to be the first to use the microscope as a tool of disease investigation. In his *Scrutinium pestis* (Rome, 1658), Kircher described the blood of plague patients as being filled with "worms" seen only under the microscope.

The greatest early microscopist was Marcello Malpighi, father of histology and founder of iconographic embryology. In 1661 Malpighi's work *De pulmonibus* defined the pulmonary anatomy of capillary anastomosis between arteries and veins.[40] In 1759 Hallwell performed the first recorded vascular repair using metal pins and thread to repair a brachial artery.[88] By 1897 Murphy had completed the first vascular anastomosis. Alexis Carrel first described the triangulation technique for vascular anastomosis in 1902. Carrel and Guthrie's work on blood vessel surgery laid the foundation for vascular and transplantation surgery.[22,50] Hopfner performed the first experimental limb replantation in dogs in 1903.

In 1921 the microscope reached the operating room (OR). Carl-Olof Nylen, an otolaryngologist, used a monocular microscope to treat patients with chronic otitis and pseudo-fistula syndrome.[41] In 1922 his chief, Holmgren, was the first to bring the binocular microscope to the OR, and Perrit introduced it to the ophthalmic world in 1946.[88] Surprisingly, the microscope was not applied to the vascular world until 1960.

The 1960s represented a period of rapid expansion and expression of microsurgery throughout the world. Microvascular surgery originated from the work of Jacobson and Suarez[59] in anastomosing vessels ranging from 1.6 to 3.2 mm in diameter. Between 1962 and 1964 Malt and McKhann[70] successfully replanted the limbs of two amputation victims. In 1963 two Chinese surgeons reportedly successfully replanted a patient's hand.[39] In 1963 Kleinert and Kasden revascularized a partial digital amputation, and in 1968 Komatsu and Tamai[63] performed the first successful thumb replantation. Peripheral nerve surgery was brought to the microsurgery arena in 1964 by a number of independent surgeons.[65,77,112]

While replantation was taking place, the world of free flap surgery began to emerge. Limb salvage surgery using replantation was paving the way for this new world of microsurgery. Goldwyn, Krizek, and Strauch and Murray all performed early experimental work on free flap surgery. In 1964 Nakayama[86] and associates reported on microsurgical transfer in a series of patients who underwent free transfer of an intestinal segment for esophageal reconstruction. Buncke, Schultz, and McLean were early pioneers in bringing microsurgery to plastic surgery.[14,16,17,75] Capt. McLean and Buncke[75] performed the first free transfer of omentum for scalp coverage at Oak Knoll Naval Hospital in 1969. In India in 1971, Antia and Buch[7] published a case in which a free, vascularized dermatofat graft based on the superior epigastric vessels was transferred to a facial contour defect. This was a buried flap, which made survival difficult to evaluate. That same year, Harii and Ohmori[52] fashioned a vascularized tube flap by anastomosing to the omental vessels. Within 2 years, Daniel and Taylor[30] and later O'Brien et al[90] separately reported the successful transfer of a free groin flap to the lower extremity. This ushered in the current era of microsurgery.

The evolution of microsurgery over the last 20 years has progressed with continued refinements and applications to many fields of surgery. Intense study continues on the physiology and pathology of small vessels and nerves. The positive and negative outcomes of their repair and transfer are a part of that refinement. Our understanding of surgical anatomy and blood supply to the skin, fascia, muscles, and bones expands exponentially, and the reconstructive ladder continues to grow. The transfer of free vascularized tissue represents the highest rung of that ladder, and microsurgery offers another possible step.

REQUIREMENTS

At present the four main requirements for microsurgery today are magnification, microinstrumentation, microsutures, and acquired skills.

Magnification

The microscope used in the present-day OR is much more advanced than those used by Nylen and Holmgren, but the principles are very similar. Classically the binocular microscope can be broken down into three parts: body, neck (arm), and head. The body contains the power and light sources. The halogen or xenon source projects a strong, even, wide-field light through a cold fiberoptic cord lighting system. The fiberoptic cord runs through the neck and enters the head. This system is designed to keep the heat-producing light source away from the surgical field.

The operating microscope head is usually a dual system. The two heads each have a binocular system attached, which allows two surgeons to operate together with the same full stereoscopic field. A beam splitter makes this binocular system possible by dividing the light produced into the different binocular tubes. The beam splitter may be used to carry light to a third binocular system or camera system. A 200-mm focal length lens is most often used in reconstructive surgery, although a 275-mm lens may be needed for better visualization in deep cavity surgery. Magnification ranges from 6 to 40×, and foot-operated focus and zoom have become the standard. Zeiss, Weck, Wild, and Leitz companies make the most frequently used microscopes.

A relatively new alternative to the operating microscope is the *ocular loupe.* Surgical loupes have magnifications ranging from 2.0× and above and are available with expanded field lenses. The range of magnification generally accepted as appropriate for microsurgery is 4.0× or higher. The advantage of loupe magnification is emphasized in head and neck reconstruction, where odd angles and deep cavity reconstruction can be common. The ocular loupe technique provides the ease of an increased visual field and allows the incorporation of a head light for these difficult reconstructions. Proponents of ocular loupes report good patency rates and advocate their use for vessels greater than 1 mm in diameter.[110]

Microinstrumentation

Microinstrumentation for the microsurgeon should be of the utmost quality and simplicity. Ideally the instruments are glare free, nonmagnetic, and ergonomic in that they are easy to handle, fit well into the hand, and are fine at the tips (Figure 14-1). The basic set consists of the following:

1. Forceps: fine tipped, smooth, sizes 2 to 5, short, long for deeper cavity work
2. Scissors: fine tipped, one smooth, one serrated; straight, curved
3. Needle holder: thin jawed, narrow shouldered, pencil grip, nonlocking
4. Microvascular clamps: adjustable double microvascular clamps (Kleinert-Kutz type); series of different-sized smooth, single, straight microvascular clamps; disposable clamps
5. Background: contrasting color (yellow, green, blue; we use yellow because of extreme contrast to suture color)
6. Vessel dilator: smooth tipped
7. Syringe: 3 ml (cc) with 26-gauge angiocatheter

Other necessary nonmicrosurgical instruments are a bipolar cautery, microclips and microclip appliers, sterile Doppler ultrasound, and a microsuction system. One micromat suction system has the suction catheter incorporated into the background matting. All these instruments require delicate care and constant cleaning throughout the case. The microinstruments should be stored with their tips resting in saline-soaked sponges and housed in a sterilized instrument box.

Microsutures

Microsutures are essential to the microsurgeon. In 1962 Chase and Schwartz[24] used 7.0 silk to repair 1.2- to 1.7-mm vessels in a dog model. In 1966 Buncke and Schultz[17] electroplated nylon, and in 1970 O'Brien et al[89] used and developed sutures that were also metallized nylon. Currently, monofilament nylon and prolene sutures are used. The suture size varies from 8.0 to 11.0, and the most common needle diameters are 75 to 135 μm. Although not yet achieved, the ideal needle size would match the suture diameter.

Microsurgical Skills

Microsurgical skills are acquired; no one is born with an ability to do microsurgery. The laboratory is the starting ground for new microsurgeons. Initially the surgeons practice under the microscope by suturing fine tubing, then progress to laboratory animals. The student must become familiar with arterial and venous anastomoses (both end-end and end-side), nerve repairs, vein grafts to bridge vessel defects, and eventually flap transfer. These technical skills are crucial in the OR.

MICROVASCULAR SURGERY

In 1902 Alexis Carrel described the end-end and end-side anastomoses and a triangulation vascular technique. These techniques, first advocated by Carrel and Guthrie in the early 1900s, were later applied to smaller vessels. In 1948 Schumacker and Lowenberg[106] anastomosed vessels measuring 3.2 mm in diameter. Later, Seidenberg et al[109] performed anastomoses in the microsurgical range but were limited by suture size and lack of magnification use. The introduction of the microscope and swedged on needles allowed the surgeon to

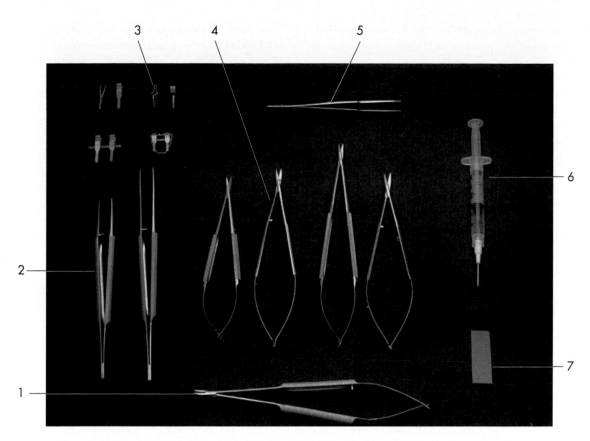

Figure 14-1. Microinstrumentation. *1*, Needle holder; *2*, forceps; *3*, microvascular clamps; *4*, scissors; *5*, vessel dilator; *6*, irrigation syringe; *7*, background.

enter the microsurgical world. In 1960 Jacobsen and Suarez[59] reported a 100% patency rate with their first microvascular repairs on vessels 1.6 to 3.2 mm in diameter. In 1962 O'Brien et al[89] were among the first to put metallized nylon to use and reported patency rates of 81% and 90% in 1-mm rabbit artery and veins, respectively. Fujimaki et al[38] demonstrated an 85% patency rate in 0.5-mm rat arteries in 1977.

As surgeons struggled with vascular suturing techniques to bring together smaller and smaller vessels, in 1956 Ansrosov[6] introduced the concept of *stapling.* In 1963, not long after Jacobsen and Suarez performed their first microvascular repair, Chase and Schwartz[24] brought the stapling system to the microvascular arena. The need for extensive mobilization of vessels, precise matching, and difficulty dealing with mismatch have limited this repair.

Vascular anastomoses incorporating vein cuffs and polyglycolic acid tubing have also been used in one variation of the *sleeve anastomosis,* which was introduced in 1978.[68] The sleeve repair, which arose from a modification of the end-end anastomosis, is used typically for mismatched veins. The smaller vessel is invaginated into the lumen of the larger vessel. The advantage of this procedure is that fewer sutures are necessary. Lauritzen[68] reported high patency rates with this technique. In contrast, Sully et al[117] found that the sleeve anastomosis was inferior to end-end repair.

More recent additions to anastomotic repair include the coupler system and the laser. A 1.5-mm absorbable polyglactin coupler has been described. The *coupler* is made up of two cuffs, which are placed on the cut end of the vessels, and an interconnecting collar. Daniel and Olding[28] reported patency rates of 100% and 88% in a rabbit model. Clinical trials have reported a single thrombosis in 20 procedures.[29] The technical difficulties with arteries and the size of vessels that can be anastomosed limit the coupler system.

Morris and Carter[83] first described the laser-assisted microvascular anastomosis. The *laser* welds the vessels together and is used in addition to a minimal number of microsutures. In 1991 Kiyoshige[62] presented the first clinical report of laser-assisted microvascular anastomosis for free tissue transfer and replantation. Patency rates have been reported to be equal to those of standard techniques, but the formation of stenosis and pseudoaneurysm has limited widespread use of the laser.[35,98,102]

Today the predominant anastomosis used in microsurgery is a microsuture technique with either an end-end or an end-side repair. The typical sutures are either monofilament nylon or prolene, and anastomosis of vessels less than 1 mm is common.

Preparation and Anastomotic Technique

The surgeon must be in a comfortable sitting or standing position to perform vascular anastomosis. Adequate support to the arms should be established at the level of the wrist or anterior forearms. This allows the intrinsic muscles of the hand to be the predominant support to the microsurgical instruments. The surgeon must be sure to use the appropriate magnification for the vessels involved. Adequate exposure of the vessels greatly enhances the success of a vascular repair.

The perivascular sheath is gently dissected off the vessels. If the ends of the vessels are traumatized, they are sharply resected. The periadventitia is cleared from the distal ends of the vessels, with care taken to ensure only the necessary amount is removed to allow for suturing. Excessive stripping is time consuming and causes devascularization of the vessels by removing the vasa vasorum.

The proximal arterial end is checked for forward flow. The lumen is inspected and any debris or clot removed, with care taken not to grasp the intima. The vessel lumen is irrigated with heparinized lactated Ringer's solution (100 U heparin/ml). The vessel is gently and atraumatically dilated. The vessels are then placed into position, with a double approximating clamp used to bring the vessel ends into proximity. With experience, single approximating clamps can be used; ideally they are located at right angles to the operator's hand. the clamp should be placed so that the vessel ends are brought into the same plane to visualize both vessel lumina, with no kinks or excessive tension on the vessels.

End-End Anastomosis

ARTERIAL. The end-end anastomosis is a technique that joins the two distal free ends of a vessel or separate vessels together, usually through a suturing procedure. This method is appropriate for most arterial and venous anastomoses. A halving, a triangulation, or a "backwall up" technique can be used to perform the end-end anastomosis (Figures 14-2 and 14-3).

We prefer the backwall up technique, which allows for visualization of each suture, ensures proper spacing, and is ideal for suturing in a cavity or when the clamp cannot be turned. The suturing commences posterocentrally, with sutures placed on each side of the first knot, working around the circumference and spacing sutures appropriately. Each suture is easier to insert than the previous suture, which gives the surgeon a psychologic advantage. In 1981 Harris et al[54] described the basic tenants of the backwall up technique to allow for visualization of the lumen throughout the entire anastomosis. This technique is useful for the novice microsurgeon and in deep cavity situations where vision is limited.

The fundamentals are the same for all suturing techniques. The needle is passed at a right angle to the vessel surface. The distance from the vessel's cut end to the needle is slightly

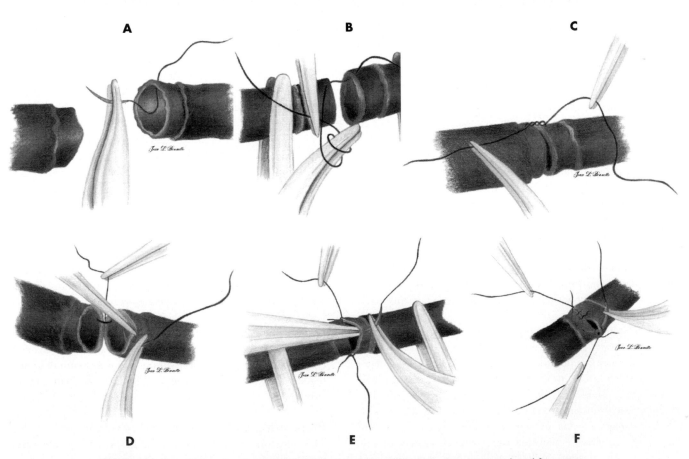

Figure 14-2. Artery or venous end-end anastomosis technique. **A,** First suture placed from outside to inside vessel. **B,** Surgeons' knot placed. **C,** Tails left for future retraction, **D,** Second suture placed 120 degrees from first. **E,** Third interrupted suture placed 120 degrees from first two sutures. **F,** Remaining sutures placed in halving technique between three retracting triangulation sutures.

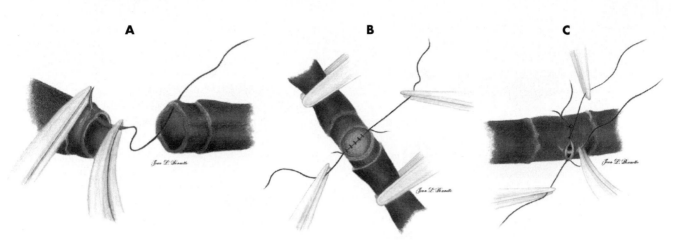

A **B** **C**

Figure 14-3. Arteriovenous end-end anastomosis: backwall up technique. **A,** Placement of single interrupted suture. **B,** Completion of backwall closure. **C,** Placement of final sutures, with visualization of lumen throughout entire anastomosis.

greater than the vessel wall thickness, which is normally less than 1 mm. The needle holder firmly grasps the needle as it passes through the vessel wall. The opposite hand holds the vessel steady with the jeweler forceps. The needle is retrieved from the vessel lumen and placed into the receiving lumen with the needle holder. The jeweler forceps is placed outside the vessel and applies counterpressure as the needle passes through the second vessel. The first suture is tied with a double loop, or surgeons' knot; the second and third are single knots. The sutures are spaced evenly, and care should be taken not to make the knots too loose or too tight. Strangling the tissue with a knot may cause vessel damage and tearing, which leads to platelet aggregation and thrombosis.

Throughout the procedure and just before the last suture is placed, the vessel lumen is irrigated with heparinized normal saline solution. Once the anastomosis is complete, the clamp is released. The distal clamp is released first and backflow checked. Leaks found at this point are repaired, and the proximal clamp is subsequently removed.

The patency is assessed by first checking the anastomosis and then the flap or replanted tissue. It is prudent to avoid early manipulation of the vessels, waiting for 3 to 5 minutes. If the vessel appears to be in spasm, lidocaine (Xylocaine) or papaverine can be applied. A patency test is performed only as a last test. The lumen is occluded distal to the anastomosis with a jeweler forceps, and the blood is emptied downstream with a second jeweler forceps. The first forceps is then released, maintaining distal compression; when the anastomosis is patent, the empty segment of vessel fills with blood. The vein is checked first and the artery second. If the patency test shows no flow, continued manipulation of a nonfunctioning anastomosis is harmful because a clot may be dislodged and the surgeon lulled into a false sense of security. The anastomosis appears patent but has a high potential for further thrombosis. As stressed by O'Brien and Morrison,[88] "The surgeon's assessment of the microvascular anastomosis is the most important measure of the likelihood of success."

VENOUS. The venous anastomosis can be a difficult repair because of the relative thinness of the vessel wall and a tendency for vein collapse during the repair. This is more evident in the laboratory because experimental animals have much thinner veins than humans. One useful technique is to inflate the collapsing vessel with the irrigation solution. An added benefit is magnification from the fluid.

The end-end anastomosis is the standard technique used for venous anastomosis. Small vessels are typically closed with interrupted sutures, but larger vessels may be closed with either an interrupted or running repair. The advantages of the running repair are (1) greater speed, (2) fewer sutures, and (3) ease of correcting size discrepancies. The greatest disadvantage is lumen narrowing. Thus the running technique should only be used with larger veins and is typically not used with smaller veins, such as those encountered in digital replantation. We prefer to use an interrupted-continuous technique for vessels larger than 1.5 mm or those with a mismatch of less than 4:1.[82]

The interrupted-continuous (triangulation) microsurgical suture technique involves the placement of three evenly spaced, interrupted sutures (Figure 14-4). The first suture is placed in the center of the backwall, and a long tail is left. The next two sutures are placed 120 degrees from the first. After placement of the third suture, the knot is tied and the needle left attached. The connected suture is used to close the open segments between the interrupted anchoring knots. As each third of vessel is closed, the running suture is tied to the tail of the interrupted suture, thereby minimizing the potential for excessive narrowing. The goal of venous anastomosis is to attain edge-to-edge approximation so that no leaks occur. Excessive tension must also be avoided. This type of repair is easy to master and is excellent for vessels with size discrepancy.

End-Side Anastomosis
The techniques of end-side anastomosis have been described by various authors.[1,12,96] The end-side anastomosis is a

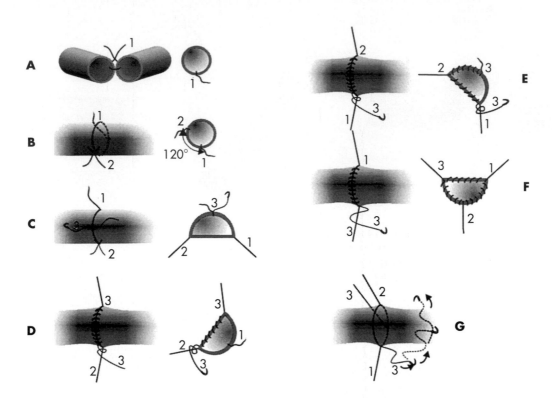

Figure 14-4. Venous interrupted continuous (triangulation) technique. **A,** Posterior interrupted suture. **B,** Second suture placed 120 degrees from first. **C,** Third suture placed 120 degrees from other sutures. **D,** Third suture run to second and tied. **E,** Running suture continued to third suture and tied. **F,** Running suture continued to first knot and tied. **G,** Anastomosis complete.

technique in which the distal free end of a vessel is joined to an opening in the side of a vessel supplying or draining a tissue. This technique is used to preserve flow to distal tissue, to avoid the effects of spasm at the anastomosis, and to eliminate the effects of size discrepancy. It is technically more demanding if done in a deep location when the clamp cannot be turned.

The end-side technique is initiated by dissecting out a proximal and distal segment of a local vessel. Proximal and distal control are established by placing clamps across the recipient vessel. An opening is made into this vessel in one of the following three ways:

1. A slit is made in the vessel with a fine scissors.
2. The Acland technique is used, with a suture placed in the recipient vessel. As the suture is pulled up, an ellipse is cut out.[1]
3. An aortic punch is used to make a circular opening in the vessel. The smallest available punch is 2.5 mm.

We prefer excising an ellipse to making a slit in the vessel, and if an aortic punch is not too large for the donor vessel, this technique is the first choice (Figure 14-5). Once the opening is established, the vessels are sutured together. The posterior wall is closed first. The left corner is established, and the suture is run to the opposite corner. Alternatively, interrupted sutures are used, starting from the left corner. The anterior wall is closed either using a running suture tracking from right to left or placing interrupted sutures. If the vessel can be flipped, the two corner sutures are placed first. In this situation, either wall can be closed first. If the donor vessel is small, the luminal diameter can be enlarged by cutting the vessel obliquely or by incorporating a T junction of a branching point.

Secondary Techniques

VASCULAR GRAFTS. Grafts are often necessary in microsurgery when a vessel deficiency exists. This is often seen in replantation surgery or in free flap reconstruction when the injury forces the anastomosis to be performed out of the zone of injury. Vein grafts are more readily available and easier to harvest than arterial grafts and have a better long-term patency rate than most microsurgical prosthetic grafts. They may be used to bridge both venous, and if reversed, arterial defects. Yasargil[130] described the early experimental use of vein grafts. Overton and Owens,[92] among others,[9,15,18] described the early clinical applications of vein grafts in replantation and flap surgery.

When choosing a vascular graft, the appropriate diameter and length are important. For small grafts the volar wrist or forearm veins are the preferred grafts. Medium-sized veins are easily harvested from the dorsum of the foot. The most often used large vein is the saphenous. Arterial grafts are less often used, but arterial grafts from nonreplantable parts or from the thoracodorsal artery, descending branch of the lateral femoral circumflex artery, and the radial artery have been described. Schneider et al,[105] using a rabbit model, determined the ideal length of a venous graft to be 35% of the relaxed recipient's

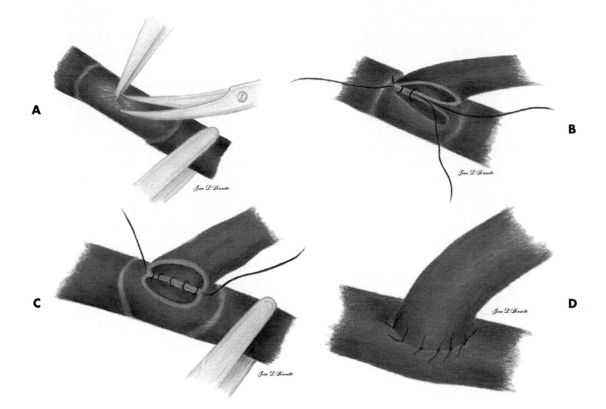

Figure 14-5. Artery or venous end-side anastomosis. **A,** Opening made in vessel wall by picking up wall and cutting out an ellipse. **B,** Posterior wall is closed first. **C,** Anterior wall closure. **D,** Anastomosis complete.

arterial defect. They found that a venous graft would contract 35% to 55% once harvested. Further findings showed that excess tension caused thrombosis, whereas any redundancy disappeared and was associated with high patency rates (Figure 14-6).

The techniques of a vascular graft harvest are relatively standard and well described by Acland.[1] First, a longitudinal incision is made over the vessel. The vessel is identified and the branches are ligated. The proximal and distal ends are clipped or sutured. The vessel is removed and flushed with heparinized lactated Ringer's solution. The proximal end is clipped and the distal end is canalized, and the vessel is hydrodilated with heparinized Ringer's solution. The hydrodilation is extremely useful because it dilates the vessel, unravels any kinks, and demonstrates leaks. We recommend marking one surface of the vessel after it has been hydrodilated to prevent twists during inset. This should especially be done with a vein graft for an arterial defect, which has a high potential for elongation and kinks.

ARTERIOVENOUS LOOPS. When a graft is required for both arterial and venous defects, a vein graft may be harvested and used to create an arteriovenous (AV) loop. The vein may be harvested locally and used in situ or transferred to distal vessels. With a locally used saphenous vein the distal end may be anastomosed to the femoral or popliteal artery in preparation for the free flap transfer. Distal transfer requires the vein to be positioned so that the valves of the vein are not obstructing

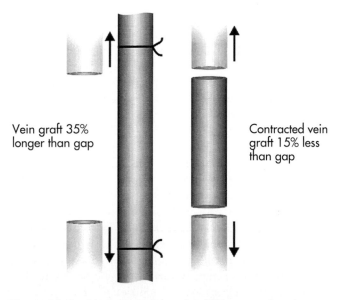

Vein graft 35% longer than gap

Contracted vein graft 15% less than gap

Figure 14-6. Ideal vein graft length is 35% greater than the gap. Even with a correction of 35%, vein grafts can contract up to 55%.

the arterial side. Once formed, the AV loop is divided at midpoint and anastomosed to the corresponding artery and vein of a transferred free flap.

Initially the use of AV loops was staged. The vessel was transferred and then allowed to mature for 10 days. After maturation the loop was divided and anastomosed to the recipient free flap. Often, however, considerable scarring and thrombosis occur in the AV loop. As do most surgeons, we prefer that the AV loop be divided at the initial setting and anastomosed to the free flap.

PROSTHETIC GRAFTS. Attempts at using prosthetic grafts in microvascular surgery have not been as successful as in vascular surgery. Experimentally, Yeh et al[131] described good early patency with human umbilical artery grafts, but the vessel wall degenerated later.

Polytetrafluoroethylene (PTFE) grafts have been used successfully in microsurgery. Early patency is satisfactory, but neointimal hyperplasia and anastomotic narrowing occur over time, leading to long-term patency problems.[56] Short segments of PTFE may be used in high-flow situations but not in low-flow states when patency is a problem. Graham et al[48] have investigated endothelial seeding of prosthetic grafts to improve patency.

Complications and Prevention
TISSUE ISCHEMIA AND NO-REFLOW PHENOMENON.
Free tissue transfer and replantation inevitably require a period of ischemia before revascularization. The amount of ischemia that tissue can tolerate depends on the tissue type and the temperature of the transferred tissue. In a review of the literature, English and Tittle[33] estimated periods of warm and cold ischemia for different tissues. Skin and subcutaneous tissue tolerate ischemia well, with excellent survival up to 6 hours for warm ischemia and 12 hours for cold ischemia. Tissues made up of fibroblast, chondroblasts, and osteoblasts are relatively resistant; specifically, bone tolerates warm ischemia up to 3 hours and cold ischemia for 24 hours. Skeletal muscle, however, begins to have irreversible damage at 4 to 6 hours of warm ischemia and ideally should be transferred after no more than 2 hours.[34,128] Muscle can tolerate cold ischemia approximately 8 hours.

Studying the reperfusion of ischemic tissue, the term *no-reflow phenomenon* was first coined by Ames et al.[4] They found that once vascular patency was established, some tissues failed to reperfuse. May et al[73] studied the effects of the no-flow phenomenon in a rabbit epigastric flap model and found that at 1 hour a decreased flow could be seen that progressed up to 12 hours after ischemia. Reversible histologic damage was noted at 4 hours and irreversible damage at 12 hours. Their data parallel the more accepted pathophysiology of no-reflow phenomenon. Initial swelling of the endothelium leads to platelet aggregation and adhesion of white cells to the endothelium. The unquenched free radical protected by the white cell mass leads to an increase in endothelial permeability. The small capillary beds are occluded, and AV shunting occurs. The end result is lack of tissue perfusion and eventual flap or replantation death.

TECHNICAL PROBLEMS. With normal vessels, vascular failure is generally caused by technical errors. Traumatic handling, high clamp pressure, poor suture placement, and vessel kinking or twisting are all preventable if a methodic,

regimented technique is used. Clamp pressure should not exceed 30 g/mm^2, and flat clamps cause less damage.[2] Damage to the vessel wall from poor suture placement and inappropriate needle technique may occur secondary to inexperience or poor visibility. This can lead to endothelial lacerations and subendothelial exposure with subsequent platelet aggregation. Collagen found in the adventitia and media appears to be one of the most sensitive activators of this platelet aggregation. Full-thickness, evenly spaced sutures should be placed to prevent this vessel damage. The vessel lumen should not be pinched by the microforceps. The suture line should be inspected before placement of the last sutures to make sure no stitch is catching the backwall.

Anatomic problems such as excessive tension from a short pedicle and size discrepancy should be identified before transferring the free flap. If the pedicle is too short or recipient vessels are not available, a venous graft or AV loop should be considered. Several methods are used to correct size discrepancy, as mentioned earlier. Minor discrepancies can be adjusted by simple dilation. Alternatively, cutting the smaller vessel obliquely will widen the lumen opening. To achieve a larger lumen, a **T** junction can be used. The vessel's distal end is opened at a branch point. Another option is to perform an end-to-side anastomosis.

VASOSPASM. The best management for vascular spasm is prevention. The patient should be warm and the surgical site well perfused. Proximal blocks (e.g., arm, epidural) tend to decrease the occurrence of spasm. If vascular spasm develops, treatments include gentle dilation or hydrodilation and topical application of 2% lidocaine, papavarine, or verapamil. Gentle dilation is performed using a dilating forceps, which has smooth narrow tips that are round in cross section. Hydrodilation is achieved using heparinized lactated Ringer's solution. Solutions of 2% lidocaine (without epinephrine), papaverine, or verapamil may be applied directly to the vessels in an attempt release the spasm pharmacologically.

Clotting Mechanism
The basic healing process of an anastomosed vessel is relatively well known.[2] Initially the anastomosis site is coated in a thin layer of platelets, which falls away over 24 to 72 hours. A pseudointima develops during this period and is replaced by a repaired endothelial lining in 7 to 10 days. It correlates that during the formation of the pseudointima the highest risk for clot formation exists.[55]

The formation of a clot at the anastomosis occurs when the intima has significant damage or when a sleeve of intimal lining is left at the cut edge of the vessel. The subendothelium and the collagen trigger platelet aggregation. The aggregation leads to the release of platelet granules and the subsequent attraction of more platelets. The granules are made up of alpha and dense types and contain von Willebrand's factor, fibrinogen, adenosine diphosphate (ADP), calcium, and serotonin. All these components play a role in the attraction of more platelets and can lead to the activation of the extrinsic clotting cascade. Anastomotic failure results from the formation a thrombus from accumulation of an occluding white clot (platelet aggregation) or red clot (fibrin rich).[23] Multiple pharmacologic agents have been used to minimize thrombus formation and prevent anastomotic failure.

HEPARIN. One of the most frequently used antithrombolytic agents is heparin. Heparin inactivates thrombin and other serine esterases in the clotting cascade (IXa, Xa, XIa, XIIa) by increasing the effect of antithrombin III. Some surgeons advocate the use of bolus heparin (5000 U) at the time of arterial anastomosis, whereas others reserve its use for emergencies. Khouri et al[60] evaluated the effects of heparin on a rat arterial anastomosis model. They concluded that a bolus of heparin given before the reperfusion inhibits the development of a thrombus. Interestingly, approximately 12% of the animals developed hematomas. A large multiinstitutional study, headed by Khouri,[61] examined the effects of multiple pharmaceutical antithrombotic agents, including heparin, dextran, and aspirin, on survival of free tissue transfers. The only agent to show a statistically significant effect was postoperative subcutaneous heparin given as deep venous thrombosis (DVT) prophylaxis.

The use of heparin has undergone many changes in plastic surgeons' and other microsurgeons' practices, with a tendency to reduce the use of heparin. Ever-changing protocols still make it difficult to generalize about use of anticoagulants. In our practice, heparin is used routinely for intraoperative irrigation of the microanastomosis. Postoperatively, heparin is given for DVT prophylaxis (5000 U subcutaneously two times a day for 5 days). In free flap surgery, heparin is given as a bolus intraoperatively (5000 to 10,000 U) if (1) a clot has developed at the anastomosis intraoperatively or (2) the free flap is redone because of anastomotic failure. Postoperatively these patients receive a heparin drip, with a goal partial thromboplastin time of 50 to 60 seconds (1.5 to 2 times normal) for 5 to 7 days. This heparinization technique is routinely used in traumatic amputations and digital replantation.

DEXTRAN. Dextran is a low-molecular-weight polysaccharide. This agent has both antiplatelet and antifibrin functions and is considered a vascular lubricant. The exact mechanism of action is unknown. Dextran's effect may be caused by the formation of a negative charge on the platelet surfaces or an inactivation of von Willebrand's factor.[8,101] Because of the antigenicity of dextran the patient is given a small test dose (less than 5 ml) of a 10% solution of Dextran-40. If no allergic reaction develops after 1 hour, the patient is given 20 to 30 ml of 10% Dextran-40 as a loading dose. This is followed by a maintenance dose of 15 to 25 ml/hour for 3 days. No tapering is required because the effects of dextran persist for hours to days after being discontinued. In our practice the routine use of dextran has been discontinued because of potential adverse effects.

We currently advocate the use of dextran only in those patients who develop anastomotic complications associated with white clot platelet aggregate. The loading dose and maintenance doses are standard, but we treat for only 3 days. If a white clot develops intraoperatively, irrigating with dextran may be helpful and is now routinely used.

ASPIRIN. Acetylsalicylic acid given at standard or low doses (325 mg) has an inhibitory effect on platelet aggregation. The antiplatelet aggregation effects are thought to be caused by blockage of thromboxane A_2 production from the cyclooxygenase pathway. The platelet cyclooxygenase enzyme is acetylated and thereby blocks the generation of prostaglandins that are converted to thromboxane A_2. These attributes of aspirin are moderately offset in theory by the inhibition of prostacyclin formation, a vasodilator. We typically administer a dose of 325 mg daily for 14 postoperative days.

FIBRINOLYTIC AGENTS. The use of fibrinolytic agents in microsurgery is controversial. Little evidence shows that local streptokinase, tissue plasminogen activator, and urokinase have efficacy in salvaging free tissue transfers.[44] Other authors have stated that if these agents are used alone, a thrombus often recurs after discontinuation.[115,116]

This literature is consistent with our belief that often the mechanical problem with the anastomosis has lead to the failure, and thus dissolving the clot does not correct the underlying problem.

MICRONEURAL SURGERY

In 1938 Sir Terrence Cawthorne ushered in the modern era of microneural surgery, using an operating microscope on the facial nerve. Before this time, great thinkers and early surgeons had discussed and performed nerve grafts and transfers. Avicenna (980-1037) actually postulated the currently used epineural repair for nerve coaptation. Fascicular repair was described approximately nine centuries later by Langley and Hashimoto.[67] In the eighteenth century, Albrecht von Haller found that nerves control muscle function, and Sir Charles Bell (1774-1842) wrote a textbook on nerves and their disorders. In 1879 Drobnik performed the first nerve transfer of the spinal accessory to the facial nerve. By the early 1900s, Sir Charles Balance, who would be considered a neurotologist today, compared nerve grafts in facial nerve deficits with nerve transfers from lower cranial nerves and found that nerve grafting was superior.[5]

The microscope opened the door to more precise coaptation and manipulation of diseased and injured nerves. In 1957 Wullstein exposed the facial nerve from the geniculate ganglion to the stylomastoid foramen. In 1961 House used a middle cranial fossa approach to the labyrinthine segment of the fallopian canal, leaving both vestibular and cochlear function intact.[113] In 1971 Smith reported the cross-facial nerve graft, and by 1981 Miehlke and Stennert detailed the use of an interpositional graft from the hypoglossal nerve to the facial nerve.[113] May et al[74] later called a similar technique the "jump graft."

Experimental data showed outstanding peripheral nerve repair results in the early 1960s, but few clinical trials have been as optimistic. The results of microneural repair are varied, and research continues. Multiple factors play a role in nerve repair and regeneration. Factors that affect nerve repair can be classified as proximal to the lesion, at the lesion, or distal to the lesion.[124]

Peripheral Nerves

A nerve cell or neuron is made up of a cell body and two extensions, the dendrite and the axon, covered by a Schwann

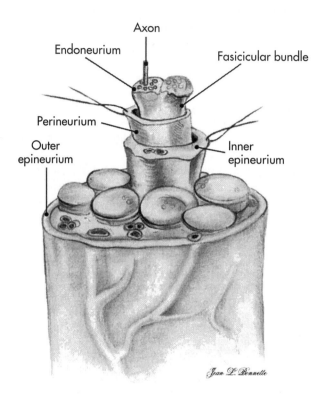

Figure 14-7. Peripheral nerve. Endonerium is between axons. Groups of axons are bundled together in fascicles. Fascicle is surrounded by perineurium, and fascicles are grouped together to form peripheral nerve. Inner epineurium is between fascicular bundles, and outer epineurium surrounds entire group of fascicles (the nerve).

sheath. The axon of one neuron communicates with the dendrite of a following neuron. This connection is termed the *synapse.* The axon is surrounded by endoneurium. Multiple axons are bundled together and are called *fascicles,* which are surrounded by the perineurium. The fascicles are grouped together to form the nerve. The fascicles are surrounded by an outer epineurium and an inner epineurium that intertwines between the fascicles. A longitudinal capillary plexus is found around each fascicle in the perineurium and around the group of fascicles in the epineurium. Therefore, with two vascular networks for each nerve fascicle, limited fascicular dissection does not devitalize the perineural system in fascicular repair[91] (Figure 14-7).

Nerve Repair

The three distinct nerve repairs are the epineural, perineural, and group fascicular repair. Each has its proponents, but no current data demonstrate that one type is better.

EPINEURAL REPAIR. The epineural repair may be used for all sizes of nerves but is the standard for small nerves. The repair is a completed using 10-0 or 11-0 sutures. This type of repair is technically simple and efficient, requires less magnification than other repairs, and does not disturb the inner contents of the nerve.

Initially the nerve is placed in a tensionless position with the fascicles aligned anatomically. The sutures are placed approximately two to three needle breadths from the cut edge. Care is taken to pass through only the outer lining of the nerve (epineurium). The first two sutures are placed approximately 160 to 180 degrees from each other. The remaining sutures are placed by first closing the front surface, then the back surface. The first two sutures are left long so they can be used to invert the nerve and allow for back surface closure (Figure 14-8).

PERINEURAL (FASCICULAR) REPAIR. The fascicular repair is technically more challenging than an epineural repair, and its superiority over an epineural repair has not been established. The fascicular repair has the theoretic advantage of

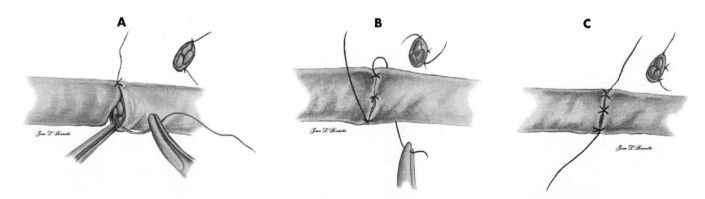

Figure 14-8. Epineural repair. **A,** Outer epineurium is sutured together with 9.0 to 11.0 nylon suture in interrupted fashion. **B,** Anterior surface is closed first. **C,** Corner sutures may be used to rotate nerve so that posterior surface of epineurium can be reapproximated.

improved coaptation of the perineural tubes, allowing for the regenerating axon to enter endoneural tubules of the distal nerve stump.

The fascicular repair is established by first identifying the fascicles in each segment and placing the nerve ends in the best possible alignment. The fascicles are then individually sutured together. Typically the fascicles are approximated using one or two 10.0 or 11.0 nylon perineural sutures (Figure 14-9).

GROUP FASCICULAR REPAIR. Group fascicular repair is typically used when the nerve is transected at a level that allows the specific branches to be identified for specific function. Jabaley[58] has reported specific indications for this type of repair. For the median nerve group, fascicular repair can be used when the transection is 2 to 3 cm distal to the elbow and from 5 cm proximal to the wrist crease to the palm. The ulnar nerve is a candidate for a group fascicular repair at approximately 7 to 8 cm proximal to the wrist crease.

The group fascicular repair is performed by suturing distinct fascicular groups together with inner epineural sutures (Figure 14-10).

Nerve Defect Repair

The ideal nerve repair is the end-end coaptation of the original nerve segments. Unfortunately, this is not always possible, and other options must be considered. Millesi's work in the 1970s

initiated the modern era of nerve grafting.[79] He performed interfascicular nerve grafting (a form of group fascicular repair) and recommended its use for defects 2 cm wide or greater in the radial, median, or ulnar nerves. Nunley et al[87] used nerve grafts in 21 patients for digital nerve defects of 1 cm or greater. With the facial nerve, grafts are considered for defects of 1.7 cm or greater or for any defect when the final repair has tension.[114,129] Facial nerve defects of 1.7 cm or less may be reapproximated by rerouting the mastoid and extratemporal portions of the nerve.

A number of techniques have been found to be viable options for reconstructing nerve deficits. The most common technique is nonvascularized nerve grafting, although vascularized nerve grafts and conduits have been described.

NONVASCULARIZED NERVE GRAFTING. Nerve grafting may be performed using an epineural, fascicular, or group fascicular repair. Fascicular or group fascicular repair is ideal for large-diameter, multifascicled nerves such as the brachial plexus nerves or sciatic nerve. Ideally the number of fascicles in the graft should be approximately the same as the nerve it is replacing. With group fascicular repair the groups are aligned and sutured together at staggered lengths.

VASCULARIZED NERVE GRAFTING. Vascularized nerve grafts reportedly have a greater number of myelinated axons and earlier regeneration than nonvascularized grafts. The technique requires the transfer of a segment of nerve with its surrounding vascular supply. The nerve is repaired in one of the three techniques discussed earlier, and a microvascular anastomosis is performed to complete the transfer. Portions of the radial nerve-artery, sural nerve-artery, ulnar nerve-artery, and deep peroneal nerve–dorsalis pedis artery complexes have been described.[10,64,100,122] No evidence indicates that this is superior to nonvascularized nerve grafts, but vascularized repair makes intuitive sense if the bed of the graft has compromised vascularity (e.g., irradiated bed).

NERVE CONDUITS. Nerves have been shown to grow through tubular conduits that bridge a gap between the nerve ends. Autogenous vein grafts are the most often used nonneural conduits and are recommended for sensory nerve defects of

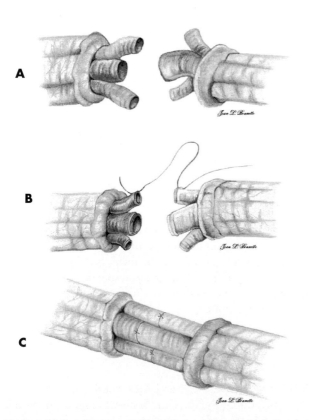

Figure 14-9. Perineural (fascicular) repair. **A,** Identification of fascicles. **B,** Alignment and suturing of fascicles. **C,** End-end repair with minimal sutures.

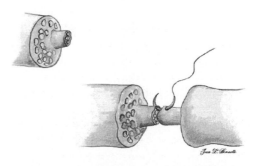

Figure 14-10. Group fascicular repair.

3 cm or less.[27] Experimentally, a variety of degradable synthetic conduits have also been described.

Factors in Nerve Coaptation Results

PROXIMAL TO SITE. The severity of the peripheral nerve injury determines the level of proximal change (axonal degeneration). Typically the degeneration proceeds to the next node of Ranvier. In severe injuries the degeneration can proceed to the anterior horn or the sensory root ganglion neuron.[47] At 24 to 48 hours the cell body swells and the reticular endothelium begins to fragment. On approximately the twelfth day after injury the cell body begins to normalize and the axoplasm flow begins. Some authors believe regeneration begins immediately, whereas others think it starts later as the cell body normalizes.[20,32] Regenerating axons grow at a rate of 1 to 3 mm/day. If the damage is at two levels or is so severe that the cell body is destroyed, nerve repair results are typically poor.[88]

AT SITE. The level of injury and the degree of surrounding tissue injury play a critical role in the regeneration of a lacerated nerve and the final functional outcome. Typically the more proximal the level of injury, the poorer the final result and the greater is the likelihood that the distal tubule has narrowed, scar has formed, and end-organ degeneration has occurred. The end result is blockage of the regenerating nerve. Furthermore, severe soft tissue injury surrounding the nerve may lead to poor blood supply and increased levels of scar tissue that can block the nerve and decrease mobility of the reintervated tissue.

The type of nerve injured plays a role in the regeneration. A pure sensory nerve or a pure motor nerve is more likely to regenerate than a mixed nerve. In a mixed nerve the regenerating axons may not travel down the appropriate sheath.

The degree or type of nerve injury also affects regeneration of a nerve. The degrees of injury described by Seddon[108] and Sunderland[118] are as follows:

1. *Neuropraxia* (Sunderland's first degree): minimal axonal disruption; complete recovery occurs within days to months.
2. *Axonotmesis* (Sunderland's second degree): total axonal disruption with wallerian degeneration; complete regeneration should occur within months.
3. *Neurotmesis* (Sunderland's third, fourth, and fifth degrees): disruption of axon, endoneurium, and possibly the perineurium and epineurium; mild to severe deficits result. Sunderland's third degree is axonal and endoneurial disruption that typically causes mild deficits. Sunderland's fourth degree is disruption of the axon, endoneurium, and perineurium that causes moderate deficits. Sunderland's fifth degree is complete disruption of all layers (complete laceration) and represents the worst prognosis.

DISTAL TO SITE. The most significant factor in nerve regeneration distal to the site of injury appears to be the end organ. Motor end plates degenerate rapidly after injury. The

muscle fibers subsequently atrophy, and scar formation begins. Motor function can return once axonal ingrowth and end-plate regeneration occurs. Two years appears to be the endpoint at which motor function is restored or lost indefinitely. Sensory regeneration appears to be more resilient, with regeneration for as long as 20 years reported.[88]

REPLANTATION

Replantation was the driving force that led to the early development of microsurgery and paved the way for free tissue transfer. In 1896 Murphy[85] opened the door for replantation when he performed the first end-end anastomosis on separated tissue. As stated earlier, Hopfner performed the first experimental dog limb replantation in 1903. In 1906 Carrel and Guthrie opened the door to composite tissue replantation and to transplantation. In 1954 the Nobel laureate Joseph Murray performed the first kidney transplantation at the Peter Bent Brigham Hospital, but a successful human replantation was not performed until 1962. A 12-year-old boy with an above-elbow amputation underwent replantation by Malt and McKhann.[70] At this same time, two Chinese surgeons reportedly successfully replanted a patient's hand.[39] In 1963 Kleinert and Kasden revascularized both a partial digital amputation and a partial above-elbow amputation. The first thumb replantation was in 1968.[63]

Once digital replantation and composite transplantation became a reality, the replantation of other tissues was inevitable. In 1976 Miller et al[78] and later Van Beek and Zook[126] replanted avulsed scalp. Tamai et al[121] performed a penile and scrotal replantation in 1977. The first reported ear replantation was by Pennington et al[95] in 1980, with an upper lip by Holtje[57] in 1984 and a nose by Tajima et al[119] in 1989. In 1985 Leuing[69] and in 1986 Frykman et al[36] reported their results of toe-to-thumb and toe-to-hand transfer. With the advent of more precise immunologic genetic engineering and pharmacologic agents, a successful extremity transplantation is on the horizon.

Indications

The indications for replantation of an amputated part have changed dramatically since the advent of this type of surgery. Initially the majority of amputated appendages were replanted without an understanding of postoperative function. Most amputated appendages now can be reattached and revascularized, but the decision to replant the amputated part must be made with an understanding of future function. Although guillotine-type amputations are ideal for replantation, the majority of amputations are crush and avulsion injuries. These injuries are more difficult to repair and have a lower percentage of survival and long-term function.

HEAD AND NECK. Head and neck injuries vary greatly in severity. Because of the dramatic aesthetic component of this anatomy and the high vascularity of the surrounding non-avulsed tissues, replantation of facial structures should be attempted. This is typically more difficult than extremity replantation, mainly because of the small, fragile, and often inadequate veins to reanastomose. Structures ideal for replantation are as follows:

1. Scalp avulsions where a large single unit is present (excellent if superficial temporal vessels are available)
2. Large nasal facial avulsions of any kind (involving one or more facial units)
3. Auricular injuries with present vessels

GENITAL. As with head and neck injuries, genital injuries are typically replanted if possible.

UPPER EXTREMITY AND DIGITS. In general, upper extremity amputations are warranted for the following:

1. Midpalm, wrist, or forearm
2. Thumb
3. Multidigit amputations
4. Digital amputations distal to insertion of superficial vessels
5. Guillotine amputations above elbow (with warm ischemia less than 6 hours)
6. Pediatric amputations

LOWER EXTREMITY. Lower extremity amputations are seldom suitable for replantation because of the extensive zone of injury in traumatic amputation. Guillotine-type amputations may be considered, however, for replantation in children and young adults. Ideally the amputation should be distal to the knee and a nonavulsing injury. Patients with traumatic injuries above the knee should be assessed for partial replantation of the amputated part, which also can be used as a free flap to produce a below-knee amputation. This has been called "spare parts surgery."[97]

Operations

The basic tenets of microvascular surgery are relatively the same as those used in free tissue transfer. The main differences involve management of the amputated part before revascularization. Initially the amputated part should be placed in a plastic bag with moist gauze and transferred with the patient. The bag should be resting in an ice bath. Once the patient's stability is confirmed, the part is removed and evaluated for adequacy for replantation. After the body parts have been evaluated and prepared for replantation, a plan of reconstruction should be established so that all members of the team understand the reconstructive goals. Our basic reconstructive plan is as follows:

1. Debridement and tissue preparation
2. Bony shortening and fixation
3. Tendon repair
4. Arterial repair
5. Venous repair
6. Nerve repair
7. Skin and soft tissue closure

DEBRIDEMENT AND TISSUE PREPARATION. During tissue preparation the body part is placed on a separate sterile field and readied for replantation. Ideally, two teams separately address the patient and the amputated part. Vessels that have been avulsed or have damaged portions should be cut back to normal tissue. The blue streaking seen in skin overlying an avulsion injury is a telltale sign of vascular intimal damage. In a rabbit avulsion injury model, Mitchell et al[80] found that the average length of vessel injury beyond the cut end was 0.8 cm but could extend as far as 4 cm. The wound edges should be debrided to viable tissue. Too much shortening of a body part can lead to muscle tendon imbalances and should be avoided if possible.

The extremities not involved with the injury should be prepared for possible vein or nerve grafts. If an amputated portion of the body is not replantable, it should be considered for "spare parts." Vein grafts, tendons, digits, and even joints often can be salvaged and used to reconstruct a more functional extremity.

BONY SHORTENING AND FIXATION AND TENDON REPAIR. With an amputated extremity or digit, bony fixation is the first step in reattachment of a severed part. Fixation is accomplished using wires, plates, lag screws, or external fixators. We prefer to use crossed and intramedullary Kirschner wires, which can be rapidly applied. The type of fixation depends on the wound, the type of rehabilitation planned, and patient compliance.

Shortening of the bones may be necessary to reapproximate good tissue, but overresecting must be avoided, since an imbalance of the tendons and muscles can develop, leading to less than optimal function. The flexor and extensor tendons are then repaired using conventional techniques.

ARTERIAL AND VENOUS REPAIRS. A tension-free repair of the vessels is the goal. If too much tension is apparent or the gap between viable vessel ends is too great, a vein graft or vascular transfer from adjacent digit should be used. Veins from the hand, foot dorsum, saphenous vein, or "spare parts" are common sources. If venous repair is not possible, Gordon et al[46] have described a 71% survival rate in digital replantations by giving systemic heparin and removing the nail beds.

The addition of leeches is another option. Leeches release *hirudin,* a selective thrombin inhibitor, and decompress venous congestion. A small pinprick is made in the skin, and the leech is applied to the site and attaches. Once the leech is completely engorged, it will release. The site continues to bleed because of hirudin's local antithrombotic effects. These patients should receive prophylactic antibiotics because *Aeromonas hydrophila* infections have been reported using leech therapy.[76] The antibiotics of choice are ciprofloxacin, tetracycline, or trimethoprim-sulfamethoxazole.

NERVE REPAIR. As stated previously, nerve repair is typically performed using an epineural technique. If a segment of a nerve is missing, an interpositional graft can be placed. The placement of a nerve graft requires a thoroughly debrided, well-vascularized bed. Severed nerves, which are found in a poorly vascularized dirty wound, may be marked with a prolene suture and repaired secondarily. Nerve grafts may be taken from nonviable amputated tissue or from any one of multiple sensory nerves, the most common being the sural nerve.

SKIN AND SOFT TISSUE CLOSURE. Closure of the skin and soft tissue requires a simple common-sense approach. The closure must be nonconstricting to prevent vascular compromise. Simple interrupted sutures are spaced widely to allow for edema. Penrose drains offer a site of drainage for traumatized tissues and prevent hematoma formation. If a large defect is present, a skin graft may be warranted or even a free tissue transfer. These decisions are made on a case-by-case basis. Godina[42] presented his data on early free tissue transfer for extremity coverage and found that early free flap surgery was superior to delayed coverage.

Outcomes

EXTREMITY. Many different approaches are used to record functional recovery. In 1972 Malt et al[71] reported functional outcomes of a major limb replantation. Chen et al[25] used a grading scale to record functional recovery of 214 replantation patients. Grade I (excellent) patients were able to return to work and had at least 60% range of motion. Grade II (good) patients could resume suitable work with 40% or more range of motion. Grade III (fair) patients were able to function in daily life but had only 30% or greater range of motion. Grade IV (poor) patients had negligible function. Most patients were grades II and III; 34% were grade I and 4% grade IV.

Tamai[120] reported an overall 88% survival with 293 replantations, of which 261 were digital. He used the same functional scale as Chen for evaluating arm and forearm amputations. For hand and digit replantations a separate grading scale considered range of motion, activities of daily life, sensation, subjective symptoms, cosmesis, and patient satisfaction. Five of the patients had arm amputations, four of whom had fair or poor results. Of 10 patients with forearm amputations, half had good or excellent results and half fair to poor results. Fourteen patients had hand amputations, and 63% had good or better results. Digital replants ranged from 39% excellent, 36% good, 13% fair, to 11% poor. Matsuda et al[72] found that 60% of their replantation patients had effective grasp, pinch, and sensation.

THUMB. The thumb is the most important digit of the hand, and every effort is made to replant an amputated thumb. Schlenker et al[104] studied the functional results of 20 replanted thumbs. They found that nine patients had two-point discrimination of less than 10 mm. The average range of motion for the metacarpophalangeal joint was 29 degrees and interphalangeal joint 35 degrees.

FREE VASCULARIZED TISSUE TRANSFER

Despite previous microvascular transfer of tissues, the report of a cutaneous flap transfer by Daniel and Taylor[30] in 1973 sparked the rapid development of free flap surgery (see earlier section on history). Initially, few flaps were available for transfer, but this new field of surgery stimulated extensive anatomic studies of blood supply to the skin and other tissues. Many different vascularized tissues are now available for microvascular reconstruction. The initial thrust of microvascular free tissue transfer 25 years ago was to obtain survival, which in recent years has been greater than 95%. Today the thrust has shifted to the refinement and increased function of the reconstruction.

Indications

The indications for the transfer of free vascularized tissue are relative. Many factors must be evaluated and are different for different sites. A reconstructive ladder is developed for each specific anastomotic site, with consideration of the defect's location, the region's native vascular supply, the wound bed, the patient's overall general health, and the reconstructive team's experience and expertise. The basic concepts of the reconstructive ladder must be understood before the surgeon can proceed with the surgical plan. The reconstructive ladder generally starts with the basic tenets of wound healing: can the defect site heal without surgical manipulation? This may be possible for small defects, and the simple approach may be the best. The next rungs of the reconstructive ladder, in ascending order of complexity, are skin graft, local flap, regional flap, and free tissue transfer.

HEAD AND NECK. Head and neck patients undergoing ablative surgery are often good candidates for free flap reconstruction if any of the following applies:

1. The operative site requires a compound flap, and considerable bone stock, or the mandibular symphysis is needed for reconstruction.
2. A large defect cannot be closed with a regional flap.
3. A multilaminated structure needs to be constructed.
4. A sensate flap is required to help restore normal function.
5. Facial reanimation surgery is being considered and may require a functional muscle flap.
6. A complex defect requires a free flap for structure and a local flap for coverage.

CHEST AND TRUNK. Patients with defects of the chest and trunk have similar indications as head and neck patients, but the number of satisfactory regional flaps available is significantly higher. Skin grafts, local flaps, and regional flaps are the mainstays of chest and neck reconstruction. Free vascularized tissue transfer is reserved for patients with no other options, with the possible exception of the patient with breast reconstruction. Free flap reconstruction for breast cancer patients has recently expanded, and many surgeons believe that free transverse rectus abdominis muscle (TRAM) reconstruction offers the best result.

UPPER EXTREMITY. Free flap reconstruction is indicated in the upper extremity when local flap options are inadequate to obtain satisfactory coverage. Other patients may require vascularized tissue transferred to an ischemic bed or request aesthetic reconstruction of a large, soft tissue defect. Composite reconstruction of major losses with similar tissue from the other extremities provides the best possible reconstruction without transplantation. Free toe, joint, toenail, and vascularized tendon transfers are frequently performed techniques.

LOWER EXTREMITY. The indications for free vascularized reconstruction of lower extremities are similar to those in other areas, that is, lack of a well-vascularized wound bed and inadequacy of the other reconstructive ladder options. Large, lower one-third tibiofibular defects typically require free tissue transfer because no suitable alternatives exist. The reason is the lack of local regional flaps, although recent reports have popularized the reverse-pedicled fasciocutaneous flaps for selected small and moderately sized defects.

The timing of free flap reconstruction of traumatic lower extremity wounds is essential to the final healing. Byrd et al[19] evaluated open tibial fractures and found that during the first 6 days after injury the wound is in an acute phase and is not yet colonized. During the next 6 weeks the wound is in a subacute phase and is colonized. Flaps transferred during this period have a higher incidence of complications because of the infectious risks. After the 6-week period the wound is in a chronic wound state. A wound with granulation tissue characterizes the chronic phase, which represents a more viable tissue bed.

We recommend debridement and flap coverage of type III tibial wounds early, within the first 6 days. If the flap closure is not possible during this time, attempted flap closure may still be considered on a case-by-case basis, but a potentially higher complication rate may result.[19,42]

Operations

The patient is prepared for free tissue transfer by first detailing the flap pattern on the patient's skin. The future position of the pedicle, its specific length, and the vascular perforators should be marked using Doppler studies. The patient's body should be positioned and prepared so a venous graft can be taken without difficulty. Once the free flap has been isolated and the recipient vessels identified, multiple steps prepare the vessels for anastomotic repair, as described earlier.

Outcomes

Mostly retrospective reports have evaluated specific variables in free tissue transfer. A recently completed, multiinstitutional prospective study evaluated a variety of factors affecting free tissue transfer outcome, tobacco use, irradiated bed, vein graft, end-end versus end-side, dextran, heparin, aspirin, and free flap type. Over 6 months, 493 free flaps were preoperatively studied and registered. The results are included in the following discussions.

AGE

The patient's age has long been thought to be a variable in free tissue transfer, but the literature suggests that advanced age alone is not an absolute contraindication to patient selection.

The patient's general health must be the determining factor for selection. Pediatric patients have outstanding free flap survival rates and few nonsurgical complications. Parry et al[93] reported a 96% free flap survival rate in children. Canales et al[21] reviewed their 16-year experience with free tissue transfer and found similar complication and survival rates between their pediatric and adult populations.

Older patients have similarly high free flap survival rates, but postoperative morbidity must be considered. Shestak and Jones[111] reported a free flap survival rate of 99% in patients ranging in age from 50 to 79. In the 94 free flaps, however, 30% developed complications. Interestingly, the majority of the complications were nonsurgical, and mortality was 5.4%. Chick et al[26] performed free tissue transfers in 31 patients over age 65, and 30 had good outcomes. Khouri et al[61] found no difference in free flap survival when extremes of age were evaluated.

IRRADIATION. Irradiated blood vessels have fragile walls, decreased smooth muscle, and endothelial dehiscence, but survival of free tissue transfer to irradiated sites is similar to that in nonirradiated sites.[48,127] Mulholland et al[84] demonstrated no significant survival difference between free flaps transferred to radiated and nonirradiated head and neck defects. In a review of 308 free flaps, poor flap survival occurred in two groups of patients: those who had undergone previous surgery and those requiring vein grafts.[107] Vein grafts were more often needed in the patients with prior surgery and radiation. Khouri et al[61] found that reconstruction of an irradiated recipient site and use of a skin-grafted free flap were significant predictors of flap failure, with increased odds of 4.2 and 11.1, respectively.

The key techniques to working in an irradiated bed are similar to those used in the patients with severe peripheral vascular disease. Guelinckx[49] offers the following recommendations for surgery on the irradiated patient:

1. Minimize dissection of recipient vessels.
2. Limit use of electrocoagulation.
3. Decrease intramural dissection by directing the microneedle from inside to outside.
4. Use the smallest gauge needle possible.
5. As always, limit clamp time and use heparinized saline flush throughout the procedure.

TOBACCO. Smoking has been shown to lead to vasospasm and poor wound healing. Nicotine, found in varying levels in tobacco, inhibits platelet aggregation and stimulates the release of catecholamines, leading to the vasoconstriction.[13,45] Random pattern flaps and random portions of pedicled flaps are known to be at a higher risk with tobacco use.

Reus et al[99] reported on a retrospective review of free flap survival in smokers and nonsmokers. Free tissue transfer survival for nonsmokers was 95% and 94% for smokers, but wound healing at the recipient site of a patient using tobacco was a significant problem. The results seen in the multiinstitutional study[61] are consistent with these authors' findings that smokers are not at a higher risk for free flap loss. Perforator free flaps, however, may be different. A 1999 prospective study found that smokers who underwent perforator flap breast reconstruction had a significant increase in reexploration and delayed healing.[51]

The findings suggest that vasoconstriction caused by nicotine may be offset by its inhibitory platelet aggregation effects. The larger vessels supplying the free flap are in equilibrium, but not the potentially less vascularized recipient bed.

We recommend that the patient stop smoking at the earliest possible date before surgery and to continue in a nonsmoking status for a minimum of 2 weeks while the anastomosis reendothelializes and the recipient wound heals.

TIME OF WOUNDING. The timing for reconstruction of wounds seems rather specific. As stated earlier, Byrd et al[19] found that a traumatic, open-fracture wound has acute, subacute, and chronic phases. During the subacute phase, 1 to 6 weeks after injury, the wound is typically colonized and represents a poor tissue bed. Godina[42] reviewed 532 patients who had undergone complex extremity wound reconstruction with free vascularized tissue. He divided patients into three groups. The first (acute) group consisted of patients who had undergone free flap coverage of a lower extremity wound in the first 72 hours. The second group was covered between 72 hours and 3 months. The final (chronic) group underwent free flap coverage from 3 months to 12.6 years. The free tissue transfer failure rate was 0.75% in the first group, 12% in the second group, and 9.5% in the final group. Postoperative infections were found in 1.5% of the acute group, 17.5% of the second group, and 6% of the chronic group.

END-END VERSUS END-SIDE ANASTOMOSES. Parsa and Spira[94] and Albertengo et al[3] found no significant difference between the patency of end-end and end-side anastomoses. Others have found that a large size discrepancy in venous anastomosis is more likely to remain patent with an end-side anastomosis. No difference is found between end-end and end-side venous anastomoses with similar vessel diameters. Godina[43] found that nine of 27 free flaps repaired with an end-end anastomosis failed, with no losses in 41 free flaps transferred with an end-side technique. Although not documented, the size discrepancy may have played a role. In 1997 Samaha et al[103] evaluated 2000 microvascular anastomoses and found no difference between end-end and end-side microvascular techniques.

We recommend end-side anastomosis when (1) size discrepancy is 4:1 or greater, (2) the only recipient option is a major vessel that supplies or drains a distal system, and (3) accessibility of a good vessel for end-end anastomosis is problematic.

VASCULAR GRAFTS. Microvenous grafts are often used in both free tissue transfer and replantation. Mitchell et al[81] studied the long-term fate of microvenous autografts and found patency rates of 98% in intraarterial grafts and 100% in intravenous grafts. The intraarterial grafts thickened due to ingrowth of smooth muscle cells from recipient artery, and a thickened neointima was created. Intravenous grafts maintained normal venous morphology. The length of the graft

does not effect the patency, as evidenced by the work of Fujikawa and O'Brien.[37] Khouri et al[61] found that intraoperative thrombosis was more common in patients requiring venous grafts, but with no increased incidence of flap failure.

MUSCLES AND NERVES. In 1976 Harii et al[53] reported the transfer of a functional gracilis muscle to a patient with facial paralysis. Since that time, many different functional muscle transfers have been reported, with outcomes reported on a case-by-case basis. The recurring theme in all these cases is the need for (1) reestablishing the resting tension of muscle, (2) proper anatomic positioning of the transferred muscle, and (3) nerve repair without tension. Even with all these factors considered, functional outcomes are extremely variable. Kuzon et al[66] reported that functional muscle transfers had significantly less normal activity compared with controls. In a rabbit rectus femoris muscle model, Terzis et al[123] found only 25% of the maximum working capacity developed after a functional muscle transfer.

"Without sensation the hand is blind."[31] This statement by Eric Moberg in 1953 has been modified to represent the oral cavity reconstruction by Urken[125] in 1995. Urken and many other authors stress the importance of oral reconstruction using sensate free flaps. The need not only to maintain oral continence but also to feel the oral cavity is essential for optimal oral function.

Boyd et al[11] compared the oral reconstruction of 16 patients, eight of whom underwent sensate radial forearm flap reconstruction; the other eight underwent nonsensate reconstruction. The two groups were compared along with the normal contralateral side of the oral cavity to the reconstructed side. The innervated radial forearm flap was statistically superior to the noninnervated flap when pain, two-point discrimination, and hot/cold sensations were tested. The normal contralateral side ranked marginally higher than the innervated radial forearm flap reconstruction, but no significant difference was found between the two.

REFERENCES

1. Acland RD: *Microsurgery: a practice manual,* St Louis, 1980, Mosby.

2. Acland RD: Microvascular anastomosis: a device for holding stay sutures and a new vascular clamp, *Surgery* 75:185, 1974.

3. Albertengo JB et al: A comparative study of flap survival rates in end-to-end and end-to-side microvascular anastomoses, *Plast Reconstr Surg* 67:194, 1981.

4. Ames A III et al: Cerebral ischemia. II. The no-reflow phenomenon, *Am J Pathol* 52:437, 1968.

5. Anderson RG: Facial nerve disorders and surgery, *Select Read Plast Surg* 8(20), 1997.

6. Androsov PI: New method of surgical treatment of blood vessel lesion, *Arch Surg* 73:902, 1956.

7. Antia NH, Buch VI: Transfer of an abdominal dermo-fat graft by direct anastomosis of blood vessels, *Br J Plast Surg* 24:15, 1971.

8. Battle J et al: Effect of dextran on factor VIII/von Willebrand factor structure and function, *Thromb Haemost* 54:697, 1985.

9. Biemer E: Vein grafts in microvascular surgery, *Br J Plast Surg* 30:197, 1977.

10. Bonney G et al: Experience with vascularized nerve grafts, *Clin Plast Surg* 11:137, 1984.

11. Boyd B et al: Reinnervated lateral antebrachial cutaneous neurosome flaps in oral reconstruction: are we making sense? *Plast Reconstr Surg* 93:1350, 1994.

12. Brennen MD, O'Brien BM: Patency rates in end to side anastomoses in the rabbit, *Br J Plast Surg* 32:24, 1979.

13. Brinson K, Chakrabarti BK: Effect of nicotine on rabbit blood platelet aggregation, *Atherosclerosis* 20:527, 1974.

14. Buncke HJ Jr, McLean DH: The advantage of a straight needle in microsurgery, 47:602, 1971.

15. Buncke HJ, Murray DE: Autogenous arterial interposition of grafts less than 1 mm in external diameter in rats. In *Transactions of the Sixth International Congress of Plastic and Reconstructive Surgery,* London, 1971, Butterworth.

16. Buncke HJ Jr, Schultz WP: Experimental digital amputation and reimplantation, *Plast Reconstr Surg* 36:62, 1965.

17. Buncke HJ Jr, Schultz WP: Total ear reimplantation in the rabbit utilizing microminiature vascular anastomoses, *Br J Plast Surg* 19:15, 1966.

18. Buncke HJ, Alpert B, Shah KG: Microvascular grafting, *Clin Plast Surg* 5:185, 1978.

19. Byrd HS, Spicer TE, Cierny G III: Management of open tibial fractures, *Plast Reconstr Surg* 76:719, 1985.

20. Cabaud HE, Rodkey WG, Nemeth TJ: Progressive ultrastructural changes after peripheral nerve transection and repair, *J Hand Surg* 7:353, 1982.

21. Canales F et al: Microvascular tissue transfer in pediatric patients: analysis of 106 cases, *Br J Plast Surg* 44:423, 1991.

22. Carrel A: The operative technique of vascular anastomoses and the transplantation of viscera, *Clin Orthop* 29:3, 1963 (English translation; published 1902).

23. Chang WHJ, Petry JJ: Platelets, prostaglandins, and patency in microvascular surgery, *J Microsurg* 2:27, 1980.

24. Chase MD, Schwartz SI: Consistent patency of 1.5 mm arterial anastomoses, *Surg Forum* 13:220, 1962.

25. Chen ZW et al: Present indications and contraindications for replantation as reflected by long-term functional results, *Orthop Clin North Am* 12:849, 1981.

26. Chick LR et al: Free flaps in the elderly, *Plast Reconstr Surg* 90:87, 1992.

27. Chiu DTW, Berish S: A prospective clinical evaluation of autogenous vein grafts used as a nerve conduit for distal sensory nerve defects of 3 cm or less, *Plast Reconstr Surg* 86:928, 1990.

28. Daniel RK, Olding M: An absorbable anastomotic device for microvascular surgery: experimental studies, *Plast Reconstr Surg* 74:329, 1984.

29. Daniel RK, Olding M: An absorbable anastomotic device for microvascular surgery: clinical applications, *Plast Reconstr Surg* 74:337, 1984.

30. Daniel RK, Taylor GI: Distant transfer of an island flap by microvascular anastomoses: a clinical technique, *Plast Reconstr Surg* 52:111, 1973.

31. Dellon AL: The sensational contributions of Erik Moberg, *J Hand Surg* 15B:14, 1990.

32. Ducker TB, Kempe LG, Hayes GJ: Metabolic background for peripheral nerve surgery, *J Neurosurg* 30:270, 1969.

33. English JM, Tittle BJ: Microsurgery: free tissue transfer and replantation, *Select Read Plast Surg* 8(11), 1997.

34. Eriksson E, Anderson WA, Replogie RL: Effects of prolonged ischemia on muscle microcirculation in the cat, *Surg Forum* 25:254, 1974.

35. Flemming AFS et al: Laser-assisted microvascular anastomosis of arteries and veins, *Br J Plast Surg* 41:378, 1988.

36. Frykman GK et al: Functional evaluation of the hand and foot after one-stage toe-to-hand transfer, *J Hand Surg* 11A:9, 1986.

37. Fujikawa S, O'Brien BMC: An experimental evaluation of microvenous grafts, *Br J Plast Surg* 28:244, 1975.

38. Fujimaki A, O'Brien BM, Kurara T, Threlfall GN: Experimental micro anastomosis of 0.4-0.5 mm vessels, 30:269, 1977.

39. Gallico GG III, McCarthy JG, editors: *Plastic surgery,* vol 7, Philadelphia, 1990, Saunders.

40. Garrison FH: *History of medicine,* ed 4, Philadelphia, 1929, Saunders.

41. Glasscock ME, Shambaugh GE, Mitchell JM, editors: *Surgery of the ear,* ed 4, Philadelphia, 1990, Saunders.

42. Godina M: Early microsurgical reconstruction of complex trauma of the extremities, *Clin Plast Surg* 13:619, 1986.

43. Godina M: Preferential use of end-to-end arterial anastomoses in free flap transfers, *Plast Reconstr Surg* 64:673, 1979.

44. Goldberg JA, Pederson WC, Barwick WJ: Salvage of free tissue transfers using thrombolytic agents, *J Reconstr Microsurg* 5:351, 1989.

45. Goodman LS, Gilman AG, Gilman A, editors: *The pharmacological basis of therapeutics,* ed 6, New York, 1980, MacMillian.

46. Gordon L et al: Partial nail plate removal after digital replantation as an alternative method of venous drainage, *J Hand Surg* 10A:360, 1985.

47. Graftstein B: The nerve cell body response to axonotomy, *Exp Neurol* 48:32, 1975.

48. Graham LM et al: Endothelial cell seeding of prosthetic vascular grafts, *Arch Surg* 115:929, 1980.

49. Guelinckx PJ: Scanning electron microscopy of irradiated recipient blood vessels in head and neck free flaps, *Plast Reconstr Surg* 74:217, 1984.

50. Guthrie CC: Some physiologic aspects of blood vessel surgery, *JAMA* 51:1658, 1908.

51. Hamdi M, Weiler-Mithoff E, Webster M: Deep inferior epigastric perforator flap in breast reconstruction: experience with first 50 flaps, *Plast Reconstr Surg* 103:86, 1999.

52. Harii K, Ohmori S: Use of the gastroepiploic vessels as recipient or donor vessels in the free transfer of composite flaps by microvascular anastomosis, *Plast Reconstr Surg* 52:541, 1973.

53. Harii K, Ohmori K, Torii S: Free gracilis muscle transplantation with microneurovascular anastomoses for the treatment of facial paralysis, *Plast Reconstr Surg* 57:133, 1976.

54. Harris GD, Finseth F, Buncke HJ: Posterior-wall first microvascular anastomotic technique, *Br J Plast Surg* 34:47, 1981.

55. Hayhurst JW, O'Brien BM: Experimental study of microvascular technique, patency rates, and related factors, *Br J Plast Surg* 28:128, 1975.

56. Hess F: History of (micro) vascular surgery and the development of small-caliber blood vessel prostheses (with some notes on patency rates and re-endothelialization), *Microsurgery* 6:59, 1985.

57. Holtje WJ: Successful replantation of an amputated upper lip, *Plast Reconstr Surg* 73:664, 1984.

58. Jabaley ME: Current concepts of nerve repair, *Clin Plast Surg* 8:33, 1981.

59. Jacobson JH, Suarez EL: Microsurgery in anastomosis of small vessels, *Surg Forum* 11:243, 1960.

60. Khouri RK et al: Thrombosis of microvascular anastomoses in traumatized vessels: fibrin versus platelets, *Plast Reconstr Surg* 86:110, 1990.

61. Khouri RK et al, International Microvascular Research Group: A prospective study of microvascular free-flap surgery and outcome, *Plast Reconstr Surg* 3:711, 1998.

62. Kiyoshige Y: CO_2 laser–assisted microvascular anastomosis: biochemical studies and clinical applications, *J Reconstr Microsurg* 7:225, 1991.

63. Komatsu S, Tamai S: Successful replantation of a completely cut-off thumb: case report, *Plast Reconstr Surg* 42:374, 1968.

64. Koshima I, Harii K: Experimental study of vascularized nerve grafts: multifactorial analyses of axonal regeneration of nerves transplanted into an acute burn wound, *J Hand Surg* 10A:64, 1985.

65. Kurze T: Micro technique in microneurological surgery, *Clin Neurosurg* 11:128, 1964.

66. Kuzon WM Jr et al: The effect of intraoperative ischemia on the recovery of contractile function after free muscle transfer, *J Hand Surg* 13A:263, 1988.

67. Langley JN, Hashimoto M: On the suture of separate nerve bundles in a nerve trunk and on internal nerve plexuses, *J Physiol (Lond)* 51:318, 1917.

68. Lauritzen C: A new and easier way to anastomose microvessels: an experimental study in rats, *Scand J Plast Reconstr Surg* 12:291, 1978.

69. Leuing PC: Thumb reconstruction using second-toe transfer, *Hand Clin* 1:285, 1985.

70. Malt RA, McKhann CF: Replantation of severed arms, *JAMA* 189:716, 1964.

71. Malt RA, Remensynder JP, Harris WH: Long term utility of replanted arms, *Ann Surg* 176:334, 1972.

72. Matsuda M, Shibahara J, Kato N: Long term results of replantation of ten upper extremities, *World J Surg* 2:603, 1978.

73. May JW Jr et al: The no-reflow phenomenon in experimental free flaps, *Plast Reconstr Surg* 61:256, 1978.

74. May M, Sobol SM, Mester SJ: Hypoglossal-facial nerve interpositional-jump graft for facial reanimation without tongue atrophy, *Otolaryngol Head Neck Surg* 104:818, 1991.

75. McLean BH, Buncke HJ Jr: Autotransplant of omentum to a large scalp defect, with microsurgical revascularization, *Plast Reconstr Surg* 49:268, 1972.

76. Mercer NSG et al: Medical leeches as sources of wound infection, *Br Med J* 294:937, 1987.

77. Michon J, Masse P: Le moment optimum de la suture nerveuse dans les plaies du membre superieur, *Rev Chir Orthop* 50:205, 1964.

78. Miller GD, Anstee J, Snell JA: The successful replantation of an avulsed scalp by microvascular anastomoses, *Plast Reconstr Surg* 58:137, 1976.

79. Millesi H: Fascicular nerve repair and interfascicular nerve grafting. In Daniel RK, Terzis JK, editors: *Reconstructive microsurgery,* Boston, 1977, Little, Brown.

80. Mitchell GM et al: A study of the extent and pathology of experimental avulsion injury in rabbit arteries and veins, *Br J Plast Surg* 38:278, 1985.

81. Mitchell GM et al: The long-term fate of microvenous autografts, *Plast Reconstr Surg* 82:473, 1988.

82. Morris DJ, Pribaz JJ: The interrupted-continuous microsurgical suture technique, *Microsurgery* 13:103, 1992.

83. Morris JR, Carter M: Laser assisted microvascular anastomosis (LAMA). Presented at the Annual Meeting of the Orthopedic Research Society, Las Vegas, 1980.

84. Mulholland S et al: Recipient vessels in head and neck microsurgery: radiation effect and vessel access, *Plast Reconstr Surg* 92:628, 1993.

85. Murphy JB: Resection of arteries and veins injured in continuity: end-to-end suture—experimental and clinical research, *Med Rec* 51:73, 1987.

86. Nakayama K: Experience with free autografts of the bowel with a new venous anastomosis apparatus, *Surgery* 55:796, 1964.

87. Nunley JA et al: Use of the anterior branch of the medial antebrachial cutaneous nerve as a graft for the repair of defects of the digital nerve, *J Bone Joint Surg* 58:209, 1976.

88. O'Brien BM, Morrison WA: *Reconstructive microsurgery,* New York, 1987, Churchill Livingstone.

89. O'Brien BM, Henderson PN, Crock GW: Metallized microsutures, *Med J Aust* 1:717, 1970.

90. O'Brien BM et al: Successful transfer of a large island flap from the groin to the foot by microvascular anastomoses, *Plast Reconstr Surg* 52:271, 1973.

91. Orenstein HH: Hand. II. Peripheral nerves and tendon transfers, *Select Read Plast Surg* 7(33), 1995.

92. Overton JH, Owens ER: The successful replacement of minute arteries, *Surgery* 68:713, 1970.

93. Parry SW, Toth BA, Elliot LF: Microvascular free-tissue transfer in children, *Plast Reconstr Surg* 81:838, 1985.

94. Parsa FD, Spira M: Evaluation of anastomotic techniques in the experimental transfer of free skin flaps, *Plast Reconstr Surg* 63:696, 1979.

95. Pennington DG, Lai AD, Pelly AD: Successful replantation of a completely avulsed ear by microvascular anastomoses, *Plast Reconstr Surg* 65:820, 1980.

96. Popov DG, Trichikova PI: A new technique for end-to-end anastomosis in microvascular surgery, *Plast Reconstr Surg* 59:444, 1977.

97. Pribaz JJ, Pelhan F: Upper extremity reconstruction utilizing spare parts. In Hosangadi A, Pederson WC, editors: *Problems in plastic and reconstructive surgery,* Philadelphia, 1993, Lippincott.

98. Pribil S, Powers SK: Carotid artery end-to-end anastomosis in the rat using the argon laser, *J Neurosurg* 63:771, 1985.

99. Reus WF III, Colen LB, Straker DJ: Tobacco smoking and complications in elective microsurgery, *Plast Reconstr Surg* 89:490, 1992.

100. Rose EH, Kowalski TA: Restoration of sensibility to anesthetic scarred digits with free vascularized nerve grafts from the dorsum of the foot, *J Hand Surg* 10A:514, 1985.

101. Rothkopf DM: The effect of dextran on microvascular thrombosis in an experimental rabbit model, *Plast Reconstr Surg* 92:511, 1993.

102. Ruiz-Razura A et al: Bursting strength in CO_2 laser–assisted microvascular anastomosis, *J Reconstr Microsurg* 4:291, 1988.

103. Samaha FJ et al: A clinical study of end-end versus end-side techniques for microvascular anastomosis, *Plast Reconstr Surg* 99:1109, 1997.

104. Schlenker JD, Kleinert HE, Tsai TM: Methods and results of replantation following traumatic amputation of the thumb in sixty-four patients, *J Hand Surg* 5:63, 1980.

105. Schneider PR, Pribaz JJ, Russell RC: Microvenous graft length determination for arterial repair, *Ann Plast Surg* 4:292, 1986.

106. Schumacker HB, Lowenberg RI: Experimental studies in vascular repair, *Surgery* 24:79, 1948.

107. Schusterman MA et al: A single center's experience with 308 free flaps for repair of head and neck cancer defects, *Plast Reconstr Surg* 93:472, 1994.

108. Seddon HJ: Three types of nerve injury, *Brain* 66:237, 1943.

109. Seidenberg B, Hurwitt ES, Carton CA: Technique of anastomosing small arteries, *Surg Gynaecol Obstet* 106:743, 1958.

110. Shenaq SM, Klebuc MJM, Vargo D: Free-tissue transfer with the aid of loupe magnification: experience with 251 procedures, *Plast Reconstr Surg* 95:261, 1995.

111. Shestak KC, Jones NF: Microsurgical free-tissue transfer in the elderly patient, *Plast Reconstr Surg* 88:259, 1991.

112. Smith JW: Microsurgery of peripheral nerves, *Plast Reconstr Surg* 33:317, 1964.

113. Smith JW: A new technique of facial reanimation. In Hueston JT, editor: *Transactions of the Fifth International Congress of Plastic and Reconstructive Surgery,* Melbourne, 1971, Butterworth.

114. Spector JG et al: Facial nerve regeneration through autologous nerve grafts: a clinical and experimental study, *Laryngoscope* 101:537, 1991.

115. Stein B, Fuster V: Antithrombotic therapy in acute myocardial infarction: prevention of venous, left ventricular and coronary artery thromboembolism, *Am J Cardiol* 64:33B, 1989.

116. Stein B et al: Antithrombotic therapy in cardiac disease, *Circulation* 80:1501, 1989.

117. Sully L, Nightingale GM, O'Brien BM, Hurley JV: An experimental study of the sleeve technique in microarterial anastomoses, *Plast Reconstr Surg* 70:186, 1982.

118. Sunderland S: *Nerves and nerve injuries,* ed 2, Edinburgh, 1978, Churchill Livingstone.

119. Tajima S, Ueda K, Tanaka Y: Successful replantation of a bitten-off nose by microvascular anastomosis, *Microsurgery* 10:5, 1989.

120. Tamai S: Twenty years' experience of limb replantation: review of 293 upper extremity replants, *J Hand Surg* 7:549, 1982.

121. Tamai S, Nakamura Y, Motomiya Y: Microsurgical replantation of a completely amputated penis and scrotum, *Plast Reconstr Surg* 60:287, 1977.

122. Taylor GI, Ham FJ: The free vascularized nerve graft: a further experimental and clinical application of microvascular techniques, *Plast Reconstr Surg* 57:413, 1976.

123. Terzis JK et al: Recovery of function in free muscle transplants using microneurovascular anastomoses, *J Hand Surg* 3:37, 1978.

124. Terzis J, Daniel RK, Terzis J, editors: *Reconstructive microsurgery,* Boston, 1977, Little, Brown.

125. Urken ML: The restoration or preservation of sensation in the oral cavity following ablative surgery, *Arch Otolaryngol Head Neck Surg* 121:607, 1995.

126. Van Beck A, Zook EG: Scalp replantation by microsurgical revascularization, *Plast Reconstr Surg* 61:774, 1978.

127. Watson KS: Experimental microvascular anastomosis in radiated vessels: a study of the patency rate and the histopathology of healing, *Plast Reconstr Surg* 63:525, 1979.

128. Wolff KD, Stiller D: Ischemia tolerance of free-muscle flaps: an NMR-spectroscopic study in the rat, *Plast Reconstr Surg* 91:485, 1993.

129. Yarbrough WG, Brownlee RE, Pillsbury HC :Primary anastomosis of extensive facial nerve defects: an anatomic study, *Am J Otol* 14:238, 1993.

130. Yasargil MG: Experimental small vessels in the dog including patching and grafting of cerebral vessels in the formation of functional extracranial shunts. In Donaghy RPM, Yasargil MG, editors: *Microvascular surgery,* St Louis, 1967, Mosby.

131. Yeh H-S et al: Human umbilical artery for microvascular grafting: experimental study in the rat, *J Neurosurg* 61:737, 1984.

CHAPTER

Lasers in Plastic Surgery

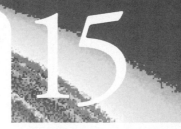

15

Bruce M. Achauer
Victoria M. VanderKam

The origin of current laser systems dates back to 1916, when Einstein proposed his theory of *l*ight *a*mplification by *s*timulated *e*mission of *r*adiation. The principles of this theory are the foundation of the laser, and from it the laser derived its name as an acronym. In the 1950s, building on Einstein's theory, Shcawlow and Townes created a device called a *maser* (*m*icrowave *a*mplification by *s*timulated *e*mission of *r*adiation), which intensified a beam of microwaves. In 1957 they decided to produce a similar device that would amplify much shorter, visible light, an *optical laser.*

Simultaneously, Theodore Maiman was working on such a device at the Hughes Corporation in California. Using a synthetic pink ruby crystal, he succeeded in producing the first *optical maser* in 1960. It amplified light rather than microwaves and was given the name *laser.* To demonstrate the power of this light beam, the millisecond pulse of light was used to drill a tiny hole through a stack of razor blades. It was reportedly suggested that the power of the laser light should be measured not in watts but in "gillettes."

In the next 4 years, laser inventions proliferated. In 1961, Java and others developed the helium-neon (HeNe) laser, and Johnson developed the neodymium:yttrium-aluminum-garnet (Nd:YAG) laser. The argon laser (blue-green visible beam) was developed in 1962 by Bennett. In 1964, Pate and colleagues developed the carbon dioxide (CO_2) laser. These lasers represent the foundation of lasers still in use.

PHYSICS OF LASERS

The basic unit of light is the *photon.* Whether discussing light generated from a bulb or that from a laser, both are composed of this basic unit. Laser energy is created by stimulated emission of radiation. When atoms achieve an "excited" state, they begin to emit photons (Figure 15-1). These atoms then collide with another excited atom, stimulating emission of yet another photon (Figure 15-2). These photons travel at the same frequency along the same axis.

Creating a laser beam requires several key components:

(1) an energy source, (2) a "lasing" medium (gas or solid state), and (3) a laser cavity (Figure 15-3). An external power source is used to excite the atoms of the lasing medium. This results in the atoms being in an excited state. These excited atoms are reflected back and forth between mirrors on the inside of the laser cavity.

Random spontaneous emission initiated as energy is delivered to the laser medium. This energy, in the form of photons, is reflected and multiplied within the laser cavity. A portion of light is passed through a partially reflective mirror, producing the laser beam. The beam is then delivered through fiberoptics or a handpiece. The resulting light has the qualities of coherence, monochromaticity, and intensity.

Properties of Lasers

The photons produced in a laser retain the beam's properties, which are frequency, wavelength, and energy. The difference lies in the organization.

Lasers have three distinct qualities that distinguish them from natural light. Light from a bulb radiates in all directions. As it disperses, the intensity decreases. Laser light does not diverge (Figure 15-4); a laser emits light in waves that are *coherent* (Figure 15-5). Coherence is the state in which all the waves of the light are spatially and temporally in phase.

Natural light comprises all colors and wavelengths in the visual band of the electromagnetic spectrum. In contrast, laser light is usually *monochromatic.* A specific wavelength is selected and then produced based on the lasing medium. This specific wavelength becomes the basis of the therapeutic effect. A wavelength is matched to the absorption spectrum of a specific tissue or structure (Figure 15-6). This allows that target to be altered or selectively destroyed.

The third way in which laser light differs from natural light is *intensity.* Photons produced by a laser are the greatest per unit area than any other form of light. This property allows for great variation in tissue effects by varying the laser's power. Effects vary from gently heating tissue with low power to causing an explosion at high powers.

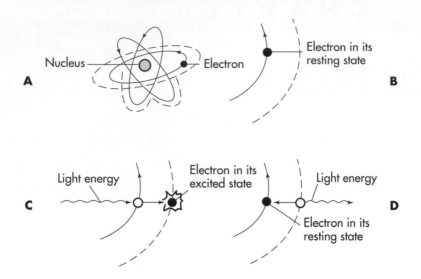

Figure 15-1. **A** and **B,** Electron in its resting state. **C,** Light energy is absorbed, causing transition of atom to excited state. **D,** Energy is released as light when electron returns to resting state.

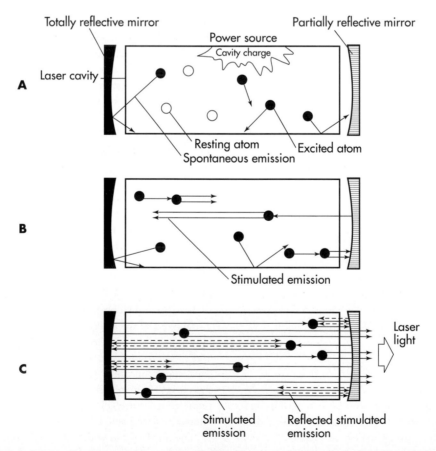

Figure 15-2. Production of laser light. **A,** Atoms are excited by external power source. **B,** As spontaneous emission increases, stimulated emission results as photons collide with other excited atoms. Mirrors reflect light back and forth, and production of light is amplified. **C,** Small portion of light is emitted from cavity.

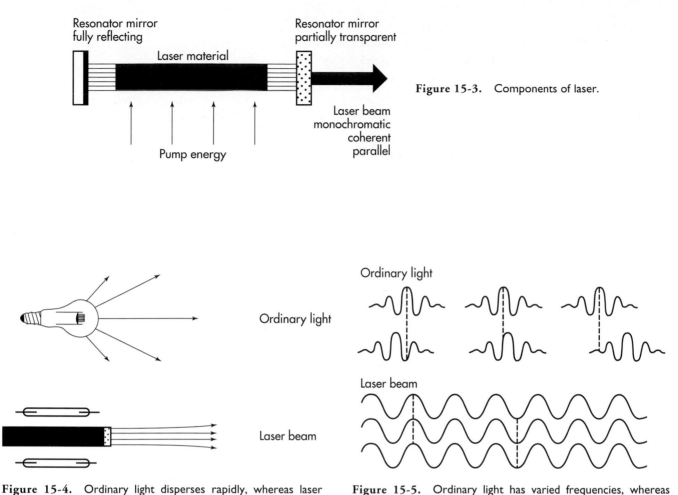

Figure 15-3. Components of laser.

Figure 15-4. Ordinary light disperses rapidly, whereas laser light does not diverge.

Figure 15-5. Ordinary light has varied frequencies, whereas laser light has fixed frequency and is coherent.

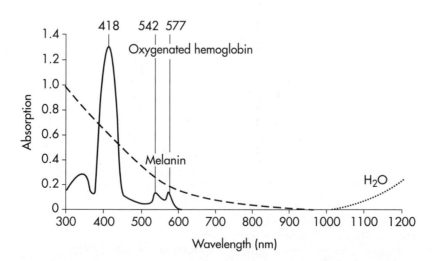

Figure 15-6. Absorption spectrum of prominent chromophores of skin: melanin, oxygenated hemoglobin, and water (H_2O). Hemoglobin has peaks at 418, 542, and 577 nm.

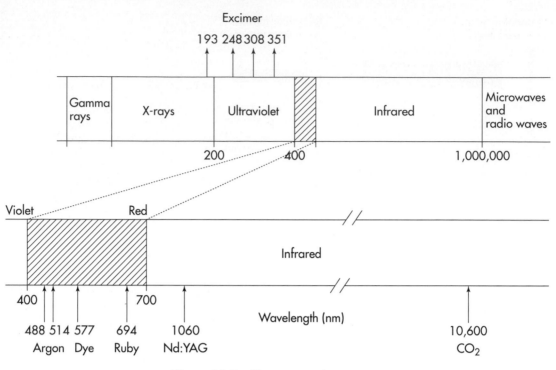

Figure 15-7. Electromagnetic spectrum.

Electromagnetic Spectrum

The electromagnetic spectrum ranges from gamma rays to radio waves (Figure 15-7). Most clinical lasers are in the visible portion (400 to 700 nm) of the spectrum. The therapeutic use of lasers depends on the energy delivered to the tissue and the mode in which it is delivered.

Mastery of a few concepts can help the surgeon to understand and effectively use laser light. These concepts are energy, power, fluence (energy density), and irradiance.

Energy is measured in joules. It is an expression of work. *Power* is expressed in watts (joules per second) and is the rate at which energy is expended as follows:

$$\text{Power density} = \text{Watts/cm}^2$$

These two parameters, energy and power, are a quantitative measure of the light emitted from a laser. Another term must be available for measuring the impact of the laser on the skin. This is *energy density,* expressed as follows:

$$\text{Energy density} = \text{power density (watts/cm}^2 \times \text{time [sec]/cm}^2)$$

By varying the laser's spot size, the energy density can be dramatically changed. For example, by cutting the spot size in half, the energy density increases by a factor of 4. To achieve the same energy density with a spot size of one-half the laser energy, output must be decreased by a factor of 4. *Fluence* and energy density are interchangeable terms.

Irradiance refers to the intensity of a continuous-wave (CW)

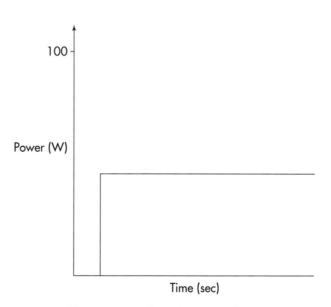

Figure 15-8. Continuous-wave laser.

laser beam and is measured in watts per square centimeter. Irradiance is inversely proportional to the square of the radius of the spot size.

MODES OF DELIVERY

Laser energy may be delivered in a variety of modes, including CW, pulsed, or Q switched. A *continuous wave* is an uninterrupted beam of light without pulses (Figures 15-8 and 15-9). In contrast, a laser may be delivered in an interrupted or

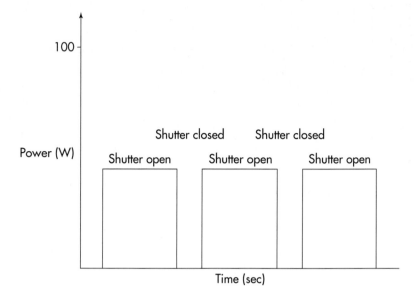

Figure 15-9. Continuous-wave laser electronically shuttered to create three pulses of equal duration.

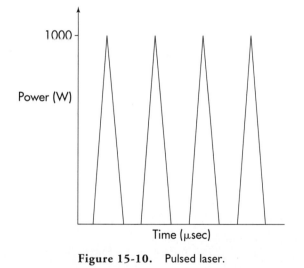

Figure 15-10. Pulsed laser.

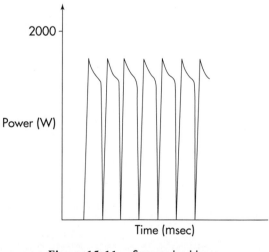

Figure 15-11. Superpulsed laser.

pulsed manner. In a *pulsed mode,* laser light is delivered in the form of single pulses or a train of pulses (Figure 15-10). In the *superpulsed mode,* pulses have extremely high peak powers with each pulse (Figure 15-11). The pulses are very brief, and the repetition rate may be varied.

Q switching is created when one of the resonating mirrors is nonreflective for an interval of pumping (Figure 15-12). The mirror is then made reflective. When this switch occurs, the stored energy in the lasing medium is emitted as a pulse of light approximately 10 billionths of a second in length.

Beam Profile

In addition to variations in the mode of delivery, the beam profile may also vary. A cross section of laser energy distribution demonstrates that the beam does not have uniform intensity (Figure 15-13). The most common beam profile is the TEM_{00}.

Skin Optics

When laser light contacts the target, the interaction depends on the wavelength and the composition of the target substance. The energy may be *reflected;* when light cannot be absorbed or

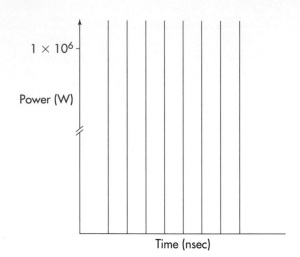
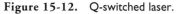

Figure 15-12. Q-switched laser.

cannot pass through (e.g., contact with metal), it bounces off. The light may be *transmitted,* such as passing through glass unchanged. The light also may be *refracted* (direction of light change) or *scattered* (light dispersed randomly). Laser light may be *absorbed* as well (Figure 15-14).

TISSUE INTERACTIONS

Thermal
Laser light creates a tissue effect once it is absorbed. The effect is primarily thermal (Figure 15-15). The extent of thermal effect is influenced by the following:

1. Absorption of the light by the chromophore
2. Diffusion of the heat to adjacent tissues

Key factors that determine the extent of thermal damage

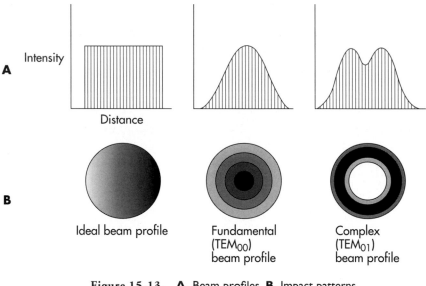

Figure 15-13. **A,** Beam profiles. **B,** Impact patterns.

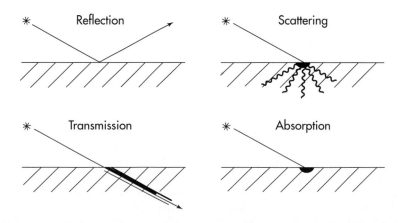

Figure 15-14. Laser light interacts with tissue in various ways. It may be reflected, scattered, transmitted, or absorbed.

are (1) energy density, (2) pulse duration, and (3) heat conduction. Thermal effects can be minimized by manipulation of these parameters.

Mechanical

A photomechanical effect may be created by laser energy. If a pulse duration that is shorter than the thermal relaxation time of the target is used, *thermoelastic expansion* will occur. This change is sudden and generates acoustic waves that damage the surrounding structures.

Selective Photothermolysis

A major breakthrough for treatment of cutaneous lesions resulted from the theory of selective photothermolysis proposed by Anderson and Parrish.[7] This theory has the following two components:

1. The wavelength of the laser specifically determines the absorption of the laser energy in the tissue.
2. The exposure time of the laser light (pulse width) limits the thermal diffusion if the pulse width is less than the thermal relaxation time of the tissues.

Thermal relaxation time is defined as the time required for a specific tissue to absorb and transmit the thermal energy of a specific wavelength. Thermal injury is based on the lateral spread of heat from the point of laser impact into the adjacent tissue. To minimize thermal injury and tissue necrosis, the appropriate pulse width is chosen. *Pulse width* is defined as the duration of the pulse. The ideal pulse width is less than the thermal relaxation time for the target tissue.

By developing lasers with wavelengths highly specific to the target tissue and with pulse widths to match thermal relaxation times of specified tissues, laser therapy has been refined. Undesirable tissue damage, which leads to delayed healing and scarring, has been minimized. When laser light passes through tissue and is absorbed by the target, the clinical result is maximized.

Research and development of lasers has concentrated on creating lasers that can be selectively absorbed by the desired target substance. These target substances are known as *chromophores* (Figure 15-16). Primary chromophores in the skin are hemoglobin, melanin, and water. Chromophores also may be from an exogenous source, such as tattoo pigments. When a particular wavelength has a predominant chromophore in the skin, it is highly absorbed by it. Minimal scatter of the laser light occurs, and the desired clinical result is maximized.

Thermally induced damage to the epidermis and papillary dermis has limited the cutaneous treatment of vascular lesions. Various cooling techniques, such as icing the lesion or cooling with chilled water, have been used.[19,23,33] These techniques result in cooling not only the skin but also the blood vessels. The thermal injury eliminated by the cooling is offset by the additional energy required to heat the blood vessel sufficiently for destruction.

Selective cooling of the skin can be accomplished with cryogen spray.[16,30,31] With short spurts of cryogen the distribution of cooling is confined to the epidermis, with the deeper vessel temperature unchanged. The vessels can then be treated effectively.

Available treatments for cutaneous pathology have expanded, with consistently favorable results. Many lasers are now available for clinical use in plastic surgery (Table 15-1).

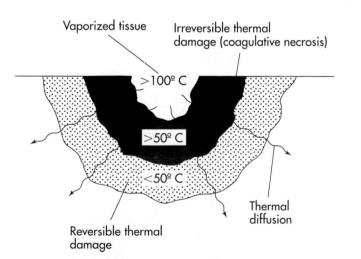

Figure 15-15. Tissue is vaporized at temperatures greater than 100° C (212° F). Irreversible thermal coagulation occurs at 50° to 100° C (122° to 212° F). At temperatures below 50° C, thermal damage is reversible.

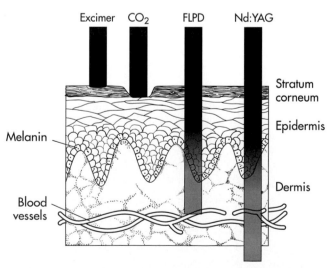

Figure 15-16. Cross section of skin showing penetration of various lasers. Excimer laser has shallow penetration, less than 100 μm. Carbon dioxide *(CO2)* laser is absorbed by water, limiting penetration to 0.1 mm. Flashlamp-pumped pulsed dye (FLPD) laser is absorbed by melanin and hemoglobin and penetrates well into skin. Nd:YAG laser penetrates deeply into skin.

Table 15-1.
Lasers Used in Plastic Surgery

LASER	WAVELENGTH (nm)	APPLICATIONS
Erbium:YAG	294	Skin resurfacing
Argon	488 and 514	Vascular lesions Coagulation of small vessels
Potassium-titanyl-phosphate:YAG	532	Excision of vascular lesions and lymphangiomas
Copper vapor	578	Vascular lesions
Flashlamp-pumped pulsed dye	585	Vascular lesions
Long pulse	595-600	Leg veins
Ruby	694	
Q switched		Decorative and traumatic tattoos
Long pulse		Hair removal
Q-switched alexandrite	755	Pulsed delivery Tattoo without scarring
Neodymium:YAG	1064	Penetration to deep vascular lesion Deep coagulation Fiberoptic delivery Sapphire tip excision
Q-switched YAG	1064	Pulsed delivery Tattoo without scarring Pigmented lesions
Carbon dioxide	10,600	Scalpel, incisional, vaporization Rhytids when used with pulsed machines or computer-generated scanning device

YAG, Yttrium-aluminum-garnet.

LASER SYSTEMS

Carbon Dioxide

The most frequently used surgical laser is the CO_2 laser. Since the advent of laser skin resurfacing, it has become even more widely used in plastic surgery. The CO_2 laser emits light in the invisible, midinfrared range of the electromagnetic spectrum. The invisible beam of the CO_2 laser is routinely coupled with an HeNe aiming beam.

CO_2 laser light cannot be delivered through fiberoptics; an articulated arm is required. Much research and effort has been expended to develop a more user-friendly delivery mode for the CO_2 laser. To date, no satisfactory alternative has been developed.

CO_2 laser light can be delivered to the tissue in several ways. The first mode developed was the continuous wave. In CW mode the laser is delivered by depression of a foot device, light is emitted through the articulated arm in a continuous beam of light, and no change in power output occurs over time.

The CW mode can be modified with a shutter system to produce pulses of light. Several advantages exist to pulsing the CO_2 laser. Primarily, a pulsed laser produces less thermal injury to the surrounding tissues. Also, a precise incision can be produced with a pulsed laser.

The CO_2 laser can also be delivered through a scanning device. This method is widely used in skin resurfacing (see Chapter 138).

Flashlamp-pumped Pulsed Dye

Dye lasers contain fluorescent dyes that are dissolved in solvents such as water or alcohol. The solvent absorbs the light at one wavelength and emits it at another.

The most common dye laser in plastic surgery is the flashlamp-pumped pulsed dye (FLPD) laser. This laser can be tuned over a wide band of the electromagnetic spectrum (400 to 1000 nm) by changing the dyes. The laser is delivered in short, single pulses at high peak powers. The 585 nm wavelength is well absorbed by hemoglobin and less well by other chromophores in the skin, particularly melanin. The pulse duration is 450 microseconds (μsec). This closely matches the thermal relaxation time of blood vessels in the dermis. These factors make the FLPD laser a viable treatment for cutaneous vascular lesions such as port-wine stains,* superficial hemangiomas,[13,34,35] and telangiectasias.

The FLPD laser can improve the pliability and the texture of burn scars. It can also decrease erythema and associated symptoms. The result is improved function and cosmesis.[6,18]

LONG-PULSE DYE LASER. The 595-nm wavelength is well established as treatment of choice for port-wine stains and various vascular lesions. It has not been effective, however, for the treatment of large-caliber vessels. To treat these vessels effectively, a longer pulse width is necessary. The long-pulse dye laser emits at 595 to 600 nm with a 1.5-millisecond pulse. Clinical studies have shown promising results for the treatment of leg veins.[20,25]

YAG Lasers

Several YAG lasers have application in plastic surgery, including the neodymium (Nd), potassium-titanyl-phosphate (KTP), and erbium (Er). The common denominator of these lasers is the YAG, a crystal of yttrium-aluminum-garnet. The YAG laser is then "doped" with an ion. *Doping* is a process whereby the YAG crystal is grown with an impurity so the crystal forms with an impurity (e.g., Nd) embedded in it.

NEODYMIUM:YAG The Nd:YAG laser is delivered through a fiberoptic system fitted with a handpiece. It emits in the invisible, near-infrared spectrum at 1064 nm. This wavelength has no specific cutaneous chromophore.

Because the Nd:YAG laser is poorly absorbed by water, hemoglobin, or melanin, its use for cutaneous lesions is limited. Because of limited cutaneous absorption, it scatters and penetrates more deeply into tissue. It has strong coagulative and hemostatic effects that can be produced to depths of 4 to 6 mm.

When diffuse thermal injury is required, the Nd:YAG laser is effective. It has been used mostly for thick, nodular port-wine stains, bulky hemangiomas, and deep vascular tumors.

The Q-switched Nd:YAG has been effective for the treatment of decorative tattoos.[27]

KTP:YAG. The KTP lasing medium emits a wavelength of 532 nm, producing a green, visible light. It is delivered through a conventional fiberoptic system. It is a good tool for oral mucosa and tongue tumors. Most recently, the KTP:YAG laser has been used intralesionally to treat bulky hemangiomas.[1,3,11]

ERBIUM:YAG. The Er:YAG laser is doped with the element erbium to produce a wavelength at 294 nm. This wavelength corresponds closely with the maximum absorption of water. The Er:YAG absorption by tissue water is about 12 times that

of the CO_2 laser. Because of the efficient absorption, very little energy is transferred in the form of heat to the surrounding tissue. A fine rim (20 to 50 μm) of thermal damage is created. Ablation is very efficient. No hemostasis occurs, and tissue splatter is significant. The wound created is similar to a mechanically induced wound.

The Er:YAG laser is recommended for skin resurfacing; superficial wrinkles and pigment irregularities can be improved. Unlike with the CO_2 laser, overall tightening is not seen after Er:YAG laser treatment. This is probably because minimal thermal damage is created, resulting in less impact on the underlying collagen. The Er:YAG may be used simultaneously with the CO_2 laser.

Q-switched Alexandrite

This solid-state laser is chromium-doped $BeAl_2O_4$ and can be tuned from 701 to 826 nm. Clinically, the Q-switched alexandrite laser is usually operated at 755 msec, with a pulse duration of 50 to 100 nm. It is recommended for tattoos, particularly green and blue pigments.[5,36]

Argon

The argon laser was one of the first lasers used in plastic surgery and was the treatment of choice for port-wine stains and other vascular lesions throughout the 1980s.[12,26] It emits two wavelengths, 488 and 514 nm. These wavelengths are absorbed by hemoglobin and melanin. The primary side effect of the thermal injury from argon laser treatment was hypertrophic scarring, so it was not recommended in children. Because of the competing chromophore, melanin, hypopigmentation was common.

The argon laser is sometimes used for thicker, nodular port-wine stains. Its use for other vascular lesions, however, has been largely supplanted by the FLPD laser (585 nm).

Copper Vapor

The copper vapor laser operates at two wavelengths, 578 (yellow) and 511 (green). The 578-nm wavelength coincides with the absorption peak of oxyhemoglobin and the 511-nm wavelength with melanin. The delivery is a quasi-CW mode composed of 20-nanosecond pulses at a frequency of 15,000 pulses per second. Because of the delivery, heat will accumulate in the tissue. To minimize the thermal effects, a scanning device can be used, or the pulses can be modified with twenty-millisecond secondary pulses.

The copper vapor laser has been used primarily for the treatment of port-wine stains and telangiectasia.

Ruby

The first laser developed was a CW ruby laser. As technology expanded, the Q-switched mode was developed, providing a higher fluence with a very short duration. The 694-nm wavelength emitted is well absorbed by melanin.

The ruby laser is effective for the treatment of both endogenous and exogenous pigmented lesions. In particular, this laser revolutionized the treatment of decorative tattoos.[15,28] It is also effective for treating traumatic tattoos[4] and a variety of pig-

---

*References 2, 14, 21, 24, 29, 32, 37, 38.

Table 15-2.
Lasers Used in Tattoo Removal

LASER (nm)	PIGMENT REMOVED
Q-switched alexandrite (755)	All colors except red and orange
Q-switched Nd:YAG (532)	Red and orange
Q-switched Nd:YAG (1032)	All colors except green, orange, and red
Q-switched ruby (694)	All colors except red and orange
Pulsed dye (510)	Red and orange

Nd:YAG, Neodymium:yttrium-aluminum-garnet.

mented lesions.[10,17,22] It remains one of the best lasers for tattoo removal (Table 15-2).

Tattoo pigment darkening has been reported after treatment attempts to remove cosmetic tattooing.[8]

LONG-PULSE. This ruby laser also emits at 694 nm, but with a longer pulse than the Q-switching mode, allowing for deeper penetration. Several manufacturers have developed this laser for hair removal. The treatment is based on the concept of selective photothermolysis. Melanin is the target chromophore.

Results of this treatment appear to be based on the melanin content in the hair shaft. Epidermal injury may lead to pigment changes because melanin is also present in the epithelial cells of the epidermis. Skin pigment changes remain the limiting factor to this technology.

SAFETY

In the hands of experienced and cautious users, lasers are very safe. General safety guidelines and manufacturer recommendations for specific lasers must be followed.

Eye protection is essential. Goggles are available for protection from each of the therapeutic wavelengths and for the most part are *not interchangeable*. Corneal shields for the patient are recommended when treatment involves the periorbital area. Goggles are essential for the physician, personnel, and patient during any laser procedure.

Limited access to the laser is achieved by posting "Laser in Use" signs at the entry of the operating arena. Keys are required for accessing the laser and should be available only to qualified personnel. Standby modes built into the machines are helpful for preventing accidental firing. Common-sense rules regarding electricity and water apply to the use of lasers.

Combustible agents should be restricted in the operating room environment. Fires involving surgical drapes and hair have been reported in oxygen-rich environments when the laser is used around the face. Endotracheal tubes can be penetrated, resulting in an explosion or fire. The anesthesiologist should be well trained in the use of lasers and emergency procedures for an endotracheal fire. A fire extinguisher should be readily available. Plume (smoke) evacuation is essential during most procedures. This is accomplished with the use of a smoke evacuator. Standard wall suction is not sufficient.

The American National Standards Institute (ANSI) has published standards for the safe use of lasers in hospitals and health care facilities. Adherence to these standards is essential to the safe use of lasers clinically.[9]

SUMMARY

A wide variety of lasers provide treatment options that were not previously available. Appropriate, safe use of lasers complements the many therapeutic treatment options available to plastic surgeons.

The use of lasers continues to expand. Plastic surgeons need to be knowledgeable about all aspects of laser therapy for cutaneous conditions to offer optimum care to their patients.

REFERENCES

1. Achauer BM, Celikoz B, VanderKam VM: Intralesional bare fiber laser treatment of hemangioma of infancy, *Plast Reconstr Surg* 101:1212, 1998.
2. Achauer BM, VanderKam VM, Padilla JF: Clinical experience with tunable pulsed-dye laser (585 nm) in the treatment of capillary vascular malformations, *Plast Reconstr Surg* 92:1233, 1993.
3. Achauer BM, Chang CJ, VanderKam VM, Boyko A: Intralesional photocoagulation (ILP) of periorbital hemangiomas, *Plast Reconstr Surg* 103:11-19, 1999.
4. Achauer BM, Nelson JS, VanderKam VM, Applebaum R: Treatment of traumatic tattoos by Q-switched ruby laser, *Plast Reconstr Surg* 93:318, 1994.
5. Alster TS: Successful elimination of traumatic tattoos by the Q-switched alexandrite (755 nm) laser, *Ann Plast Surg* 34:542, 1995.
6. Alster TS, Nanni CA: Pulsed dye laser treatment of hypertrophic burn scars, *Plast Reconstr Surg* 102:2190, 1998.
7. Anderson RR, Parrish JA: Selective photothermolysis: precise microsurgery by selective absorption of pulsed radiation, *Science* 2:12, 1988.
8. Anderson RR, Geronemus R, Kilmer SL, et al: Cosmetic tattoo ink darkening, *Arch Dermatol* 129:1010, 1993.
9. ANSI Z 136.3 Standard: *For the safe use of laser in health care facilities*, Toledo, Ohio, 1996, Laser Institute of America.
10. Apfelberg DB: Argon and Q-switched YAG laser treatment of nevus of Ota, *Ann Plast Surg* 35:150, 1995.

11. Apfelberg DB: Intralesional laser photocoagulation–steroids as an adjunct to surgery for massive hemangiomas and vascular malformations, *Ann Plast Surg* 35:133, 1995.

12. Apfelberg DB, Maser MR, Lash H: Review of usage of argon and carbon dioxide lasers for pediatric hemangiomas, *Ann Plast Surg* 12:353, 1984.

13. Ashinoff R, Geronemus RG: Capillary hemangioma and treatment with the flashlamp-pumped dye laser, *Arch Dermatol* 127:202, 1991.

14. Ashinoff R, Geronemus RG: Flashlamp-pumped pulsed dye laser for port-wine stains in infancy: early versus later treatment, *J Am Acad Dermatol* 24:467, 1991.

15. Ashinoff R, Geronemus RG: Rapid response of traumatic and medical tattoos to treatment with the Q-switched ruby laser, *Plast Reconstr Surg* 91:841, 1993.

16. Chang CJ, Anvari B, Nelson JS: Cryogen spray cooling for spatially selective photocoagulation of hemangiomas: a new methodology with preliminary clinical reports, *Plast Reconstr Surg* 102:459, 1998.

17. Chang CJ, Nelson JS, Achauer BM: Q-switched ruby laser treatment of oculodermal melanosis (nevus of Ota), *Plast Reconstr Surg* 5:784, 1996.

18. Dierickx C, Goldman MP, Fitzpatrick RE: Laser Treatment of erythematous/hypertrophic and pigmented scars in 26 patients, *Plast Reconstr Surg* 95:84, 1995.

19. Dreno B, Patrice T, Litoux P, Barriere H: The benefit of chilling in argon-laser treatment of portwine stains, *Plast Reconstr Surg* 75:42, 1985.

20. Garden JM, Bakus AD: Treatment of leg veins with high energy pulsed dye laser, *Laser Surg Med Suppl* 8:34, 1996.

21. Garden JM, Polla LL, Tan OT: The treatment of port wine stains by the pulsed dye laser: analysis of pulsed duration and long term therapy, *Arch Dermatol* 124:889, 1988.

22. Geronemus RG: Q-Switched ruby laser therapy of nevus of Ota, *Arch Dermatol* 128:1618, 1992.

23. Gilchrest BA, Rosen S, Noe JM: Chilling port wine stains improves the response to argon laser therapy, *Plast Reconstr Surg* 69:278, 1982.

24. Goldman MP, Fitzpatrick RE, Ruiz-Esparza J: Treatment of port-wine stains (capillary malformation) with the flashlamp-pumped pulsed dye laser, *J Pediatr* 122:717, 1993.

25. Grossman MC, Bernstein LJ, Kauvar ANB, et al: Treatment of leg veins with a long pulse tunable dye laser, *Laser Surg Med Suppl* 8:35, 1996.

26. Hobby LW: Further evaluation of the potential of the argon laser in the treatment of strawberry hemangiomas, *Plast Reconstr Surg* 71:481, 1982.

27. Kilmer SL, Anderson RR: Clinical use of the Q-switched ruby and the Q-switched Nd:YAG (1064 nm and 532 nm) lasers for treatment of tattoos, *J Dermatol Surg Oncol* 19:330, 1993.

28. Kilmer SL, Lee MS, Grevelink JM, et al: The Q-switched Nd:YAG laser (1094 nm) effectively treats tattoos: a controlled, dose-response study, *Arch Dermatol* 129:971, 1993.

29. Morelli JG, Weston WL: Pulsed dye laser treatment of port-wine stains in children. In Tan OT, editor: *Management and treatment of benign cutaneous vascular lesions,* Philadelphia, 1992, Lea & Febiger.

30. Nelson JS, Milner TE, Anvari B, et al: Dynamic epidermal cooling during pulsed laser treatment of port-wine stain: a new methodology with preliminary clinical evaluation, *Arch Dermatol* 131:695, 1995.

31. Nelson JS, Milner TE, Anvari B, et al: Dynamic epidermal cooling in conjunction with laser-induced photothermolysis of port wine stain blood vessels, *Laser Surg Med* 19:224, 1996.

32. Reyes BA, Geronemus R: Treatment of port-wine stains during childhood with the flashlamp-pumped pulsed dye laser, *J Am Acad Dermatol* 23:1142, 1990.

33. Rosen S, Noe JM: Chilling portwine stains improves the response to argon laser therapy, *Plast Reconstr Surg* 69:278, 1982.

34. Scheeper JH, Quaba A: Does the pulsed tunable dye laser have a role in the management of infantile hemangiomas? Observations based on 3 years' experience, *Plast Reconstr Surg* 95:305, 1995.

35. Sherwood KT, Tan OT: The treatment of capillary hemangiomas with the flashlamp-pumped dye laser, *J Am Acad Dermatol* 22:136, 1990.

36. Stafford TJ, Lizek R, Boll J, Tan OT: Removal of colored tattoos with the Q-switched alexandrite laser, *Plast Reconstr Surg* 95:313, 1995.

37. Tan OT, Morrison P, Kurban AK: 585 nm for the treatment of portwine stains, *Plast Reconstr Surg* 86:1112, 1990.

38. Tan OT, Sherwood K, Gilchrest BA: Treatment of children with port-wine stains using the flashlamp-pulsed tunable dye laser, *N Engl J Med* 320:416, 1989.

CHAPTER

Endoscopic Plastic Surgery

16

Felmont F. Eaves III

HISTORY

Although endoscopies have a long history, endoscopic surgical techniques have found widespread use within plastic surgery only in the last decade. The term *endoscope,* derived from the Greek *endon* (within) and *skopein* (to examine), can be applied to virtually any instrument used to examine internal body spaces. In the first known "endoscopic" procedures, Hippocrates II (460-375 BC) described the use of rectal speculas. The Arabian physician Abulkasim (936-1013) used reflected light to illuminate the cervix, and in 1515 Aranizi used a water-filled glass sphere to focus sunlight within the nasal cavity.[25]

The first tubelike endoscope was described in 1805 by Bozzini to view the bladder. Further development of endoscopic techniques during the nineteenth century focused primarily on cystoscopy. Laparoscopic procedures were developed in the first decade of the twentieth century.[20] Although these early techniques did not receive widespread acceptance, endoscopy has become a valuable tool with wide clinical use in a variety of specialties during the latter part of the twentieth century. Several key developments have led to this incorporation of endoscopic techniques into plastic surgery.

The earliest endoscopes were rigid and relatively fragile and until 1914 used internal light sources.[3] In 1952 the "cold light" fiberglass source was introduced, reducing the risk of burns inherent with earlier light sources.[11] In 1953 Hopkins introduced the rod-lens endoscope, heralding the modern era of endoscopic surgery.[20] The Hopkins rod endoscope replaced the thin, fragile lenses of early endoscopies with elongated, rod glass lenses with small intervening air spaces. This new design was much more durable and allowed a clearer and brighter view from internal reflectance. The Hopkins rod endoscope is still widely used today and is the endoscope of choice for the vast majority of endoscopic plastic surgical procedures (Figure 16-1). Although flexible fiberoptic endoscopes were developed about the same time and have also found widespread nonsurgical use, their fragility and expense have limited their surgical applications.[12]

Although the Hopkins rod system led to increased use of the endoscope for gynecologic, orthopedic, and other procedures, the need for the surgeon to view the operative field directly through the eyepiece created an ergonomic challenge and excluded other members of the operating team from viewing the procedure. The introduction of the computer-chip video camera in the 1980s corrected this deficiency. With the endoscope coupled to a video camera, the surgical image could be displayed on a large monitor that could be comfortably positioned for the surgeon and that also allowed assistants, technicians, and the anesthesia team to follow the operation's progress. The surgeon was no longer physically linked to the eyepiece, thus improving mobility of the surgeon and the endoscope. The image could be recorded for documentary or teaching purposes. Together with the Hopkins rod endoscope, the incorporation of video technology set the stage for the development of endoscopic plastic surgery.

Although the first report of subcutaneous endoscopic plastic surgery dates to 1984, when Teimourian and Kroll[26] viewed subcutaneous tissues after liposuction, the potential of endoscopic plastic surgery was not widely appreciated until the explosive development of laparoscopic cholecystectomy in the late 1980s. Thereafter, endoscopic surgical techniques for both aesthetic and reconstructive surgery were developed at multiple centers around the world. Endoscopy in plastic surgery thus offers promising possibilities but still requires development and critical analysis.

POTENTIAL BENEFITS

The indications for endoscopic technique in plastic surgery are directly related to its potential benefits. The reduction of morbidity from laparoscopic procedures suggests that similar benefits can be derived for plastic surgical patients. Because the endoscope can allow visualization of deep tissue structures through small incisions, reduction of scarring is the most obvious and easily documented benefit of most endoscopic plastic surgical procedures. Scar reduction can be profound, as with a pedicled endoscopic latissimus dorsi harvest, in which no back incision is placed (using instead an existing breast incision, with 100% scar reduction), or with endoscopic brow or neck lifts, in which scarring is reduced approximately 90%. A broader reduction in morbidity is possible, however, because of the decrease in incision length, limitation of dissection, and

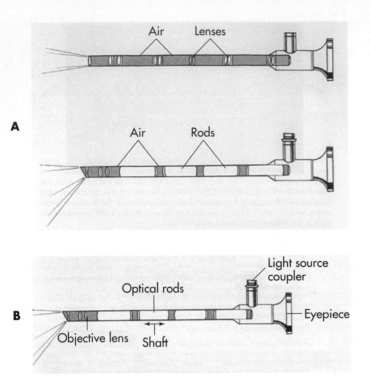

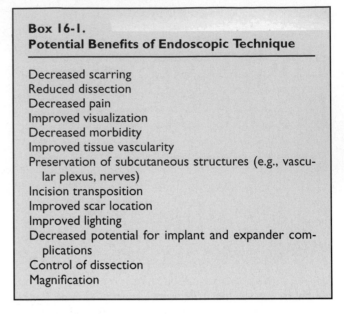

Box 16-1.
Potential Benefits of Endoscopic Technique

Decreased scarring
Reduced dissection
Decreased pain
Improved visualization
Decreased morbidity
Improved tissue vascularity
Preservation of subcutaneous structures (e.g., vascular plexus, nerves)
Incision transposition
Improved scar location
Improved lighting
Decreased potential for implant and expander complications
Control of dissection
Magnification

Figure 16-1. **A,** Early endoscopes had interspersed lenses with relatively wide gaps with air (above). The Hopkins rod endoscope (below) reverses these relationships, with longer glass rods interspersed with relatively narrow spaces, creating an endoscope which is more durable and has a brighter image. **B,** Cross section of the Hopkins rod endoscope. Light enters the endoscope through the light source coupler which is located superiorly on the neck of the endoscope. The light is channeled through fiberoptic fibers to emerge at the distal end of the scope, often in a crescent shape terminus. The light is reflected off of the operative field, and some of the reflected light is gathered in the objective lens, which can be angled in relationship to the axis of the endoscope as is necessary. The light travels back through the rod-lens system to the neck of the endoscope where it can be focused on the eyepiece. In general use, the eyepiece is coupled to a video camera for viewing on a large screen monitor. In many systems the eyepiece is removed and the camera couples directly to the endoscope. (**A** and **B** from Bostwick J, Eaves FF, Nahai F: *Endoscopic Plastic Surgery.* Quality Medical Publishing. St. Louis, 1995, with permission).

optimized tissue vascularity. These benefits are more difficult to document (Box 16-1).

The technical benefits of endoscopic techniques are generally related to improved visualization or transposition of incisions. Because endoscopes are connected to a powerful light source, the level of illumination is generally excellent. In addition, the lens structure and large monitor provide significant magnification, even allowing microsurgical anastomoses. These factors allow the operative space, or *operative cavity,* to be clearly seen, aiding structure identification and control of dissection. A prime example is endoscopic transaxillary augmentation. Although the axillary incision may not be significantly shortened, the procedure is greatly aided by full visualization of the subpectoral cavity, allowing careful and

complete dissection of the pectoralis major muscle origins as well as direct, complete hemostasis. In essence, the endoscope converts this procedure from a closed, blind operation to one with a visualization and control of dissection that rival other techniques.[1,22]

Because endoscopes are elongated, they can be placed through incisions distant to the site of actual dissection. This allows incisions to be moved for aesthetic purposes (e.g., from back to axilla for free latissimus dorsi harvest) or to reduce complications (e.g., locating incisions distant to site of expander, reducing risk of extrusion or exposure).

APPLICATIONS AND INDICATIONS

The application of endoscopic technique in plastic surgery are extremely broad and involve both aesthetic and reconstructive procedures, adult and pediatric patients, and virtually all anatomic regions (Box 16-2). The specific indications for any given plastic surgical procedure are not generally governed by whether endoscopic techniques are used. Rather, *after* a patient has been deemed a candidate for a plastic surgical procedure, *then* determination is made as to whether an endoscopic technique could be helpful.

The description of indications for endoscopic technique for all procedures is beyond the scope of this chapter. Certain key factors in selecting patients and procedures can be outlined, however, and can be of great assistance to the plastic surgeon. These indications can be described through a series of questions.

1. *Is skin resection, transfer, or harvest an unnecessary part of this operation?* The determination of the importance of skin changes to the success of the operation is the single greatest factor determining the applicability of endoscopic technique. In some operations, incisions function solely to provide exposure to deeper tissues, and thus the skin acts as a conduit.

Examples include excision of deep neoplasms or tissues, augmentation mammoplasty, and harvest of muscle flaps. In such procedures, where the skin is not modified, endoscopic techniques may have the theoretic advantages of reduced scarring, morbidity, or complications. In other procedures, however, such as musculocutaneous flap harvest, manipulation of skin is an integral part of the procedure and will determine the length, shape, and location of the incisions. In most of these procedures, endoscopy is of no assistance.

In other procedures the impact of skin on the success of the operation is less clear and concrete, depending instead on individual patient characteristics and desires. The endoscopic abdominoplasty is a good example of such intermediate procedures. Some patients have significant skin excess and laxity, and the success of abdominal rejuvenation and recontouring depends largely on skin removal and transposition. Other patients, however, may have excellent skin quality and do not require skin resection, but exposure of the musculofascial layer is necessary to correct diastasis recti abdominis or hernia. These latter patients may be excellent candidates for endoscopic repair, which may be combined with liposuction.[4,7,10]

Often the importance of skin manipulation on the success of the procedure remains unresolved. For instance, although many surgeons believe that the results from an endoscopic brow lift rival those from open techniques, others contend that skin excision is necessary for optimal fixation and longevity. Therefore some surgeons use traditional "open" techniques in older patients with obvious skin laxity, reserving endoscopic techniques for younger patients.[30]

2. *Can the procedure be performed as well or better using endoscopic technique compared with open technique?* In other words, is the corollary "open" procedure technically feasible through limited incisions, and can it be performed in a reasonable time? In many instances the answer greatly depends on the surgeon's experience. For example, after a brief learning period, many surgeons are comfortable in their ability to identify and resect glabellar muscle during an endoscopic brow lift at a level consistent with open technique. On the contrary, although an endoscopic microsurgical anastomosis can be safely performed in expert hands, this is beyond the experience of most plastic surgeons using endoscopic techniques.

3. *Will endoscopic techniques allow sound surgical and oncologic principles to be followed?* The use of endoscopic techniques must not violate standard surgical principles. For example, the transaxillary biopsy of a suspicious breast mass could allow tumor spread along the optical cavity and would be contraindicated. Fortunately, most endoscopic procedures closely follow their open counterparts using the same dissection planes and methods. It is only the mechanism of exposure and visualization that changes.

4. *Is scar reduction possible?* If a procedure performed in a standard open manner has a long incision, the use of endoscopic techniques offers the potential for scar reduction. Many procedures, from aesthetic surgery of the face to harvest of the sural nerve and saphenous vein, demonstrate such potential. If a scar already exists in the surgical field, however,

---

Box 16-2.
Applications and Indications for Endoscopic Plastic Surgery

TECHNICAL
Tissue harvest
Tissue release
Mass excision
Cavity development
Tissue repair and plication
Scar reduction
Foreign body removal

SPECIFIC
Brow lift
Procerus and corrugator muscle resection
Removal of frontal osteomas
Removal of subcutaneous masses
Placement of tissue expanders
Malar and subperiosteal facelift
Facelift
Neck lift
Release of torticollises
Flap harvest
    Pedicled latissimus dorsi muscle
    Free latissimus dorsi muscle
    Rectus abdominis muscle
    Gracilis muscle
    Omental
    Jejunal
    Colonic
    Peritoneal
    Scapular fascia
Hardware removal
Expander placement
Augmentation mammoplasty
Breast reconstruction
    Expander placement
    Secondary procedures
    Latissimus dorsi muscle harvest
    Transverse rectus abdominis muscle vascular delay
    Revisional procedures
Rhinoplasty
Reduction mammoplasty
Breast mass excision
Axillary dissection
Capsulectomy
Capsulotomy
Capsulorrhaphy
Implant inspection
Nerve harvest
Vein harvest
Pedicle inspection
Abdominoplasty
Hernia repair
Flap vascular delay
Diagnostic procedures (e.g., nasopharyngoscopy)
Facial and other fractures
Sinus turbinectomy
Microsurgical anastomosis

or if the scar is already minimal, the potential for improvement is significantly less.

5. *Will incision transposition be helpful?* The length of the endoscope offers the potential to move the access incision, or port, through which it is placed some distance from the area of dissection. This can be done (1) to position the resultant scar in a more aesthetically acceptable location, (2) to reduce the potential for injury to regional structures (e.g., nerves), or (3) to fulfill functional needs (e.g., prevention of expander extrusion). For example, a subcutaneous lesion of the forehead region can be resected endoscopically, allowing the resultant scar to lie within the scalp rather than the forehead. Another example is to reposition the scar for latissimus dorsi harvest from the back to the axilla.[28] Since most expander extrusions occur through the incision used for placement, the endoscope can be used to transpose the scar to a more distant site to decrease the likelihood of this complication. In this case, endoscopic techniques may still be applicable even with an existing scar.[24]

6. *Will the endoscope facilitate visualization?* Improvement in surgical visualization may make the endoscope valuable for a plastic surgical procedure even with no reduction in scarring. The endoscopic transaxillary augmentation is one such procedure. Through an axillary incision that is similar in size to that used for open dissection, the endoscope completely illuminates the subpectoral pocket and projects this clear, magnified image onto the monitor. Freed from working by blunt dissection only, the surgeon now has complete control of the subpectoral dissection, tailoring it to the needs of the specific patient. Hemostasis can now be obtained through direct electrocautery application, in contrast to the blind application of pressure.

7. *Does a reasonable chance exist to reduce morbidity?* With an operation that already has low morbidity, less benefit may be gained from the application of endoscopic techniques than in applications where morbidity is higher.

8. *Does endoscopic technique fit the patient's preference?* This indication, patient preference, must be applied with caution; as with most new techniques, endoscopy is inherently appealing to most patients. If asked, "Would you like the procedure with the long scar or an endoscopic procedure?" the patient's response is uniformly predictable. As seen from the previous indication issues, however, endoscopy may not be in the patient's best interest.

In certain cases, however, patient preference should be actively sought for purposes of procedure selection; abdominoplasty candidates represent one example. In the patient with good skin quality (e.g., elasticity preserved, no scares or striae), small to moderate fat excess, and diastasis recti abdominis, a variety of surgical options may allow successful abdominal recontouring surgery. If the diastasis is minimal, liposuction alone may provide a significant improvement in contour. An endoscopic abdominoplasty, combining liposuction with endoscopic repair of the diastasis recti, may be indicated and performed through incisions limited to the pubic region and the umbilicus.[4] A more traditional abdominoplasty technique could also provide excellent improvement in contour, although with significantly greater scarring. The open technique, however, using direct removal of skin, may lead to improved "tightness" of the abdominal skin and may help rejuvenate adjacent areas such as the thighs,[19] whereas the endoscopic procedure, without skin resection, cannot provide these benefits. Such options should be explained in full and patients

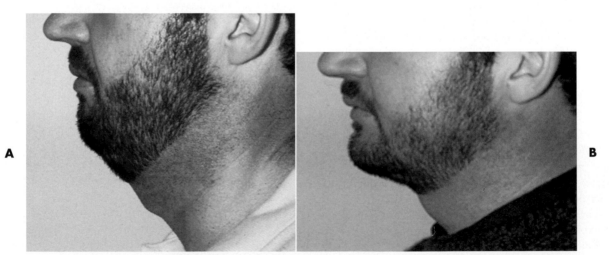

Figure 16-2. **A,** Preoperative view of male patient for endoscopic neck lift. In males, concern for scarring in the pre- and post-auricular locations and beard pattern disturbance may be expressed. Endoscopic techniques represent one option in such patients. **B,** Postoperative view of patient after endoscopically assisted neck lift. A 2-centimeter submental incision allowed direct exposure of the central platysma for plication. Excepting for a small (0.5 millimeter) access incision behind the ear lobe, there is no pre- or post-auricular scarring and the facial hair pattern is not altered. An endoscopic approach may be particularly appropriate to the neck area because restoration of a youthful cervicomental angle helps accommodate slight or apparent excesses of central neck skin. (Photos courtesy F Nahai and F Eaves)

allowed to choose. The patient who wants maximum improvement in skin tightening should choose an open technique. If the patient is more concerned about the resultant scarring than maximizing skin tightness, the endoscopic approach may be preferable.

The endoscopic neck lift is a second example where patient preference may play a particularly prominent role (Figure 16-2). An endoscopic approach can be successfully used in patients with moderate fat excess in whom central platysmal plication is desired but who may benefit from a wider dissection than conveniently provided through a central, submental incision. As with abdominoplasty patients, these neck rejuvenation patients represent a spectrum of morphology and have a choice of appropriate procedures. A full, open neck lift provides greater tightening of the skin but with a longer scar. An endoscopic neck lift, performed through small submental and posterior scalp ports, offers significant benefit with greatly reduced scarring. This option may be particularly beneficial in the younger patient or in the male who wants to avoid preauricular and postauricular scarring.[8]

When the answer to each of questions 1 to 3 and at least one of questions 4 to 8 is "yes," endoscopic technique may be appropriate for the patient and procedure considered.

CONTRAINDICATIONS

Endoscopic techniques are contraindicated if the answer to any of the first three questions is "no" or if no reasonably perceived benefits exist. Endoscopy is also contraindicated if the surgeon has not had adequate training in endoscopic techniques or is unfamiliar with the open equivalent to the surgery. Prolongation of the operative procedure to accommodate endoscopic techniques, especially in light of the patient's physical condition, may represent a contraindication. Endoscopy is contraindicated when adequate instrumentation and technical assistance are unavailable.

INFORMED CONSENT

The ability to understand properly the risks, benefits, and alternatives of any procedure not only is the patient's right but also represents the bond of communication between surgeon and patient. Informed consent for endoscopic techniques should involve a discussion of both the general procedure and the endoscopic issues. Thus, for the patient considering brow and forehead rejuvenation, the discussion must include the risks, benefits, and alternatives of the brow lift by traditional means as well as the specifics of endoscopic technique. Patients are informed of any risks that may be unique to endoscopic techniques and should be informed that, if necessary, intraoperative conversion to a standard open incision may be undertaken to control bleeding, facilitate dissection, or optimize results.

Since an endoscopic procedure often parallels its sister open technique in most ways, the conversation does not focus on the use of endoscopy. Rather, endoscopy should be presented as one of the tools available to the surgeon to address the patient's particular needs and desires. Recommending the proper operation is much more important than whether or not endoscopy is used.

SURGICAL TECHNIQUE

The description of all currently used endoscopic plastic surgical techniques is beyond the scope of this chapter. This section describes several key concepts, however, covering the basics of endoscopic procedures. The next section describes endoscopic augmentation mammoplasty, a common procedure. The reader is referred to chapters covering specific procedures and comprehensive textbooks on endoscopic surgery.

Optical Cavity

For the general, orthopedic, or thoracic surgeon, specific body cavities (e.g., peritoneal cavity, pleural space) can be used for endoscopic visualization and tissue dissection. Most endoscopic plastic surgical procedures, however, are done in the soft tissues, where no such naturally occurring cavities exist, requiring instead both dissection to create a space and an external mechanism to hold the space open. The development, maintenance, and utilization of this space, known as the *optical cavity,* represent one of the most fundamental concepts of endoscopic surgery. This space permits separation of the endoscope from the tissues, allowing clear visualization and room to maneuver the endoscope and dissecting instruments as well as to manipulate the tissues involved.

Depending on the area of the body being examined or treated, the optical cavity can be one of several types[1] (Table 16-1). These types differ based on the mechanism of support for the optical cavity and whether they are dissected or naturally occurring. Although each type may be used in endoscopic plastic surgery, type IV is encountered most often and is used for virtually all face, neck, breast, and extremity surgery.

RETRACTION. The most common method used to support and maintain the optical cavity for endoscopic surgical procedures is internal retraction, usually in the form of an endoscopic retractor or cannula (Figure 16-3). Although they vary in size and configuration, these instruments share the following components:

1. The endoscopic retractor or cannula is rigid so that it can apply an upward, elevating force on the roof of the optical cavity.
2. These devices have a channel through which the endoscope is inserted. This channel serves to support and stabilize the endoscope as well as properly orient it to the area of the optical cavity being dissected.
3. These instruments have a blade or extension so that the point of retraction can be located forward of the endoscope's tip, optimizing both retraction and visualization.

To modify the visual field further, the endoscope can generally be advanced (providing a close-up view) or retracted (providing a wide-angle view) within the channel. Endoscopic retractors generally have a handle separated from the channel-blade assembly, but with endoscopic cannulas the sheath-endoscope complex is held directly without the use of a separate handle. Other components can be added, such as channels to allow irrigation or suction of the scope and cavity, locking rings or couplers to stabilize the endoscope, and grooves to stabilize light cords.[5]

Regardless of the specific design elements, endoscopic retractors and cannulas are used in much the same way.

Table 16-1.
Types of Optical Cavities

TYPE	SPACE	SUPPORT	EXAMPLES
I	Potential	Hyperbaric medium	Laparoscopy
II	Potential	Existing (e.g. bony) normobaric	Thoracoscopy
III	Existing	Varied	Nasoendoscopy, arthroscopy
IV	Requires dissection	Mechanical	Endoscopic face, breast, and trunk procedures

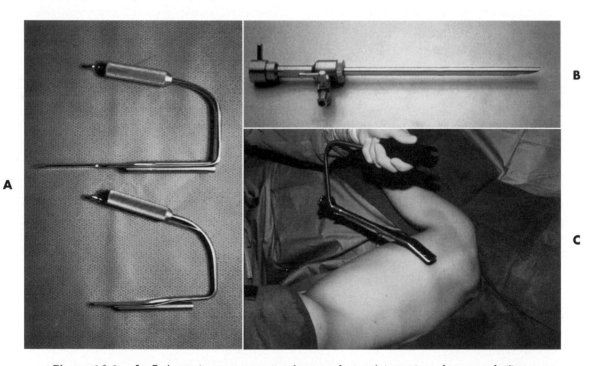

Figure 16-3. **A,** Endoscopic retractors can be manufactured in various forms to facilitate endoscopic plastic surgical procedures in varying anatomical regions. All retractors have in common a handle, support structure, and blade in combination with a sheath into which the endoscope is inserted. The blade length can be modified to address optical cavities of different sizes. For example, the longer blade of the upper retractor helps expose the larger optical cavity encountered during endoscopic abdominoplasty, and the shorter blade is more ergonomic for breast procedures (both retractors, Olympus America, Lake Success, New York). Both retractors use the same thirty degree Hopkins rod endoscope. **B,** Endoscopic cannulas are retractors without separate handles that operate in smaller optical cavities. Like handled retractors, they have a protective sheath into which the endoscope is placed. Instead of having a separate blade assembly, cannulas generally have a small projecting tip at the distal end that functions in retraction and optical cavity maintenance. **C,** Specialized retractor modifications can be created for unusual anatomical constraints. In this example, a bend is applied to the end of a long endoscopic retractor that allows the blade to slide more easily around the curvature of the lateral chest wall. This greatly assists in harvest of the latissimus dorsi muscle for breast reconstruction. Using this modification, often the entire muscle can be harvested through a skin-sparing mastectomy incision.

Inserted into the optical cavity, the blade or extension end is placed against the margin of the cavity and the retractor is lifted, often with a "toeing-in" motion. The angle created from the elevation is compensated by the use of a 30-degree, down-viewing endoscope, generally providing a forward field of view. Thus, in one motion and with a single hand, the operator uses the retractor-scope complex to open the optical cavity, provide retraction, and orient the endoscope. The retractor-endoscope complex can be shifted and repositioned frequently to optimize retraction and visualization as dissection proceeds.

Endoscopic cannulas are most often used in smaller optical cavities, such as in the endoscopic brow lift or carpal tunnel release. These smaller optical cavities generally have tighter tissue walls and do not require a wider blade for support. The wider blades of the endoscopic retractor are quite useful, however, in the larger optical cavities used in breast and trunk surgery or when the roof of the optical cavity is quite lax, as in the endoscopic neck lift.

INSUFFLATION. Although internal retraction has emerged as the most common method of supporting the optical cavity for endoscopic plastic surgery, other techniques have proved useful in certain cases. Insufflation, the most common of these methods, involves placing carbon dioxide gas into the optical cavity under pressure to distend the optical space. Insufflation is often used for laparoscopic surgery and thus is the method of choice for plastic surgical techniques such as harvest of the omentum or other intraabdominal procedures.[21,23] Some surgeons prefer to use insufflation outside the main body cavities, as in the endoscopic latissimus dorsi harvest.[28]

Unlike retraction, insufflation does require an airtight seal around all incisions separating the optical cavity and the exterior so that the proper pressure can be maintained. This is usually accomplished by the use of valved cannulas and may limit the ability to place curved instruments into the optical cavity. Insufflation also carries a risk of subcutaneous emphysema and other potential complications not associated with the retraction methods.

OTHER METHODS. Some surgeons have found surgical balloons to be efficient tools to help develop and maintain the optical cavity for a variety of endoscopic surgical procedures.[17,18,27] These balloons are disposable devices that can help dissect tissue planes to expand the optical cavity.

Other, less frequently used methods include externally applied retraction, such as with sutures.

Basic Approach

Despite the wide variety of anatomic areas and techniques addressed, a common sequence of steps can be outlined for most endoscopic plastic surgical procedures. Understanding these logical steps helps the plastic surgeon apply existing techniques and design procedures to address individual patient needs.

Before beginning any endoscopic procedure, it is advisable to confirm that the endoscopic equipment is in good working order by making sure a clear image is present on the monitor. The choice of anesthesia for endoscopic plastic surgical procedures varies depending on the specific operation but in general parallels the choices made for the corresponding open (nonendoscopic) procedure.

PROVIDE ACCESS. The first step in any endoscopic procedure involves the planning and placement of access incisions, or ports, through which the endoscope and any necessary instruments can be placed. The following factors influence the placement of access incision sites:

1. The port(s) must provide effective access to the optical cavity. This requires that the port be neither too close nor too distant to the area of dissection and thus within the *effective range* of the endoscope.
2. The path of dissection from the access incision should not place any vital structures at risk. For example, an incision high in the temporal scalp would not be a safe location to dissect the midface in a subcutaneous plane because the frontal branch of the facial nerve would be placed at risk.
3. The surgeon should use the port to approach the area of dissection from an acceptable angle to perform the required dissection. An incision in the central hairline region, for example, provides a good angle of exposure to the procerus and corrugator muscles as well as the supraorbital and supratrochlear nerves during foreheadplasty. An incision in the supraauricular scalp, however, would not provide good exposure.
4. The access incisions should be positioned in aesthetically and functionally acceptable locations. The hair-bearing scalp, the axilla, and the umbilicus are excellent port locations if the other requirements are met.

INITIATE DISSECTION. The second step is initial optical cavity dissection, which produces a limited optical cavity for insertion of the endoscope and retractor. Depending on the characteristics of the optical cavity, this initial dissection can constitute a lesser or greater portion of optical cavity dissection.

In the subperiosteal endoscopic foreheadplasty, for example, the central access incisions are carried down directly to the frontal bone. Without inserting the endoscope, a periosteal elevator is placed through the incision, and the majority of the central forehead area dissection is completed without internal visualization. After the endoscope is inserted, little area remains to dissect; rather, the endoscope is used to guide release at the supraorbital rim and address the glabellar musculature.

In the endoscopic abdominoplasty, however, only a small initial optical cavity is created under direct vision, and the endoscope is inserted early in the procedure. The majority of the optical cavity dissection is completed under endoscopic visualization.

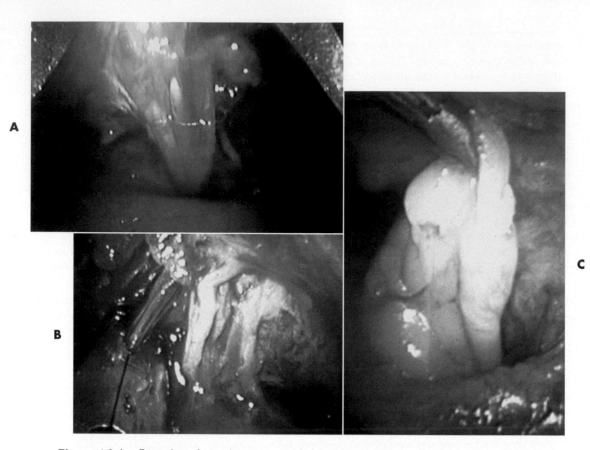

Figure 16-4. Examples of visualization provided by the endoscope. In Figure 16-4, **A,** the supraorbital nerve is clearly seen in a subperiosteal view during endoscopic brow lift. In certain instances, dissection of the corrugator muscles is necessary to fully expose this neurovascular bundle (Figure 16-4, **B**). In the facial region, relatively small anatomical structures such as the buccal fat pad (Figure 16-4, **C**) are clearly seen.

PROVIDE VISUALIZATION. The third step is to achieve the necessary visualization of the optical cavity. For many procedures, this involves only the insertion and upward retraction of the endoscope-retractor complex. Generally, inserting the retractor or cannula empty, followed by insertion of the endoscope, prevents body fluid from clouding the distal lens of the endoscope. The endoscope can then be adjusted by advancing or withdrawing it slightly within its sheath to optimize the view (Figure 16-4).

If balloons or insufflation are used, these steps generally precede placement of the endoscope. If insufflation is used, usually the access incision is closed around a valved laparoscopic cannula to create a tight seal after initial optical cavity dissection and before insufflation.

COMPLETE DISSECTION. With the endoscope inserted and the optical cavity maintained, the optical cavity dissection is completed. As mentioned previously, this may constitute the majority of the endoscopic operating time, as in the endoscopic abdominoplasty. In the latissimus dorsi harvest, development of the dual supramuscular and submuscular cavities largely mobilizes the muscle for transfer. The

instruments used will vary depending on the tissues and procedure; they include rigid elevators, endoscopic scissors, and endoscopic suction-cautery instruments, as well as traditional instruments.

MANIPULATE TISSUES. With the optical cavity fully developed, the next step is to complete any necessary endoscopic tissue manipulation. This may involve release or removal of muscle, harvest of tissue, removal of masses, plication or repair, and other steps, depending on the operation's goals (Figure 16-5).

Concurrently, hemostasis of the entire endoscopic dissection is achieved, usually through the use of an endoscopic electrocautery instrument. Any necessary implant, expander, or other hardware (e.g., fixation plates) is placed at this point (Figure 16-6).

CLOSE INCISION. The final step in an endoscopic procedure is closure of the access incision. Since these incisions are small, this portion of an endoscopic procedure is generally accomplished more quickly than that of parallel open procedures. Drains may or may not be used, depending on the specific procedure and the surgeon's approach.

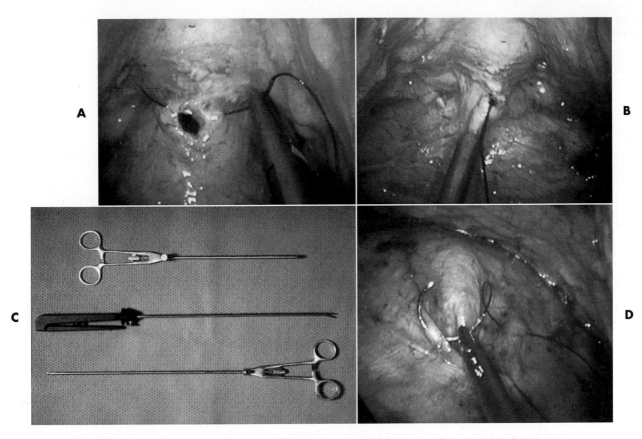

Figure 16-5. In endoscopic abdominoplasty the steps of dissection and tissue manipulation may be mixed. In Figure 16-5, **A,** an umbilical hernia has been exposed during development of the optical cavity. Repair proceeds at that time by placement of sutures to close the defect. Tying can be completed by use of an endoscopic knot pusher as seen in Figure 16-5, **C.** The use of in-line needle holders, see Figure 16-5, **C,** greatly facilitates placement of such repair sutures. After the umbilical hernia is repaired, the remainder of the optical cavity can be dissected up to the level of the xyphoid and plication of the rectus sheaths completed (Figure 16-5, **D**), again using the in-line instrumentation.

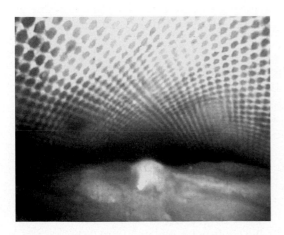

Figure 16-6. Endoscopic visualization can be used to inspect the entire operative site before closure. In this instance, the endoscopic view confirms the back of the tissue expander is appropriately positioned and there is no bleeding within the optical cavity.

SUBPECTORAL TRANSAXILLARY AUGMENTATION MAMMOPLASTY

The transaxillary approach to augmentation mammoplasty is an accepted technique with the initial advantage of an incision far from the breast. Although the transaxillary route can be used for either subglandular[2] or subpectoral[13,15,22] positioning of implants, I prefer the subpectoral route because of the following:

1. Lower anticipated rates of capsular contracture
2. Improved mammography
3. Increased soft tissue coverage over superior aspect of the implant

The transaxillary route has been used since 1973[14] and subpectorally since 1982.[29] As originally described, however, the technique required blunt and blind dissection of the subpectoral pocket, and the implants tended to be superiorly displaced. In addition, hemostasis is more difficult to achieve because of the lack of visualization and direct access.

Endoscopic techniques were developed to maintain the desirable remote incision yet allow full visualization of the subpectoral pocket to improve control and increase predictability. Ho[13] first described an endoscopic transaxillary procedure in 1993 using two axillary incisions and infusion of a 1.5% glycine irrigation solution in the optical cavity. With the development of the endoretractor system at Emory, the procedure was developed without insufflation of gas or fluid,[9] which remains my preferred technique. Endoscopic techniques are also described for inframammary and periareolar incisions and may be of some benefit, although these approaches may be more cumbersome than the transaxillary route.[1] The transaxillary route also provides an optical exposure at right angles to the muscle, whereas other approaches may visualize the muscle "on end."

A transumbilical approach has likewise been advocated by some, although as originally described, this was amenable only to subglandular augmentation.[16] In this technique the endoscope is used to confirm the plane of dissection, but the dissection itself is completed using expanders.

Disadvantages of the transaxillary endoscopic technique relate primarily to increased instrumentation requirements compared with open techniques and an inability to directly address the significant ptosis, as can be done through a periareolar approach. In addition, reoperation through the axillary incision, although possible, is considerably more difficult than from other breast access incisions.

Patient Evaluation

Because of the increased control of dissection, the use of endoscopic techniques has expanded the role of the transaxillary route for augmentation mammoplasty such that most women considering augmentation are potential candidates for this procedure. It is especially beneficial in the patient with a small nipple-areolar complex diameter or a poorly defined inframammary fold, in whom neither periareolar nor inframammary approaches are optimal. It can be used for subglandular or subpectoral implant positioning and for virtually any implant style or composition.

Endoscopic techniques are not indicated in patients who prefer an alternate route or who have significant ptosis when an alternate approach might allow simultaneous or delayed mastopexy incorporating the same incision.

Anatomy

The breast is a subcutaneous glandular structure that primarily overlies the fascia of the pectoralis major muscle, although the inferolateral aspect of the breast overlies the serratus anterior muscle. The breast receives its blood supply from the thoracoacromial trunk via pectoral branches, from anterolateral perforating vessels of the intercostal vessels, and medially from perforators of the internal mammary system. Sensory innervation is supplied by anteromedial and anterolateral intercostal nerve branches, with sensory innervation to the nipple-areola complex originating primarily from the third through fifth levels. Several of the anteromedial branches are divided during release of the medial pectoralis major origins. The rich cross-innervation of the nipple-areolar complex, however, allows preservation of sensibility as long as some anterolateral branches are preserved.

The intercostobrachial cutaneous nerve, which originates from the second intercostal nerve, courses laterally through the axilla to provide sensory innervation to the upper inner arm. This branch is at risk during transaxillary dissection, however, since it lies deep within the axilla. Dissecting superficially toward the lateral pectoral border prevents injury. The medial and lateral pectoral nerves are also close to the area of dissection during transaxillary augmentation. The medial pectoral nerve either perforates the pectoralis minor muscle in route to the pectoralis major or curves around its lateral border. The medial pectoral nerve can be injured during endoscopic transaxillary augmentation, although the resulting partial denervation actually minimizes postoperative pectoralis major activity. The lateral pectoral nerve, lying medial to the medial branch, is situated high and near the clavicle and therefore is at minimal risk during subpectoral pocket dissection.

The pectoralis major muscle has origins from costal, sternal, and clavicular bone and cartilage (Figure 16-7). During endoscopic transaxillary augmentation the costal origins and inferior sternal origins are divided to allow the implant to lie properly within the pocket and to minimize muscular animation.

Patient Preparation

The general preparations for a transaxillary endoscopic augmentation parallel those for any elective augmentation in terms of history and physical examination, mammography, and preoperative instructions. The procedure can be performed using either general anesthesia or intravenous sedation with local anesthesia.

Markings of a prominent axillary crease are made to locate the axillary incision. Both the existing and the desired inframammary fold levels can be marked with the patient in an upright position. Perioperative antibiotics are given.

Operative Procedure

The patient is placed on the operative table in a supine position with the arms padded and abducted to 90 degrees. After anesthesia is achieved, the breast and axillary regions are prepped and draped. Local anesthetic with epinephrine is injected into the axillary incision site. If intravenous sedation is being used, a breast block with the same anesthetic agent is completed. The endoscopic cart is positioned at the foot of the operating table so that it can be viewed during dissection of either breast without repositioning, and the camera, light cords, and electrocautery are connected. The picture on the monitor is focused against clean, white surgical gauze, and image coloration is balanced using the "white balance" button of the camera box. The endoscope itself is heated in a warm water bath. Antifogging solution may be used to minimize fogging of the lens.

ACCESS INCISION AND TUNNEL (Figure 16-8). The axillary incision is then made in the marked fold, usually extending from the anterior edge of the hair-bearing axilla posteriorly for 2.5 to 3.0 cm (about 1 inch). Skin hooks are placed, and dissection is turned toward the lateral pectoral border using a spreading-scissors technique. The pectoral muscle is pinched between the fingers of the nondominant hand, and with the scissors tips closed, the instrumentation is bluntly advanced to the muscle's deep surface. With the subpectoral space entered, the scissors are opened to widen the channel through the lateral pectoral fascia. Using this spreading motion decreases bleeding of the access tunnel and dilates this channel to allow easy placement of the endoscopic retractor. The index finger may be inserted to sweep any loose areolar tissue away from the tunnel and to evaluate the adequacy of the tunnel's diameter. If the access incision and tunnel will not easily admit the surgeon's finger, they will also constrict placement of the endoscopic retractor, endoscope, and suction-cautery instruments. Palpable fascial bands may be lysed digitally to widen the channel as necessary.

POCKET DISSECTION. With the access incision and tunnel completed, allowing exposure of the subpectoral space, initial pocket dissection is completed bluntly. The endoscope can be inserted at this point, but gently sweeping the subpectoral pocket first will open the space more widely. Aggressive blunt pocket dissection is avoided, however, since this generally causes bleeding and staining of the tissues, which will impede the endoscopic view. Instead, the medial and inferior pocket dissection is completed with electrocautery dissection under endoscopic visualization. The exception is the most lateral aspect of the implant pocket that overlies the serratus anterior muscle, where blunt dissection with a large urethral sound or other appropriate dissector will easily release the lateral pocket. Although electrocautery dissection can address this lateral area,

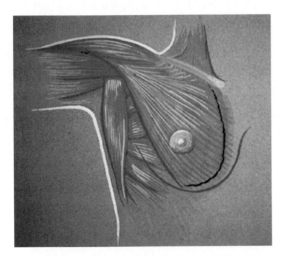

Figure 16-7. Areas for potential muscle release during endoscopic subpectoral augmentation mammaplasty. The costal origins of the pectoralis major are generally fully released from the level of the nipple extending inferiorly and laterally. Above the level of the nipple, full thickness division of the muscle is avoided, although partial dissection may allow improved development of cleavage.

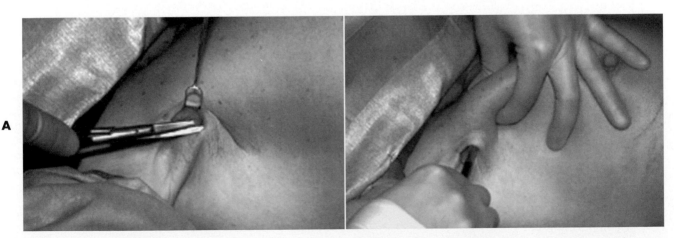

Figure 16-8. **A,** Spreading scissors dissection is generally used to open the access tunnel and allow atraumatic insertion of endoscopic instruments. **B,** By elevating the pectoralis major in the nondominant hand, an instrument is inserted into the subpectoral space.

the risk of anterolateral intercostal nerve branch injury is increased compared with using blunt dissection.

The initial pocket dissection is now completed. The implant pocket is limited inferiorly and medially, however, by the lower sternal and costal origins of the pectoralis major muscle and overlying fascia. Failure to release these origins adequately will cause the implant to be situated superiorly on the chest wall and will lead to accentuated animation of the augmented breast with pectoral contraction. The endoscope, however, allows full visualization and complete release of these attachments in a controlled dissection; the impetus for the endoscopic procedure is therefore improved control of the inframammary fold dissection and position.

MUSCLE DIVISION AND RELEASE (Figure 16-9). The endoscopic breast retractor is placed into the subpectoral pocket. A 10-mm, 30-degree, down-viewing endoscope is slid into the holding cannula underneath the retractor blade. The endoscope is advanced into the cavity while the retractor is elevated, allowing clear visualization of the deep surface of the pectoralis major muscle against the chest wall. The costal cartilages, external intercostal muscles, and pectoralis minor muscle can be visualized deeply. To orient themselves to the exact area visualized, surgeons use the position of the hand holding the retractor, the transilluminated light from the endoscope, or manual compression of the tissues from either internal or external surfaces. The area for muscle division is thus defined, and surgical release proceeds.

In most patients the pectoralis major muscle is released from the level of the nipple medially downward and then laterally until the lateral margins are free. This can be accomplished with laser or ultrasonic dissection. A curved, 5-mm suction-cautery instrument is used most often. The muscle is released 5 to 10 mm above the level of the chest wall, allowing better control of bleeding perforating vessels and preventing their retraction below the level of the intercostal muscles. The release continues until the pectoral fascia is exposed, and in most cases this plane is divided as well.

Superiorly, a limited, partial muscle division can be accomplished as necessary to prevent a "step-off" of the pocket. The full dissection of the pocket can be confirmed by inserting a blunt dissector, ensuring that the pocket matches the level marked preoperatively. The pocket is carefully inspected for adequacy of release and hemostasis, and all instruments are withdrawn.

SIZERS AND IMPLANTS. Implant sizers are generally placed after endoscopic dissection. This confirms that the pocket dissection matches the implant's dimensions, with the optimal implant size chosen. If small areas of the pocket appear to be irregular, the blunt dissector can be used to dilate the pocket in that area, since the tougher muscle dissection has been

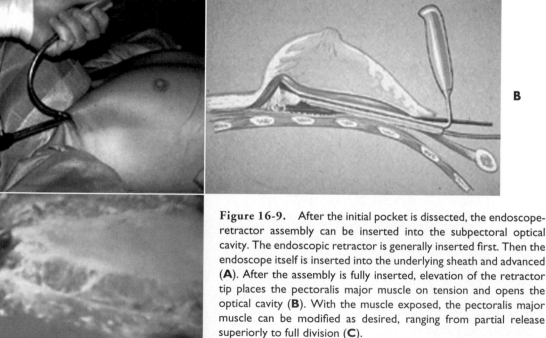

Figure 16-9. After the initial pocket is dissected, the endoscope-retractor assembly can be inserted into the subpectoral optical cavity. The endoscopic retractor is generally inserted first. Then the endoscope itself is inserted into the underlying sheath and advanced (**A**). After the assembly is fully inserted, elevation of the retractor tip places the pectoralis major muscle on tension and opens the optical cavity (**B**). With the muscle exposed, the pectoralis major muscle can be modified as desired, ranging from partial release superiorly to full division (**C**).

completed and only subcutaneous tissue is being addressed. Conversely, the sizer can be removed and the endoscope and retractor reinserted to adjust the pocket. This is especially helpful when larger pocket modifications are required or in the inferomedial region near the xyphoid, where the soft tissue attachments are quite tenacious. In either case the back of the operating table is elevated to allow inspection of the sizer in an upright position after any modifications are completed. The definitive implant size and fill are then chosen.

The sizers are removed and the implants placed in the normal manner. Smooth, textured, round, anatomic, saline, gel, and alternative-fill implants all can be placed through an axillary approach, although the access incision might need to be enlarged slightly to allow insertion and positioning of textured implants. The choice of implants is therefore not contingent on the transaxillary route. Rather, patient breast morphology, adequacy of soft tissue coverage, implant availability, and surgeon and patient preferences will determine the choice. Smooth saline implants rolled and placed in an uninflated position are the easiest to insert through this route. The implants should be handled according to the manufacturer's recommendations, and thus endoscopes or sharp instruments are not reinserted into the implant pocket after the implant is inserted.

Final inspection with the patient upright confirms the surgical result. If adjustable implants are used, the fill tubes are removed and the axillary incision closed with absorbable suture (Figure 16-10).

Postoperative Care

Postoperative care after endoscopy transaxillary augmentation parallels that of any other augmentation procedure. A light dressing is placed over the axillary incision and a surgical bra is placed. The patient is prescribed postoperative analgesics and antibiotics. Warnings are given for hematoma, although the author has not encountered this clinically to date. The patient is usually examined on the first postoperative day and then 1 and 2 weeks after surgery. The use of implant displacement exercises may be encouraged when smooth implants are used and when tolerated by the patient (Figure 16-11).

Secondary Procedures

To date, secondary procedures after endoscopic transaxillary augmentation procedures have been infrequent but have included capsulorrhaphy in one patient. Capsulectomy and capsulotomy can be performed through this route using the endoscope, although complete capsulectomy can be technically challenging[6] (Figure 16-12). Replacement of deflated implants is generally quite simple through this route. If delayed mastopexy or more extensive revisional surgery were to become necessary, an alternate incision approach might be indicated.

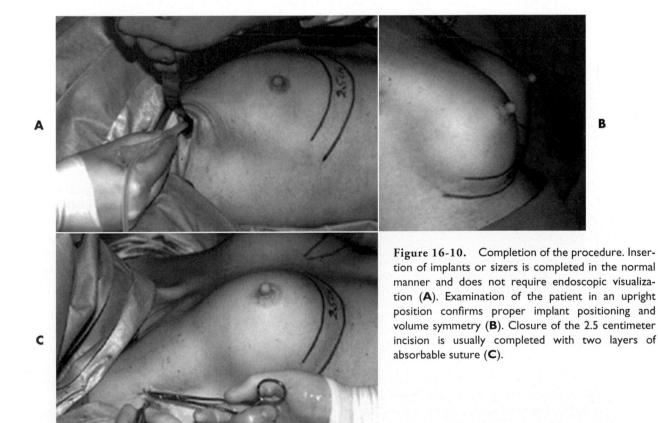

Figure 16-10. Completion of the procedure. Insertion of implants or sizers is completed in the normal manner and does not require endoscopic visualization (**A**). Examination of the patient in an upright position confirms proper implant positioning and volume symmetry (**B**). Closure of the 2.5 centimeter incision is usually completed with two layers of absorbable suture (**C**).

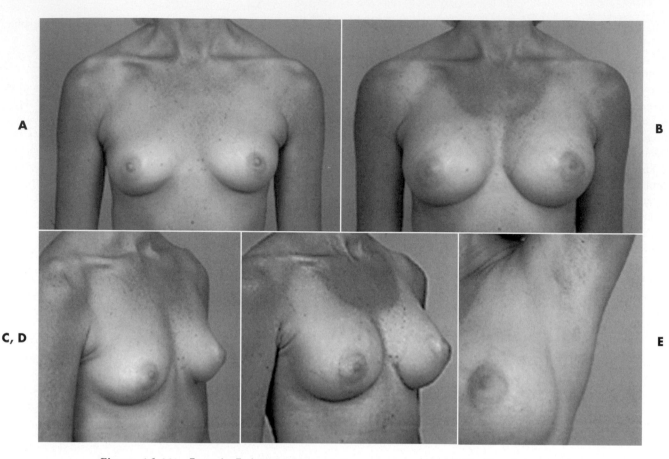

Figure 16-11. Example: Endoscopic augmentation seen preoperatively (**A**, **C**) and nine months after (**B**, **D**) endoscopic transaxillary subpectoral augmentation with a smooth saline implant. The axillary scar is minimally visible (**E**).

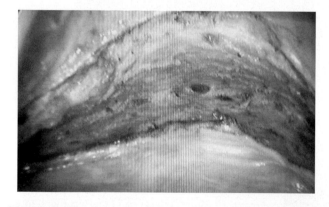

Figure 16-12. Intraoperative view of endoscopic capsulectomy. The light color and high level of light reflection in the implant pocket make visualization quite clear. A portion of the capsule has been removed.

OUTCOMES

Because endoscopic plastic surgery has been commonplace for less than a decade, many techniques, especially those involving more advanced reconstructive procedures, are still being developed and refined. Instrumentation continues to be improved, especially those tools specific to plastic surgery, such as retractors and dissecting instruments. Although endoscopic techniques are increasingly used in plastic surgery, this developmental status also means that objective outcomes for endoscopic surgery are lacking for many, if not most, procedures. In addition, all endoscopic procedures cannot be judged solely as a group; only certain procedures will prove to be effective.

Data are lacking because most early endoscopic procedures were primarily aesthetic, and assessment of results and comparison with open techniques tend to be difficult and subjective. An exception is the large volume of data available on endoscopic carpal tunnel release, although controversy remains concerning the optimal surgical technique. Some complications would be expected to be lower with endoscopic techniques (e.g., skin loss in facelift, alopecia with brow lift).

Safety and Complications

Because endoscopic plastic surgery differs significantly from traditional open techniques, certain complications may be unique to endoscopy. Since most endoscopic techniques are designed to mirror their corresponding open procedures, however, the same complications could also be anticipated as seen with open techniques.

In general, endoscopic techniques appear to be safe. In a review of 1005 patients undergoing 1200 endoscopic plastic surgical procedures at the Emory Clinic, overall complications were low (5.2% of patients, 3.8% of procedures). Reoperations were 2%, although this number would be expected to increase over time. No deaths occurred, and no complications appeared specific to endoscopic technique. Complications seemed to mirror the types and frequencies of complications seen in the corresponding open technique. This range of complications relates favorably to general rates of complication; for example, in this same series, the rate of hematoma after endoscopic facelift was 1%, significantly less than that seen with traditional open techniques.

Certain endoscopic-specific complications (i.e., those that would not be expected to occur with corresponding open technique) appear to be secondary to the use of electrocautery dissection. A burn of the inframammary fold after endoscopic transaxillary augmentation mammoplasty and a burn of the glabellar region have been reported. In such cases, extreme thinness of the skin is a warning to the surgeon to exercise caution. To limit such complications, an assistant should monitor the skin directly rather than observing the monitor during endoscopic dissection. If the dissection becomes too thin, the color of the transilluminated light from the endoscope will change from pink to white and the intensity will increase, providing a warning.

Another type of electrocautery injury specific to endoscopic surgery relates to breaks in insulation along the shaft of the long endoscopic devices. If such a break occurs, injury might result within the access tunnel (e.g., burn to the chest wall deeply with transaxillary augmentation) or to the skin of the access incision, either directly or through contact with a metallic retractor.

Other possible complications with endoscopic techniques that have not been widely reported include subcutaneous emphysema from insufflation and skin burns secondary to direct contact with light source cables.

For some specific procedures, data concerning complications in endoscopic techniques and comparison with open procedures are beginning to emerge. A survey of the faculty of the University of Alabama at Birmingham in 1994 showed that the endoscopic brow procedure was the most common endoscopic procedure performed. Of 305 reported cases, major complications occurred in 3.4% of cases and included six hematomas, one transcutaneous electrical burn, and four frontal branch pareses. Minor complications were reported in 9.5% of patients and included brow asymmetry (four), early recurrence of rhytids (seven), glabellar skin contour deformity (four), and alopecia (10). In 47 patients undergoing endoscopic subgaleal brow lift, two had hematomas, three had seromas, two developed transient nerve paresis, and four had unsatisfactory brow position. The Emory series of 305 brow lifts reported no hematomas, six transient frontal branch pareses (all resolved by 6 weeks postoperatively), and one glabellar depression (minor). Similarly, in this early series, 200 endoscopic facelifts had a 2% hematoma rate and no major nerve injuries, and 67 facelifts had a 1.4% hematoma rate. Endoscopic brow surgery, although sometimes associated with minor alopecia

at access and fixation incision sites, generally has fewer problems with alopecia and decreased sensibility of the scalp than open techniques.

The early data again appear to support the use of endoscopic technique as safe and effective in breast surgery. In the first report of endoscopic transaxillary augmentation, Ho[13] reported on 20 patients using a 1.5% glycine irrigation solution for optimal cavity maintenance, with only one intraoperative hematoma. In 35 patients undergoing transaxillary endoscopic augmentation, no hematomas, infections, or intraoperative complications occurred using a retractor-mounted endoscopic system. Transumbilical augmentation also has a relatively low rate of complications, with Johnson and Christ[16] reporting problems in only four patients: one with intraoperative bleeding and conversion to open technique, one with early implant deflation by 24 hours postoperatively, and two with subpectoral implant positioning requiring conversion to open technique. Others have reported low complication rates for endoscopic breast inspection procedures.

Some early data are also available for endoscopic abdominoplasty. The group at the University of Alabama at Birmingham has reported that complications occurred in 31 of 54 patients (57.4%), although the majority of these were minor complications and included two conversions to open technique, 20 patients with prolonged edema, eight seromas, and one plication suture rupture. The Emory group reported on 40 patients, with two infections and two seromas. Faria-Correa[10] reported that seromas occurred in 12 of 54 patients undergoing endoscopic abdominoplasty, without mention of additional complications.

Aesthetic Results

As with an analysis of complications, data on aesthetic outcomes for endoscopic surgery are limited, especially given the number of procedures that must be independently evaluated and compared with open techniques. As instrumentation and techniques are refined, it is anticipated that outcomes may be further improved and refined.

Economic Issues

The cost of endoscopic equipment and the potential for prolonged operative times, especially early in a surgeon's endoscopic experience, suggest that an economic analysis would be beneficial in defining the role of endoscopy in plastic surgery. For procedures performed within the hospital or surgery center operating room, much of the required equipment is already easily accessible. Thus, with the endoscopic cart and electronics readily available, the only additional instrumentation required is specific hand devices. Some operating rooms may place a separate charge on the use of endoscopic equipment. On the other hand, the surgeon performing these procedures in the office operating suite needs to obtain video-electronic instrumentation as well, at a cost of several thousand dollars. This cost must be offset against the anticipated frequency of use.

SUMMARY

Endoscopic technologies offer great potential for scar reduction and improved control of dissection through limited incisions in selected patients, and endoscopic procedures have become established in several areas of plastic surgery. Because the technology is still relatively new, long-term data on efficacy and comparisons to standard open procedures are not yet available. The study of these factors promises to further define the role of endoscopy in plastic surgery.

REFERENCES

1. Bostwick J, Eaves FF, Nahai F: *Endoscopic plastic surgery,* St Louis, 1995, Quality Medical Publishing.

2. Chajchir A, Benzaquen I, Sagnono N, Lusicic N: Endoscopic augmentation mammoplasty, *Aesthetic Plast Surg* 18:377-382, 1994.

3. Cohen MR: Culdoscopy vs peritoneoscopy, *Obstet Gynecol* 31:30, 1968.

4. Core CB, Mizgala C, Bowen JC III, Vasconez LO: Endoscopic abdominoplasty with repair of diastasis recti and abdominal wall hernia, *Clin Plast Surg* 22:707-722, 1995.

5. Eaves FF, Bostwick J, Nahai F: Instrumentation and setup for endoscopic plastic surgery, *Clin Plast Surg* 22:591-603, 1995.

6. Eaves FF, Bostwick J, Nahai F, et al: Endoscopic techniques in aesthetic breast surgery: augmentation, mastectomy, biopsy, capsulotomy, capsulorrhaphy, reduction, mastopexy, and reconstructive techniques, *Clin Plast Surg* 22:683-695, 1995.

7. Eaves FF, Nahai F, Bostwick J: Endoscopic abdominoplasty and endoscopically assisted miniabdominoplasty, *Clin Plast Surg* 23:599-616, 1996.

8. Eaves FF, Nahai F, Bostwick J: The endoscopic neck lift, *Operative Tech Plast Reconstr Surg* 2:145-151, 1995.

9. Eaves FF, Price CI, Bostwick J, et al: Subcutaneous endoscopic plastic surgery using a retractor-mounted endoscopic system, *Perspect Plast Surg* 7:1-22, 1993.

10. Faria-Correa MA: Endoscopic abdominoplasty, mastopexy, and breast reduction, *Clin Plast Surg* 22:723-745, 1995.

11. Fourestier N, Gladu A, Bulmiere J: Perfectionnments, an L'endoscopic medicale: realisation bronchoscopique, *Presse Med* 60:1292, 1952.

12. Hirschwitz BI: A personal history of the fiberscope, *Gastroenterology* 76:864, 1979.

13. Ho LCY: Endoscopic assisted transaxillary augmentation mammoplasty, *Br J Plast Surg* 46:332-336, 1993.

14. Hoehler J: Breast augmentation: the axillary approach, *Br J Plast Surg* 26:373-376, 1973.

15. Howard PS, Oslin BD, Moore JR: Endoscopic transaxillary submuscular augmentation mammoplasty with textured saline breast implants, *Ann Plast Surg* 37:12-17, 1996.

16. Johnson GW, Christ JE: The endoscopic breast augmentation: the transumbilical insertion of saline-filled breast implants, *Plast Reconstr Surg* 92:801-808, 1993.

17. Karp NS, Bass LS, Kasabian AK, et al: Balloon assisted endoscopic harvest of the latissimus dorsi muscle, *Plast Reconstr Surg* 100:1161-1167, 1997.

18. Koh KS, Park S: Endoscopic harvest of sural nerve graft with balloon dissection, *Plast Reconstr Surg* 101:810-812, 1998.

19. Lockwood T: High lateral tension abdominoplasty with superficial fascial system suspension, *Plast Reconstr Surg* 96:184, 1996.

20. Marlow J: History of laparoscopy, optics, fiberoptics, and instrumentation, *Clin Obstet Gynecol* 19:261, 1976.

21. Miller MJ, Robb GL: Endoscopic technique for free flap harvesting, *Clin Plast Surg* 22:755-773, 1995.

22. Price CI, Eaves FF, Nahai F, et al: Endoscopic transaxillary subpectoral breast augmentation, *Plast Reconstr Surg* 94:612-619, 1994.

23. Restifo FJ, Ahmed SS, Rosser J, et al: TRAM flap perforator ligation and the delay phenomenon: development of an endoscopic/laparoscopic delay procedure, *Plast Reconstr Surg* 101:1503-1511, 1998.

24. Saltz R, Anger AJ, Arnaud E: Endoscopic expansion surgery. In Ramirez OM, Daniel RK, editors: *Endoscopic plastic surgery,* New York, 1996, Springer-Verlag.

25. Semm K: *Atlas of gynecological laparoscopy & hysterectomy,* Philadelphia, 1977, Saunders (translated by A Rice).

26. Teimourian B, Kroll S: Subcutaneous endoscopy in suction lipectomy, *Plast Reconstr Surg* 74:708-711, 1984.

27. Van Buskirk ER, Khouri RK, Torre F, Pena JA, et al: Endoscopic balloon assisted pre-peritoneal repair of abdominal wall laxity, *Plast Surg Forum* 20:442-443, 1997.

28. Van Buskirk ER, Rehnke RD, Montgomery RL, et al: Endoscopic harvest of the latissimus dorsi muscle using the balloon dissection technique, *Plast Reconstr Surg* 99:899-903, 1997.

29. Watanabe K, Tsurukiyi K, Fugui Y: Subpectoral transaxillary method of breast augmentation in orientals, *Aesthetic Plast Surg* 6:231-236, 1982.

30. Wolfe SA: Discussion, *Plast Reconstr Surg* 100:1044-1046, 1997.

CHAPTER 17

Anesthesia

Kathleen J. Welch

Marina D. Bizzarri-Schmid

Lawrence Tsen

In 1846 Oliver Wendell Holmes introduced the term *anesthesia* to describe the state of drug-induced "senselessness" in patients undergoing surgical procedures.[34] The duties of anesthesiologists and anesthetists have become more complex and certainly involve more than mere induction of the state of anesthesia. Anesthesiologists now deliver sophisticated intensive medical care during the entire perioperative period, beginning with patient evaluation and preparation before surgery, continuing with control over physiologic functions during surgery, and finishing with postoperative critical care and pain management. Therefore the words "perioperative medicine" more accurately describe the scope of today's anesthesia specialists. In addition, anesthesiologists have expanded their duties to include management of operating rooms, preadmitting test centers, pain centers, conscious sedation credentialing, and intensive care and postanesthesia care units.

CONSCIOUS SEDATION

Plastic surgeons must be familiar with the practice of conscious sedation. A survey of aesthetic plastic surgeons revealed that local anesthesia with intravenous (IV) sedation was employed for office surgery without an anesthesiologist or nurse anesthetist about one third of the time.[10]

Conscious sedation lies on a dose-dependent continuum ranging from minimal sedation to general anesthesia. During conscious sedation, patients' ability to maintain their airway independently and continuously is preserved, along with their ability to respond appropriately to a verbal command or tactile stimulation (Table 17-1). By contrast, during unconscious sedation, patients are unable to respond purposefully and may exhibit only a reflex withdrawal from a tactile or painful stimulus. Unconscious sedation is accompanied by a partial loss of protective airway reflexes and cardiopulmonary function. Deeply sedated patients approach a state of general anesthesia accompanied by complete loss of protective reflexes, including

inability to maintain their airway independently. Therefore unconscious sedation is best administered by an anesthesia specialist.

Conscious sedation, or the preferred term *sedation-analgesia*, may be provided by nonanesthesiologists.[1] Individuals responsible for administering sedatives and analgesics must be familiar with the clinical pharmacology of these medications and their potential interactions. Since the primary complication of sedation-anesthesia is related to respiratory and cardiovascular depression, at least one person capable of establishing a patent airway, maintaining ventilation and oxygenation, and initiating basic life support should be present. This may be either the individual monitoring the patient or the surgeon performing the procedure, provided that surgeon can discontinue the procedure and attend to the patient's cardiorespiratory function in an emergency. Most importantly, an individual with advanced life support skills should be immediately available.

In some patients the need for deep sedation may not be obvious until the procedure has been attempted unsuccessfully. Rather than administer "just a bit more" sedation-analgesia, the assistance of an anesthesiologist should be enlisted. Also, surgeons tend to perform invasive procedures on elderly patients or those with significant medical problems using "local with sedation" rather than the procedure-appropriate anesthetic, general anesthesia. These patients may suffer needlessly increased surgical stress, hypoventilation, and excessive postoperative sedation. With the present system of improved preoperative patient preparation, monitoring devices, anesthesia equipment, and pharmaceuticals, a general anesthetic might be considered more than it was years ago when anesthesia risk was greater. The requirements for anesthesia should be realistically assessed preoperatively, when an anesthesia consultation may be useful.

An anesthesiologist is recommended for monitoring the underlying disease process and the undesired effects of sedation in higher risk patients, called *monitored anesthesia care* (MAC). Patients at greatest risk during conscious sedation are (1) those

Table 17-1.
Conscious versus Unconscious Sedation

FACTOR	CONSCIOUS SEDATION	UNCONSCIOUS SEDATION
Patient	Mood altered Cooperative	Unconscious Unable to cooperate
Protective airway reflexes	Intact	Obtunded
Vital signs	Stable	Labile
Anesthetic action	Local anesthesia: analgesia	Pain eliminated centrally
Risk of perioperative complications	Low	High

Modified from Kallar SK, Dunwiddle WC: In Wechtler BV, editor: *Problems in anesthesia,* Philadelphia, 1988, Lippincott.

with extremes of age; (2) those with concomitant cardiopulmonary, hepatic, renal, or central nervous system disease; (3) smokers; (4) alcohol or illicit drug abusers; (5) patients with a prior adverse outcome with sedation or general anesthesia; and (6) those with increased likelihood of airway obstruction during sedation (morbid obesity, sleep apnea, atypical airway anatomy).

The American Society of Anesthesiologists[1] (ASA) has published guidelines for nonanesthesiologists.* Monitoring and drugs used for conscious sedation are discussed further in the section on sedation and analgesia.

OFFICE ANESTHESIA

A census survey of members of the American Society for Aesthetic Plastic Surgery in 1992 found that more than 50% of respondents performed 50% of surgeries or more in their office.[10] Twenty-eight percent of respondents always or almost always performed aesthetic surgery in their office, whereas 39% never or almost never did this.

Office-based surgeries will continue to increase because the office setting may be the most cost-effective approach to surgical procedures, as well as more time-efficient for surgeons. Also, most patients scheduled for cosmetic surgery prefer the office setting over the hospital.[41] With this growth, appropriate considerations must be given to patient safety, especially administration of anesthetics in the office setting. Several states, including Florida, California, and New Jersey, have passed legislation regarding standards in office surgery and anesthesia. The New Jersey standards are the most defined and detailed to date and include regulations on machines, monitoring, equipment maintenance, and personnel. The goal is that office-based surgery and anesthesia must be safe and

meet acceptable standards. The minimal standards of care should be no different than those expected in hospitals or ambulatory surgery centers.

Essentials for office-based anesthesia include the following[22]:

1. Safe, reliable source of oxygen and ability to deliver positive-pressure ventilation via Ambu bag or anesthesia machine
2. Emergency airway equipment (e.g., oronasal airways, laryngoscopes, endotracheal tubes, laryngeal mask airways, tracheotomy kits)
3. Suction apparatus powerful enough to clean airway of secretions or vomitus
4. Reliable monitors with backup power
5. Defibrillator
6. Resuscitative drugs

Service checks and maintenance of equipment must be documented. The responding emergency medical services (EMS) team must be located and their estimated response time documented. The local EMS policy and protocols should be reviewed regarding responsibilities at a scene when a physician is present. Finally, the local hospital emergency room director should be contacted and informed that anesthesia services will be provided in the community.[22]

As with the operating room (OR), the recovery area needs to be properly equipped and staffed. Both recovery and discharge criteria should be suitable for specific patients and procedures. A staff member should be responsible for monitoring the recovery of patients and another readily available and capable of treating complications. Emergency procedures for cardiopulmonary resuscitation (CPR) and management of medical problems during office surgery should be reviewed at frequent, consistent intervals.[9] An office policy manual for employees should be developed and quality improvement (QI) data collected.

The ASA physical status classification remains a major factor in patient selection for office-based surgery (Table 17-2). Typ-

*Available from the ASA, 520 N. Northwest Highway, Park Ridge, IL 80088-2573.

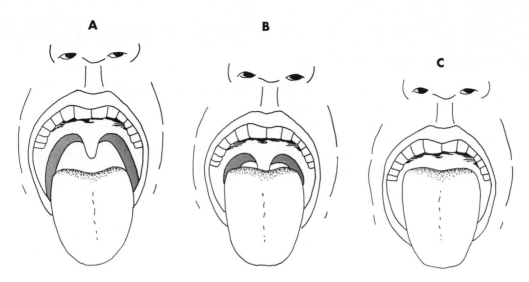

Figure 17-1. Classification of airway. **A,** Class I: uvula, faucial pillars, and soft palate visible. **B,** Class II: faucial pillars and soft palate visible. **C,** Class III: only soft palate visible. (From Longnecker DE, Tinker JA, Morgan GE: *Principles and practice of anesthesiology,* ed 2, St Louis, 1998, Mosby.)

Table 17-2.
American Society of Anesthesiologists (ASA) Physical Status Classification

CLASS	DESCRIPTION
I	Healthy patient
II	Mild-moderate systemic disease; no functional limitation
III	Severe systemic disease; definite functional limitation
IV	Severe systemic disease that is constant threat to life
V	Moribund patient unlikely to survive 24 hours with or without surgery

ically, patients appropriate for office surgery and anesthesia are either healthy (ASA I) or have mild systemic disease (ASA II). A review of closed claims involving anesthesia morbidity and mortality in dental offices suggests that preexisting conditions (e.g., obesity, cardiac disease, epilepsy, chronic obstructive pulmonary disease) require serious attention, especially if an anesthesiologist is not present.[17] Advances in anesthesia equipment and machines and development of safer, shorter-acting medications may broaden the patient population appropriate for office procedures.

PREOPERATIVE ASSESSMENT

The preoperative evaluation is an essential part of anesthetic management and includes the patient's history and physical examination, relevant laboratory tests, prior anesthetic history, time and nature of last oral intake, and consultation with the appropriate medical specialists based on the patient's medical condition. Only after obtaining such information can anesthesia risk be determined and an anesthetic plan formulated. This is discussed with the patient and reflected in the signed informed consent.

Likewise, nonanesthesiologists must preoperatively evaluate and obtain consent from patients when providing sedation and analgesia. An anesthesiologist should be consulted for patients at potential risk for airway obstruction or cardiorespiratory depression during conscious sedation. Patients at risk are (1) those with airway abnormalities, such as abnormal craniofacial anatomy, limited head and neck range of motion, or an airway classification of III (Figure 17-1); (2) those with a prior history of difficult intubation or fiberoptic intubation; (3) morbidly obese patients; (4) those with a known history of obstructive sleep apnea; (5) those with a previous adverse outcome under sedation or general anesthesia; and (6) those classified as an ASA III or greater.[25]

In the past, preoperative testing consisted of batteries of tests ordered as screens for asymptomatic illness, but this is neither cost-effective nor medically necessary.[2] Ordering preoperative tests should be based on the patient's age and preexisting medical condition; specifically, tests should optimize the patient's current condition for surgery. Table 17-3 lists a current recommendation for preoperative tests. Preoperative laboratory testing and electrocardiograms (ECGs) are valid for 1 year unless medical conditions or age warrant otherwise. These guidelines for preoperative testing are fairly conservative and most likely will be amended as standards evolve.

The importance of preoperative fasting must be clearly communicated to the patient (Table 17-4). Since airway reflexes are impaired in proportion to the degree of sedation rendered, even patients receiving only sedation-analgesia must fast to minimize the risk of pulmonary aspiration. Despite fasting, factors that delay gastric emptying, such as intestinal obstruction, obesity, diabetes, pain, trauma, and pregnancy, place the patient at an increased risk for aspiration. Such patients are considered to have a "full stomach," and unless

they have only minimal sedation, their airways require protection by a cuffed endotracheal tube.[5]

TYPES OF ANESTHESIA

The choice of anesthesia, whether general anesthesia (GA), regional (or local) anesthesia (RA), or MAC, depends on the type and length of surgery, the patient's physical and psychologic status, the patient's position during the surgery, and the surgeon's needs. Patients who are highly motivated to avoid GA might tolerate complicated procedures performed under RA or MAC. At other times, GA may be required for simple, office-based surgery if the patient is apprehensive. In general, patients undergoing major reconstruction require GA.

Sedation and Analgesia

Sedation-analgesia is often used to diminish a patient's anxiety and discomfort during surgery performed under local infiltration and peripheral nerve block techniques. When an anesthesiologist is involved, the goal of MAC is to ensure patient safety as well as comfort. Therefore the same level of monitoring is required during a MAC as during GA or RA.

Basic monitoring includes assessment of level of consciousness, pulmonary ventilation by capnography (end-tidal carbon dioxide), pulse oximetry, blood pressure, heart rate, and continuous ECG. Also, during sedation-analgesia, supplemental oxygen should be given to increase the oxygen reserve in the lungs. This provides a margin of safety should apnea or airway obstruction occur. This advantage is lost, however, if pulmonary ventilation is not monitored independently. The goal is to identify a ventilation problem and correct it before it leads to hypoxemia and potential brain damage, cardiac arrest, or death.

The optimal route for administration of sedative-analgesic drugs during conscious sedation is the IV route because the lag time from administration to effect is the shortest. This allows titration to the desired anesthetic effect while minimizing the risk of oversedation, with possible respiratory and cardiovascular depression. The endpoint for titration of sedative-analgesic drugs during conscious sedation is the patient's verbal acknowledgment of comfort and relaxation, along with stable vital signs. The patient should remain cooperative and comfortable, with airway reflexes intact.

A wide variety of drugs can be used to provide sedation and analgesia (Box 17-1). The most frequently used agents for IV sedation in the office setting for cosmetic surgical procedures are midazolam (82%), fentanyl (60%), diazepam (57%), meperidine (46%), barbiturates (43%), ketamine (43%), and propofol (37%).[10]

In about one third of surgeries, sedation-analgesia was not administered by a nurse anesthetist or anesthesiologist. At our institution, only the benzodiazepines (diazepam, midazolam), opioid analgesics (meperidine, morphine, fentanyl) and opiate agonist/antagonist (butorphanol) are approved for use by nonanesthesiologists credentialed in conscious sedation

Table 17-3.
Current Recommendations for Preoperative Laboratory Tests*

AGE (yr)	MALES	FEMALES
<40	None	Pregnancy test†
40-49	Hct, ECG	Hct, pregnancy test†
50-64	Hct, ECG	Hct, ECG
>75	Hct, ECG, CXR	Hct, ECG, CXR

Hct, Hematocrit; *ECG*, electrocardiogram; *CXR*, chest radiograph.
*At Brigham and Women's Hospital, Boston; for asymptomatic healthy patients undergoing peripheral surgery involving minimal blood loss
†If patient is uncertain about her pregnancy status.

Table 17-4.
Fasting Protocol

PATIENT GROUP	SOLIDS AND NONCLEAR LIQUIDS* (hr)	CLEAR LIQUIDS (hr)
Adults	6-8, or none after midnight†	2-3
Children‡		
>36 mo	6-8	2-3
6-36 mo	6	2-3
<6 mo	4-6	2

Modified from American Society of Anesthesiologists: *Anesthesiology* 84:459-471, 1996.
*Includes milk, formula, and breast milk (high fat content may delay gastric emptying).
†No data have established whether fasting for 6 to 8 hours is equivalent to an overnight fast.
‡Unless contraindicated, pediatric patients should be offered clear liquids until 2 to 3 hours before surgery to minimize risk of dehydration.

(Table 17-5). The benzodiazepines are used for anxiolysis, amnesia, and sedation. The opioids are administered to provide analgesia.

Midazolam and *fentanyl* are ideal agents for IV sedation because both have a rapid onset of action, allowing for easy titration to effect, and a short half-life. Both drugs have a steep dose-response curve, however, so they must be administered in small, incremental doses. The dose must be reduced in patients with preexisting cardiac or pulmonary disease, particularly when given in combination, because midazolam and fentanyl exert a synergistic cardiorespiratory depressive effect. Likewise, in patients with hepatorenal disease, the total dose must be reduced because of impaired drug metabolism and excretion. The short duration of action of midazolam and fentanyl, however, is secondary to redistribution from the brain to other tissues, such as muscle and fat. Thus metabolism becomes important only with larger cumulative doses. Patients with comorbidities, especially ASA III or greater, may be extremely sensitive to the effects of these drugs.

Flumazenil and *naloxone* are specific antagonists to benzodiazepines and narcotic analgesics, respectively (Table 17-6). Their administration is indicated in an oversedated or overnarcotized patient who is hypoxemic and when airway control and positive-pressure ventilation are difficult. Reversal agents should be administered cautiously because they have potentially adverse effects. Rather, patients who become hypoxemic or apneic during sedation-analgesia should (1) receive supplemental oxygen, (2) be encouraged or stimulated to breathe deeply, and (3) receive positive-pressure ventilation if spontaneous ventilation is inadequate.[1] Also, patients given reversal agents must be monitored for a longer period postoperatively (up to 2 hours) to ensure that resedation does not recur, since these drugs' duration of action may be shorter than that of the agonist drug.

Postoperative monitoring of all patients in the recovery phase is important to recognize cardiorespiratory depression, especially since the patient is no longer experiencing surgical stimulation.

Regional Anesthesia

RA includes local infiltration, peripheral nerve blocks, and central neuroaxial blocks (spinal, epidural, and candal anesthesia). It can be supplemented with IV sedation or light GA. RA offers a safe alternative for patients in whom GA may be undesirable. Patients may be reluctant to have RA because of concerns about complications or awareness of OR activities. Surgeons may be concerned about inadequate anesthesia or the time required to achieve surgical anesthesia. Anesthesiologists often prefer RA for themselves. Advantages of RA include attenuation of the stress response, postoperative analgesia, and avoidance of GA.

Early practitioners, such as John S. Lundy, Sir Robert Macintosh, and George W. Crile, espoused the idea of "balanced" anesthesia, that is, a combination of RA and GA.[6]

RA dates back to ancient times, when ice and pressure were used to produce numbness. The "refrigeration" technique was described by Severino in the 1600s and was used as recently as World War II.[6] Modern RA began in 1884 with the introduction of cocaine into clinical practice by Carl Koller, an ophthalmology resident in Vienna. Koller showed that cocaine produced loss of sensation when applied to the corneas of laboratory animals. This discovery was demonstrated publicly on an ophthalmology patient on Sept. 15, 1884. Cocaine, a crystalline alkaloid derived from coca leaves and isolated in 1860, proved to be highly addictive and dangerous. Fatalities associated with its use prompted the search for safer local anesthetics. Procaine represented a major advance and became the main local anesthetic for decades after its introduction in 1905.

The ideal local anesthetic is nontoxic, potent, and stable in solution. Local anesthetics belong to two major groups, esters and amides (Table 17-7). The *ester group* comprises derivatives of benzoic acid (cocaine) and paraaminobenzoic acid (PABA; procaine, chlorprocaine, tetracaine, benzocaine). They are hydrolyzed by plasma pseudocholinesterase. Allergic reactions to the ester local anesthetics are most likely in response to PABA, and therefore these anesthetics should be avoided in patients with PABA sensitivity. Chloroprocaine has been implicated in cases of neurotoxicity and back pain thought to be related to the solution stabilizers sodium metabisulfite and ethylenediaminetetraacetic acid (EDTA), respectively.

The *amide group* was introduced with the discovery of lidocaine in 1948. Prilocaine, mepivacaine, etidocaine, bupivacaine, and ropivacaine are the other amide local anesthetics. The amides are anilides or quinolines. True allergic reactions to this class of local anesthetics are exceedingly rare. Patients

---

Box 17-1.
Drugs Used for Sedation and Analgesia

OPIOID AGONIST ANALGESICS
Alfentanil (Alfenta)
Fentanyl (Sublimaze)
Hydromorphone (Dilaudid)
Meperidine (Demerol)
Morphine sulfate
Oxymorphone (Numorphan)
Sufentanil (Sufenta)

OPIOID AGONIST/ANTAGONIST ANALGESICS
Nalbuphine (Nubain)
Butorphanol (Stadol)

SEDATIVE-ANXIOLYTICS
Diazepam (Valium)
Hydroxyzine (Vistaril)
Lorazepam (Ativan)
Midazolam (Versed)

SEDATIVE-HYPNOTICS
Propofol (Diprivan)
Thiopental (Pentothal)

SEDATIVE-ANALGESIC
Ketamine (Ketalar)

Table 17-5.
Guidelines for Intravenous Administration of Sedative-Analgesic Medications*

AGENT	TITRATION DOSE	TYPICAL DOSE†	DYNAMICS/CLEARANCE	SPECIAL CONSIDERATIONS‡
BENZODIAZEPINES				
Midazolam (Versed)	0.25-0.5 mg May repeat after 2 min to achieve desired effect	0.007-0.04 mg/kg 0.2-2.5 mg	Onset: 1-5 min Peak: 2 min Duration: 15-60 min Clearance: hepatic	Water soluble; less pain and irritation than with diazepam. Reduce dose by one-third when used with narcotics or in elderly patients.
Diazepam (Valium)	0.25-1.0 mg May repeat after 5 min to achieve desired effect	0.1-0.7 mg/kg 2-5 mg	Onset: 1-2 min Peak: 3-5 min Duration: 60-90 min Clearance: hepatic/renal	Venoirritating; administer into large vein. Contraindicated in adult narrow-angle and open-angle glaucoma. Has active metabolites; use with caution in patients with hepatorenal disease. Reduce dose by one-third when used with narcotics or in elderly patients.
NARCOTICS				
Fentanyl (Sublimaze)	12.5-25 µg May repeat in 2-3 min	1-2 µg/kg 25-100 µg	Onset: immediate Peak: 5-15 min Duration: 30-60 min Clearance: hepatic	Reduce dose when given with benzodiazepines or in elderly patients. May cause muscle rigidity, especially truncal, and bradycardia.
Morphine sulfate	1-2 mg May repeat in 5-10 min	0.05-0.1 mg/kg 1-3 mg	Onset: 5 min Peak: 20 min Duration: 3-4 hr Clearance: hepatic/renal	Reduce dose when given with benzodiazepines or in elderly patients. May release histamine (hives over IV site).
Meperidine (Demerol)	12.5-25 mg May repeat in 2-3 min	0.5-1 mg/kg 25-50 mg	Onset: 5-10 min Peak: 5-7 min Duration: 1-2 hr Clearance: hepatic/renal	Reduce dose when given with benzodiazepines. Contraindicated in patients receiving monoamine oxidase inhibitors. Anticholinergic effects may cause tachycardia and delirium, especially in elderly patients.
NARCOTIC AGONIST/ANTAGONIST				
Butorphanol (Stadol)	0.25-0.5 mg May repeat in 2-3 min	1-2 mg	Onset: 2-3 min Peak: 30-60 min Duration: 3-4 hr Clearance: hepatic/renal	Patients physically dependent on narcotics may withdraw because of antagonist properties. Reduce dose by one-half in elderly patients, with twice the interval for repeat dose.

*Currently approved at Brigham and Women's Hospital for conscious sedation in adults by nonanesthesiologists.
†Dosages should be based on ideal body weight and not actual body weight.
‡Practitioners should refer to other sources for complete list of side effects and contraindications.

Table 17-6.
Flumazenil and Naloxone: Guidelines for Intravenous Administration

AGENT	ACTION	DOSE*	DYNAMICS/ CLEARANCE	SIDE EFFECTS†
Flumazenil (Romazicon)	Reverses sedative effects of benzodiazepines	0.2 mg over 15 sec May repeat in 1 min to obtain desired effect Maximum dose of 1 mg	Onset: 1 min Peak: 2-6 min Duration: 45-90 min Clearance: hepatic	Seizures Cardiac dysrhythmias Dizziness Agitation
Naloxone (Narcan)	Reverses opioid-induced respiratory depression	Titrate 0.04 mg Repeat every 2 min to desired effect If no response after 0.4 mg, seek assistance and question diagnosis	Onset: 2 min Peak: 5-15 min Duration: 45-90 min Clearance: hepatic	Nausea and vomiting Tachycardia Hypertension Pulmonary edema Ventricular dysrhythmias

*Dosages should be based on ideal body weight and not actual body weight.
†Practitioners should refer to other sources for complete list of side effects and contraindications.

Table 17-7.
Local Anesthetics

AGENT	DOSE (mg/kg)*	DURATION (min)
ESTERS		
Procaine (Novocain)	14	60-90
Chloroprocaine (Nesacaine)	10	30-60
Tetracaine (Pontocaine)	1.5	
AMIDES		
Lidocaine (Xylocaine)	7†	90-200
Mepivacaine (Carbocaine)	7†	120-240
Prilocaine (Citanest)	10	120-240
Bupivacaine (Marcaine)	1-2	180-600
Ropivacaine (Naropin)	1-2	180-600
Etidocaine (Duranest)	2-4	180-600

Modified from Moore DC, Bridenbaugh LD, Thompson GE, et al: *Anesthesiology* 47:263-268, 1977.
*Manufacturer-suggested dose limits for perineural (extravascular and extrathecal) use. This table in no way implies that these dosages are safe or absolute maxima.
†With 5 µg/ml of 1:200,000 epinephrine.

Table 17-8.
Bicarbonate Doses for Local Anesthetic Solutions

BICARBONATE (mEq)	LOCAL ANESTHETIC (ml)
1	Chloroprocaine (30)
1	Lidocaine (10)
0.1	Bupivacaine (10)

with impaired liver function may have delayed clearance of these drugs, which are metabolized in the liver.

Local anesthetics (weak bases) reversibly prevent nerve conduction by blocking sodium channels. The local anesthetic molecules exist in anionic (nonionized) and cationic (ionized) form. The anionic form penetrates the nerve membrane. Commercially prepared solutions of local anesthetics are acidic and thus contain more cationic than anionic molecules. The addition of sodium bicarbonate to the solution increases the proportion of anions, thereby increasing the onset of the block (Table 17-8). Furthermore, the addition of bicarbonate decreases the discomfort associated with dermal or subcutaneous injection.[26]

The duration of action of local anesthetic agents is related primarily to their degree of protein binding, since local anesthetics are believed to act by binding to a protein receptor in the sodium channel. The greater protein binding of a specific agent presumably results in a longer period of sodium channel blockade and a longer duration of anesthesia. Tetracaine, bupivacaine, and etidocaine are more highly bound to protein, and their duration of action is two to four times longer than their homologous compounds (procaine, mepivacaine, and lidocaine, respectively). Increased duration of action of a local anesthetic can be achieved by increasing the total dosage or by adding a vasoconstrictor such as epinephrine, which decreases the rate of vascular absorption, allowing more local anesthetic molecules to diffuse to the nerve membrane.

The vascular absorption of local anesthetic agents is related to the injection site, dosage, addition of vasoconstrictor agent, and specific agent employed. The plasma concentration of local anesthetics is highest after intercostal nerve blockade and the lowest after subcutaneous infiltration. The decreasing order for effective vascular absorption is intercostal, paracervical, caudal, epidural, brachial plexus, subarachnoid, and subcutaneous.

Contraindications to RA include patient refusal, severe coagulopathy, infection at the site of injection, compartment syndrome, and history of an allergic reaction to local anesthetics. Complications of RA may be immediate or may arise postoperatively. Immediate complications can result from central nervous system and cardiovascular system drug reactions or neurovascular injury from the nerve block. Delayed reactions include infection, chemical and immunologic reactions, direct or indirect trauma, and headache after dural puncture. Post–dural puncture headaches can progress to cranial nerve damage and should be treated aggressively with IV and oral fluids and analgesics, avoiding aspirin and nonsteroidal antiinflammatory drugs (NSAIDs), which inhibit platelet function. The anesthesia team should be contacted. If conservative measures do not relieve the headache, the patient might be a candidate for an epidural blood patch.

Tumescent Anesthesia

A special application of local infiltration anesthesia is the tumescent technique for liposuction surgery. Tumescent anesthesia is the subcutaneous injection of a large volume of dilute local anesthetic solution with epinephrine. The advantages of tumescent anesthesia for liposuction surgery are (1) profound local anesthesia, (2) decreased surgical blood loss, (3) reduced IV fluid requirements, and (4) enhanced anesthetic results.[21]

The tumescent anesthetic solution consists of a 0.05% to 0.1% lidocaine with epinephrine at a 1:1 million to 1:2 million dilution in normal saline (Table 17-9). Sodium bicarbonate is added to neutralize the solution's acidity and thus decrease the pain associated with injection. Triamcinolone is added to reduce postoperative soreness by decreasing swelling and inflammation. Finally, the liter bags of normal saline are stored in a blanket warmer at 40° C (104° F) and removed just before the anesthetic solution is mixed.[21] Warming reduces the discomfort associated with infusion of the anesthetic solution.[15]

In general the volume of tumescent solution injected is twice that of the volume of fat aspirated. Klein[21] and Ostad et al[31] have reported the safe use of high doses of lidocaine, 33 mg/kg and 55 mg/kg, respectively. This is five to eight times the manufacturer's recommended maximum safe dose

Table 17-9.
Tumescent Anesthetic Solution

AGENT	AMOUNT	CONCENTRATION
Lidocaine	500-1000 mg	0.05%-0.1%
Epinephrine	0.5-1 mg	1:2 to 1:1 million*
Sodium bicarbonate	10 mEq	
Triamcinolone	10 mg	
Normal saline	1000 ml	

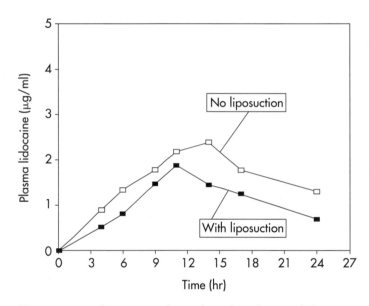

Figure 17-2. Comparison of time-dependent changes of plasma lidocaine levels with subcutaneous infiltration of 2625 mg lidocaine (35 mg/kg) in 5.25 L anesthetic solution in 75-kg woman using tumescent technique both with and without liposuction. (From Klein J: *Plast Reconstr Surg* 92:1089, 1993.)

of lidocaine with epinephrine. Factors responsible for the safety of tumescent anesthesia may include (1) dilute solution of lidocaine, (2) slow rate of administration, (3) relatively avascular subcutaneous tissue, (4) lipid solubility of lidocaine, (5) vasoconstriction from epinephrine, and (6) compression of the vasculature from the large volume infused.[3] The slow rate of administration of tumescent anesthetic solution (50 to 150 ml/min) and the relatively avascular subcutaneous compartments tumesced (abdomen, flanks, buttocks, hips, and thighs) are also important factors. Faster rates of injection and more vascular compartments injected may lead to unsafe blood levels of local anesthetic.

The safety of tumescent anesthesia initially, was thought to result from a significant portion of lidocaine being removed during liposuction. In Klein's study, however, lidocaine absorption was not significantly altered by liposuction (Figure 17-2).[21] Peak plasma lidocaine concentration occurred about

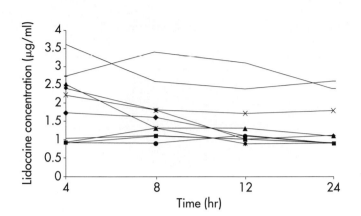

Figure 17-3. Serial plasma lidocaine levels measured over 24 hours. (From Ostad A, Kageyama N, Moy RL: *Dermatol Surg* 22:921-927, 1996.)

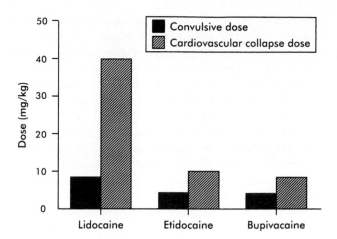

Figure 17-4. Relationships between doses of lidocaine and bupivacaine that cause toxic response in central nervous system and doses that produce cardiovascular collapse. (From Longnecker DE, Tinker JA, Morgan GE: *Principles and practice of anesthesiology*, ed 2, St Louis, 1998, Mosby.)

Table 17-10.
Plasma Lidocaine Concentration and Toxicity

CONCENTRATION (μg/ml)	EFFECTS
3-5	Drowsiness, dizziness, lightheadedness
5-9	Muscle fasciculations, tinnitus, paresthesias
8-12	Seizures, coma
20	Respiratory arrest
24	Cardiac arrest

12 to 15 hours after injection. Ostad et al used a higher dose of lidocaine and a faster rate of injection, and the peak plasma lidocaine levels occurred sooner, 4 to 8 hours after injection (Figure 17-3).[31] Although both studies reporte4d no cases of objective local anesthetic systemic toxicity, some patients had subjective symptoms of drowsiness, dizziness, and lightheadedness (Table 17-10).

The local anesthetic effect of lidocaine injected by the tumescent technique has a longer duration of action than normally expected. Therefore no need exists to use a longer-acting and potentially more cardiotoxic local anesthetic such as bupivacaine (Figure 17-4). Patients undergoing tumescent liposuction should be in good health, with no impaired cardiovascular, hepatic, or renal function.

General Anesthesia

GA renders a patient unconscious and insensitive to stimulation. The exact mechanism of action of general anesthetic agents is still unknown. Substances with very different molecular structure can induce GA. In the early twentieth century, Meyer and Overton noted that the potency of a general anesthetic is related to its solubility in olive oil; this is known as the Meyer-Overton rule. Later, Ferguson suggested that thermodynamic activity and potency were interrelated. Currently, three theories explain where general anesthetics work: the lipid bilayer, neurotransmitter receptor proteins, or lipid-protein juncture.

The objectives of GA—unconsciousness, amnesia, analgesia, and muscle relaxation—can be achieved with inhalational or IV anesthetic agents. For maintenance of general anesthesia, a combination of the two usually is employed, reducing the need for and potential toxicity of a large dose of a single anesthetic.

The phases of general anesthesia are induction, maintenance, and emergence. In the pediatric population, inhalational inductions are preferred, whereas in adults, IV inductions are the norm. The two most common IV induction agents, thiopental and propofol, are potent short-acting hypnotics that can cause cardiovascular depression in a dose-dependent manner. When avoiding cardiovascular depression is an issue, other hypnotic drugs such as etomidate, which has minimal cardiovascular effects, or ketamine, which has sympathomimetic effects, may be employed.

Inhalational agents include nitrous oxide, isoflurane, enflurane, halothane, desflurane, and sevoflurane. *Nitrous oxide* (N_2O) is a stable, inorganic compound that is not metabolized in the body and is relatively insoluble in blood. It is used primarily as a supplement to other inhalational agents or IV medications. N_2O has rapid uptake during induction and rapid elimination. This property can cause diffusion hypoxemia if the patient is given room air instead of supplemental oxygen to breathe after surgery. N_2O can expand into air-filled cavities and support combustion. It should be avoided in patients with marginal oxygenation, pneumothorax, pneumopericardium, or bowel obstruction and in those undergoing tympanic membrane closure.

The other inhalational agents are halogenated hydrocarbons, each with specific advantages and disadvantages. *Halothane* produces a smooth inhalational induction but is known to predispose to dysrhythmias and hepatotoxicity. *Enflurane* has a lower potential for myocardial sensitization but produces fluoride ions, which may lead to nephrotoxicity. *Isoflurane* undergoes minimal biotransformation but is eliminated slowly.

Desflurane and seroflurane are newer inhalational agents. They have the advantage of rapid uptake and elimination, making them particularly suitable for ambulatory surgery. *Desflurane* has a pungent odor that may be unsuitable for patients with an irritable airway. *Sevoflurane* produces smooth, rapid inhalational induction but may cause renal injury when used at low flows for long periods.

GA with spontaneous or controlled ventilation may be performed with a mask, a laryngeal mask airway (LMA), or an endotracheal (ET) tube. Mask anesthesia is suitable for short operations that involve no encroachment on or near the airway. It is contraindicated in any patient at increased risk for aspiration (e.g., obese, full stomach). The LMA, introduced by Brain in 1983, allows for more control of the airway, does not require a muscle relaxant for insertion, and causes less stimulation than ET intubation (Figure 17-5). It is used extensively for operations of medium length and for patients who cannot be intubated. The same restrictions for mask anesthesia apply to the LMA; damage to the uvula and other oropharyngeal structures has been reported. GA with an ET tube is the standard for long, complicated procedures. The ET tube protects the airway and provides positive-pressure ventilation.

Patients with craniofacial abnormalities, facial trauma, upper body burns, head and neck tumors, hemangiomas, severe rheumatoid arthritis, ankylosing spondylitis, obesity, or facial anomalies may be difficult to ventilate by mask and to intubate. The patient and OR staff should be prepared for fiberoptic intubation with the patient awake. The plan should be nonthreatening to the patient, with emphasis on comfort and safety. The patient should receive a nonparticulate antacid, an antisialogogue, an antiemetic such as metoclopramide, and topical anesthesia of nasopharynx and oropharynx. Sedatives and analgesics are important adjuncts to the local anesthesia; their judicious use will relax the patient without significant respiratory depression. The fiberoptic scope and light source should be in the OR and tested before the intubation attempt. Small ET tubes presoftened in sterile saline should be checked and ready.

In patients with abnormal airway anatomy, fiberoptic intubation is usually the safest, most prudent way to proceed. The surgical team must be psychologically and technically

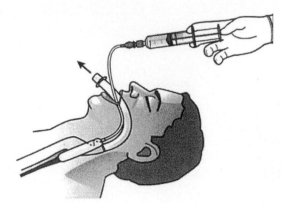

Figure 17-5. Laryngeal mask airway (LMA). Without holding tube of LMA, cuff is inflated with recommended volume of air. LMA may protrude slightly on inflation of cuff. (From Longnecker DE, Tinker JA, Morgan GE: *Principles and practice of anesthesiology,* ed 2, St Louis, 1998, Mosby.)

prepared to perform a tracheostomy if the intubation attempt fails and the patient cannot be ventilated. Occasionally a patient may appear to have normal anatomy and prove to be very difficult to intubate and ventilate. Allowing the patient to wake up and breathe spontaneously is the safest approach. The team may decide to proceed with fiberoptic intubation or to postpone surgery, as determined by the degree of difficulty, the patient's trauma, and the surgical urgency (Figure 17-6).

IV access can be challenging in patients undergoing reconstructive surgery who have had multiple previous procedures. Scarring in burn patients, limited sites in mastectomy patients, and anticipated use of a radial artery graft can make IV access difficult. To minimize patient anxiety and to maximize the chance of finding a vein, the patient may be given oral diazepam (2.5 to 10 mg) or intramuscular midazolam (5 mg/ml), and the potential sites may be treated with a thin layer of nitroglycerin paste, if the patient's blood pressure is not too low. These modalities require 10 to 15 minutes but are useful if the IV cannula can be placed painlessly in a calm patient. The patient should be monitored while the midazolam and nitropaste are taking effect.

PATIENT POSITIONING

Positioning the patient for surgery must accommodate the surgeon's needs and not put the patient at risk for injury. Proper positioning will expedite surgery by providing good exposure of the surgical site and will minimize the risk of complications. Improper positioning can cause injuries to the integument, muscles, bones, neurovascular bundles, and eyes. Patients with diabetes, obesity, arthritis, osteoporosis, spinal cord injuries, burns, and connective tissue disorders are more vulnerable to position injuries. Changes in position can result in major circulatory and respiratory changes. Anesthetized patients cannot complain; therefore, whenever possible, the surgeon must ascertain that the patient is comfortable in the anticipated position before induction of anesthesia.

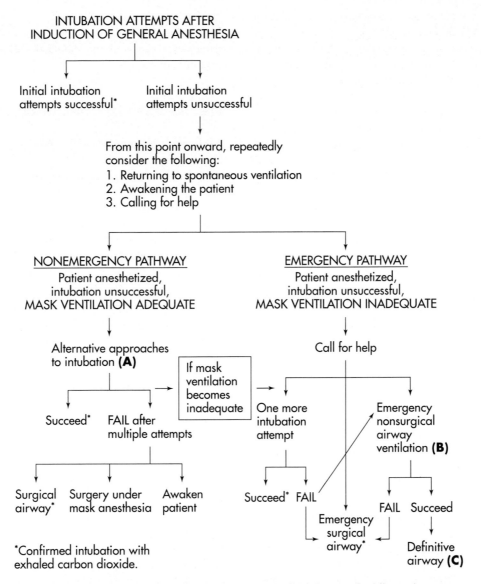

Figure 17-6. Difficult airway algorithm. Options include the following: **A,** different laryngoscope blades, awake intubation, "blind" oral or nasal intubation, fiberoptic intubation, intubating stylet or tube changer, light wand, retrograde intubation, surgical airway access; **B,** transtracheal jet ventilation, laryngeal mask ventilation, combined esophageal-tracheal ventilation; **C,** spontaneous ventilation, tracheotomy, endotracheal intubation. (Modified from American Society of Anesthesiologists Task Force on Management of the Difficult Airway: *Anesthesiology* 78:597, 1993.)

The common positions are supine, prone, lateral decubitus, and lithotomy. The *supine position* is generally well tolerated, although pulmonary functional residual capacity is decreased. Complications may occur from (1) traction on the brachial plexus; (2) pressure on the radial nerve, ulnar nerve, long saphenous vein, and dorsalis pedis artery; (3) hyperextension of the knee; and (4) pressure on bony prominences. Injuries can be avoided by not abducting the arms above 85 degrees, padding arm boards and all bony prominences, making sure the patient's legs are not crossed, and periodically relieving the pressure by lifting parts of the body prone to pressure necrosis.

The *prone position* poses many more problems. Achieving this position may be difficult and hazardous for the patient and for the OR staff if the patient is very large or obese. Some anesthesiologists advocate intubation with local anesthesia followed by patients moving themselves into the correct position. GA is usually induced on a stretcher, then the patient is turned prone onto the operating table. The stretcher should be adjustable so that the head-down position can be achieved if regurgitation should occur during induction. Before the turn, the eyes should be protected with a sterile ophthalmic ointment, closed, covered, and rechecked after the turn. No pressure must be exerted on the eyes to prevent retinal artery occlusion, which can cause postoperative visual loss. Lubrication for the eyes is important because lacrimation is decreased under GA. The ET tube must be very carefully secured, preferably with benzoin, tape, and tie, since accidental extubation could be catastrophic. The breath sounds should be rechecked immediately after the turn to rule out endobronchial intubation or dislodgment of the ET tube. The head should be cushioned on a foam donut and maintained in as neutral a position as possible, with the ears and nose checked for folding. The arms should be parallel to the operating table either above the head or at the sides. Rolls should be placed under the thorax; the breasts, nipples, and male genitalia should be free of pressure. Frequent lifting of the head can alleviate pressure. Compression boots help prevent venous pooling.

The *lateral decubitus position* is associated with cardiorespiratory changes. Compression of the dependent lung results in loss of lung volume. Combined inequalities in functional residual capacity, distribution of inhaled gas, and pulmonary blood flow lead to ventilation/perfusion mismatch. These alterations are more pronounced in the patient on positive-pressure ventilation. The blood supply to the head may be impeded by rotation of the neck. The areas at greatest risk are the head, ear, brachial plexus, upper arm, and common peroneal nerve. The head should be supported on a foam donut at an appropriate height to avoid stretching the brachial plexus and to protect the ear. A roll under the upper rib cage will also protect the brachial plexus. The upper arm should be supported on a padded armrest and the lower extremities separated with a pillow.

The *lithotomy position* puts the patient at risk for injury to the brachial plexus hips, back, knees, arms, and fingers. Proper positioning in the stirrups will alleviate pressure and traction on the lower extremities. Placing the arms at the patient's side puts the fingers at risk for a crushing injury when the foot of the bed is raised. Therefore the upper extremities should be carefully secured on padded arm boards abducted less than 90 degrees.

The *Trendelenburg position,* first described by Meyer in 1885 for gynecologic surgery, involves tilting the operating table so that the head is lower than the pelvis. This facilitates surgery by shifting the abdominal contents away from the surgical site. The upward movement of the viscera may impinge on pulmonary circulation and ventilation. This position is not well tolerated in awake patients because of subjective and objective respiratory difficulty. Anesthetized obese patients may experience too great a decrease in functional residual capacity to be maintained in this position for long. Cardiovascular effects are complex. In normotensive patients, preload may increase, but systemic vascular resistance may decrease. In hypotensive patients, afterload may decrease, preload may not change, and cardiac output may fall. Central baroreceptors exposed to increased venous pressure may cause a fall in systemic vascular resistance. Intraocular pressure rises in proportion to the patient's angle. The Trendelenburg position is often used in conjunction with the supine and lithotomy positions. The upper and lower extremities, eyes, and ET tube should be rechecked after the operating table is tilted head down. Brachial plexus injury may occur if the arms rotate cephalad. A corneal abrasion may occur if the eyes are open. The ET tube can slip into the right mainstem bronchus or out of the larynx.

Positioning the patient properly can be time consuming and difficult. Attention to detail is imperative and may prevent major complications. The operating table should be appropri-ate for the patient's weight and tested for proper function. Precautions to avoid injury to the brachial plexus, peripheral nerves, eyes, ears, and skin should be followed for all patients, regardless of position.[23]

SPECIAL PATIENT CONSIDERATIONS

Malignant Hyperthermia

Malignant hyperthermia (MH) is a syndrome in which a patient develops life-threatening hyperthermia. The exact mechanism and incidence are unknown, although myoplasmic calcium is increased. MH is usually transmitted as an autosomal dominant trait but may also be passed as a recessive gene. It can be triggered by depolarizing muscle relaxants, general anesthetics, and stress. Previous anesthesia may have been uneventful. The episode may occur immediately after induction of anesthesia or after surgery. Early signs include hypercarbia and tachycardia. Discontinuing potent inhaled anesthetic agents, aggressive treatment with dantrolene (an intracellular muscle relaxant), and efforts to cool the patient are critical because MH can be fatal.[23]

Autonomic Hyperreflexia

Patients with chronic spinal cord injury may have debridement of sores or wound closure. Physicians should be aware of the phenomenon of autonomic hyperreflexia, which occurs in about 85% of patients with lesions above the sixth thoracic vertebra (T6). Patients with lesions above T6 experience loss of the inhibitory influence of cortical fibers on spinal reflexes initiated by afferent impulses from visceral and peripheral sensory fibers. Severe hypertension can develop and lead to cerebral hemorrhage and death. Treatment consists of α-adrenergic receptor antagonists, ganglionic blockers, or direct-acting vasodilators. Patients at risk for autonomic hyperreflexia should be treated as though they have normal sensation below the level of the lesion. Spinal or general anesthesia will block the response to surgical stimulation, thereby decreasing the likelihood of autonomic hyperreflexia. Succinylcholine, a depolarizing muscle relaxant, should be avoided because hyperkalemia may result.[23]

Burns

Patients with acute burns are in a hypermetabolic state, have increased vascular permeability, and may have inhalation injuries. Aggressive airway and fluid management are essential. Succinylcholine must be avoided after the fourth day because fatal hyperkalemia may result. These patients are at risk for hypothermia, so the OR must be kept warm (80° to 82° F, about 27° C) at all times. IV fluids must be warmed. Blood loss can be extensive, especially with eschar excision (about 200 ml/1% body surface area excised), so blood should be in the OR in a cooler before induction.

Cosmetic Surgery

A smooth emergence from anesthesia and a stress-free postoperative course are critical to an optimal outcome after cosmetic surgery. It is important to minimize coughing, bucking, and retching on emergence. These events may increase tension on suture lines, risking disruption such as in an abdominoplasty, and may increase incisional bleeding through an associated increase in venous pressure and systemic arterial pressure.

To achieve the previous goals, we prefer to avoid GA and use RA, such as thoracic epidural anesthesia for cosmetic breast surgery.[24] When GA is necessary, intubation should be avoided when feasible. If intubated, patients should breathe on their own toward the end of the procedure and be extubated while still anesthetized. If patients are at risk for aspiration or have a potentially difficult airway to ventilate by mask or intubate, they should be extubated as soon as arousable. Before extubation, we may titrate in small doses of fentanyl, which is an excellent antitussive agent, or give IV lidocaine to minimize reaction to the ET tube.

Postoperative nausea and vomiting must be prevented. In general, all patients receive an antiemetic before emergence. Since pain and opioid pain medication can cause postoperative nausea and vomiting, use of local anesthetics at the operative site is important. Nonopioid analgesics such as acetaminophen are useful adjuvants for treating postoperative pain. We do not use NSAIDs in the acute postoperative period because of their potential for increasing bleeding at incisional sites. Despite good pain control, some patients, especially those with preoperative hypertension, are still at risk for postoperative hypertension. They should be appropriately managed with an antihypertensive agent such as labetalol.

Flaps

The intraoperative management of patients having a flap transfer, especially a free flap requiring microvascular anastomoses, necessitates keeping the patient warm and well hydrated to minimize peripheral vasoconstriction, which might impair graft perfusion. Also, vasoconstrictors such as phenylephrine, which is a direct-acting α-adrenergic agonist, should not be used to treat hypotension. A better choice is ephedrine, which restores systemic blood pressure, primarily by increasing cardiac output.

Multiple Comorbidities

The choice of the optimal anesthetic for patients with multiple, active disease processes is a complex question with no simple answer. For example, although pulmonary function may be better after RA than GA, a heavy smoker with extensive chronic obstructive pulmonary disease may have a chronic cough and excessive need to clear sputum, which could preclude a regional or local anesthetic during a delicate plastic surgical procedure.[32] Similarly, a patient with significant mitral regurgitation may benefit from the afterload reduction provided by a spinal or epidural anesthetic, but the coexisting aortic stenosis may not allow the patient to tolerate this decrease. Such situations are controversial and best discussed with all the involved parties, including primary care practitioners and consultants, and resolved on a case-by-case basis.

Nausea and Vomiting

Postoperative nausea and vomiting have important patient comfort, surgical, and cost implications. Overall incidence varies from 20% to 30%, depending on such factors as type and location of surgery and choice of anesthesia[40] (Box 17-2). In plastic surgery, increased intraabdominal pressure from emesis may precipitate bleeding and disruption of suture lines.

Since the cause and treatment of nausea and vomiting are multifactorial, data must be interpreted with caution. The incidence appears to be less with RA, including thoracic epidural, than with GA for breast surgery.[24,40] This may result from blockade of inhibitory spinal reflex arcs, increases in gastrointestinal blood flow, or less pushing on the stomach by ventilated lungs. With GA the choice of anesthetic drugs may have an important impact on nausea and vomiting; after propofol administration, the incidence was as low as 7%, whereas with desflurane and N_2O anesthesia, the incidence was as high as 71%.[42]

Antiemetic drugs have had varying success (Box 17-3). Although droperidol and metoclopramide are often used, newer agents that antagonize the serotonin type 3 receptor (5-HT3), such as ondansetron, have been advocated for intractable nausea and vomiting. Other serotonin antagonists are currently under clinical investigation.

Box 17-2.
Factors Influencing Nausea and Vomiting

PATIENT
Age: higher incidence (peak 11-14 yr) in pediatric than adult patients
Gender: higher incidence (2-3 times) in female than male adults
Obesity
History of motion sickness
History of previous postoperative nausea
Anxiety
Gastroparesis (e.g., patients with diabetes mellitus, neuromuscular disorders, gastrointestinal obstruction, or chronic cholecystitis)

ANESTHESIA
Premedication with opioids
Gastric distention (e.g., face mask ventilation)
Anesthetic techniques: general anesthesia (N_2O/narcotic/muscle relaxant > inhalational > IV propofol) > regional anesthesia

SURGERY
Pain, especially visceral or pelvic
Narcotic pain medication
Procedure
    Gynecologic (laparoscopy)
    Breast
    Head and neck
    Stomach, duodenum, gallbladder

Box 17-3.
Antiemetic Drugs

ANTICHOLINERGICS
Atropine
Scopolamine

ANTIHISTAMINES
Dimenhydrinate
Hydroxyzine
Cyclizine
Diphenhydramine

PHENOTHIAZINES
Chlorpromazine
Promethazine
Prochlorperazine
Perphenazine

BUTYROPHENONES
Haloperidol
Droperidol*

BENZAMIDES
Metoclopramide*
Domperidone

SEROTONIN ANTAGONISTS
Ondansetron*
Granisetron
Tropisetron
Dolasetron

*Intravenous agents frequently used for prevention and treatment of postoperative nausea and vomiting.

OUTCOMES

Anesthesia today is incredibly safe and helps make possible even the most complex surgical techniques on the most unstable patients. Interestingly, outcome studies directly and indirectly reflect its safety. Directly, they demonstrate a continuing and significant reduction in anesthetic mortality. Indirectly, as anesthesia has became safer, studies allow more introspection, and their focus has shifted from intraoperative mortality to perioperative morbidity.

Perioperative Morbidity and Mortality

From the mid-1950s to the 1980s, anesthetic outcome studies focused on mortality and major morbidity. The development and use of pulse oximetry and capnography in the 1980s allowed for the detection of hypoxemia and hypoventilation, respectively, and revolutionized the practice of anesthesia.[11] These monitors were first introduced into the anesthetic practice standards at Harvard in 1985, and today most developed countries have guidelines for intraoperative safety that include these advances.[8,13] These guidelines are partly responsible for the reduction from 1:75,700 to 1:244,000 severe anesthetic accidents.[4,12]

With improvements in the overall safety of intraoperative anesthesia and health care demands now linked to medical economics, studies changed the focus to perioperative concerns: patient satisfaction, pain control, length of stay, and overall costs.

Regional versus General Anesthesia

Controversy surrounds whether RA or GA is better for patient outcomes. Unfortunately, many studies have difficulties with their experimental design, including uneven distribution of sick patients, small sample size, unclear descriptions, and inadequate anesthetic management.[16] Also, fewer studies still focus on plastic surgical procedures.

Of specific interest to the plastic surgeon, however, is the relationship between the type of anesthesia and thromboembolic responses to surgery. RA has been demonstrated to decrease significantly the incidence of thromboembolic phenomenon; these changes in blood flow and rheodynamics may have implications for tissue flaps. Studies have focused on each stem of Virchow's triad, including the flow of blood, the nature of the endothelial cells, and the nature of the blood itself. The flow of blood and measurements of arterial inflow, venous emptying rate, and venous capacity are all significantly higher in patients under epidural anesthesia than under GA, with the improvement in flow most pronounced at the conclusion of and after surgery, when the clotting stimulus is maximal.[29]

The impact of endothelial wall damage has been minimized by local anesthetics, which reduce the adhesion of leukocytes to blood vessel walls by stabilizing the cell membranes of both blood and endothelial cells.[28] In addition, a decreased capacity for factor VIII activation, increased levels of plasminogen and plasminogen activators (which break down clot), and decreased inhibitors of fibrinolysis have been demonstrated with the use of epidural anesthesia.[7] Although some of these studies suggest that these antithrombogenic effects require continued epidural anesthesia postoperatively, these benefits may occur even if spinal anesthesia is used only intraoperatively.[7,36,37]

Preemptive Anesthesia

The recently introduced concept of preemptive, or *preincisional*, analgesia refers to the prevention or treatment of pain using measures initiated before the injury or noxious stimulus.[39] Mendell[27] coined the word "wind-up" more than 30 years ago, demonstrating that repetitive stimulation of C fibers resulted in a progressive increase in dorsal horn cell activity (i.e., sensitization of spinal cord neurons). GA at best produces only partial suppression of noxious stimuli. RA, by contrast, has produced more positive results.[30] Studies comparing patients who received regional techniques, including preoperative versus postincisional lumbar epidural and femoral blocks, showed lower analgesic requirements postoperatively.[19,33]

Preemptive effects are not limited to patients who have had a centrally active regional anesthetic; those with peripheral local anesthetic infiltration benefit as well.[14] Interestingly, the peripheral effect may be more significant: GA with preincisional local anesthesia was superior to spinal anesthesia, and both were

---

Box 17-4.
Types of Analgesic Drugs

Nonopioid: aspirin, acetaminophen
Nonsteroidal antiinflammatory: ibuprofen, ketorolac
Opioid: codeine, oxycodone, hydromorphone, meperidine, morphine, fentanyl
Opioid agonist-antagonist: nalbuphine, butorphanol
Local anesthetic: lidocaine, bupivacaine
Sedative: ketamine
Adjuvant: α_2-adrenergic agonists (e.g., clonidine), phenothiazines

---

superior to GA alone in terms of pain with movement or wound pressure and longer periods to first analgesia request.[38]

Postoperative Analgesia

Treatment of postoperative pain has important implications beyond patient comfort; beneficial effects on perioperative morbidity and mortality also have been demonstrated. With peripheral vascular graft survival, which may have application to flaps and graft placements in plastic surgery, sufficient postoperative analgesia enhanced survival and resulted in improved convalescence and reduced hospital stay.[20]

The route of postoperative analgesia has important implications. Systemic administration of intramuscular or IV opioids, even the newer ones, does not result in satisfactory analgesia.[3] In an analysis of published comparative trials, patient-controlled analgesia (PCA) pump systems provided greater analgesic efficacy and patient satisfaction than conventional intermittent analgesia. PCA also reduced the length of hospital stay. No change in the incidence of adverse effects was noted.[3]

A current trend is the shift from unimodal to multimodal treatment of postoperative pain. By taking advantage of the additive or synergistic effects of using two or more classes of analgesics, pain control can be optimized while using lower doses of each drug (Box 17-4). The use of lower doses in turn minimizes unwanted side effects from each class of drug. Preliminary data support the effectiveness of multimodal pain therapy, but more studies are needed to determine the optimal combination in specific procedures.[20]

SUMMARY

Anesthesia outcome studies may be summarized by the changes in mortality caused by changes in anesthesia care reported by Sharrock et al.[35] In comparisons of two 5-year periods, the major differences in anesthesia were (1) predominant use of epidural anesthesia both intraoperatively and postoperatively,

(2) more frequent use of perioperative invasive hemodynamic monitoring and pulse oximetry, and (3) establishment of postanesthesia care units. The mortality rate decreased from 0.39% (23 of 5874 patients) to 0.10% (10 of 9685 patients). Although a direct relationship between anesthesia care and improved outcome cannot be drawn from these observations, the study emphasized the role of anesthesia monitoring and management, its importance for surgery, and potential applications to plastic surgery.

REFERENCES

1. American Society of Anesthesiologists: Practice guidelines for sedation and analgesia by non-anesthesiologists, *Anesthesiology* 84:459-471, 1996.
2. Bader AM, Pothier M: Preoperative assessment clinics: organization and goals, *Anesth Analg Samba Suppl,* July 1997, pp 1-6.
3. Ballantyne JC, Carr DB, Chalmers TC, et al: Postoperative patient-controlled analgesia: meta-analysis of initial randomized controlled trials, *J Clin Anesth* 5:182-193, 1993.
4. Beecher HK, Todd DP: A study of the deaths associated with anesthesia and surgery based on a study of 599,548 anesthetics in ten institutions 1948-1952, inclusive, *Ann Surg* 140:2-35, 1954.
5. Benumof JL: *Airway Management: principles and practice,* St Louis, 1996, Mosby.
6. Brown DL: *Regional anesthesia and analgesia,* Philadelphia, 1996, Saunders.
7. Christopherson R, Beattie C, Frank SM, et al: Perioperative morbidity in patients randomized to epidural or general anesthesia for lower extremity vascular surgery, *Anesthesiology* 79:422-434, 1993.
8. Cooper JB, Newbower RS, Kitz RJ: An analysis of major errors and equipment failures in anesthetic management: considerations for prevention and detection, *Anesthesiology* 60:34-42, 1984.
9. Courtiss EH, Kanter MA: The prevention and management of medical problems during office surgery, *Plast Reconstr Surg* 85:125-136, 1990.
10. Courtiss EH, Goldwyn RM, Joffe JM, Hannenberg AA: Anesthetic practices in ambulatory anesthetic surgery, *Plast Reconstr Surg* 93:792-801, 1994.
11. Eichhorn JH: Influence of practice standards on anaesthesia outcome. In *Bailliere's Clinical anaesthesiology,* ed 6, Bailliere Tindall. 1992, London.
12. Eichhorn JH: Prevention of intraoperative anesthesia accidents and related severe injury through safety monitoring, *Anesthesiology* 70:572-577, 1989.
13. Eichhorn JH, Cooper JB, Cullen DJ, et al: Anesthesia practice standards at Harvard: a review, *J Clin Anesth* 1:55, 1988.
14. Ejlersen E, Andersen HB, Eliasen K, Mogensen T: A comparison between preincisional and postincisional lidocaine infiltration and postoperative pain, *Anesth Analg* 72:495-498, 1992.
15. Fialkor JA, McDougall EP: Warmed local anesthetic reduces pain on infiltration, *Ann Plast Surg* 36:11-13, 1996.

16. Gelman S: General versus regional anesthesia for peripheral vascular surgery, *Anesthesiology* 79:415, 1993.

17. Jastak TJ, Peskin RM: Major morbidity or mortality from office anesthesia procedures: a closed-claim analysis of 13 cases, *Anesth Prog* 38:39-44, 1991.

18. Kallar SK, Dunwiddle WC: Conscious sedation. In Wechtler BV, editor: *Problems in anesthesia,* Philadelphia, 1988, Lippincott.

19. Katz J, Clairoux M, Kavanagh BP: Pre-emptive lumbar epidural anaesthesia reduces postoperative pain and patient-controlled morphine consumption after lower abdominal surgery, *Pain* 59:395-403, 1995.

20. Kehlet H: Postoperative pain relief: a look from the other side, *Reg Anesth* 19:369-377, 1994.

21. Klein J: Tumescent technique for local anesthesia improves safety in large volume liposuction, *Plast Reconstr Surg* 92:1085-1098, 1993.

22. Koch ME, Goldstein RC: The office anesthesiologist as a perioperative manager: safety, outcomes and practice recommendations, *Anesth Analg Samba Suppl,* July 1997, pp. 17-24.

23. Longnecker DE, Tinker JA, Morgan GE: *Principles and practice of anesthesiology,* ed 2, St Louis, 1998, Mosby.

24. Lynch EP, Welch KJ, Carabuena JM, Eberlein TJ: Thoracic epidural anesthesia improves outcome after breast surgery, *Ann Surg* 222:663-669, 1995.

25. Mallampati R, Gatt S, Gugino L, et al: A clinical sign to predict difficult tracheal intubation: a prospective study, *Can Anaesth Soc J* 32:429-434, 1985.

26. McKay W, Morris R, Mushlin P: Sodium bicarbonate attenuates pain on skin infiltration with lidocaine, with or without epinephrine, *Anesth Analg* 66:572-576, 1987.

27. Mendell LM: Physiological properties of unmyelinated fiber projections to the spinal cord, *Exp Neurol* 16:316-322, 1966.

28. Modig J: Thromboembolism and blood loss, *Reg Anesth* 7:284-288, 1982.

29. Modig J, Marmberg P, Karlstrom G: Effect of epidural versus general anaesthesia on calf blood flow, *Acta Anaesth Scand* 24:305, 1980.

30. O'Connor TC, Abram S: Inhibition of nociception-induced spinal sensitization by anesthetic agents, *Anesthesiology* 82:259-266, 1995.

31. Ostad A, Kageyama N, Moy RL: Tumescent anesthesia with a lidocaine dose of 55 mg/kg is safe for liposuction, *Dermatol Surg* 22:921-927, 1996.

32. Pederson T, Viby-Mogensen J, Ringsted C: Anaesthetic practice and postoperative pulmonary complications, *Acta Anaesth Scand* 36:812-818, 1992.

33. Ringrose NH, Cross MJ: Femoral nerve block in knee joint surgery, *Am J Sports Med* 12:398-402, 1984.

34. Robinson V: *Victory over pain: a history of anesthesia,* New York, 1946, Schuman.

35. Sharrock NE, Cazan NE, Hargett MJ, et al: Changes in mortality after total hip and knee arthroplasty over a ten year period, *Anesth Analg* 80:242-248, 1995.

36. Thorburn J, Louden JR, Vallance R: Spinal and general anaesthesia in total hip replacement: frequency of deep venous thrombosis, *Br J Anesth* 52:1117-1121, 1980.

37. Tuman K, McCarthy RJ, March FJ, et al: Effects of epidural anesthesia and analgesia on coagulation and outcome after major vascular surgery, *Anesth Analg* 73:696-704, 1991.

38. Tverskoy M, Cozacov C, Ayache M, et al: Postoperative pain after inguinal herniorrhaphy with different types of anesthesia, *Anesth Analg* 70:29-35, 1990.

39. Wall PD: The prevention of postoperative pain, *Pain* 33:289-290, 1988.

40. Watcha M, White PF: Postoperative nausea and vomiting, *Anesthesiology* 77:162-184, 1992.

41. Williams J: Plastic surgery in an office surgical unit, *Plast Reconstr Surg* 52:513-519, 1973.

42. Wrigley SR, Fairfield JE, Jones RM, Black AE: Induction and recovery characteristics of desflurane in day case patients: a comparison with propofol, *Anaesthesia* 46:615-622, 1991.

Transplant Immunology and Allotransplantation

W. P. Andrew Lee
J. Peter Rubin

HISTORY

The use of allogeneic or xenogeneic tissue to replace human body parts has been the subject of myth throughout history. A notable legend describes the miraculous efforts of Saints Cosmos and Damian in removing the gangrenous leg of a church servant and replacing it with the limb of a deceased Moor.[1] Human skin allograft was described as early as 1871 by Pollock[2] and later by Lexer in 1911, establishing that skin grafts transplanted between humans would not be permanently accepted.[3]

The Nobel Prize–winning work by Sir Peter Medawar in the 1940s and 1950s made important contributions to our basic understanding of transplantation immunology. Using skin grafts between different strains of rodents, Medawar demonstrated that the primary immune response to allografts was prolonged ("primary rejection"), but the response to a skin graft applied after rejection of a prior graft would be greatly accelerated ("second set reaction"). In addition, Medawar showed that the response to foreign antigens is donor specific and that rodents could become tolerant to the tissue of a specific allogeneic donor.[4] These three principles of immunology—recognition of nonself, memory, and specificity—laid the groundwork for clinical transplantation.

Gorer is credited with identifying *major histocompatibility complex* (MHC) antigens in animals, providing a basis for the specificity of tissues from an individual.[5] Dausset later identified MHC antigens in humans, calling them *human leukocyte antigens* (HLAs).[6]

Barker and Billingham proved the importance of an afferent arc in the process of rejection.[7] They transplanted donor skin grafts to skin flaps connected by vessels and lymphatics or by vessels alone. Grafts on beds connected only by vessels were not recognized by the host, whereas grafts on beds with lymphatic drainage were rejected normally. Interestingly, the grafts on beds without lymphatic drainage were rejected when a second donor graft was applied to another site on the same animal. This showed that the efferent limb of the rejection arc is vascular.

The age of human allograft transplantation was ushered in by the first successful kidney transplant between identical twins in 1955 by Murray et al.[8]

DEFINITIONS

A *graft* is composed of tissues separated completely from the donor bed. It depends on the ingrowth of vessels from the recipient bed for survival. A vascularized graft, or *flap,* remains attached to donor blood supply or becomes revascularized via microvascular anastomoses to recipient vessels.

Tissue transplanted within the same individual is termed an *autograft.* A graft exchanged between genetically identical individuals (e.g., inbred mice or identical human twins) is an *isograft.* Tissue transplanted between genetically different individuals of the same species is an *allograft* (or homograft). An interspecies graft is called a *xenograft.* A graft placed in the same anatomic location from which it originated in the donor is an *orthotopic transplant,* whereas a graft placed in a different anatomic location is a *heterotopic transplant.*

This chapter focuses on allograft tissues.

MAJOR HISTOCOMPATIBILITY COMPLEX

The most important antigens contributing to allograft rejection are the MHC antigens. The MHC proteins are encoded in a gene complex on the short arm of chromosome 6 and have different nomenclature among species: HLA in humans, SLA in swine, H-2 in mice, and RT1 in rats. MHC genes are expressed in a codominant fashion, with one *haplotype,* or set of alleles, inherited from each parent.

There are two major classes of MHC genes. *Class I* genes encode a transmembrane glycoprotein complex with a polymorphic, 44-kD heavy chain consisting of three extracellular domains (a1, a2, a3). The a1 domain is highly variable and contains sites for antigen binding. The heavy chain is stabilized by noncovalent binding to a lighter chain referred to as β_2-microglobulin. The three distinct genetic loci for the class I antigens in the human are HLA-A, HLA-B, and HLA-C. Class I antigens are expressed on nearly all nucleated cells and serve as the primary target for cytotoxic (CD8+) T lymphocytes.

Class II MHC genes encode two noncovalently bound transmembrane proteins, a 34-kD alpha chain and a 29-kD beta chain. The three class II loci in humans are HLA-DR, HLA-DP, and HLA-DQ.[9] Class II antigens are expressed primarily on vascular endothelium and cells of hematopoietic stem cell origin, such as lymphocytes and macrophages.

Both class I and class II molecules have a specific site at which foreign peptide antigens can be presented after they have been processed by the cell.[10-13] Tissue distribution is not the same in all species; humans, pigs, and monkeys express class II antigens on endothelial cells, whereas rodents and many other large species do not.[14] Matching of HLA-A, HLA-B, and HLA-DR has been found to be the most important factor in determining long-term renal allograft survival.[15]

Other Transplant Antigens

In addition to the MHC antigens, the three other classes of surface proteins are ABO blood group proteins, minor histocompatibility antigens, and skin-specific antigens.

The *blood group antigens* are important in clinical transplantation because they are expressed on vascular endothelial cells. Patients with type A or type B blood develop natural antibodies to the other protein, whereas patients with type O blood develop natural antibodies to *both* type A and B proteins. Although ABO antigens will not stimulate cell-mediated rejection, a brisk antibody-mediated attack can rapidly lead to graft failure.[16]

Minor histocompatibility antigens are self-originating peptides presented by the MHC complexes. Siblings (other than identical twins) with a completely matched MHC profile still differ with respect to minor antigens because of allelic variation of the genes encoding for those proteins. Although minor antigens stimulate a cell-mediated response, they will not do so in a primary in vitro test. Graft rejection caused by minor antigens alone often proceeds at a slower rate.[17]

Skin-specific antigens (Sk antigens) are tissue-specific proteins that can cause graft rejection by a cell-mediated response. Consequently, skin is one of the most difficult tissues to which transplantation tolerance can be induced.[18]

CELLS OF IMMUNE RESPONSE

A number of cells with varied but interconnected functions participate in the process of graft rejection. They work together to effect two main arms of the immune reaction: the humoral response and the cell-mediated response.

Antigen-presenting cells (APCs) are of lymphoid origin and nonspecifically bind antigen and process it into smaller fragments *(epitopes)* that can be presented on the surface membrane in special configurations. APCs include macrophages, monocytes, histiocytes, Langerhans' cells (skin), Kuppfer's cells (liver), and dendritic cells. In addition to presenting antigen to other cells of the immune system, APCs, especially macrophages, assist in immune regulation by secreting soluble, peptide signaling agents called *cytokines.*[19,20]

B lymphocytes produce soluble antibodies and thus support the humoral arm of the immune response. Through rearrangement of a highly variable genetic region during immune development, antibodies are produced that can bind countless millions of different epitopes. Each B cell is programmed to produce antibodies with only a single specificity. When stimulated, the specific B cell will divide and produce generations of clones that become antibody secreting plasma cells.

T lymphocytes have a central role in coordinating the immune response, forming the cell-mediated arm of the immune response. Each T cell expresses a T-cell receptor (TCR) capable of binding antigen. As with B-cell development, T cells undergo rearrangement of genes coding for a hypervariable region on the receptor proteins. This allows a body's population of T cells to respond to a nearly limitless array of foreign antigens, with each individual T cell capable of binding one specific antigen. The TCR is a 90-kD heterodimer composed of an alpha chain encoded on chromosome 14 and a beta chain encoded on chromosome 7. The TCR is actively acquired in the thymus during ontogeny, with cells binding to self-antigens eliminated in the process.

Associated with the TCR is a set of five nonvariable transmembrane proteins referred to as *CD3* (CD, cluster of differentiation). The CD3 complex participates in the assembly of the TCR and serves as a marker for T cells. Another set of antigens, either *CD4* or *CD8,* is also associated with the TCR. T cells are thus divided into two major subsets, depending on whether CD4 or CD8 is present.

CD4 cells are termed *T helper cells,* and CD8 cells are *T cytotoxic cells.* CD4 cells regulate the immune response through the secretion of cytokines. CD8 lymphocytes bind cells expressing foreign antigen and kill them directly by releasing cytotoxic granules in the local environment. CD8 cells are thought to have a suppressor role as well.[21,22]

Natural killer cells (NK cells) are lymphocytes that differ from T cells and B cells because they respond without requiring MHC binding or presensitization to antigen.[23] Identified by their ability to lyse certain tumor cells nonspecifically in vitro, NK cells may have a role in tumor surveillance in vivo.[24] They may also serve to eliminate cells that fail to express normal-self MHC proteins.

T-Cell Binding and Activation

Although the TCR is capable of binding antigen, it cannot recognize the target molecule by itself.[25] The TCR can only bind antigen if it has been processed and presented by an APC, along with the MHC; thus it recognizes the MHC complex, together with the target antigen. This limitation of binding is referred to as *MHC restriction.* CD4 (helper) T cells can only bind antigen presented with MHC class II molecules, whereas CD8 (cytotoxic) T cells recognize antigen along with MHC class I proteins. The T helper cell is most critical to the immune response because its activation results in the

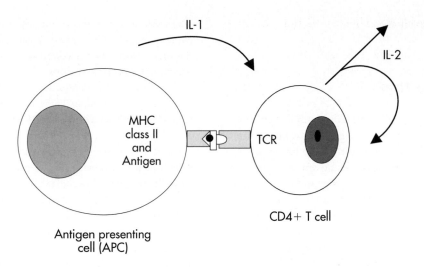

Figure 18-1. Initial events in T-cell activation. Antigen-presenting cell *(APC)* processes foreign antigen and displays it in association with major histocompatibility complex *(MHC)* class II. CD4 T cell (T helper) binds to MHC with T-cell receptor *(TCR)*. APC produces interleukin-1 *(IL-1)*, which stimulates the T cell to produce interleukin-2 *(IL-2)*. IL-2 acts to self-stimulate T cell and stimulate other T cells in region.

production of cytokines that are necessary for the function of many other immune cells.

Binding of a CD4 cell to an APC that expresses target antigen, together with MHC class II molecules, initiates a predictable cycle of intercellular communication. The APC is stimulated to produce the cytokine *interleukin-1* (IL-1), which is a powerful chemoattractant, a primary mediator in the acute-phase reaction, and a potent activator of lymphoid cells. The T cell, in turn, secretes *interleukin-2* (IL-2), which is a required stimulant for differentiation and proliferation of T cells (Figure 18-1). The IL-2 produced by the bound T cell has autocrine function by binding to newly expressed self IL-2 receptors. Secreted IL-2 also has paracrine function that affects other T cells in the region such as CD8 cells, which require IL-2 for activation but do not produce it themselves.

As CD4 cells become further activated, they secrete IL-4 and IL-5, which stimulate the maturation and proliferation of B lymphocytes. Furthermore, evidence indicates that two subsets of CD4 cells, *TH1* and *TH2,* function to enhance alloreactivity and to stimulate antibody production by B cells, respectively. With such a central role by CD4 cells in cell signaling, it is easy to understand the severely compromised immune response from the loss of host CD4 function secondary to human immunodeficiency virus (HIV) infection.[26-29]

Recognition of Transplant Antigens

With allogeneic tissue, foreign antigens can be recognized by host T cells after being processed by *host* APCs and presented in the context of self-MHC. This is termed *indirect presentation.* Host T cells also can directly recognize donor MHC on *donor* APCs, termed *direct presentation.* This mechanism helps to explain the more vigorous response to allograft tissue than that to foreign peptides aloe.[30]

Graft Rejection

Clinically, rejection of allogeneic tissue can proceed at different levels of intensity for different tissues. The common component for rejection of any graft is inflammation. This may manifest as a loss of graft function with local and systemic signs of inflammation. Several distinct clinical syndromes of graft rejection with different time courses have been noted. These syndromes differ with regard to the underlying primary immunologic process.

Hyperacute rejection occurs almost immediately after perfusion of the allograft with host blood. It is the result of preformed antibodies, either to ABO blood group proteins or to donor MHC, enacting a rapid attack on the donor tissue. Complement activation results in destruction of vascular endothelial cells, induces rapid thrombosis of vessels, and amplifies the inflammatory signal. Standard pretransplant screening should detect preformed antibodies, making hyperacute rejection a rare clinical entity. Many mammals possess preformed antibodies to other species, which is a major obstacle to xenotransplantation.[31]

Acute rejection takes place days to weeks after transplantation and occurs with rapid onset. This T-cell–mediated response is characterized by fever, graft tenderness and edema, and loss of function. Interstitial lymphocytic infiltration is seen on microscopic examination. Severe forms of acute rejection also may include a humoral attack on the graft, resulting in a vasculitis.[32]

Chronic rejection is an indolent process occurring months to years after transplantation. It is characterized by a progressive loss of tissue architecture, with fibrosis and mononuclear cell infiltration. The etiology is not well understood but may be multifactorial, and immunosuppression may slow the process. Chronic rejection also may result from the cumulative effect of damage to the graft from ischemia during transplantation, graft infection, or drug toxicity.

IMMUNOLOGIC TESTING

Methods are available to predict the compatibility of donor tissue to a particular recipient. The greatest value of these clinical tests is to exclude recipients who would be expected to manifest a hyperacute rejection to a specific donor organ.

Blood group typing is an important first step in determining transplant compatibility. An ABO mismatch will result in certain failure because of preformed antibodies.[33] Although it is possible to transplant type O donor tissue into type A or type B recipients, the limited supply of donor organs in the United States makes this practice uncommon.

HLA typing is used to match organs with potential recipients. Serologic methods are employed to type HLA-A, HLA-B, and HLA-DR. A heterozygous individual with a complete match at all these loci is referred to as a *six-antigen match*. For renal allografts, HLA matching has been shown to affect graft survival. Kidneys transplanted from HLA-identical siblings have a 3-year success rate that exceeds 90%, and parent-to-child grafts have an 82% survival. Cadaveric kidney grafts have a 70% 3-year survival rate.[34] MHC class II matching is more important than class I matching for renal transplantation, whereas the reverse appears to be true for liver transplantation. This would suggest differences in mechanisms of graft rejection for different tissues.[35]

Serologic tissue typing has certain limitations. An HLA antigen can be identified only if it is being sought with a specific antibody. For example, if only a single HLA-DR phenotype is identified in donor tissue, the individual could be either homozygous for that allele or heterozygous with an unrecognized HLA-DR antigen. Also, this method of testing fails to type the other class II antigens, HLA-DP and HLA-DQ.

Crossmatching is a test that detects the presence of preformed donor-specific antibodies in the serum of a particular recipient. It represents the definitive screening measure before transplantation. In this lymphocytotoxicity assay, donor lymphocytes are incubated with recipient serum and complement. Cell viability is then assessed by a dye exclusion technique. A positive crossmatch, indicated by lysis of the donor lymphocytes, suggests that a hyperacute reaction is likely to occur. One pitfall of this test, however, is that organ-specific antibodies may be missed if those antigens are not expressed on the lymphocytes being evaluated.

Antibody screening is another modality used in clinical transplantation. Serum from prospective transplant recipients is routinely tested in a lymphocytotoxicity assay against a panel of cells from different donors with known HLA antigens. The percentage of panel cells lysed reflects the degree of *panel-reactive antibody* (PRA), demonstrating HLA antibodies in an individual's serum. A high PRA suggests that a patient is unlikely to have a negative crossmatch. These data are used in determining organ allocation when the tissue must be transplanted quickly. Individuals are likely to have a high PRA if they have been sensitized by previous transplantation, pregnancy, or blood transfusions.

CLINICAL IMMUNOSUPPRESSION

With the exception of transplants between identical twins, allografts in humans will fail unless the immune system is partially inhibited. Even HLA-identical siblings will eventually reject each other's tissue because of minor antigen differences. Measures to inhibit the immune system are usually prescribed in combination for greatest efficacy.

Adrenocorticosteroids represent the most basic measure available to produce clinical immunosuppression. Steroids bind to an intracellular receptor and form a complex that then interacts with deoxyribonucleic acid (DNA) to affect transcription. Steroids function to downregulate all T-cell functions, including cytokine production, and to inhibit chemotaxis and phagocytosis by macrophages and neutrophils. Both the initial cellular response to foreign antigen and the signals that serve to amplify the process of inflammation are reduced. Steroids are used in concert with other immunosuppressants to prevent allograft rejection. The complications of steroids are well known and include hypertension, hyperglycemia, osteoporosis, and peptic ulcer disease.[36-38]

Azathioprine (Imuran) is a purine analog based on a modification of 6-mercaptopurine (6-MP). Once converted to its active form (6-MP ribonucleoside) by the liver, azathioprine interferes with nucleic acid synthesis by blocking the enzymes that convert inosine to adenosine and guanosine monophosphate. Blocking this key biosynthetic pathway results in inhibition of the differentiation and proliferation of lymphocytes. Both cellular immunity and humoral immunity are downregulated. Nonspecific effects on all rapidly dividing cells can result in severe leukopenia. In addition, hepatic toxicity may occur with azathioprine.[39]

Methotrexate is a folic acid antagonist that inhibits the enzyme dihydrofolate reductase and prevents the formation of tetrahydrofolic acid, a key component in the synthesis of DNA and ribonucleic acid (RNA). Like azathioprine, methotrexate is an antimetabolite.

The introduction of *cyclosporine* in 1972 has greatly advanced the field of organ transplantation, since it provides effective immunosuppression without significant marrow depression. Produced by a fungus, this cyclic peptide inhibits the production of IL-2 at the level of transcription, thereby blocking T-cell differentiation and proliferation. Nephrotoxicity is the most frequent adverse reaction.[40]

FK-506, a macrolide antibiotic, is a potent immunosuppressive agent that is also derived from a fungus. It inhibits IL-2 production and the expression of IL-2 receptors on T lymphocytes. FK-506 is new to the clinical arena and is currently undergoing human trials. Major side effects identified include nephrotoxicity and anorexia with weight loss.[41-43]

Antibodies are often employed in clinical transplantation. *Antilymphocyte globulins* (ALGs) are polyclonal antibodies to human lymphocytes produced in animals. This nonspecific mixture of antibodies coats and deactivates T cells in vivo. Monoclonal antibodies are also used. *OKT3* is a monoclonal antibody directed specifically at the CD3 receptor present on all T cells. It is given to combat episodes of acute rejection.[44]

Radiation is another method that can produce clinical immunosuppression by interfering with lymphocyte replication and division. Total lymphoid irradiation, originally developed for the treatment of Hodgkin's disease, has been used successfully in both experimental and clinical transplantation.[45,46]

Immunologic Tolerance

Tolerance refers to the state of immunologic acceptance or unresponsiveness of the recipient to the donor allograft.[4] Induction of tolerance allows transplantation without the need for prolonged immunosuppression. Acceptance or tolerance of one's own tissues first develops in utero, along with an immunologic ability to recognize foreign tissue. Medawar exploited this phenomenon in his original experiments.

The production of the tolerant state in an adult can be achieved experimentally by various methods. A combination of total body irradiation to remove mature recipient T cells followed by donor bone marrow infusion before transplantation induces a state of *chimerism*. (The term *chimera* is derived from the Greek mythologic figure comprised of the parts of different animals.) The chimeric host then develops an immune system that is tolerant of both donor and host antigens. A further refinement is the use of total lymphoid irradiation, in which the marrow cavities of long bones in mice are protected during irradiation, thus producing a state of mixed chimerism.[47,48] These animals accept donor skin grafts while rejecting third-party grafts.

Another method of achieving transplant tolerance involves intrathymic injection of donor cells. These cells survive in the immunologically "privileged" thymus, resulting in production of maturing T cells that are tolerant of the donor alloantigen.[49-51] All these methods are referred to as *central mechanisms* of tolerance induction.

Peripheral methods of tolerance induction include suppression of the donor MHC antigens by antibodies, which prevent the donor leukocytes from stimulating the lymphocyte cascade in the recipient. Donor-specific blood transfusions have also been used to increase graft survival, supposedly by presenting MHC antigens in a limited way and inducing a state of T-cell anergy rather than activation.[52] Other methods of peripheral tolerance induction include donor APC depletion or modification and use of anti-CD4 antibody to block helper T-cell function.[53] These peripheral methods of tolerance induction have not been as effective as the central mechanisms.

Induction of tolerance holds exciting promise for the plastic and reconstructive surgeons in transplantation of limb tissue allografts without prolonged immunosuppression.

ALLOTRANSPLANTATION OF TISSUES

Bone

The use of frozen bone allograft has become a common practice for the reconstruction of long bone defects, with an estimated annual volume of more than 200,000 procedures in the United States.[54] These are used as intercalary grafts to bridge diaphyseal defects or as osteochondral grafts to provide an articular surface. Although autogenous bone is still the material of choice for many defects, bone allografts have clear advantages in selected patients, such as the size and shape of graft and the lack of donor site morbidity. In addition to long bone repair, bone allografts are being used in hand and craniofacial surgery.

Frozen bone allografts are fundamentally different from other solid organ transplants. Not primarily vascularized, they are devoid of living cells and serve as a mineral scaffold that becomes resorbed and replaced by host bone through a process known as *creeping substitution.* Immunosuppressive drugs are not necessary because the graft antigenicity is greatly diminished, if not eliminated. An inflammatory response is initiated at the graft surface by the host, which is usually followed by union at the graft-host interface. Resorption of the allograft then proceeds with replacement by recipient-derived bone, followed by a final remodeling phase in graft incorporation.[55]

This same process occurs with autografts,[56] but it progresses at a much slower rate with allografts.[57] Biopsies of frozen half-joint knee allografts demonstrate presence of viable bone starting at 12 months. Fibrocartilage was noted on the articular surface at 12 months, but islands of hyaline cartilage were not seen until 7 years.[58] In a histologic study of retrieved massive human allografts, host repair involved only 20% of the graft at 5 years.[59]

Tissue banks process and store bone allografts. The bone grafts are excised in an operating room under sterile conditions and can be removed from the donor up to 24 hours postmortem. Soft tissue, periosteum, and marrow are removed, and the bone is exposed to a glycerol solution before controlled freezing at −80° to −100° C and storage in liquid nitrogen. The bone grafts may also be freeze-dried in a vacuum chamber, a process lasting 14 to 16 days. Freeze-dried grafts may be stored at room temperature and require rehydration in saline before use.

Gamma irradiation and ethylene oxide are often used as adjunctive measures to ensure sterilization of the specimens. Donor serum is tested for transmissible diseases at the time of harvest. The risk of disease transmission is quite small, with only isolated case reports of hepatitis B and HIV infection after bone allografting.[60-63] At least 30,000 Gy of gamma radiation is necessary to eliminate completely the HIV virus from a fresh-frozen allograft.[64]

Only slight variations in strength have been observed in frozen bone specimens. Freeze drying, however, can result in significant decreases in bending and torsional strength, especially when combined with exceedingly high doses of gamma radiation.[65]

With regard to the immunogenicity of bone allografts, experimental models in animals reveal that *vascularized* allografts undergo rejection of the cellular elements mediated by class I and class II MHC antigens.[66-68] For frozen allografts that are not primarily vascularized, the mechanical and thermal obliteration of cellular elements greatly reduces but does not uniformly eliminate the host immune response. Friedlaender et al[69] found that nine of 44 human allograft placements resulted in the formation of donor-specific anti-HLA antibodies by the recipient, suggesting that HLA antigens can survive the freezing process. The significance of this humoral response is unclear, since eight of the nine patients who developed antibodies had a favorable clinical result.

The use of frozen bone allografts has been associated with a 25% to 35% overall rate of complications within 3 years postoperatively, including infection, nonunion, and fracture.[70] Graft infection occurred in 13.3% of 75 patients[71] and 11.7% of 283 patients.[72] Graft removal was required, and many patients underwent amputation. The incidence of fractures in long bone allografts after tumor resection is approximately 16%, occurring 28 months on average after surgery. Fracture is a less serious complication than infection, with most grafts amenable to salvage with internal fixation.[73]

In craniofacial and hand surgery the relatively small bony defects encountered often justify the donor site morbidity necessary for an autogenous graft. Applications for allograft, however, have been explored in these fields.

Epker et al[74] used freeze-dried bone allografts in a series of 18 patients undergoing midfacial advancements. Despite an infection rate of 22%, which necessitated partial graft removal, osteotomies healed in all patients treated. Zhe and Tingchun[75] reported the successful use of a frozen split-rib allograft as a tray for autogenous bone chips in a small series of mandibular reconstruction. Kline and Rimer[76] used a similar composite of autogenous bone fragments in a freeze-dried allogeneic bone casing to treat 58 patients with mandibular, maxillary, and zygomatic defects. Three patients with graft infections failed to heal, whereas the other 55 patients had a successful result. Two of the three patients with graft infections underwent successful healing of a second composite graft system after a 4-month waiting period.

Bauer et al[77] used freeze-dried allograft bone to treat 12 patients with enchondromas of the hand and compared the results with a control group of 16 patients treated with autogenous iliac crest grafts. Hospital stay was significantly shorter in patients with allograft, and clinical outcomes between the two groups were comparable over an average follow-up time of 34.6 months.

Upton and Glowacki[78] reported a series of 12 patients treated with 26 demineralized bone grafts for hand defects (12 metacarpal, 14 phalangeal), including enchondromas and congenital deformities. Nine patients were children, and many had refused autografts because they had previously undergone massive bone graft harvesting for craniofacial reconstruction. All patients were discharged on the first postoperative day and followed for an average of 50 months. No infections, nonunions, or other complications occurred.

Time to healing was no different than in patients with autogenous grafts, and all patients in this series were remobilized within 3 months.

Smith and Brushart[79] used 12 frozen allografts for metacarpal reconstruction in seven pediatric and three adult patients with traumatic or congenital defects. Nine patients in this series received intercalary grafts after distraction lengthening of the metacarpal. Union occurred at 23 of 24 bony interfaces, and 9 of 10 patients had improved function on long-term follow-up. No infections or fractures were noted.

Carter et al[80] used frozen scaphoid allograft to replace the proximal half of the scaphoid in eight patients with avascular necrosis, proximal nonunion, or unreconstructable fragments. Union was achieved in all scaphoids, with no episodes of infection. Six patients showed good clinical function during follow-up ranging from 8 to 30 months. Two patients, however, encountered graft failure.

Larger allografts have also been used in the upper extremity for reconstruction of distal radius[81] and elbow.[82,83] The results of these allografts do not appear as favorable as the smaller grafts in the hand.

Cartilage

Isolated chondrocytes express HLA antigens and elicit immune responses. The extracellular matrix that surrounds the chondrocytes, however, is only weakly antigenic.[84] This partly protects the chondrocytes from recognition by the host immune system. Cartilage allograft, usually with irradiation pretreatment, has been used to augment the facial skeleton. Despite good initial results in many patients,[85] long-term data suggest a high rate of resorption.[86] Given the variable clinical results, it is unclear whether cartilage allograft offers any advantages for facial contouring.

Another potential application for cartilage allograft is improving the function of damaged joints. Viable chondrocytes that produce proteoglycan have been demonstrated in biopsies of fresh osteochondral grafts in humans.[87] Mahomed et al[88] used small fragments of fresh osteochondral allografts to resurface traumatic defects of the knee joint in young patients. Success rates, based on functional and radiographic assessment, were 75% at 5 years, 64% at 10 years, and 63% at 14 years. The long-term survival of these grafts is encouraging.

Skin

Skin allografts have been employed in plastic surgery, primarily in the treatment of burn victims. A survey of U.S. burn center directors revealed that 12% of all admitted patients in 1992 were treated with skin allografts, with 69% of burn unit directors preferring fresh to cryopreserved skin.[89] In addition to the risk of transmission of hepatitis and HIV, clinically significant cytomegalovirus (CMV) infections have been reported in burn patients after cadaveric skin transplants.[90]

Although effective for burn wound coverage, fresh skin allografts are rejected in approximately 14 days.[91] This led to the use of immunosuppression in an attempt to prolong graft survival. In 1975 Burke et al[92] successfully used azathioprine to extend the survival of skin allografts in three pediatric patients with burns over 80% to 90% of body surface area. The grafts were harvested from either mother or father after HLA typing. All three children maintained the allograft long enough to undergo wound coverage with skin autograft. Antithymocyte globulin (ATG) was also used to achieve prolongation of skin allograft survival in burn patients.[93,94] When cyclosporine became available, Achauer et al[95] reported its effectiveness in prolonging the survival of mixed donor and cadaveric skin in a severely burned patient.

The risks of exogenous immunosuppression in the already immunocompromised burn patient prompted interventional strategies directed at the graft itself. In one clinical model, epidermal Langerhans' cell activity in split-thickness cadaver skin grafts was suppressed by ultraviolet B (UVB) radiation. These cells would otherwise serve as potent APCs and accelerate the host T-cell response.[96,97] Other investigators have transplanted skin allografts and stripped the more antigenic epidermis from the graft after initial graft take. A successful composite graft was then created by placing autologous epidermis[98] or autologous cultured keratinocytes[99,100] on the dermal allograft. Preservation with glycerol reduces the antigenicity of skin allografts and prolongs their survival.[101] Glycerol-treated grafts have been used in burn centers as coverage for burn wounds before autografting[102] or as composite grafts overlying widely meshed autografts.[103]

The potential for disease transmission has lead to the development of tissue-engineered skin replacements that utilize allograft tissues in a more controlled manner. One clinical model uses a dermal matrix that is processed to remove all cellular elements. Similar to cadaver skin that is stripped of the epidermis after grafting, the acellular dermal matrix will support an overlying autologous split-thickness skin graft.[104] Acellular dermal grafts are available commercially in the United States under the trade name AlloDerm (Life Cell Corporation, Woodlands, Texas).

Another model uses a tissue-engineered, living, allogeneic dermal construct. Tested in the United States under the name Dermagraft (Advanced Tissue Sciences, La Jolla, Calif), this material consists of human neonatal dermal fibroblasts seeded onto a synthetic mesh. The fibroblasts secrete extracellular matrix and have a low antigenicity, allowing long-term use in the host.[105] It has compared favorably with skin allograft as a temporary cover for severe burn wounds.[106,107]

Clinical trials are also being conducted with a bilayer, allogeneic, living-skin equivalent. Apligraf (organogenesis) is composed of a type I bovine collagen matrix seeded with allogeneic human fibroblasts and overlayed with allogeneic human keratinocytes. When applied to surgical wounds in nonburn patients, this material had an 80% initial rate of survival, with no overt signs of inflammation or rejection. At 3 months, 55% of patients appeared to have 100% take of the allograft. Tests for anti-HLA antibodies in the serum of recipients were negative. The long-term fate of these grafts has not yet been determined.[108] Apligraf has been approved by the FDA for the treatment of venous stasis ulcers. Approval for treatment of burns, diabetic ulcers, and pressure sores is pending.

Nerve

Although autogenous nerve is considered the material of choice for nerve grafting, in some clinical situations the amount of available autograft is not sufficient for reconstruction. Peripheral nerve allograft has been shown in animal models to be highly antigenic, with expression of MHC class I and class II proteins by Schwann cells.[109,110] Survival of donor Schwann cells can be maintained by administration of cyclosporine, but host immunosuppression may be necessary for only a limited period. As wallerian degeneration occurs in the nerve grafts, the donor Schwann cells form a scaffold to guide host axonal regeneration. Once the regenerated axons have traversed the graft, withdrawal of immunosuppression results in rejection of donor Schwann cells and replacement by host Schwann cells.[111]

The clinical experience with peripheral nerve allograft has been limited. Mackinnon and Hudson[112] reported two cases of successful transplantation of fresh cadaveric nerve allograft with temporary cyclosporine treatment. In the first case, cable grafts were used to bridge a 23-cm defect of the sciatic nerve in an 8-year-old trauma patient. Cyclosporine was discontinued at 2 years. Sensory regeneration occurred, with diminished light touch and pain sensation returning in the peroneal and posterior tibial nerve distributions, but no motor function returned. In the second case a traumatic 20-cm gap in the posterior tibial nerve of a 12-year-old boy was repaired with nerve allograft. Cyclosporine was used for 17 months. Similar to the previous case, this patient developed protective sensibility in the distribution of the grafted nerve.[113]

These cases demonstrate that nerve allograft may be a treatment alternative in carefully selected patients.

Limb

The need for limb allografts in patients with congenital absence or traumatic loss has been apparent from the time of Saints Cosmos and Damian. The modern advent of microvascular surgery has made transplantation of vascularized limb tissues technically feasible. The ability to transplant limb tissue allografts would revolutionize the field of reconstructive surgery.

Allograft survival has been achieved experimentally with various immunosuppressive regimens.[114-124] Normal wound healing and bony growth occur after experimental transplantation.[122,125-127] Return of neuromuscular function has been observed in limb allografts of animals treated with immunosuppression,[124,128] including those of nonhuman primates.[129,130] The tissue components of a limb allograft (e.g., skin, subcutaneous tissue, muscle, bone, blood vessels) possess different antigenic mechanisms, and rejection varies in timing and intensity.[68] Techniques that selectively decreased the antigenicity of component parts were found to prolong allograft survival.[131,132]

Tolerance to limb tissue allografts without immunosuppression has been induced by neonatal or in utero exposure to donor antigens experimentally.[133,134] Genetic matching achieved allograft tolerance after only a short course of cyclosporine in a large-animal model.[135]

FUTURE TRANSPLANTATION

Despite experimental successes, use of chronic, toxic immunosuppression to achieve transplantation of limb tissue allograft is difficult to justify clinically. Development of effective regimens to induce host tolerance without prolonged immunosuppression is therefore essential to alter the risk/benefit ratio. Such regimens may involve site-specific immunosuppression directed at the graft, monoclonal antibodies that block a particular step in the rejection cascade, exposure to donor antigen before transplant, or appropriate matching of MHC antigens between donor and recipient.

Further experimental investigation is needed to define better the mechanism of limb allograft rejection and to achieve long-term tolerance in a large-animal model. With such a foundation in basic science, transplantation of limb tissue allograft may represent the next frontier in plastic surgery.[136]

REFERENCES

1. Danilevicius Z: Cosmos and Damian: the patron saints of medicine in art, *JAMA* 201:1021, 1967.
2. Pollock GD: Cases of skin grafting and skin transplantation, *Trans Clin Soc Lond* 4:37, 1871.
3. Gibson T: Zoografting: a curious chapter in the history of plastic surgery, *Br J Plast Surg* 8:234, 1955.
4. Billingham RE, Brent L, Medawar PB: Actively acquired tolerance of foreign cells, *Nature* 172:603, 1952.
5. Gorer PA, Kaliss N: Studies on the genetic and antigenic basis of tumour transplantation: linkage between a histocompatibility gene and "fused" in mice, *Proc Biol Soc Lond* 135:499, 1948.
6. Dausset J: Iso-leuco-anticorps, *Acta Haematol* 20:156, 1958.
7. Barker CF, Billingham RE: The role of regional lymphatics in the skin homograft response, *Transplantation* 5:962, 1967.
8. Murray JE, Merrill JP, Harrison JH: Renal homotransplantation in identical twins, *Surg Forum* 6:432, 1955.
9. Bodmer JG, Marsh SGE, Parham P, et al: Nomenclature for factors of the HLA system, *Hum Immunol* 28:326, 1990.
10. Hughes AL, Yeager M: Molecular evolution of the vertebrate immune system, *Bioessays* 19:777, 1997.
11. Gill T Jr, Salgar SK, Yuan XJ, Kunz HW: Current status of the genetic and physical maps of the major histocompatibllity complex in the rat, *Transplant Proc* 29:1657, 1997.
12. Salter-Cid L, Flajnik MF: Evolution and developmental regulation of the histocompatibility complex, *Crit Rev Immunol* 15:31, 1995.
13. Kasahara M, Flajnik MF, Ishibashi T, Natori T: Evolution of the major histocompatibility complex: a current overview, *Transplant Immunol* 3:1, 1995.
14. Pescovitz MD, Sachs DH, Lunney JK, Hsu SM: Localization of class II MHC antigens on porcine renal vaculature endothelium, *Transplantation* 37:627, 1984.
15. Hors J, Busson M, Bouteiller AM, et al: Dissection of the respective importance of HLA-A, B, DR matching in 3,789 prospective kidney transplants, *Transplant Proc* 19:687, 1987.
16. Oriol R: Tissular expression of ABH and Lewis antigens in humans and animals: expected value of different animal models in the study of ABO-incompatible organ transplants, *Transplant Proc* 19:4416, 1987.
17. Lai PK, Waterfield JD, Gascoigne NR, et al: T-cell responses to minor histocompatibility antigens, *Immunology* 47:371, 1982.
18. Steinmuller D, Wachtel SS: Transplantation biology and immunogenetics of murine skin-specific (Sk) alloantigens, *Transplant Proc* 12:100, 1980.
19. Schmitz J, Radbruch A: Distinct antigen presenting cell-derived signals induce TH cell proliferation and expression of effector cytokines, *Int Immunol* 4:43, 1992.
20. Sherry B, Horii Y, Manogue K, et al: Macrophage inflammatory proteins 1 and 2: an overview, *Cytokines* 4:117, 1992.
21. Davis MM, Lyons DS, Altman JD, et al: T cell receptor biochemistry, repertoire selection and general features of TCR and Ig structure, *Ciba Found Symp* 204:94, 1997.
22. von Boehmer H, Fehling HJ: Structure and function of the pre–T cell receptor, *Annu Rev Immunol* 15:433, 1997.
23. Durantez A, de Landazuri MO, Silva A, et al: Comparison of the cytotoxic activities of different human lymphoid tissues, *J Clin Lab Immunol* 2:59, 1979.
24. Brittenden J, Heys SD, Ross J, Eremin O: Natural killer cells and cancer, *Cancer* 77:1226, 1996.
25. Zinkernagel R, Doherty P: H-2 compatibility requirement for T-cell mediated lysis of target cells infected with lymphocytic choriomeningitis virus: different cytotoxic T-cell specificities are associated with structures encoded for in H-2K or H-2D, *J Exp Med* 141:1427, 1975.
26. Fulcher DA, Basten A: B-cell activation versus tolerance: the central role of immunoglobulin receptor engagement and T-cell help, *Int Rev Immunol* 15:33, 1997.
27. Lanzavecchia A: Understanding the mechanisms of sustained signaling and T cell activation, *J Exp Med* 185:1717, 1997.
28. Margulies DH: Interactions of TCRs with MHC-peptide complexes: a quantitative basis for mechanistic models, *Curr Opin Immunol* 9:390, 1997.
29. Qian D, Weiss A: T cell antigen receptor signal transduction, *Curr Opin Cell Biol* 9:205, 1997.
30. Sherwood R, Brent L, Rayfield L: Presentation of alloantigens by host cells, *Eur J Immunol* 16:569, 1986.
31. Platt JL, Bach FH: The barrier to xenotransplantation, *Transplantation* 52:937, 1991.
32. Miltenberg A, Meijer-Paape M, Weening J, et al: Induction of antibody-dependent cellular cytotoxicity against endothelial cells by renal transplantation, *Transplantation* 48:681, 1989.
33. Wilbrandt R, Tung KS, Deodhar SD, et al: ABO blood group incompatibility in human renal homotransplantation, *Am J Clin Pathol* 51:15, 1969.
34. Terasaki PI, Cecka JM, Gjertson DW, Takemoto S: High survival rates of kidney transplants from spousal and living unrelated donors, *N Engl J Med* 333:333, 1995.
35. Knechtle SJ, Kalayolu M, D'Alessandro AM, et al: Histocompatibility and liver transplantation, *Surgery* 114:667, 1993.

36. Di Stefano R, Scavuzzo M, Pietrabissa A, et al: Effect of immunosuppressive regimens on neutrophil chemotaxis, *Transplant Proc* 26:2861, 1994.

37. Hricik DE, Almawi WY, Strom TB: Trends in the use of glucocorticoids in renal transplantation, *Transplantation* 57:979, 1994.

38. Veith FJ, Koerner SK, Sprayregen S, et al: Corticosteroids in clinical and experimental lung transplantation, *Transplant Proc* 7:99, 1975.

39. Elion GB: The pharmacology of azathioprine, *Ann NY Acad Sci* 685:400, 1993.

40. Kahan BD: Cyclosporine, *N Engl J Med* 321:1725, 1989.

41. Klintmalm GB: Clinical use of FK 506 in liver transplantation, *Transplant Proc* 28:974, 1996.

42. Shapiro R: Tacrolimus (FK-506) in kidney transplantation, *Transplant Proc* 29:45, 1997.

43. Wagner K, Herget S, Heemann U: Experimental and clinical experience with the use of tacrolimus (FK506) in kidney transplantation, *Clin Nephrol* 45:332, 1996.

44. Norman DJ: Rationale for OKT3 monoclonal antibody treatment in transplant patients, *Transplant Proc* 25(suppl 2):1, 1993.

45. Najarian JS, Ferguson RM, Sutherland DER, et al: Fractionated total lymphoid irradiation as preoperative immunosuppression in high risk renal transplantation: clinical and immunological studies, *Ann Surg* 196:442, 1982.

46. Slavin S, Fuks Z, Strober S, et al: Transplantation across major histocompatibility barriers after total lymphoid irradiation, *Transplantation* 28:359, 1979.

47. Auchincloss H Jr, Sachs DH: Mechanisms of tolerance in murine radiation bone marrow chimeras. II. Absence of non-specific suppression in mature chimeras, *Transplantation* 36:442, 1983.

48. Sharabi Y, Sachs DH: Mixed chimerism and permanent specific transplantation tolerance induced by a non-lethal preparative regimen, *J Exp Med* 169:493, 1989.

49. Alfrey EJ, Wang X, Lee L, et al: Tolerance induced by direct inoculation of donor antigen into the thymus in low and high responder rodents, *Transplantation* 59:1171, 1995.

50. Gritsch H, Glaser R, Emery D, et al: Induction of tolerance to pig antigens in mice grafted with fetal pig thymus and liver grafts, *Transplantation* 57:906, 1994.

51. Cober SR, Randolph MA, Lee WPA: Skin graft survival following intrathymic injection of donor bone marrow, *J Surg Research* 85:204, 1999.

52. Opelz G, Terasaki PL: Improvement of kidney-graft survival with increased numbers of blood transfusions, *N Engl J Med* 299, 1978.

53. Morel P, Vincent C, Cordier G, et al: Anti-CD4 monoclonal antibody administration in renal transplanted patients, *Clin Immunol Immunopathol* 56:311, 1990.

54. Friedlaender G: Bone allografts: the biological consequences of immunological events, *J Bone Joint Surg* 73A:1119, 1991 (editorial).

55. Stevenson S, Horowitz M: The response to bone allograft, *J Bone Joint Surg* 74A:939, 1992.

56. Burchardt H: Biology of bone transplantation, *Orthop Clin North Am* 18:187, 1987.

57. Delloye C, Verhelpen M, D'Hemricourt J, et al: Morphometric and physical investigations of segmental cortical bone autografts and allografts in canine ulnar defects, *Clin Orthop* 282:273, 1992.

58. Salenius P, Holmstrom T, Koskinen EV, Alho A: Histological changes in clinical half-joint allograft replacements, *Acta Orthop Scand* 53:295, 1982.

59. Enneking W, Mindell E: Observations on massive retrieved human allografts, *J Bone Joint Surg* 73A:1123, 1991.

60. Hardin CK: Banked bone, *Otolaryngol Clin North Am* 27:911, 1994.

61. Malinin TI, Martinet OV, Brown MD: Banking of massive osteoarticular and intercalary bone allografts: 12 years' experience, *Clin Orthop* 197:44, 1985.

62. Scarborough NL: Current procedures for banking allograft human bone, *Orthopedics* 15:1161, 1992.

63. Tomford WW, Mankin HJ, Friedlaender GE, et al: Methods of banking bone and cartilage for allograft transplantation, *Orthop Clin North Am* 18:241, 1987.

64. Fideler BM, Vangsness CT Jr, Moore T, et al: Effects of gamma irradiation on the human immunodeficiency virus: a study in frozen human bone–patellar ligament–bone grafts obtained from infected cadavera, *J Bone Joint Surg* 76A:1032, 1994.

65. Pelker RR, Friedlaender GE, Markham TC: Biomechanical properties of bone allografts, *Clin Orthop* 174:54, 1983.

66. Horowitz M, Friedlander G: Induction of specific T-cell responsiveness to allogenic bone, *J Bone Joint Surg* 73A:1157, 1991.

67. Gotfried Y, Yaremchuk M, Randolph M, Weiland A: Histologic characteristics of acute rejection in vascularized allografts of bone, *J Bone Joint Surg* 69A:410, 1987.

68. Lee WPA, Yaremchuk MJ, Pan YC, et al: Relative antigenicity of components of a vascularized limb allograft, *Plast Reconstr Surg* 87:401, 1991.

69. Friedlaender GE, Strong DM, Sell KW: Studies on the antigenicity of bone. II. Donor-specific anti-HLA antibodies in human recipients of freeze-dried allografts, *J Bone Joint Surg* 66A:107, 1984.

70. Mankin H: Complications of allograft surgery. In Friedlaender G, Mankin H, Sell K, editors: *Osteochondral allografts: biology, banking, and clinical applications,* Boston, 1983, Little, Brown.

71. Dick HM, Strauch RJ: Infection of massive bone allografts, *Clin Orthop* 306:46, 1994.

72. Lord CF, Gebhardt MC, Tomford WW, Mankin HJ: Infection in bone allografts: incidence, nature, and treatment, *J Bone Joint Surg* 70A:369, 1988.

73. Berrey BH Jr, Lord CF, Gebhardt MC, Mankin HJ. Fractures of allografts: frequency, treatment, and end-results, *J Bone Joint Surg* 72:825, 1990.

74. Epker BN, Friedlaender G, Wolford LM, West RA: The use of freeze-dried bone in middle-third face advancements, *Oral Surg Oral Med Oral Pathol* 42:278, 1976.

75. Zhe C, Tingchun W: Reconstruction of mandibular defects with composite autologous iliac bone and freeze-treated allogeneic rib grafts, *J Oral Maxillofac Surg* 40:29, 1982.

76. Kline SN, Rimer SR: Reconstruction of osseous defects with freeze-dried allogeneic and autogenous bone: clinical and histologic assessment, *Am J Surg* 146:471, 1983.

77. Bauer RD, Lewis MM, Posner MA: Treatment of enchondromas of the hand with allograft bone, *J Hand Surg* 13A:908, 1988.

78. Upton J, Glowacki J: Hand reconstruction with allograft demineralized bone: twenty-six implants in twelve patients, *J Hand Surg* 17A:704, 1992.

79. Smith RJ, Brushart TM: Allograft bone for metacarpal reconstruction, *J Hand Surg* 10A:325, 1985.

80. Carter PR, Malinin TI, Abbey PA, Sommerkamp TG: The scaphoid allograft: a new operation for treatment of the very proximal scaphoid nonunion or for the necrotic, fragmented scaphoid proximal pole, *J Hand Surg* 14:1, 1989.

81. Smith RJ, Mankin HJ: Allograft replacement of distal radius for giant cell tumor, *J Hand Surg* 2A:299, 1977.

82. Urbaniak J, Aitken M: Clinical use of bone allografts in the elbow, *Ortho Clin North Am* 18:311, 1987.

83. Kay RM, Eckardt JJ: Total elbow allograft for twice-failed total elbow arthroplasty: a case report, *Clin Orthop* 303:135, 1994.

84. Herman J, Dennis M: Polydispersity of human articular cartilage proteoglycan antigens, *J Rheumatol* 3:390, 1976.

85. Kridel RW, Konior RJ: Irradiated cartilage grafts in the nose: a preliminary report, *Arch Otolaryngol Head Neck Surg* 119:24, 1993.

86. Welling D, Maves M, Shuller D, Bardach J: Irradiated homologous cartilage grafts: long-term results, *Arch Otolaryngol Head Neck Surg* 114:291, 1988.

87. Czitrom AA, Langer F, McKee N, Gross AE: Bone and cartilage allotransplantation: a review of 14 years of research and clinical studies, *Clin Orthop* 208:141, 1986.

88. Mahomed MN, Beaver RJ, Gross AE: The long-term success of fresh, small fragment osteochondral allografts used for intraarticular post-traumatic defects in the knee joint, *Orthopedics* 15:1191, 1992.

89. Greenleaf G, Hansbrough JF: Current trends in the use of allograft skin for patients with burns and reflections on the future of skin banking in the United States, *J Burn Care Rehabil* 15:428, 1994.

90. Kealey GP, Aguiar J, Lewis RW, et al: Cadaver skin allografts and transmission of human cytomegalovirus to burn patients, *J Am Coll Surg* 182:201, 1996.

91. Amos D, Siegler H, Southworth J: Skin graft rejection between subjects genotyped for HL-A, *Transplant Proc* 1:342, 1969.

92. Burke J, May J, Albright N, et al: Temporary skin transplantation and immunosuppression for extensive burns, *N Engl J Med* 290:269, 1974.

93. Delmonico F, Cosimi A, Russell P: Temporary skin transplantation for the treatment of extensive burns, *Ann Clin Res* 13:373, 1981.

94. Burke J, Quinby W, Bondoc C, et al: Immunosuppression and temporary skin transplantation in the treatment of massive third degree burns, *Ann Surg* 182:183, 1975.

95. Achauer BM, Hewitt CW, Black KS, et al: Long-term skin allograft survival after short-term cyclosporin treatment in a patient with massive burns, *Lancet* 1(8471):14, 1986.

96. Alsbjorn BF: Langerhans cell depleted allograft skin on excised burns, *Lancet* 1(8333):1106, 1983 (letter).

97. Alsbjorn BF: Clinical results of grafting burns with epidermal Langerhans' cell depleted allograft overlay, *Scand J Plast Reconstr Surg Hand Surg* 25:35, 1991.

98. Heck EL, Bergstresser PR, Baxter CR: Composite skin graft: frozen dermal allografts support the engraftment and expansion of autologous epidermis, *J Trauma* 25:106, 1985.

99. Cuono C, Langdon R, McGuire J: Use of cultured epidermal autografts and dermal allografts as skin replacement after burn injury, *Lancet* 1(8490):1123, 1986.

100. Langdon RC, Cuono CB, Birchall N, et al: Reconstitution of structure and cell function in human skin grafts derived from cryopreserved allogeneic dermis and autologous cultured keratinocytes, *J Invest Dermatol* 91:478, 1988.

101. Hoekstra MJ, Kreis RW, du Pont JS: History of the Euro Skin Bank: the innovation of preservation technologies, *Burns* 20(suppl 1):S43, 1994.

102. Hussmann J, Russell RC, Kucan JO, et al: Use of glycerolized human allografts as temporary (and permanent) cover in adults and children, *Burns* 20(suppl 1):S61, 1994.

103. Horch R, Stark GB, Kopp J, Spilker G: Cologne Burn Centre experiences with glycerol-preserved allogeneic skin. Part I. Clinical experiences and histological findings (overgraft and sandwich technique), *Burns* 20(suppl 1):S23, 1994.

104. Wainwright DJ: Use of an acellular allograft dermal matrix (AlloDerm) in the management of full-thickness burns, *Burns* 21:243, 1995.

105. Hansbrough JF, Morgan J, Greenleaf G, Underwood J: Development of a temporary living skin replacement composed of human neonatal fibroblasts cultured in Biobrane, a synthetic dressing material, *Surgery* 115:633, 1994.

106. Purdue GF, Hunt JL, Still JM Jr, et al: A multicenter clinical trial of a biosynthetic skin replacement, Dermagraft-TC, compared with cryopreserved human cadaver skin for temporary coverage of excised burn wounds, *J Burn Care Rehabil* 18:52, 1997.

107. Hansbrough JF, Mozingo DW, Kealey GP, et al: Clinical trials of a biosynthetic temporary skin replacement, Dermagraft-Transitional Covering, compared with cryopreserved human cadaver skin for temporary coverage of excised burn wounds, *J Burn Care Rehabil* 18:43, 1997.

108. Eaglstein W, Iroindo M, Laszlo K: A composite skin substitute (Graftskin) for surgical wounds: a clinical experience, *Dermatol Surg* 21:839, 1995.

109. Ansselin AD, Pollard JD: Immunopathological factors in peripheral nerve allograft rejection: quantification of lymphocyte invasion and major histocompatibility complex expression, *J Neurol Sci* 96:75, 1990.

110. Ishida O, Ochi M, Ikuta Y, Akiyama M: Peripheral nerve allograft: cellular and humoral immune responses of mice, *J Surg Res* 49:233, 1990.

111. Midha R, Mackinnon SE, Becker LE: The fate of Schwann cells in peripheral nerve allografts, *J Neuropathol Exp Neurol* 53:316, 1994.

112. Mackinnon SE, Hudson AR: Clinical application of peripheral nerve transplantation, *Plast Reconstr Surg* 90:695, 1992.

113. Mackinnon SE: Nerve allotransplantation following severe tibial nerve injury: case report, *J Neurosurg* 84:671, 1996.

114. Arai K, Hotokebuchi T, Miyahara H, et al: Limb allografts in rats immunosuppressed with FK506. I. Reversal of rejection and indefinite survival, *Transplantation* 48:782, 1989.

115. Black KS, Hewitt CW, Fraser LA, et al: Composite tissue (limb) allografts in rats. II. Indefinite survival using low-dose cyclosporine, *Transplantation* 39:365, 1985.

116. Doi K: Homotransplantation of limbs in rats: a preliminary report on an experimental study with non-specific immunosuppressive drugs, *Plast Reconstr Surg* 64:613, 1979.

117. Fealy MJ, Umansky WS, Bickel KD, et al: Efficacy of rapamycin and FK 506 in prolonging rat hind limb allograft survival, *Ann Surg* 219:88, 1994.

118. Fritz WD, Swartz WM, Rose S, et al: Limb allografts in rats immunosuppressed with cyclosporin A, *Ann Surg* 199:211, 1984.

119. Furnas DW, Black KS, Hewitt CW, et al: Cyclosporine and long-term survival of composite tissue allografts (limb transplants) in rats, *Transplant Proc* 15(suppl 1):3063, 1983.

120. Goldwyn RM, Beach PM, Feldman D, et al: Canine limb homotransplantation, *Plast Reconstr Surg* 37:184, 1966.

121. Hewitt CW, Black KS, Fraser LA, et al: Composite tissue (limb) allografts in rats. I. Dose-dependent increase in survival with cyclosporine, *Transplantation* 39:360, 1985.

122. Hotokebuchi T, Arai K, Takagishi K, et al: Limb allografts in rats immunosuppressed with cyclosporine: as a whole-joint allograft, *Plast Reconstr Surg* 83:1027, 1989.

123. Lance EM, Inglis AE, Figarola F, Veith FJ: Transplantation of the canine hind limb: surgical technique and methods of immunosuppression for allotransplantation, *J Bone Joint Surg* 53A:1137, 1971.

124. Press BH, Sibley RK, Shons AR: Limb allotransplantation in the rat: extended survival and return of nerve function with continuous cyclosporin/prednisone immunosuppression, *Ann Plast Surg* 16:313, 1986.

125. Hotokebuchi T, Arai K, Arita C, et al: Limb allografts in skeletally immature rats with cyclosporine: behavior of the growth plate, *Transplant Proc* 21:3183, 1989.

126. Lee WPA, Pan Y-C, Kesmarky S, et al: Experimental orthotopic transplantation of vascularized skeletal allografts: functional assessment and long-term survival, *Plast Reconstr Surg* 95:336, 1995.

127. Yaremchuk MJ, Sedacca T, Schiller AL, May JW Jr: Vascular knee allograft transplantation in a rabbit model, *Plast Reconstr Surg* 71:461, 1983.

128. Guzman-Stein G, Shons AR: Functional recovery in the rat limb transplant model: a preliminary study, *Transplant Proc* 19:1115, 1987.

129. Daniel RK, Egerszegi EP, Samulack DD, et al: Tissue transplants in primates for upper extremity reconstruction: a preliminary report, *J Hand Surg* 11:1, 1986.

130. Hovius SER, Stevens HP, Van Nierop PW, et al: Replantation of the radial side of the hand in the rhesus monkey, anatomical and functional aspects: a preliminary study of composite tissue allografting, *J Hand Surg* 17B:651, 1992.

131. Lee WPA, Randolph MA, Weiland AJ, Yaremchuk MJ: Prolonged survival of vascularized limb tissue allografts after donor irradiation, *J Surg Res* 59:578, 1995.

132. Lee WPA, Yaremchuk MJ, Manfrini M, et al: Prolonged survival of vascularized limb allografts from chimera donors, *Plast Surg Forum* 11:51, 1988.

133. Butler PEM, Randolph MA, Van de Water AP, Lee WPA: Neonatal induction of tolerance to skeletal tissue allografts without immunosuppression, *Plast Reconstru Surg* (in press).

134. Rubin JP, Cober SR, Butler PEM, et al: Induction of transplantation tolerance in swine by utero injection of allogeneic bone marrow cells, *Transplantion* (in press).

135. Lee WPA, Rubin JP, Cober S, et al: Use of a swine model in transplantation of vascularized skeletal tissue allografts, *Transplant Proc* 30:2743, 1998.

136. Lee WPA, Butler PEM: Transplant biology and applications to plastic surgery. In Aston SJ, Beasley RW, Thorne CHM, editors: *Grabb and Smith's Plastic surgery*, ed 5, Philadelphia, 1997, Lippincott-Raven.

CHAPTER 19

Biomaterials

Myron Spector

As in other surgical specialties, plastic surgery has been revolutionized by implantable devices. These advances have been largely based on biomaterials science and engineering. Materials have been used for the fabrication of permanent implants to replace diseased, injured, or congenitally absent tissues and to restore tissue function.

In the future, however, materials will play a different role in plastic surgery. Materials will also be used for the fabrication of temporary, absorbable implants to facilitate the regeneration of tissue. This new role for materials is associated with novel therapeutic approaches associated with tissue engineering.

HISTORY AND OVERVIEW

The changing role for materials in plastic surgery can be considered through the various eras of the discipline. The 1930s through the 1970s might be considered the "Age of Devices." During these years a wide variety of implants were developed for treating myriad problems. These devices revolutionized plastic surgery and were fabricated from relatively few materials: stainless steel, cobalt-chromium alloy, polymethylmethacrylate (PMMA), and silicone.

Selection criteria for materials in implants were (1) strength, (2) biocompatibility, and (3) degradation resistance. The latter two specifications were often combined and referred to as "inertness." Materials proposed initially for implants in plastic surgery and for other surgical applications were generally shown to display this property in nonmedical uses, especially metallic materials. Advantages and disadvantages of materials for specific applications often were determined only after their introduction into the clinic. Materials commended for a particular clinical application because of one favorable property were found to fail because of a deficiency in another property.

The 1980s and 1990s might be considered the "Age of Biomaterials." New materials were introduced for the refabrication of devices already in clinical use to improve their performance. Also, the development of other materials led to new types of implants.

Titanium alloy was introduced as an alternative to cobalt-chromium alloy for fabrication of components with lower stiffness to reduce bone loss associated with stress shielding.

Synthetic calcium phosphate materials were introduced as bone graft substitute materials. Research was also initiated on carbon fiber–reinforced polymer composite materials to replace metals in devices with even lower stiffness. Absorbable polymers were developed to produce biodegradable devices for fracture fixation and other applications.

Also during these decades, however, the limitations of permanent biomaterials and devices became apparent, largely as a result of clinical experience and follow-up. Device failure from specific deficiencies of materials prompted the search for new substances that might improve the performance and extend the longevity of these devices.

More recently, a new class of the absorbable materials has been developed to augment or replace graft materials for defects in bone and certain soft tissues. These materials include different forms of absorbable polymers used in devices for fracture fixation, as well as calcium phosphate substances and collagen materials. In many respects these absorbable substances and the experience with transplants in many surgical specialties have served as the foundation for the imminent "Age of Tissue Engineering." Currently, porous absorbable synthetic and natural polymers are being investigated as scaffolds to be seeded with cells in vitro for the production of tissue in the laboratory or for the preparation of implants to facilitate tissue regeneration in vivo.

We also seem to be on the threshold of the "Age of Gene Therapy." Although experiments are investigating the efficacy of injecting gene fragments alone, it is likely that absorbable materials may be effectively employed as delivery systems for these genes. Also, the ex vivo transfection of cells with selected genes is certain to combine gene therapy with tissue engineering. Laboratory findings have been promising, but much work remains before the benefit/risk ratio of gene therapy for specific indications can be assessed.

Selection and development of a material for a specific indication are based on the following (Figure 19-1):
1. The device's function
2. The device's effect on the body
3. The body's effect on the implant

Issues related to the attachment of tissue to the implant (i.e., incorporation of the device into the body) also are important.

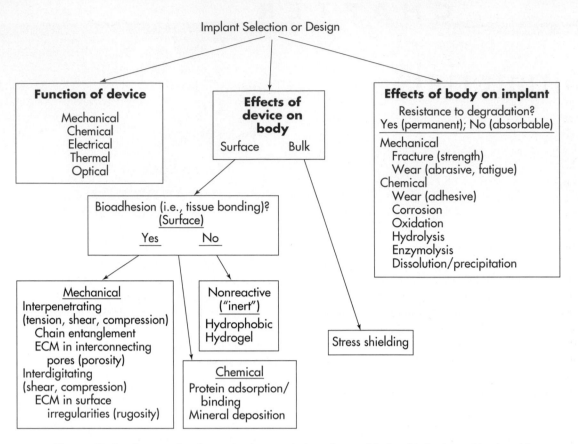

Figure 19-1. Issues related to selection or design of materials for fabrication of implantable devices. *ECM,* Extracellular matrix.

This chapter provides a framework for understanding the composition and properties of the wide variety of materials used for implantable devices in plastic surgery as they impact the biologic response to these implants. Additional background on biomaterials science and engineering can be found in a recent text.[89]

COMPOSITION AND PROPERTIES

The term *biomaterials* generally refers to synthetic and treated natural materials employed in the fabrication of implantable devices that are used to replace or augment tissue or organ function. An understanding of the physical properties of these materials is important for the judicious implementation of implants and provides for a realistic expectation of clinical performance.

The physical properties of materials result from their chemical makeup. Therefore an understanding of the molecular structure and chemical bonding of biomaterials can provide the basis for understanding the physical properties.[63]

Metals

In metals, closely packed arrays of positively charged atoms are held together in a loosely associated "cloud" of free electrons. The essential features of the metallic bond are that (1) it is nondirectional and (2) the electrons are freely mobile. The metals most often used for the fabrication of implantable devices are stainless steel, cobalt-chromium alloys, and titanium and titanium alloy. The specific members of these families used as biomaterials are usually identified by a designation provided by the American Society for Testing and Materials (ASTM).

The *stainless steels,* as with all steels, are iron-based alloys. *Chromium* is added to improve the corrosion resistance through the formation of a chromium oxide surface layer; at least 17% chromium is required for the term *stainless* to be used. *Carbon* and *nickel* are employed as alloying elements to increase strength. The most common type of stainless steel used for implants is 316L (American Iron and Steel Institute designation; ASTM F-138), containing 17% to 19% chromium, 13% to 15.5% nickel, and less than 0.03% carbon.

Surgical *cobalt-chromium alloy* is a cobalt-based system with chromium added for increased corrosion resistance. Its composition contains 27% to 30% chromium and 5% to 7% molybdenum. Tungsten is added to the wrought alloy to enhance ductility.

Titanium and its alloy, with 6% aluminum and 4% vanadium (Ti-6Al-4V), are used for their excellent corrosion resistance and their modulus of elasticity, which is approximately one-half that of stainless steel and cobalt-chromium alloys. This lower modulus results in devices with lower stiffness, which may be advantageous in certain applications, such as implants in bone because they will result in less stress shielding of bone. The alloy of titanium has much better material properties than the pure titanium. Problems with titanium are its severe notch sensitivity and poor wear resistance.

The mechanical properties of any material are linked to its *ultrastructure*. Any processing treatment that alters the phase structure, grain size, or grain orientation of a metal will affect the material properties. Mechanically deforming a metal beyond its yield stress will produce, in addition to a shape change, a material with increased yield and ultimate stresses and a higher endurance limit. Because this process, called *cold working*, results in permanent deformation, the resultant material is less ductile than the initial material.

Casting is the pouring of molten metal into a mold to produce a specific shape on cooling. Voids and other flaws are a major problem with casting. *Forging* is a process by which a blank of metal is heated and pressed into a die by the application of a large, single force. This produces a part with fewer defects than a casting. *Annealing* is essentially heating for prolonged periods to allow stress relaxation and grain reorganization and growth. *Hot isostatic pressing* is a newer technology involving the consolidation of metal powder into a fine-grained material under high temperature and pressure. These and other processing methods have been developed to produce parts of complex shape with the highest degree of mechanical integrity.

Metallic materials have certain properties that make them ideal for load-bearing applications. They can maintain very high strength under the aggressive aqueous environment in the body. The *biocompatibility* of metallic materials is related to their corrosion resistance.

STAINLESS STEELS. Many alloys and grades of alloys are identified as commercial stainless steels. Only the iron-chromium-nickel alloys are used as biomaterials. Unalloyed iron, carbon steels, and alloyed carbon steels cannot be used because they corrode in oxygenated saline solutions.

Despite their very good corrosion resistance, stainless steels are subject to several other corrosion processes, including crevice, pitting, intergranular, and stress corrosion. These processes can profoundly degrade the mechanical strength of the alloy and can lead to the release of metallic ions into the surrounding tissue, with undesirable biologic consequences (see later discussion).

Alloying with chromium generates a protective, self-regenerating oxide film that resists perforation, has a high degree of electrical resistivity, and thus provides a major protection against corrosion. Formation of the chromium oxide "passivation" layer is facilitated by immersion of the alloy in a strong nitric acid solution. The nickel imparts more corrosion resistance and outstanding fabricability. The molybdenum addition provides resistance to pitting corrosion. Other alloying elements facilitate manufacturing processes.

The presence of carbon in stainless steel is undesirable. Under certain conditions the carbon segregates from the major elements of the alloy, taking with it a substantial amount of chromium in forming chromium carbide precipitates. Local depletion of chromium deprives those zones of corrosion resistance, and since the carbides form most frequently at the alloy crystal interfaces, the resultant corrosion occurs selectively in the intercrystalline paths. Certain grades of stainless steel (e.g., F-138) have a maximum of only 0.03% carbon to reduce the formation of these carbides.

Another feature of the stainless steels relates to the presence of inclusions, which can serve as flaws or cracks that can be propagated by cyclic loading—the process of *fatigue failure*. To increase resistance to fatigue failure, certain grades of steel are available with smaller and more widely spaced inclusions.

COBALT-CHROMIUM ALLOYS. As with stainless steels, the chromium content of this alloy generates a highly resistive, passive film that contributes substantially to corrosion resistance. The cobalt-chromium-molybdenum (Co-Cr-Mo) alloy (F-75) has superior corrosion resistance to the F-138 stainless steel, particularly in crevice corrosion, and has an extensive history of biocompatibility in human implantation.

Co-Cr-Mo devices are currently produced by hot isostatic pressing, which results in parts with more favorable strength characteristics than results from casting processes. In the hot isostatic pressing process the liquid alloy is atomized to powder. Loose powder is consolidated to a void-free solid, resulting in a part reasonably close in shape to the ultimate device. The preformed part is finished by machining and polishing. The resulting structure has a very fine, alloy crystal size and very fine, uniform dispersion of carbide particles. The availability of the high-strength varieties and their superior corrosion resistance and biocompatibility make them excellent choices for high-stress applications.

Cobalt-chromium-titanium-nickel (Co-Cr-Ti-Ni) alloy (ASTM F-90) is very different from the F-75 alloy, with which it is often confused. This alloy can be hot forged and cold drawn and is not used in the cast form. In clinical practice it is used to make wire and internal fixation devices (e.g., plates, intramedullary rods, screws).

UNALLOYED TITANIUM AND TITANIUM ALLOY. Titanium and its alloys are of particular interest for biomedical applications because of their outstanding biocompatibility. In general, their corrosion resistance significantly exceeds that of the stainless steels and the cobalt-chromium alloys. In saline solutions at near-neutral pH the corrosion rate is extremely small, with no evidence of pitting, intergranular, or crevice corrosion. Data from in vivo animal experimental models and from human sources indicate superior biocompatibility.

So-called unalloyed titanium actually is alloyed by the level of oxygen dissolved into the metal. In large amounts, oxygen embrittles titanium and its alloys, but in small, regulated amounts it helps control the yield strength of the materials. ASTM F-67 is a specification for oxygen providing 345 megapascals (MPa) of yield strength in grade III and 485 MPa of minimum yield strength in grade IV. Other elements in unalloyed titanium include nitrogen, 0.07% (maximum); carbon, 0.15% (maximum); hydrogen, 0.015% (maximum); and iron, 0.35% (maximum). Any excess of these elements may degrade the performance of the basic material.

Unalloyed titanium is used less frequently than the alloy for implants but is available in various configurations, such as plain wire for manufacturing purposes. In addition, it is used to produce porous coatings for certain designs of total joint replacement prostheses.

ASTM F-136 specifies a titanium alloy with a content of 5.5% to 6.5% aluminum, 3.5% to 4.5% vanadium, 0.25% iron (maximum), 0.05% nitrogen (maximum), 0.08% carbon (maximum), 0.0125% hydrogen (maximum), and 0.1% other (maximum 0.4% total). Developed by the aircraft industry as one of several high-strength titanium alloys, this particular formulation has a yield strength reaching 1110 MPa. The ASTM F-136 specification limits the oxygen to an especially low level of 0.13% maximum. This is also known in the industry as the *extra low interstitial* (ELI) grade. Limiting the level of oxygen improves the mechanical properties of the material, particularly increasing its fatigue life.

One interesting feature of titanium and its alloys is the low modulus of elasticity of 100 gigapascals (GPa), as compared with 200 GPa for the cobalt-chromium alloys. This feature leads to their use in plates for internal fixation of fractures. Some have found that the lower stiffness of these plates may decrease the severity of bone stress shielding, which results in osteopenia under these devices.

One of the weaknesses of titanium is poor wear resistance. This problem apparently relates to the mechanical stability of the passive film covering the alloy's surface. On a carefully polished surface, the film is highly passive but mechanically weak.

Permanent and Absorbable Synthetic and Natural Polymers

Polymers consist of long chains of covalently bonded molecules characterized by the repeated appearance of a monomeric molecular unit. They can be produced de novo by the polymerization of synthetic monomers or prepared from natural polymers isolated from tissues. Most synthetic and natural polymers have a carbon backbone. Bonding among polymer chains results from the much weaker secondary forces of hydrogen bonds or van der Waal's forces. Covalent bonding among chains, referred to as *cross-linking,* can be produced in certain polymer systems.

Physical entanglements of the long polymer chains, the degree of crystallinity, and chemical cross-linking among chains play important roles in determining polymer properties. The molecular bonding of the backbone of the polymer can be designed to undergo hydrolysis or enzymatic breakdown, thus allowing for the synthesis of absorbable, as well as permanent, devices.

Polymeric materials are generally employed for the fabrication of implants for soft tissue applications that require a greater degree of compliance than can be achieved with metals. They have also been shown to be of value as implants in bone for indications that would also benefit from their lower modulus of elasticity, as well as the ability of some to be polymerized in vivo and adapt to defects of complex shape. For some indications the radiolucency of polymeric materials may be an important benefit. Because of the limited strength and wear resistance of polymers, the load-bearing requirements of the applications must be considered.

POLYMETHYLMETHACRYLATE. PMMA is used in a self-curing form as a filling materials for defects in bone and as a grouting agent for joint replacement prostheses.[35] It can be shaped in vivo while in a dough stage before complete polymerization, and thus a custom implant is created for each use. Its purpose is more even redistribution of stress on the surrounding bone.

Often referred to as "bone cement," when PMMA is employed for joint arthroplasty, it acts as a grout to support the prosthesis rather than a glue; it has minimal adhesive properties. The time-dependent properties of PMMA during curing require an understanding of its handling characteristics. Immediately after mixing, the low viscosity permits interdigitation with cancellous bone. Viscosity rises quickly once the chemical setting reaction begins, requiring that the prosthesis be accurately positioned and stationary to achieve maximum fixation.

The chemical toxicity of the methylmethacrylate monomer and the heat generated during polymerization must be considered when using PMMA. Its brittle nature after curing and low fatigue strength make PMMA vulnerable to fracture under high mechanical loading. Also, wear debris is produced when other, harder materials rub against PMMA.

Although the adjunctive use of PMMA to stabilize pathologic fractures of diaphyseal bones has become routine, its implantation about the cervical spine has been limited because of the exothermic reaction during the curing process. Bone-cement interfacial temperatures of 60° to 65° C (140° to 149° F) during total knee arthroplasty and of 80° to 90° C (176° to 194° F) during total hip arthroplasty have been reported. These temperatures are of sufficient magnitude to cause degradation of protein. The adverse effects of such temperatures on the cerebrospinal fluid and spinal cord can be avoided by the following:

1. Precooling the soft tissues and bone
2. Placing the cement on the dorsal aspect of the intact lamina
3. Applying precooled Gelfoam over exposed dura

In this way, acrylic cement and wire fixation of pathologic fractures of the cervical spine can be performed safely to allow early mobilization of patients with limited life expectancies.

SILICONE. Silicones are polymers with a backbone comprised of alternating silicon and oxygen atoms and organic side groups bonded to the silicon through covalent bonding with the carbon atom.[61] One form of silicone typically used for the fabrication of implants is *polydimethylsiloxane* (PDMS). In PDMS, methyl (CH_3) side groups are covalently bonded to the silicon atom. PDMS can be used in the following three forms:

1. A fluid comprising linear polymers of varying molecular weight (i.e., chain length)
2. A cross-linked network referred to as a *gel*
3. A solid elastomer comprising a highly cross-linked gel filled with small particles of silica.

Silica is another silicon-containing molecule, silicon dioxide. PDMS elastomers contain a noncrystalline silica particle 7 to 22 nm in diameter that has been surface-treated to facilitate chemical bonding of the particle to the PDMS gel. Addition of the silica particle to a highly cross-linked PDMS gel is done to modify the mechanical properties of the elastomer. In certain cases, such as the PDMS elastomeric shell for silicone-filled breast implants, the elastomer may contain side groups of phenyl (C_6H_5) or trifluoropropyl ($CF_3CH_2CH_2$) instead of the methyl groups to better contain the PDMS fluid.

In evaluating the performance of silicone implants, the role of each form of PDMS in the device must be considered. Attributing specific biologic responses to individual components of a silicone device is complicated by the implant's many molecular forms of silicone.

POLYETHYLENE. Ultrahigh-molecular-weight polyethylene (UHMWPE) has a very low frictional coefficient against metal and ceramics and is therefore used as a bearing surface for joint replacement prostheses.[13,62] Moreover, the wear resistance of UHMWPE is lower than that of other polymers investigated for this application. Low strength and creep, however, present potential problems.

The term *polyethylene* refers to plastics formed from polymerization of ethylene gas. The possibilities for structural variation in molecules formed by this simple repeating unit for different factors (e.g., molecular weight, crystallinity, branching, cross-linking) are so numerous and dramatic with such a wide range of attainable properties that polyethylene truly refers to a subclass of materials. The earliest type of polyethylene was made by reacting ethylene at high (20,000 to 30,000 pounds per square inch) pressure and temperatures of 200° to 400° C with oxygen as a catalyst. Such material is referred to as *conventional,* or *low-density,* polyethylene.

Much polyethylene is produced now by newer, low-pressure techniques using aluminum-titanium (Ziegler) catalysts. This is called *linear* polyethylene due to the linearity of its molecules, in contrast to the branched molecules produced by high-pressure processes. The linear polymers can be used to make high-density polyethylene by means of the higher degree of crystallinity attained with the regularly shaped molecules. Typically, molecular weight is not significantly different between the low-density and high-density varieties (e.g., 100,000 to 500,000).

If the low-pressure process is used to make extremely long molecules (i.e., UHMWPE), however, the result is remarkably different. This material, with a molecular weight of 1 to 10 million, is less crystalline and less dense than high-density polyethylene and has exceptional mechanical properties. It is extremely tough and is remarkably wear resistant; a 0.357-magnum bullet fired from 25 feet bounces back from a 1-inch-thick slab of UHMWPE. The material is used in very demanding applications (e.g., ore chutes in mining equipment) and is the most successful polymer used in total joint replacements. It far outperforms the various acrylics, fluorocarbons, polyacetals, polyamides, and polyesters tried for such purposes.

ABSORBABLE POLYMERS

Synthetic. Absorbable polymers have been used in plastic surgery for decades in the form of absorbable sutures.[4] More recently this class of materials has been investigated for the application of resorbable devices, including fracture fixation implants and scaffolds for tissue engineering. The principal issues associated with the implementation of absorbable polymers as implants include the following:

1. Mechanical properties (e.g., strength)
2. Degradation rate
3. Biologic response to the degradation products.

One of the classes of polymers used frequently for the fabrication of absorbable implants is the alpha-hydroxy acids, including L-lactic acid, glycolic acid, and dioxanone. These molecules normally are used in their polymeric forms: poly-L-lactic acid (PLLA), polyglycolic acid (PGA), and polydioxanone. Copolymers of lactic and glycolic acids are also frequently employed.

A particular class of polyester undergoes breakdown as a result of the hydrolytic scission of the ester bond. The access of water to this bond in PGA is much greater, resulting in a more rapid degradation rate compared with that occurring with PLLA, which has a bulkier CH_3 side group instead of the H atom in PGA. The copolymer of polylactic and polyglycolic acid can be designed to have an intermediate degradation rate. Although most breakdowns of these polymers are caused by hydrolytic scission, nonspecific enzymatic action is also involved.

Factors that affect the rate of breakdown of these polymers include (1) the relative amount of monomers composing the copolymers, (2) the degree of crystallinity, and (3) the surface area. These polymers are normally broken down to natural body components excreted in the urine or exhaled. The process of degradation involves the gradual decrease in the average molecular weight of the polymer as hydrolysis proceeds. At some point the molecular weight decreases to the extent that the polymer becomes soluble in the aqueous environment, and a bolus release of the molecules occurs. Depending on the mass of the implanted device, the concentration of the molecules may elicit an inflammatory response.[108]

Natural. Myriad devices are fabricated from *collagen,* the principal structural protein of the body.[117] The collagen molecule comprises three tightly coiled helical polypeptide chains. In vivo the collagen molecule, *tropocollagen,* is assembled to form fibrils, which in turn assume various orientations and configurations to form the architecture of various tissues. The wide array of properties of tissues that make up collagen, from dermis to musculoskeletal tissues and including articular cartilage, meniscus, and ligament, is caused by differences in the chemistry, density, and orientation of the fibrils formed from the collagen molecule.

Collagen is soluble in specific solutions in which the chains can become disentangled to produce gelatin. Collagen can be isolated from tissue and purified through the use of several agents: acids, alkalis, enzymes, and salt. Treatment in acid results in the elimination of acidic proteins and glycosaminoglycans, which cause dissociation of the collagen fibrils. A similar effect can be achieved using alkaline extraction with the removal of basic proteins. Proteolytic enzymes that cleave the telopeptides, which serve as natural cross-linking agents for collagen, allow for the dissolution of collagen molecules and aggregates in aqueous solutions. Salt extraction leads to the removal of newly synthesized collagen molecules and certain noncollagenous molecules, thus facilitating the disaggregation of collagen fibrils.

Collagen's solubility in an acidic medium facilitates its extraction from tissues and reprocessing into biomaterials. Several factors are critical determinants of the properties of reconstituted collagen biomaterials. The degree of denaturation or degradation of the collagen structures isolated from tissue will affect the mechanical properties. These properties will also be affected by the degree to which the material is subsequently cross-linked.

An important biologic property related to collagen's molecular structure is the *collagen-induced blood platelet aggregation.* The quarternary structure of collagen resulting from the periodic aggregation of the collagen molecules has been well documented. Methods for isolating and purifying collagen fibrils result in the preservation or destruction of this quarternary structure and are used to produce either hemostatic or thromboresistant biomaterials. Another factor relates to the removal of soluble components that might serve as antigens. The immunogenicity can be reduced to clinically insignificant levels by chemically modifying the antigen molecules.

A wide variety of methods have been employed for the fabrication of collagen sutures, fleeces for hemostasis, and spongelike materials for scaffolds in tissue engineering.

Ceramics

Ceramics are typically three-dimensional arrays of positively charged metal ions and negatively charged nonmetal ions, often oxygen. The ionic bond localizes all the available electrons in the formation of a bond. Network organization ranges from highly organized, crystalline, three-dimensional arrays to amorphous, random arrangements in glassy materials.

Ceramics may be the most chemically inert implant materials currently in use. Their relatively low tensile strength, high modulus, and brittleness, however, limit their applications. Current techniques allowing the formation of ceramic coating on metallic substrates have revitalized interest in ceramics for hard-tissue applications.

ALUMINUM OXIDE. Aluminum oxide has been found of value for the articulating components of total joint arthroplasties because of its high wear resistance and its low coefficient of friction when prepared in congruent, polished geometrics. The brittle nature of alumina remains a detriment.

CALCIUM PHOSPHATES AND HYDROXYAPATITE. Calcium-based ceramics, closely related to the naturally occurring hydroxyapatite in bone, have generated great interest in recent years. Their ability to bond directly to bone and their osteoconductive capability promise to enhance biologic fixation of implant devices. Hydroxyapatite is only slightly resorb-

able and is used in both dense and porous forms as a permanent implant. Tricalcium phosphate is bioabsorbable to varying degrees, depending on formulation and structure. Many calcium phosphate materials are currently undergoing investigation as bone graft substitute materials (see later discussion).

Composite Materials

Composite materials are combinations of two or more materials and usually involve more than one material class (e.g., metals, polymers, ceramics). They are used to achieve a combination of mechanical properties for specific applications. Composite technology, much of it developed for the aerospace industry, is beginning to make its way into biomedical materials. Carbon fiber–reinforced polymers are being investigated as substitutes for metals. The advantage is that devices with comparable strength but with significantly lower stiffness can be produced. Moreover, these types of composite devices are radiolucent.

BIOLOGIC RESPONSE TO BIOMATERIALS

The biological processes composing the tissue response are affected by the following implant-related factors[99]:

1. "Dead space" created by presence of the implant
2. Soluble agents released by the implant (e.g., metal ions, polymer fragments)
3. Insoluble particulate material released from the implant (e.g., wear debris)
4. Chemical interactions of biologic molecules with the implant's surface
5. Alterations in the strain distribution in tissue caused by (a) mismatch in the modulus of elasticity between the implant and surrounding tissue and (b) movement of the implant relative to adjacent tissue as a result of the absence of mechanical continuity

Study of the tissue response to implants requires methodology capable of measurements at the molecular, cellular, and tissue levels (Figure 19-2). *Time* is an important variable because of the critical temporal relationship between the molecular and cellular protagonists of the biologic reactions. Also, implant-related factors act on the biologic responses with different time constants. The dynamic nature of implant-tissue interactions requires that the final assessment of tissue compatibility be qualified by the time frame in which it has been evaluated.

The tissue response to an implant is the cumulative physiologic effect of the following[100]:

1. Modulation of the acute wound healing response to the surgical trauma of implantation and presence of the implant (Figure 19-3)
2. Subsequent chronic inflammatory reaction associated with presence of the device
3. Remodeling of surrounding tissue as it adapts to presence of the implant

In addition, the healing and stress-induced adaptive remodeling responses of different tissues to the same implant can vary greatly.

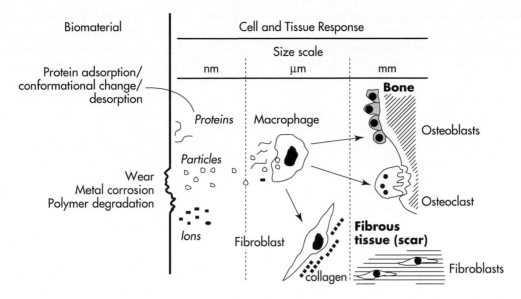

Figure 19-2. Interactions among moieties released by implants, biologic molecules, cells, and tissues.

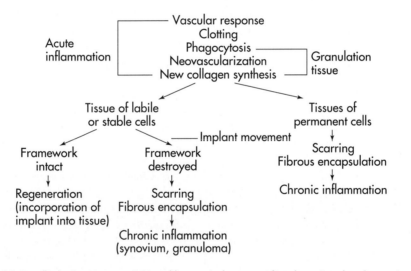

Figure 19-3. Biologic processes initiated by surgical trauma of implantation that determine tissue response to implantable devices.

The biologic response elicited by an implant involves the healing and remodeling characteristics of the four basic types of tissue: connective tissue, muscle, epithelium, and nerve. The characteristics of the parenchymal cells in each type of tissue can provide a basis for understanding the tissue response to an implant. The following characteristics of an implant site are determinants of the biologic response:

1. Vascularity
2. Nature of the parenchymal cell with respect to its capability for mitosis and migration, because these processes determine the regenerative capability of the tissue
3. Presence of regulatory cells, such as macrophages and histiocytes
4. Effect of mechanical strain, associated with deformation of the extracellular matrix, on the behavior of the parenchymal cell

Surgical wounds in avascular tissue (e.g., cornea, inner third of meniscus) will not heal because of the limited potential for the proliferation and migration of surrounding parenchymal cells into the wound site. Gaps between an implant and surrounding avascular tissue will remain indefinitely. Implant sites in vascular tissues where the parenchymal cell is incapable of mitosis (e.g., nerve tissue) will heal by scar formation in the gap between the implant and surrounding tissue. Moreover, adjacent cells that have died as a result of the implant surgery will be replaced by fibroblasts and scar tissue.

Normal Local Tissue Response

WOUND HEALING. The tissue that forms around implants is the result of the influence of the device on (1) the wound healing response initiated by the surgical trauma of implantation (Figure 19-3) and (2) subsequent tissue remodeling.

Implantation of a medical device initiates a sequence of cellular and biochemical processes that lead to healing by *secondary intention,* that is, healing by the formation of granulation tissue within a defect, as opposed to the healing of an incision, or, healing by *primary intention.*

The first phase of healing in vascularized tissues is inflammation. This is followed by a reparative phase, the replacement of the dead or damaged cells by healthy cells. The pathway of the reparative process depends on the regenerative capability of the cells composing the injured tissue (i.e., the tissue or organ into which the implant has been placed).

Cells can be distinguished as labile, stable, or permanent based on their capacity to regenerate. *Labile cells* continue to proliferate throughout life, replacing cells that are continually being destroyed. Epithelial and blood cells are examples of labile cells, as are cells of splenic, lymphoid, and hematopoietic tissues.

Stable cells retain the capacity for proliferation, although they do not normally replicate. These cells can undergo rapid division in response to a variety of stimuli and can reconstitute the tissue of origin. Stable cells include the parenchymal cells of all the glandular organs of the body (e.g., liver, kidney, pancreas), mesenchymal derivatives (e.g., fibroblasts), smooth muscle cells, osteoblasts and chondrocytes, and vascular endothelial cells.

Permanent cells cannot reproduce themselves after birth. Examples are nerve cells.

Tissues comprised of labile and stable cells can regenerate after surgical trauma (Figure 19-3). The injured tissue is replaced by parenchymal cells of the same type, often leaving no residual trace of injury. Tissues comprised of permanent cells, however, are repaired by the production of fibrocollagenous scar. Despite the capability of many tissues to undergo regeneration, destruction of the tissue stroma remaining after injury or constructed during the healing process will lead to formation of scar. The biologic response to materials therefore depends on the influence of the material on the inflammatory and reparative stages of wound healing.

The following types of questions need to be addressed when assessing the "biocompatibility" of materials:

Does the material yield leachables or corrosion products that interfere with the resolution of inflammation initiated by the surgical trauma?

Does the presence of the material interfere with the stroma required for the regeneration of tissue at the implant site?

A number of systemic and local factors influence the inflammatory-reparative response. Systemic influences include age, nutrition, hematologic derangements, metabolic derangements, hormones, and steroids. Although the prevailing "conventional wisdom" is that elderly persons heal more slowly than young people, few control data and animal experiments support this theory. Nutrition can have a profound effect on the healing of wounds. Prolonged protein starvation can inhibit collagen formation, and high-protein diets can enhance the rate of tensile strength gained during wound healing. Local influences that can affect wound healing include infection, inadequate blood supply, and presence of a foreign body.

FIBROUS TISSUE INTERFACE. The implant creates a dead space in tissue that attracts macrophages to the implant-tissue interface.[96] These cells are attracted to the prosthesis as they are to any dead space (e.g., bursa, joint space), presumably because of certain microenvironmental conditions (e.g., low oxygen, high lactate). In this regard it is not clear why macrophages are absent from the surface of osseointegrated implants (see following discussion).

Macrophages and the scar's fibroblasts form synovial tissue, which can be considered the chronic inflammatory response to implants, unless the device is apposed by osseous tissue (i.e., osseointegrated).[101] This process is often termed *fibrous encapsulation.*[27,54] The presence of regulatory cells such as macrophages at the implant-tissue interface can profoundly influence the host response to a device because these cells can release proinflammatory mediators if irritated by the movement of the device or substances released from the biomaterial.[3] The inflammatory response of the synovial tissue around implants is comparable to the inflammation that can occur in the synovium lining any bursa (e.g., bursitis); thus the response to implants has been termed *implant bursitis.*[101]

RESPONSE TO IMPLANTS IN BONE. Wound healing governs the makeup of the tissue that forms around implants. Because it can regenerate, bone should be expected to appose implants in osseous tissue and form within the pore spaces of porous coatings. Is this bone bonded in any way to the implant? Bonding of a prosthesis to bone would enhance its stability, limiting the relative motion between the implant and bone. In addition, bonding might provide a more favorable distribution of stress to surrounding osseous tissue.

Bonding and Osseointegration. Bonding of bone to an implant can be achieved by mechanical or chemical means. Interdigitation of bone with PMMA bone cement or with irregularities in implant topography and bone ingrowth into porous surfaces can yield interfaces capable of supporting shear and tensile as well as compressive forces. These types of *mechanical bonding* have been extensively investigated and are reasonably well understood.

Chemical bonding of bone to materials may result from molecular (e.g., protein) adsorption and bonding to surfaces with subsequent bone cell attachment. This phenomenon has undergone intensive investigation in recent years but is not yet as well understood as mechanical bonding.

The term *osseointegration* has been used to describe the presence of bone on the surface of an implant with no histologic intervening nonosseous (e.g., fibrous) tissue. All implants in bone should become osseointegrated unless the bone regeneration process is inhibited.

Bone Ingrowth. The bone ingrowth into a porous-surface coating on an implant leads to an interlocking bond that can stabilize the device. In order for the porous material to accommodate the cellular and extracellular elements of bone, the average pore diameter should be greater than about 100 μm.

The bone ingrowth process proceeds in two stages. First, surgical trauma of implantation initially leads to the regeneration of bone throughout the pores of the coating. Second, mechanical stress–induced remodeling leads to resorption of bone from certain regions of the implant and continued formation and remodeling of bone in other regions.

Chemical Bonding of Bone to Biomaterial. Previous investigations have provided evidence of bone bonding to many different types of calcium phosphate materials, calcium carbonate substances, and calcium-containing "bioactive" glasses. Chemical bonding was evidenced by the high strength of the implant-bone interface, which could not be explained by a mechanical interlocking bond alone. In addition, electron microscopy has shown that no identifiable border exists between these calcium-containing implants and adjacent bone.

Many recent studies have investigated the bonding of bone to one particular calcium phosphate mineral, hydroxyapatite. This was chosen because of its relationship to the primary mineral constituent of bone; natural bone mineral is a calcium-deficient *carbonate apatite*. Experiments have been performed on both hydroxyapatite-coated metallic implants and on particulate and block forms of the mineral used as bone substitute materials. Histology of specimens shows that a layer of new bone approximately 100 µm in thickness covers most of the hydroxyapatite surface within a few weeks of implantation and remains indefinitely. This layer of bone is attached to the surrounding osseous tissue by trabecular bridges.

In studying the mechanism of bone bonding, researchers have found that within days of implantation, *biologic apatites* precipitate (from body fluid) onto the surface of the calcium-containing implants. These biologic apatites are comparable to the carbonate apatite of bone mineral. Proteins probably adsorb to this biologic mineral layer, thereby facilitating bone cell attachment and the production of osteoid directly onto the implant. This osteoid subsequently undergoes mineralization, as it does normally in osteogenesis, thus forming a continuum of mineral from the implant to the bone. The bone cell responds to the biologic apatite layer that has formed on the implant and not directly to the implant itself.

Recent studies have shown that this biologic apatite layer forms on many different calcium phosphate substances, explaining why bone-bonding behavior has been reported for many different types of calcium phosphate materials. The clinical value of this phenomenon will depend on the following:
1. For coatings, how well these substances can be bonded to implants
2. For bone graft substitute materials, their strength, modulus of elasticity, and ability to be resorbed

The finding that bone can become chemically bonded to certain biomaterials, however, is a significant advance in understanding the implant-bone interface.

IMPLANT-INDUCED ALTERATIONS. The presence of the implant can alter the stress distribution in the extracellular matrix and thereby reduce or increase the strains experienced by the constituent cells. Many studies have demonstrated immobilization-induced atrophy of certain tissues resulting from the decrease in mechanical strains. Loss of bone mass around stiff femoral stems and femoral condylar prostheses of total hip and knee replacement devices has been associated with the reduced strains resulting from stress shielding. Hyperplasia and hypertrophy of tissue have also occurred, in which mechanical strains have increased due to the presence of an implant.

CRITERIA FOR TISSUE RESPONSE. The in vivo assessment of tissue compatibility of biomaterials requires that certain criteria be implemented for determining the acceptability of the tissue response relative to the intended application of the material or device. The biomaterial or device should be considered biocompatible only in this context. Every study involving the in vivo assessment of tissue compatibility should provide a working definition of biocompatibility.

Biomaterials and devices implanted into bone can become apposed by the regenerating osseous tissue and thus can be considered compatible with bone regeneration. Altered bone remodeling around the device caused by stress shielding, with a net loss of bone mass (i.e., osteopenia), could lead to the assessment that the material or device is not compatible with normal bone remodeling. When the implant is surrounded by fibrous tissue, macrophages appearing on the material's surface are the expected response to the dead space produced by the implant. The synovial tissue thus produced might be considered an acceptable response relative to the material's chemical compatibility. Using the thickness of the scar capsule around implants alone as a measure of biocompatibility is problematic because it can be influenced by tissue movement at the site relative to the implant.

The cellular and molecular makeup of tissue and the interactions among these components are complex. Criteria for assessing certain features of the biocompatibility of biomaterials and devices should focus on specific aspects of the biologic response. Importantly, materials yielding acceptable tissue compatibility in one site of implantation might yield unfavorable results in another site.

Degeneration of Biomaterial-Tissue Interface

As noted earlier, the wound healing response initially establishes the tissue characteristics of the implant-tissue interface. Several agents can initiate degenerative changes in the interface tissue. Other agents probably act as promoters to stimulate the production of proinflammatory mediators that stimulate tissue degradation and potentiate the failure process.

Of the many factors affecting the implant-tissue interface, two of the most important are motion of the prosthetic component and particulate debris. It is difficult, however, to determine the causal relationships between these factors and implant failure from studying only the end-stage tissue. Other histopathologic findings and laboratory studies indicate that metal ions and immune reactions might play roles in the degenerative processes leading to prosthesis loosening in certain patients. Systemic diseases and drugs used to treat the disorders could also contribute to the breakdown of the implant-bone interface.

Finally, interindividual differences in genetically determined cellular responses might explain why prostheses fail in some patients with a low mechanical risk factor for failure.

EFFECTS OF IMPLANT MOVEMENT. Movement of the implant relative to the surrounding tissue can interfere with the wound healing response by disrupting the granulation tissue. With bone implants this relative movement, if excessive, can destroy the stroma required for osseous regeneration, and a fibrous scar results.

Another important effect of implant motion is the formation of a bursa within connective tissue, in which shearing and tensile movement has led to disruption of tissue continuity and formation of a void space or sac (lined by synovial-like cells). Therefore the tissue around prosthetic components that are removed because of loosening might display features of synovial-like tissue. The presence of synovial cells (macrophage and fibroblast-like cells) is important because they could be activated by other agents, such as particulate debris, to produce proinflammatory molecules. The process of activation of this tissue might be similar to that occurring in inflammatory joint synovium or bursitis.

Previous studies explain how prosthetic motion leads to the formation of the synovial-like tissue by showing that "synovial lining is simply an accretion of macrophages and fibroblasts stimulated by mechanical cavitation of connective tissue."[36] These findings are based on experiments in which the mechanical disruption of connective tissue was produced by injection of air and fluid into the subcutaneous space of animals.[94] The resulting sac was initially described as a "granuloma pouch." Later studies demonstrated that the membrane lining the pouch displayed the characteristics of synovium, and this tissue was referred to as "facsimile synovium."[36]

Prosthetic motion can also contribute to wear of the prosthetic component abrading against the bone cement sheath or surrounding bone. This generates increased amounts of particulate debris, which might contribute to activation of the macrophages and synovial-like cells at the implant-tissue interface.

EFFECTS OF IMPLANT-DERIVED PARTICLES. Particulate debris can be generated from the abrasion of the implant against surrounding tissue. The potential for wear is greater with materials or devices rubbing against a hard surface such as bone and with the articulating components of joint replacement prostheses. This particulate debris can induce changes in the tissue around the implants. Adverse responses have been found to both metallic and polymeric particles.

The biologic reactions to particles are related to (1) particle size, (2) quantity, (3) chemistry, (4) topography, and (5) shape. Although the role that each of these factors play in the biologic response is unclear, particle size appears to be particularly important. Particles small enough to be phagocytosed (less than 10 μm) elicit more of an adverse cellular response than larger particles.

Particulate metallic particles (e.g., cobalt-chromium alloy) can induce rapid proliferation of macrophages and focal degeneration of synovial tissues.[49] Animal investigations and histopathologic studies of tissues from human subjects have suggested that titanium alloy is more "biocompatible" than cobalt-chromium alloys. Therefore researchers assumed that titanium particulate debris would be less problematic than particles of cobalt-chromium alloy. Histology of pigmented tissue surrounding titanium implants has generally revealed considerably fewer macrophages and multinucleated foreign body giant cells than around cobalt-chromium alloy particles and polymeric particulate debris. However, titanium alloy particles generated by the abrasion of femoral stems against bone cement in human subjects can cause histiocytic and lymphoplasmacytic reactions to the metallic particles.[1] Titanium particles have also been found to cause fibroblasts in culture to produce elevated levels of prostaglandin E_2 (PGE_2). These findings show that adverse effects may occur with the biologic response to titanium particles as well as to cobalt-chromium alloy particulate debris.

Many investigations evaluating the histologic response to polyethylene and PMMA particles in animals and in tissue recovered from revision surgery have revealed the histiocytic response to these polymer particles. This macrophage response can also lead to bone resorption.

Synovial cells also respond to calcium-containing ceramic particles.[79] Local leukocyte influx, proteinase, PGE_2, and tumor necrosis factor (TNF) levels have been measured after injection of calcium-containing ceramic materials into the "air-pouch model" described earlier. TNF was detected in significant amounts after injection of the ceramics. These substances also caused elevated leukocyte counts and increased levels of proteinase and PGE_2. Substances with surface chemistries that elicit a beneficial tissue response (e.g., bone bonding) when implanted in bulk form can cause destructive cellular reactions when present in particulate form.

Investigations indicate that most biomaterials, when present in particulate form in a size range small enough to be phagocytosed (less than 10 μm), can elicit a biologic response that could cause the bone resorption that initiates and promotes the loosening process. This degenerative process has been referred to as *small-particle disease*.

METALLIC IONS. Animal and human investigations have revealed elevated levels of metal ions in subjects with certain types of implants (e.g., total joint replacement prostheses). The mechanisms of metal ion release are still being studied, and results often vary when determining the concentration of specific metal ions in tissues and fluids. Metal in ionic form is often not distinguished from that present as particles, which confounds interpretation of results.

Serum and urinary chromium levels increase in patients who have undergone conventional cemented cobalt-chromium alloy hip replacement.[6] An attempt to determine the valency of chromium as either +3 (III) or +6 (VI) from the metal ion concentration in a blood clot was not successful. This experiment was based on erythrocytes displaying a unidirectional uptake of Cr (VI) while effectively excluding Cr (III). The distinction of the valency of chromium is important because Cr (VI) is much more biologically active than Cr (III).

Unfortunately, our knowledge of the local and systemic biologic and clinical sequelae of metal ion release has not significantly advanced over the past several years. Addition of cobalt ions in the form of cobalt fluoride solutions to the media of synovial cells can stimulate their production of neutral proteinases and collagenase.[37] These findings may be relevant to tissue degradation (e.g., osteolysis) around implants, since metal ions could activate synovial cells in the surrounding synovial tissue to produce agents that promote tissue degeneration.

DISEASES AND DRUGS. Implant failure has not been well correlated with disease states and drugs used to treat the disorders. Some observations indicate that antiinflammatory agents, as well as certain anticancer drugs, can reduce the amount of bone formation around devices in the early stages of wound healing after implantation. Little is known, however, about the role of these and other agents on tissue remodeling and degeneration at the biomaterial-tissue interface.

Systemic Response to Particulate Debris

Local and regional lymphadenopathy caused by wear particles released from implants is becoming increasingly recognized as a possible complication with certain prostheses. Particles generated by mechanical wear of prostheses can leave the site of the implant via the lymphatics and become engulfed by macrophages within local and regional lymph nodes. Accumulation of cells containing particles causes enlargement of the lymph node and the characteristic histologic appearance of sinus histiocytosis.[44]

Distension and prominence of the lymphatic sinuses result from large numbers of (1) histiocytes derived from the cells that line the sinuses or (2) macrophages derived from circulating monocytes. Multinucleated giant cells, resulting from the fusion of macrophages or histiocytes, may also be found in the dilated sinuses.

Accumulation of polyethylene, PMMA, and metal particles in lymph nodes draining joints replaced with prostheses has been found in animal[69,112] and human studies.[7,14,47,57] Some have reported lymphadenopathy in surgical patients.[44,86,95]

With joint replacement prostheses, synovial macrophages readily engulf particles released into the joint space. When the production of particulate debris exceeds the phagocytic capacity of synovial macrophages, excess particles enter lymphatic vessels.[114] Evidence indicates that macrophages laden with particles can also gain entry to the lymphatics.[46] Macrophages present within lymph nodes endocytose free particles traveling within the lymphatic system. A steady influx of wear debris causes these macrophages to accumulate within the sinus of the lymph node.[14] Over several years, macrophages with particles may become so abundant that they cause dilation of nodal sinuses and nodal enlargement. As mentioned, accumulation of histiocytes or macrophages within lymph node sinuses is described pathologically as sinus histiocytosis.

SYSTEMIC MIGRATION OF PARTICLES. Numerous studies report the migration of particles, released from implants, to lymph nodes and many organs. The spread of particles from silicone elastomer and liquid droplets (e.g., from breast implants) is well documented.[104] The translocation of these particles results from the following:

1. Migration through soft tissues
2. Entry into the lymphatic system
3. Direct entry into the vascular system.

Silicone particles have been found to migrate from breast implants through soft tissue to sites as distant as the groin.[20] The finding of silicone lymphadenopathy in axillary lymph nodes is common in patients with breast implants.[105] The hematogenous dissemination of silicone to viscera has also been reported as a result of soft tissue injection of the material.[104] In the orthopedic literature, silicone lymphadenopathy has become a common finding in patients receiving finger joint prostheses made of silicone elastomer.[24]

Reports documenting dissemination of particles in the lymphatic system from total joint prostheses are mounting, suggesting that this phenomenon may be more common than previously thought. Several animal studies have documented lymphatic spread of polyethylene particles to regional nodes.[69,112] Bos et al[14] recently provided evidence from human autopsies that polyethylene, PMMA, and metal particles released from stable total hip replacements spread to inguinal, parailiac, and paraaortic lymph nodes as early as 1½ years after implantation of the prosthesis.

Sinus histiocytosis in association with wear particles of polyethylene has been an incidental finding in lymph nodes biopsied at revision arthroplasty[29] and in the staging of prostate[7,44] and breast cancer.[86] Adenopathy related to an implant is not limited to total hip and knee replacement prostheses. Axillary histiocytic lymphadenopathy was reported in association with polyethylene wear particles from a total shoulder replacement.[86]

CLINICAL IMPLICATIONS. Lymphadenopathy secondary to the accumulation of wear particles in sinus macrophages may make the appropriate diagnosis difficult, especially when malignancy is suspected. For example, a 19-year-old man had right inguinal pain and a 3-cm² palpable mass 3 years after a right total knee replacement following resection of an osteosarcoma.[95] The lymph node was biopsied to evaluate for suspected metastatic recurrence of osteosarcoma. Histologic examination revealed sinus histiocytosis caused by metal particles released from the knee prosthesis. The patient had no evidence of malignancy.

The ultimate fate of particles released from total joint prostheses is unknown. A recent report suggests that metallic particles from orthopedic prostheses may pass through the lymphatics and gain a systemic distribution.[57]

Immune Reactions and Genetic Determinants

Two patients matched for gender, age, weight, activity level, and other factors that might affect prosthesis performance often have very different outcomes. This suggests that immune reactions or genetically determined responses might play a role in the failure of prostheses in some patients.

Immune responses include antibody and cell-mediated reactions and activation of the complement system. Certain metal ions can behave as haptens, which can trigger an immune response when complexed with serum proteins. The cell types that might be expected to occur at sites of antibody and cell-mediated reactions, however, are not often found in tissue retrieved. These cells include lymphocytes and plasma cells. The finding of occasional lymphocytic infiltrates in tissue around implants does not provide enough information. Immune reactions to polymeric materials (e.g., silicone) have also been suggested as the cause of certain systemic diseases, but mechanisms for such a response, as well as its prevalence, remain in question. Much more work is necessary to determine the role of immune reactions in the response to implantable devices.

Previous studies have demonstrated that many biomaterials can activate (cleave) certain molecules (C3 and C5) in the complement system and thereby stimulate the alternative pathway of the immune response. Complement activation by biomaterials may play a role in adverse reactions to certain devices. Again, however, additional studies are required.

One form of cell-mediated immune reaction associated with implants that has been studied is the *delayed hypersensitivity response*. "Metal allergy" has been incriminated as the cause of failure in certain patients,[72] but results are not yet definitive. "The incidence of metal sensitivity in the normal population is high, with up to 15% of the population sensitive to nickel and perhaps up to 25% sensitive to at least one of the common sensitizers Ni, Co, and Cr. The incidence of metal sensitivity reactions requiring premature removal of an orthopedic device is probably small (less than the incidence of infection). Clearly there are factors not yet understood that caused one patient but not another to react."[71]

A similar situation exists with respect to sensitivity reactions to polymeric materials, including bone cement (PMMA). The monomer of PMMA is a strong skin sensitizer.[70] Failure of cemented devices, however, has not yet been correlated with a hypersensitivity response in patients.

No clear etiology exists for prosthesis loosening in some patients, and in others with multiple risk factors for failure the prosthesis functions well. Therefore some suggest that genetic determinants may be responsible for loosening.

One investigation has shown interindividual differences in the in vitro cytokine and PGE_2 production by lipopolysaccharide-stimulated macrophages.[77] HLA-DR$_2$-positive individuals and first-degree relatives were found to be low responders. Such studies suggest that in certain individuals, genetic determination might affect the degree to which cells in the tissue around prostheses can be activated to produce proinflammatory agents that stimulate tissue degradation. Additional studies could help identify patients who might be high responders to prosthetic motion and particulate debris and therefore at high risk for prosthesis failure.

Carcinogenicity

Chromium and nickel are known carcinogens, and cobalt is a suspected carcinogen. Therefore the release of these metal ions into the human body from implants might raise some concern.

Fortunately, reports of neoplasms around implanted devices (e.g., total joint replacement prostheses) have been few. Although no causal relationship has been shown, the index of suspicion is high enough to warrant serious investigation through epidemiologic and other studies. The use of porous coated metallic devices (e.g., noncemented total joint replacement prostheses with large surface area) in younger patients has added to the concern about the long-term clinical consequences of metal ion release.

The relationship of metallic ion release to oncogenesis[12] and reports of neoplasms around orthopedic implants have been reviewed.[68] Differences in the tumor types, time to appearance, and type of prosthesis confound attempts to associate the neoplasm with the implant materials and released moieties.

In an epidemiologic investigation in New Zealand, more than 1300 total joint replacement patients were followed to determine the incidence of tumors at remote sites.[43] The incidence of neoplasms in the lymphatic and hemopoietic systems was found to be significantly greater than expected in the decade after arthroplasty. Importantly, the incidence of cancer of the breast, colon, and rectum was significantly less than expected. The investigators acknowledged that although the association might be an effect of the prosthetic implants, other mechanisms, particularly drug therapy, require consideration.

Somewhat similar results were obtained from another study of the cancer incidence in 443 patients who had total hip replacement (McKee-Farrar) between 1967 and 1973 and were followed through 1981. The risk of leukemias and lymphomas increased, whereas the risk of breast cancer decreased. The authors concluded that the local occurrence of cancer associated with Co-Cr-Mo prostheses indicates that "chrome-cobalt-alloy plays some role in cancerogenesis (sic)."[109]

Bacterial Infection

Under certain circumstances, biomaterial surfaces can provide favorable substrates for the colonization of bacteria. The adherence of bacteria to solid surfaces is facilitated by their production of a biofilm. The *biofilm* is a complex structure comprising bacterial cells encapsulated in a polymeric matrix. The detailed composition of the matrix has yet to be determined. Certain biomaterials may favor the production and adherence of a biofilm, and certain material characteristics may predispose to bacterial colonization. Studies are underway to understand these processes.

BIOMATERIAL FAILURE

Potential causes of failure of implanted devices include the following:

1. Deficiencies in design of the device for a particular patient
2. Surgical problems (e.g., problematic orientation and excessive surgical trauma leading to problems in wound healing)
3. Host abnormalities and diseases
4. Infections
5. Biomaterial fracture, wear, and corrosion

In what cases has the failure of the biomaterial initiated the failure of the device? It is difficult to determine whether breakdown of one or more biomaterials used in the fabrication of a particular prosthesis was the primary cause of the system failure or secondary to other factors. Diagnostic imaging methods such as radiography and computed tomography rarely provide evidence of biomaterial failure early enough for it to be identified as the primary cause of implant failure. Recovery of the device and surrounding tissue at revision surgery provides limited information about the initiating causes of failure.

All the materials used to fabricate devices have finite "fatigue lives" (i.e., failure as a result of cyclic loading). Unfortunately, the endurance limit for many implantable devices or the magnitude of the applied stress is not known. How does the device's serviceable life relate to the patient's longevity.

The introduction of the "supermetals" virtually eliminated concerns about breakage of metallic devices. Corrosion can occur, but only rarely is it the initiating cause of device failure. Wear, however, is clearly the principal cause of failure in certain articulating devices (e.g., joint replacement prostheses) and can occur to some extent in soft tissue implants.

Breakdown of a biomaterial does not necessarily cause the immediate failure of a device. In fact, biomaterial failure might be considered an ongoing process. It becomes clinically important when it is the initiating cause of failure or accelerates a degenerative process initiated by other factors.

Wear

Wear is generally defined as the loss of material from solid surfaces as a result of mechanical action. Several mechanisms can contribute to wear. In each case, fracture through the substance (i.e., loss of cohesive bonding) must occur for a fragment of the material to be removed from the surface. The three main mechanisms of wear are (1) adhesive wear, (2) abrasive wear, and (3) fatigue wear.

Adhesive wear occurs when the force of adhesion between contacting surfaces exceeds the cohesive force within one of the materials. When two surfaces come into contact, atomic bonding can occur between the materials (Figure 19-4 and Table 19-1). Generally, when the surfaces separate, this bond is broken. In some cases, however, this bond strength exceeds the strength of the atomic bonding in one of the two contacting materials. When the two surfaces separate, fracture occurs within the material, leading to loss of a transferred fragment.

In adhesive wear the amount of material lost is generally directly proportional to the applied load and to the distance slid. In many material systems the amount of wear is inversely proportional to the hardness of the surface being worn away. These relationships are incorporated in the following equation:

$$V_{adh} = \frac{kWL}{H}$$

V_{adh} is volume of adhesive wear, and k is a dimensionless wear coefficient related to the probability of particle formation, or the fraction of adhesive junctions that eventually produces wear particles; k is generally less than 0.1 (i.e., only one of 10 adhesive junctions results in a wear particle). W is the load perpendicular to the surface; L is the distance through which the surfaces slid; and H is the indention hardness of the softer material.

Abrasive wear results when asperities on one material plow material from a softer contacting surface (Figure 19-4). The loss of material that occurs as two surfaces contact is referred to as *two-body wear*. When a third substance is interposed between the two surfaces, the process is *three-body wear*. The following equation has been used to evaluate the volume of material lost in abrasive wear:

$$V_{abr} = \frac{WL}{H\, p \tan \Theta}$$

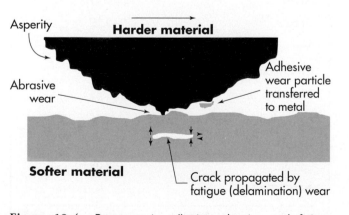

Figure 19-4. Processes in adhesive, abrasive, and fatigue (delamination) wear.

Table 19-1. Wear Processes

TYPE	MECHANISM	PART SIZE
Adhesive	Chemical adhesion	nm to μm
Abrasive (two body)	Plowing of asperity through softer material	μm
Abrasive (three body)	Entrapment and plowing of particle	μm
Fatigue (delamination)	Propagation of subsurface cracks to surface by cyclic compression, tension, or shear	μm to mm

V_{abr} is the volume of abrasive wear, and Θ is one-half the included angle of the asperity of the harder material plowing through (i.e., abrading) the softer material. Tan Θ is very small for sharp aperities, leading to high wear volume.

Fatigue wear results from repeated loading of contacting surfaces. The cyclic stresses initiate or propagate surface or subsurface cracks (Figure 19-4). This process eventually leads to the loss of relatively large fragments of material.

The term *fretting wear* is used to describe the loss of material from contacting surfaces undergoing oscillatory tangential displacement of small magnitude (micrometers). The loss of material from fretting wear is the result of adhesive or abrasive wear.

Another form of wear involves the process of corrosion. The oxide passivation layer on metals may be lost as a result of a wear process. The removal of this film may accelerate the corrosion process and lead to alterations in the oxide layer. These alterations may include an increase in rugosity (surface roughness), which can promote abrasive wear of the opposing surface.

Corrosion

Whereas wear is the loss of solid fragments from surfaces as a result of mechanical action, corrosion is release of ions and compounds as a result of chemical action. Relatively little is known about the mechanisms underlying the corrosion of nonmetallic substances. The following discussion focuses on corrosion of metallic substances.

Although they are relatively inert, metals are soluble in aqueous solutions. Metal leaves the solid metallic state to form aqueous cations in electrolyte solutions ($M^{n+}_{aqueous}$ in following reaction). *Passivation,* the formation of an insoluble salt (oxide) on pure metals and metal alloys, inhibits metal egress and thus inhibits corrosion. This layer serves to protect the metal by insulating it from the electrolyte solution. A chromium oxide passivation layer forms on stainless steel and cobalt-chromium alloy. A titanium oxide layer forms on titanium and titanium alloys.

The *electrochemical series* (or galvanic series) of metals rates the relative tendencies of metal ions to go into solution (Table 19-2). This classification of metals, however, does not consider the effect of an oxide layer on the metal's surface. The electrochemical series shows that metallic elements such as gold are relatively insoluble, whereas substances such as titanium and aluminum, when present in pure elemental form, are relatively soluble (and active). When these same reactive metallic elements are covered by their oxide layers, however, these metals tend much less to go into aqueous solution.

Titanium is a more active element than chromium; titanium and its alloys form oxide passivation layers more rapidly than do substances containing chromium (i.e., cobalt-chromium alloy and stainless steel). Although an active metal such as titanium forms its oxide passivation layer spontaneously in any environment containing oxygen, however, the strength of adhesion of the oxide layer to the underlying titanium metal is not as great as that of the chromium oxide layer to its metal substrate. In addition, the chromium oxide passivation film is more dense than the titanium oxide layer.

The following reaction describes the ion transfer $M^{n+}_{aqueous}$ into solution (i.e., the corrosion) that occurs when a metal is immersed in an electrolyte solution. Electrons, freed as the metal ions enter solution from one region of the specimen (the anode), travel to other regions of the same specimen, making those areas cathodic. If the metallic sample is connected to (e.g., touching) another metal specimen with less of a tendency for corrosion, the second metallic specimen becomes the cathode (Figure 19-5). Corrosion of the anode can be accelerated by increasing the rate of reaction at the cathode.

Anodic reaction

$$M \rightarrow M^{n+}_{aqueous} + ne^{-}_{metal}$$

Cathodic reactions

Reduction of dissolved oxygen

$$\frac{n}{2}\left(\frac{1}{2}O_2\right) + \frac{n}{2}H_2O + ne^{-}_{metal} \rightarrow nOH^{-}_{aqueous}$$

Reduction of hydrogen ions

$$nH^{+} + ne^{-} \rightarrow \frac{n}{2}H_2$$

Table 19-2.
Electrochemical Series of Metals with Normal Electrode Potentials*

METAL	ELECTRODE POTENTIAL (V)
NOBLE END	
Gold	+1.45
Platinum	+1.20
Silver	+0.80
Copper	+0.34
Hydrogen	0.00
Molybdenum	−0.20
Nickel	−0.25
Cobalt	−0.28
Iron	−0.44
Chromium	−0.73
Titanium	−1.63
Aluminum	−1.66
Magnesium	−2.37
Lithium	−3.05
ACTIVE END	

*Measured in volts at 25° C (77° F), referred to hydrogen as zero.

The mechanisms controlling corrosion processes relate to factors that favor either the anodic reaction or the cathodic reactions. Factors that assist electron transfer from the metal would facilitate the anodic reaction, whereas changes in oxygen concentration at sites along the metallic surface would facilitate the cathodic reaction.

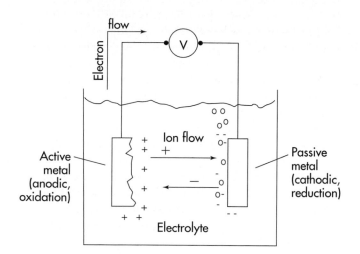

Figure 19-5. "Concentration cell" depicting types of reactions in corrosion of metals.

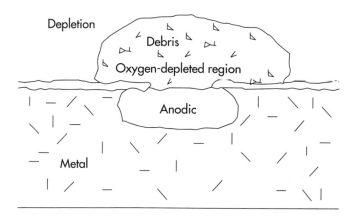

Figure 19-6. Propensity of oxygen-deleted regions to corrosion on metallic surfaces.

The mechanisms of corrosion referred to as *pitting, crevice,* and *depletion* relate to situations in which oxygen is relatively depleted at certain sites on a metal implant (Figure 19-6). These sites take on an anodic character, favoring metal ion release. Salts can accumulate at the sites of scratches produced by instruments at insertion. The depletion of oxygen at these sites can lead to corrosion, resulting in pitting of the surface. The low oxygen concentration at the bottom of the pits favors continuing corrosion.

Crevices formed at the sites where components are joined (e.g., in modular components of prostheses or at screw-plate junctions) also create a microenvironment favorable to corrosion as a result of depleted oxygen (Figure 19-7). The depletion of oxygen can also occur under plaques of biologic debris on the surface of devices, thus also predisposing to a so-called concentration cell corrosion mechanism.

Another basic mechanism of corrosion can occur when dissimilar metals touch. The tendencies of electrons to move from the more active metal to the more noble metal causes the former to become anodic, thereby producing conditions that would favor accelerated corrosion. This mechanism of corrosion has been referred to as *galvanic, two-metal, mixed-metal,* or *couple corrosion.* The degree of galvanic corrosion depends on the electrochemical nature of the two metals and the relative areas of contact and surfaces exposed to the solution.

The term *galvanic corrosion* is derived from an observation made by Galvani in 1791 as he was investigating the susceptibility of nerves to irritation. He found that if a rod of brass contacted the frog's foot while a silver rod contacted the spinal cord, the leg muscles contracted when the free ends of the rods touched. In 1800 Volta confirmed that the force that provoked the contraction was electrical in nature. The electric current generated by contact of dissimilar metals in an electrolyte solution is referred to as *galvanic current.*

In certain situations the breakdown of material is caused by mechanical and chemical processes acting in concert. These mechanochemical processes include (1) fretting corrosion, (2) stress corrosion, and (3) metallic transfer (with subsequent galvanic corrosion).

Fretting corrosion is a process in which abrasive wear is accompanied by corrosion. The protective oxide layer on the

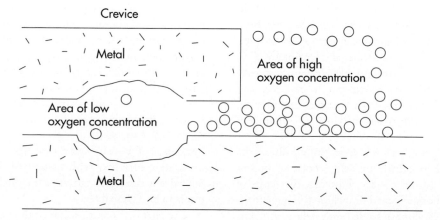

Figure 19-7. Crevices in which oxygen concentration is lower than that around metallic device are predisposed to corrosion.

metal is removed by abrasive wear. The new passivation layer that forms after abrasion is not as durable or chemically inert as the original layer, thereby making the metal more susceptible to corrosion. Stainless steel and cobalt-chromium alloys are susceptible to fretting corrosion. This form of corrosion often occurs between screw heads and bone plates.

Stress corrosion is the process by which the presence of an electrolyte decreases the strength of the metal. Microcracks develop at anodic areas of the metallic device as the result of corrosion processes. These cracks propagate under applied stress. The tips of these microcracks are at a more highly strained state than surrounding metal and are more susceptible to corrosion, which contributes to crack propagation.

As dissimilar metals come in contact, *metallic transfer* of small fragments of the softer metal can occur to the harder one. As these two metals remain in contact, galvanic corrosion processes may develop. Therefore implants should be handled with instruments made of the same metal as the device.

Several methods are available to assess the predisposition of metals to corrosion. A simple method involves weighing the specimen after exposure to corrosive environments and assaying the bathing electrolyte solution for corrosion products. An electrochemical method that has been valuable in characterizing the potential of metals to corrode is *anodic polarization.* In this experimental procedure the test metal is the anode of an electrolytic cell. An increasing voltage is applied between it and a reference cathode (usually platinum). The *current density* (current divided by cross-sectional area of the anode) is a measure of the corrosion rate of the anodic metal in the particular electrolyte used.

Table 19-2 shows the electrochemical potentials and tendency for corrosion (i.e., current density) for the orthopedic alloys. The current density for titanium alloy is significantly less than that of the cobalt-chromium alloy and stainless steel, indicating that titanium and its alloys have much less of a tendency for corrosion. Because the release of metal depends on surface area, a greater amount of metal is released from porous metal specimens.

BIOMATERIALS FOR TISSUE ENGINEERING

The wound healing process in many types of lesions in connective tissues does not lead to spontaneous regeneration; the end result is often a dysfunctional scar. Recent research has shown that some cells can proliferate and maintain their phenotype when cultured on certain two-dimensional substrates or in specific three-dimensional porous matrices and gels in vitro. This has formed the basis for tissue engineering, with the promise of forming tissues in vitro for subsequent implantation.

Initially, "tissue engineering" was used principally to describe tissue produced in culture by cells seeded in porous absorbable matrices.[55] More recently, however, the scope of tissue engineering has been widened to include the implementation of porous matrices, alone or seeded with cells, as implants to facilitate tissue regeneration in vivo. This enfranchises decades of investigation of wound healing and treatments implementing absorbable implants.

In Vivo Versus In Vitro Strategies

Just as they are the three components of tissue, the matrix, cells, and soluble regulators are primary elements in strategies to engineer tissue in vivo or in vitro for subsequent implantation. Decisions about which elements might be required for regeneration of tissue in vivo can be guided by an understanding of the deficits of the natural (i.e., spontaneous) healing processes that prevent regeneration.

An advantage of tissue synthesis in vitro is the ready ability to examine the material as it is formed and to make certain measurements to establish its functions before implantation. A disadvantage, particularly in the production of tissues that must play a load-bearing role, is the absence of a physiologic mechanical environment during the formation of the tissue in vitro. Mechanical force serves as a critical regulator of cell function and can profoundly influence the architecture of tissue as it is forming.[21,93] Because the mechanical environment extant during formation of most load-bearing tissue in vivo is not well understood, it is not yet possible to recreate such an environment in vitro during the engineering of most tissues.

Another disadvantage in the formation of load-bearing tissue outside the body is the necessary incorporation of the tissues after implantation, which requires that the engineered tissue be mechanically coupled to the surrounding structures. Union of the implanted tissue with the host organ requires remodeling (degradation and new tissue formation) at the interfaces of the implant with the host tissues. Remodeling of implanted tissue engineered in vitro is essential for its functional incorporation. This demonstrates the benefit of de novo regeneration in vivo, with the incorporation occurring as the tissue is being formed.

Thus, for certain tissues, an effective strategy may be to facilitate tissue formation in vivo, under the influence of the physiologic mechanical environment. One disadvantage of this approach, however, is that the regenerating tissue may be dislodged or degraded by the mechanical forces normally acting at the site, before it is fully formed and incorporated.

Matrices

Matrices for engineering bone and soft connective tissues have included synthetic and natural calcium phosphates[51,60] and many synthetic (e.g., polylactic acid,[25,76] PGA,[40,56]) and natural polymers (e.g., collagen,[81,102] fibrin[48,52]). Material used in the fabrication of matrices for engineering tissue in vitro or used as implants to facilitate generation in vivo must have the necessary microstructure and chemical composition to accommodate parenchymal cells and their functions. In this regard a porous structure is generally needed. The required percentage of porosity and the pore diameter, distribution, and orientation may vary with tissue type. Moreover, because the objective is the regeneration of the original tissue, the scaffold needs to be absorbable.

The chemical composition of the matrix is important with respect to its influence on cell adhesion and the phenotypic expression of the infiltrating cells. The degradation rate of the material generally may be determined based on the rate of new tissue formation and the normal period for tissue remodeling at the implantation site. It is important to consider the effects of moieties released during matrix degradation on the host and regenerating tissue.

A matrix can play the following roles during the process of regeneration in vivo:

1. The matrix can structurally *reinforce* the defect site to maintain the shape of the defect and prevent distortion of surrounding tissue. For example, cysts that form in the subchondral bone underlying the articulating surfaces of joints can lead to collapse of the joint surface.
2. The matrix can serve as a *barrier* to the ingress of surrounding tissue that may impede the process of regeneration. The concept of guided tissue regeneration is based in part on the prevention of overlying gingival tissue from collapsing into the periodontal defect.[32]
3. The matrix can serve as a *scaffold* for migration and proliferation of cells in vivo or for cells seeded in vitro.
4. The matrix can serve as an *insoluble regulator* of cell function through its interaction with certain integrins and other cell receptors.

One class of properties that is likely to play an especially important role in the engineering of load-bearing tissues is mechanical properties. Design specifications for several bone graft substitute materials have included the strength of the matrix material, with the principal objective of employing high-strength substances for immediate load bearing. Synthetic calcium phosphate ceramics were implemented as matrix materials to facilitate bone regeneration in vivo.[17,33]

Besides possessing high strength, however, some of these materials also have a high modulus of elasticity, making them extremely stiff structures. The disadvantage of this extreme stiffness is that the presence of the material greatly alters the distribution of mechanical forces in surrounding tissue and thus adversely affects the stress-induced remodeling of neighboring bone. Because many materials of this class of matrix are essentially nonresorbable, the adverse effects on remodeling will persist indefinitely. This remodeling can result in osteopenic regions around the implanted site, increasing the risk of fracture. Further complications can arise because conventional methods for treatment of such fractures are likely to be difficult, since the high density of the material precludes drilling and sawing procedures. Revision surgical procedures at sites implanted with these substances may require their complete removal.

Based on these considerations, the materials used should match the modulus of elasticity of the tissue at the implant site. Thus the makeup and properties of the extracellular matrix (ECM) should be considered in selecting or designing a scaffold for tissue engineering.

One design approach has been to employ matrices that serve as analogs of the ECM of the tissue to be engineered.[119] This concept recognizes that the molecular composition and architecture of the ECM display chemical and mechanical properties required by the parenchymal cells and the physio-

logic demands of the tissue. For scaffolds in regeneration of bone, this approach has led to the use of natural bone mineral produced by removing the organic matter of bovine bone.* The calcium-deficient carbonated apatite, which constitutes the mineral phase of bone, and the unique microstructure of the ECM of bone are determined by the organic template of collagen and the initial release of calcium phosphate–containing vesicles from osteoblasts. This largely explains why bone mineral cannot be replicated in the laboratory.

Several synthetic and natural polymers have been used in the development of implants for the treatment of lesions in soft connective tissues. For example, with cartilage defects, PGA and PGA-polylactic acid blends[30,106] and natural polymers, including fibrin,[48] collagen gel[110] and sponge,[102] and hyaluronan,[58] have been seeded with chondrocytes in studies in vitro and in vivo.

The approach of using analogs of ECM as implants for the regeneration of the soft connective tissue and nerve has employed porous collagen-glycosaminoglycan (GAG) copolymers. Regeneration of dermis in animals and human subjects[18,115,116,118] and reconnection of axons of cells in ruptured peripheral nerves in rats[23,116,120] require certain tissue-specific pore characteristics and degradation rate. To produce these materials, collagen is precipitated from acid dispersion in the presence of chondroitin-6-sulfate.[119] The suspended coprecipitate suspension is injected into a silicone tube (3.8 mm inside diameter), or it is spread on a pan for immersion into a coolant bath and freeze-dried, to produce a porous architecture. The matrices are then exposed to a dehydrothermal treatment or to ultraviolet light for cross-linking and sterilization. Additional cross-linking can be achieved using aldehydes or other cross-linking agents. These collagen-GAG matrices are nominally 95% porous and can be produced with an average pore diameter of 30 to 120 μm.

CALCIUM PHOSPHATE AND BONE GRAFT SUBSTITUTE MATERIALS. Although some polymers have been investigated as matrices to be used as implants to facilitate bone regeneration, most materials comprise calcium-containing substances. Calcium sulfate[88] and tricalcium phosphate[19,31,78,84] were two of the calcium-containing substances first implemented as bone graft substitute materials. These materials undergo physiochemical dissolution relatively quickly, disappearing in days to weeks in some cases.

Some question remains, however, about the rate at which these materials become absorbed by the body. Differences may be related to variations in the composition and structure and the different physiologic characteristics of the implant sites and animal models. Tricalcium phosphate often undergoes physiochemical dissolution at a rate that precludes the precipitation of biologic apatite and subsequent bone formation on its surface. The dissolving surface does not allow for protein adsorption and cell attachment.

Work with hydroxyapatite began in the mid-1970s.[34,50] Many studies focused on the use of hydroxyapatite in dense

*References 10, 11, 26, 51, 53, 75, 83, 98, 113.

and porous forms of block and particles.[45] The increasing interest in bone graft substitute materials has advanced our understanding of the bone response to these substances. Mechanisms underlying the bone bonding associated with incorporation of these substances in osseous tissue are beginning to be revealed (see earlier discussion).

The mechanism of breakdown of calcium phosphates in vivo is not fully understood. The appearance of macrophages and multinucleated foreign body giant cells around some types of calcium phosphates suggest that particles might provoke the activation of phagocytes, which in turn might stimulate other cells and an inflammatory response. Agents produced by these cells could accelerate the degradation process.

Although generally considered a nonresorbable material, synthetic hydroxyapatite has also been found to undergo physicochemical dissolution, albeit at a very slow rate. Because it is only slightly soluble in biologic fluid, synthetic hydroxyapatite substances can functionally be considered as long-lasting implants, especially when they are incorporated into bone.

CARTILAGE ENGINEERING. Natural and synthetic materials have been employed as scaffolds for implantation in defects of cartilage. With articular cartilage defects, matrices have been used alone or seeded with cells before implantation. Nonresorbable materials that have been studied include carbon fiber mesh[15,74] and spongelike constructs of polytetrafluoroethylene[2,73] and polyester.[73]

Concern about the effects of the permanent scaffold on the mechanical performance of regenerated cartilage has focused on resorbable substances as matrices. These include fibrin,[48,87] collagen gels,[111] collagen sponges,[9,41,42,85,102] PGA,[39,97,107] and polylactic acid.[25,30,97]

Questions remain as to the most suitable chemical composition and pore structure in the fabrication of a cell-seeded implant to treat defects in the articular surface. The substance should have a composition that maintains the chondrocyte phenotype and a pore structure that accommodates cell infiltration. Furthermore, the scaffold must be mechanically stable enough to be surgically manipulated for implantation. Because of the poor surgical handling characteristics of gels, spongelike matrices may be preferred.

Insoluble type I collagen matrices have been successful in animal models to improve healing of cartilage defects.[9,85,102] Complete regeneration was not achieved, however, and the reparative tissue consisted of fibrous and fibrocartilaginous substances, with some hyaline cartilage. Recent work has investigated the behavior of adult canine articular chondrocytes in vitro in matrices comprising collagen-GAG copolymers made from types I and II collagen.[82]

PERIPHERAL NERVE REGENERATION. One focus of experimental efforts to promote and improve peripheral nerve regeneration across gaps has been guiding the axonal growth cone to the distal stump. The proximal and distal nerve ends are encased in a tube[103]—a *nerve guide* or nerve channel—in a procedure referred to as "fascicular tubulization"[28,91] and "entubulation repair."[67] This approach is analogous to strategies

employed to facilitate regeneration of certain connective tissues, including bone,[80] periodontium,[32] and tendon.[64] The lesion is isolated from the negative influence of surrounding tissues, particularly as they collapse into the defect, while wound-derived trophic factors are maintained in the lesion site. With nerve the tube also serves as a guide for axonal elongation. Many synthetic and natural resorbable tubes, as well as silicone, have been investigated for this application.[8]

Silicone tubulization of nerve gaps has been the standard experimental model for many years[59,65] and has been shown to improve regeneration compared with defects that were not contained with a tube. In clinical use, however, the silicone tubes have presented problems for long-term recovery. Silicone tubes typically have become encapsulated with fibrous tissue, which has led to constriction of the nerve, necessitating surgery to remove the tube.

Several previous studies have investigated the performance of biodegradable tubes fabricated from type I collagen. Archibald et al[5] obtained the most extensive longitudinal data for nonhuman primate peripheral nerve repair. Their 3½-year study demonstrated that repair of a 5-mm gap in the monkey median nerve with a collagen tube had similar results to autograft repair.

Despite the promising results obtained using tubular nerve guides, incomplete regeneration and the desire to accelerate the process have prompted the investigation of soluble factors and insoluble regulators (matrices) placed within the tubes before implantation.[8] It has been hypothesized that these substances may (1) provide more specific directional orientation for the axons, (2) enable haptotaxis, and (3) act as growth and trophic factors.[38] Materials investigated as promoters of nerve regeneration in tubes include laminin,[8,67] gelatin with ACTH4-9,[90] type I collagen precipitate,[66,92] fibronectin,[66] and skeletal muscle basal lamina grafts.[16] The results of these efforts have been mixed; some substances did improve regeneration, whereas others actually impeded it. A recent study reported results of a collagen-GAG–filled tube that were comparable to an autograft in a rat model.[22]

Future of Biomaterials for Tissue Engineering

Tissue engineering may solve a number of compelling clinical problems in dentistry not adequately addressed using permanent replacement devices. The challenge will be to select the optimal combination of matrix, cells, and soluble regulators for a particular clinical problem.

For many connective tissues of the musculoskeletal system, with microstructures that reflect the mechanical environment, it may be more advantageous to regenerate the tissue in vivo than to engineer the tissue fully in vitro for subsequent implantation. The porous material that will serve as the matrix to facilitate this regeneration must have certain pore characteristics, chemical constituents, and mechanical properties. One approach has been to employ substances that serve as analogs of the ECM for the tissue to be regenerated.

With bone, natural bone mineral (anorganic bone) has been efficacious in several experimental animal and clinical studies. For selected indications in which the supply of endogenous precursor cells has been compromised by disease or prior surgical procedures, it may be necessary to seed the matrix before implantation with exogenous cells or to use the matrix as a delivery vehicle for growth or differentiation factors.

REFERENCES

1. Agins HJ, Alcock NW, Bansal M, et al: Metallic wear in failed titanium-alloy total hip replacements, *J Bone Joint Surg* 70A:347-356, 1988.

2. Ahfeld SK, Larson RL, Collins HR: Anterior cruciate reconstruction in the chronically unstable knee using an expanded polytetrafluoroethylene (PTFE) prosthetic ligament, *Am J Sports Med* 15:326-330, 1987.

3. Anderson JM, Miller KM: Biomaterial biocompatibility and the macrophage, *Biomaterials* 5:5-10, 1984.

4. Andriano KP, Pohjonen T, Tormala P: Processing and characterization of absorbable polylactide polymers for use in surgical implants, *J Appl Biomat* 5:133-140, 1994.

5. Archibald SJ, Shefner J, Krarup C, Madison RD: Monkey median nerve repaired by nerve graft or collagen nerve guide tube, *J Neurosci* 15:4109-4123, 1995.

6. Bartolozzi A, Black J: Chromium concentrations in serum, blood clot and urine from patients following total hip arthroplasty, *Biomaterials* 6:2-8, 1985.

7. Bauer TW, Saltarelli M, McMahon JT, Wilde AH,: Regional dissemination of wear debris from a total knee prosthesis: a case report, *J Bone Joint Surg* 75A:106-111, 1993.

8. Bellamkonda R, Aebischer P: Tissue engineering in the nervous system. In Bronzino JD, editor: *Biomedical engineering handbook,* Boca Raton, Fla, 1995, CRC Press.

9. Ben-Yishay A, Grande DA, Schwartz RE, et al: Repair of articular cartilage defects with collagen-chondrocyte allografts, *Tiss Engr* 1:119-133, 1995.

10. Benezra V, Hobbs LW, Spector M: Ultrastructure and architecture of bone mineral and synthetic bone substitutes revealed by low-voltage high-resolution SEM. Presented at the 23rd Annual Meeting of the Society for Biomaterials, New Orleans, 1997.

11. Berglundh T, Lindhe J: Healing around implants placed in bone defects treated with Bio-Oss, *Clin Oral Implants Res* 8:117-124, 1997.

12. Black J: Metallic ion release and its relationship to oncogenesis. In Fitzgerald RHJ, editor: *The Hip, Proceedings of the Thirteenth Open Scientific Meeting of the Hip Society,* St Louis, 1985, Mosby.

13. Bobyn JD, Spector M: Polyethylene. In *Encyclopedia of materials, science, and engineering,* New York, 1987, Pergamon.

14. Bos I, Johannisson R, Löhrs U, et al: Comparative investigations of regional lymph nodes and pseudocapsules after implantation of joint endoprostheses, *Path Res Pract* 186:707-716, 1990.

15. Brittberg M, Faxen E, Peterson L: Carbon fiber scaffolds in the treatment of early knee osteoarthritis, *Clin Orthop* 307:155-164, 1994.

16. Bryan DJ, Miller RA, Costas PD, et al: Immunocytochemistry of skeletal muscle basal lamina grafts in nerve regeneration, *Plast Reconstr Surg* 92:927-940, 1993.

17. Bucholz RW, Carlton A, Holmes RE: Hydroxyapatite and tricalcium phosphate bone graft substitutes, *Orthop Clin North Am* 30:49-67, 1987.

18. Burke JF, Yannas IV, Quinby WC, et al: Successful use of a physiologically acceptable artificial skin in the treatment of extensive burn injury, *Ann Surg* 194:413-428, 1981.

19. Cameron HU, Macnab I, Pilliar RM: Evaluation of a biodegradable ceramic, *J Biomed Mater Res* 11:179-186, 1977.

20. Capozzi A, DuBou R, Pennisi VR: Distant migration of silicone gel from a rupture breast implant, *Plast Reconstr Surg* 62:302, 1978.

21. Carter DR, Orr TE: Skeletal development and bone functional adaptation, *J Bone Miner Res* 7:389-395, 1992.

22. Chamberlain LJ, Yannas IV, Hsu H-P, et al: Collagen-GAG substrate enhances the quality of nerve regeneration through collagen tubes up to the level of autograft, *Exp Neurol* 154:315-329, 1998.

23. Chang AS, Yannas IV, Perutz S, et al: Electrophysiological study of recovery of peripheral nerves regenerated by a collagen-glycosaminoglycan copolymer matrix. In Gebelein CG, editor: *Progress in biomedical polymers,* New York, 1990, Plenum.

24. Christie AJ, Weinberger KA, Dietrich M: Silicone lymphadenopathy and synovitis: complications of silicone elastomer finger joint prostheses, *JAMA* 237:1463-1464, 1977.

25. Chu CR, Coutts RD, Yoshioka M, et al: Articular cartilage repair using allogeneic perichondrocyte-seeded biodegradable porous polylactic acid (PLA): a tissue-engineering study, *J Biomed Mater Res* 29:1147-1154, 1995.

26. Clergeau L, Danan M, Clergeau-Guerithault S, Brion M: Healing response to anorganic bone implantation in periodontal intrabony defects in dogs. Part I. Bone regeneration: a microradiographic study, *J Periodontol* 67:140-149, 1996.

27. Coleman DL, King RN, Andrade JD: The foreign body reaction: a chronic inflammatory response, *J Biomed Mater Res* 8:199-211, 1974.

28. Colin W, Donoff RB: Nerve regeneration through collagen tubes, *J Dent Res* 63:987-993, 1984.

29. Corrin B: Silicone lymphadenopathy, *J Clin Pathol* 35:901-902, 1982.

30. Coutts R, Yoshioka M, Amiel D, et al: Cartilage repair using a porous polylactic acid matrix with allogenic perichondrial cells. Presented at the 40th Annual Orthopedic Research Society Meeting, New Orleans, 1994.

31. Cutright DE, Bhaskar SN, Brady JM, et al: Reaction of bone to tricalcium phosphate ceramic pellets, *Oral Surg* 33:850-856, 1972.

32. Dahlin C, Linde A: Bone formation by guided tissue regeneration. In Glimcher MJ, Lian JB, editors: *The chemistry and biology of mineralized tissue,* New York, 1988, Gordon and Breach Science.

33. Damien CJ, Parsons JR: Bone graft and bone graft substitutes: a review of current technology and applications, *J Appl Biomat* 2:187-208, 1991.

34. deGroot K: *Bioceramics of calcium phosphates,* Boca Raton, Fla, 1983, CRC Press.

35. Donkerwolcke M, Burny F, Muster D: Tissues and bone adhesives: historical aspects, *Biomaterials* 19:1461-1466, 1998.

36. Edwards JCW, Sedgwick AD, Willoughby DA: The formation of a structure with the features of synovial lining by subcutaneous injection of air: an in vivo tissue culture system, *J Pathol* 134:147-156, 1981.

37. Ferguson GM, Watanabe S, Georgescu HI, Evans CH: The synovial production of collagenase and chondrocyte activating factors in response to cobalt, *J Orthop Res* 6:525-530, 1988.

38. Fields RD, Le Bleu JM, Longo FM, Ellisman MH: Nerve regeneration through artificial tubular implants, *Prog Neurol* 33:87-134, 1989.

39. Freed LE, Grande DA, Lingbin Z, et al: Joint resurfacing using allograft chondrocytes and synthetic biodegradable polymer scaffolds, *J Biomed Mater Res* 28:891-899, 1994.

40. Freed LE, Vunjak-Novakovic G, Langer R: Cultivation of cell-polymer cartilage implants in bioreactors, *J Cell Biochem* 51:257-264, 1993.

41. Frenkel SR, Toolan B, Menche D, et al: Chondrocyte transplantation using a collagen bilayer matrix for cartilage repair, *J Bone Joint Surg* 79B:831-836, 1997.

42. Fujisato T, Sajiki T, Liu Q, Ikada Y: Effect of basic fibroblast growth factor on cartilage regeneration in chondrocyte-seeded collagen sponge scaffold, *Biomaterials* 17:155-162, 1996.

43. Gillespie WJ, Frampton CMA, Henderson RJ, Ryan PM: The incidence of cancer following total hip replacement, *J Bone Joint Surg* 70B:539-542, 1988.

44. Gray MH, Talbert ML, Talbert WM, et al: Changes seen in lymph nodes draining the sites of large joint prostheses, *Am J Surg Pathol* 13:1050-1056, 1989.

45. Grote JJ, Kuypers W, de Groot K: Use of sintered hydroxyapatite in middle ear surgery, *ORL J Otorhinolaryngol Relat Spec* 43:248-254, 1981.

46. Harmsen AG, Muggenburg BA, Snipes MB, Bice DE: The role of macrophages in particle translocation from lungs to lymph nodes, *Science* 230:1277-1280, 1985.

47. Heilmann K, Diezel PB, Rossner JA, Brinkmann KA: Morphological studies in tissues surrounding allorthroplastic joints, *Virchows Arch Pathol Anat Hist* 306:93-106, 1974.

48. Hendrickson DA, Nixon AJ, Grande DA, et al: Chondrocyte-fibrin matrix transplants for resurfacing extensive articular cartilage defects, *J Orthop Res* 12:485-497, 1994.

49. Howie DW, V-Roberts B: The synovial response to intraarticular cobalt-chrome wear particles, *Clin Orthop* 232:244-254, 1988.

50. Jarcho M, Kay JF, Gumaer KI, et al: Tissue, cellular and subcellular events at a bone-ceramic hydroxyapatite interface, *J Bioengineering* 1:79-92, 1977.

51. Jensen SS, Aaboe M, Pinholt EM, et al: Tissue reaction and material characteristics of four bone substitutes, *Int J Oral Maxillofac Implants* 11:55-66, 1996.

52. Kerenyi G: Properties and applications of Bioplast, an absorbable surgical implant material from fibrin, *Biomaterials* 1:30-32, 1980.

53. Klinge B, Alberius P, Isaksson S, Johsson J: Osseous response to implanted natural bone mineral and synthetic hydroxylapatite ceramic in the repair of experimental skull defects, *J Oral Maxillofac Surg* 50:241-249, 1992.

54. Laing PG, Ferguson AB, Hodge ES: Tissue reaction in rabbit muscle exposed to metallic implants, *J Biomed Mater Res* 1:135-149, 1967.

55. Langer R, Vacanti JP: Tissue engineering, *Science* 260:920-926, 1993.

56. Langer R, Vacanti JP, Vacanti CA, et al: Tissue engineering: biomedical applications, *Tiss Engr* 1:151-161, 1995.

57. Langkamer VG, Case CP, Heap P, et al: Systemic distribution of wear debris after hip replacement: a cause of concern? *J Bone Joint Surg* 74B:831-839, 1992.

58. Larsen NE, Lombard KM, Parent EG, Balazs EA: Effect of hylan on cartilage and chondrocyte cultures, *J Orthop Res* 10:23-32, 1992.

59. LeBeau JM, Ellisman MH, Powel HC: Ultrastructural and morphometric analysis of long-term peripheral nerve regeneration through silicone tubes, *J Neurocytol* 17:161-172, 1988.

60. LeGeros RZ, Bautista C, Styner D, et al: Comparative properties of bioactive bone graft materials. In Wilson J, Hench LL, Greenspan D, editors: *Bioceramics,* New York, 1995, Elsevier Science.

61. LeVier RR, Harrison MC, Cook RR, Lane TH: What is silicone? *Plast Reconstr Surg* 92:163-167, 1992.

62. Li S, Burstein AH: Ultra-high molecular weight polyethylene, *J Bone Joint Surg* 76A:1080-1090, 1994.

63. Litsky AS, Spector M: Biomaterials. In Simon SR, editor: *Orthopaedic basic science,* Park Ridge, Ill, 1994, American Academy of Orthopaedic Surgeons.

64. Louie LK, Yannas IV, Spector M: Development of a collagen-GAG copolymer implant for the study of tendon regeneration. In Mikos AG, Murphy RM, Bernstein H, Peppas NA, editors: *Biomaterials for drug and cell delivery,* Pittsburgh, 1994, MRS.

65. Lundborg G, Gelberman RH, Longo FM, et al: In vivo regeneration of cut nerves encased in silicone tubes, *J Neuropathol Exp Neurol* 41:412-422, 1982.

66. Madison R, Sidman RL, Nyilas E, et al: Nontoxic nerve guide tubes support neovascular growth in transected rat optic nerve, *Exp Neurol* 86:448-461, 1984.

67. Madison RD, Silva CD, Dikkes P, et al: Peripheral nerve regeneration with entubulation repair: comparison of biodegradable nerve guides versus polyethylene tubes and the effects of a laminin-containing gel, *Exp Neurol* 95:378-390, 1987.

68. Martin A, Bauer TW, Manley MT, Marks KE: Osteosarcoma at the site of total hip replacement, *J Bone Joint Surg* 70A:1561-1567, 1988.

69. Mendes DG, Walker PS, Figarola F, Bullough PG: Total surface hip replacement in the dog, *Clin Orthop* 100:256-264, 1974.

70. Merritt K: Role of medical materials, both in implant and surface applications, in immune response and in resistance to infection, *Biomaterials* 5:47-53, 1984.

71. Merritt K, Brown SA: Biological effects of corrosion products from metals. In Fraker A, editor: *Corrosion and degradation of implant material,* Philadelphia, 1985, American Society for Testing and Materials.

72. Merritt K, Rodrigo JJ: Immune response to synthetic materials, *Clin Orthop* 326:71-79, 1996.

73. Messner K, Gillquist J: Synthetic implants for the repair of osteochondral defects of the medial femoral condyle: a biomechanical and histological evaluation in the rabbit knee, *Biomaterials* 14:513-521, 1993.

74. Minns RJ, Muckles DS, Donken JE: The repair of osteochondral defects in osteoarthritic rabbit knees by use of carbon fibre, *Biomaterials* 3:81-86, 1982.

75. Mitchell SL, Villars PA, Orr TE, Spector M: Compressive properties of cancellous bone defects in a rabbit model treated with natural bone mineral and synthetic HA. Presented at the 21st Annual Meeting of the Society for Biomaterials, San Francisco, 1995.

76. Miyamoto S, Takaoka K, Okada T, et al: Evaluation of polylactic acid homopolymers as carriers for bone morphogenetic protein, *Clin Orthop* 278:274-285, 1992.

77. Molvig J, Baek L, Christensen P, et al: Endotoxin-stimulated human monocyte secretion of interleukin 1, tumor necrosis factor alpha, and prostaglandin E_2 shows stable interindividual differences, *Scand J Immunol* 27:705-716, 1988.

78. Mors WA, Kaminski EJ: Osteogenic replacement of tricalcium phosphate ceramic implants in the dog palate, *Arch Oral Biol* 20:365, 1977.

79. Nagase M, Baker DG, Schumacher HR Jr: Prolonged inflammatory reactions induced by artificial ceramics in the rat air pouch model, *J Rheum* 15:1334-1338, 1988.

80. Narang R, Wells H: Osteogenesis within polyethylene implants at fracture gaps, *Oral Surg Oral Med Oral Pathol* 39:203-209, 1975.

81. Natsume T, Ike O, Okada T, et al: Porous collagen sponge for esophageal replacement, *J Biomed Mater Res* 27:867-875, 1993.

82. Nehrer S, Breinan HA, Ramappa A, et al: Matrix collagen type and pore size influence behaviour of seeded canine chondrocytes, *Biomaterials* 18:769-776, 1997.

83. Nentwig G-H, Gassner A: 2.5 years of clinical experience in the therapy of cystic alveolar defects with a spongious bovine hydroxyapatite material. In Heimke G, editor: *Bioceramics,* Cologne, German Ceramic Society, 1990.

84. Nery EB, Lynch KL: Preliminary clinical studies of bioceramic in periodontal osseous defects, *J Periodontol* 49:523-527, 1978.

85. Nixon AJ, Sams AE, Lust G, et al: Temporal matrix synthesis and histologic features of a chondrocyte-laden porous collagen cartilage analogue, *Am J Vet Res* 54:349-356, 1993.

86. O'Connell JX, Rosenberg AE: Histiocytic lymphadenitis associated with a large joint prosthesis, *Am J Clin Pathol* 99:314-316, 1993.

87. Paletta GA, Arnoczky SP, Warren RF: The repair of osteochondral defects using an exogenous fibrin clot, *Am J Sports Med* 20:725-731, 1992.

88. Peltier LF: The use of plaster of Paris to fill defects in bone, *Clin Orthop* 21:1-31, 1961.

89. Ratner BD, Hoffman AS, Schoen FJ, Lemons JE, editors: *Biomaterials science: an introduction to materials in medicine,* San Diego, 1996, Academic Press.

90. Robinson PH, van der Lei B, Hoppen HJ, et al: Nerve regeneration through a two-ply biodegradable nerve guide in the rat and the influence of ACTH4-9, *Microsurgery* 12:412-419, 1991.

91. Rosen JM, Hentz VR, Kaplan EN: Fascicular tubulization: a cellular approach to peripheral nerve repair, *Ann Plast Surg* 11:397-411, 1983.

92. Rosen JM, Padilla JA, Nguyen KD, et al: Artificial nerve graft using glycolide trimethylene carbonate as a nerve conduit filled with collagen compared to sutured autograft in a rat model, *J Rehabil Res Dev* 29:1-12, 1992.

93. Rubin CT, Lanyon LE: Osteoregulatory nature of mechanical stimuli: function as a determinant for adaptive remodeling in bone, *J Orthop Res* 5:300-310, 1987.

94. Selye H: Use of "granuloma pouch" technic in the study of antiphlogistic corticoids, *Proc Soc Exp Biol Med* 82:328-333, 1953.

95. Shinto Y, Uchida A, Yoshikawa H, et al: Inguinal lymphadenopathy due to metal release from a prosthesis, *J Bone Joint Surg* 75B:266-269, 1993.

96. Silver IA: The physiology of wound healing. In Hunt TK, editor: *Wound Joint healing and wound infection,* New York, 1984, Appleton-Century-Crofts.

97. Sittinger M, Reitzel D, Dauner M, et al: Resorbable polyesters in cartilage engineering: affinity and biocompatibility of polymer fiber structures to chondrocytes, *J Biomed Mater Res* 33: 57-63, 1996.

98. Spector M: Anorganic bovine bone and ceramic analogs of bone mineral as implants to facilitate bone regeneration, *Clin Plast Surg* 21:437-444, 1994.

99. Spector M, Lalor PA: In vivo assessment of tissue compatibility. In Ratner BD, Hoffman AS, Schoen FJ, Lemons JE, editors: *Biomaterials science: an introduction to materials in medicine,* San Diego, 1996, Academic Press.

100. Spector M, Cease C, Xia T-L: The local tissue response to biomaterials, *CRC Crit Rev Biocompat* 5:269-295, 1989.

101. Spector M, Shortkroff S, Hsu H-P, et al: Synovium-like tissue from loose joint replacement prostheses: comparison of human material with a canine model, *Semin Arthritis Rheum* 21:335-344, 1992.

102. Speer DP, Chvapil M, Volz RG, Holmes MD: Enhancement of healing in osteochondral defects by collagen sponge implantation, *Clin Orthop* 144:326-335, 1979.

103. Suematsu N: Tubulation for peripheral nerve gap: its history and possibility, *Microsurgery* 10:71-74, 1989.

104. Travis WD, Balough K, Abraham JL: Silicone granulomas: report of three cases and review of the literature, *Hum Pathol* 16:19-27, 1985.

105. Truong LD, Cartwright J, Goodman MD, Woznicki D: Silicone lymphadenopathy associated with augmentation mammaplasty, *Am J Surg Pathol* 12:484-491, 1988.

106. Vacanti CA, Kim W, Upton J, et al: Tissue engineered composites of bone and cartilage using synthetic polymers seeded with two cell types. Presented at the 39th Annual Orthopedic Research Society Meeting, San Francisco, 1993.

107. Vacanti CA, Kim WS, Schloo B, et al: Joint resurfacing with cartilage grown in situ from cell-polymer structures, *Am J Sports Med* 22:485-488, 1994.

108. Vert M, Pascal C, Chabot F, Leray J: Bioresorbable plastic materials for bone surgery. In Hastings GW, Ducheyne P, editors: *Macromolecular biomaterials,* Boca Raton, Fla, 1984, CRC Press.

109. Visuri T, Koskenvuo M: Cancer risk after McKee-Farrar total hip replacement, *Acta Orthop Scand* 60:25, 1989.

110. Wakitani S, Goto T, Pineda SJ, et al: Mesenchymal cell-based repair of large, full-thickness defects of articular cartilage, *J Bone Joint Surg* 76A:579-592, 1994.

111. Wakitani S, Kimura T, Hirooka A, et al: Repair of rabbit articular surfaces with allograft chondrocytes embedded in collagen gel, *J Bone Joint Surg* 71B:74-80, 1989.

112. Walker PS, Bullough PG: The effects of friction and wear in artificial joints, *Orthop Clin North Am* 4:275, 1973.

113. Wetzel AC, Stich H, Caffesse RG: Bone apposition onto oral implants in the sinus area filled with different grafting materials, *Clin Oral Implants Res* 6:155-163, 1995.

114. Willert H-G, Semlitsch M: Reactions of the articular capsule to wear products of artificial joint prostheses, *J Biomed Mater Res* 11:157-164, 1977.

115. Yannas IV: Certain biological implications of mammalian skin regeneration by a model extracellular matrix, *Cutan Dev Aging Repair* 18:131-139, 1989.

116. Yannas IV: Regeneration of skin and nerves by use of collagen templates. In Nimni ME, editor: *Biotechnology,* vol III, *Collagen,* Boca Raton, Fla, 1989, CRC Press.

117. Yannas IV: Natural materials. In Ratner BD, Hoffman AS, Schoen FJ, Lemons JE, editors: *Biomaterials science: an introduction to materials in medicine,* San Diego, 1996, Academic Press.

118. Yannas IV, Burke JF, Orgill DP, Skrabut EM: Wound tissue can utilize a polymeric template to synthesize a functional extension of skin, *Science* 215:174-176, 1982.

119. Yannas IV, Lee E, Orgill DP, et al: Synthesis and characterization of a model extracellular matrix that induces partial regeneration of adult mammalian skin, *Proc Nat'l Acad Sci USA* 86:933-937, 1989.

120. Yannas IV, Orgill DP, Silver J, et al: Regeneration of sciatic nerve across 15 mm gap by use of a polymeric template. In Gebelein CG, editor: *Advances in biomedical polymers,* New York, 1987, Plenum.

Flaps

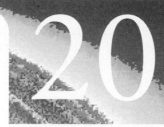

Jeffrey D. Smith
Julian J. Pribaz

A *flap* is a surgically developed segment of mobile tissue that remains attached to a portion of its original blood supply. Although in its simplest form a flap consists of skin and subcutaneous tissue, any layer of tissue may be raised with its blood supply and referred to as a flap. Thus there are skin flaps, fascial flaps, muscle flaps, bone flaps, omental flaps, and others. The *pedicle* is the base by which the flap is attached and includes the blood supply. The pedicle may also include other tissues, such as skin, subcutaneous tissue, fascia, and muscle.

Many different classification schemes exist for flaps. Flaps containing more than one tissue layer are *composite flaps* and are described by the type of tissue contained in the flaps. Fasciocutaneous, musculocutaneous, osteocutaneous, osteomusculocutaneous, omental, jejunal, and gastro-omental-jejunal are examples of composite flaps. Flaps also may be classified by the method of transfer, such as advancement, transposition, rotation, interpolation, jumping, or waltzing, or by their proximity to the defect, such as local or distant. Finally, flaps may be characterized by their blood supply. *Free flaps* are distinguished by their dependence on a vascular anastomosis at the recipient site. A *graft,* on the other hand, survives on the blood supply at the recipient site without the benefit of a surgically created vascular anastomosis.

This chapter addresses the specific topic of reconstruction with pedicled flaps.

HISTORY

Surgical reconstruction with flaps has been performed for more than 2000 years. Susruda Samhita (600 BC) is usually attributed with the earliest recorded applications of pedicle flaps in the face and forehead for nasal reconstruction.[84] Interestingly, the Kanghiara family of India has reportedly performed pedicled forehead flap reconstruction of nasal defects since 1000 BC.[15] In 1597 Tagliacozzi,[77] writing in *De Curtorum Chirurgia,* provided a classic description of nasal reconstruction using a tubed pedicle flap from the arm (Figure 20-1). These early flaps were

discovered empirically and performed without a clear understanding of why and how they worked. In particular, the importance and relevance of the blood supply was not appreciated. Consequently, adherence to fairly rigid length-to-width ratios in their planning and execution was mandated. These early flaps also posed management problems. They were fashioned without anesthesia or antibiotics and were not closed on their undersurface, leaving an open wound. In 1920 Gillies[27] described the innovation of the *tubed* pedicle flap, which protected against infection, and made the pedicle less vulnerable to twisting and kinking, "enormously improving" its blood supply.

The modern understanding of flap reconstruction is based primarily on the knowledge of the blood supply to the skin. Interestingly, the English physician William Harvey did not propose the current theory of circulation until 1628. Harvey's theory proposed that the heart is the center of the circulation and that blood must return to the heart. This theory was in contradiction to Galen's universally accepted theory of "circulation," in which blood was produced in the intestine and distributed by both veins and arteries to be consumed peripherally. In 1660, 3 years after Harvey's death, Marcello Malpighi used a microscope to see the capillaries, the microscopically thin blood vessels that formed the needed connection between the arteries and veins, proving Harvey's theory. This was the first tryst between microscopy and microvasculature, about 300 years before microsurgery and free flaps.

Historically, some breakthroughs in the descriptions of flaps were not appreciated until much later. Some have been rediscovered and further developed to provide invaluable reconstructive options. Tagliacozzi's work was not really exploited in Europe until nearly 200 years after the 1597 publication, when a popular London magazine reported on the Indian method for nasal reconstruction.[26] Shortly thereafter, the method first appeared in the American literature in an 1837 article by Warren[85] (Figure 20-2). In 1898 Monks[53] first reported a one-stage island pedicle flap based on the superficial temporal artery to resurface the lower eyelid (Figure 20-3). In 1863 John Wood described the groin flap,[6] which was not utilized until 1972, when McGregor and Jackson[49] reintroduced and popularized this flap. Jacques Joseph,[34] relying on work by Manchot[44] from 1889, described deltopectoral flaps as "vascular pattern" flaps in 1931. In 1965 Bakamjian[2] described a large deltopectoral flap for pharyngeal reconstruc-

tion. Tanzini[78] described the latissimus dorsi flap for breast reconstruction in 1906. At the same time the influential William S. Halsted (1852-1922) was popularizing the radical mastectomy for breast cancer and discouraging reconstruction. As a result, Tanzini's pioneering methods were largely forgotten.[15]

Many advances have come together to bring flaps to their current state (Table 20-1). Some of the advances that influenced the relatively recent explosion of knowledge and reconstructive options include the birth of anesthesia in 1846, Lister's concept of antisepsis between 1861 and 1869, the clinical challenges of World Wars I and II, and the advent of surgical microscopy. Presumably, advances in the fields of gene transfer, tissue engineering, organogenesis, and transplantation represent the new frontier. Nevertheless, it is interesting to wonder how much further advanced plastic surgery might be if some of these discoveries had been appreciated and further developed from their initial inception.

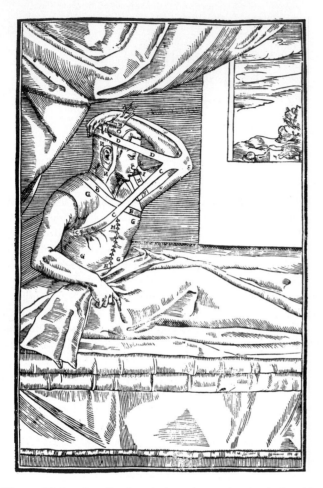

Figure 20-1. Arm flap for nasal reconstruction, as depicted by Tagliacozzi in 1597.

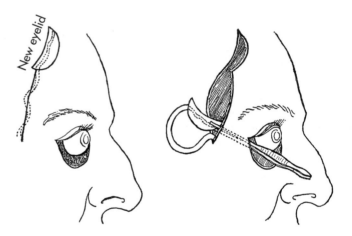

Figure 20-3. First one-stage island pedicle flap. (From Monks GH: *Boston Med Surg J* 139:385, 1898.)

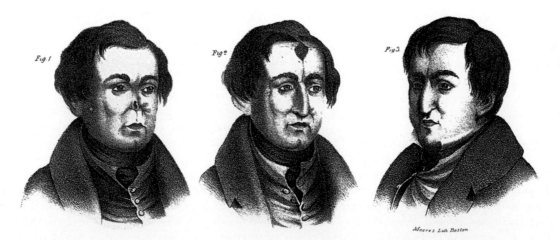

Figure 20-2. First American report of forehead flap for nasal reconstruction. (From Warren JM: *Boston Med Surg J* 16(5), 1837.)

Table 20-1.
Timeline of Flap Development and Important Contributing Advances

YEAR	SOURCE	EVENT
1000 BC	Kanghiara family of India	Pedicled forehead flap for nasal reconstruction
700 BC	Susruta Samhita	Pedicled flap for nasal reconstruction
25 BC	Celsus (25 BC-50 AD)	Advancement flaps
600 AD	Paulus Aegineta	Originator of modern plastic surgery
700	Arab scholars	Translate Susruta Samhita
1450	Gutenberg (Gensfleisch)	Invents printing press
1543	Vesalius, Andreaus	*De Humani Corporis Fabrica*
1597	Tagliacozzi	Pedicled arm flap for nasal reconstruction
1657	Harvey	Describes heart as center of circulation
1660	Malpighi	Identifies capillaries, proving Harvey's theory
1756	Herziel	Lip-switch flap (Sweden)
1794	*Gentleman's Magazine*	Reintroduces Indian forehead flap to England
1814	Carpue	Forehead flap (37 minutes) for nasal reconstruction
1817	Cooper	First successful reported skin graft
1818	Von Graefe	Introduces term *plastic*
1837	Horner	Z-plasty
1846	Morton	Anesthesia
1861	Lister	Antisepsis
1862	Wood	Performs groin flap
1889	Manchot	Cutaneous territories based on blood supply
1893	Spalteholz	Describes fasciocutaneous blood supply to skin
1898	Monks	First single-stage island pedicle flap
1906	Tanzini	Latissimus dorsi flap for breast reconstruction
1908	Carrel	Describes method of vascular anastomosis
1914	World War I	Beginning of plastic surgery as specialty
1918	Filatov/Gillies	Tubed pedicle flaps
1918	Esser	Describes V-Y advancement flap
1919	Davies	First American plastic surgery textbook
1930	Ragnell	Begins plastic surgery at Karolinska Institute
1936	Salmon	*Arteres de la peau*
1937	Blair	Father of American Board of Plastic Surgery
1955	Murray	Renal homograft
1963	Goldwyn et al	First free flap (groin flap in dog)

Continued

Table 20-1.
Timeline of Flap Development and Important Contributing Advances—cont'd

YEAR	SOURCE	EVENT
1965	Bakamjian	Deltopectoral flap
1966	Buncke et al	Hallux-to-hand transplantation in monkey
1973	Daniel/Taylor	First successful free flap transfer in human
1973	McGregor/Jackson	Reintroduce groin flap
1977	Ger	Muscle flap
1977	McCraw	Musculocutaneous flaps
1981	Ponten	Fasciocutaneous flap
1981	Mathes/Nahai	Classification of muscle flaps
1987	Taylor	Angiosomes

APPROACH TO PATIENT AND DEFECT

The management of defects presenting to the reconstructive surgeon requires careful assessment and planning. In 1564 Ambroise Paré described some surgical principles that are still applicable: to take away what is superfluous, to restore to their places things that are displaced, to separate these things that are joined together, and to supply the defects of nature.[50] Traditionally, defect repair has been approached using a "reconstructive ladder," an orderly progression from simple to complex solutions, from direct closure to local and regional flaps, and then to microvascular free flaps (Figure 20-4).

As microvascular reconstruction has become more reliable, other factors such as donor site morbidity and functional outcome assume a more primary role and render the ladder a less useful construct. The approach to evaluation and repair of a tissue defect on the most simplistic level involves an inventory of what is available weighed against what can be spared in light of the tenable reconstructive options. Robin Hood's tissue apportionment principle, or "robbing Peter to pay Paul," exemplifies this concept. Millard,[50] drawing on years of experience in his *Principlization of Plastic Surgery,* defines 33 principles, including the Robin Hood principle, to guide repair of defects. Adequate repair requires a careful analysis of the defect and assessment of specific tissue deficiencies. Such an analysis must take into account the following:

1. Location and size of defect
2. Functional and aesthetic consequences of original defect
3. Potential donor site defect
4. Vascularity of surrounding tissue
5. Presence of exposed structures
6. Natural history of problem
7. Cost of care
8. Potential complications

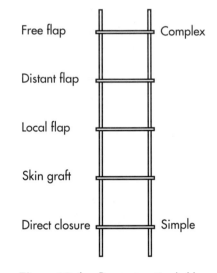

Figure 20-4. Reconstructive ladder.

9. Patient expectations
10. Impact on patient's quality of life

Outcome studies are needed to facilitate decision making in all these areas.

FLAP PHYSIOLOGY

The blood flowing to the skin not only provides oxygen to support metabolism but also performs important thermoregulatory and immunologic functions.

Blood Supply of Skin

An appreciation of the blood supply to the skin is essential because it defines the flap and is central to understanding how flaps can be moved. A rich network of vessels, whose density and size vary from site to site, feeds the skin. The blood supply

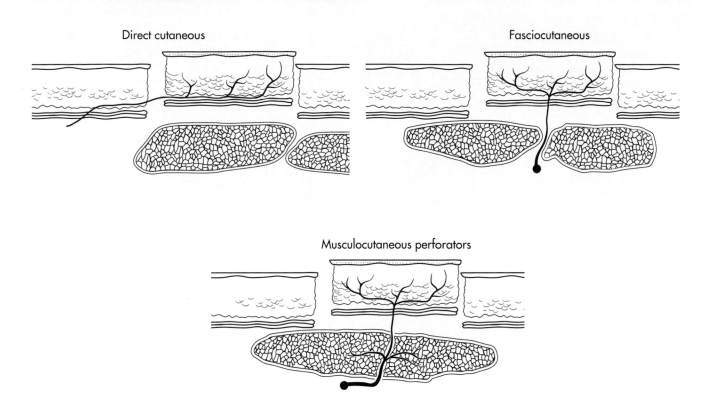

Figure 20-5. Patterns of blood supply to the skin: direct cutaneous pedicle, fasciocutaneous pedicle, musculocutaneous pedicle. (From Mathes S, Nahai F: *Reconstructive Surgery: Principles, anatomy and technique,* London, 1997, Churchill Livingstone.)

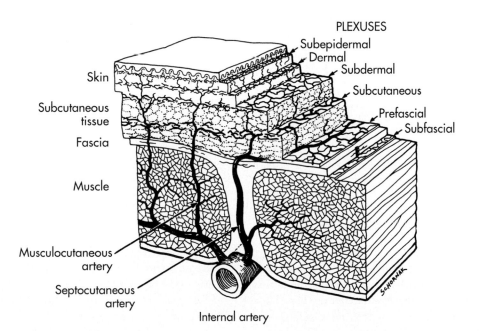

Figure 20-6. Vascular plexuses of the skin. (From Daniel RK, Kerrigan CL: In McCarthy JG, editor: *Plastic surgery,* Philadelphia, 1990, Saunders.)

to the skin arises from fasciocutaneous vessels, musculocutaneous perforators, or direct cutaneous arteries (Figure 20-5). These vessels supply a *deep plexus* located at the junction of the subcutaneous tissue and the deep dermis and a *superficial plexus* at the junction of the papillary and reticular dermis (Figure 20-6). Cormack and Lamberty[15] organize the arterial anatomy

of skin flaps partly into categories of a direct cutaneous system, a fasciocutaneous system, and a musculocutaneous system of vessels. They graphically depict the flaps that can be raised while relying on each category of vessels (Figure 20-7).

Before the blood supply to the skin was understood, most flaps were random, and their design was based on empirically

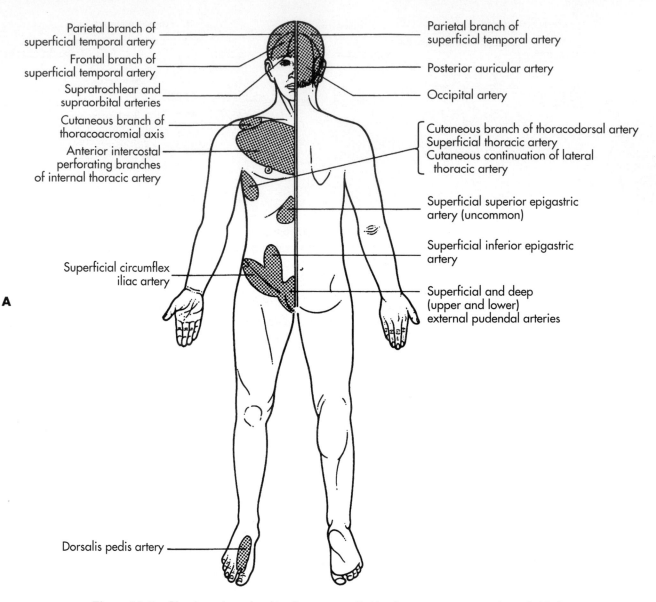

Parietal branch of
superficial temporal artery

Frontal branch of
superficial temporal artery

Supratrochlear and
supraorbital arteries

Cutaneous branch of
thoracoacromial axis

Anterior intercostal
perforating branches
of internal thoracic artery

Superficial circumflex
iliac artery

Dorsalis pedis artery

A

Parietal branch of
superficial temporal artery

Posterior auricular artery

Occipital artery

Cutaneous branch of thoracodorsal artery
Superficial thoracic artery
Cutaneous continuation of lateral
thoracic artery

Superficial superior epigastric
artery (uncommon)

Superficial inferior epigastric
artery

Superficial and deep
(upper and lower)
external pudendal arteries

Figure 20-7. Blood supply to the skin: **A,** areas supplied by direct cutaneous arteries, suitable for raising axial pattern flaps. (From Cormack GC, Lamberty BGH: *The arterial anatomy of skin flaps,* ed 2, London, 1994, Churchill Livingstone.) *Continued*

established length-to-width ratios. For example, it was known that in the head and neck, flaps with a 4:1 or 5:1 ratio could be raised safely because of the rich blood supply in this area. In contrast, a 1:1 ratio was safe for a lower extremity flap. These tenets were slowly dismissed in favor of a more sophisticated system based on the cutaneous blood supply. In 1970 Milton[52] denounced the inflexible application of length-to-width ratios. The concept that flap survival depended on blood supply and not on flap width was actually appreciated before the turn of the twentieth century.[27,53] In fact, it was noted that flaps could be raised with no base at all, dividing skin on all sides and leaving only the direct cutaneous blood supply.

Early work defining the blood supply to the skin included that of Manchot,[44] a German anatomist, who in 1889 topographically depicted cutaneous vascular territories served by named arteries that he identified through dissection of cadavers. The French surgeon-anatomist Salmon[72] further developed Manchot's concepts in the 1936 publication *Arteres de la peau* by obtaining radiographs subsequent to the intraarterial injection of contrast into cadavers, demonstrating with greater detail the skin's blood supply. In 1893 Spalteholz[75] described vessels that traveled in the fascial septa to supply the skin and those that also supply muscle before penetrating the fascia to supply the skin, providing the anatomic basis for fasciocutaneous and musculocutaneous flaps. These early studies depict the blood supply on an anatomic basis and do not provide information about potential vascular territories or how blood flow may vary in vivo in a dynamic situation.

In the manner of Manchot and Salmon, Taylor et al[80-82]

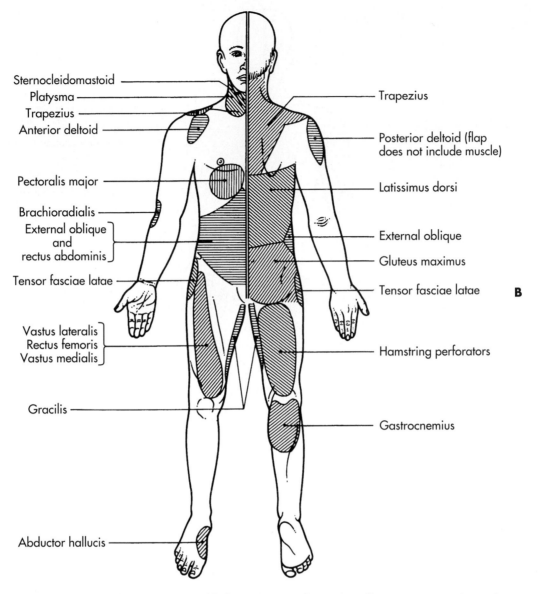

Figure 20-7, cont'd. **B,** Areas suitable for raising musculocutaneous flaps. *Continued*

have performed the most extensive recent vascular studies of the periphery. It is interesting to compare the figures depicting the blood supply to the skin from Manchot, Salmon, and Taylor (Figure 20-8). Taylor and Palmer[82] developed the *angiosome* concept to depict the three-dimensional composite tissue block that is supplied by an artery and its vein. Although depicting blood flow on an anatomic basis, they also have described changes that occur dynamically, explaining how these composite blocks interact under various conditions. Each angiosome can be subdivided into an arteriosome and a venosome for the arterial and venous territories. Each angiosome is connected to adjacent angiosomes by *true anastomoses* or reduced-caliber "choke" vessels (Figure 20-9). These *choke vessels* may dilate to the caliber of true anastomoses in certain situations,

such as when a flap is delayed. Furthermore, Taylor and Minabe[81] note that these choke anastomoses clearly define the vascular territories and are what Salmon referred to as "retiform anastomoses." The accompanying venous connections, called *oscillating veins,* are avalvular and can flow in either direction.

This work has had tremendous conceptual and clinical impact. It has helped to develop new flaps by defining safe three-dimensional anatomic boundaries that may include one or more angiosomes, since tissue within adjacent angiosomes can usually be included safely if desired, particularly if carried on a traversing muscle. The identification of choke vessels has also provided a better understanding of the delay phenomenon. The oscillating veins may be important in understanding how reverse-flow flaps work by allowing blood to bypass

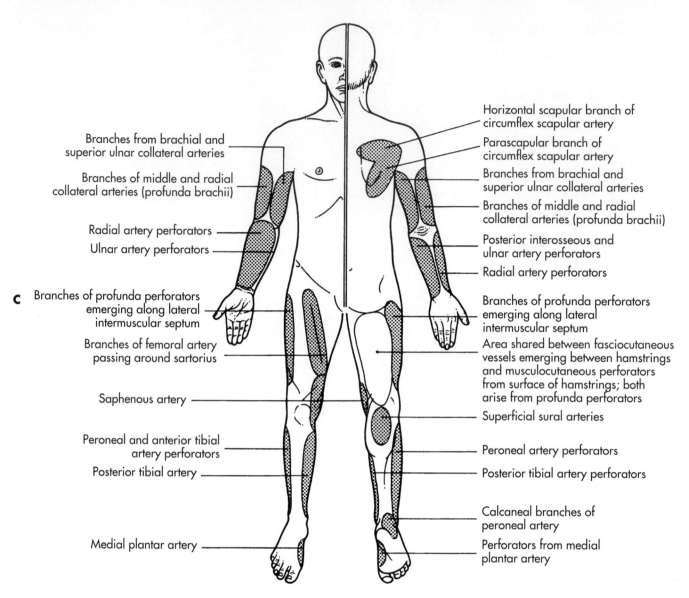

Figure 20-7, cont'd.   C, Areas suitable for raising fasciocutaneous flaps. (From Cormack GC, Lamberty BGH: *The arterial anatomy of skin flaps,* ed 2, London, 1994, Churchill Livingstone.)

valvular segments (Figure 20-10). Box 20-1 lists several important anatomic concepts.[79,81] Taylor's work has given plastic surgeons a better understanding of flap blood supply, which will further increase the number and types of flaps that can be raised and improve the safety of raising and transferring these flaps.

Regulation of Blood Flow

Extrinsic and intrinsic factors impinge on the vasculature to regulate blood flow to the skin. These factors can be divided into those that are predominantly a function of (1) the vessel, (2) the circulating elements in the blood, and (3) the interaction between the two. It is beyond the scope of this chapter to discuss this in great detail, but some important facts should be noted. The endothelial cell clearly plays the central role in maintenance of hemostasis and consequently in the viability of the flaps that are created. Also, nitric oxide (NO) is

the final common mediator for many substances that exert an effect on the vessel wall. Table 20-2 summarizes some of the factors that modulate blood flow, classified by their propensity for vasoconstriction or dilation and whether they are local or systemic agents.[17] Beta-adrenergic stimuli, cholinergic stimuli, bradykinin, histamine, prostaglandin E_1 (PGE_1), prostacyclin (PGI_2), hypoxia, acidosis, and hyperthermia are noted as vasodilators. Alpha-adrenergic stimuli, serotonin, thromboxane A_2 (TXA_2), hypothermia, and myogenic distention play a role in vasoconstriction. It is now known that intact endothelium, which is capable of producing nitric oxide, is necessary for the vasodilatory effects of acetylcholine. When no intact endothelium exists, there is a net vasoconstrictive effect of acetycholine.[25] Serotonin, thrombin, adenosine diphosphate (ADP), and histamine all cause vasodilation by stimulating NO release. Furthermore, studies in the human forearm suggest that a continuous basal release of NO is an important

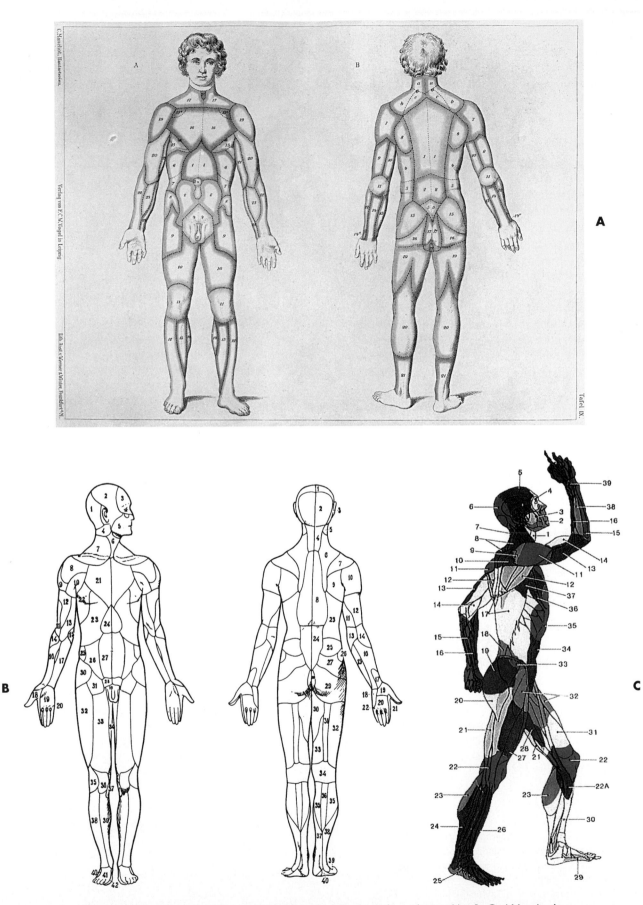

Figure 20-8. Dermal territories defined by their blood supply, as depicted by **A,** Carl Manchot's *die hautartien des menschlichen körpus* (1889), **B,** Michel Salmon's *arteres de le peau* (1936), and **C,** Taylor's angiosomes of body (1987). (**A** and **B** from Cormack GC, Lamberty BGH: *The arterial anatomy of skin flaps,* ed 2, London, 1994, Churchill Livingstone; **C** from Taylor GI, Palmer JH: *Br J Plast Surg* 40:113, 1987.)

determinant of resting vascular resistance.[83] When a NO inhibitor was infused, the resting flow decreased substantially.

Other humoral vasoactive substances also contribute to the regulation of blood flow. *Endothelins* are a group of endothelially synthesized polypeptides that exert a direct vasoconstrictive effect independent of NO.[87]

Myogenic control is an important regulatory mechanism in which arteriolar smooth muscle reacts to increased intraluminal pressure by contracting. This mechanism is prominent in arterioles smaller than 100 microns (μ) and tends to maintain normal flow despite increased pressure.[59]

The sympathetic nervous system provides direct innervation to vessels and is, if indirectly, one of the most important contributors to a baseline vascular tone. This tone appears to be largely a function of the flow through normally occurring shunts or arteriovenous (AV) anastomoses. Studies on the effect of sympathectomy on extremity perfusion in a canine model confirm this by showing an increase in nonnutritive blood flow suggestive of an effect on the level of the AV anastomosis.[16] Another important facet of the regulation of blood flow is the interaction between the vessel wall and the blood elements. Specifically, through direct or indirect trauma, endothelial cell loss or dysfunction may occur and lead to thrombosis and ischemia. With an ischemia reperfusion cycle, the reperfusion results in the formation of reactive oxygen metabolites and a reduction in NO production. The resulting

effects include increased neutrophil adhesion and vasoconstriction. The adherence of neutrophils to the endothelial surface through various cell surface adhesion molecules is the first step in neutrophil-mediated tissue injury during reperfusion.[40]

Poiseuille's law is often used to describe the energy loss in vessels as a function of vessel length, radius, and blood

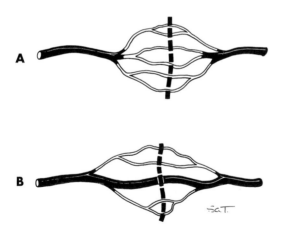

Figure 20-9. Schematic representation of "choke" anastomoses **(A)** and true anastomoses **(B).** (From Taylor GI: In Aston SJ, Beasley RW, Thorne CHW, editors: *Grabb and Smith's Plastic surgery,* ed 5, Philadelphia, 1997, Lippincott-Raven.)

Box 20-1.
Important Anatomic Concepts Associated with Flaps, Vascularity, and Angiosomes

1. The vascular architecture of the integument and the deep tissues is an unbroken network of interconnecting vessel arcades.
2. The vessels follow the connective tissue framework of the body.
3. The vessels radiate from fixed to mobile areas. If the skin over a muscle is mobile, the supply from the muscle will be tenuous.
4. A parallel relationship exists between tissue mobility and the size and density of supplying vessels. Where tissues are mobile, the vessels are large and widely spaced; where tissues are fixed, the vessels are small and closely spaced.
5. The territory of each adjacent artery obeys the law of equilibrium. For example, if one vessel or territory is large, its partner is small.
6. Vessels tend to have a constant destination but may have a variable origin. This is true between individuals of the same species and between different species.
7. Vessels course with nerves.
8. Vessel size and orientation are a product of tissue growth and differentiation. Thus developmental expansion and surgical tissue expansion are similar and depend on the ability of vessels to lengthen and hypertrophy.
9. The anatomic territory of each tissue in the adjacent angiosome can usually be captured safely.
10. Most muscles span across two or more angiosomes and are supplied by each territory, allowing one to capture the skin island from one angiosome by muscle supplied in an adjacent territory.

Modified from Taylor GI, Minabe T: *Plast Reconstr Surg* 89:181, 1992.

Figure 20-10. Composite diagram of integument and underlying muscle *(shaded),* illustrating superficial *(S)* and deep *(D)* venous systems and their interconnections. Small arrows depict choke *(C)* vessels. (From Taylor GI: In Aston SJ, Beasley RW, Thorne CHW, editors: *Grabb and Smith's Plastic surgery,* ed 5, Philadelphia, 1997, Lippincott-Raven.)

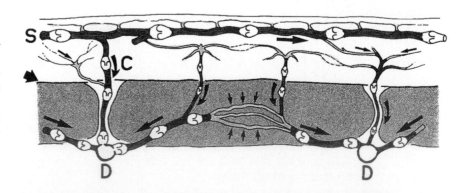

viscosity. The law is intended to apply to steady nonpulsatile laminar flow in a straight cylinder with rigid walls. Flap anatomy and physiology do not conform to these prerequisites and exemplify the difficulty of (1) developing a meaningful mathematical description of the blood supply at the level of the microcirculation and (2) predicting the impact of altering variables, such as hematocrit. Haynes showed that hematocrit has little influence on the flow rate through small-diameter tubes approaching the size of capillaries (6 μ), where the relative viscosity changes little between hematocrits of 10% and 70%. At the capillary level the highly deformable red blood cell easily traverses 3-μ to 4-μ pores, whether few or many corpuscles are present. Furthermore, the other effects of bleeding, such as increased cardiac output and alteration in composition of blood constituents, confound in vivo studies on the effect of hematocrit on random flap survival.[15] Also, when hypoxic tissue may already be present, the imagined rheologic benefits of a low hematocrit must be weighed against decreased oxygen delivery.

Many factors from different systems contribute to the regulation of blood flow. Our recent understanding of the central and active role of the endothelial cell may create new opportunities for improving flap survival.

Pharmacologic Manipulation of Flaps
Many approaches to pharmacologic flap manipulation have been attempted to make a flap more robust before transfer or to salvage a struggling flap. No conclusive studies show a clear benefit with the use of any adjunctive treatment, including vasodilators, rheologic agents, prostaglandins or prostaglandin inhibitors, free radical scavengers, allopurinol, and steroids. No consensus exists on the efficacy of these methods of pharmacologic intervention, and few, if any, are used routinely.

Some substances are known to be injurious to flaps. A large body of data supports the adverse effects of nicotine on flaps. Nicotine is a vasoconstrictive substance repeatedly shown to have an adverse effect on the random, nonaxial portion of the flap rather than at the site of a microvascular anastomosis.[70]

FLAP CLASSIFICATION

Flaps may be classified according to their proximity to the defect (e.g., local or distant), method of flap movement, type of vascularity, composition of tissue transposed, or method of manipulation before transfer. It is helpful to consider each of these schemes because all are instructive and useful, emphasize different characteristics of flaps, and underscore relevant anatomy, physiology, and technical aspects of flap reconstruction (Table 20-3).

Methods of *movement* include advancement, transposition, rotation, interpolation, pedicled, jumping, waltzing, and free. Flaps often are described by their proximity and then further delineated by their method of movement; thus local flaps

---

Table 20-2.
Systemic and Local Factors Affecting Blood Supply to Skin

NERVOUS	HUMORAL	METABOLIC	PHYSICAL
VASOCONSTRICTORS			
Alpha-adrenergic	Norepinephrine		Viscosity
Serotinergic	Epinephrine		Hypothermia
	Serotonin		Myogenic reflex
	Prostaglandin F$_2$		
	Thromboxane A$_2$		
	Endothelins		
VASODILATORS			
Beta-adrenergic	Nitric oxide	Hypoxia	Hyperthermia
Cholinergic	Bradykinin	Acidosis	Sympathectomy
	Histamine	Hypercarbia	
	Prostacyclin		
	Adenosine diphosphate		
	Prostaglandin		
	Thrombin		

Modified from Daniel RK, Kerrigan CL: In McCarthy JG, editor: *Plastic surgery*, Philadelphia, 1990, Saunders.

Table 20-3.
Classification Schemes of Flaps

SCHEME	TYPES
Proximity to defect	Local
	Distant
Method of movement	Advancement
	Rotation
	Transposition
	Interpolation
	Jumping
	Waltzing
	Free
Composition	Cutaneous
	Fasciocutaneous
	Musculocutaneous
	Osteocutaneous
	Omental
	Visceral
Specialized	Sensory
	Innervated muscle
	Tendon
	Hair bearing
	Gut
Blood supply	Random
	Axial pattern
	Fasciocutaneous
	Musculocutaneous
Manipulation before transfer	Delay
	Expansion
	Prefabrication
	Prelamination

may be advanced, transposed, rotated, or interpolated into nearby defects, whereas distant defects require pedicled, tubed, jumping, waltzing, or free flaps.

Flaps may also be classified by their *blood supply.* The blood supply to the transferred tissue may be direct or indirect. If direct, the vessel may be a direct cutaneous artery, and the flap may be referred to as an axial or arterial pattern flap. Alternately, the flap may originate from subjacent muscle perforators, giving rise to a musculocutaneous or perforator flap. Also, the flap may travel through the fibrous septa or fasciae between the muscles, giving rise to a fasciocutaneous flap (see Figure 20-5).

Flaps may be characterized by their *tissue composition.* Simple flaps contain only skin, whereas composite flaps contain multiple tissue types, such as skin, fat, fascia, muscle, and bone. *Specialized flaps* contain structures to fulfill certain needs, such as innervated muscle for movement, sensory nerves

for sensation, or conduit flaps for flow-through perfusion of distal structures.

An additional category involves *flap manipulation* before transfer. It includes flap delay, tissue expansion (a form of delay), flap prefabrication, and flap prelamination. *Flap prefabrication* involves the transfer of a vascular pedicle containing the artery, its venae comitantes, and surrounding adventia with or without fascia or small amount of muscle into the area to be neovascularized. After maturation the tissue surrounding the implanted vascular pedicle can be raised as a flap and transferred locally or as a free flap. This technique has been useful for creating thin flaps at a distant site, especially in the burn patient for head and neck reconstruction.

Flap prelamination, a term initially coined by Pribaz and Fine,[63] is used when composite tissue reconstruction is desired but no ideally suited donor site exists. In this two-stage procedure the first stage involves preparing the donor site by grafting additional surfaces (e.g., skin, mucosa), adding structural support (e.g., cartilage graft), and using tissue expansion, if necessary. The second stage involves the flap transfer, either local or free.

Local Tissue Advancement

Reconstructive surgeons primarily have confronted cutaneous defects that are managed most simply with local tissue rearrangements. These local tissues are moved into the defect by a process of advancement, transposition, rotation, or interpolation. These flaps, which depend on a random blood supply carried in the subcutaneous, subdermal, dermal, or subepidermal plexuses, have been used for centuries. Although random, their design, orientation, and extent of undermining should be based on the known blood supply arising from underlying muscle and fascia. These flaps rely on skin elasticity and excess to permit undermining and movement of skin and subcutaneous tissue into a defect.

ADVANCEMENT FLAPS. Advancement flaps have been performed for over 2000 years and were described by Celsus (25 BC).[12] The tissue adjacent to a defect may be mobilized and stretched in a straight line to close a defect without any rotation about a pivot point. Examples of advancement flaps include the single-pedicle advancement flap, bipedicle advancement flap, and V-Y and Y-V advancement flaps.

The *single-pedicle advancement flap* is raised as a square or rectangle by making two parallel incisions along the sides of a defect, then undermining the subcutaneous tissue (Figure 20-11). The elasticity of the skin is then used to stretch the flap into the defect. To facilitate the advancement, triangles may be excised from the tissues adjacent to the base of the flap, or small backcuts may be made into the base of the flap to provide the so-called pantographic expansion. Backcuts narrow the pedicle and must be done judiciously. A small Z-plasty may also be performed at the flap base to achieve greater advancement; this must be done with special caution as well because it also narrows the pedicle.

A more versatile type is the *V-Y advancement flap,* which relies on the mobility of the subcutaneous layer. In 1918

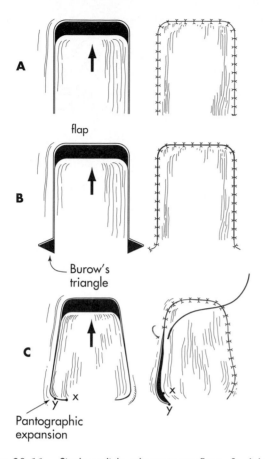

Figure 20-11. Single-pedicle advancement flaps. **A,** Advancement flap. **B,** Excising Burow's triangle of skin laterally to equalize flap length and adjacent wound edge. **C,** "Pantographic" expansion. (From Aston SJ, Beasley RW, Thorne CHW, editors: *Grabb and Smith's Plastic surgery,* ed 5, Philadelphia, 1997, Lippincott-Raven.)

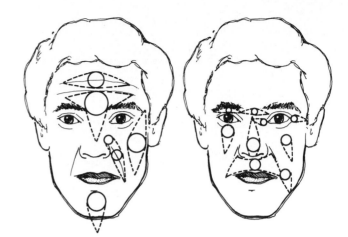

Figure 20-12. V-Y flaps for face. (From Zook EG, Van Beek AL, Russell RC, Moore JB: *Plast Reconstr Surg* 65:786, 1980.)

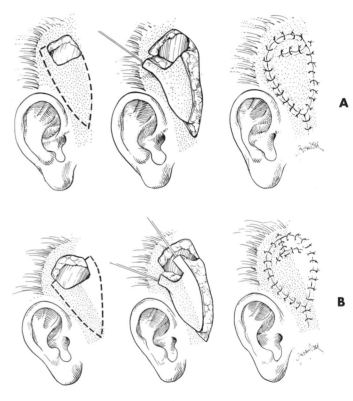

Figure 20-13. Extended Y-V flaps: **A,** single; **B,** double. (From: Pribaz JJ, Chester CH, Barrall DT: *Plast Reconstr Surg* 90:275, 1992.)

Esser[21] originally described the method of using an island skin flap, ideally with an identifiable artery. This was a triangular flap that was raised by making two intersecting incisions in the tissue adjacent to a defect. The incisions made through the dermis and the subcutaneous tissues are bluntly mobilized and left attached to the subcutaneous pedicle. A deeper dissection of the subcutaneous tissue only occurs at the distal end of the flap adjacent to the defect. This type of advancement flap is suitable in areas where mobile subcutaneous tissue is abundant with a rich blood supply. These flaps are most useful on the face, especially over the cheeks, nasolabial areas, upper lips, and glabellar regions[90] (Figure 20-12).

A modification of the V-Y advancement flap is the *extended V-Y advancement flap,* in which a transposition flap is added to one or both ends of a V-Y advancement flap that is larger than the defect.[62] This is subsequently advanced, and the extended portion is rotated onto the end of the flap to increase its length and usefulness. Single and double extended V-Y advancement flaps have been used in the temporal and forehead regions and over the nose. These flaps have less subcutaneous fat and are less mobile than the cheek areas. The extensions on the V-Y flaps enable complex defects to be closed adequately. The

rotation of the extended portion of these flaps, however, may lead to the tissue distortion seen with other rotation and transposition flaps (Figure 20-13).

A variation of the V-Y advancement flap is the *Y-V advancement flaps,* which may be used in serial fashion for release of scar contractures. The Y limb cuts across the scar contracture, and the adjacent V flap is advanced into the area of scar release (Figure 20-14).

Another type is the *bipedicle advancement flap,* an extremely useful flap for reconstructing longitudinal defects of the extremities. An incision is made parallel to the longitudinal

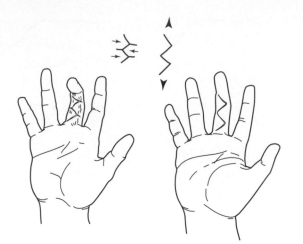

Figure 20-14. Serial Y-V advancement flaps for scar contracture release.

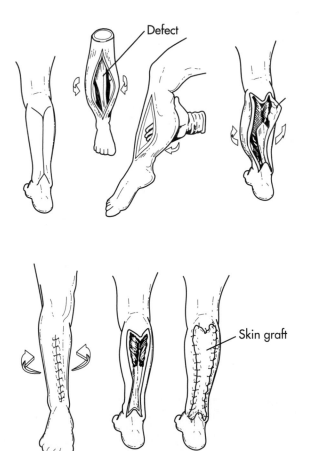

Figure 20-15. Bipedicle flap. (From Hartwell SW Jr: In Strauch B, Vasconez LO, Hall-Findlay ED, editors: *Grabb's Encyclopedia of flaps*, ed 2, Philadelphia, 1998, Lippincott-Raven.)

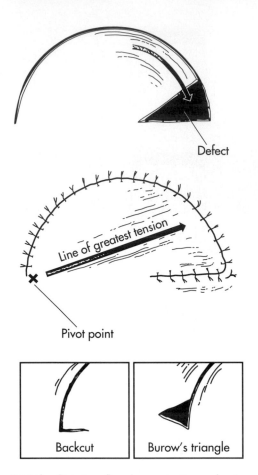

Figure 20-16. Rotation flap demonstrating reduction of tension by backcut or Burow's triangle. (From Aston SJ, Beasley RW, Thorne CHW, editors: *Grabb and Smith's Plastic surgery*, ed 5, Philadelphia, 1997, Lippincott-Raven.)

defect, making sure that the bases and center of the bipedicle flap are not narrowed. The flap is undermined and advanced into the defect. The resulting donor defect may be skin grafted, or a primary skin closure may be achieved by further mobilization of the skin adjacent to the flap incision (Figure 20-15).

ROTATION FLAPS. Rotation and transposition flaps rotate about a pivot point. A rotation flap is a semicircular flap raised from the edge of a triangular defect. The tissue is undermined and rotated about a pivot point to close a triangular defect. If the arc of rotation is kept long, the donor site can be closed primarily by distributing the tension along the suture line. The greatest tension in this flap occurs from the pivot point to the proximal edge of the defect. If the tension is too great, a backcut may be made from the pivot point along the base of the flap judiciously so as not to narrow the base of the flap and thereby decrease the blood supply to the flap. Another way of reducing the tension is to excise a triangle of skin adjacent to the pivot point, which does not narrow the base of the flap and only minimally reduces the tension (Figure 20-16). Rotation flaps are most often used to close scalp defects and sacral pressure sores (Figure 20-17).

Another type of rotation flap frequently used to reconstruct small tissue defects on the nose is the *bilobed flap*. As described by Esser,[21] each flap was the same size, and the lobes were

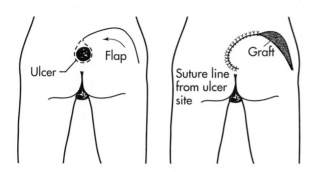

Figure 20-17. Rotation flap for sacral decubiti. (From Griffith BH: In Strauch B, Vasconez LO, Hall-Findlay ED, editors: *Grabb's Encyclopedia of flaps,* ed 2, Philadelphia, 1998, Lippincott-Raven.)

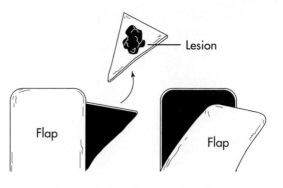

Figure 20-19. Transposition flap.

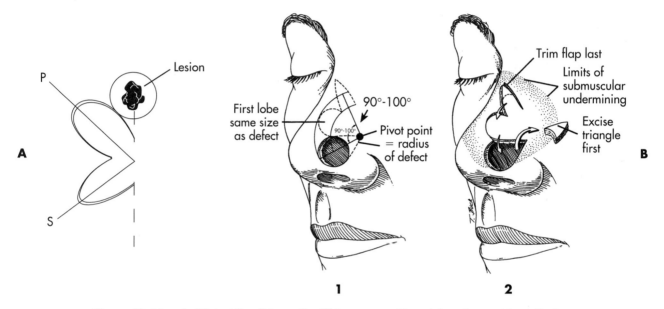

Figure 20-18. A, Bilobed flap. Primary flap *(P)* is transposed into defect after excision of lesion. Secondary flap *(S)* is transposed into defect left by primary flap. Donor area of secondary flap is closed primarily. **B,** Zitelli's design of bilobed flap. (**B** from Burget GC, Menick FJ: *Aesthetic reconstruction of the nose,* St Louis, 1994, Mosby.)

oriented 90 degrees to each other. Zimany[88] modified this in 1953 by designing the second flap smaller than the first flap. Zitelli[89] kept the second flap smaller and reduced the angle between the two flaps to approximately 50 degrees, preventing buckling and large dog ears. This flap is used when sufficient tissue laxity is available to close the donor site primarily. When used in distal nasal reconstruction, the defect should be less 1.5 cm in diameter. The primary flap is the same size as the adjacent defect, and a second flap adjacent to the primary flap is about half the width of the primary flap. The primary flap then rotates into the defect, the secondary flap rotates into the primary flap donor site, and the secondary flap donor site is closed primarily (Figure 20-18).

TRANSPOSITION FLAPS. A transposition flap is a rectangular or square area of skin and subcutaneous tissue that is raised on three sides and transferred laterally into an adjacent defect. The pivot point is located at the base distal to the defect (Figure 20-19). A backcut at this pivot point will reduce the

tension, but it will also narrow the flap base and therefore should be done judiciously. Care is needed in designing these flaps because the end of the flap should extend beyond the defect, since transposition results in some loss of length, so that the tip of the flap can be transferred into the defect without undue tension. The resulting donor defect can either be closed with a skin graft or, if the surrounding tissues are lax, by a direct suture after local undermining and mobilization.

LIMBERG FLAPS. The Limberg flap (1946) is a type of transposition flap used to close a rhomboid defect.[41] The flap design is very precise, with the rhomboid defect having angles of 60 and 120 degrees (Figure 20-20). The flap is designed by extending the short axis of the defect into the adjacent area where there is loose skin. The length of the extension is equal to the short diagonal of the defect. The third limb of the flap is then drawn parallel to the edge of the defect, and the flap is undermined and transposed into the defect.

For larger defects, corresponding flaps can be raised on each side of the defect so that, theoretically, four Limberg flaps can be designed for any rhomboid defect. A double-rhomboid flap can be used for closing longer defects, whereas a triple-rhomboid can be applied to circular defects after conversion to a hexagon (Figure 20-21). This latter application is useful for closing defects of the scalp.

DUFOURMENTAL FLAPS. A modification of the Limberg flap was described by Dufourmentel[20] in 1962. This more complex closure provides a larger flap to fill the defect and relies on the looseness of the surrounding skin to close the resulting donor defect. This flap is used to fill rhomboidlike defects with angles that are not necessarily 60 and 120 degrees and with diagonals or sides that may be unequal. In designing this flap, a line is drawn as a continuation of the short diagonal, and another line is drawn as a continuation of one of the sides, typically at the obtuse angle. These two lines form an angle that, when bisected, is the edge of the flap. The length of the edge should equal the length of the side, and an incision parallel to the long axis allows the flap to be raised (Figure 20-22).

Z-PLASTY FLAPS. One of the most basic types of transposition flap is the Z-plasty, described by Fricke[24] in 1829 and Horner[31] in 1837, in which two adjacent triangular flaps are transposed into each other's defect, lengthening the central incision. The function of Z-plasties is to lengthen tight contracted scars or to change the direction of scars or displaced tissue (Figure 20-23, *A*). The classic Z-plasty comprises a central member, which runs along the scar or tissue that needs to be lengthened, and two limbs oriented at 60 degrees to the central member, with each of the three parts being equal in length. Although the angle between the limbs and the central member may vary between 30 and 90 degrees, the force

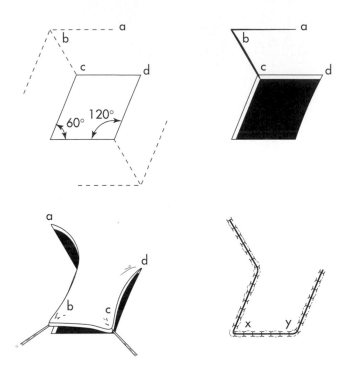

Figure 20-20. Limberg flap. Line *bc* is an extension of the short axis. Flap *abcd* is moved into the defect.

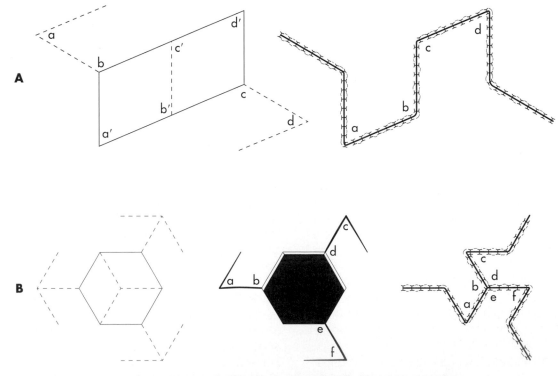

Figure 20-21. **A,** Double-rhomboid flap. **B,** Triple-rhomboid flap.

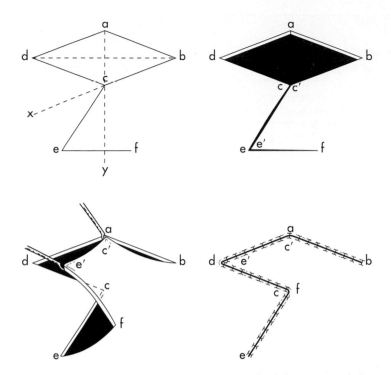

Figure 20-22. Dufourmental flap. The short diagonal *ac* and side *bc* are extended to *y* and *x*. The angle *xcy* is bisected with line *ce* (*ce* length equals *bc* length). A line *(ef)* is then drawn parallel to long diagonal *db*. The flap, *bc'e'f* is then transposed. Mobilization of *dce* may facilitate closure at donor site. (From Jackson IT: *Local flaps in head and neck reconstruction,* St Louis, 1985, Mosby.)

required to close the wound increases with an increase in the angle. Increasing that angle increases the gain in length. In practice, 60 degrees is typically the greatest angle that will allow both lengthening in the direction of the central member and transposition of the newly created triangles.

The theoretic gain in length can be calculated for the various angles, but the variability in the elastic properties of the skin may cause the actual gain to be more or less. A number of authors have reported on the actual disparity within a series of Z-plasties between the calculated and the realized gain in length. Table 20-4 shows the theoretic gain in length for Z-plasties constructed with different angles. Grabb[30] reported on a series of Z-plasties in which the actual and calculated gains were compared. The actual gains were the same as the calculated gains in 40%, greater in 10%, and less in 50%. The gains from a Z-plasty depend on the ability of the skin in the base of the flaps to accommodate to the new position. That is, laxity or elasticity must be sufficient in the direction perpendicular to the central member to allow the flaps to transpose, or a Z-plasty may not be possible.

An increase in length may also be achieved by increasing the length of the central member (Figure 20-23, *B*). The disadvantage of increasing the length of the central member is the correspondingly larger scar that results. Multiple Z-plasties may be arranged serially so that they create a longer central member when added together (Figure 20-23, *C*). The gain in length, however, is actually less than a single longer central member, although the scar is also smaller.[30]

Double-opposing Z-plasties have been used for correction of epicanthal folds.[13] Other multiple Z-plasties include the

four-flap Z-plasty originally described by Berger,[4] in which the triangular flaps created by a Z-plasty with limbs at 90 degrees are divided, each creating two smaller flaps (Figure 20-24). There are also well-described five-flap (double-opposing) and six-flap Z-plasties (Figure 20-25).

The Z-plasty is often used to lengthen scar contractures, as occur across flexion creases, congenital skin webs (e.g., pterygium colli), and circumferential or U-shaped scars; to lengthen the lip in cleft lip repair; and to change the direction of scars or displaced tissues (e.g., eyebrow).

INTERPOLATION FLAPS. The interpolation flap is a racquet-shaped flap in which a distal skin paddle is supplied by a direct cutaneous vascular pedicle that has been dissected from surrounding structures. This flap is then transposed into a nearby defect. The dissected pedicle may pass above or below the intervening skin bridge. Monks' eyelid flap, a composite forehead flap based on the superficial temporal artery, which was tunneled subcutaneously to resurface the lower eyelid, is an early example of an interpolation flap.[53] This type of flap is also known as a *composite island flap* (Figure 20-26). It also includes the standard median forehead flap routinely used in nasal reconstruction.

Distant Transfer

For more extensive and distant defects when local and regional tissue were not adequate, innovative surgeons developed several methods for transferring tissue to a distant site, including the pedicle flap, the tubed pedicle flap, jumping flaps, and waltzing flaps. As depicted in *De Curtorum Chirurgia,* these

Table 20-4. Theoretic Gain in Length for Z-plasty Constructed at Different Angles	
ANGLES OF Z-PLASTY (DEGREES)	**THEORETIC GAIN IN LENGTH (%)**
30-30	25
45-45	50
60-60	75
75-75	100
90-90	120

Modified from Grabb WC, Smith JW, editors: In *Plastic surgery*, ed 3, Boston, 1979, Little, Brown.

flaps were identified by trial and error throughout history and were not refined until the last 150 years. It became apparent that certain flaps were more reliable and could be raised beyond the predicted length-to-width ratios of more traditional flaps because these flaps contained an AV pedicle within them, allowing the flap to be raised more safely.

Bakamjian's utilization of the larger deltopectoral flap for pharyngeal reconstruction[2] has its roots in the work of Manchot[44] (1889) and of Joseph[34] (1931), who described the deltopectoral flap as a *vascular pattern flap*. In 1863 Wood described a groin flap that was based on the superficial inferior epigastric artery and that was used to treat severe contractures on the dorsum of a young female patient's hand and forearm.[6] In 1972 McGregor and Jackson[49] redescribed the groin flap as an axial pattern flap, fashioned along the course of the superficial circumflex iliac artery. Further refinements of axial flaps led to the pedicle flaps and island flaps. In 1920 Gillies[27] noted that a flap could be made longer if a vessel were

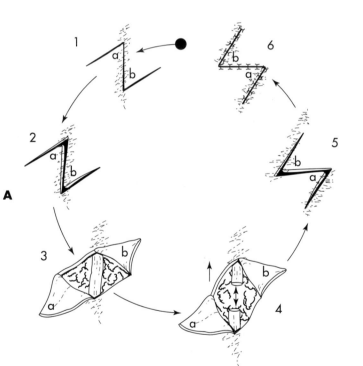

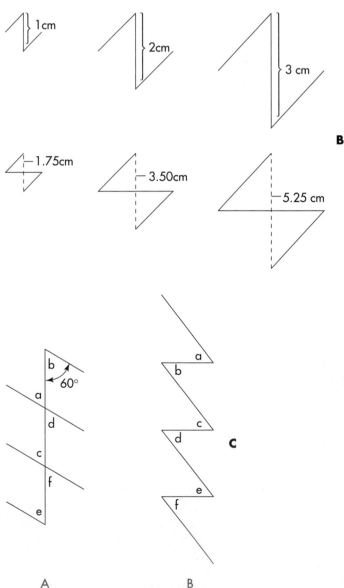

Figure 20-23. **A,** Z-plasty technique. *1,* Central limb designed along scar. Both limbs are equal in length. Angles *a* and *b* are 60 degrees. *2* and *3,* Flaps are incised and elevated. *4,* Release of deeper portion of scar. *5,* Transposition of triangular flaps. *6,* Wounds approximated. Note lengthening and new direction of scar. **B,** Greater gain in length with Z-plasty as length of central limb is increased. Lower row shows theoretic linear increase. **C,** Multiple Z-plasty technique. *A,* Design. *B,* Final appearance after transposition of flaps. Preferred technique for revision of long scars, especially on face. (From McCarthy JE, editor: *Plastic surgery*, Philadelphia, 1990, Saunders.)

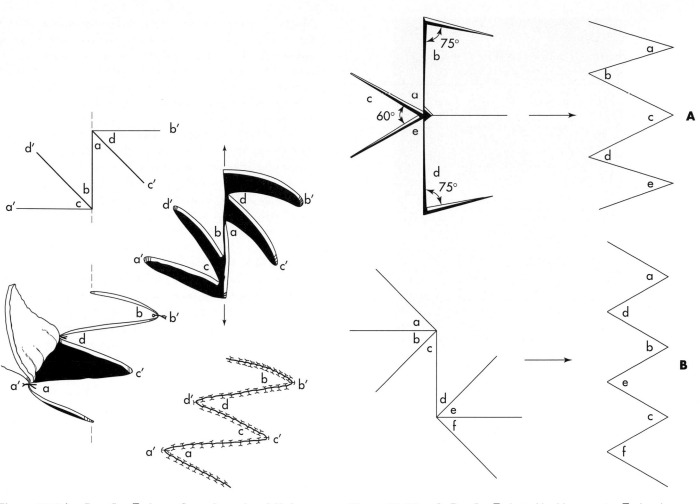

Figure 20-24. Four-flap Z-plasty. Central member *(ab)* drawn along area desired to be lengthened. Line *aba'* 90°, *cd'* bisects this angle. Line *a* meets *c̄; a'* add meets *c̄d'*.

Figure 20-25. **A,** Five-flap Z-plasty (double-opposing Z-plasty). **B,** Six-flap Z-plasty.

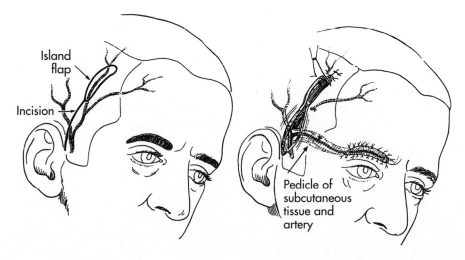

Figure 20-26. Interpolation (composite island) flap. (From McCarthy JG, editor: *Plastic surgery,* Philadelphia, 1990, Saunders.)

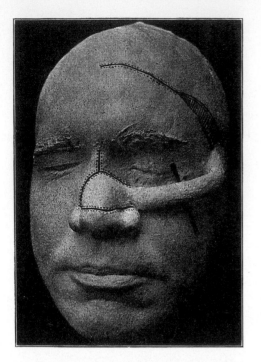

Figure 20-27. Gillies tubed pedicle flap nasal reconstruction. (From Gillies HD: *NY Med J* 111:1, 1920.)

contained in its base. This was the recipe for an *axial pattern flap,* a flap that contains a direct cutaneous vessel running in its longitudinal axis. After these initial descriptions a resurgence in anatomic studies of the blood supply to the skin and underlying structures led to a vast increase in the number and variety of axial flaps, which were safer and resulted in improved reconstruction.

TUBED PEDICLE FLAPS. Tubed pedicle flaps were very important historically but are seldom used today (Figure 20-27). Further developments of the tubed pedicle occurred earlier in the twentieth century with the work of Gillies and Filatov, who performed extensive reconstructions with tubed pedicle flaps, working out the ways in which these were transferred in stages, with intermediate wrist carriers.[27] These flaps involve multiple stages; the surgeon begins by incising and delaying flaps in areas with an abundance of tissue, eventually forming this flap into a tube. After the tube has matured, one end of the tube can be divided and sutured to an intermediate carrier, such as the wrist, and allowed to heal to the carrier. After adequate vascular connections have been made, the other end of the tube can be detached and the flap then brought to its final destination and partially inset, leaving it attached to the wrist carrier. Once healed in place, the flap is separated from the carrier and partially inset. Several other stages are generally needed to revise the flap in its new location. These flaps are largely of historic interest today because free tissue transfers have superseded them (Figure 20-28).

DISTANT PEDICLE FLAPS. Distant pedicle flaps are still widely used, mainly for extremity reconstruction. The most common pedicle flap for upper extremity reconstruction is the *groin flap* described by McGregor and Jackson[49] (Figure

20-29). This is an axial flap based on the superficial circumflex iliac vessels. A large flap can be raised from this relatively mobile area in the groin, allowing for primary closure of the donor defect and providing a large flap that can be used to resurface the hand. After 3 weeks, adequate vascular connections have been made between the flap and the hand, allowing the pedicle to be divided.

Pedicle flaps may also be raised from the trunk. These are often smaller and random flaps. Smaller pedicle flaps may also be used for reconstructing smaller defects on the fingertips. These include the cross-finger flaps and thenar flaps, which are staged pedicle flaps. In the lower extremity, cross-leg flaps may occasionally be indicated, although today they have been supplanted by free tissue transfers.

FREE FLAPS. Free flaps are currently the most commonly used method for reconstructing distant defects. Historically, refined knowledge of the vascular supply to the skin and subjacent structures and the concomitant development of microsurgery ushered in the era of free tissue transfer. In 1902 Carrel[10] described the anastomosis of blood vessels. In 1962 Jacobson and Suarez[33] described the microsurgical anastomosis of vessels. In 1963 Goldwyn et al[29] described the first successful free transfer in dogs. The initial experience with clinical microsurgery was with replantation of severed parts. Buncke et al[7] performed a toe-to-hand transfer in the rhesus monkey in 1966. In 1968 Komatsu and Tamai[38] replanted a severed thumb. In 1969 Cobbett[11] performed a toe-to-hand transfer to replace an amputated thumb. It then became apparent that these newly developed axial flaps could be raised on their feeding blood vessels as island pedicle flaps, which could be detached and reattached using these same techniques. Groin flaps were transferred to the neck in rats.[76]

The first attempted cutaneous free flap was reported by Kaplan, Buncke, and Murray[35] in 1973, but this survived only 3 weeks. The first successful free tissue transfer in a human was actually a kidney transplantation between monozygotic twins in 1954.[56] Daniel and Taylor[18] reported the first successful non–solid organ free tissue transfer in 1973. From a practical standpoint, these are axial flaps that are carefully dissected on their vascular pedicle, which is subsequently divided and reanastomosed microsurgically to appropriate vessels at the recipient site. Any axial flap may be raised as a free flap, and an expanding array of skin and subcutaneous tissue, fasciocutaneous, muscle, myocutaneous, osteomyocutaneous, omental, and other intestinal flaps may be used to reconstruct distant defects in a single stage.

Tissue Composition

Any type of tissue with an intact blood supply may be raised as a flap and used in reconstruction. Further descriptions of these individual flaps are provided in the respective chapters dealing with these anatomic areas.

Further vascular studies of the skin and underlying structures led to the understanding of the relationships among the blood supply of the skin, fascia, and muscle. This led to the development of muscle, musculocutaneous, fascial, and fasciocutaneous flaps. In 1893, Spalteholz[75] outlined the anatomy of

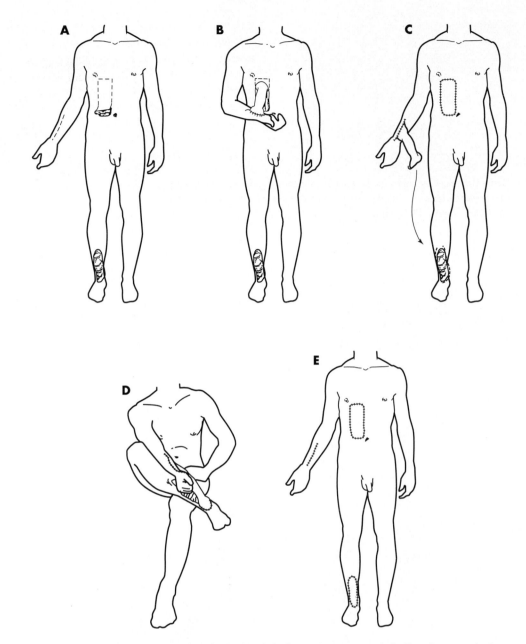

Figure 20-28. Stages in transfer of tubed pedicle flap with arm carrier. **A,** Flap design with chest donor and wrist carrier sites identified. **B,** Flap attached to arm carrier. **C,** Arm carrier maintains viability of chest flap for transfer. **D,** Flap attached to lower extremity defect. **E,** Flap base division and final flap inset. (From Mathes S, Nahai F: *Reconstructive surgery: principles, anatomy and technique,* London, 1997, Churchill Livingstone.)

the cutaneous blood supply, describing vessels that travel in the fascial septa to supply the skin and those that also supply muscle before penetrating the fascia to supply the skin. In 1968 Hueston and McConchie[32] described a compound pectoral flap, clinically demonstrating that the underlying muscle could perfuse a paddle of skin. In 1977 McCraw et al[47] described vascular territories of several new musculocutaneous units with proper dimensions and arcs of rotation. Mathes and Nahai[45] developed a classification scheme for the blood supply to muscle. In 1981 Ponten[61] described a clinical series of 23 fasciocutaneous flaps for lower extremity reconstruction. In 1984 Cormack and Lamberty[14] devised a classification system for fasciocutaneous flaps. These newly described flaps could be used as local and regional flaps based on their vascular pedicles, or they could be detached and transferred microsurgically.

MUSCLE, MUSCULOCUTANEOUS, AND PERFORATOR FLAPS. The appreciation that the muscles and the overlying tissues receive a predictable axial blood supply was a major milestone in the evolution of flap reconstruction. Mathes and Nahai[45] studied different muscle groups and provided a classification of the different patterns of vascular anatomy, which they divided into five groups (Figure 20-30 and Table 20-5). *Type I* flaps have a single pedicle; *type II* flaps have a dominant pedicle and one or more minor pedicles; *type III* flaps have two dominant pedicles; *type IV* flaps have a

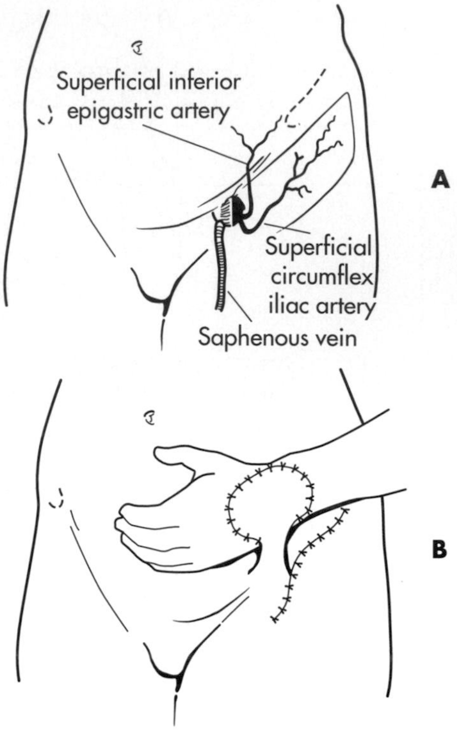

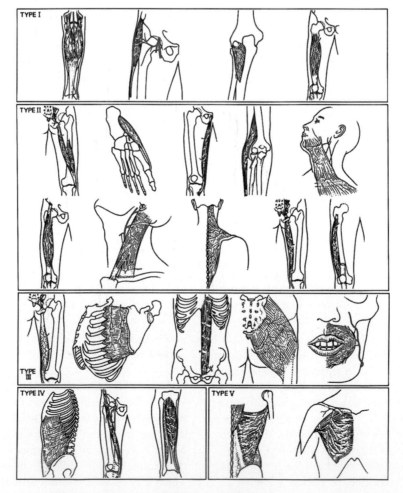

Figure 20-29. Groin flap. **A,** Key anatomic landmarks with design and vascular supply. **B,** Transfer of flap to cover distant hand defect with tubing of intervening pedicle. (From McCarthy JG, editor: *Plastic surgery,* Philadelphia, 1990, Saunders.)

Figure 20-30. Classification and examples of muscle flaps. (From Cormack GC, Lamberty BGH: *The arterial anatomy of skin flaps,* ed 2, London, 1994, Churchill Livingstone.)

Table 20-5.
Classification and Examples of Musculocutaneous (Myocutaneous) Flaps

TYPE	DESCRIPTION	EXAMPLES
I	One vascular pedicle	Anconeus Gastrocnemius Tensor fasciae latae Vastus intermedius
II	One dominant pedicle and one or more smaller pedicles	Biceps femoris Rectus femoris Soleus Sternocleidomastoid Temporalis Trapezius
III	Two dominant pedicles	Gluteus maximus Rectus abdominis Semimembranosus Serratus anterior
IV	Segmental pedicles	Extensor hallucis longus Sartorius Vastus medialis
V	One dominant pedicle and several smaller segmental pedicles	Pectoralis major Latissimus dorsi

Modified from: Cormack GC, Lamberty BGH: *The arterial anatomy of skin flaps,* ed 2, London, 1994, Churchill Livingstone.

segmental blood supply; and *type V* flaps have a single dominant pedicle with secondary segmental pedicles. Muscle flaps are unique because of the following:

1. Their bulk can be used to fill large defects.
2. They are malleable and conform to the contours of an irregular or complex wound.
3. They confer some ability to resist infection at the recipient site because of their vascularity, which is much greater than the blood supply to the skin. For example, several studies have described their salutary effect on osteomyelitis.

The transfer of a muscle flap results in some diminished function at the donor site, a clinical area that needs to be carefully evaluated with outcomes research. Recently, several studies have functionally evaluated various muscle (e.g., latissimus dorsi) donor sites.

Further study of the vascular anatomy of these flaps led to further refinement as surgeons realized that the muscle itself was not needed as long as the perforating vessels of the skin and subcutaneous tissues were preserved. This led to the development of *perforator flaps,* which have been shown to be reliable, but which involve a more tedious dissection of the pedicle through the substance of the muscle to the deeper source vessels.[1,5,38] Beneficial byproducts of these new developments are the possibility of raising reliable thinner flaps for reconstruction and the potential decrease in donor site morbidity.

Finally, when muscle flaps are used, they may also be transferred as a functional unit by coapting a motor or sensory nerve of the flap to an appropriate nerve at the recipient site. This is typically performed in conjunction with a cross-facial nerve graft for facial reanimation or in transverse rectus abdominis myocutaneous (TRAM) flap breast reconstruction for protective sensation.

FASCIOCUTANEOUS FLAPS. Depending on the site, many cutaneous and fasciocutaneous flaps are now available for reconstruction. The vascularity and reliability of each flap have been evaluated. Appreciation of the anatomy, especially of the underlying blood supply, is essential for the safe raising and transfer of these flaps. The advantages, disadvantages, special characteristics, and limitations of each flap and the resulting donor defect must also be considered when planning reconstruction. The resulting defect may be closed primarily by direct suture due to the mobility of the surrounding tissues. Alternatively, skin grafting or a second flap (e.g., rotational) may close the donor site.

Anatomic studies of the skin's blood supply also led to the description of many large fasciocutaneous flaps from tissues with deep fascia, such as the trunk and extremities. Ponten,[61] in 1981, first described fasciocutaneous flaps in the lower extremity (type A in the Cormack and Lamberty scheme). Cormack and Lamberty[14] classified these flaps into three different subgroups and further described their vascular anatomy (Figure 20-31). These are large, safe flaps containing no muscle and are based on an axial blood supply coming from deeper source vessels in the septa between muscle groups.

OTHER TISSUES. The *omentum* is another type of axial flap that may be raised as a pedicle flap based on the right or left gastroepiploic vessels and used for extraperitoneal reconstruction (e.g., chest wall, intrathoracic, and back defects). This flap can also be detached and transferred as a free flap for distant reconstruction where a large raw surface needs to be covered. After transfer, the defect is covered with a split-thickness skin graft. When used as a pedicle flap, various methods have been described by Das[19] and others to open up the arcades and lengthen the omentum to extend its reach well into the lower extremities. As a free flap, the greater omentum has also been used to neovascularize ischemic areas, such as in the upper and lower extremities, where conventional vascular surgical bypass procedures were not possible. The omental flap has also been used as a lymphatic conduit over scarred areas (e.g., groin) associated with lymphedema of the extremity.

Free tissue transfers can also be performed with segments of small and large intestine as well as from the greater curvature of the stomach, with or without the omentum, for reconstruction of the upper aerodigestive tract.

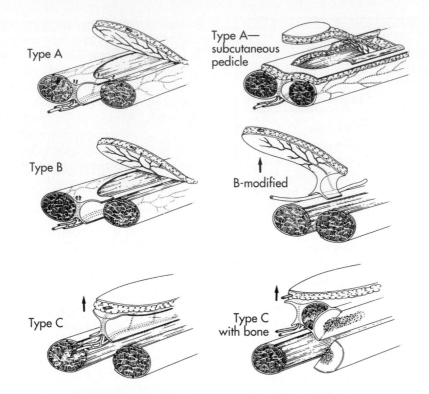

Figure 20-31. Classification of fasciocutaneous flaps. Type A flaps contain several axial fasciocutaneous vessels that enter its base. An example is the "super flap" described by Ponten. Type B flaps are supplied by a single fasciocutaneous perforator. An example is the parascapular flap. Type C flaps are supplied by multiple Sm perforators, which pass along a fascial septum between muscles. An example is the radial forearm flap, a.k.a., the Chinese screen flap. (From: Cormack GC, Lamberty BGH: *The arterial anatomy of skin flaps,* ed 2, London, 1994, Churchill Livingstone.)

COMPOSITE FLAPS. Tissues other than skin, fascia, and muscle may be required for more complex reconstruction, and thus composite flaps may be used. The blood vessels that supply the overlying muscle and skin also supply adjacent bone, nerve, and joints. Thus composite flaps may be raised as osseous flaps, osteocutaneous flaps, osteomusculocutaneous flaps, and sensory flaps. Free joints may also be raised as axial flaps and subsequently transferred as free flaps. Entire subunits, such as double toes, toe pulp, toenail and bone, and toe joints, may all be raised as composite flaps to reconstruct specific defects in the upper extremity. Vascularized tendon grafts and vascularized nerve grafts have been described and transferred to reconstruct specific defects.

Blood Supply

Flaps may also be classified by their blood supply (see earlier discussion). Several interesting applications of flaps depend on the unique utilization of their vascular anatomy.

REVERSE-FLOW FLAPS. Reverse-flow flaps are also known as *distal pedicle flaps* or *reverse–axial pattern flaps.* Not all distally based flaps are reverse flow, since perforating vessels spread out radially in the subcutaneous tissues. Thus a flap may be oriented such that flow is antegrade and yet the pedicle may be based proximally, distally, medially, or laterally. These flaps are created when the proximal blood supply is divided, leaving only its distally based pedicle to provide perfusion and venous drainage, essentially reversing flow in the vessels (Figure 20-32). This follows Taylor's angiosome concept. If the flap encroaches on an adjacent angiosome, however, the blood flow is reversed. The arterial supply typically depends on the presence of choke vessels to exploit the potential connection of one arteriosome to an adjacent arteriosome.[82] The venous valves that normally prevent retrograde flow are bypassed through macrovenous and microvenous connections, avalvular segments that Taylor called oscillating veins. These venous connections can take several days to compensate fully, and the flap often experiences a transient period of venous hypertension.

Reverse-flow flaps exemplify how flaps were developed empirically before any understanding of the blood supply or how they work. A number of examples exist, including a distally based radial forearm fasciocutaneous flap, a posterior interosseous flap, and a reversed first dorsal metacarpal artery flap useful in hand reconstruction. In the lower extremity, distally based sural fasciocutaneous flaps based on perforators from the peroneal artery, as well as reversed flexor hallucis longus flaps based on retrograde flow through the peroneal artery[65] itself, are useful for foot and ankle reconstruction.

VENOUS FLAPS. Venous flaps are a type of free flap created by making a direct AV anastomosis. These flaps are unreliable

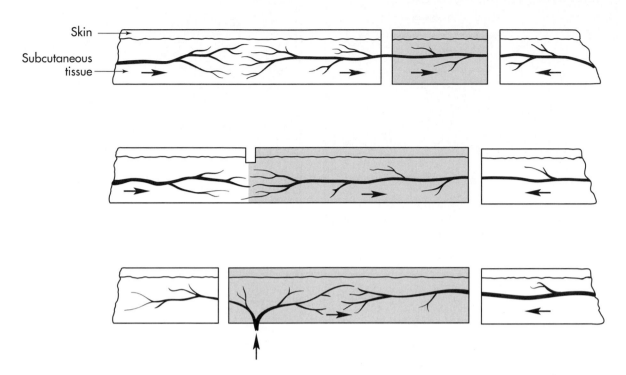

Skin →
Subcutaneous tissue →

Figure 20-32. Reverse-flow flaps. (From Cormack GC, Lamberty BGH: *The arterial anatomy of skin flaps,* ed 2, London, Churchill Livingstone.)

and have a variable rate of survival and a potential for the complications concomitant with an AV fistula. Although exactly how they work is unclear, it is generally believed that venous flaps have a better survival rate if they are fashioned as flow-through flaps.

Flow-through free flaps are another potential modification of a free flap where the vascular pedicle not only nourishes the flap covering the defect but also acts as a conduit. These are useful for revascularizing tissue distal to a defect.

SUPERCHARGING

Supercharging is a method of augmenting the blood supply to a large pedicled flap that may extend beyond the boundary of a single pedicle by performing a microvascular anastomosis to a secondary or distal pedicle in that flap. It is most often used for superiorly based unipedicle TRAM flaps, in which the ligated deep inferior epigastric artery and vein are anastomosed to vessels in the axilla, neck, or chest. This method takes advantage of the deep inferior epigastric artery being the dominant vessel in this flap and better able to support the most distal random portion (zone IV). Supercharging may be employed as an alternative to a double-pedicle TRAM flap to decrease donor site morbidity. It may also be used to salvage a jeopardized flap.

Yamamoto et al[86] reviewed 50 TRAM flaps, some of which were unipedicled and others augmented or supercharged. They concluded that the incidence of flap site complications was significantly less in the augmented group than in the

unipedicled group. Although not necessary in all TRAM flap reconstructions, supercharging is clearly beneficial in some carefully selected patients.

FLAP MANIPULATION BEFORE TRANSFER

Flap Delay

With further evolution and refinement of flap transfer, various techniques have been described in which the flap may be modified before its transfer. One such technique is flap delay. Delay is typically accomplished surgically, but pharmacologic interventions that are believed to have an effect similar to surgical delay are also used and referred to as *pharmacologic delay.* Surgical delay may be done to increase vascularity, thereby increasing the length and reliability of the flap. These techniques were used frequently before the description and use of axial flaps, fasciocutaneous flaps, musculocutaneous flaps, and free flaps. Although used less often today, surgical delay has many potential applications because it may be used adjunctively to lengthen flaps all over the body.

Hamilton first described the principle of flap delay in 1854.[67] Although not called "delay," Tagliacozzi surgically delayed his upper arm flap in the sixteenth century, saying that he wanted to make the flap "firm and robust"[15] (Figure 20-33). In his description of tubed pedicle flaps in 1920, Gillies[27] also relied on surgical delay. In 1965 Milton[51] performed classic experiments in the pig, comparing ventrally based flaps using differing methods of flap delay: a bipedicle flap, an L-shaped incision and corresponding undermining, a

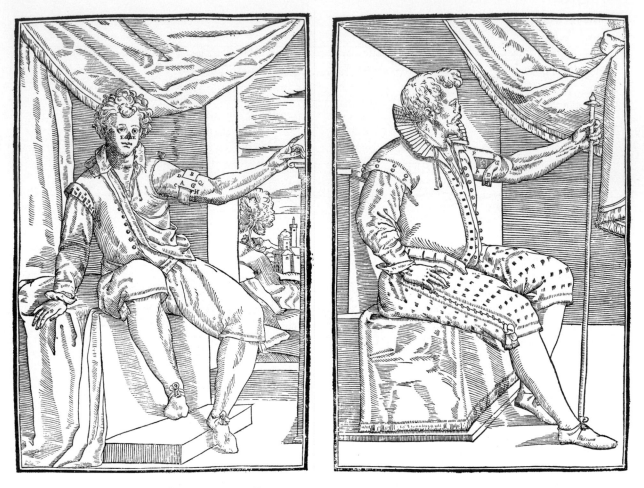

Figure 20-33. Flap delay, as depicted by Tagliacozzi in 1597.

U-shaped flap with corresponding undermining, and a simple U-shaped incision with no undermining. Milton demonstrated that the bipedicle delay technique provided the best results (Figure 20-34).

A typical process of flap delay involves raising a rectangular flap on two sides, essentially creating a bipedicle flap. One week later the third side is divided; division of the third side may also be done in two stages 3 days apart. Eventually, between day 10 and 14, the flap is raised based on the blood flow from the single remaining intact side. Increased flap length survival may range from 60% to 100%. Recommendations for the timing of delay vary from several days to several weeks. Lopez et al,[42] using immunohistochemical methods, showed that the number and size of capillaries increased in delayed flaps from 48 hours to a maximum at 7 days. They believed that the greatest benefit is derived by 7 days. Pang et al[59] showed that blood flow in delayed flaps increased within 2 days, reached a plateau after day 3, and showed no change between day 4 and 14.

The mechanism by which flap delay works has not been completely elucidated and involves many factors. Apparently the benefit is derived from (1) an alteration in the sympathetic tone secondary to a sympathectomy, (2) an increase in vascularity of the flap with possibly a reorientation of the vessels and formation of new vessels, (3) the dilation of choke

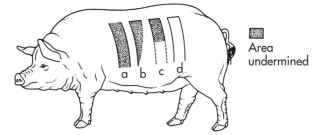

Figure 20-34. Early experiment of delayed flaps in the pig. (From Milton SH: *Br J Plast Surg* 22:244, 1965.)

vessels, and (4) the possibility of conditioning or hardening to ischemia by metabolic alterations.

A significant contributor to flap ischemia in the immediate postelevation phase is the hyperadrenergic state that results from creation of the flap. It is postulated that division of the sympathetic nerves results in a release of noradrenaline from the nerve endings, causing a transient hyperadrenergic state.[60] Several authors have published data that suggest that surgical or pharmacologic delay, which ameliorates this postelevation hyperadrenergic state, resulted in improved flap survival. Isoxsuprine, a direct vascular smooth muscle relaxant, has been shown to produce the delay pahenomenon in rats.[22]

Pearl[60] has presented a coherent conceptualization of the role of the hyperadrenergic state and its relationship to delay. Specifically, an initial postelevation hyperadrenergic state lasts up to 30 hours and results in vasoconstriction, predominantly affecting the precapillary sphincters and reducing nutrient blood flow to the flap. In the distal, random end of a freshly elevated flap, decreased nutrient flow coupled with decreased inflow from elevation may lead to ischemia. In a bipedicle delayed flap, however, the inflow is not as greatly compromised during this period of vasoconstriction and the tissues are able to endure the transient hyperadrenergic state. Finseth and Cutting's work[23] supports this concept. They maintain that delay results in vasodilation secondary to sympathectomy, with increased nutrient blood flow. They evaluated flap delay by dividing artery alone, vein alone, nerve alone, artery and vein, or artery, vein, and nerve. All these combinations resulted in improved flap survival in their rat model. Division of vein alone gave the least benefit, whereas division of all three structures gave the greatest delay benefit.

Other factors involved in the delay phenomenon result in increased blood flow and are independent of sympathectomy. Anatomic studies have shed some light on the changes associated with the delay phenomenon. An increase in the number and size of vessels and a change in their orientation, favoring vessels parallel to the long axis of the flap, have been demonstrated experimentally.[73] The work by Taylor and others is important because it provides a framework on which to conceptualize blood flow anatomically and dynamically. This facilitates flap planning and contributes to an understanding of the mechanism and effects of delay. These authors have demonstrated experimentally that the maximal anatomic effect on the arterial side, secondary to surgical delay, is at the level of the choke vessels that link adjacent vascular territories. Clinically, this is the area of a flap that is most likely to undergo necrosis, with demarcation at the zone of the choke vessels. Anatomically, these vessels increase appreciably in size in response to delay. A sequential increase in size of the choke vessel occurs during the delay period, with a rapid increase in size between 48 and 72 hours. Also, tissue expansion is a form of delay with demonstrable vessel hypertrophy.[9,54,80]

Delay also has many effects on tissue metabolism, utilization of substrates (e.g., oxygen, glucose), and balance of the products of arachidonic acid. Murphy et al[55] showed that in a rat model, thromboxane and PGF_2 were transiently increased and then returned to normal, with a blunted increase compared with controls when the delayed flaps were ultimately raised. This was in the setting of an increase in PGE_2 in the delayed flaps. The authors concluded that inflammatory mediators are an important component of the delay process.

Current applications of delay include TRAM flap reconstruction of the breast in high-risk patients (e.g., obesity, smoking, history of radiation, requirement for large flap). A recent study of delay performed in high-risk patients as outpatient surgery, followed by a TRAM flap, showed increased diameter and flow of the superior epigastric artery and decreased flap necrosis.[69] Some novel applications of the delay process are more pertinent to free tissue transfer in the setting of arterialized venous flaps and prefabricated flaps.[8,43]

Tissue Expansion

Another modification increasingly used in reconstruction is preliminary tissue expansion before flap transfer. Although the concept of stretching skin for closure dates back to Celsus (25 BC),[12] Neumann[57] is credited with the first modern report of this technique in 1957. Radovan[68] broadened its clinical application to breast reconstruction in 1976. Expansion is achieved by inserting a silicone bag beneath the flap and serially injecting saline over time, often waiting 3 to 5 days between injections. Tissue expansion has the beneficial effects of the delay process, stimulates angiogenesis, and provides overall thinning of the flap, which may be advantageous for reconstruction. Also, the use of tissue expansion enables a larger flap to be harvested and may allow for direct closure of the resulting donor defect. The base of the expander generally needs to be 2 to 2.5 times the size of the defect. Expanders are contraindicated in poorly vascularized areas and in the presence of infection.

Flap Prelamination and Prefabrication

In an effort to further improve reconstruction, techniques for manipulation of flaps before transfer have also been described. This includes the prelamination of flaps to create a multilayered flap before transfer. The concept of *flap prelamination* has recently been introduced into the reconstructive literature and has further increased the repertoire of reconstructive options. This involves the insertion of other tissue layers into a flap before transfer. These maneuvers are usually done for modifying a flap used in head and neck reconstruction, especially for the central part of the face, which consists of specialized tissues with multiple surfaces, all of which need to be addressed in the reconstructive process. Thus the surgeon is not limited by natural flaps. This has led to the possibility of custom designing flaps that are thinner or have special characteristics that would enhance the specific reconstruction. Gillies and Millard[28] lined midline forehead flaps with skin and cartilage grafts before pedicle transfer for total nasal reconstruction. Baudet et al[3] and Pribaz et al[66] have used prelamination techniques on the forearm for total nasal and central facial reconstruction.

Another area of flap manipulation is the total introduction of a new blood supply to an area of tissue, termed *flap prefabrication*. As noted earlier, this involves the transfer of a vascular pedicle containing the artery, its venae comitantes, and the surrounding adventia with or without fascia or small amount of muscle into the area to be neovascularized. After 6 weeks, by a process of inosculation and neovascularization, the tissue surrounding the implanted vascular pedicle can be raised as flap and transferred either locally or distantly as a free flap. This technique has been useful for creating thin flaps at a distant site, especially in the burn patient for head and neck reconstruction. It has also been used in the head and neck to create a pedicled flap that would have better color and texture for facial reconstruction. Flaps with special characteristics, such as hair-bearing flaps, can also be prefabricated by this technique.[64]

FLAP MONITORING

Methods to facilitate monitoring of the flap vary greatly in complexity and invasiveness. They are used primarily with free tissue transfer and thus are addressed only briefly here. Assessment of the flap begins with a clinical evaluation of temperature, color, capillary refill, and bleeding with puncture. The flap and surrounding tissues should also be assessed to identify a possible problem extrinsic to the flap, such as a hematoma, a seroma, kinking, or compression from positioning or dressings. Assessment of temperature, color, and capillary refill is subjective and prone to error. Bleeding from stab wounds can be a useful in identifying a problem and determining whether it is predominantly arterial or venous.[36]

More formal tests to assess blood flow and viability include chemical tests such as the use of vital dyes, nuclear medicine studies, and use of specific sensors (e.g., oxygen pressure probes, laser Doppler, temperature probes). Fluorescein can be useful when injected intravenously at a dose of 1.5 mg/kg; an ultraviolet light is used to check for fluorescence at approximately 20 minutes.[48] Fluorescein has the disadvantages of requiring at least 20 minutes to perform, being able to assess only the exposed portion of the flap, being able to be repeated only every 8 hours, being associated occasionally with nausea and rarely with anaphylaxis, and tending to underestimate flap perfusion. Instruments are available to quantify the amount of fluorescein in the skin, allowing administration of smaller doses and more frequent assessment of flap viability.

OUTCOME STUDIES

Outcome studies are becoming increasingly relevant as the demand for quality in health care increases. Outcomes also allow plastic surgeons to state clinical results objectively in regard to cost, quality of life, patient satisfaction, and practice patterns. Since flap reconstruction is a relatively new area of research, there are more questions than answers, and many studies focus only on some functional aspect, not addressing quality of life or cost-benefit analysis.

In an early important outcomes study of flap reconstruction, Russell et al[71] performed a functional evaluation of latissimus dorsi donor sites. They evaluated the cosmetic and functional problems associated with free and pedicled muscle and myocutaneous flaps. All patients had a contour defect at the donor site. Most patients displayed mild to moderate shoulder weakness and loss of motions, which improved over several months. More than 95% of the patients were satisfied with the outcome and would recommend the operation to others.

Serletti and Moran[74] compared the costs and outcomes of free versus pedicled TRAM flaps. They found no significant difference in many variables for their 125 patients, including duration of hospital stay, return to work, strength, symmetry, and patient satisfaction. They saw no difference between the two groups with respect to perioperative complications. There was a difference in the complication rate between surgeons who performed microsurgical procedures infrequently versus more skilled surgeons. The authors stated that a surgeon's comfort level with the procedure should be a factor in the decision process.

In one of the few prospective outcome studies in this area, Kind et al[37] discussed the functional outcome in the abdominal wall after TRAM flap reconstruction. At 6 weeks postoperatively, the patients who had a unilateral pedicled TRAM flap were able to generate significantly less torque than the free TRAM group, 58% versus 87%, respectively. At 6 months, however, there was no significant difference, with torque generation at 89% and 93% for pedicled and free, respectively.

Additional outcomes data will help the plastic surgeon to deliver a higher quality of care commensurate with the current economy of health care.

SUMMARY

Plastic and reconstructive surgery has a rich history that is well represented by the historic events surrounding the utilization and development of flaps. This topic also is an excellent example of the tremendous breadth and depth of this surgical specialty, which affects all other medical specialties and spans all age groups, disabilities, and tissue types. Flap reconstruction is a bridge between normal and abnormal and thus is an excellent lens through which to view these issues and their disparity, similarity, utility and necessity.

Tagliacozzi's utilization of flap delay 400 years ago is a good example of the technical feats that have been accomplished over the years in the context of the medical knowledge at that time, especially since such procedures were performed without anesthesia. Flap advances are a testament to humankind's pursuit of knowledge and tremendous capacity to flourish under adversity. Many of these developments have occurred recently, and many more are on the horizon.

REFERENCES

1. Allen RJ, Treece P: Deep inferior epigastric perforator flap for breast reconstruction, *Ann Plast Surg* 32:32, 1994.
2. Bakamjian VY: A two-stage method for pharyngoesophageal reconstruction with a primary pectoral skin flap, *Plast Reconstr Surg* 36:173, 1965.
3. Baudet J, Pelissiet P, Casoli V: 1984-1994: ten years of skin flaps, *Ann Chir Plast Esthet* 40:597, 1995.
4. Berger P: Autoplastic par dedoublement de la palmure, et echange de lambeaux. In Berger P, Banzet S: *Chirurgie orthopedic*, Paris, 1904, Steinheil.

5. Blondell PN, Boeckx WD: Refinements in full breast reconstruction: the free bilateral deep inferior epigastric perforator flap anastomosed to the internal mammary artery, *Br J Plast Surg* 47:495, 1994.

6. Boo-Chai K: John Wood and his contribution to plastic surgery: the first groin flap, *Br J Plast Surg* 30:9, 1977.

7. Buncke HJ, Buncke CM, Schulz WP: Immediate Nicoladoni procedures in the rhesus monkey, or hallux-to-hand transplantation, utilising microminiature vascular anastomoses, *Br J Plast Surg* 19:332, 1966.

8. Byun JS, Constantinescu MA, Lee WP, May JW Jr: Effects of delay procedures on vasculature and survival of arterialized venous flaps: an experimental study in rabbits, *Plast Reconstr Surg* 96:1650, 1995.

9. Callegari PR, Taylor GI, Caddy CM, Minabe T: An anatomic review of the delay phenomenon. I. Experimental studies, *Plast Reconstr Surg* 89:397, 1992.

10. Carrel A: La technique operatoire des anastomoses vasculaires et la transplantation des viscere, *Lyon Med* 98:859, 1902.

11. Cobbett JR: Free digital transfer: report of a case of transfer of a great toe to replace an amputated thumb, *J Bone Joint Surg* 51B:677, 1969.

12. Converse JM: Introduction to plastic surgery. In *Reconstructive plastic surgery,* Philadelphia, 1977, Sanders.

13. Converse JM, Smith B: Naso-orbital fractures and traumatic deformities of the medial canthus, *Plast Reconstr Surg* 8:147, 1966.

14. Cormack GC, Lamberty BGH: A classification of fascio-cutaneous flaps according to their patterns of vascularization, *Br J Plast Surg* 37:80, 1984.

15. Cormack GC, Lamberty BGH: *The arterial anatomy of skin flaps,* ed 2, London, 1994, Churchill Livingstone.

16. Cronenwett JL, Zelenock GB, Whitehouse WM Jr, et al: The effect of sympathetic innervation on canine muscle and skin blood flow, *Arch Surg* 118:420, 1983.

17. Daniel RK, Kerrigan CL: Principles and physiology of skin flap surgery. In McCarthy JG, editor: *Plastic surgery,* Philadelphia, 1990, Saunders.

18. Daniel RK, Taylor GI: Distant transfer of an island flap by microvascular anastomoses, *Plast Reconstr Surg* 52:111, 1973.

19. Das SK: Use of the omentum in reconstructive surgery. In Barron JN, Saad MN, editors: *Operative plastic and reconstructive surgery,* vol 1, London, 1980, Churchill Livingstone.

20. Dufourmentel E: Le fermeture des pertes de substance cutane limites "le lambeau de rotation en L pour losange," *Ann Chir Plast Surg* 7:61, 1962.

21. Esser JFS: In Burget GC, Menick FJ: *Aesthetic reconstruction of the nose,* St Louis, 1994, Mosby.

22. Finseth F, Adelberg MG: Experimental work with isoxsuprine for prevention of skin flap necrosis and for treatment of the failing flap, *Plast Reconstr Surg* 63:94, 1979.

23. Fineseth F, Cutting C: An experimental neurovascular island flap for the study of the delay phenomenon, *Plast Reconstr Surg* 61:412, 1978.

24. Fricke JCG: *Bildung neuer Augenlider (Blepharoplastik) nach Zerstorung und dadarch hervorgebrachter Answartwendung derselben,* Hamburg, 1829, Perthes & Basser.

25. Furchgott RF, Zawadzki JV: The obligatory role of endothelial cell in the relaxation of arterial smooth muscle by acetylcholine, *Nature* 288:373, 1980.

26. *Gentleman's Magazine:* A communication to the editor (1794). In McCarthy JG, editor: *Plastic surgery,* Philadelphia, 1990, Saunders.

27. Gillies HD: The tubed pedicle in plastic surgery, *NY Med J* 111:1, 1920.

28. Gillies HD, Millard DR: *The principles and art of plastic surgery,* Boston, 1957, Little, Brown.

29. Goldwyn RM, Lamb DL, White WL: An experimental study of large island flaps in dogs, *Plast Reconstr Surg* 31:328, 1963.

30. Grabb WC: Basic techniques of plastic surgery. In Grabb WC, Smith JW, editors: *Plastic surgery,* ed 3, Boston, 1979, Little, Brown.

31. Horner WE: Clinical report on surgical department of the Philadelphia Hospital, *Am J Med Sci* 21:105, 1837.

32. Hueston JT, McConchie IH: A compound pectoral flap, *Aust NZ J Surg* 38:61, 1968.

33. Jacobson JH, Suarez EL: Microvascular surgery, *Dis Chest* 41:220, 1962.

34. Joseph J: Nasenplastik und Sontige Gesichtsplastik nebst einem Anhang veber Mammaplastik und einige weit—Operationen aus dem Gebiete der aussen Karper Plastic, Leipzig, 1931, Verlag Kaplitzsch.

35. Kaplan EN, Buncke HJ, Murray DE: Distant transfer of cutaneous island flaps in humans by microsurgical techniques, *Plast Reconstr Surg* 52:301, 1973.

36. Kerrigan CL, Daniel RK: Monitoring acute skin-flap failure, *Plast Reconstr Surg* 71:519, 1983.

37. Kind GM, Rademaker AW, Mustoe TA: Abdominal wall recovery following TRAM flap: a functional outcome study, *Plast Reconstr Surg* 99:417, 1997.

38. Komatsu S, Tamai S: Successful replantation of a completely cut-off thumb, *Plast Reconstr Surg* 42:374, 1968.

39. Koshima I, Soeda S: Inferior epigastric artery skin flaps without rectus abdominis muscle, *Br J Plast Surg* 42:645, 1989.

40. Lefer AM, Tsao PS, Lefer DJ, et al: Role of endothelial dysfunction in the pathogenesis of reperfusion injury after myocardial ischemia, *FASEB J* 5:20, 1991.

41. Limberg AA: *Mathematical principles of local plastic procedures on the surface of the human body,* Leningrad, 1946, Government Publishing House for Medical Literature.

42. Lopez JLA, Nieto CS, Garcia PB, Ortega JMR: Evaluation of angiogenesis in delayed skin flaps using a monoclonal antibody for the vascular endothelium, *Br J Plast Surg* 48:479, 1995.

43. Maitz PK, Pribaz JJ, Duffy FJ, Hergrueter CA: The value of the delay phenomenon in flap prefabrication: an experimental study in rabbits, *Br J Plast Surg* 47:149, 1994.

44. Manchot C: Die Hautarterien des Menschlicher Korpers, *Lepzig,* 1889, Vogel.

45. Mathes SJ, Nahai F: Classification of the vascular anatomy of muscles: experimental and clinical correlation, *Plast Reconstr Surg* 67:177, 1981.

46. Mathes S, Nahai F: *Reconstructive surgery: principles, anatomy and technique,* London, 1997, Churchill Livingstone.

47. McCraw JB, Dibbell DG, Carraway JH: Clinical definition of independent myocutaneous vascular territories, *Plast Reconstr Surg* 60:341, 1977.

48. McCraw JB, Myers B, Shanklin KD: The value of fluorescein in predicting the viability of arterialized flaps, *Plast Reconstr Surg* 60:710, 1977.

49. McGregor IA, Jackson IT: The groin flap, *Br J Plast Surg* 25:3, 1972.

50. Millard DR: *Principalization of plastic surgery,* Boston, 1986, Little, Brown.

51. Milton SH: The effects of delay on the survival of experimental studies on pedicled skin flaps, *Br J Plast Surg* 22:244, 1965.

52. Milton SH: Pedicled skin flaps: the fallacy of the length:width ratio, *Br J Surg* 57:50, 1970.

53. Monks GH: The restoration of the lower eyelid by a new method, *Boston Med Surg J* 139:385, 1898.

54. Morris SF, Taylor GI: The time sequence of the delay phenomenon: when is a surgical delay effective? An experimental study, *Plast Reconstr Surg* 95:526, 1995.

55. Murphy RC, Lawrence WT, Robson MC, Heggers JP: Surgical delay and arachidonic acid metabolites: evidence for an inflammatory mechanism: an experimental study in rats, *Br J Plast Surg* 38:272, 1985.

56. Murray JE, Merrill JP, Harrison JH: Renal homotransplantation in identical twins (surgical forum). In *Proceedings of the 41st Clinical Congress of the ACOS,* Chicago, 1955.

57. Neumann CG: The expansion of an area of skin by progressive distribution of a subcutaneous balloon, *Plast Reconstr Surg* 19:124, 1957.

58. Oien AH, Aukland K: A mathematical analysis of the myogenic hypothesis with special reference to the aurtoregulation of renal blood flow, *Circ Res* 52:241, 1983.

59. Pang CY, Forest CR, Negligan PC: Augmentation of blood flow in delayed random skin flaps in the pig: effect of length of delay period and angiogenesis, *Plast Reconstr Surg* 78:68, 1986.

60. Pearl RM: A unifying theory of the delay phenomenon: recovery from the hyperadrenergic state, *Ann Plast Surg* 7:102-112, 1981.

61. Ponten B: The fasciocutaneous flap: its use in soft tissue defects of the lower leg, *Br J Plast Surg* 34:215, 1981.

62. Pribaz JJ, Chester CH, Barrall DT: The extended V-Y flap, *Plast Reconstr Surg* 90:275, 1992.

63. Pribaz JJ, Fine NA: Prelamination: defining the prefabricated flap—a case report and review, *Microsurgery* 15:618, 1994.

64. Pribaz JJ, Fine N, Orgill DP: Flap prefabrication in the head and neck: a ten year experience, *Plast Reconstr Surg* 103:808-820, 1999.

65. Pribaz JJ, Orgill DO: Reverse peroneal flaps: two surgical approaches, *Ann Plast Surg* 33:17, 1994.

66. Pribaz JJ, Weiss DD, Mulliken JM, Eriksson E: Prelaminated free flap reconstruction of complex central facial defects, *Plast Reconstr Surg* 104:357-365, 1999.

67. Prince D: Plastics: a new classification and brief exposition of plastic surgery. In Strauch B, Vasconez LO, Hall-Findlay ED, editors: *Grabb's Encyclopedia of flaps,* ed 2, Philadelphia, 1998, Lippincott-Raven.

68. Radovan C: Adjacent flap development using expandable silastic implant. Presented at the annual ASPRS meeting, Boston, 1976.

69. Restifo RJ, Ward BA, Scoutt LM, et al: Timing magnitude and utility of surgical delay in TRAM flap. II. Clinical studies, *Plast Reconstr Surg* 99:1217, 1997.

70. Reus WF III, Colen LB, Straker DJ: Tobacco smoking and complications in elective microsurgery, *Plast Reconstr Surg* 89:490, 1992.

71. Russell RC, Pribaz J, Zook EG, et al: Functional evaluation of latissimus dorsi donor site, *Plast Reconstr Surg* 78:336, 1986.

72. Salmon M: *Arteres de la peau,* Paris, 1936, Masson.

73. Seitchik MW, Kahn S: The effects of delay on the circulatory efficiency of pedicled tissue, *Plast Reconstr Surg* 33:16, 1964.

74. Serletti JM, Moran SL: Free versus the pedicled TRAM flap: a cost comparison and outcome, *Plast Reconstr Surg* 100:1418, 1997.

75. Spalteholz W: Die Vertheilung der Blutgefasse in der Haut, *Arch Anat,* 1893.

76. Strauch B, Murray DE: Transfer of composite graft with immediate suture anastomosis of its vascular pedicle measuring less than 1 mm in external diameter using microsurgical techniques, *Plast Reconstr Surg* 40:325, 1967.

77. Tagliacozzi G: *De curtorum chirurgia per institione,* vol 2, Venice, 1597.

78. Tanzini I: Sporo il nito nuova processo di aupertoziane della menuelle, *Riforme Med* 22:757, 1906.

79. Taylor GI: The blood supply to the skin. In Aston SJ, Beasley RW, Thorne CHW, editors: *Grabb and Smith's Plastic surgery,* ed 5, Philadelphia, 1997, Lippincott-Raven.

80. Taylor GI, Corlett RJ, Caddy CM, Zelt RG: An anatomic review of the delay phenomenon. II. Clinical applications, *Plast Reconstr Surg* 89:408, 1992.

81. Taylor GI, Minabe T: The angiosomes of mammals and other vertebrates, *Plast Reconstr Surg* 89:181, 1992.

82. Taylor GI, Palmer JH: The vascular territories (angiosomes) of the body: experimental study and clinical applications, *Br J Plast Surg* 40:113, 1987.

83. Vallance P, Collier J, Moncada S: Effects of endothelium-derived nitric oxide on peripheral arteriolar tone in man, *Lancet* 2:997, 1989.

84. Wallace AF: History of plastic surgery, *J R Soc Med* 71:834, 1978.

85. Warren JM: Rhinoplastic operation, *Boston Med Surg J* 16(5), 1837.

86. Yamamoto Y, Nohira K, Sugihara T, et al: Superiority of the microvascularly adjusted flap: analysis of 50 transverse rectus abdominis myocutaneous flaps for breast reconstruction, *Plast Reconstr Surg* 97:79-83, 1996.

87. Yanagisawa M, Kurihara H, Kimura S, et al: A novel potent vasoconstrictor peptide produced by vascular endothelial cells, *Nature* 332:411, 1988.

88. Zimany A: The bilobed flap, *Plast Reconstr Surg* 11:424, 1953.

89. Zitelli JA: The bilobed flap for nasal reconstruction, *Arch Dermatol* 125:957, 1989.

90. Zook EG, Van Beek AL, Russell RC, Moore JB: V-Y advancement flap for facial defects, *Plast Reconstr Surg* 65:786, 1980.

PART II

GENERAL RECONSTRUCTIVE SURGERY

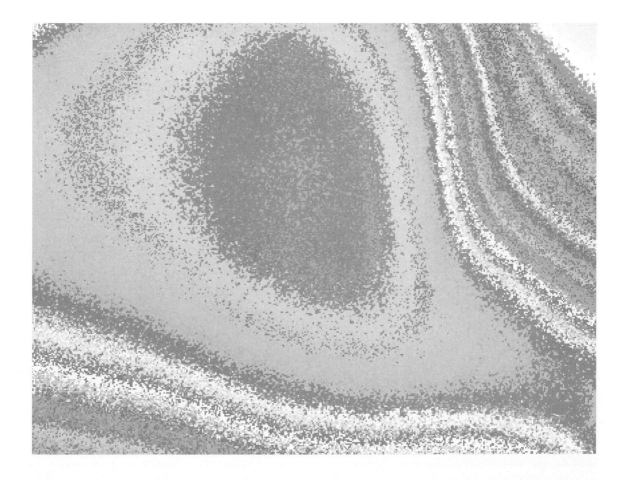

CHAPTER

Benign and Premalignant Skin Conditions

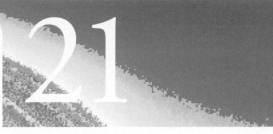

David Netscher
Melvin Spira
Victor Cohen

INTRODUCTION

This chapter discusses a wide spectrum of conditions, including pigmented skin lesions and deeper dermal pathology. Vascular tumors are specifically excluded. The lesions discussed can be broadly classified according to their tissue of origin: (1) *epidermis* (including melanocyte system), (2) *epidermal appendages* (hair structures, sebaceous glands, apocrine and eccrine glands), or (3) *dermis*.

INDICATIONS

Treatment of these skin conditions may be ablative or nonablative. Diagnostic biopsy may be required before definitive treatment can be performed. Biopsy may be therapeutic if, for example, excisional or shave biopsy totally eradicates the lesion. The indications for treatment of benign or premalignant skin conditions therefore depend on the following factors:

1. *Natural history of the lesion.* To advise a patient on treatment options, the surgeon must understand the potential for malignant transformation of such lesions as congenital nevus, actinic keratosis, Bowen's tumor, and nevus sebaceus of Jadassohn. Some lesions generally regarded as benign may be destructive in nature. For example, rapid enlargement with a subsequent deforming scar may occur with a keratocanthoma and its resolution.

2. *Lesion size.* Ablation of very large or diffusely disseminated lesions may be impractical, even in the presence of malignant potential, as with a giant congenital pigmented (bathing trunk) nevus or with multiple dysplastic nevi. On the other hand, diffuse actinic keratoses may be more practically treated by topical application of 5-fluorouracil than by surgical excisions, and a large congenital nevus may be more

satisfactorily treated by expansion of surrounding tissues and excision than by multiple serial excisions.

3. *Functional disturbances.* Early treatment may be required for benign lesions that compromise function by their size alone (e.g., larger cysts in eyelids or fingers). Such lesions may also compress nerve structures or have the potential for infection. Infected or abscessed inclusion cysts require incision and drainage, followed by definitive excision of the sac lining. Simple seborrheic keratoses irritated or traumatized by clothing (e.g., brassiere straps, collars) may need to be shaved.

4. *Anatomic location and cosmesis.* A patient or surgeon may elect to treat a lesion because of poor cosmetic appearance. For example, a periocular lesion may be cosmetically unsightly, and a subungual verruca not only disturbs nail growth function but is also ugly. Also, a surgeon may choose *not* to ablate a lesion for cosmetic reasons. For example, wide resection and skin grafting of a congenital nevus in a cosmetically exposed area may ultimately result in a worse cosmetic appearance than the untreated lesion. In certain critical areas, ablation may result in serious functional disturbance, and the surgeon may elect to treat the lesion by observation alone.

5. *Masked malignancy.* A surgeon may choose to excise congenital nevi in the scalp region because surveillance of this site for cancer development is difficult. A cutaneous horn, although not premalignant itself, may arise from an underlying squamous carcinoma and disguise its presence.

The surgeon then selects treatment method based on the following:

1. Lesion diagnosis and potential for malignant transformation
2. Location and size of lesion (to determine practicality of ablation)
3. Depth of skin involvement

Many epidermal lesions can be treated by shaving or curettage. These forms of treatment, where indicated, have an advantage over elliptic excision, since the deeper dermal layers are not violated and the likelihood of adverse scarring is minimized.

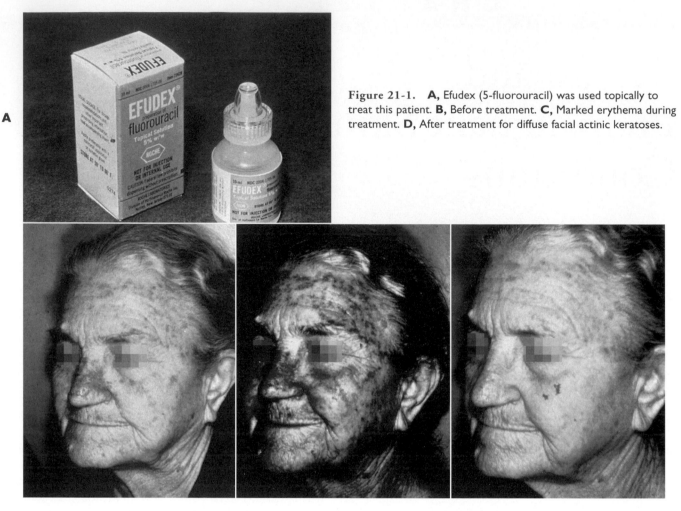

Figure 21-1. **A,** Efudex (5-fluorouracil) was used topically to treat this patient. **B,** Before treatment. **C,** Marked erythema during treatment. **D,** After treatment for diffuse facial actinic keratoses.

A

B   **C**   **D**

OPERATIONS

After discussing treatment options, this section describes various benign and premalignant skin conditions, with greater detail on appropriate treatments available for each.

TYPES OF TREATMENT

Patient Observation and Surveillance

If ablation is not feasible or possible for whatever reason, periodic clinical examination with follow-up photographs assists in detecting potential malignant transformation. Such a course may be chosen when total excision of a large congenital nevus is impractical, when a patient has multiple dysplastic nevi, or when certain syndromal conditions (e.g., xeroderma pigmentosum, basal cell nevus syndrome) with a high risk for development of cutaneous malignancy are present.

Topical Medications

Diffusely spread conditions with malignant potential may be best treated by topically applied 5-fluorouracil. The typical

regimen is 4 weeks of twice-daily application of 2% 5-fluorouracil solution on a cotton-tipped applicator to cover the area; a face cream is applied daily for 2 weeks thereafter (Figure 21-1).

Bowen's lesions and basal cell or squamous cell cancers are not amenable to 5-fluorouracil treatment. Verrucae may be treated by topical application of podophyllin or keratolytic agents such as salicylic acid.

Curettage

The 5-mm curet (curette) is the size most often used, although curets as small as 2 mm are available. The hollow ring curet offers superior visibility and control over the true spoon-shaped curet used by orthopedists for cutaneous surgery. Curettage is performed after adequate local anesthesia. The procedure yields material for histologic examination and allows safe removal of superficial lesions with minimal scarring.

After curettage, hemostasis may be achieved by light electrocautery. The curetted area is cleansed daily and covered with antibiotic ointment and a light dressing.

Lesions especially amenable to treatment by curettage include actinic and seborrheic keratoses and verruca vulgaris.

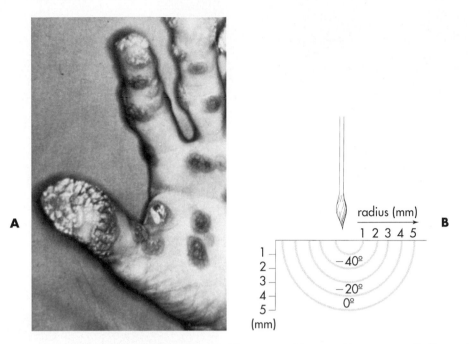

Figure 21-2. **A,** Verrucae on fingers are probably most suitably treated by curettage. **B,** Tapered cotton-tipped applicator dipped in liquid nitrogen is applied to lesion treated by cryotherapy. Cells are killed within outward-spreading freezing wave.

Curettage is an excellent treatment for subungual verrucae, leaving virtually no residual nail deformity (Figure 21-2, *A*). The nail plate is removed, and with loupe magnification the curet can identify a clear cleavage plane along the deep surface of the verruca.

Cryosurgery

Cryosurgery is the destruction of tissue by the application of intense cold in which all cells within the freezing wave are killed (Figure 21-2, *B*). Liquid nitrogen is ideal for removing warts, superficial keratoses, and actinic lentigines. It should be used with caution, however, in areas where peripheral nerves may be immediately subjacent. Permanent freeze damage to nerves may result from careless liquid nitrogen treatment of lesions on the fingers or over the olecranon. This technique must be limited to clearly benign lesions because no material is obtained for pathology.

A cotton-tipped applicator is used, with the cotton teased out and tapered. The applicator is dipped into a thermos of liquid nitrogen and applied to the lesion. As the liquid nitrogen runs down the applicator, the skin at the applicator tip turns white and the ice front spreads outward; application should cease when the area of visible freezing extends just beyond the lesion. The rate of delivery of liquid nitrogen can be adjusted by altering the degree of saturation and the applicator angle.

Cryosurgery causes little pain and rarely requires anesthesia. Occasionally a patient may experience pain for up to 24 hours posttreatment and may require analgesia. Although the aesthetic results are usually excellent, hypopigmentation may result, and cryotherapy is used with caution in dark-skinned patients.

Electrosurgery

Electrosurgery refers to tissue destruction by the conversion of electrical energy into heat through tissue resistance. An office hyfrecator is an adequate electrosurgical instrument for small cutaneous lesions and may be used to destroy seborrheic keratoses, skin tags, lentigines, and spider nevi.

Biopsy

SHAVE BIOPSY. This removes the portion of skin elevated because of the exophytic nature of the disease process, the manner of injection of local anesthetic, or the technique of tissue stabilization, which involves pinching the skin between thumb and index finger above the plane of the surrounding tissue (Figure 21-3). Shave biopsy is appropriate for conditions such as seborrheic or actinic keratoses and warts, in which characteristic histologic changes are expected in the epidermis or papillary dermis. Shave biopsies are not suitable for neoplasms that clinically appear to infiltrate the dermis or for pigmented lesions with even slight clinical suspicion of melanoma.

PUNCH BIOPSY. This may be either incisional or excisional, resulting in partial or complete removal of the lesion, depending on its size. Punch biopsy is performed with a circular cutting instrument, available in sizes ranging from 1.5 to 6 mm; 3 mm and 4-mm punches are most often used.

The biopsy site is cleansed with alcohol, and local anesthetic is injected into the deep dermis. When the circular punch incision reaches subcutaneous fat, the punch is removed. Shallow biopsies are subject to misinterpretation and must be avoided. The small cylinder of tissue is then gently lifted, and

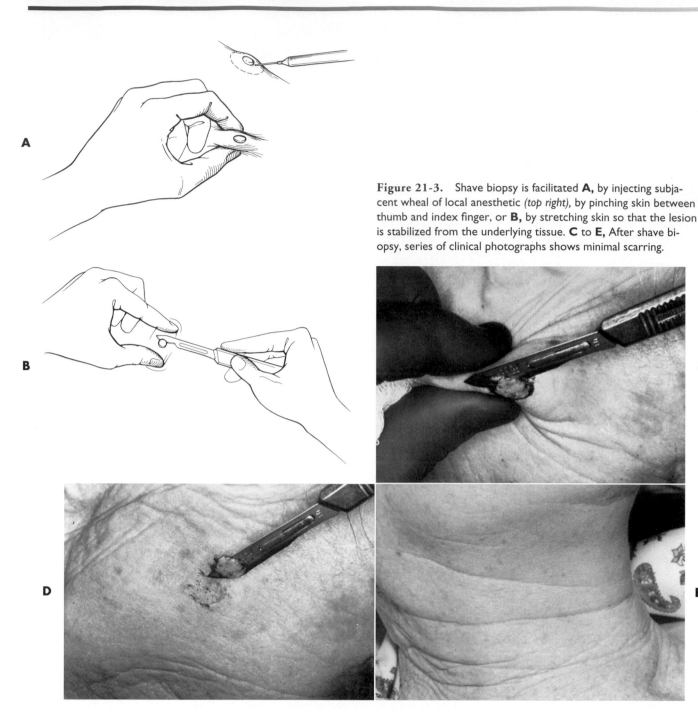

Figure 21-3. Shave biopsy is facilitated **A,** by injecting subjacent wheal of local anesthetic *(top right),* by pinching skin between thumb and index finger, or **B,** by stretching skin so that the lesion is stabilized from the underlying tissue. **C** to **E,** After shave biopsy, series of clinical photographs shows minimal scarring.

its base transected at the level of the subcutaneous tissue with a small iris scissors (Figure 21-4).

After a 3-mm excisional punch biopsy, hemostasis is achieved by pressure or light cautery. Sutures are not placed, and a very favorable cosmetic appearance results from cicatricial contracture to a tiny dimple. Sampling error is minimized by carefully choosing which portion of a lesion to biopsy. A pigmented lesion suspected of being a melanoma should not be biopsied but should undergo an excision that encompasses the entire lesion, with margins of 1 to 2 mm.

ELLIPTIC INCISIONAL/EXCISIONAL BIOPSIES. When a lesion is large enough to make excisional biopsy impractical, incisional biopsy with a margin of normal adjacent skin can

provide a histologic diagnosis before definitive therapy is planned. As long as subsequent excision is performed in a timely manner for histologically proven malignant conditions, prior incisional biopsy does not alter the natural history of melanoma or other cutaneous malignancies. Incisional biopsies for larger, deeper dermal lesions should generally be oriented longitudinally on extremities so that the resulting scar (which may have to be excised later) does not interfere with the possible need for compartmental excision of a malignant soft tissue sarcoma.

Excisional biopsy of lesions is usually done in an elliptic fashion so that linear closure can be performed along the line of least skin tension. Excess skin of the "dog ear" is excised (Figure 21-5, *A*). If the line of least skin tension is difficult to

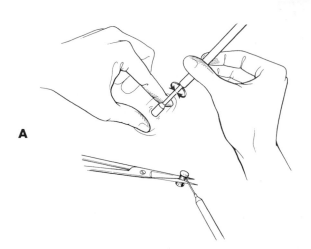

A

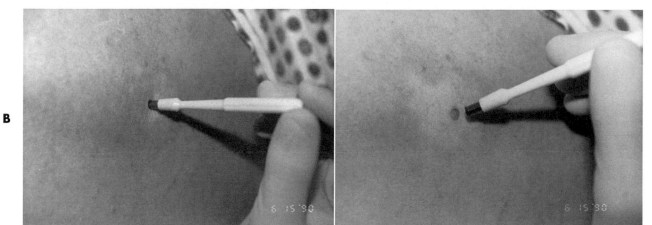

Figure 21-4. **A,** Steps in obtaining punch biopsy. **B** and **C,** Some small cutaneous lesions may be completely excised with appropriate-size punch.

B

C

A

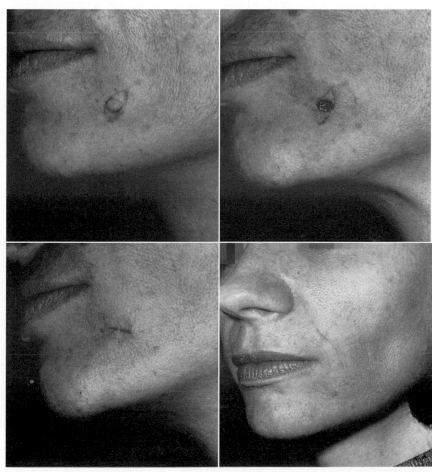

Figure 21-5. **A,** Method of excision of "dog ear." **B** to **E,** Planned elliptic excision is marked out and noted to be 90 degrees to excision indicated by lines of least tension. Once lesion excised as exact circle, resulting gaping ellipse is then sutured, with good cosmetic result.

D

E

determine, the lesion may simply be excised precisely around its perimeter with an appropriate margin. The wound will then gape into an ellipse, indicating the line of least skin tension. The ellipse and its "dog ears" can then be excised to facilitate linear wound closure (Figure 21-5, *B* to *E*).

Scissors Removal

Benign pedunculated lesions (e.g., acrochordons, polypoid nevi) are readily snipped off with scissors.

More Complex Excisions

MOHS' MICROGRAPHIC SURGERY. This is seldom required for the treatment of benign lesions. Certain widespread Bowen's lesions, however, may be best treated by Mohs' surgery to allow evaluation of the surgical margins with optimum conservation of noninvolved tissue (Figure 21-6).

TISSUE EXPANSION. Lesions with large surface areas may be most satisfactorily treated by placement of tissue expanders, which allow later excision and coverage with adjacent tissue of similar quality. This technique is frequently used in the treatment of giant congenital nevi.

FACIAL COSMETIC PROCEDURES. Diffuse facial lesions may be debulked by a rhytidectomy procedure. For example, the appearance of a patient with cutaneous lesions of von Recklinghausen's disease (neurofibromatosis) diffusely distributed over the face may be improved by wide undermining and excision of large areas of involved skin using facelift techniques.

EPIDERMAL TUMORS

Verruca Vulgaris (Wart)

Verruca vulgaris is caused by the papovavirus and is transmissible by direct contact or by autoinoculation. Histologically, hyperkeratosis, acanthosis, and parakeratosis are seen. Various treatment modalities are suitable, including application of topical irritants, cryotherapy, excision, or laser ablation.

If the wart is shaved to the level of the surrounding epidermis and inspected with magnification loupes, a discrete edge is seen. The entire wart can then be sharply curetted from surrounding normal epidermis. Since the basal epidermal layer is not invaded, reepithelialization occurs rapidly. Subungual

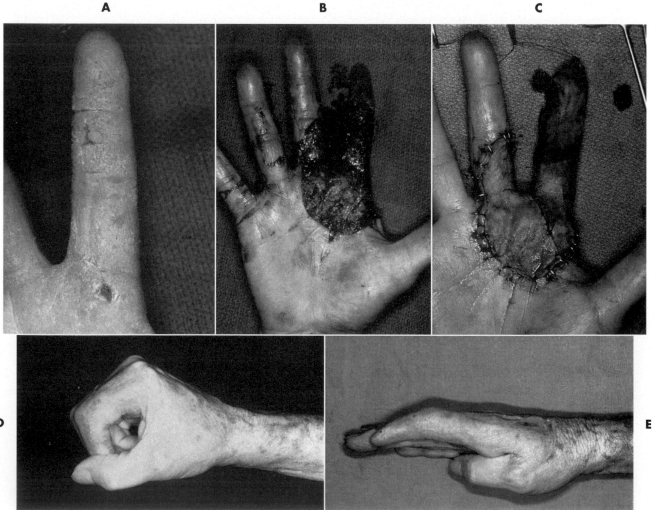

Figure 21-6, A-E. Bowen's lesion of fingers excised by Mohs' micrographic surgery. Immediate split-thickness skin grafting was performed.

warts can be similarly treated after removal of sufficient overlying nail plate to gain access to the wart.

Seborrheic Keratosis

Seborrheic keratoses are seen in older patients (Figure 21-7). Growth and depth of pigmentation are directly related to sun exposure. These lesions are covered by a greasy scale and characteristically appear to have been stuck on the skin surface; they do not undergo malignant transformation. Seborrheic keratoses occur predominantly on the central areas of the body, the chest, back, neck, face, scalp, and proximal extremities. Irritation of these lesions by clothing or other trauma results in increased keratinization.

A variant lesion *(dermatosis papulosa nigra)* is seen in black individuals. These lesions occur most frequently on the upper cheeks and are small, pedunculated, and heavily pigmented with minimal keratosis.

Treatment of seborrheic keratoses takes advantage of their superficiality and includes curettage, shave biopsy, or application of liquid nitrogen, with minimal scarring.

Keratoacanthoma

Keratoacanthoma is a benign, self-limited epithelial tumor, usually occurring in sun-exposed areas, which closely resembles squamous cell carcinoma both clinically and histologically. A firm, erythematous papule appears initially and rapidly enlarges up to 2 cm or more in diameter over 2 to 8 weeks (Figure 21-8). The central umbilicated portion of the lesion is filled with a keratinous plug (Figure 21-9).

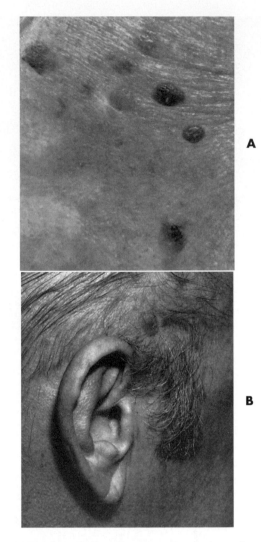

Figure 21-7, A and **B.** Greasy scaling lesions that have "pasted-on" appearance are typical of seborrheic keratoses.

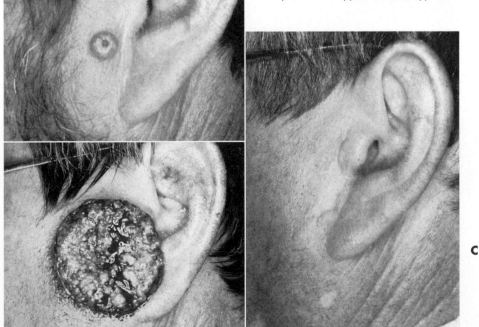

Figure 21-8. This patient with preauricular keratoacanthoma **(A)** shows its natural evolution through rapid enlargement **(B)** to involution and cicatricial healing over 19-week period **(C).**

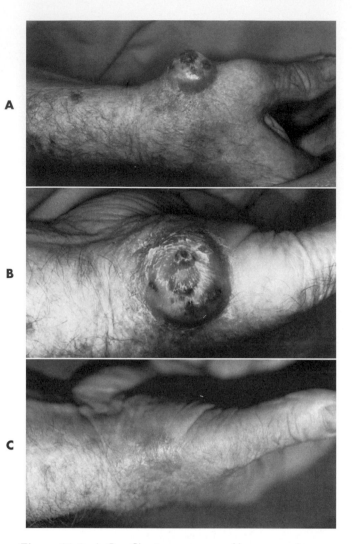

Figure 21-9, A-C. Classic appearance of keratoacanthoma on hand with central keratinous plug. After shave excision, healing resulted in good cosmetic and functional outcome.

These large lesions, although often indurated, are freely movable over the underlying structures. A regressive phase then begins, during which the central plug is expelled, spontaneous resolution occurs, and the lesion heals with a scar. Keratoacanthoma is believed to arise from a proliferation of pilar epithelium, and the evolution and regression of the lesion are thought to be related to the hair cycle.

Occasionally, keratoacanthomas have an aggressive course with metastasis and cannot be distinguished from squamous cell carcinoma. In such cases it is difficult to know whether the cause of confusion was mistaken diagnosis; the histopathologic interpretation of keratoacanthoma may be problematic. The usual cause of difficulty in histologically differentiating keratoacanthoma from squamous cell carcinoma is a biopsy that fails to include the entire breadth of the lesion and its central core.

The treatment for keratoacanthoma is complete excision, especially when the lesion is first recognized and small. The linear scar after excision is more satisfactory than the scar after spontaneous resolution, particularly in such critical cosmetic areas as the nasal ala, where cicatricial healing may result in significant deformity. The similarities between keratoacanthoma and squamous cell carcinoma may dictate excisional biopsy. If the lesion is already quite large, spontaneous resolution may yield a more favorable cosmetic appearance than excision of the widely proliferating lesion.

Cutaneous Horn

Cutaneous horns arise from underlying epidermal lesions and are usually actinic keratoses (Figure 21-10). Although these lesions are not considered premalignant, up to 10% of patients with cutaneous horns have underlying squamous carcinomas. Cutaneous horns only rarely arise from basal cell carcinomas.

Other underlying epidermal lesions may be keratoacanthoma, sebaceous adenoma, or Kaposi's sarcoma. Accurate determination of the underlying pathology requires excision of the lesion with a 1-mm to 2-mm margin of normal skin. Subsequent treatment depends on the nature of the underlying lesion.

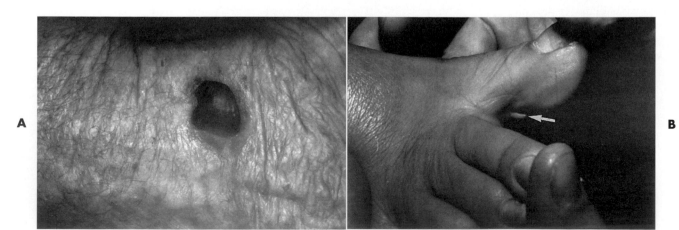

Figure 21-10. Cutaneous horns on hand **(A)** and foot **(B)**.

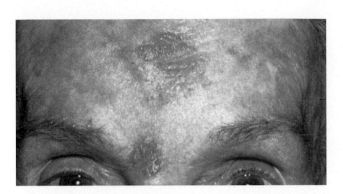

Figure 21-11. Actinic keratoses of forehead.

Actinic Keratosis

Actinic keratosis is the most frequently occurring premalignant cutaneous condition. Also called *senile keratosis* and *solar keratosis,* these lesions are rough and scaly with discrete, usually erythematous borders; they range in color from yellow to dark brown (Figure 21-11). Histologic examination of an actinic keratosis lesion reveals extensive hyperkeratosis and sharply defined areas of parakeratosis. The granular layer is usually absent, and involved epidermal cells are more eosinophilic than the normal adjacent epidermal cells, with an atypical cellular pattern of budding proliferation extending into the epidermis.

Actinic keratoses must be differentiated from other hyperkeratotic lesions that may occur with chronic eczematoid dermatitis, psoriasis, Bowen's disease, and Paget's disease. They usually occur in genetically susceptible people (generally, older males of Celtic ancestry) on sun-exposed sites such as the face, the lower lip, the back of the hands, the forearms, neck, and bald scalp.

Arsenical (arsenic) keratosis occurs secondary to exposure to inorganic arsenic compounds and usually manifests on the palms and soles.

Although it has been suggested that squamous cell carcinoma develops in 20% of patients with facial actinic keratoses, the true incidence of malignant transformation is probably much lower. We generally prefer an elliptic surgical excision, particularly for larger, nodular lesions, so that the tissue can be carefully evaluated microscopically. Liquid nitrogen, superficial curettage, and light electrocautery are also acceptable modes of treatment, especially for smaller lesions. Topical 5-fluorouracil is useful for diffuse facial lesions when surgical therapy is impractical. Lesions resistant to 5-fluorouracil treatment may contain foci of squamous cell carcinoma.

Bowen's Disease

Bowen's disease is a chronic disorder involving cutaneous hyperkeratotic lesions (Figure 21-12). These represent intraepidermal squamous cell carcinoma (carcinoma in situ); 10% of these lesions become invasive after many years. Invasive squamous cell carcinoma arising from Bowen's disease is more aggressive than carcinoma developing from actinic keratoses, and metastatic disease occurs in at least one third of patients.

Bowen's disease occurs in older patients of fair complexion. Chronic sun exposure and arsenic exposure are etiologically related to its development. In many patients, however, no etiologic factors are evident; approximately half of Bowen's disease lesions arise in sun-exposed areas and half in areas covered by clothing. The lesions are irregular plaques with thickened, hyperkeratotic surfaces and are usually erythematous. They must be differentiated from superficial basal cell carcinoma, actinic keratosis, Paget's disease, psoriasis, lichen simplex chronicus, verrucae, eczematous lesions, and chronic fungal infections (Figure 21-12, *A*).

Surgical excision with a margin of normal tissue is the most effective treatment. Because of the deep follicular involvement of Bowen's lesions, curettage and topical application of 5-fluorouracil are frequently followed by recurrence. Mohs' micrographic surgical techniques may be helpful.

Erythroplasia of Queyrat

Erythroplasia of Queyrat is essentially Bowen's disease of the mucous membranes. Lesions occur most often on the glans penis and adjacent mucosal skin in uncircumcised males and less often on the female vulva. The lesion surface is velvety and brightly erythematous. The rate of malignant transformation is higher than in Bowen's disease. Biopsy diagnosis is required and followed by conservative excision.

Paget's Disease

Paget's disease is an eczematous lesion of the nipple and areola that is also found in extramammary areas. Extramammary Paget's disease occurs in both sexes but is more common in older women; it is found primarily in the anogenital region, principally on the vulva. It may also occur on the scrotum, in the perianal region, and in the axillae where apocrine glands are located.

Biopsy is necessary to differentiate Paget's disease from psoriatic and eczematous conditions. Microscopically, large, round Paget cells lie within the epidermis; these cells have large nuclei and abundant pale-staining cytoplasm. Mucin stains differentiate these cells from the cells of Bowen's disease and those of malignant melanoma.

Paget's disease of the breast without a palpable mass requires excision and has an excellent prognosis. Treatment for Paget's disease of the breast with a palpable lump is similar to that for other breast carcinomas, as is the prognosis. Wide and deep excision is employed for extramammary Paget's disease, with a careful search for underlying carcinoma. Paget cells may be identified outside the clinical limits of the lesion, and an adequately wide excision will reduce the possibility of recurrence. Mohs' micrographic surgery may be indicated. The prognosis for extramammary Paget's disease is much less favorable when an underlying carcinoma is present.

Other Epidermal Conditions

The following lesions require total excision to provide cure.

Giant condyloma acuminatum presents as a fungating growth, usually on the prepuce of an uncircumcised male. The lesion is locally destructive, resulting in ulceration and urethral

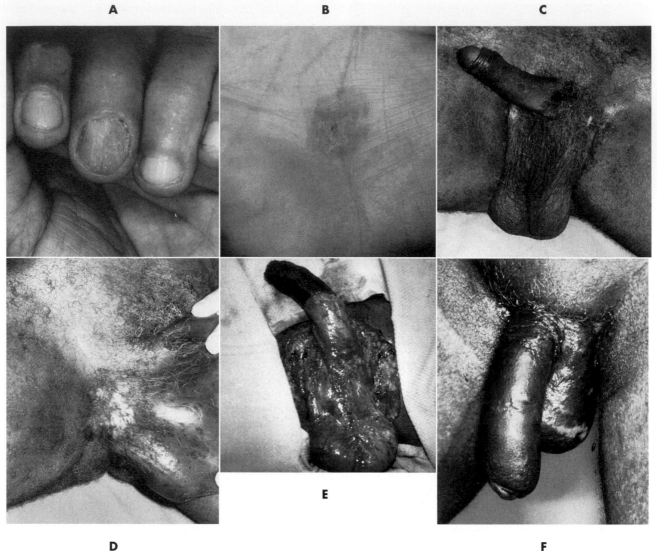

Figure 21-12. **A,** Bowen's disease of the paronychium and nail bed may be confused with chronic fungal infection. **B,** Chronic scaling patch of Bowen's disease affecting palm. **C** to **F,** Perineal Bowen's disease that required wide excision and skin grafting.

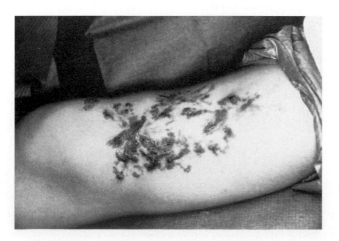

Figure 21-13. Porokeratosis of Mibelli.

fistulas, and may transform into a verrucous squamous cell carcinoma.

Epidermodysplasia verruciformis consists of wartlike lesions on the face, neck, hands, feet, and trunk. These are caused by the human papillomavirus (HPV-3, HPV-5) and degenerate into squamous cell carcinomas. T-cell formation is defective.

Porokeratosis is an hereditary condition characterized by disseminated annular plaques with sharply raised, horny borders (Figure 21-13). Approximately 13% of these lesions transform into basal and squamous cell carcinomas. The most common type is porokeratosis of Mibelli.

Epithelial Cysts

Most epidermal cysts (inclusion or keratinous cysts) arise from occluded pilosebaceous follicles, although some arise from traumatic displacement of epidermal cells into the dermis

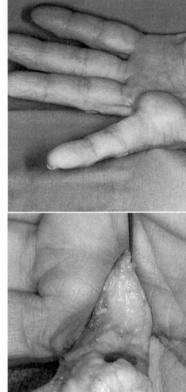

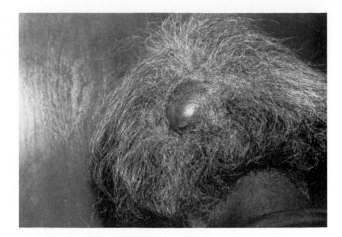

Figure 21-15. Pilar cyst on occipital area of scalp.

Figure 21-14. **A,** Epidermal inclusion cyst of hand. **B,** Intraoperative exposure of cyst.

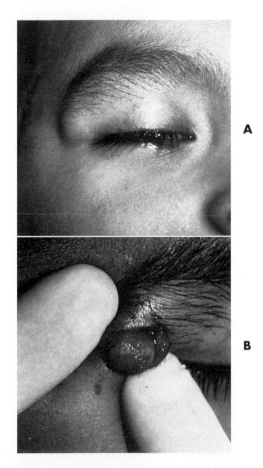

Figure 21-16. **A,** Dermoid cyst at lateral brow. **B,** Excision of dermoid cyst.

(Figure 21-14). The skin is elevated over the underlying lesion and adherent to it; a small keratin-filled punctum, representing the orifice of the plugged pilosebaccous follicle, may be seen. Epidermal cysts are asymptomatic but may become secondarily infected.

The preferred treatment for epidermal cysts is excision to include the entire epidermal lining. Even small numbers of cells, if left behind, may result in recurrence.

Pilar cysts occur in the scalp, derived from the outer root sheath of a hair follicle (Figure 21-15). Pilar cysts are clinically indistinguishable from epidermal inclusion cysts although the two can be differentiated histologically. Treatment consists of excision to include the sac lining.

Milia are tiny (1-mm to 2-mm) epidermal cysts that usually occur on the face (eyelids, cheeks, forehead). They may occur de novo or may follow skin trauma, such as burns or dermabrasion. Posttraumatic milia are usually self-limited. Treatment, when required, consists of lightly incising the top of the lesion and expressing the contents.

Dermoid cysts on the face are usually present at birth and are found subcutaneously along the lines of embryonic fusion, most often at the lateral brow (Figure 21-16). Treatment is by excision. *Midline dermoids* require preoperative computed tomography (CT) scan to define their anatomic extent because they frequently communicate with the central leptomeninges.

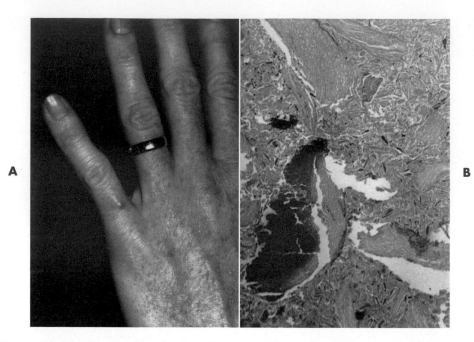

Figure 21-17. A, Nondescript, firm dermal nodule on the finger. **B,** Histology reveals pilomatricoma with foci of calcification.

TUMORS OF EPIDERMAL APPENDAGES

These lesions form a large group of relatively rare tumors that often present as dermal nodules. They require excisional biopsy for diagnostic purposes and cannot otherwise be differentiated from each other. A few lesions in this category, such as nevus sebaceus of Jadassohn, present very characteristic clinical appearances. Although that particular lesion has malignant potential, most benign tumors of epidermal appendages are not premalignant. Some, such as trichoepithelioma and syringoma, may be numerous and scattered over a large area, making excision impractical.

Pilar Differentiation

Pilomatricoma, or *calcifying epithelioma of Malherbe,* occurs as a solitary tumor, usually on the face, neck, or upper extremities of children and young adults (Figure 21-17). The clinical appearance is of a nondescript, firm dermal nodule usually approximately 0.5 cm in diameter. Foci of calcification and even of ossification may be seen histologically. Treatment consists of surgical excision.

Tricholemmoma usually occurs as a solitary facial papule. Rarely, multiple tricholemmomas occur as part of Cowden disease, which is characterized by keratoses on the distal extremities, mucosal papillomas and fibromas, and internal organ involvement, including thyroid, gastrointestinal tract, ovaries, and breasts, with an associated high incidence of breast carcinoma.

Trichoepithelioma may occur as solitary or multiple lesions (Figure 21-18). The multiple form is inherited as an autosomal dominant disorder; 2-mm to 5-mm, firm, flesh-colored coalescing papules develop in the early years of life, concentrated in the nasolabial folds over the nose, forehead, upper lip,

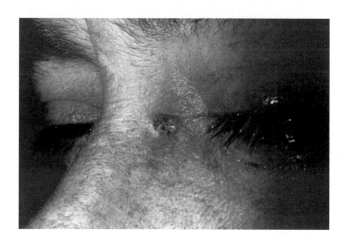

Figure 21-18. Solitary trichoepithelioma.

and eyelids. These lesions must be clinically differentiated from adenoma sebaceum, syringoma, basal cell nevus syndrome, and neurofibromatosis.

Any method of removal is usually curative for solitary lesions, but eradication of multiple trichoepitheliomas is more difficult.

Sebaceous Gland Differentiation

Nevus sebaceus of Jadassohn is usually present at birth and gradually enlarges (Figure 21-19). The most common sites are the scalp, face, and neck, and, more rarely, the trunk and limbs. The lesion in young patients consists of a patch of alopecia with a smooth surface and yellow-brown waxy appearance; it thickens with puberty and becomes verrucous with papillomatous projections. As the patient ages, some lesions develop new nodular proliferations.

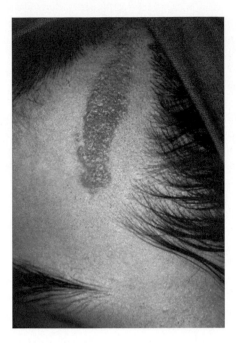

Figure 21-19. Nevus sebaceus.

Nevus sebaceus of Jadassohn is a hamartomatous conglomerate of large sebaceous glands associated with heterotopic apocrine glands and defective hair follicles. It is called an *organoid nevus* because it involves the entire skin organ and numerous skin adnexa. Late lesions have the potential for development into other benign or malignant adnexal tumors, such as apocrine carcinoma; 10% to 15% of late lesions develop into basal cell carcinoma. Complete excision before puberty is recommended.

Sebaceous adenoma may manifest as a nondescript solitary lesion. Adenoma sebaceum, associated with tuberous sclerosis, is an angiofibromatous proliferation and not a true sebaceous adenoma. Multiple sebaceous tumors of the face, scalp, and trunk, together with multiple keratoacanthomas, may be associated with numerous internal malignancies (which may precede appearance of skin lesions) in Torre's syndrome.

Sweat Gland Differentiation

These tumors show great diversity, and classification is confusing. Multiple vesicular lesions occur with *eccrine hidrocystoma* and *syringoma;* treatment is necessary only for cosmetic reasons and may be accomplished electrosurgically. Eccrine hidrocystoma usually occurs on the faces of older women and may be exacerbated by heat and sweating. Syringomas, which usually appear during puberty, also occur primarily in women, especially on the face, eyelids, neck, and upper anterior chest.

Other lesions, such as *cylindroma, eccrine spiradenoma,* and *eccrine poroma,* are most frequently solitary lesions occurring as firm, flesh-colored papules. Treatment consists of surgical excision.

TUMORS OF MELANOCYTE SYSTEM

Arising from Nevus Cells

Nevi are the most common tumors in humans. Few are present at birth, but they begin appearing soon after birth, reach their greatest incidence in young adults, and regress with age. Most nevi in younger patients are junctional; by adulthood, most are intradermal.

Junctional nevi exhibit nevus cell nests confined to the dermoepidermal junction, whereas *intradermal nevi* demonstrate these nests in the dermis alone; *compound nevi* have nevus cells in both locations (Figure 21-20). The junctional component in both junctional and compound nevi may transform into malignant melanoma, although such transformation is rare. Malignant transformation is suggested in a lesion by the following:

1. Spontaneous ulceration and bleeding
2. Enlargement and darkening
3. Spread of pigment from lesion into surrounding skin
4. Pigmented satellite lesions
5. Inflammatory changes without trauma
6. Pain and itching

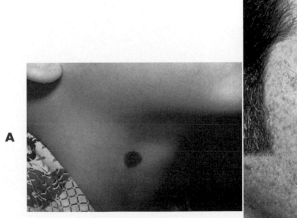
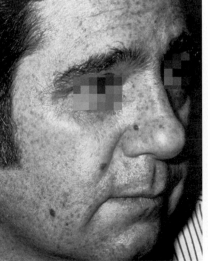

Figure 21-20. A, Junctional nevus on lateral aspect of neck. **B,** Multiple intradermal nevi in nasolabial region and on nasal ala.

TREATMENT. The majority of nevi require no treatment except cosmetic removal when the patient so desires. Simple excision is the treatment of choice. Although these lesions should be completely excised, no evidence suggests that incompletely removed nevi will undergo malignant transformation. The microscopic differentiation of a recurrent nevus is distinctive.

Any nevus suspected of malignant transformation must be totally excised to permit careful histologic examination of its full depth. A full-thickness incisional biopsy is permissible for diagnostic purposes in a larger nevus suspected of malignant change. This will not alter the lesion's natural history if melanoma is confirmed, provided that definitive surgical ablation follows shortly.

Palmar and plantar nevi had been thought to be especially prone to malignant transformation, but this view has changed. The overall incidence of palmar and plantar nevi is in 10% of the young adult population, making routine excision of nevi in these locations both impractical and unnecessary.

HALO NEVUS. This nevus has a depigmented halo surrounding a central nevus (Figure 21-21). A halo around a lesion may more rarely be associated with malignant melanoma. Halo nevi occur primarily in children and young adults, usually on the back.

When the diagnosis is in question, complete excision with histologic examination is indicated.

SPINDLE AND EPITHELIOID CELL NEVUS. Also called *benign juvenile melanoma* and *Spitz nevus,* this lesion has a close histopathologic resemblance to melanoma. The color ranges from pink to purplish red, and a minority are pigmented. These nevi are elevated, firm nodules that may reach 1 to 2 cm in size. The incidence of malignant transformation is no greater than with other compound nevi.

Treatment is total excision.

CONGENITAL NEVUS. Congenital nevi have a reported incidence of malignant transformation of approximately 12% (Figure 21-22). Transformation is to malignant melanoma and usually occurs in childhood.

When feasible, treatment of giant congenital nevi is total excision, usually in stages, with or without tissue expansion. Besides preventing melanoma development, excisional surgery can significantly improve a child's appearance. In areas where excision is not feasible, periodic cancer surveillance and biopsy of any suspicious areas must be done.

DYSPLASTIC NEVUS SYNDROME. Both sporadic and familial varieties of this syndrome may occur. The lesions are multiple atypical nevi ranging in number from 10 to greater than 100, occurring most often on the upper trunk. A characteristic lesion measures approximately 1 cm in diameter and has an irregular outline and variegated colorations of brown, black, and pink. The lesion appears flat but has a palpable dermal component. The microscopic appearance is

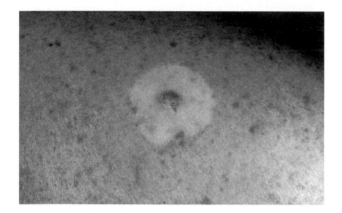

Figure 21-21. Halo nevus on back (nodular central lesion must be biopsied to exclude melanoma).

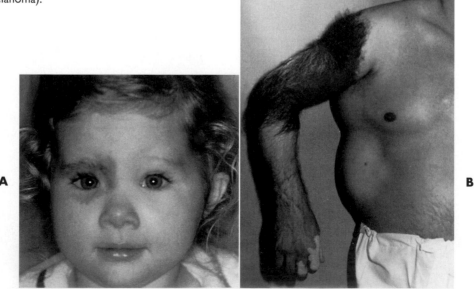

Figure 21-22. A, Periocular congenital hairy nevus. **B,** Giant hairy nevus on arm.

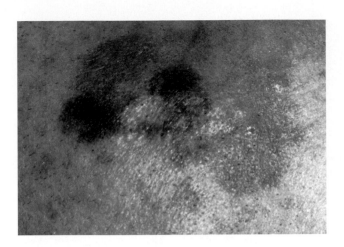

Figure 21-23. Irregularly mottled appearance of lentigo maligna.

also characteristic. Atypical melanocytes are large cells with a spindle or epithelioid cell configuration. The papillary dermis shows fibroplasia and new vessel formation, and a dermal lymphocytic response is present.

It is impractical to excise all these lesions. Excision of a representative lesion serves to confirm the pathologic diagnosis of dysplastic nevi. Patients with dysplatic nevus syndrome should be carefully observed, and suspicious lesions should be excised.

LENTIGO MALIGNA. Also called *Hutchinson's melanotic freckle,* this lesion occurs in elderly patients in sun-exposed areas of the face and extremities (Figure 21-23). It is a melanoma in situ with a slow radial growth phase of 10 to 15 years. The lesion is typically irregularly mottled with shades of brown and black. Both erythema and whitish areas of regression are present. Transformation to melanoma occurs in 30% to 50% of lesions, heralded by the appearance of nodules within the lentigo maligna (vertical growth phase).

Treatment is by excision. An extremely large, wide lesion may require preliminary incisional biopsy for diagnosis.

Arising from Melanocytes

LENTIGINES (FRECKLES). These multiple small, flat, pigmented lesions result from increased melanocytic activity. They are benign, and treatment is not necessary. If desired, they may be destroyed by light electrodesiccation or the application of liquid nitrogen.

Multiple lentigines syndrome, or *LEOPARD syndrome* (*l*entigines, *e*lectrocardiographic conduction defects, *o*cular hypertelorism, *p*ulmonary stenosis, genital *a*bnormalities, growth *r*etardation, sensorineural *d*eafness) is inherited as an autosomal dominant trait. The lesions associated with LEOPARD syndrome are numerous small, dark macules distributed especially over the neck and trunk; café au lait spots may also be present.

BLUE NEVUS. This nevus results from arrested migration of dermomelanocytes in embryonic life and is a solitary lesion often present at birth (Figure 21-24, *A*). A blue nevus is a dark, firmly rounded nodule that usually does not exceed 1 cm in diameter. Rare malignant transformation of cellular blue nevi is described. Treatment is surgical excision.

NEVUS OF OTA. This is a unilateral proliferation of dermomelanocytes in the distribution of the first and second branches of the trigeminal nerve (Figure 21-24, *B*). Most nevi of Ota have been reported among Oriental patients, and approximately 80% are found in female patients. The lesions typically have poorly defined margins and consist of a bluish black discoloration affecting the skin of the eyelid and adjacent face and forehead. The sclera and conjunctiva may show a similar discoloration, as may the tympanum, auditory canal, and mucous membranes of the nose and mouth.

Specific treatment is not needed. A similar anomaly involving the deltoid region is called the *nevus of Ito.*

MONGOLIAN SPOT. This is a variably sized, bluish black patch over the lower back and buttocks in infants. Usually present at birth, mongolian spots are more common in Asians and blacks and are rare among whites.

These lesions generally regress in early childhood, and treatment is not indicated.

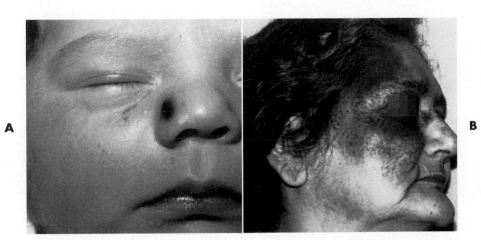

Figure 21-24. **A,** Blue nevus on nose of infant. **B,** Nevus of Ota.

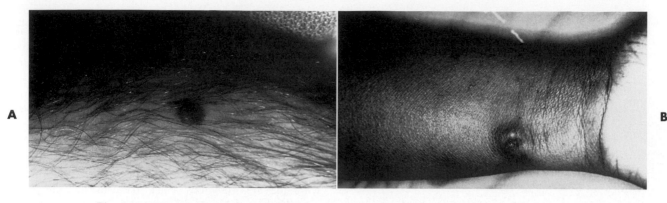

Figure 21-25. **A,** Firm, brownish dermal papule is a dermatofibroma. **B,** Dermatofibromas may show central "umbilication."

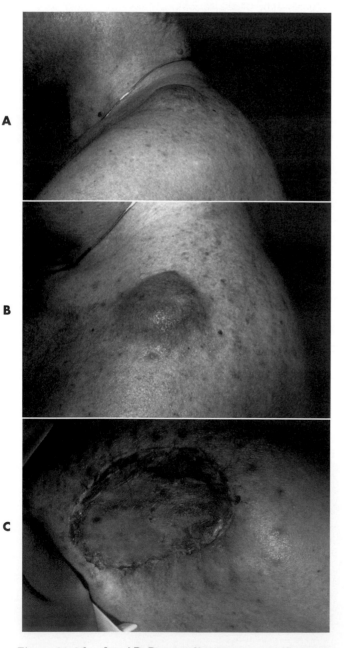

Figure 21-26. **A** and **B,** Dermatofibrosarcoma protuberans on shoulder. **C,** Treatment by wide local excision and skin grafting.

TUMORS OF MESODERMAL ORIGIN

Mesodermal lesions form a complex group of tumors of varying presentation, a few of which are highlighted here.

Acrochordon

Acrochordon *(skin tag)* is a common papillomatous lesion that usually has onset in middle adult life. These are multiple, fleshy, skin-colored tags occurring predominantly on the neck, upper chest, and axilla. Larger lesions may be pedunculated, and the only symptoms result from local irritation. An occasional lesion may be twisted and become infarcted.

Treatment is accomplished with tangential scalpel removal or with scissors.

Dermatofibroma

Dermatofibroma is a common lesion appearing as a papule or nodule, generally on the extremities, although other areas may be involved (Figure 21-25). Dermatofibromas are usually solitary, but 20% of patients may demonstrate more than one lesion. The lesion is a slow-growing, firm dermal papule attached to the overlying skin but freely movable in relation to the subcutaneous tissues.

Dermatofibromas vary in size from a few millimeters to 1 to 2 cm and may exhibit a depressed central umbilication. Occasionally they may be dark brown and clinically confused with malignant melanoma.

When indicated, simple excision is the treatment of choice.

Dermatofibrosarcoma Protuberans

Dermatofibrosarcoma protuberans is considered a malignant form of fibrohistiocytic tumor despite that metastasis is virtually unknown (Figure 21-26). The lesion exhibits a marked tendency toward recurrence. Deep infiltration into subcutaneous fat and even skeletal muscle may occur.

Dermatofibrosarcoma protuberans typically arises in the dermis of the trunk and proximal extremities and is more common in men, with a peak incidence in the third decade of life. The lesion initially appears as a firm, plaquelike nodular lesion affixed to the overlying skin but moving freely

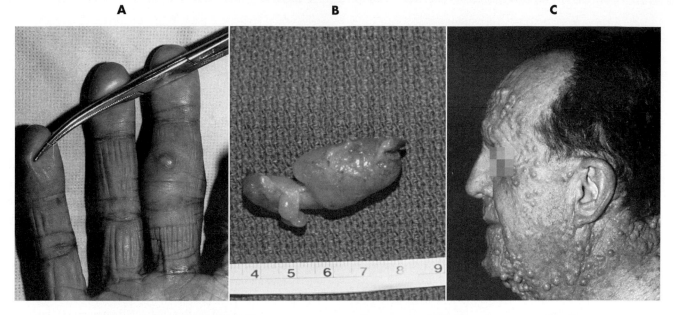

Figure 21-27. **A** and **B,** Solitary cutaneous neurofibroma on middle finger appears as dermal nodule. **C,** Multiple neurofibromas of von Recklinghausen's disease.

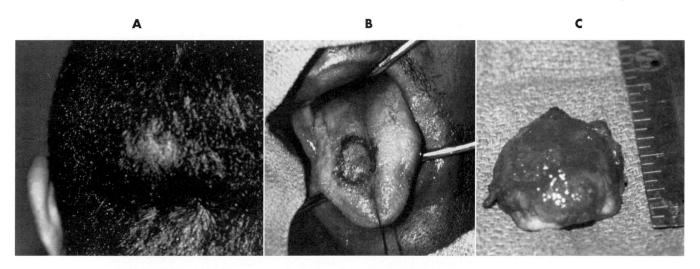

Figure 21-28. Multiple granular cell myoblastomas. Patient has lesions on occipital scalp **(A)** and tongue **(B). C,** Excised tongue lesion.

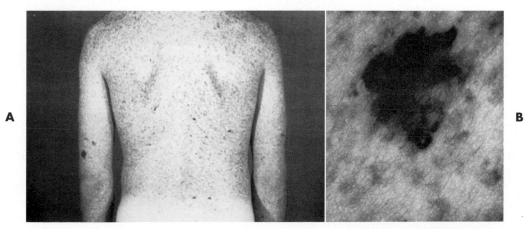

Figure 21-29. A, Patient with xeroderma pigmentosum developed multiple melanomas. **B,** Closeup of lesion. (Courtesy Don Gard, MD.)

over the deeper tissues. Color ranges from brown to a bluish red. The size may remain unchanged for years before a rapid growth phase forms a multinodular mass more than 5 cm in diameter.

Successful treatment of dermatofibrosarcoma protuberans requires wide and deep local excision. Skin grafting is usually needed to cover the resulting defect. Patients must be followed carefully in anticipation of recurrence.

Neurofibroma

Neurofibromas may exist as solitary tumors or as multiple neurofibromas *(von Recklinghausen's disease)*. *Neurofibromatosis* is an uncommon hereditary condition characterized by neurofibromas within the skin and subcutaneous tissue. The peripheral and cranial nerves are also involved, with associated café au lait spots (Figure 21-27).

Granular Cell Tumor

Granular cell myoblastoma has an uncertain histologic origin but appears to be a tumor derived from the Schwann sheath (Figure 21-28). It is most common in the fourth to sixth decades and occurs more frequently in the black population. Approximately one third of these lesions occur on the tongue and one half over the head and neck region. They are located primarily in the skin and subcutaneous tissue, although deeper tissues (e.g., lung, gastrointestinal tract, heart) may also be involved.

Although the lesions are usually solitary, multiple granular cell tumors manifest in approximately 10% of patients. Approximately 3% of granular cell tumors are malignant and can metastasize. Treatment consists of surgical excision.

Infantile Digital Fibromatosis

Recurring digital fibrous tumor of childhood arises within the first year of life, with one third of such tumors present at birth. These lesions occur almost exclusively on the hands and feet. The nodules are generally poorly circumscribed and may be single or multiple. They are usually asymptomatic, although they may cause functional impairment and joint deformity.

Approximately 60% of patients experience tumor recurrence after surgical excision. These lesions do not metastasize and may occasionally regress spontaneously; therefore, when functional impairment or joint deformity is not present, observation is a reasonable alternative after histopathologic confirmation of the diagnosis. If surgery is elected, the tumor should be removed completely to diminish the risk of recurrence.

SYNDROMAL CONDITIONS

Xeroderma Pigmentosum

Xeroderma pigmentosum is a genodermatosis characterized by an autosomal recessive defect in which the deoxyribonucleic acid (DNA) repair mechanism for ultraviolet light–induced damage is impaired; the skin and eyes are intolerant of ultraviolet light. The skin appears normal at birth, but with the earliest exposure to sunlight, an exaggerated sunburn reaction occurs. Pigmentation changes occur with repeated sun exposure, giving the appearance of intensely pigmented freckles (Figure 21-29). The skin subsequently thickens, and cutaneous and subcutaneous atrophy ultimately occur, particularly around the eyes, nose, and mouth. The eyes become painfully sensitive to light and tear excessively early in the disease.

Patients with more severe xeroderma pigmentosum exhibit progressive neurologic deterioration that leads to "xerodermic idiocy." Many patients develop multiple malignant epithelial tumors and melanomas during the first decade of life and frequently die in the second decade.

The prognosis remains dismal, and no specific treatment exists. The use of sun-protective clothing and topical sunscreens and an indoor lifestyle are the most effective preventive measures. A child with this condition must be monitored frequently to detect and treat malignant cutaneous lesions.

Basal Cell Nevus Syndrome (Gorlin's Syndrome)

The typical nevi of basal cell nevus syndrome are reddish brown, papular, and variously sized (Figure 21-30). They appear in most patients after puberty and may number from a few to many thousands. These lesions may become invasive basal cell carcinomas.

The principal features of the syndrome are multiple basal cell carcinomas scattered throughout the body, jaw cysts, skeletal abnormalities (e.g., bifid ribs, scoliosis, brachymetacarpalism, overdeveloped supraorbital ridges), broad nasal root, hypertelorism, palmar and plantar pits, calcification of falx cerebri, and occasional neurologic abnormalities (e.g., mental impairment, medulloblastoma).

Other Syndromes

Bazex syndrome (paraneoplastic acrokeratosis) is inherited as an X-linked dominant trait and consists of follicular atrophoderma with multiple basal cell carcinomas, hypotrichosis, and hypohidrosis.

Haber's syndrome, dyskeratosis congenita, and Rothmund-Thomson syndrome are also associated with skin cancers. *Haber's syndrome* is a familial variant of Bowen's disease consisting of a rosacea-like eruption of the face and Bowen's lesions on the covered areas of the body.

NONHEMANGIOMATOUS VASCULAR LESIONS

Pyogenic Granuloma

Pyogenic granuloma is a proliferation of capillaries arising at the site of trauma (Figure 21-31). An associated infection may occur, but the condition is not an infectious process. Pyogenic granulomas have a pliable surface and bleed easily. They occur most often on the face and distal extremities, probably because of the higher incidence of minor trauma at these sites.

Pyogenic granulomas may be excised. Smaller lesions may be destroyed with electrosurgery, carbon dioxide laser, or silver nitrate cautery. Incompletely removed lesions may recur.

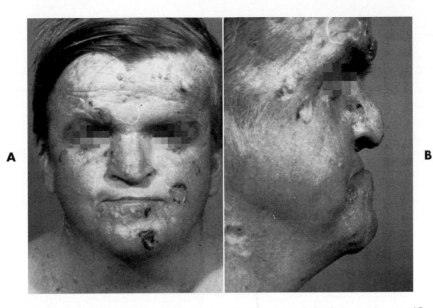

Figure 21-30. A and **B,** Patient with classic facial features of Gorlin's syndrome. (Courtesy Don Gard, MD.)

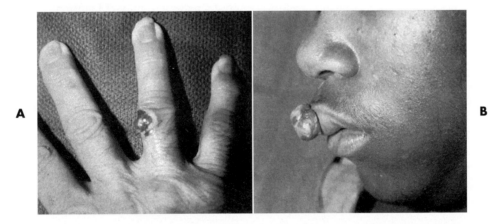

Figure 21-31. A, Pyogenic granuloma on finger. **B,** Pyogenic granuloma of upper lip after child fell off bicycle and accidentally bit lip.

Glomus Tumor

Glomus tumors arise from specialized arteriovenous shunts that circumvent the normal capillary bed (Figure 21-32). These tumors are derived from smooth muscle cells and are usually solitary, occurring in the nail beds and somewhat less frequently on the pulp of the fingertips. Other anatomic sites may also be affected. Glomus tumors are tender, blue-red papules that are subject to spontaneous, sharp, episodic radiating pain and are sensitive to temperature change. Multiple lesions are less frequently painful than solitary lesions.

Treatment consists of surgical excision. Resection of subungual lesions requires loupe magnification to minimize damage to the nail bed and allow anatomic resuturing of the exploratory longitudinal nail bed incision.

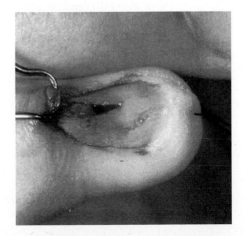

Figure 21-32. Subungual glomus tumor is excised by removing nail plate and exploring nail bed through longitudinal incision.

OUTCOMES

Central to outcome analysis of treatment for benign and premalignant skin conditions is the accuracy of clinical diagnosis. Many benign lesions are excised because of their disfiguring nature or because of a functional problem, such as exposure to shaving trauma or irritation by clothing. Many lesions are excised for diagnostic purposes.

A study involving the removal of more than 2000 skin lesions under local anesthesia by a senior plastic surgeon revealed two thirds of the lesions to be benign.[4] Of suspected benign lesions, 97% were found on histology not to be malignant. Only 65% of the lesions removed were correctly clinically identified preoperatively; 35% of those lesions suspected of malignancy were benign. One quarter of all malignant lesions with positive margins were initially not regarded as malignant. In summary, benign lesions were usually correctly assessed, but a few malignant lesions would have been missed without aggressive intervention. Surgical acumen cannot be expected to be flawless and was only two-thirds correct in this study.

As a rule, outcome for smaller benign lesions revolves around the potential for adverse scarring. Although a nevus in the presternal or shoulder region may be a cosmetic embarrassment to a female patient when she wears certain clothing styles, elliptic surgical excision must be weighed against the potential for hypertrophic scarring, which is particularly likely to develop in these areas (Figure 21-33). The deeper an ablation extends into the dermis, the greater the propensity for hypertrophic scarring. Superficial lesions such as seborrheic keratoses, which have a totally benign course, are best treated by shave excision, curettage, or liquid nitrogen, all of which leave virtually no visible scar.

POTENTIAL FOR MALIGNANCY

For larger lesions with malignant potential, outcome analysis must focus on the likelihood of adverse scarring versus malignant transformation. Adult patients or minor patients and their parents must understand these considerations, especially when infants with giant congenital nevi are treated.

For example, congenital nevi have an overall reported incidence of malignant transformation of 12%. Such melanoma transformation usually occurs in childhood. On the other hand, a huge bathing trunk nevus may require excision that leaves unsightly, massive skin-grafted areas. Fully excising such nevi may not be possible when rectal and vaginal extension occur.

Conversely, a periocular nevus may be in a prominently unaesthetic location and also have known malignant potential. Such a lesion may be excised and the resulting defect resurfaced with retroauricular full-thickness skin grafts (or even by preexpanding the retroauricular donor area to obtain larger skin grafts), thus achieving good aesthetic and functional results. Other lesions with invasive malignant potential have already been discussed. These include dysplastic nevi, nevus sebaceus of Jadassohn, giant condylomata, actinic keratoses, and Bowen's disease.

The type of treatment chosen and thus the anticipated outcome depend on (1) diffuseness of tumor involvement, (2) practicality of excision versus an alternative form of treatment (e.g., topical chemotherapy), (3) anatomic location, and (4) risk of malignant transformation. The high risk of aggressive metastatic behavior if a Bowen's lesion becomes an invasive cancer warrants wide excision or Mohs' micrographic surgery in areas where excessively wide excision may produce adverse functional or aesthetic results.

Locally invasive lesions such as digital fibromatoses and dermatofibrosarcoma protuberance must be widely excised (when indicated in the former) to minimize recurrence. Incomplete excision of simple nevi and congenital nevi may lead to "recurrence" and initial concern of malignant transformation, although an experienced pathologist can differentiate a benign residual lesion from malignancy. Congenital nevi may often invade into the deep subcutaneous tissues and even into fascia. Pigment may not be observed at these deeper levels, but residual nevus cells may later develop into islands of pigmented cells (Figure 21-34).

When larger lesions involve the hand, the surgeon must consider not only the cosmetic consequences of adverse

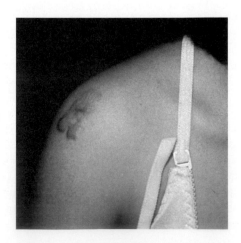

Figure 21-33. Hypertrophic scarring on shoulder after excision of benign cutaneous lesion.

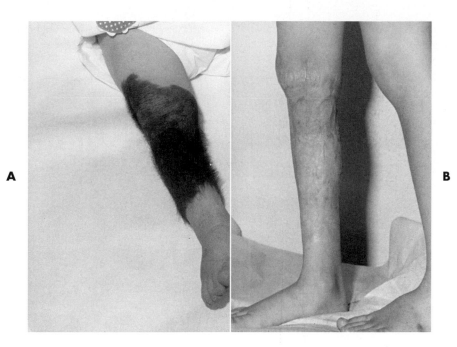

Figure 21-34. **A,** Congenital hairy nevus on leg of infant. Lesion was fully excised down to fascia and skin grafted. **B,** Eight years later, islands of pigmentation have developed because residual microscopic nevus cells have remained.

scarring from excisional treatment, but also the functional consequences of stiffness and loss of range of motion. The therapeutic decision must consider the depth of the skin lesion, its natural history if left untreated, and its anatomic location.

RECONSTRUCTION RESULTS

Almost no literature deals with aesthetic, psychologic, and functional outcomes of reconstructive efforts after tumor excision. Most outcome studies that evaluate aesthetic and functional outcome of facial reconstructions are either anecdotal or retrospective. None uses standardized quality of life or functional outcome instruments. These studies are more appropriate for malignant lesions, in which larger ablative defects are encountered than with benign cutaneous lesions. Prospective outcome evaluations are clearly an avenue for further study.

The more common reconstructions with evaluated outcomes involve nasal, lip, and oromandibular areas, three sites where function and aesthetics are crucially interwoven. One study evaluated the success of a turn-in flap to provide internal nasal lining.[8] Of 18 patients, 89% (16) had total flap viability, and 94% (17) reported normal nasal function. Other studies evaluated outcome of forehead flap nasal reconstruction.[9] Retrospective, subjective, functional, and aesthetic evaluations by three surgeons and their patients supported the predictability of good outcome using this particular form of nasal reconstruction.

Free microvascular tissue reconstruction for oropharyngeal and oral cavity defects has been shown to provide improved functional outcome. The fewer complications seem to justify its use over pedicle soft tissue transfer despite a slightly increased treatment cost. Total lip reconstruction is fraught with difficulty.

The general consensus is that staged reconstruction, using local tissues wherever possible, provides improved aesthetic appearance and functional oral competence compared with single-stage microvascular reconstructions.

REFERENCES

1. Arndt KA, Leboit PE, et al, editors: *Cutaneous medicine and surgery: an integrated program in dermatology,* Philadelphia, 1996, Saunders.

2. Burge S, Colver G, Lester R: *Simple skin surgery,* ed 2, Cambridge, Mass, 1996, Blackwell.

3. Gard D: Nonpigmented premalignant lesions of the skin, *Clin Plast Surg* 14:413-421, 1987.

4. Hallock GG: Prospective study of the accuracy of the surgeon's diagnosis in removal of 2000 skin lesions. Presented at the 76th Annual Meeting of American Association of Plastic Surgeons, Portland, 1997.

5. Harris AO, Levy ML, Goldberg LH, Stal S: Nonepidermal and appendageal skin tumors, *Clin Plast Surg* 20:115-130, 1993.

6. Moschella SL, Hurley HJ, editors: *Dermatology,* ed 3, Philadelphia, 1992, Saunders.

7. Netscher DT, Anous M, Spira M: Premalignant skin tumors, basal cell carcinoma, and squamous cell carcinoma. In Cohen M, editor: *Mastery of plastic and reconstructive surgery,* Boston, 1994, Little, Brown.

8. Park SS, Cook TA, Wang TD: The epithelial "turn-in" flap in nasal reconstruction, *Arch Otolaryngol Head Neck Surg* 121:1122-1127, 1995.

9. Quatela VC, Sherris DA, Rounds MF: Esthetic refinements in forehead flap nasal reconstruction, *Arch Otolaryngol Head Neck Surg* 121:1106-1113, 1995.

10. Stal S, Goldberg L: Nonexcisional therapy for benign skin lesions, *Clin Plast Surg* 14:237-242, 1987.

11. Tsue TT, Desaytnikova SS, Deleyiannis FW, et al: Comparison of cost and function in reconstruction of the posterior oral cavity and oropharynx: free versus pedicled soft tissue transfer, *Arch Otolaryngol Head Neck Surg* 123:731-737, 1997.

12. Williams EF, Setzen G, Mulvaney MJ: Modified Bernard-Burow cheek advancement and cross-lip flap for total lip reconstruction, *Arch Otolaryngol Head Neck Surg* 122:1253-1258, 1996.

CHAPTER 22

Malignant Skin Conditions

Marc H. Hedrick

H. Peter Lorenz

Timothy A. Miller

INTRODUCTION

Skin carcinoma is the most common human cancer. More than 700,000 new cases are diagnosed annually; 77% are basal cell carcinomas, 20% squamous cell carcinomas, and 3% melanomas and rare tumors.[8] Furthermore, the incidence and mortality rates of these cancers are increasing in the United States.[17] An annual increase of 3% to 7% has been noted in whites, and the number of cases doubled between 1970 and 1986.[4] Squamous cell and basal cell carcinomas grow deliberately, typically progressing from small, easily managed lesions with high cure rates to larger lesions with less certain outcomes.

INDICATIONS

Sun exposure has been shown to be the major environmental cause of both basal and squamous cell carcinoma (Box 22-1). More than 80% of nonmelanoma skin cancers are found on sun-exposed areas (e.g., head, arms, hands). The incidence increases in populations living closer to the equator.

Nonvisible ultraviolet B (UVB) energy (290 to 320 nm) is the most carcinogenic spectrum of light. Epidemiologic data have shown that extended periods in the sun and most importantly "sun burning" are more important in the development of basal cell carcinoma than chronic sun exposure.[12] Some have implicated the decrease in thickness of the ozone layer to explain the increasing incidence of skin cancer.

Besides sun exposure, several well-documented genetic and biophysical traits are associated with an increased susceptibility to developing skin cancer (Box 22-2). Melanin granules in the skin and dark skin coloring appear to be photoprotective.

PATHOPHYSIOLOGY

The pathophysiology of skin cancer is unknown but likely multifactorial. The multistep hypothesis of carcinogenesis provides a plausible explanation.[1] First, *initiation* occurs in the form of a genetic mutation that permanently alters the host genome. This alteration is not sufficient for transformation alone but confers a latent growth advantage to the mutated cell and its progeny. Next, tumor *promotion* results from epigenetic changes in the cell's environment that are broadly mitogenic to all cells. Finally, *progression* occurs when further genetic alterations are caused by increasing genetic instability, ultimately resulting in the transformed, malignant phenotype.

Ultraviolet (UV) radiation produces characteristic changes to deoxyribonucleic acid (DNA) that are typically corrected by native repair mechanisms. Failure to repair these erroneous sequences allows their propagation during DNA replication. UV-related mutations have been linked to mutations of the p53 tumor suppressor gene. In 56% of basal cell carcinomas and in 26% of basal cell tumors, mutations were noted in both p53 alleles.[1] Furthermore, the presence of p53 protein seems to correlate with the aggressiveness of the basal cell carcinoma.[5]

Besides the direct mutagenic effects of UV light on the genome, UV radiation may also negatively affect the host-tumor relationship by producing an immunosuppressive effect in the host. This is thought to result from depletion of Langerhans' cells in the epidermis and stimulation and production of suppressor T-cell subpopulations. This may hinder the host's ability to detect and kill mutated or transformed cells.

In addition to UVB radiation from sunlight, a past history of therapeutic radiation treatment has been associated with the development of cutaneous malignancies. Although radiotherapists now are more precise in the indications and dosing of radiation, patients who received therapeutic radiation 20 to 30 years ago remain at risk. Patients with chronic radiation dermatitis (e.g., erythema, atrophy, alopecia, telangiectasia, pigmentation change, actinic keratosis) may develop squamous carcinoma.

Box 22-1.
Etiologic Factors for Skin Cancer

Sun exposure (ultraviolet B radiation)
Previous radiation therapy with radiation dermatitis
Chemical exposure (e.g., coal tar, petroleum products, arsenic)
Chronic ulceration and inflammation
Genetic predisposition (fair skin)
Xeroderma pigmentosum
Immunosuppression

Box 22-2.
Biophysical Risk Factors for Skin Cancer

Male gender
White race
Celtic origin
Sunburn easily
Increasing age
Blue eyes
Fair complexion

Box 22-3.
Histologic Patterns and Variants of Basal Cell Carcinoma

UNDIFFERENTIATED
Nodular-ulcerative
Superficial
Pigmented
Morpheaform (sclerosing)
Fibroepithelioma
Giant cell

DIFFERENTIATED
Adenoid
Basosquamous
Keratotic
Clear cell
Infundibulocystic
Glandular differentiated subtypes

UNCERTAIN DIFFERENTIATION
Adamantinoid
Granular cell

Data from Nguyen AV, Whitaker DC, Frodel J: *Otolaryngol Clin North Am* 26:37-56, 1993.

Squamous cell carcinoma can also develop at sites of chronic inflammation, such as nonhealing ulcers (e.g., burn scar, pressure sore, venous or arterial insufficiency ulcer), and at chronic sinus sites from osteomyelitis.[16] These cancers typically occur on nonexposed areas and appear many years after the start of the original process. Frequently a delay in diagnosis occurs, and these lesions present as poorly differentiated tumors with lymphatic spread. When squamous cell carcinoma is present in a chronic burn ulcer, it is termed *Marjolin's ulcer.* Although mainly of historic interest because of improvements in the workplace safety, chemical exposure (e.g., coal tar, petroleum products, arsenic) may predispose exposed individuals to squamous carcinoma.[17]

BASAL CELL CARCINOMA

Basal cell carcinoma typically presents as a sporadically occurring tumor, but several syndromic causes have also been described.

Basal cell nevus syndrome (Gorlin's syndrome) is transmitted in an autosomal dominant manner with a low penetrance. Its cause has been traced to a mutation in a putative tumor suppressor gene located at 9q23.1-q31. Mutations at this locus may have implications for sporadic basal cell carcinoma as well; 50% of nonsyndromic basal cell carcinomas exhibit a mutation at this locus. The primary manifestations of basal cell nevus syndrome, in addition to carcinoma, are odontogenic keratocysts, dyskeratosis, pitting of the palms and soles, intracranial calcifications, and other anomalies. Basal cell carcinoma was reported in 76% of 118 patients with Gorlin's syndrome. The average age of onset was 20 years, and the face and back were primarily affected.[28]

Bazex syndrome is also an autosomal dominant disorder resulting in multiple small basal cell carcinomas of the face, usually first noticed in adolescence or young adulthood. It may also result in "ice pick" marks on the extremities and hypotrichosis. *Rombo syndrome* is an autosomally inherited disorder also associated with basal cell carcinoma. These syndromes tend to occur later in life, around 35 years of age, and are associated other skin conditions and hypotrichosis. Finally, other inherited disorders, such as xeroderma pigmentosum, albinism, linear unilateral basal cell nevus, and nevus sebaceus of Jadassohn, have been associated with an increased risk of developing basal cell carcinoma.

The gross and microscopic morphology of basal cell carcinoma varies. Five major gross morphologic types of basal cell carcinoma exist: (1) nodular-ulcerative, (2) pigmented, (3) superficial, (4) morpheaform, and (5) fibroepithelioma. Rarer variants have also been reported (Box 22-3).[19]

Nodular-ulcerative basal cell carcinoma is most common and begins as a small, slowly enlarging papule with pearly edges and telangiectasias. Central ulceration (rodent ulcer) may occur when the tumor grows and replaces the epidermis. Most nodular-ulcerative tumors behave predictably and exhibit slow growth. They rarely display aggressive growth and invade local structures.

Pigmented basal cell carcinoma is similar to the nodular-ulcerative type. It has brown pigmentation, however, and is often misdiagnosed grossly as malignant melanoma.

Superficial basal cell carcinoma occurs as single or multiple patches that are indurated and scaly. Grossly, they may be

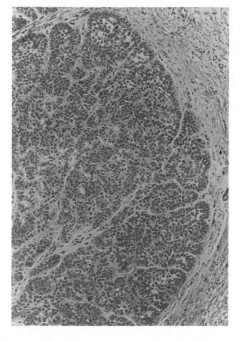

Figure 22-1. Histologic appearance of well-differentiated basal cell carcinoma.

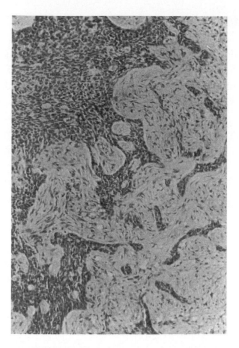

Figure 22-2. Histologic appearance of more aggressive basal cell carcinoma with fibrous tissue component (sclerosing).

ringed by a raised, pearly border that slowly expands. Superficial ulceration or crusting may occur centrally, resembling eczema, psoriasis, or tinea.

Morpheaform, or *sclerosing,* basal cell carcinoma is the most aggressive of the clinical subtypes. These lesions appear as flat or slightly depressed, yellowish plaques with indistinct borders. Ulceration is rare but is typically located on the face.

Fibroepithelioma is a variant of basal cell carcinoma first described by Pinkus. These lesions are typically raised and moderately firm with an erythematous and smooth surface. They typically occur on the lower trunk, especially on the lumbosacral region.[19]

Histologically, basal cell carcinoma exhibits lobules, nests, cords, or strands of tumor cells extending from the basal layer of the epidermis. The classic histologic pattern is cellular, with peripheral palisading of cells that are clustered and separate from the stroma (Figure 22-1). The tumor cells contain large, hyperchromatic nuclei but are nonanaplastic in appearance and resemble the nuclei of epidermal basal cells. They may have a large nucleus/cytoplasm ratio.

Basal cell carcinomas can be divided histologically into differentiated and undifferentiated subtypes (Box 22-3). Several histologic patterns may exist in a single tumor. Two major factors influence the histologic appearance of a basal cell carcinoma: (1) relative differentiation and proliferating ability of its cells and (2) nature of the stromal response evoked. Nodular-ulcerative lesions and the syndromic basal cells have variable degrees of differentiation. In contrast, the other four subtypes are not typically differentiated.

Morpheaform (sclerosing) basal cell carcinoma is notable for its dense desmoplastic reaction around the tumor. Typically the tumor cells are surrounded by type IV collagen containing basement membrane. This stroma surrounds

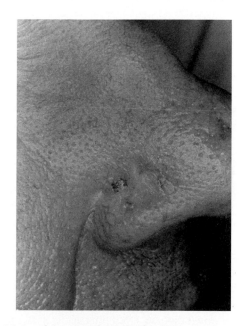

Figure 22-3. Sclerosing (morpheaform) basal cell carcinoma of nose with poorly defined demarcation of tumor–normal skin junction.

epithelial elements that have fewer cells, often in "spikes" (Figure 22-2). Molecular and ultrastructural studies of this tumor have suggested a variety of potential factors explaining its increased virulence, such as decreased basement membrane continuity, type IV collagenase production, and diminished amyloid production.

In general, patients with more aggressive tumors, based on histologic appearance, initially have lesions in which the distinction between normal skin and tumor may be more difficult (Figure 22-3).

SQUAMOUS CELL CARCINOMA

Squamous cell carcinoma has uniform gross and microscopic morphology, unlike that of basal cell carcinoma. Squamous cell carcinoma appears as sharply defined, erythematous plaques with elevated borders. As invasion deepens, the borders elevate further, and the lesions appear as painless, firm, red nodules with scaling, ulceration, and horn formation. Carcinoma in situ lesions are reddish with slightly raised borders.

Histologically, squamous carcinoma in situ is characterized by atypical squamous cells completely replacing the epidermis. In actinic keratosis the atypical cells only partially replace the epidermis. A lymphocytic infiltrate is usually present in the superficial dermis.

Invasion is defined as atypical keratinocyte migration through the basement membrane into the dermis. These cells are pleomorphic, have multiple mitoses, and are dyskeratotic, with horn pearls consisting of concentric layers of squamous cells with central keratinization. They range in histologic grade from well differentiated to poorly differentiated, depending on their resemblance to normal cells.

In addition, histologic evidence of perineural invasion may herald a more aggressive lesion. The pseudoglandular and spindle cell types are variants of squamous cell carcinoma. Verrucous carcinomas are a slow-growing variant characterized by their fungating appearance and can be deeply invasive without metastasis.

Skin cancers, particularly squamous cell carcinoma, may occur in several precursor lesions. These lesions help identify patients at risk for later development of either basal cell carcinoma, squamous cell carcinoma, or melanoma (Table 22-1).

Actinic Keratosis

Actinic keratoses are rough, scaly, erythematous plaques present on chronically exposed skin of the forehead, nose, cheeks, neck, and superior pinna. Mild tenderness usually is present. Because these lesions represent a risk factor for nonmelanoma skin cancer (basal or squamous cell), these patients should be closely followed. The progression rate for a single actinic keratotic lesion to squamous cell carcinoma is estimated to be 1 in 1000 per year.[18]

Signs of conversion to carcinoma include an increase in thickness, induration, and ulceration, with a rapid increase in size. These lesions should be biopsied at their base. Histopathology shows keratinocyte atypia limited to the epidermis, usually only the basal layer, and no invasion into the dermis. These lesions may also spontaneously regress if the patient limits sun exposure. Up to 25% per year may regress, but they typically recur at the same site after substantial reexposure.

Treatment ranges from continued observation to destructive ablation. Single lesions can be destroyed with liquid nitrogen cryotherapy. Diffuse involvement is best treated with topical medications such as 5-fluorouracil, masoprocol, or retinoids.[30] Treatment with isotretinoin (Retin-A), chemical

Table 22-1. Precursor Lesions and Cancer Risk	
PRECURSOR LESION	**CANCER RISK**
Actinic keratosis	1 : 1000 per year
Bowen's disease	5% develop dermal invasion
Human papillomavirus	Unknown

Data from Sober AJ, Burstein JM: *Cancer* 75(suppl 2):645-650, 1995.

peeling, and carbon dioxide (CO_2) laser resurfacing may reduce the risk of further development of cutaneous malignancy in these sun-damaged patients.[3,31]

Bowen's Disease

Squamous cell carcinoma in situ has been referred to as Bowen's disease and predominantly occurs in older patients.[30] These lesions are erythematous with raised, well-defined borders and a scaly appearance that may be confused with psoriasis. They have an indolent history with years of slow growth. When located on the penis, this lesion is termed *erythroplasia of Queyrat.*

Histopathologically, atypia of the full thickness of the epidermis occurs without dermal invasion. Progression to squamous carcinoma is slow, but 5% of lesions show dermal invasion with metastatic potential.

Treatment of Bowen's disease generally requires complete excision both for definitive diagnosis to rule out invasion and for cure. If surgical excision is not performed after biopsy, ablation can be done with cryotherapy or electrodesiccation and curettage.

Keratoacanthoma

Keratoacanthoma is a rapidly growing lesion with either a benign or a malignant phenotype. Grossly and histologically, it resembles squamous cell carcinoma. Its ambivalent nature, however, is manifested by rapid initial growth over several weeks, typically followed by a latent period, then a period of regression, each lasting several weeks as well.

Keratoacanthomas have been termed *deficient squamous cell carcinomas* because they tend to regress spontaneously, but they may occasionally progress to invasive or metastatic squamous cell carcinoma.[13] The cause of this regression is unknown but may be immunologically mediated.[20]

Because of malignant potential and frequent confusion with squamous cell carcinoma, we recommend complete excision of keratoacanthoma and histologic evaluation.

Human Papillomavirus

Human papillomavirus (HPV) has been found in patients with Bowen's disease and with epidermodysplasia verruciformis, both of which are associated with squamous cell carcinoma.[30]

Immunocompromised patients with human immunodeficiency virus (HIV) and immunosuppressed transplant patients also have an association with HPV and squamous cell carcinoma. These groups require aggressive sun protection and frequent surveillance.

OPERATIONS

Various techniques have been used to treat basal and squamous cell carcinomas. Almost any of these may be used in a certain setting to achieve acceptable results. The surgeon's choice of technique for a particular lesion may be based on a series of factors, including the following:

1. Personal bias and experience
2. Level and type of training
3. Accessibility to operative facilities or equipment
4. Patient preference

Selection of treatment should always be based primarily on a thorough knowledge of all modalities. The surgeon should select the method that best achieves the two major goals of treatment: (1) eradication of the tumor and (2) aesthetic and functional reconstruction.

EXCISION

Surgical excision is the most common technique used for treating basal and squamous cell carcinomas. Its advantages are simplicity, versatility, and speed. It can be used in essentially all locations of the body and on lesions of any size.

Since approximately 80% of basal and squamous cell carcinomas are small and can be closed primarily, excisional biopsy and primary closure are frequently appropriate for both biopsy and treatment and can be performed in a single office visit. The lesion should be resected as an ellipse, with its long axis along Langer's lines. The tissue specimen should be marked according to its original orientation in situ, placed in fixative, and sent to the pathologist for evaluation of margins.

For larger lesions or those with a questionable diagnosis, punch or shave biopsies may be appropriate. Cytologic analysis may also be useful to confirm the diagnosis in large or multiple lesions.[6] For pigmented lesions with malignant melanoma in the differential diagnosis, a complete excisional biopsy should be performed to allow proper histologic staging.

For both squamous and basal cell carcinomas, clear surgical margins are essential. Multiple frozen sections should be used on all but the most straightforward lesions to ensure complete excision.

After excising the specimen, we obtain additional margin(s) of 1 to 2 mm in all directions and submit these for frozen-section evaluation (Figure 22-4). These fragments of tissue can be excised at the margin of resection, as identified at specific points based on their orientation relative to an

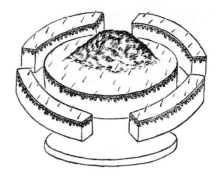

Figure 22-4. Biopsy technique for skin malignancies. Central portion of lesion is excised with 1-mm margin and is sent as a permanent section. Subsequent margins are taken separately, based on imaginary superimposed clock, and are sent for frozen-section evaluation. Further resection before reconstruction is guided by frozen-section results.

imaginary clock placed on the wound (e.g., 12 to 3 o'clock, 3 to 6 o'clock). The deep margin should also be marked separately and submitted. We use silver nitrate rather than ink to mark the border of interest in all our specimens. It leaves a thin layer of red-brown pigment that will not wash off and is easily visible histologically. Further resection can be performed in precise locations as indicated by the frozen-section results.

With extremely large tumors or when margins are difficult to clear, the surgeon should perform the tumor excision with careful marking of the margins, then cover the wound with petroleum gauze until the final pathologic result is known. If the wound is in an area that should be closed promptly, such as the medial or lateral canthal areas, it can be temporarily covered with a skin graft. Definitive reconstruction can then be performed when the margins are known conclusively to be clear. This is inconvenient for the patient and surgeon, and every effort should be made to clear the margins and reconstruct the lesion at the original procedure.

The optimal surgical margin is not known. Nguyen et al[19] recommend margins of 2 to 10 mm, depending on the size of the lesion and the histologic subtype. Wolf and Zitelli[32] recommend a minimum margin of 4 mm to eradicate more than 95% of tumors greater than 2 cm. They were able to construct a tumor eradication curve based on margin and tumor size in 117 primary basal cell cancers.

Although the planned surgical margin is an important consideration, it is still arbitrary and not a histologically clear margin. Therefore, frozen-section analysis must be used to confirm clear margins histologically in all but the most straightforward cases.

MOHS' SURGERY

Mohs' chemosurgery was first described in 1941 by Frederic Mohs, who used zinc chloride paste on tumors as a means of evaluating surgical margins. Currently, Mohs' technique uses a frozen-section technique that allows the immediate examination of microscopic margins.

The technique of Mohs' surgery involves obtaining tumor-free margins in three planes. Careful, fresh tissue techniques are used to obtain immediate feedback from positive margins, if present, in each of three dimensions. A positive margin is then subjected to reexcision until that margin is cleared. This is particularly useful for infiltrative basal cell carcinomas, which have fingerlike projections emanating from the tumor. These projections may be missed by less directed excision of tissue.

Mohs' surgery yields excellent results for skin cancers. It is a time-consuming, expensive, and tedious procedure, however, and may require postponing complicated reconstructions, which is inconvenient for the patient and surgeon.[16]

Indications for Mohs' surgery for basal cell carcinoma are poorly defined because of a lack of randomized studies. Clearly, however, Mohs' surgery provides excellent results with recurrent tumors. Furthermore, tumors with an aggressive histologic subtype with infiltrative features or those in critical anatomic locations may be best treated with Mohs' or a direct excisional technique that carefully examines each margin.

Lesions in which the risk of significant functional loss increases with each 1 mm of margin taken may benefit most from Mohs' surgery. Lesions of the medial canthal region and the alar rim are frequent candidates. On other head and neck areas the functional and aesthetic results do not change significantly by preserving 1 or 2 extra mm of potentially normal skin. Therefore Mohs' surgery is of little benefit in these areas, and its higher marginal cost is not justified compared with simple excision.

LASER EXCISION

Reports continue to describe the use of lasers to treat skin cancers. The most common use involves the CO_2 laser, which emits nonvisible infrared light that is absorbed by the water present in all tissues. The CO_2 laser has been used in two ways.

In the *focused mode* the CO_2 laser is used to coagulate or excise tissue. The major benefit is the laser's ability to coagulate blood vessels during dissection and potentially reduce bleeding. Significant blood loss, however, is rarely a consideration in the excision of these lesions. Also, the thermal damage may hinder preparation and evaluation of microscopic margins and may alter the success of certain methods of reconstruction (e.g., skin grafting). The CO_2 laser may also be used in a *unfocused mode* to vaporize small tumors.

No randomized trials show any clear advantage to the laser for the treatment of basal cell carcinoma.[9]

NONOPERATIVE THERAPY

Radiation Therapy

Radiation therapy may be an effective treatment for some patients with basal cell carcinoma. It is particularly indicated in older patients who may be too ill to tolerate a general anesthetic and who have little risk of late development of radiation-induced skin cancers. Radiation may also be useful in areas where it may be difficult to obtain a negative margin or to perform reconstruction (e.g., periorbital, nasal, periauricular).

The surgeon must consider potential complications of radiation, such as dry eye, xerostomia, epilation, lacrimal duct scarring, skin necrosis, and poor wound healing. In addition, histologically negative margins cannot be obtained using radiation.

Before radiation therapy, a confirmatory biopsy is typically required to establish the histologic diagnosis. The subsequent treatment regimen generally uses 4000 to 6000 cGy in 10 to 30 fractions, depending on the tumor, and typically requires multiple patient visits.

Chemotherapy

5-FLUOROURACIL. 5-FU is a chemotherapeutic agent used topically for the treatment of basal cell carcinoma. It is applied until the lesion becomes red and ulcerated. The lesion typically sloughs and then heals over the ensuing 1 to 2 months while normal adjacent tissue remains uninjured.

The success of 5-fluorouracil treatment depends on contact between the agent and the tumor. Therefore its usefulness in large nodular or infiltrative lesions is limited. Tumors measuring 5 to 20 mm may show good responses to treatment.

Topical 5-fluorouracil is formulated in a hydrophilic base in concentrations of 5% to 20%. Application to the lesion, including a small margin of normal tissue, is typically performed at night and covered. Treatment is usually continued for 4 to 12 weeks.[14]

ISOTRETINOIN AND OTHER VITAMIN A–BASED TREATMENTS. An increased susceptibility to carcinogenesis in epithelium is known to be increased by vitamin A deficiency and inhibited by high dietary levels of retinoids.[2] Retinoids have been shown in vivo to have antineoplastic effects, possibly by restoring normal cellular differentiation and maturation. Topical in vivo retinoic acid treatment causes marked epithelial thickening, with an increase in the number of cell layers expressing markers of differentiation.[2]

Oral isotretinoin is not effective in the prevention of basal cell carcinomas.[25] Clinically, actinic keratoses regress with topical retinoid therapy, which may be enhanced by cotreatment with 5-fluorouracil. Other evidence suggests that topical retinoids may be useful in the prevention of basal cell carcinoma.[11]

INTERFERON-α. Preliminary studies have shown interferon-α to be effective in the treatment of nodular-ulcerative and superficial basal cell carcinomas. Its mechanism of action appears to be related to a nonspecific activation of macrophages and natural killer cells in the area of the tumor, increasing the magnitude of the host's antineoplastic response.[14]

Phototherapy

Photodynamic therapy is a relatively new modality for the treatment of basal cell carcinoma. An inactive photosensitizer is administered and accumulates in the tissue of interest. Light is then delivered to the tumor, photoactivating the sensitizer, which in turn converts molecular oxygen to free radicals that are tumoricidal (oncolytic).

Because of the widespread photosensitization to the patient, phototherapy is not currently useful for treating isolated tumors. It may have a role, however, in the treatment of patients with widespread disease (e.g., Gorlin's syndrome).[24]

Cryosurgery and Electrosurgery

The use of physical energy to treat basal cell carcinoma may yield excellent cure rates in properly selected patients. Patients who have nodular-ulcerative or superficial tumors that are small (5 to 15 mm) with well-defined borders, in locations where wound contraction will provide an acceptable functional and aesthetic outcome, are good candidates for cryosurgery or electrosurgery.

Cryosurgery typically uses liquid nitrogen (−195.6° C), which is applied rapidly with a spray device or wand. An intracellular temperature of −40° C is required for cell destruction. Thermocouples placed at the tumor base may be used to ensure adequate heat loss.

Electrosurgery uses manual curettage of the tumor, followed by the application of electrical energy, such as through electrocautery.

When using these techniques, the wounds are covered with antibiotic ointment and allowed to heal by secondary intention. Margins cannot be inspected for residual cancer using these methods.[14]

OUTCOMES

Since basal and squamous cell carcinomas are rarely fatal, survival should not be used to measure treatment success. Rather, complete tumor eradication and functional and aesthetic reconstruction are the goals of treatment.

Tumor control is best determined by recurrence rate, but unfortunately, several factors make this parameter difficult to evaluate. Various methods have been used to determine recurrence rates; when comparing separate outcome studies, the surgeon must be cognizant of the statistical method used. Although not always used, the life table or Kaplan-Meier method best approximates the actual recurrence rate and is the preferred means for reporting recurrence rates.[29]

The surgeon also must consider length of follow-up. Because most recurrences appear 1 to 4 years after therapy, at least a 5-year follow-up period should be used.

Finally, reliable prospective and randomized data are difficult to obtain because of the following:

1. Number of successful treatments available
2. Difficulty in controlling and comparing treatment-related variables
3. Specialty biases and preferences for certain treatments

To assess accurately the treatment outcome for basal cell carcinoma, patients at risk to fail therapy should be identified. Randle[22] has identified characteristics of patients at high risk for recurrence (Box 22-4).[25]

Skin cancers on the midface, particularly around the nose and ears, are more likely to recur (Figure 22-5). The location of these tumors near the embryonic lines of fusion may facilitate deeper tumor spread. Furthermore, surgeons are less willing to obtain wide margins in these areas. Large cancers, often an indication of neglect and denial, are also more likely to recur. In a Cleveland Clinic study of basal cell carcinomas treated by a variety of techniques, 46% of tumors greater than 2 cm were recurrent, whereas only 13% of those less than 2 cm were recurrent.[26]

As noted earlier, the morpheaform variety behaves much more aggressively and has the greatest recurrence rate of the various histologic subtypes. Subclinical tumor extension in morpheaform basal cell carcinoma is three times that in nodular-ulcerative forms.[27] Recurrence rates of tumors with histologic features of sclerosis (morpheaform) and infiltration as well as features of both basal and squamous carcinoma are several times higher than for nodular forms (12% to 30%

Box 22-4.
Risk Factors for Recurrence of Basal Cell Carcinoma

Long duration
High-risk area (e.g., midface, ear)
Large size
Aggressive histologic features (e.g., morpheaform type, perineural invasion)
Neglected tumor
Inadequately treated or recurrent disease
History of radiation exposure

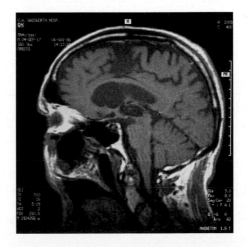

Figure 22-5. Sagittal magnetic resonance image shows extensive squamous cell carcinoma of cheek invading left maxillary sinus and growing along infraorbital nerve and into orbital floor.

versus 1% to 6%).[21] This is a result of the fingerlike projections emanating from the central tumor mass, which may extend several millimeters into surrounding normal tissue.

Table 22-2 details a reasonable approach to estimating margins preoperatively.

Squamous cell carcinoma lesions larger than 3 cm and with anaplasia are substantially more difficult to cure because of the tendency for lymphatic spread and distant metastases (Figure 22-6). Some authors recommend at least 3-cm margins for these lesions, especially if located on the trunk or extremities, as often occurs.

The type of treatment can significantly affect recurrence. Unfortunately, the literature has little meaningful randomized data regarding the best methods of treatment for particular tumor patterns. Julian and Bowers[10] did report a prospective study of Mohs' surgery for basal cell carcinoma. In 228 basal cell carcinomas treated, the 5-year recurrence rate was 3.8%. The authors noted high cure rates in difficult and recurrent tumors treated with Mohs' surgery.

Any technique that includes surgical excision of the tumor, careful histologic examination of the margins, and reexcision of positive margins yields cure rates of approximately 95% for primary tumors. This should be considered the standard of care for basal cell carcinoma.

Acceptable cure rates can also be obtained with other forms of therapy. For example, small truncal lesions can be adequately treated with cryotherapy or curettage and electrosurgery.

Radiation therapy, although reasonable in certain cases, should not be relied on as a first-line treatment for basal cell carcinoma. The surgeon should carefully consider its many limitations. Radiation carries the risk of inducing further injury to already actinically damaged skin, thereby increasing the risk of future malignant cutaneous transformation and altering the tumor-host relationship.[16] Damaging effects to the skin also make future treatment and reconstruction of recurrent lesions significantly more difficult.

A positive margin after definitive resection represents a significant dilemma for the surgeon and patient. We recommend obtaining clear margins in the operating room. Occasionally, however, the surgeon may encounter a reconstructed patient who has an untreated positive margin. Management of this patient has been the source of considerable debate in the literature.

In patients with microscopically positive margins, the wound scar can be excised and usually closed primarily. Recurrence typically occurs within the first 2 years after the initial resection.[7] If recurrent tumor is present grossly, larger

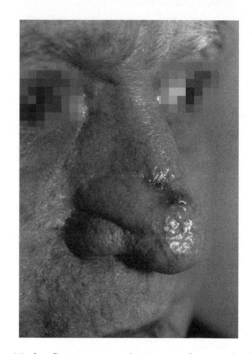

Figure 22-6. Recurrent erythematous, firm, and ulcerated squamous cell carcinoma of lateral nasal wall and dorsum in 68-year-old patient 1½ years after initial resection and reconstruction with superiorly based nasolabial flap.

Table 22-2.
Planning Surgical Margins for Primary Excision of Basal Cell Carcinoma

TUMOR TYPE	AREA*	ANTICIPATED MARGIN (MM)	FROZEN SECTION
Solid, circumscribed			
<2 cm	Noncritical	5-10	No
>2 cm	Noncritical	5-10	Yes
<1 cm	Critical	2-3	Yes
>1 cm and <2 cm	Critical	3-5	Yes
>2 cm	Critical	5-10	Yes
Morpheaform or aggressive subtype	Any	7-10	Yes
Other histologic subtypes	Individualized	Individualized	

*Noncritical areas include trunk, upper arms, and legs; critical areas include face, head, hands, feet and perineum.

margins are indicated, which may include tissue previously used to reconstruct the defect. If the lesion is on the face, a more complex and larger flap reconstruction is required, with a greater potential for donor site morbidity. A poor aesthetic outcome is more likely in this patient.

Proponents of observing the surgical site without reexcision in the patient with a positive margin note that fewer than half these patients with basal cell carcinoma will have a recurrence. Those favoring reexcision, however, consider a 30% recurrence rate for observation too high. They suggest than eventual control of the disease may require more radical surgery than would be required if done immediately.

Richmond and Davie[23] recommend immediate reexcision based on a retrospective review of 23 recurrences in 60 patients. They noted a mean recurrence time of almost 3 years. The combination of a positive, deep, and lateral margin was more prevalent in recurring lesions.

Liu et al[15] reported a series 67 patients with a microscopic margin who were observed after resection; 21 had local recurrences. In a cost analysis of treatment versus observation, the authors noted only a small cost savings to patients treated with postoperative radiation therapy compared with those observed. Because they showed no difference in ultimate local control, the authors suggest observation for these patients, primarily to avoid the morbidity of unnecessary treatment.

Functional outcome can be studied by analyzing the success of meeting the reconstructive goals and avoiding complications (Box 22-5). From a functional perspective, an open skin wound permits water and protein fluid loss and is at risk for infection. An open wound is also painful and inconvenient for the patient and family. Therefore residual wounds after skin cancer excision should be primarily closed or reconstructed, if possible.

Skin grafts typically heal with a color and texture mismatch that may be very noticeable on the face. Contour differences often occur with skin grafts and result in unappealing shadowing that accentuates the graft–normal skin boundary. Composite grafts of skin, fat, and cartilage, usually taken from the ear or another well-camouflaged area, may provide both contour and wound closure with minimal donor morbidity.

Properly conceived flaps also typically provide improved color and texture matches relative to skin grafts, although they may require donor site dissections onto aesthetically critical areas. Local facial flaps generally are reliable reconstructive options. Arterial or venous insufficiency and flap loss occur infrequently with most of these flaps.

Clearly, significant opportunity and need exist for further investigations of clinical outcomes in malignant skin conditions. Specifically, a prospective randomized comparison of Mohs' surgery to other treatment modalities, especially to simple excision and with careful attention to pathologic margins, would be helpful. A need also exists for further clinical research into the functional and aesthetic results of each treatment modality. Because of the inherent difficulties in standardizing measures for aesthetic and functional outcomes, however, clinically meaningful data will be difficult to obtain.

Box 22-5.
Potential Complications after Treatment of Skin Malignancies

Tumor cells at resection margin
Gross tumor recurrence after resection
Hypertrophic scar
Keloid development
Skin color mismatch
Skin texture difference
Skin contour deformity
Flap loss (partial or whole)
Loss of function (e.g., eyelid loss with degradation in tear production)

REFERENCES

1. Buzzell RA: Carcinogenesis of cutaneous malignancies, *Dermatol Surg* 22:209-215, 1996.

2. Craven NM, Griffiths CE: Retinoids in the management of non-melanoma skin cancer and melanoma, *Cancer Surv* 26:267-288, 1996.

3. Craven NM, Griffiths CE: Topical retinoids and cutaneous biology, *Clin Exp Dermatol* 21:1-10, 1996.

4. Dahl E, Aberg M, Rausing A, et al: Basal cell carcinoma: an epidemiologic study in a defined population, *Cancer* 70:104-108, 1992.

5. De Rosa G, Staibano S, Barra E, et al: p53 protein in aggressive and non-aggressive basal cell carcinoma, *J Cutan Pathol* 20:429-434, 1993.

6. Derrick EK, Smith R, Melcher DH, et al: The use of cytology in the diagnosis of basal cell carcinoma, *Br J Dermatol* 130:561-563, 1994.

7. Dubin N, Kopf AW: Multivariant risk score for recurrence of cutaneous basal cell carcinomas, *Arch Dermatol* 119:373-375, 1983.

8. Fleming ID, Amonette R, Monaghan T, et al: Principles of management of basal and squamous cell carcinoma of the skin, *Cancer* 75(suppl 2):699-704, 1995.

9. Geronemus R, Ashinoff R: Lasers in the treatment of skin cancer, *Clin Podiatr Med Surg* 9:599-615, 1992.

10. Julian CG, Bowers PW: A prospective study of Mohs' micrographic surgery in two English centres, *Br J Dermatol* 136:515-518, 1997.

11. Kligman AM: Tretinoin (Retin-A) therapy of photoaged skin, *Compr Ther* 18:10-13, 1992.

12. Kricker A, Armstrong BK, English DR, et al: Does intermittent sun exposure cause basal cell carcinoma? A case-control study in Western Australia, *Int J Cancer* 60:489-494, 1995.

13. Krunic AL, Garrod DR, Smith NP, et al: Differential expression of desmosomal glycoproteins in keratoacanthoma and squamous cell carcinoma of the skin: an immunohistochemical aid to diagnosis, *Acta Derm Venereol* 76:394-398, 1996.

14. Limmer BL, Clark D: Nonsurgical management of primary skin malignancies, *Otolaryngol Clin North Am* 26:167-183, 1993.

15. Liu FF, Maki E, Warde P, et al: A management approach to incompletely excised basal cell carcinomas of skin, *Int J Radiat Oncol Biol Phys* 20:423-428, 1991.

16. Luce EA: Oncologic considerations in nonmelanotic skin cancer, *Clin Plast Surg* 22:39-50, 1995.

17. Marks R, Kopf AW: Cancer of the skin in the next century, *Int J Dermatol* 34:445-447, 1995.

18. Marks R, Rennie G, Selwoog TS: Malignant transformation of solar keratoses to squamous cell carcinoma in the skin: a prospective study, *Lancet* 1:795-797, 1988.

19. Nguyen AV, Whitaker DC, Frodel J: Differentiation of basal cell carcinoma, *Otolaryngol Clin North Am* 26:37-56, 1993.

20. Patel A, Halliday GM, Cooke BE, et al: Evidence that regression in keratoacanthoma is immunologically mediated: a comparison with squamous cell carcinoma, *Br J Dermatol* 131:789-798, 1994.

21. Preston DS, Stern RS: Nonmelanoma cancers of the skin, *N Engl J Med* 327:1649-1662, 1992.

22. Randle HW: Basal cell carcinoma: identification and treatment of the high-risk patient, *Dermatol Surg* 22:255-261, 1996.

23. Richmond JD, Davie RM: The significance of incomplete excision in patients with basal cell carcinoma, *Br J Plast Surg* 40:63-67, 1987.

24. Roberts DJ, Cairnduff F: Photodynamic therapy of primary skin cancer: a review, *Br J Plast Surg* 48:360-370, 1995.

25. Robinson JK, Salasche SJ: Isotretinoin does not prevent basal cell carcinoma, *Arch Dermatol* 128:975-976, 1992 (editorial).

26. Roenigk RK, Ratz JL, Bailin PL, et al: Trends in the presentation and treatment of basal cell carcinomas, *J Dermatol Surg Oncol* 12:860-865, 1986.

27. Salasche SJ, Amonette RA: Morpheaform basal-cell epitheliomas: a study of subclinical extensions in a series of 51 cases, *J Dermatol Surg Oncol* 7:387-394, 1981.

28. Shanley S, Ratcliffe J, Hockey A, et al: Nevoid basal cell carcinoma syndrome: review of 118 affected individuals, *Am J Med Genet* 50:282-290, 1994.

29. Silverman MK, Kopf AW, Grin CM, et al: Recurrence rates of treated basal cell carcinomas. Part 1. Overview, *J Dermatol Surg Oncol* 17:713-718, 1991.

30. Sober AJ, Burstein JM: Precursors to skin cancer, *Cancer* 75(suppl 2):645-650, 1995.

31. Trimas SJ, Ellis DA, Metz RD: The carbon dioxide laser: an alternative for the treatment of actinically damaged skin, *Dermatol Surg* 23:885-889, 1997.

32. Wolf DJ, Zitelli JA: Surgical margins for basal cell carcinoma, *Arch Dermatol* 123:340-344, 1987.

CHAPTER

Melanoma

23

Steven D. Macht

INTRODUCTION

Melanoma constitutes only 2% of all cancers.[1] It is increasing in epidemic proportions, however, and is now second in frequency to lung cancer in women.[2] The incidence of melanoma appears to be doubling every 8 to 10 years (Figures 23-1 and 23-2).[3] In 1925 the incidence was 1.1 cases per 100,000 population; in 1975 this was as high as 6.2.

Melanoma is now the leading cause of death of all skin diseases.[4-6] Approximately 40,000 new cases can be anticipated in the next year. The tumor may arise from almost any organ. The skin is the site most easily observed, however, and the most common site of presentation.[7,8]

INDICATIONS

The exact cause of melanoma is not known, but a combination of sun exposure and genetic predisposition

appears to be important.[9] Supporting the genetic theory is the increased incidence in *xeroderma pigmentosum,* a chronic progressive disease inherited as an autosomal recessive trait.[10] Tumor development is likely from actinic damage superimposed on a deoxyribonucleic acid (DNA) repair problem.[11] Approximately 3% of patients will develop melanoma in their lifetime, which is significantly greater than the general population.

The *B-K (dysplastic) mole syndrome,* or *familial atypical multimole melanoma* (FAMM) *syndrome,* also supports the genetic theory.[12-15] This is an autosomal dominant condition named after the first two families identified with this condition.[16] When this is present, melanoma is predictable. Patients often have multiple, large, irregular-appearing dysplastic nevi throughout their body.[17] Other inherited risk factors include inability to tan and fair skin color.

Excessive sun exposure is supported by the finding of increased incidence of melanoma in reference to latitude.[18] Populations in the United States and Australia demonstrate a much higher incidence in areas closer to the sun.[19] A history of at least one severe sunburn is often found in the melanoma patient population.[20] This is most likely to have occurred more than 20 years earlier. Initially, this increased incidence of

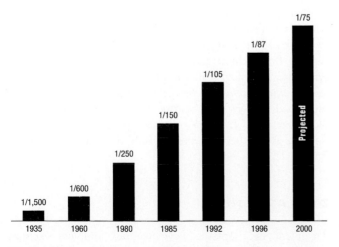

Figure 23-1. Increase in incidence (lifetime risk) of melanoma since 1935 in United States. (From Rigel DS: *CA* 46:196, 1996.)

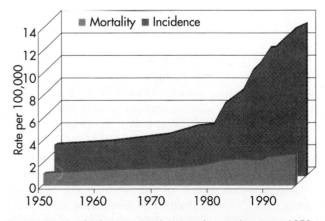

Figure 23-2. Melanoma incidence and mortality since 1950 in United States. Expected mortality did not materialize, which many theories have great difficulty explaining. (From Rigel DS: *CA* 46:197, 1996.)

tumors paralleled that of basosquamous cancers of the skin and prompted the actinic theories of causation.[21]

Despite all these epidemiologic findings, however, many inconsistencies persist. Similar latitudes and increase in altitude do *not* appear to lead to an increase in tumors. Constant outdoor exposure is *less* of a risk factor than intermittent exposure. Several countries have a higher incidence of melanoma in parts of the country that are *farther* from the equator. Nearly one half of melanomas occur on parts of the body that are not routinely exposed to sun. Researchers have theorized that the immune suppression caused by intense ultraviolet radiation exposure about 20 years earlier may be the trigger mechanism.[22-24]

Other causes, such as chemical induction, trauma, or hormonal stimulation, have been postulated.[25,26] The presence of melanoma on the soles of the feet supports the trauma theory. Chemical exposure is only anecdotally supported by petrochemical exposure.[27,28] Hormonal stimulation as a factor is supported by the occurrence or exacerbation of melanoma during pregnancy or with exogenous estrogen sources.[29] A darkening of nevi typically occurs during pregnancy.[30] Several growth factors have been isolated and implicated as the cause of melanoma, including epidermal, nerve, insulin-like, fibroblast, platelet derived, and transforming growth factor beta, (EGF, NGF, IGF, FGF, PDGF, TGF-β).[31]

CLINICAL PRESENTATION

Clinically, melanomas can be best described as irregular in color, irregular in outline, and irregular in surface topography.[33] The American Cancer Society (ACS) uses the ABCD rule to describe melanoma: *a*symmetric lesions (i.e., when cut, one half does not resemble the other half), *b*order irregularity, *c*olor variability, and *d*iameter greater than 6 mm.[34,35]

Despite all these descriptions, a subgroup of tumors still defy clinical recognition.[36] A clinician need not be 100% accurate in the diagnosis, but knowing when to biopsy is important and possibly lifesaving. Frequently the melanoma has shown a history of change, such as an increase in size, elevation, or color.[37] Occasionally, itching may be the only presenting symptom.

The variable color has been described as the "red, white, and blue" sign caused by the light reflection from melanin at different levels in the dermis *(Tyndall effect)* (Figure 23-3). Some lesions may be relatively uniform in color, primarily dark brown or black. Any suspicious lesion should be excised for biopsy.

Melanoma can present anywhere on the body, but the lower extremity in women and the truncal region in men are the most common sites.[38,39] Only one-half arise from preexisting nevi. The great majority of melanomas are clinically obvious and, again, typically have a history of change.[40] Inherited traits (e.g., fair skin color, inability to tan) are also factors.

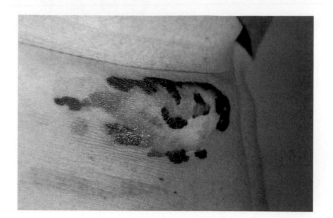

Figure 23-3. Large melanoma on flank arising from congenital nevus demonstrates "red, white, and blue" sign (Tyndall effect). Lesion is present at varying depths, irregularly reflecting light back at different wavelengths.

Significant changes have occurred in the presentation of melanoma and its natural history.[41-46] With its increasing incidence, lesions are now thinner, less invasive, less likely to be ulcerated, and more curable. Apparently, the site distribution has not changed much over the years, but the absolute number of cases has drastically increased. Although the number of cases has drastically increased, the mortality has not increased as much as would be expected. This has led some to theorize that lesions in a more "benign" form are being categorized as melanoma.

In any event, general risk factors, as mentioned earlier, include an individual or family history of melanoma, history of dysplastic nevi, fair complexion, blistering sunburn, or time spent outdoors between the ages of 10 and 24. The propensity to sun burn, as well as the number of clinically atypical nevi, particularly those greater than 2 cm, seems important, along with a history of nonmelanocytic skin cancer, such as basal cell and squamous cell carcinoma (BCC, SCC).[47]

All these factors have been well known in the past. A patient's inability to tan over a lifetime or the direct effect of a severe sunburn is not known to be the cause. Dysplastic nevi often present a confusing problem to physicians, particularly the patient who is diagnosed with "a dysplastic nevus" based on a single biopsy report. The report may even suggest the architectural pattern suggesting the FAMM syndrome. Pathologists debate whether they can identify such lesions with accuracy. Statistically, the patient's risk is predicated on (1) past history of melanoma (personal or blood relative), (2) type of mole pattern displayed, (3) number of such lesions, and (4) only then, histology of the isolated lesion.

DYSPLASTIC NEVI

Treatment of dysplastic nevi requires complete excision whenever possible, including any residual "atypical melano-

Table 23-1.
Distinguishing Features Among Normal and Dysplastic Nevi and Melanoma

FEATURE	NORMAL NEVI	DYSPLASTIC NEVI	MELANOMA
Size	>6 mm	Often >7 mm	Often >6 mm
Uniformity	Homogenous	Heterogenous	Heterogenous
Number	Few (10-40)	Often many normal nevi (50-100)	Usually 1
Perimeter	Regular	Irregular, indistinct	Irregular
Color	Uniform	Usually variegated	Usually variegated
Hue	Tan, brown	Tan, brown, black, red	Tan, brown, black; red, white, blue
Shoulder	Uncommon	Almost always	Often
Symmetry	Symmetric	Symmetric	Asymmetric
Elevation	Macular to nodular	Usually papular to plaque centrally	Papular to nodular
Hypertrichosis	Uncommon	None	None
Erosion/ulcer	None	None	May be present
Location	Usually trunk > limbs	Usually trunk > limbs > head	Male: trunk > limbs Female: limbs > trunk
Symptoms	Usually none	Usually none	Often
Change	Slow then stable	Slow then stable	Faster, continuous
Surrounding skin	Normal	Normal	May have satellites

cytic hyperplasia." The National Cancer Institute (NCI) has categorically stated that the cure rate is 100% for dysplastic nevi. These lesions must be distinguished from other nevi and malignant melanoma (Table 23-1).

When deciding treatment for patients with a diagnosis of "dysplastic nevus," the physician must assess the degree of risk.[48] The terminology is very difficult to correlate with clinical behavior, and patient risks may range from a high likelihood of developing melanoma to no greater risk than the population at large. Unfortunately, little correlation exists between the clinical appearance and the pathologic grading. At one point, the terminology "nevus with architectural disorder" was promoted at a National Institutes of Health (NIH) Consensus Conference; however, this has not become popular usage.[49]

Patients with a personal or family history of melanoma and those with many large irregular moles primarily on the trunk are at high risk and merit frequent surveillance (Table 23-2).[50-52] Generally, excision with a 1-mm to 2-mm rim of normal tissue is sufficient. The degree of dysplasia, however, does not seem to correlate the chance of developing melanoma as long as the lesion is completely excised. Alternately, if a patient has a single lesion with severe dysplasia and the area is completely excised, the risk of other lesions also becoming atypical may not increase.[53]

The state of the art is changing, and clinicians are attempting to follow guidelines acceptable to physicians, patients, and insurers. Generally, excisional biopsy is a minor procedure for any single, remotely suspicious lesion. On the other hand, a patient may have large irregular nevi, a first-degree relative with melanoma, and a diagnosis of melanoma in situ or true melanoma. These patients require close monitoring after suspicious lesions are excised. Generally these patients are followed by a dermatologist as well. Biopsies are performed as necessary. Full-body photographs are often helpful, or suitable computer imaging.[54]

Table 23-2.
Types of Dysplastic Mole Syndrome*

TYPE	DESCRIPTION
A	No personal or family history of melanoma moles uncommon in family
B	No personal or family history of melanoma moles common in family
C	Personal or family history of melanoma moles uncommon in family
D1	Personal or family history of melanoma moles common in family
D2	Two or more family members with melanoma moles common in family

*Risk increases in descending order listed here. For example, if patient has single dysplastic nevus and no other personal history of or relatives with melanoma, risk is comparable to that of general population (very small). Conversely, if patient has either personal history of or first-degree relative with melanoma, risk increases.
Modified from Green MH, Clark WH, Tucker DM, et al: *N Engl J Med* 312:91-97, 1985.

CONGENITAL NEVI

Congenital nevi are defined as those present at birth. Unfortunately, no clear histologic definition exists, and many nevi present at birth are not sufficiently pigmented to be visible. All congenital nevi are predisposed toward malignant change, even in childhood. This is recognized for larger lesions, but the precise risk is unknown for smaller lesions.[55] Larger lesions, arbitrarily defined as 20 cm², should be excised and the defect reconstructed with local flaps, tissue expansion, or grafts as needed. Researchers dispute the exact age at which this should be accomplished, but many suggest 6 to 24 months.[56,57]

Management of smaller nevi has been controversial.[58] The NIH Consensus Conference suggested that insufficient evidence exists to recommend removal of all congenital nevi.[49] A history of change, increased pigmentation, elevation, or growth should cause concern. Aesthetic consideration is also a valid indication for surgical excision.

Asymptomatic nevi can be followed safely until the child can undergo excision with local anesthesia. Nevi with the "bathing trunk" distribution, also known as "stocking glove" lesions, require treatment. Reconstruction can be formidable.[59-61]

The term *juvenile melanoma* requires clarification.[62,63] Microscopically, melanoma is most often confused with the Spitz nevus.[64] This is a smooth, pinkish tan, elevated lesion often found in children. The *Spitz nevus* is benign and has no predilection toward malignancy but unfortunately has been referred to as "juvenile melanoma."[65-68] This lesion may be confused with true melanoma, prompting the statement that melanoma

may be present in children but never metastasizes until puberty.[69-71]

Melanoma can occur in children and may be lethal, whereas the Spitz nevus is benign. When cited in a pathologic report, juvenile melanoma requires clarification.[72-75] Causing even more confusion is the report of a Spitz nevus metastasizing to only one lymph node. This rare entity may represent synchronous presentation of lesions on skin and node.

GROWTH PATTERNS

Four general growth patterns have been described for melanoma: (1) superficial spreading, (2) nodular, (3) lentigo maligna, and (4) acral lentiginous (acro lentiginous (acrolentiginous).[40,71]

Superficial spreading melanoma is the most common pattern (70% to 80% in most studies)[76] (Figure 23-4). These lesions usually are slow growing and may have variable color. The growth phase is described by Clark et al[14] as occurring in a radial fashion and "lacking a propensity to metastasize."

Nodular melanoma is the second most common group (20%) (Figure 23-5). These are aggressive tumors and develop more rapidly than the superficial spreading type. They usually

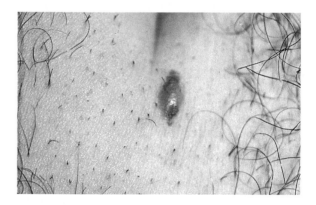

Figure 23-4. Lesions with history of recent change (enlarging) are becoming slightly darker. Biopsy indicates superficial spreading melanoma.

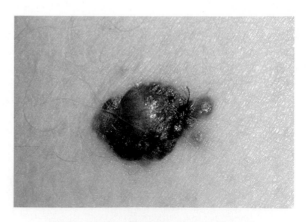

Figure 23-5. Typical nodular melanoma.

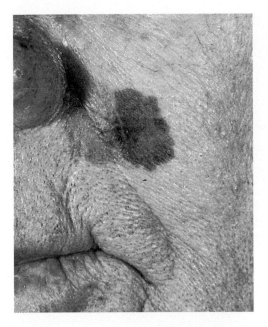

Figure 23-6. Lentigo maligna melanoma.

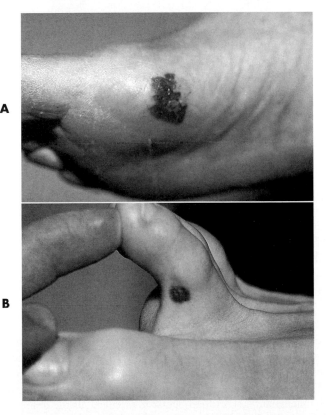

Figure 23-7. Acrolentiginous melanoma (ALM). **A,** Most typical presentation in black patients. Palms and depigmented area of soles are usually affected. **B,** ALM between toes. Note that all ALMs occur on extremities, but not all extremity lesions are ALMs.

occur in uninvolved skin but may also arise from preexisting nevi. They exhibit the vertical growth phase, become aggressive very early, and are the most virulent type of tumors. Fortunately, these are the most typically appearing melanomas and least likely to be missed.

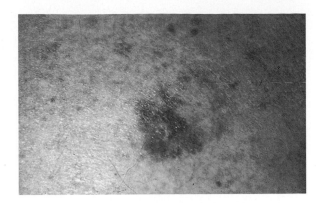

Figure 23-8. Minimally pigmented lesion but also melanoma. About 5% to 7% of lesions may defy visual recognition. Listening to patient's description of change facilitates diagnosis.

Lentigo maligna melanoma may be a somewhat different entity but still has a propensity to metastasize (Figure 23-6). Usually these lesions present as pigmented changes on sun-damaged skin.[77] These are typically large lesions with border irregularities, including notching. Often the face is involved, presenting a challenging surgical problem, particularly with reconstruction.

Acrolentiginous melanoma (ALM) is usually found on the palms, soles, or on the nail bed (Figure 23-7). Not all plantar or volar melanomas are acrolentiginous, except in darker-complected patients. They usually are large, affect patients 50 to 60 years old, and evolve slowly. Because ALM lesions often occur beneath the nail bed, the diagnosis is often delayed. Biopsy requires removal of the nail. The distribution of involvement is usually the big toe and thumb in most patients, although other extremity sites are well described.

Some minimally pigmented lesions defy visual recognition (Figure 23-8).

SUSPICIOUS LESIONS

Excisional biopsy is recommended for lesions that are 2 cm or less in diameter. In larger lesions, because of difficulties with pathology, my group's practice is to remove as much tissue for biopsy as possible in an office setting.[78-82] Shave biopsies are discouraged, and the entire lesion should be preserved for the pathologist. Generally the thickest portion of the growth, the most typical part and the transition zone from normal to abnormal, provides the best chance of an accurate diagnosis. Frozen-section analysis is used in some countries but generally is not recommended for primary melanoma.

If the tumor persists at the base of the specimen, the exact thickness may never be known.[83-85] Repeat biopsy at the same site never provides accurate information. Interestingly, repeat biopsy usually shows no evidence of tumor because of the immune reaction.

Once the diagnosis is made, patients are evaluated and staged as with other malignancies. The American Joint Committee on Cancer (AJCC) has designated the TNM system to have four stages[86] (Table 23-3).

Table 23-3.
Stages of TNM* Classification System for Melanoma

STAGE	DESCRIPTION
IA	Localized melanoma ≤0.75 mm thick or level II (T1, N0, M0)
IB	Localized melanoma >0.75 to 1.50 mm thick or level III (T2, N0, M0)
IIA	Localized melanoma >1.5 to 4.00 mm thick or level IV (T3, N0, M0)
IIB	Localized melanoma >4.00 mm thick or level V (T4, N0, M0)
III	Limited nodal metastases involving only one regional lymph node basin, movable nodes, and <5 cm in diameter; or negative regional nodes and presence of < five in-transit metastases beyond 2 cm from primary site (any T, N1, M0)
IV	Advanced regional metastases, defined as involvement of more than one regional lymph node station; regional nodes ≥5 cm in diameter or fixed or ≥ five in-transit metastases or any in-transit metastases beyond 2 cm from the primary site with regional node involvement (any T, N2, M0); or any distant metastases (any T, any N, M1 or M2)

T, Primary tumor; N, nodal involvement; M, distant metastasis.

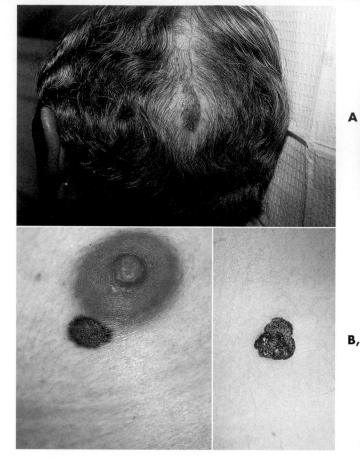

Figure 23-9. Several lesions may be mistaken for melanoma. **A,** Blue nevus of scalp. **B,** Dysplastic nevus of breast. **C,** Hemangioma.

After tissue is biopsied and the diagnosis of melanoma made, further evaluation is indicated. The information on the pathology report is only significant for stage I disease. Melanoma can metastasize to the skin from other sites (including other skin areas) and can be very difficult to distinguish from primary disease. Several lesions have been mistaken for melanoma, such as the blue nevus, dysplastic nevus, and hemangioma (Figure 23-9).

Pathology Report

First, the diagnosis should be made using histopathologic parameters. Special stains, such as S-100 and HMB-45, may be used to assist in determining whether the cells are melanocytic. HMB-45 seems to be a more specific marker than S-100.[87] Both can be used in primary and metastatic lesions. Other radiolabeled monoclonal antibodies have been used experimentally and appear more useful in metastatic disease (or locoregional).[88]

Once the diagnosis is made, some assessment or prognosis should be made. This initial biopsy specimen provides the most important factor in assessing prognosis for stage I disease. Historically, the level of invasion, as originally described by Menart and Herd and later popularized by Clark,[89] was assigned five levels, varying from in situ to invasion of subcutaneous fat (Figure 23-10).

Because of the difficulty in determining the level of the capillary-reticular dermal junction and the reproducibility of results, the *Breslow technique* of tumor thickness has become the standard.[90] This measurement is in millimeters of tumor thickness at the thickest portion of the biopsy. The clinician measures from the top of the granular cell layer to the base of the malignant cell with an ocular micrometer. If the lesion is ulcerated, the base of the ulcer is used for the measurement.[91]

Other histologic factors, such as mitosis, atypia of nuclei, nesting of cells, neural invasion, and the inflammatory cell population, are important factors in fine-tuning the original prognosis.[92] Other authors have proposed a prognostic index, or an array of cytologic factors, to assist in establishing risk.[93] Patients are then categorized into low-, intermediate-, and high-risk groups, depending on thickness measurements.[94] Less than 1 mm in thickness is considered low risk, greater than 3 to 4 mm is considered high, and varying studies have

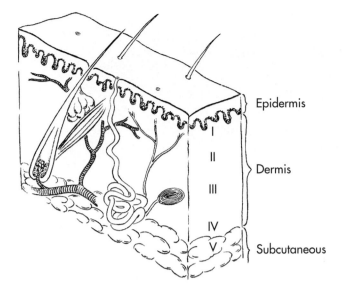

Figure 23-10. Cross section of skin showing histopathologic stages of typical melanoma.

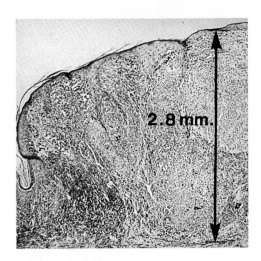

Figure 23-11. Biopsy sections for melanoma should be cut 2 to 3 mm in thickness.

placed others to move the upper end slightly to correspond with institutional data.[95,96] For lesions less than 0.76 mm in thickness, the ultimate long-term disease-free status is near 100%.[97,98]

Since tumor measurement is so important, my group obtains the slides and sends them for an independent second opinion. Tissue processing is also essential. If the number of step-cut sections is small, the deepest part of the biopsy is more likely to be missed. Generally, sections should be cut 2 to 3 mm in tissue diagnosed or suspected of melanoma. Occasionally the tissue block should be requested (Figure 23-11).

As noted, the Breslow technique appears to be the most reliable and reproducible method available at this time (Figure 23-12). A potential for error exists, however, specifically in areas adjacent to adnexal structures (e.g., hair follicles). Invagination of the epidermal-dermal junction appears to drag tumor cells deeper into the dermis, even though the tumor is still in the radial growth phase. Other problems occur when melanoma exists within a benign nevus. The clinician should measure thickness of only the tumor cells, ignoring the nevus cells. Dense inflammatory cell infiltrates may also obscure the thickness measurement. Other errors may occur with beveling of tissue or fixation artifact. The shaved biopsy is the most frequent problem; when tumor cells arise at the base, the clinician may never be certain of the true tumor thickness. In such situations the Clark level or other factors should be taken into consideration in formulating a treatment plan.

Both the Clark and Breslow techniques are subject to problems with sampling errors. Neither technique is valid in the presence of recurrent or metastatic disease; in these areas, level and thickness measurements may not accurately predict prognosis. Regression, ulceration, desmoplastic tumors, and amelanotic melanomas are controversial and may fare worse than equally thick lesions. Tumors on the back, arm, neck, and

scalp (BANS) may represent a more unfavorable group of tumors. Lentigo maligna melanoma, or melanotic freckle of Hutchinson, may be less virulent than tumors of comparable thickness. Conflicting literature exists.[99]

DNA analysis using flow cytometry to determine aneuploidy has been demonstrated in lesions greater than 3 mm in thickness.[100] This experimental technique is used more often in breast cancer but may eventually apply to all cancers. Computer analysis of color photographs is another experimental technique that may show promise. *Dermatoscopy,* or visualization of lesions in situ, is also being attempted, but any patient with a lesion that warrants this technique probably should have a biopsy.

My group's series of more than 200 cases resulted in measurement differences in 25% to 30% of cases. Some were less significant than others, but knowing the discrepancies is helpful.

PATIENT EVALUATION AND METASTATIC WORKUP

After the diagnosis and assessment of risk, the patient should have a total-body skin examination, including the scalp[101] (Figure 23-13). This examination should include palpation of the neck, axillae, and inguinal lesions for adenopathy and of other organs for organomegaly.[102-104]

With the recent increase in melanomas, synchronous tumors have also increased. Atypical or "dysplastic" lesions may be seen elsewhere on the body. Any patient with a single melanoma has a 600 to 900 times greater risk for developing another primary melanoma compared with the general population. Patients with numerous nevi, mainly on the trunk, large, and variegated in color, may be photographed using a "dysplastic mole series." This is a total-body photograph of 32 color

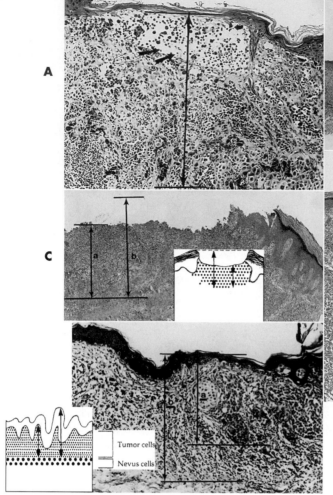

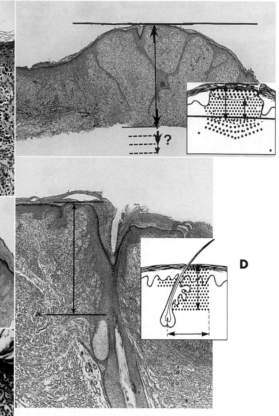

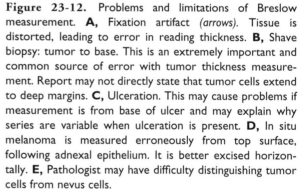

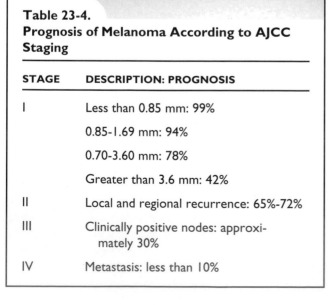

Figure 23-12. Problems and limitations of Breslow measurement. **A,** Fixation artifact *(arrows).* Tissue is distorted, leading to error in reading thickness. **B,** Shave biopsy: tumor to base. This is an extremely important and common source of error with tumor thickness measurement. Report may not directly state that tumor cells extend to deep margins. **C,** Ulceration. This may cause problems if measurement is from base of ulcer and may explain why series are variable when ulceration is present. **D,** In situ melanoma is measured erroneously from top surface, following adnexal epithelium. It is better excised horizontally. **E,** Pathologist may have difficulty distinguishing tumor cells from nevus cells.

Table 23-4.
Prognosis of Melanoma According to AJCC Staging

STAGE	DESCRIPTION: PROGNOSIS
I	Less than 0.85 mm: 99%
	0.85-1.69 mm: 94%
	0.70-3.60 mm: 78%
	Greater than 3.6 mm: 42%
II	Local and regional recurrence: 65%-72%
III	Clinically positive nodes: approximately 30%
IV	Metastasis: less than 10%

5×7 photographs that allow the examiner and patient to observe changes more easily.[105-108]

As mentioned, the workup, other than liver function tests and radiography, provides an extremely low yield. If a patient has palpable adenopathy and a lymph node dissection is planned, extending computed tomography (CT) of the chest to include the supraclavicular region and neck or extending the abdominal CT to include the femoral triangle may prove useful. Nonpalpable adenopathy (greater than 0.6 cm) may be demonstrated with CT scans or magnetic resonance imaging (MRI). Monoclonal antibodies and gallium scans are used experimentally for metastatic screens. Technetium localization of lymphatic drainage for sentinel node biopsy is not indicated in therapeutic node dissection. Positron emission tomography (PET) scans are experimental but seem to be effective in identifying metastasis (Table 23-4).

MELANOMA OF THE SKIN (ICD-O 173 With Histologic Type 872–879)

Data Form for Cancer Staging

Patient identification
Name _____
Address _____
Hospital or clinic number _____
Age _____ Sex _____ Race _____

Institutional identification
Hospital or clinic _____
Address _____

Oncology Record

Anatomic site of cancer _____
Chronology of classification* [ ] Clinical-diagnostic (cTNM)
                               [ ] Surgical-evaluative (sTNM)
Date of classification _____

Histologic type† _____ Grade (G) _____
[ ] Postsurgical resection–pathologic (pTNM)
[ ] Retreatment (rTNM)   [ ] Autopsy (aTNM)

Definitions: TNM Classification

Primary Tumor (T)

[ ] TX No evidence of primary tumor (unknown primary or primary tumor removed and not histologically examined)

[ ] T0 Atypical melanocytic hyperplasia (Clark Level I); not a malignant lesion

[ ] T1 Invasion of papillary dermis (Level II) or 0.75-mm thickness or less

[ ] T2 Invasion of the papillary–reticular-dermal interface (Level III) or 0.76- to 1.5-mm thickness

[ ] T3 Invasion of the reticular dermis (Level IV) or 1.51- to 4.0-mm thickness

[ ] T4 Invasion of subcutaneous tissue (Level V) or 4.1 mm or more in thickness or satellite(s) within 2 cm of any primary melanoma

Nodal Involvement (N)

[ ] NX Minimum requirements to assess the regional nodes cannot be met.

[ ] N0 No regional lymph node involvement

[ ] N1 Involvement of only one regional lymph node station; node(s) movable and not over 5 cm in diameter or negative regional lymph nodes and the presence of less than five in-transit metastases beyond 2 cm from primary site

[ ] N2 Any one of the following: (1) involvement of more than one regional lymph node station; (2) regional node(s) over 5 cm in diameter or fixed; (3) five or more in-transit metastases or any in-transit metastases beyond 2 cm from primary site with regional lymph node involvement

Distant Metastasis (M)

[ ] MX Minimum requirements to assess the presence of distant metastasis cannot be met.

[ ] M0 No known distant metastasis

[ ] M1 Involvement of skin or subcutaneous tissue beyond the site of primary lymph node drainage
        Specify _____

[ ] M2 Visceral metastasis (spread to any distant site other than skin or subcutaneous tissues)
        Specify _____

Type of Lesion

[ ] Lentigo maligna   [ ] Radial spreading
[ ] Nodular   [ ] Acral lentiginous
                           [ ] Unclassified

*Use a separate form each time a case is staged.
†See reverse side for additional information.

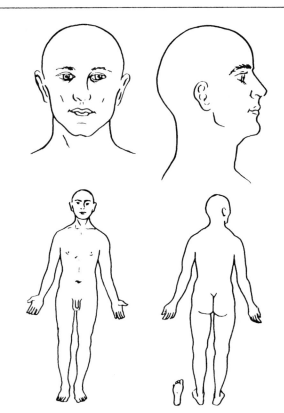

Indicate on diagrams primary tumor and regional nodes involved.

Depth of Invasion
[ ] Level I (not a melanoma and further characterization is not necessary)
[ ] Level II   [ ] Level IV
[ ] Level III   [ ] Level V
Other description _____
Maximal thickness (mm) _____
Site of primary lesion (check diagram)
_____
Extent of primary lesion (include all pigmentation)
_____
Size in greatest diameter _____ . cm

Characteristics

[ ] Ulceration
[ ] Other _____

Examination by _____ M.D.
Date _____

American Joint Committee on Cancer

Figure 23-13. American Joint Commission on Cancer's melanoma data form. (From Beahrs OH, Myers MY, editors: *Manual for staging of cancer*, Philadelphia, 1983, Lippincott.) *Continued*

Stage Grouping

[ ] Stage IA   T1, N0, M0
[ ] Stage IB   T2, N0, M0
[ ] Stage IIA   T3, N0, M0
[ ] Stage IIB   T4, N0, M0
[ ] Stage III   Any T, N1, M0
[ ] Stage IV   Any T, N2, M0
                 Any T, any N, M1 or M2

Staging Procedures

A variety of procedures and special studies may be employed in the process of staging a given tumor. Both the clinical usefulness and cost efficiency must be considered. The following suggestions are made for staging of malignant melanoma:

Essential for staging

1. Complete physical examination
2. Pathologic study of surgically removed material, including depth of invasion and thickness of primary tumor
3. Chest roentgenogram
4. Known residual tumor at primary site if present

May be useful for staging or patient management

1. Multichemistry screen
2. Gallium scan
3. Bone scan
4. Liver–spleen scan
5. CT scans
6. Brain scans
7. Performance status (Karnofsky or ECOG)

Primary Tumor (T)

Both the depth of invasion and the maximum measured thickness determine the T-classification and should be recorded. When the depth of invasion and the thickness do not match the categories of T-classification, whichever of the two is greatest should take precedence.

Regional Nodes (N)

The regional nodes are related to the region of the body in which the tumor is located; such first station nodes are as follows:

1. For head and face: preauricular, cervical
2. For neck and upper chest wall: cervical (anterior–posterior), supraclavicular, axillary
3. For chest wall, anterior and posterior, and arms above elbow: axillary
4. For hands and upper extremities below the elbow: epitrochlear or axillary
5. For the abdominal wall, anterior and posterior, and lower extremities above the knee: femoral inguinal nodes (groin)
6. For the feet and below the knees: popliteal or femoral inguinal nodes (groin)

Histopathology

Types of malignant melanoma: lentigo maligna (Hutchinson's) with adjacent intraepidermal component of radial spreading type (superficial spreading), without adjacent intraepidermal component (nodular), and unclassified.

Both the depth of invasion (Clark) and the thickness of the tumor (Breslow) have been shown to have prognostic significance and both parameters should be reported by the pathologist.

Five levels of the skin have been designated for identification of depth of invasion:

[ ] Level I (epidermis to epidermal–dermal interface). Lesions involving only the epidermis have been designated level I. These lesions are considered to be "atypical melanocytic hyperplasia" and are not included in the staging of malignant melanoma, *for they do not represent a malignant lesion*.
[ ] Level II (papillary dermis). Invasion of the papillary dermis does not reach the papillary–reticular dermal interface.
[ ] Level III (papillary–reticular dermis interface). Invasion involves the full thickness of, fills, and expands the papillary dermis; it abuts upon but does not penetrate the reticular dermis.
[ ] Level IV (reticular dermis). Invasion occurs into the reticular dermis but not into the subcutaneous tissue.
[ ] Level V (subcutaneous tissue). Invasion moves through the reticular dermis into the subcutaneous tissue.

Histologic Grade

[ ] G1   Well differentiated
[ ] G2   Moderately well differentiated
[ ] G3–G4   Poorly to very poorly differentiated

Postsurgical Resection–Pathologic Residual Tumor (R)

Does not enter into staging but may be a factor in deciding further treatment

[ ] R0   No residual tumor
[ ] R1   Microscopic residual tumor
[ ] R2   Macroscopic residual tumor
          Specify _____

Performance Status of Host (H)

Several systems for recording a patient's activity and symptoms are in use and are more or less equivalent as follows:

AJCC	Performance	ECOG Scale	Karnofsky Scale (%)
[ ] H0	Normal activity	0	90–100
[ ] H1	Symptomatic but ambulatory; cares for self	1	70–80
[ ] H2	Ambulatory more than 50% of time; occasionally needs assistance	2	50–60
[ ] H3	Ambulatory 50% or less of time; nursing care needed	3	30–40
[ ] H4	Bedridden; may need hospitalization	4	10–20

Figure 23-13, cont'd.   For legend see previous page.

OPERATIONS

SURGICAL TREATMENT

Wide surgical excision remains the treatment of choice for cutaneous melanoma. Debate still exists as to the exact size of margins, removal of fascia, the method of reconstruction, use of lymphadenectomy, and adjuvant therapy (e.g., chemotherapy, limb isolation, limb perfusion, immunotherapy with interferon).[109,110]

Stages I and II: Low-Risk Lesions

Handley[111] recommended 5-cm margins based on the finding of tumor cells within 5 cm of satellite lesions that were "in transit" rather than primary tumors (Figure 23-14). This went largely unchallenged until the 1970s, when Breslow and Macht[96] suggested that thin melanomas (stage I) were curable with smaller, more conservative margins. Handley's reference was to a lesion that would be categorized as stage II or III tumor by the AJCC classification.

The gold standard of a prospective randomized study using concurrent controls with comparable groups did not exist until 1988, when Veronesi et al[112] demonstrated the safety of a 1-cm margin for lesions 2 mm thick or less. Because of late local recurrences, the recommendation was reduced to 1-cm margin for tumors 1 mm thick. No such studies have been done exclusively for high-risk lesions.[113]

Stage I: High-risk Lesions

Wide excision remains controversial for thicker lesions (Figure 23-15). Advocates cite the increasing incidence of local recurrence with narrow margins in this patient group. The finding of atypical melanocytes several centimeters around the primary tumor suggests the benefit of wider excision. The reason for wider margins is to prevent local recurrences. It is unlikely that isolated cells in transit to a site greater than 5 cm are in transit to a regional lymph node or are affected by a more radical excision. Sacrificing a vital structure such as the ear or nose is not indicated, but when a deeply ulcerating lesion presents at that location, patient and surgeon may have little choice.

Input by the patient is always helpful, and customizing difficult clinical situations is important. If tumors recur, the question most often may be why the more aggressive procedure was not done. Clearing the area of the atypical melanocytic hyperplasia should be attempted regardless of the excision's width.

The use of Mohs' surgery remains controversial. Identifying atypical melanocytes even in stained sections is sometimes difficult; frozen sections seem even more problematic. Since local recurrences have been demonstrated to occur more frequently in the direction of lymphatic drainage, my group's practice is to excise slightly more tissue in the direction of the nodal basin (i.e., an "eccentric" ellipse rather than a circular excision) (Figure 23-15). The depth is to fascia, unless sacrificing the fascia assists in reconstruction.

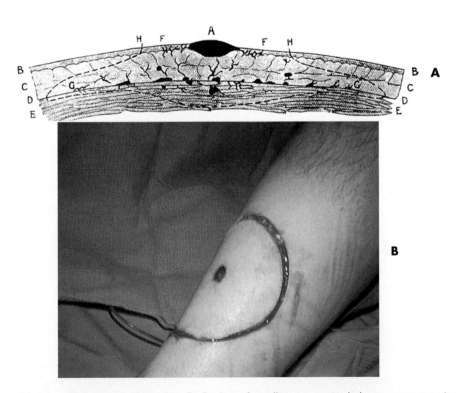

Figure 23-14. **A,** Diagram of Handley. **B,** Finding of satellite metastasis led surgeons to excise 5-cm margins for more than 80 years.

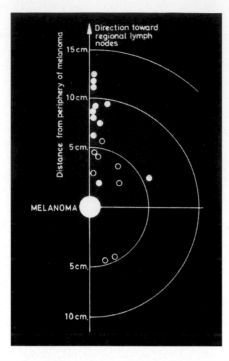

Figure 23-15. Wide excision should be "eccentric," including more normal tissue closer to nodal drainage area.

Box 23-1.
Reconstructive Options in Melanoma Patients

1. Healing by secondary intention
   a. Not recommended
   b. Obvious deformity from wound contraction and contracture, along with prolonged opening of area
   c. Comparable to older "toilet" procedure for breast carcinoma
2. Graft
   a. Split-thickness skin graft: readily available; virtually unlimited supply but aesthetically unsatisfactory on most locations
   b. Full-thickness skin graft: consideration for head and neck tumors; primarily for elderly patient population
   c. All are important options but are usually aesthetically inferior to flaps
3. Skin flaps
   a. Local advancement flap
   b. Transposition flap
   c. Rotation flap
   d. Myocutaneous flaps or muscle flaps with split-thickness skin graft
   e. Microvascular free tissue transfer

Generally we attempt to excise approximately 1 cm of normal skin for each millimeter of tumor thickness with modification.[96,114] When indicated, all traces of atypical melanocytic hyperplasia margins are reexcised. We are rarely unable to clear the margins to normal skin.

Certain areas require special mention, especially subungual, digital, and web lesions. Classically, digital melanomas require amputation, usually at the ray level. Recently, with the benefit of thickness measurements, surgeons have been better able to define high-risk and low-risk tumors. In the absence of bone invasion or satellitosis, distal interphalangeal disarticulation is adequate. Treating web space involvement of the fingers or toes depends on the tumor's thickness. Thin lesions require only small margins. High-risk lesions require ray amputations[115-117] (see later discussion).

RECONSTRUCTION

Early authors suggested that melanoma defects are best reconstructed with a skin graft to identify tumor recurrence at an earlier age and improve survival by reexcision. The ideal study does not exist, but several publications have retrospectively indicated the safety of flap coverage. My recommendation is to offer the patient the best reconstructive option available (Box 23-1).

Most cases can be reconstructed by primary closure, local advancement flap, transposition flap, myocutaneous flap, or free tissue transfer if necessary.[118] Skin grafts are rarely used because of the many, more reasonable choices. The typical split-thickness skin graft has a mediocre appearance (Figure 23-16). It is important to note that local recurrences are possible and that wider reexcision may be required. If a skin graft is chosen, the patient should be shown photographs preoperatively because expectations may be unrealistic. Plastic surgeons are uniquely qualified in creative reconstructive procedures that are designed not to compromise the extirpative portion of the primary tumor.[119]

As with other oncologic surgeries, the procedure includes both the extirpative portion and the reconstruction. The great majority of tumors seen are very thin and can be excised and primarily closed. As the thickness increases and the excision margins are also increasing, creative methods are required. The usual list of reconstructive options range from allowing the wound to heal by secondary intention (not recommended) to microvascular free tissue transfer.

Several routine local flap procedures can be performed to obviate the need for a skin graft (Figure 23-17). Besides their aesthetic differences, sflap reconstructions are usually less morbid procedures than skin grafts (Figure 23-18). Examples are the rhomboid flap (Figures 23-19 to 23-21), forehead flap (Figure 23-22), nasolabial flap (Figure 23-23), and frontalis flap (Figure 23-24).[120] Generally these options are reviewed preoperatively with the patient and are performed at the same time of tumor removal. If a patient can visualize a satisfactory outcome, the postoperative course is likely to be more satisfactory.

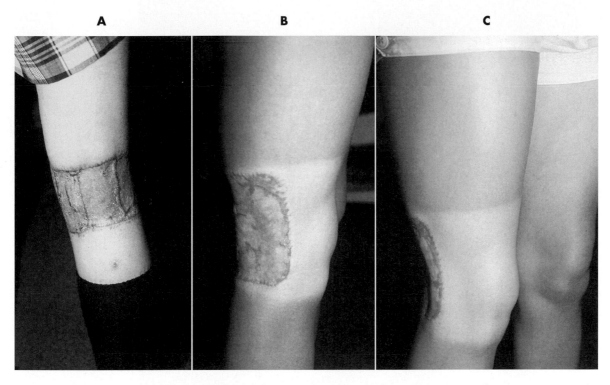

Figure 23-16. Typical appearance of split-thickness skin graft at various times after surgery. **A,** early; **B,** few weeks; **C,** several years.

LYMPHADENECTOMY

No dispute surrounds the use of a therapeutic lymph node dissection (LND). If documented tumor or palpable disease is identified within a nodal basin, LND is indicated. Fine-needle aspiration is advised to confirm the diagnosis. Classified as a therapeutic LND, the removal for staging purposes is always a valid indication. Prognosis will vary if, for example, greater than three lymph nodes are positive or capsular invasion exists.

For lesions less than 1.5 mm the survival rate is greater than 90% in 5 years; the chance of finding occult metastasis within nodes is so small that little justification exists for LND.[121] For lesions between 1.5 and 4.0 mm in thickness, several retrospective studies indicate a 15% to 25% improved disease-free survival rate with prophylactic LND.

Two prospective, randomized, controlled studies failed to show benefit with LND, although both had significant shortcomings.[122,123] Subsets of patients with tumors 1.5 to 4.0 mm in thickness, however, appeared to have increased survival. Unfortunately the number of patients was insufficient to make this statistically significant, and repeat studies are in progress. Differences in ulceration and other skewing problems, such as the preponderance of females and the variability from country to country, leaves the question unanswered.

My group suspects that subgroups of patients may benefit from elective LND. We do not know how to identify this group prospectively, and we cannot determine how many "unnecessary" LNDs are needed to help a single patient.[122,124] At the very least, however, a prophylactic LND stages the patient in a more accurate way than without an LND.[125]

Newer studies document increased survival if lymph node involvement is microscopic rather than palpable.[126,127] Conceptually, proponents of LND cite the advantage of finding "occult" tumor foci compared with treating the patient with palpable disease.[128] Clearly the quantitative number of tumor cells must be less than microscopic, nonpalpable disease.[129] Since the U.S. Food and Drug Administration (FDA) approved interferon, the value of nodal status has increased greatly.

As a reasonable compromise between elective LND and observation, the sentinel node biopsy has been used along with lymphoscintigraphy (see following discussion). This allows the nodal status to be determined without a full LND. If such a node turns up positive, the completed LND is performed either immediately or in the near future.

Sentinel Node Biopsy and Lymphoscintigraphy

Preoperative use of technetium isotope infiltrated circumferentially around the primary lesion assists in determining which nodal basin drains the area.[130] The concept is based on the observation that the biologic behavior of melanoma is such that most of the virulent lesions will behave in a *carcinomatous* manner, that is, recur at the local primary site or at the draining lymphatic basin.[131] This encompasses between 80% to 90% of treatment failures (not total patients). The remainder may behave in a *sarcomatous* manner, possibly without all the locoregional recurrences, and present in lung, liver, brain, or bone without sign of local disease.

As a further complication, of all melanoma recurrences or treatment failures, approximately 80% will become known within 2 years after the diagnosis is made. The remaining 20%

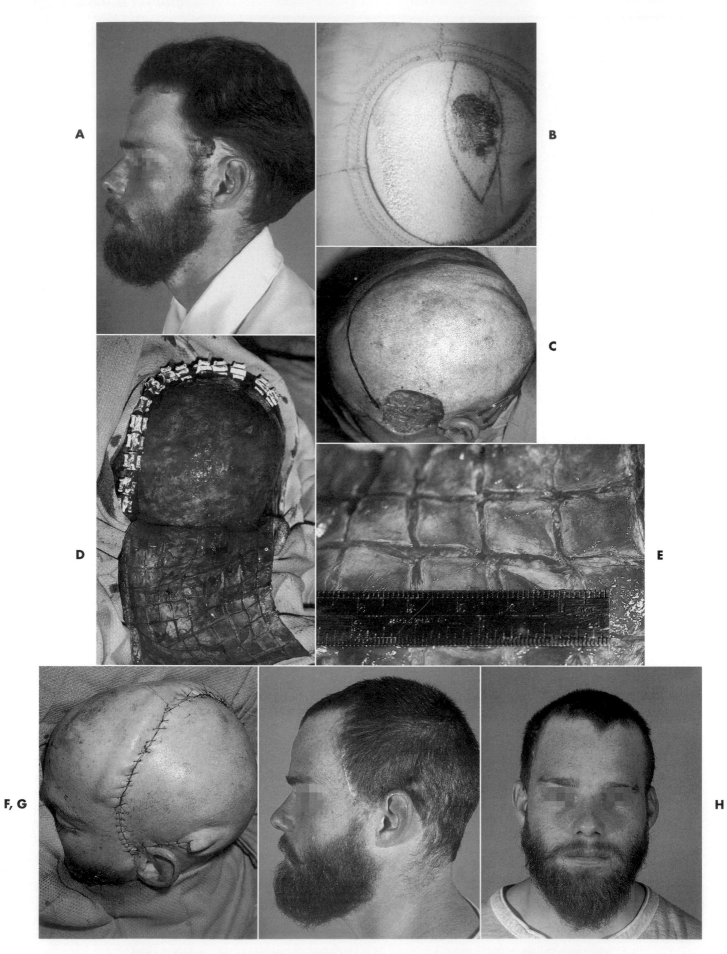

Figure 23-17. **A** to **H,** Thick, 5.5-mm lesion on preauricular area in 27-year-old male. Reconstruction used galeal scoring and local advancement.

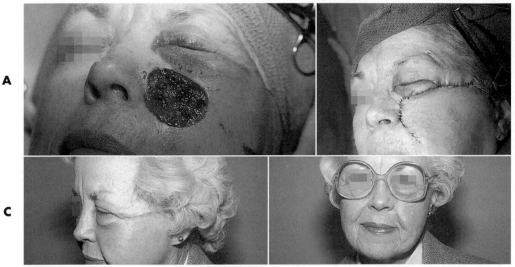

Figure 23-18. **A** to **D,** Excision and results in 64-year-old female with melanoma in situ. Reconstruction used "reverse" facelift flap, advancing tissue anteriorly. Keeping scars within "aesthetic units" is helpful.

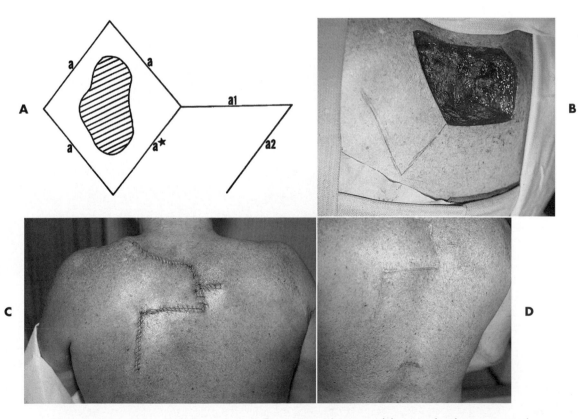

Figure 23-19. Rhomboid flap and result. Recurrent melanoma widely excised and reconstructed with single rhomboid flap.

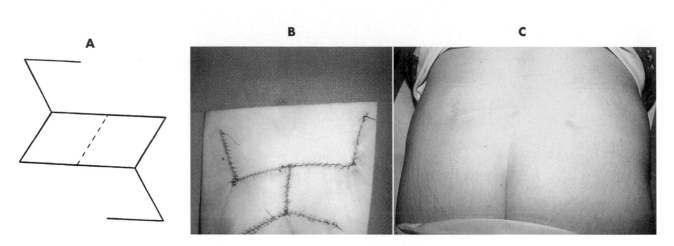

Figure 23-20. **A** and **B,** Double rhomboid flap and result. Large amelanotic melanoma resected. **C,** Double–rhomboid flap reconstruction of lower back. Advantages over skin grafts are obvious.

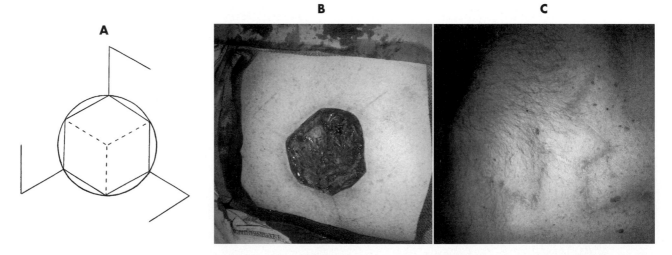

Figure 23-21. **A** to **C,** Triple rhomboid flap and result. This flap feeds tissue to defect from all directions.

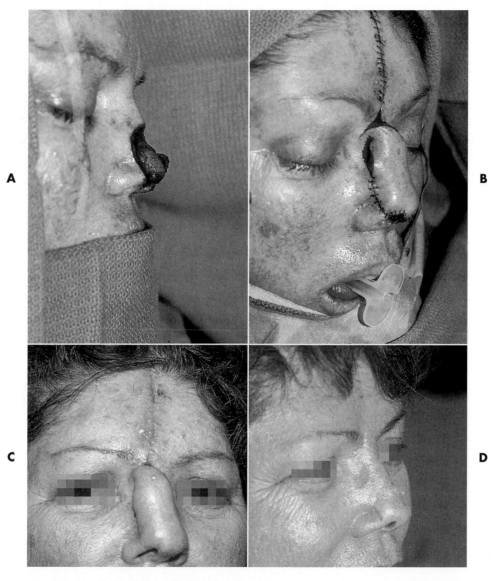

Figure 23-22. A to **D,** Large resection of melanoma in situ by dermatologist and result. Reconstruction with staged forehead flap.

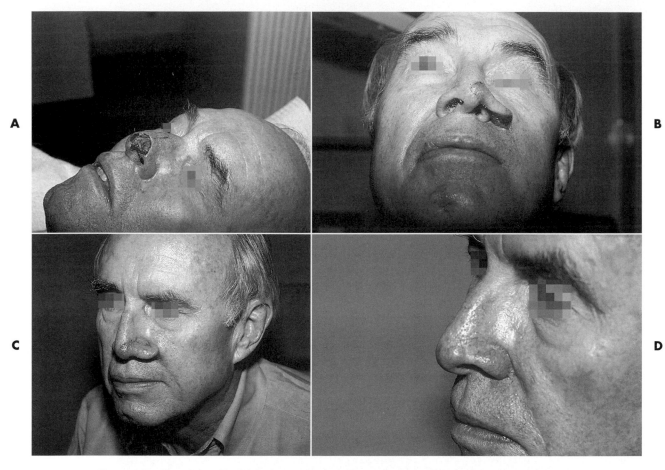

Figure 23-23. A to **D,** Melanoma of nasal tip excised in 70-year-old male and result. Reconstruction with outside nasolabial flap. Flap is divided and inset at 5 days. Blend of tissue is difficult to obtain with other techniques; flap acts as "supercharged" skin graft. Flap tip is thinned aggressively at initial procedure. Pedicle blood flow ensures safety. Because tip tissue is so thin, revascularization occurs rapidly.

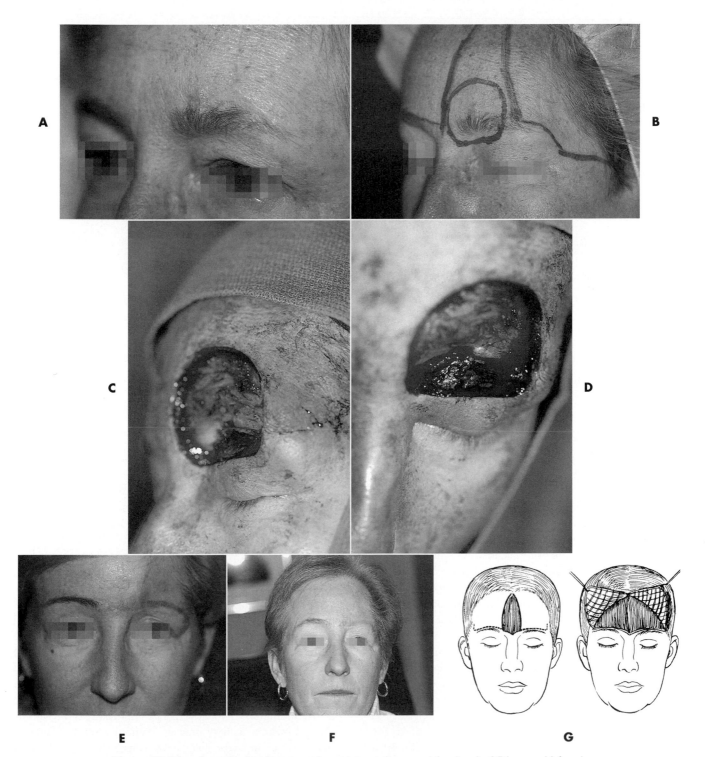

Figure 23-24. **A** to **G,** Amelanotic melanoma in eyebrow and forehead of 54-year-old female after incomplete prior excision. Wide excision with lymphoscintigraphy and sentinel node biopsy. Reconstruction with frontalis scoring and advancement.

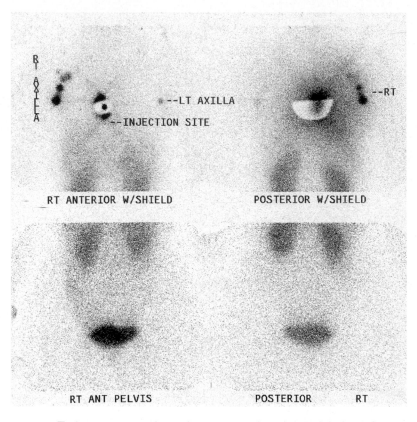

Figure 23-25. Technetium scan obtained preoperatively indicates lymphatic flow is to both axillary node groups, with no uptake in internal mammary group.

of failures appear to be evenly distributed over the ensuing 20 years or more. Statistical data may be obtained from extrapolating this finding, but the bizarre immunologic aspects are poorly understood and require more investigation.

The mapping of the sentinel node is performed by first obtaining a preoperative technetium scan[132,133] (Figure 23-25). This is either done the morning of surgery or at another time before the procedure. With technetium infiltrated around the primary lesion, the radionucleotide is tracked in the draining nodal basin, providing the surgeon with direction as to the nodal basin on which to concentrate.[134] With this information the surgeon can determine precise location of the sentinel node using one or a combination of techniques.

During the surgical procedure a vital lymphangiogram blue dye (Lymphozurin) is infiltrated intradermally around the primary tumor site. This allows the material to be tracked to the appropriate lymph node basin. By using direct visualization of the dye and the gamma probe (Neoprobe or Navigator), the single lymph node within the basin can be identified, then biopsied. If negative, the procedure is completed; if positive, the complete LND is performed with oncologic consultation for interferon.[135]

Many intermediate variations of this technique exist, and preoperatively the surgeon may obtain the scan and use either vital dye alone or the gamma probe itself. It is hoped that this technique will prevent the morbidity of LND. If an occult tumor is found, the patient is upgraded to at least stage III disease and then becomes a candidate for a more complete metastatic workup and adjuvant therapy. Interferon-α, once the mainstay of treatment for stage III disease, is no longer routine. The total number of lymph nodes that are positive can affect prognosis (less than three, approximately 40% to 50%), as can nodal size and wall integrity.

My experience with this technique has demonstrated limited value. An "educated guess" of the lymph draining area, especially when done close to the initial biopsy, may demonstrate the inflammatory hyperplastic node, which also acts as a sentinel marker. Use of this technique should be considered experimental. Extremity melanoma benefits less from these the sentinel node biopsy techniques (not node biopsy) because of the surgeon's ability to predict the location of the "sentinel node." Without question, knowledge of the exact nodal basin (when more than one may be affected) is advantageous. Our initial findings in a patient with a parasternal breast melanoma showed bilateral axillary drainage without a trace of internal mammary or supraclavicular tracer (Figure 23-26). The vital guide technique has virtually no associated complications; however, we had a patient who retained color for more than 1 year after injection.

Recent studies have used the polymerase chain reaction (PCR) technique to identify high-risk "negative" lymph nodes.[136] At present this is controversial and is performed as an immunologic test on lymph nodal tissue removed during the

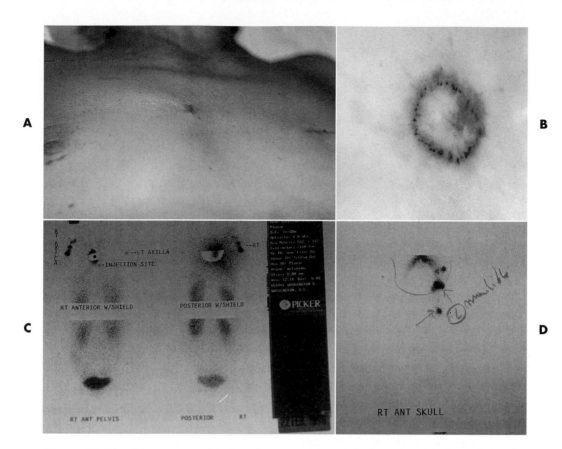

Figure 23-26. At surgery, combination of gamma probe and dye is used to identify sentinel node. Blue lymphangiogram dye (Lymphazurin) is placed in dermis around primary lesion, as is done with technetium. **A,** Parasternal site of primary melanoma. **B,** Lymphazurin injection around primary site. **C** and **D,** Technetium scans indicate bilateral axillary sentinel lymph nodes.

sentinel node biopsy. Clinical correlation is far from complete, and further work is in progress. This test seems to lack specificity and may not consider the normal melanocytes occasionally found in lymph nodes.

SURGICAL ADENECTOMY

A modified radical neck dissection is typically used for melanoma. Preservation of the sternocleidomastoid muscle, jugular vein, and spinal accessory nerve are important benefits to the patient without compromising outcome.[137]

Studies have indicated the safety of this technique. Most of the literature refers to its use with squamous carcinoma of the head and neck area, but melanoma has been examined as well. Our practice is to include the jugular vein in the dissection to facilitate the procedure. This results in minimal morbidity in unilateral neck dissection, saves operating time, and otherwise is comparable to the modified neck dissection.[138-140]

Technique

A modified radical neck dissection for a sided block of tissue in a specimen extends from just beneath the mandibular border to the clavicle (Figure 23-27). The posterior border of dissection is the trapezius muscle; anteriorly the "strap" muscles (sternohyoid and sternothyroid muscles) limit the dissection. After skin flaps are elevated deep to the platysma muscle, the contents within these landmarks are removed and blocked. In modified cases the sternocleidomastoid muscle and spinal accessory (eleventh cranial) nerve are spared. My preference is to start with the McPhee parallel, horizontal incision and create submuscular planes below the platysma muscle.[141,142] This tissue may be adequately retracted with a pair of 2-cm (¾-inch) Penrose drains.

Usually the dissection is started inferiorly and proceeds superiorly. It is helpful to suture peg the two heads of the inferior origin of the sternocleidomastoid muscles on the clavicle. After the LND is completed, reapproximation of the muscle heads to the sternum and clavicle is sometimes difficult. Careful attention is paid to the carotid sheath; if the carotid artery remains without a protective covering, the sternocleidomastoid muscle is used to ensure more complete coverage.[143-145] Alternatively, a dermal graft can be used.

Complications

Complications in all modified radical neck dissections include injury to nerves and vessels, wound drainage, airway obstruction, ear embolism, carotid sinus syndrome, fever, mediastinitis, subcutaneous emphysema, pneumothorax,

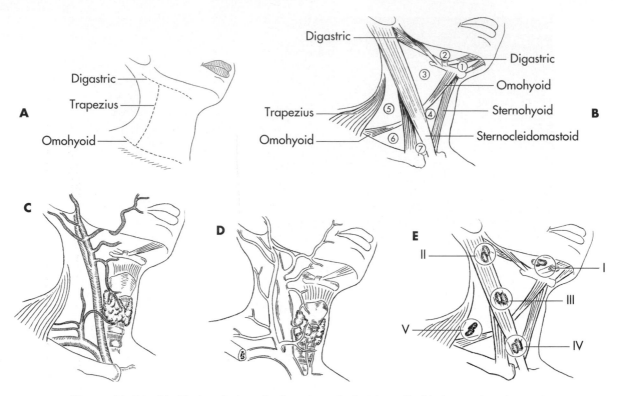

Figure 23-27. Modified radical neck dissection. **A,** Incisions. **B,** Neck muscles. Anatomic triangles: *1,* submental; *2,* submandibular; *3,* carotid; *4,* muscular; *5,* posterior; *6,* supraclavicular; *7,* lesser supraclavicular fossa. **C,** Carotid arterial supply. **D,** Venous supply. **E,** *I* to *V,* Lymph nodes.

lymphatic chylous fistulas, increased cerebral venous pressure (with bilateral), and neurologic problems.

For lymph node dissections, complications are related to the nerve and vascular injuries and include hemorrhage and infection.

Seroma lymphocele and lymphatic fistulas may be more severe and prolonged in neck surgery. Perioperative masses and drainage mandates repeat surgery for ligation of the thoracic duct or its lesser counterpart contralaterally. Any single cranial nerve disruption may be tolerable, but disruption of two is disabling. Preoperative counseling is important.

Intraoperative bleeding behind the clavicle may require clavicular osteotomy and reflection of the ribs to gain access to the branches of the subclavian artery. A thoracic surgeon must be consulted. If the jugular vein is lost at the proximal portion, emergent patient positioning is important to minimize an embolism. Should the cranial portion break loose, compression with Gelfoam would tamponade this low-pressure system. Flap necrosis is rare if the platysma muscle and skin flap are taken as a unit; when the tumor is close to the skin and muscle is left to be resected with the specimen, however, necrosis can be anticipated. Smokers are particularly vulnerable.

A vertical component to the McPhee incision provides excellent exposure and minimally compromises the aesthetic benefits of this incision. Closure of all wounds over closed-suction drainage facilitates postoperative recovery.

AXILLARY LYMPH NODE DISSECTION

Axillary LND is performed in the usual supine position with an axillary roll under the patient's shoulder anteriorly with the arm slightly hyperextended.[146,147]

Technique

My preference is to use a horizontal incision just below the hair-bearing area and running in the horizontal plane (Figure 23-28). The flaps created in this dissection are the same as those with mastectomy and other LNDs. The pectoralis and latissimus dorsi muscles in the axilla are close together. The procedure deviates from axillary dissections in that I attempt wider dissection in the direction of the primary lesion, most often the arm. This may include cautious dissections slightly caudad to the axillary vein.

Lymphedema after axillary LND performed for melanoma is much less serious than that after mastectomy. Most likely, fewer lymphatic channels are disrupted when the LND is performed alone rather than with a mastectomy.

The flaps are extended from the pectoralis major muscle to the latissimus dorsi posteriorly. The dissection starts from anterior to posterior by dissecting the fascia off the pectoralis major and then the pectoralis minor muscles along the full length of the lateral muscle border but reflecting this laterally and upward to expose the axillary vein. When the venous level is encountered, the dissection is then carried immediately above the vein, ligating

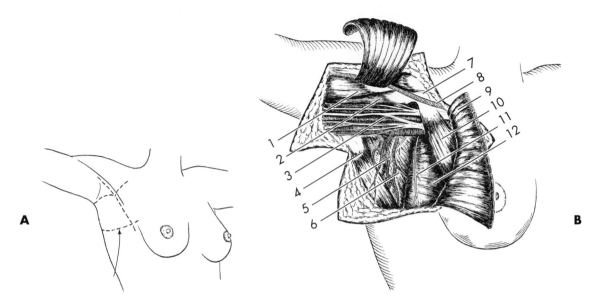

Figure 23-28. Axillary node dissection. **A,** Incisions. Arrow indicates author's preference just below hair-bearing area. **B,** Anatomic landmarks: *1*, biceps brachii muscle; *2*, coracobrachialis muscle; *3*, axillary artery, vein, and nerve; *4*, latissimus dorsi muscle; *5*, thoracodorsal artery and nerve; *6*, subscapularis muscle; *7*, coracoid process; *8*, cephalic vein; *9*, pectoralis major muscle; *10*, pectoralis minor muscle; *11*, long thoracic nerve; *12*, serratus anterior muscle.

appropriate tributaries as the dissection is carried further out to the axilla. The clavipectoral fascia is incised, and venous dissection continues with positive identification of the nerve to the serratus anterior muscle and thoracodorsal nerves. Once this is completed, some branches of the intercostobrachial muscle are usually sacrificed, but they may be preserved if visible.

The remaining dissection is completed and hemostasis obtained, with closure over Hemovac drains.[148]

Complications

Prolonged drainage and hemorrhage are the most common complications with axillary LND.[149,150] Lymphedema should be minimal, but attention to minimizing trauma to the extremity is important. Preventing infection, either by squeezing blood pressures or drawing blood from the arm, decreases the risk of further dimunition of lymphatic channels in the arm. Medially, in thin patients, pneumothorax may occur if dissection is done between the ribs, skeletonizing the muscle too vigorously.

FINGER AND TOE AMPUTATION

With the advent of Breslow thickness measurements, amputations of fingers or toes became less common.[116] Lesions must also be categorized according to the degree of risk. If less than 1.0 mm is considered as low risk and greater than 4 mm as high risk, a more conservative approach may be used. Any patient with melanoma invading the bone of a finger or toe should have a ray amputation.[117] Lesser lesions can be adequately treated with interphalangeal disarticulation. Web space lesions may require removal of even more tissue. Excision and grafting can usually be performed (Figure 23-29).

INGUINAL-FEMORAL (GROIN) LYMPH NODE DISSECTION

It is important to distinguish between superficial and deep LNDs.[151-154] *Superficial* LND usually indicates that a block of tissue is removed below the inguinal ligament in the femoral triangle. *Radical groin* or *groin* LND usually indicates disruption of the inguinal ligament and dissection proximally and even retroperitoneally and to the obturator-ilial hypergastric and periaortic nodes if necessary. The following technique refers to the superficial groin or femoral LND (Figure 23-30).

The skin incision is made as a lazy S over the course of the neurovascular bundle. The four-sided block of tissue extends from the gracilis muscle medially to the abductor muscle mass laterally, the inguinal ligaments superiorly, and the crossing of

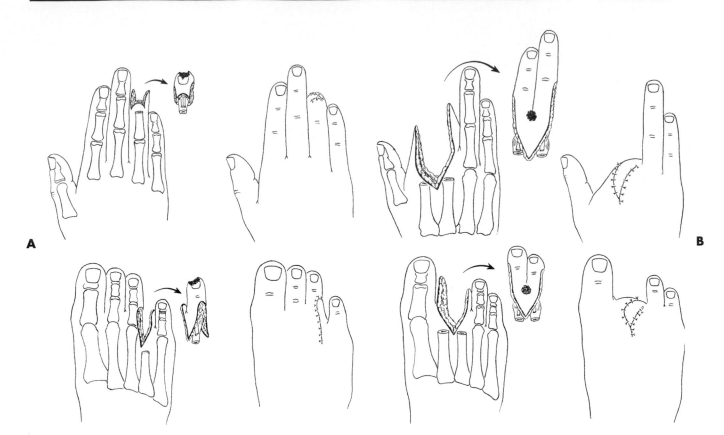

Figure 23-29. **A,** Single-finger/toe amputation. **B,** Double-finger/toe amputation: If tumor is subungual and has not invaded bone, interphalangeal disarticulation is acceptable. Web invasion requires wide skin excision. Amputation is indicated only if deeper structures are invaded. Same criteria apply to foot. Single-toe amputation may be preferable to graft.

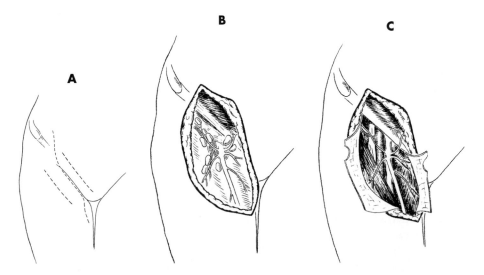

Figure 23-30. Superficial inguinal lymph node dissection. **A,** Incisions. **B,** Nodes. **C,** Flaps.

the two structures at this inferior base. The external skin flap is raised in the subcutaneous plane, and the deep margin is completed with the skeletonizing of the femoral artery and vein. The saphenous vein in the saphenofemoral junction must be doubly ligated and secured because it becomes elevated and undergoes pressure with ambulation. When the vessels are skeletonized, the sartorius muscle is transposed over the

neurovascular bundle and sutured to the inguinal ligament for protection.

In all patients the node of Cloquet is identified and biopsied; if this is negative, proximal disease is unlikely. Conversely, if this node shows micrometastasis, further extension of the dissection should be made to clear the node group proximal to the positive tumor. Some believe if this node of Cloquet is positive, the chance of cure is so small that deep node dissection is unwarranted.[155] Others have demonstrated that cures are possible and removal of gross tumor is warranted. Our experience has confirmed this latter finding, and patients with positive nodes can be long-term survivors.

Complications

The most common problem postoperatively relates to wound disruption and exposure of vessels if care is not taken to transpose the sartorius muscle over the femoral artery.[156] Lymphedema for the superficial LND is uncommon and usually transient. Compression stockings and early ambulation help with mobilization and limiting stasis.[157]

MANAGEMENT OF METASTATIC DISEASE

Melanoma has been documented to metastasize to almost every organ in the body. The prognosis is related to (1) the length of time from primary diagnosis until metastasis, (2) the number of sites involved, (3) the presence of brain involvement, and (4) involvement of other vital organs.[158,159] Local recurrence many years after the diagnosis and within 5 cm of the primary tumor has a more favorable prognosis than multiple lung, liver, or bone metastases.

Since melanoma appears to have symbiotic relationship with the immune system, surgical removal of lesions is indicated when feasible. Many patients have demonstrated improved survival over the long term with tumor removal. Craniotomy may be indicated, particularly with solitary lesions. Thoracotomy and lobectomy should also be considered. In general, patients with these solitary metastases do better than those with metastasis to other, nonvisceral sites.

Metastasis in patients may remain stable for months or even years without treatment, but progression is usually the rule. Patients should be restaged at frequent intervals as indicated. Melanoma, more so than any other tumor that metastasizes, often responds to new and unique treatments. It is extremely difficult to assess a single patient's prognosis. Virtually every physician treating this condition has patients who have done well (against all odds) for years and years.[160,161]

Generally, treatment options for systemic metastases consist of (1) surgery, (2) radiation therapy, (3) chemotherapy, (4) limb perfusion with or without hypothermia, (5) interlesional therapy, and (6) systemic immunotherapy. Surgery is the treatment of choice with solitary lesions and a low-risk patient, particularly with lesions on the skin, although other visceral organs, including lung and groin, should also be considered.[162]

Radiation therapy has long been believed to be ineffective with melanoma. Recent work, however, with adjustment of the fractionation dose, has shown significant response to merit consideration.[163]

Chemotherapy and Limb Perfusion

Generally the preferred chemotherapeutic agents are dacarbazine (DTIC), melphalan (L-phenylalanine mustard, L-PAM) with platinum, and carmustine.[164] Virtually all agents have

demonstrated a 15% to 30% partial response rate in experimental trials.

Intralesional therapy and systemic immunotherapy are experimental treatments and are changing rapidly.

The limb isolation/perfusion technique has been present since the 1960s and remains controversial. The procedure provides high-dose chemotherapy under high oxygenation and significant pressure. Minimal toxicity occurs because the limb is isolated from the systemic circulation through a tourniquet. The studies using this technique have not clearly demonstrated the benefit as an adjuvant therapy.[165-167]

The limb perfusion technique originally developed as an outgrowth of extracorporeal circulation with the membrane oxygenator used in the early 1950s. The other leg is excluded from systemic circulation with the use of vascular occlusion and rubber tourniquets placed on the skin surface. The patient is heparinized and perfused with high-dose chemotherapy, six to ten times the routine dose for 1 hour. Blood temperature is kept at 40° C (104° F). This technique is most useful to palliate limb removal. Most often, L-PAM or platinum is delivered with oxygenated blood under high perfusion pressures. Experimentally the hyperthermia has been demonstrated to improve chemotherapeutic uptake of tumor cells.

The combination of high tissue oxygen pressure, elevated perfusion pressure, heparin, and isolation of the tumor has advantages. Recent work has suggested that the addition of tissue necrosis factor (TNF) is also beneficial. The palliative benefits are well documented, but the adjuvant use remains controversial.

The complications are usually related to the chemotherapeutic agent leaking into the systemic circulation and include leukopenia, thrombocytopenia, and anemia. Moderate edema and nerve weakness are most often temporary adverse effects.

OUTCOMES

LONG-TERM FOLLOW-UP

Any patient with a diagnosis of melanoma requires long-term follow-up. Patients are at risk of developing another primary tumor, which will have an independent prognostic risk rate depending on its thickness measurement. Recurrences of metastasis most often present within 2 years and then may be found after 30 years from the initial presentation.

Routinely, skin examination with palpation of lymph nodes is performed with early chest radiography and SMA-12 analysis with complete blood count. Patients should be aware of the variable presentation of melanoma and participate in the surveillance. They are advised regarding the implications of sun exposure and its minimization.

PREVENTION

Chronic exposure to the sun causes pigment alterations, wrinkling, actinic keratoses, basosquamous carcinoma, and

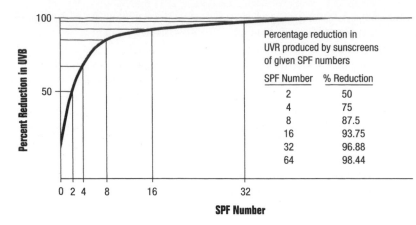

Figure 23-31. Sun protection factor *(SPF)* numbers and reduction in ultraviolet B *(UVB)* radiation. *UVR,* Ultraviolet radiation. (From Marks R: *CA* 46:212, 1996.)

Table 23-5.
Melanoma Recurrence Rates and Resection Margin, with Poor Correlation Between Width and Recurrence

AUTHOR	DATE	TUMOR (mm)	EXCISION MARGIN (cm)	PATIENTS	RECURRENCE
Breslow and Macht	1977	<0.76	0.1-3.5	66	0
Kelly	1984	In situ	<0.5	3	3 (100%)
McLoed	1985	In situ	0.5-1.0	105	0
Roses	1983	In situ	>1.0	115	0
	1983	>1.0	3.5	365	24 (6.5%)
Cascinelli et al	1980	>1.0	>3	497	16 (3.2%)
Golomb	1983	>1.0	>3	223	5 (2.2%)
Schmoeckel et al	1983	>1.0	>3	105	3 (2.9%)
Goldman	1980	>1.0	3-5	160	0
Das Gupta	1977	>1.0	5	150	10 (7%)
Milton	1977	>1.0	5	224	4 (2%)

*Patients not stratified according to incidence and proximity of atypical melanocytic hyperplasia.
When performed, wide excision should be "eccentric," including more normal tissue closer to nodal drainage area.

melanoma. About one-half the sun's energy is visible light and infrared energy; 6% is ultraviolet (UV) light, which is not visible. The UV band is broken further into UVA and UVB light.

Although once thought to be harmless, recent work has shown that UVA radiation can damage collagen and other cells in the skin. Because these rays are shorter, they are able to penetrate deeper, and the extent of damage to the tissue is not yet known. Unlike UVB, UVA light is constant all day and is not filtered by glass or the ozone layer. UVA radiation may be a greater cancer risk than previously thought.

UVB radiation has always been considered to be responsible for the "bad" burning rays known to induce changes in cells. The strongest rays occur between 10 AM and 2 PM and seem to be the source of cancer, sunburn, erythema, and tanning. Interestingly, the body has only two ways of responding to this form of trauma: (1) thickening and forming keratoses to help protect the body from further injury or (2) tanning to increase the melanocyte population and protect the deeper layers of skin. Clear-skinned, nontanning people are more susceptible to the damaging effects.

Sunscreens initially protected only against UVB rays. Now most offer sun protection against both UVB and UVA radiation. Minimization of sun exposure is always recommended. Most commercially available sunscreens consist of paraaminobenzoic acid (PABA) esters, benzophenomens, cinnamates, salicylates, and anthracytes. Another subgroup consists of physical sunblocks. These are comprised of pulverized forms of zinc oxide or titanium oxide.

The commonly used *sun protection factor* (SPF) provides a general guideline as to the efficacy of the agent (Figure 23-31). It compares the minimal time needed to produce skin erythema compared with not using the agent. In other words, a SPF of 15 would take 15 times longer to obtain the same redness; if a patient became red in 10 minutes while unprotected, wearing a 15 SPF agent would require 150 minutes.

These agents only lengthen the period it takes to absorb the harmful rays. No agent protects with prolonged exposure. Patients must be aware that (1) application 1 hour before sun exposure helps bind the sunblock on the skin and improves efficacy and (2) reapplication is needed. No minimal safe dose exists, even though the exact cause-and-effect relationship regarding melanoma remains obscure. Agents that are above 15 to 18 SPF have a mechanical makeup that help shields the patient; the chemical block only is effective up to this level.

RECURRENCE

Many studies indicate that melanoma recurrence rates are not as predictable as might have been hoped (Table 23-5).

REFERENCES

1. Koh HK: Cutaneous melanoma, *N Engl J Med* 325:171, 1991.
2. McLeod GR, David NC, Little JH, et al: Melanoma in Queensland, Australia: experience in the Queensland Melanoma Project. In Balch CM, Milton GW, editors: *Cutaneous melanoma: clinical management and treatment results worldwide,* Philadelphia, 1985, Lippincott.
3. Parker SL, Tong T, Bolden S, Wingo PA: Cancer statistics, 1996, *CA* 46:5, 1996.
4. Katz L, Den-Tuvla S, Steinitz R: Malignant melanoma of the skin in Israel: affect of migration. In Magnus K, editor: *Trends in cancer incidence,* Washington, DC, 1982, Hemisphere.
5. Greene A: Incidence in reporting of cutaneous melanoma in Queensland, *Aust J Dermatol* 23:105, 1982.
6. Eldh J, Beryd B, Suurkula M, et al: Melanoma in Sweden: experience at the University of Goteborg. In Balch CM, Milton GW, editors: *Cutaneous melanoma: clinical management and treatment results worldwide,* Philadelphia, 1985, Lippincott.
7. Lee JAH: The causation of melanoma. In Balch CM, Milton GW, editors: *Cutaneous melanoma: clinical management and treatment results worldwide,* Philadelphia, 1985, Lippincott.
8. Lee JAH: Melanoma and exposure to sunlight, *Epidemiol Rev* 4:110, 1982.
9. Elwood IB, Koh HK: Etiology, epidemiology, risk factors, and public health issues of melanoma, *Curr Opin Oncol* 6:179, 1994.
10. Lambert WC, Kuo H, Lambert MW: Xeroderma pigmentosum, *Dermatol Clin* 13:169, 1995.
11. Wallace DC, Exton LA, McLeod GRC: Genetic factors in malignant melanoma, *Cancer* 27:1262, 1971.
12. Clark WH Jr, Reimer RR, Greene M, et al: Origin of familial malignant melanomas from heritable melanocytic lesions: the B-K mole syndrome, *Arch Dermatol* 114(5):732, 1978.
13. Elder DE, Goldman LI, Goldman SC, et al: Dysplastic nevus syndrome: a phenotypic association of sporadic cutaneous melanoma, *Cancer* 46:1787, 1980.
14. Clark WH Jr, Elder DE, Guerry D IV, et al: A study of tumor progression: the precursor lesions of superficial spreading and nodular melanoma, *Hum Pathol* 15:1147, 1984.
15. Clark WH Jr, Elder DE, Guerry DW: Dysplastic nevi in malignant melanoma. In Farmer ER, Hood AF, editors: *Pathology of skin,* East Norwalk, Conn, 1990, Appleton & Lange.
16. Tucker M, Fraser M, Goldstein A, et al: Organic risk of melanoma and other cancers in melanoma-prone families, *J Invest Dermatol* 100:350, 1993.
17. Lynch HT, Frischot BC III, Lynch J, et al: Family studies of malignant melanoma and associated cancer, *Surg Gynecol Obstet* 141:517, 1975.
18. Newell GR: Is ultraviolet irradiation the sole cause of melanoma? *Melanoma Lett* 5:4, 1987.
19. Garbe C, Buttner T, Weiss J, et al: Risk factors for developing cutaneous melanoma and criteria for identifying persons at risk: multi-center case-control study of the Central Malignant Melanoma Registry of the German Dermatologic Society, *J Invest Dermatol* 102:695, 1994.
20. Kopf A, Marghoob A, Slade J, et al: Basal and squamous cell carcinomas: risk factors for cutaneous malignant melanoma (abstract A). Presented at the Sixth World Congress on Cancers of the Skin, Buenos Aires, 1995.
21. Kripke ML: Ultraviolet radiation and immunology: something new under the sun, *Cancer Res* 54:6102, 1994.
22. Crombie IK: Variation of melanoma incidence with latitude in North America and Europe, *Br J Cancer* 40:774, 1979.
23. Elwood JM, Gallagher RP: Site distribution of malignant melanoma, *Can Med Assoc J* 128:1400, 1983.
24. Rigel DS, Kopf AW, Friedman RJ: A rate of malignant melanoma in the U.S.: are we Making an Impact? *Am Acad Dermatol* 176:1050, 1987.
25. Vogelstein B, Kinsler KW: The multi-step nature of cancer, *Trends Genet* 9:138, 1993.
26. Kripke ML, Fisher LS: Immunologic parameters of ultraviolet carcinogenesis, *J Natl Cancer Inst* 57:211, 1976.
27. Groh JJ, Govemet J, Aymes D, et al: Count of benign melanocytic nevi as a major indication of risk of nonfamilial melanoma, *FSM Cancer* 69:387, 1990.
28. MacKie RM, Freudenberger T, Aitchison TC: Personal risk factor chart for melanoma, *Lancet* 2:487, 1989.
29. Evans RN, Kopf AW, Lew RA, et al: Risk factors for the development of malignant melanoma. I. Review of case-control study, *J Dermatol Surg Oncol* 14:393, 1988.

30. Garbe C, Buttner T, Weiss J, et al: Associated factors in the prevalence of more than fifty melanocytic nevi, atypical melanocytic nevi and actinic lentigines: multi-center case-control study of the Malignant Melanoma Registry of the German Dermatologic Society, *J Invest Dermatol* 102:700, 1994.

31. Baserga R: Oncogenes and the strategy of growth factors, *Cell* 79:927, 1994.

32. Brobell A, Rapaport D, Wells R, et al: Multiple primary melanomas: implications for screening and follow-up programs for melanoma, *Ann Surg Oncol* 4(1):19, 1997.

33. Friedman RJ, Regel DS, Kopf AW: Early detection of melanoma: the role of physician examination and self-examination of the skin, *CA* 35:130, 1985.

34. Mackie RN: *An illustrated guide to the recognition of early malignant melanoma,* Edinburgh, 1986, Blackwood, Pillans and Wilson.

35. Keefe M, Dick DC, Wakeel RA: A study of the value of the seven point checklist in distinguishing benign pigmented lesions from melanoma, *Clin Exp Dermatol* 15:167, 1990.

36. Cassileth BR, Clark WH Jr, Lusk EJ, et al: How well do physicians recognize melanoma and other problem lesions? *J Am Acad Dermatol* 14:555, 1986.

37. Koh HK, Miller DR, Geller AC, et al: Who discovers melanoma? patterns from a population-based survey, *J Am Acad Dermatol* 26:914, 1992.

38. Grin CM, Kopf AW, Welkovich B, et al: Accuracy in the clinical diagnosis of malignant melanoma, *Arch Dermatol* 126:763, 1990.

39. Berwick M, Begg CB, Fine JA, et al: Screening for cutaneous melanoma by skin self-examination, *J Natl Cancer Inst* 88:17, 1996.

40. Guerry D, Synnestvedt M, Elder DE, Schultz D: Lessons from tumor progression: the invasive radial growth phase of melanoma is common, incapable of metastasis, and indolent, *J Invest Dermatol* 100:S342, 1993.

41. Giles GG, Armstrong BK, Burton RC, et al: Has mortality from melanoma stopped rising in Australia? Analysis of trends between 1931 and 1994, *BMJ* 312:1121, 1996.

42. Armstrong BK: Epidemiology of malignant melanomas: intermittent or total accumulated exposure to the sun? *J Dermatol Surg Oncol* 14:835, 1988.

43. Pehamberger H, Bender M, Knollmayer S, Wolfe SK: Immediate effects of a public education campaign on prognostic features of melanoma, *J Am Acad Dermatol* 29:106, 1993.

44. Cooke KR, Skegg DC, Fraser J: Socioeconomic status, indoor and outdoor work, and malignant melanoma, *Int J Cancer* 34:57, 1984.

45. Burton RC, Armstrong BK: Recent incidence trends imply a non-metastasizing form of invasive melanoma, *Melanoma Res* 4:107, 1994.

46. Lee JA, Strickland D: Malignant melanoma: social status and outdoor work, *Br J Cancer* 41:757, 1980.

47. Miim MC, Barnhill RL, Sober AL, Hernandez MH: Precursor lesions of melanoma: do they exist? *Semin Surg Oncol* 8:358, 1994.

48. Greene MH, Clark WH Jr, Tucker MA, et al: High risk of malignant melanoma in melanoma-prone families with dysplastic nevi, *Ann Intern Med* 102:458, 1985.

49. National Institutes of Health: Consensus Development Conference statement on treatment of early melanoma, *Am J Dermatopathol* 15:34, 1993.

50. Lynch HT, Fishot BC III, Lynch JF: Familial atypical multiple mole, melanoma syndrome, *J Med Genet* 15:352, 1979.

51. Lynch HT, Fusaro RM, Kimberling WJ, et al: Familial atypical multiple mole melanoma (FAMMM) syndrome: segregation analysis, *J Med Genet* 20:342, 1983.

52. Kramer KH, Tucker MA, Tarone R, et al: Risk of cutaneous melanoma in dysplastic nevus syndrome types A & B, *N Engl J Med* (letter) 315:615, 1986.

53. Albert OS, Rhodes AR, Silber AJ: Dysplastic melanocytic nevi and cutaneous melanoma: markers of increased melanoma risk for affected persons and blood relatives, *J Am Acad Dermatol* 22:69, 1990.

54. Rhodes AR, Weinstock MA, Fitzpatrick TB, et al: Risk factors for cutaneous melanoma: a method of recognizing predisposed individuals, *JAMA* 258:3146, 1987.

55. Moss ALH, Briggs JC: Cutaneous malignant melanoma in the young, *Br J Cancer* 39:537, 1986.

56. Williams ML, Pennena R: Melanoma, melanocytic nevi and other melanoma risk factors in children, *J Pediatr* 124:833, 1994.

57. Kaplan E: The risk of malignancy in large congenital nevi, *Plast Reconstr Surg* 53:421, 1974.

58. Trozak D, Rowland W, Hu F: Metastatic malignant melanoma in prepubertal children, *Pediatrics* 55:191, 1975.

59. Pratt CB, Palmer MK, Thatcher N, et al: Malignant melanoma in children and adolescence, *Cancer* 47:392, 1980.

60. Smith K, Barrett T, Skelton H, et al: Spinal cell and epithelioid cell nevi with atypia and metastases (malignant Spitz nevus), *Am J Surg Pathol* 13:931, 1989.

61. Maldonado RR, Tamayo L, Leterza AM, et al: Giant pigmented nevi: clinical histopathologic and therapeutic considerations, *J Pediatr* 120:906, 1991.

62. Barnhill R, Flotte T, Fleischi M, et al: Cutaneous melanoma and atypical Spitz tumors in childhood, *Cancer* 76:1833, 1995.

63. Spitz S: Melanomas of childhood, *Am J Pathol* 24:591, 1948.

64. Boddie AW, Smith JJL, McBride CM: Malignant melanoma in children and young adults: effect of diagnostic criteria on staging and end results, *South Med J* 71:1074, 1978.

65. Lerman R, Murray D, O'Hara J, et al: Malignant melanoma of childhood: a clinicopathologic study and report of twelve cases, *Cancer* 25(2):436, 1970.

66. Kate PS, Ronan SG, Feucht KA, et al: Melanoma in childhood and adolescence: clinical and pathologic features of forty-eight cases, *J Pediatr Surg* 28:217, 1993.

67. Temple W, Mulloy R, Alexander F, et al: Childhood melanoma, *J Pediatr Surg* 267:135, 1991.

68. Allen AC, Spitz S: Malignant melanoma: a clinicopathological analysis of the criteria for diagnosis and prognosis, *Cancer* 145(6):1, 1953.

69. Ceballos PI, Maldonado RR, Mihm MC: Melanoma in children, *N Engl J Med* 332:656, 1995.

70. Mehregan AH, Mehregan DA: Malignant melanoma in childhood, *Cancer* 71:4096, 1993.

71. Baader W, Kropp R, Tapper D: Congenital malignant melanoma, *Plast Reconstr Surg* 90:53, 1991.

72. Davidoff AM, Cirrincione MS, Seigler HF: Malignant melanoma in children, *J Surg Oncol* 1:271, 1994.

73. Reintgen DS, Vollmer R, Seigler HF: Juvenile malignant melanoma, *Surg Gynecol Obstet* 168:249, 1989.

74. Rao BN, Hayes FA, Pratt CD, et al: Malignant melanoma in children: its management and prognosis, *J Pediatr Surg* 25:198, 1990.

75. Melanik MK, Urdaneta LF, Al-Jurf AS, et al: Malignant melanoma in childhood and adolescence, *Am Surg* 52:142, 1985.

76. Clark WH Jr, Bernardino EA, et al: The histogenesis and biologic behavior of primary human malignant melanomas of the skin, *Cancer Res* 29:705, 1969.

77. Clark WH, Mihm MC Jr: Lentigo maligna and lentigo maligna melanoma, *Am J Pathol* 55:39, 1969.

78. Landthaler M, Braun-Falco O, Leito A, et al: Excisional biopsy in the first therapeutic procedure vs. primary wide excision of malignant melanoma, *Cancer* 64:1612, 1989.

79. Bart RS, Kopf AW: Techniques of biopsy of cutaneous neoplasms, *J Dermatol Surg Oncol* 5:979, 1979.

80. Harris MN, Gunport SL: Biopsy technique for malignant melanoma, *J Dermatol Surg* 1:24, 1975.

81. Braun-Falco O, Korting HC, Konz B: Histological and cytological criteria in the diagnosis of malignant melanomas by cryostat sections, *Virchows Arch Pathol Anat* 393:115, 1981.

82. Maissy-Roberts E, Ackerman AB: A critique of techniques for biopsy of clinically suspected malignant melanomas, *Am J Dermatol Pathol* 4:791, 1982.

83. Nield DV, Saad NN, Khoo TK, et al: Tumor thickness in malignant melanoma: the limitations of frozen section, *Br J Plast Surg* 41:403, 1988.

84. Davis NC, Little JH: The role of frozen section in the diagnosis and management of malignant melanoma, *Br J Surg* 61:505, 1974.

85. Zitelli JA, Moy RL, Abell E: The reliability of frozen sections and the evaluation of surgical margins for melanoma, *J Am Acad Dermatol* 24:102, 1991.

86. Beahrs OH, Meyers MH, American Joint Committee on Cancer: *Manual for staging of cancer*, Philadelphia, 1983, Lippincott.

87. Palazzo J, Duray PH: Typical dysplastic congenital and Spitz nevi: a comparative immunohistochemical study, *Hum Pathol* 20:341, 1989.

88. Carrel S, Johnson JP: Immunologic recognition of malignant melanoma by autologous T-lymphocytes, *Curr Opin Oncol* 5:383, 1993.

89. Clark WH Jr: A classification of malignant melanoma in man correlated with histogenesis and biologic behavior. In Montagna W, Hu F, editors: *Advances in biology of the skin: the pigmentary system*, London, 1967, Pergamon.

90. Breslow A: Thickness, cross-sectional areas and depth of invasion in the prognosis of cutaneous melanoma, *Ann Surg* 172:902, 1970.

91. Worth AJ, Gallagher RP, Elwood JM, et al: Pathologic prognostic factors for cutaneous malignant melanoma: the Western Canada Melanoma Study, *Int J Cancer* 43:370, 1989.

92. Balch CN, Cascinelli N, Dirzewiecki KT, et al: A comparison of prognosis factors worldwide. In Balch CM, Houghton AN, Milton GW, et al, editors: *Cutaneous melanoma,* ed 2, Philadelphia, 1992, Lippincott.

93. Balch CM, Murad TM, Soong S-J, et al: A multi-factorial analysis of melanoma: prognostic histopathologic features comparing Clark's and Breslow's staging methods, *Ann Surg* 188:732, 1978.

94. Cascinelli N, Morabito A, Bufalino R, et al: Prognosis of stage I melanoma of the skin: WHO Collaborating Centers for Evaluation of Methods of Diagnoses and Treatment of Melanoma, *Int J Cancer* 26:733, 1980.

95. Day CL Jr, Lew RA, Mihm MC Jr, et al: The natural breakpoint for primary-tumor thickness in clinical stage I melanoma, *N Engl J Med* 305:1155, 1981, (letter).

96. Breslow A, Macht SD: Optimal size of resection margin for thin cutaneous melanoma, *Surg Gynecol Obstet* 145:691, 1977.

97. Veronesi U, Cascinelli N, Adamus J, et al: Thin-staged primary cutaneous malignant melanoma: comparison of excision with margins of one to three centimeters, *J Med* 318:1159, 1988.

98. Breslow A, Macht SD: Evaluation of prognosis of stage I cutaneous melanoma, *Plast Reconstr Surg* 61:342, 1979.

99. Day CL Jr, Sober AJ, Kopf AW: A prognostic model for clinical stage I melanoma of the upper extremity: the importance of anatomic subsites in predicting recurrent disease, *Ann Surg* 193:436, 1981.

100. Kheir SA, Bines SB, Vonroenn JH, et al: Prognostic significance of DNA aneuploidy in stage I cutaneous melanoma, *Ann Surg* 207:455, 1988.

101. Khansur T, Sanders J, Das S: Evaluation of staging work-up in malignant melanoma, *Arch Surg* 124:847, 1989.

102. Ardizzoni A, Grimaldi A, Repetto L, et al: Stage I-II melanoma: the value of metastatic work-up, *Oncology* 44:87, 1987.

103. Au F, Maier W, Malmud L, et al: Preoperative nuclear scans in patients with melanoma, *Cancer* 53:2095, 1984.

104. Panussopoulos D, Liesmann G, et al: Scintiscans in the evaluation of patients with malignant melanoma, *Surg Gynecol Obstet* 149:574, 1979.

105. Evans R, Bland K, McMurtery M, et al: Radionuclide scans not indicated for clinical stage I melanoma, *Surg Gynecol Obstet* 150:532, 1980.

106. Roth JA, Eilber F, Bennett L, et al: Radionuclide photoscanning: usefulness in preoperative evaluation of melanoma patients, *Arch Surg* 110:1211, 1975.

107. Buzaid A, Sandler A, Mani S, et al: Role of computed tomography in the staging of primary melanoma, *J Clin Oncol* 11:638, 1993.

108. Zartman G, Thomas M, Robinson W: Metastatic disease in patients with newly diagnosed malignant melanoma, *J Surg Oncol* 35:163, 1987.

109. Balch CM, Murad TM, Soong S-J, et al: Tumor thickness as a guide to surgical management of clinical stage I melanoma patients, *Cancer* 43:883, 1979.

110. Urist MM, Balch CM, Milton GW: Surgical management of the primary melanoma. In Balch CM, Milton GW, editors: *Cutaneous melanoma: clinical management and treatment results worldwide,* Philadelphia, 1985, Lippincott.

111. Handley WF: The pathology and melanotic growth in relation to their operative treatment, *Lancet* I:927, 1907.

112. Veronesi U, Cascinelli N, Adamus J, et al: Primary cutaneous melanoma 2 mm or less in thickness: results of a randomized study comparing wide with narrow surgical excision—a preliminary report, *N Engl J Med* 318:1159, 1988.

113. Balch CH, Urist MM, Karakousis CP, et al: Efficacy of 2-cm surgical margins for intermediate thickness melanomas (1-4 mm): results of a multi-institutional randomized surgical trial, *Ann Surg* 218:262, 1993.

114. Bagly FH, Cady B, Lee A, et al: Changes in clinical presentation and management of malignant melanoma, *Cancer* 47:2126, 1981.

115. Veronesi U, Cascinelli N: Narrow excision (1-cm margin): a safe procedure for myocutaneous melanoma, *Arch Surg* 126:438, 1991.

116. Cosimi AB, Sober AJ, Mihm MC: Conservative surgical management of superficially invasive cutaneous melanoma, *Cancer* 53:1256, 1984.

117. Harris M, Shapiro R, Roses D: Malignant melanoma: primary surgical management (excision and node dissection) based on pathology and staging, *Cancer* 75:715, 1995.

118. Ariyan S: Plastic and reconstructive surgery in melanoma patients. In Balch CM, editor: *Surgical approaches to cutaneous melanoma,* Basel, 1985, Karger.

119. Grabbe WC: Basic techniques in plastic surgery. In Grabbe WC, Smith JW, editors: *Plastic surgery,* ed 3, Boston, 1979, Little, Brown.

120. Tolhurst DE, Haesecker B, Zeeman RJ: The development of the fasciocutaneous flap and its clinical applications, *Plast Reconstr Surg* 71:595, 1983.

121. Koh H, Sober A, Day CJ, et al: Prognosis of clinical stage I melanoma patients with positive elective regional node dissection, *J Clin Oncol* 4:1238, 1986.

122. Varonesi U, Adamus J, Bandiera DC, et al: Inefficacy of immediate node dissection in stage I melanoma of the limbs, *N Engl J Med* 297:627, 1977.

123. Sim FH, Taylor WF, Pritchard DJ, et al: Lymphadenectomy in the management of stage I malignant melanoma: a prospective randomized study, *Mayo Clin Proc* 61:697, 1986.

124. Reintgen DS, Albertini J, Berman C, et al: Accurate nodal staging of malignant melanoma, *Cancer Control* 2:405, 1995.

125. Balch CM, Soong S-J, Bartolucci AA, et al: Efficacy of an elective regional lymph node dissection of 1-4 mm thick melanomas for patients sixty years of age and younger, *Ann Surg* 224:255, 1996.

126. Veronesi U, Adamus J, Bandiera DC, et al: Delayed regional lymph node dissection in stage I melanoma of the skin of the lower extremities, *Cancer* 49:2420, 1982.

127. Milton GW, Shaw HM, McCarthy WH, et al: Prophylactic lymph node dissection in clinical stage I cutaneous malignant melanoma: results of surgical treatment in 1319 patients, *Br J Surg* 69:108, 1982.

128. Reintgen DS, Cox EB, McCarty KS Jr, et al: Efficacy of elective lymph node dissection in patients with intermediate thickness primary melanoma, *Ann Surg* 98:379, 1983.

129. Uriest MM, Balch CM, Soong S-J, et al: Head and neck melanoma in 536 clinical stage I patients: a prognostic factors analysis and results of surgical treatment, *Ann Surg* 200:769, 1984.

130. Meyer CM, Lucklitner ML, Logic JR, et al: Technetium-99m sulfur-colloid cutaneous lymphoscintigraphy in the management of truncal melanoma, *Radiology* 131:205, 1979.

131. Reintgen DS, Cruse CW, Berman C, et al: An orderly progression of melanoma nodal metastases, *Ann Surg* 220:759, 1994.

132. Morton DL, Wen DR, Wong JH, et al: Technical details of intraoperative lymphatic mapping for early stage melanoma, *Arch Surg* 127:392, 1992.

133. Albertini J, Cruse CW, et al: Intraoperative Radiolymphoscintigraphy improved sentinel lymph node identification in melanoma patients, *Ann Surg* 223:17, 1996.

134. Heller R, Becker J, Wassalle J, et al: Detection of occult lymph node metastases in malignant melanoma, *Ann Plast Surg* 28:74, 1992.

135. Alex JC, Weaver DL, Fairbank JT, et al: Gamma-probe-guided lymph node localization in malignant melanoma, *Surg Oncol* 2:303, 1993.

136. Shivers SC, Wang W, et al: Molecular staging of malignant melanoma: correlation with clinical outcome, *JAMA* 280(16):1410, 1998.

137. Turkula LD, Woods JE: Limited or selective nodal dissection from malignant melanoma of the head and neck, *Am J Surg* 148:446, 1984.

138. Schuller DE, Reiches NA, Hamaker RC, et al: Analysis of disability resulting from treatment including radical neck dissection or modified neck dissection, *Head Neck Surg* 6:551, 1983.

139. Storm SK, Eilber FR, Sparks FC, et al: A prospective study of parotid metastases from head and neck cancer, *Am J Surg* 134:115, 1977.

140. Dunn EJ, Kent T, Hines J, et al: Parotid neoplasms: a report of 250 cases and review of the literature, *Ann Surg* 84:500, 1976.

141. O'Brien CJ, Coates AS, Petersen-Schaefer K, et al: Experience with 998 cutaneous melanomas of the head and neck over thirty years, *Am J Surg* 162:310, 1991.

142. Byers RN: The role of modified neck dissection and the treatment of cutaneous melanoma of the head and neck, *Arch Surg* 121:1338, 1986.

143. Fisher SR, Cole TB, Seigler HF: Application of posterior neck dissection in treating malignant melanoma of the posterior scalp, *Laryngoscope* 93:760, 1983.

144. Simmons JN: Malignant melanoma of the head and neck, *Am J Surg* 124:45, 1972.

145. Fisher SR: Cutaneous malignant melanoma of the head and neck, *Laryngoscope* 99:822, 1989.

146. Chretien P, Kercham A, Hoye R, Sample W: Axillary dissection with preservation of the pectoralis major muscle, *Ann Surg* 173:554, 1971.

147. Haagensen C, Feind C, Herter F, et al: *The lymphatic in cancer,* Philadelphia, 1972, Saunders.

148. Yonemoto R, Thompson W, Byron R, Riihimaki D: Complete axillary node dissection with preservation of the pectoralis major muscle, *Arch Surg* 103:578, 1971.

149. Karakousis C, Hena M, Emrich L, Driscoll D: Axillary node dissection in malignant melanoma: results and complications, *Surgery* 108:10, 1990.

150. Harris M, Gumport S, Maiwandi H: Axillary lymph node dissection for melanoma, *Surg Gynecol Obstet* 135:936, 1972.

151. Vordermark JS, Jones BM, Harrison DH: Surgical approaches to block dissection of the inguinal lymph node, *Br J Plast Surg* 38:321, 1985.

152. Karakousis CP, Driscoll DL: Groin dissection in malignant melanoma, *Br J Surg* 81:1771, 1994.

153. Karakousis CP, Driscoll DL, Rose B, et al: Groin dissection in malignant melanoma, *Ann Surg Oncol* 1:271, 1994.

154. Sterne GD, Murray DS, Grimley RP: Ilioinguinal block dissection for malignant melanoma, *Br J Surg* 82:1057, 1995.

155. Karakousis CP, Emrich LJ, Driscoll DL, et al: Survival after groin dissection for malignant melanoma, *Surgery* 109:119, 1991.

156. Abraham V, Ravi R, Shrivastava BR: Primary reconstruction to avoid wound breakdown following groin block dissection, *Br J Plast Surg* 45:211, 1992.

157. Karakousis CP: Complications of lymphadenectomy: prophylaxis in management. In Balch CM, editor: *Surgical approaches to cutaneous melanoma,* New York, 1985, Karger.

158. Bowsher WG, Taylor BA, Hughes LE: Morbidity, morality and local recurrence following regional node dissection for melanoma, *Br J Surg* 73:906, 1986.

159. Calabro A, Singletary SE, Balch CM: Patterns of relapse in 1,001 consecutive patients with melanoma nodal metastases, *Arch Surg* 124:1051, 1989.

160. Overett TK, Shiu MH: Surgical treatment of distant metastatic melanoma: indications and results, *Cancer* 56:1222, 1985.

161. Feun LG, Gutterman J, Burgess MA, et al: The natural history of resectable metastatic melanoma (stage IV A), *Cancer* 50:1656, 1982.

162. Harwood AR: Conventional fractionated radiotherapy for 51 patients with lentigo maligna and lentigo maligna melanoma, *Int J Radiat Oncol Biol Phys* 9:1019, 1983.

163. Thames HD, Withers HR, Peters LJ, Fletcher GH: Changes in early and late radiation responses with altered dose fractionation: implications for dose survival relationships, *Int J Radiat Oncol Biol Phys* 8:219, 1982.

164. Hill GJ II, Moss SE, Golomb FN, et al: DTIC and combination therapy for melanoma. III. DTIC (NSC 45388) Surg Adjuvant Study COG Protocol 7040, *Cancer* 47:2556, 1981.

165. Kremetz ET, Ryan RF, Carter RD, et al: Hyperthermic regional perfusion for melanoma of the limbs. In Balch CM, Milton GW, editors: *Cutaneous melanoma: clinical management and treatment results worldwide,* Philadelphia, 1985, Lippincott.

166. Stehlin JF Jr, Smith JL Jr, Jing B, et al: Melanomas of the extremities complicated by in-transit metastases, *Surg Gynecol Obstet* 122:3, 1966.

167. Treidman L, McNeer G: Prognosis with local metastases and recurrence in malignant melanoma, *Ann NY Acad Sci* 100:123, 1963.

CHAPTER

Thermal Burns

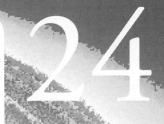

Warren L. Garner

INTRODUCTION

Burn injuries range from inconsequential epidermal injuries to lethal combinations of soft tissue and pulmonary destruction. An estimated 2 million people sustain thermal burns yearly, about 70,000 of whom require hospital treatment. About a quarter of these patients have major burn injuries that require treatment in a burn center.

Scald burns are the most common type of burn injury, about half of which occur in children. The kitchen is the most common site for these injuries. *Flame burns* are more serious and result in most burn unit admissions. House fires, automobile accidents, and work-related injuries are common causes.

Thermal burns are accidental and often devastating, and preventive efforts have significantly reduced burn injuries and deaths. These efforts include programs to place and maintain smoke detectors (e.g., Change Your Clock, Change Your Battery), programs teaching children how to respond to burning clothes (e.g., Stop, Drop, and Roll), and programs to turn down the thermostat on water heaters. The use of smoke detectors to prevent smoke inhalation and thermal burns has been particularly successful, with an estimated 80% decrease in mortality and a 74% decrease in injuries from residential fires.[27]

INDICATIONS

FUNCTION OF SKIN

The anatomic structure of the skin is designed to perform various functions (Box 24-1). The *epidermis* is the upper or outer layer. Basal keratinocytes undergo repetitive division and differentiation to form a continuously renewing cornified layer. This is the site where the body maintains the barrier between the internal self and the outside world. The stratum corneum provides protection against invasion by microorganisms and prevents the loss of fluids.

The *dermis* is composed of structural proteins, collagen and proteoglycans, and is interspersed with fibroblasts and capillaries. Embedded within the dermis are skin appendages, hair follicles, sebaceous glands, and sweat glands. These contain reservoirs of epidermal cells, which are the sources of epidermal injury and regeneration. The collagen structure of the skin provides toughness and the biomechanical properties of stretch and creep. The subcutaneous layer allows the skin to be loosely attached to the underlying fascia. This increases mobility and is extremely important in areas where motion is essential for function.

Thermal damage to the skin results in loss of these functions. Loss of the stratum corneum allows microorganisms to invade the body. Because many burn patients are also immunosuppressed, infection is a serious concern and frequent complication. Thus topical antibiotic dressings are needed to control pathogens on the wound surface. In addition, the Langerhans' cells in the epidermis that mediate the usual immune response to infection are lost. This impairs immune function at a time of increased risk of infection.

Loss of the epidermal barrier also increases fluid losses and therefore fluid requirements; this continues until the wound is reepithelialized, not only during initial resuscitation. The loss of dermis and subcutaneous tissue in a deeper injury results in a wound with limited ability to resist the normal forces of wound contraction and increased attachments between the skin and underlying structures. Mobility can be easily lost or impaired in these patients.

PATHOPHYSIOLOGY OF BURN INJURY

Local Response

Tissue injury after thermal trauma results from several factors. Most tissue is lost from heat coagulation of the protein within the tissue. The final tissue loss, however, is progressive and results from release of local mediators, changes in blood flow, tissue edema, and infection.

These initial events were first described by Jackson in 1947 (Figure 24-1). The area of irreversible tissue destruction was termed a *zone of coagulation*. An area of decreased perfusion

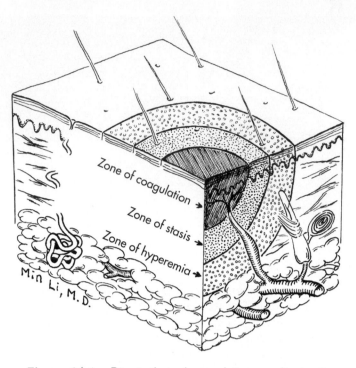

Figure 24-1. Direct thermal coagulation results in tissue necrosis, or zone of coagulation. Zone of hyperemia is adjacent to normal tissue and represents tissue response to injury with increased blood flow. Between these two zones, perfusion is marginal in zone of stasis. Inadequate fluid resuscitation results in thrombosis of vessels and tissue necrosis, leading to progressive injury.

Box 24-1.
Functions of Skin

- Provide barrier between internal tissues and outside environment
- Prevent infection
- Prevent fluid loss
- Initiate immune response
- Provide sensation
- Regulate temperature
- Synthesize vitamin D

---

surrounding this was called a *zone of stasis* and a *zone of hyperemia.* These latter zones were considered to be "at risk," but with optimal resuscitation and care, the patient might recover and heal. Without this treatment, marginal blood flow in the zone of stasis would decrease, and progressive necrosis would result in increased tissue loss. At the time of Jackson's description, this scheme was the basis for initial burn resuscitation.

In general, degree of injury is related to the temperature and duration of exposure to the burning agent. In practical terms, scald burns induced by boiling water are usually less severe than those induced by flame or oil. Such information is useful in predicting the prognosis of indeterminate injuries.

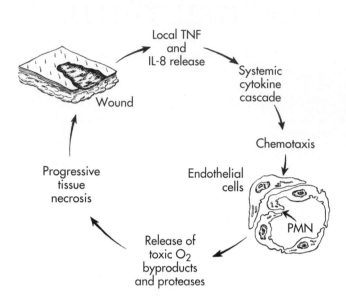

Figure 24-2. Release of numerous inflammatory mediators from injured tissue, including tumor necrosis factor *(TNF)* and interleukin-8 *(IL-8)*. These mediators induce a systemic inflammatory response, with migration and activation of polymorphonuclear neutrophil *(PMN)* into injured tissue. This causes patients to demonstrate hyperdynamic physiology. Release of oxygen metabolites, proteases, and other byproducts by activated neutrophils can cause additional tissue damage and result in progressive tissue necrosis.

Several specific mediators are present in acute burn wounds. Researchers have found various prostaglandin derivatives in burn wounds and suggested a role for an imbalance between vasoconstrictive and vasodilatory prostanoids in tissue loss in the zone of stasis and in edema. Activation of the complement and coagulation systems results in thrombosis within the microvasculature and the release of histamine and bradykinin, increasing capillary leak and tissue edema, and serotonin, causing vasoconstriction.[13] Oxygen radicals also have a role in this pathophysiology.[38] Investigators have documented both increased lipid peroxidation products after burn injury and decreased tissue edema and damage after treatment with antioxidants.[12]

Recent research has increased our understanding of the events that lead to progressive tissue loss during these first hours after burn injury (Figure 24-2). First, there is a significant release of inflammatory cytokines, such as tumor necrosis factor (TNF) and interleukins (IL-1, and IL-8), from thermally injured tissue.[15,19,26] These mediators activate leukocytes, increase chemotaxis into the wound, and upregulate cell surface adherence receptors *(integrins)* on both neutrophils and endothelial cells. The hypothetic pathophysiology is that neutrophils respond with chemotaxis into injured tissues, adhere to "sticky" capillary endothelium, and then migrate into the injured tissues.[5,28] Because these cytokines prime the neutrophils, the cells are more likely to degranulate, releasing proteases and toxic oxygen byproducts and inducing increased injury.

Several experimental studies have supported these proposed relationships by showing that blocking these events with antibodies against various integrins increases perfusion within the injured tissue and decreases tissue loss.[30] The conclusion is that some progressive tissue injury after a burn is neutrophil mediated. Unfortunately, clinically useful interventions are not yet available to prevent this process, largely because decreased neutrophil activity wound substantially increase the risks of infection.[35]

Although our knowledge is increasing about events in the burn wound, most therapeutic interventions to limit injury and its progression have not been effective. Early, effective fluid resuscitation maintains perfusion to areas at risk. Inadequate resuscitation results in progressive tissue loss. Animal studies have documented the value of interventions in altering the pathophysiology just described, often decreasing the amount of tissue loss. It is necessary to intervene before or at the time of injury, however, which prevents the use of these interventions in most clinically relevant situations.

Systemic Response

The fluid loss into the wound and release of cytokines into the systemic circulation result in a characteristic systemic response to thermal injury. *Hypovolemia* is the immediate consequence of fluid loss, resulting in decreased perfusion and oxygen delivery. Blood volume must be maintained by fluid resuscitation to prevent progressive tissue loss in the burn and distant organ dysfunction. Some patients, particularly those with large burns, also have vasoconstriction and cardiac dysfunction. The release of catecholamines, vasopressin, and angiotensin has been implicated as a cause for the vasoconstriction.[3,7] Decreased myocardial contractility appears to be mediated by the inflammatory cytokine TNF.[11]

In general the initial period after burn injury is hypodynamic. During the subsequent hours to days the hemodynamic response becomes hyperdynamic. This period is characterized by marked increases in cardiac output, low systemic vascular resistance, and a pathologic inability to respond to hypovolemia with vasoconstriction.

Significant changes in many other systems may accompany these events. Loss of red blood cells results from membrane damage and increased fragility. Acute respiratory failure is common with large burns, even without inhalation injury. Evaporative loss of water from the burn wound can induce significant cooling and, in association with loss of vasoconstrictive ability, cause hypothermia. A catabolic response includes a profound increase in resting energy expenditure, resulting in glycolysis and gluconeogenesis through the breakdown of muscle (Cori cycle).

Bacterial Translocation

The burn injury and resulting cytokine cascade cause a marked increase in metabolic rate. When nutritional support is insufficient to respond to this need, a catabolic response develops.

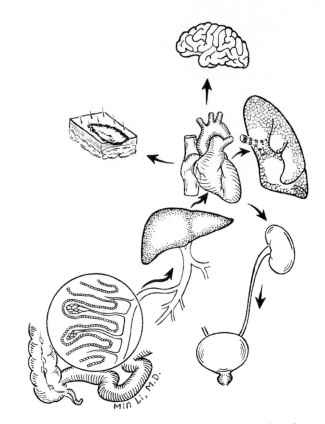

Figure 24-3. Greatly increased metabolic needs and inadequate enteral nutrition can result in intestinal villous atrophy. Bacteria present within gut lumen can translocate into portal circulation, resulting in altered hepatic, renal, pulmonary, or other organ functions and multisystem organ failure.

This may result in intestinal villous atrophy, particularly if the nutrition is not delivered enterally.

Deitch et al[10] have described a syndrome decreased bowel mucosal integrity, capillary leak, and decreased mesenteric blood flow that can result in bacterial translocation into the portal circulation. These bacteria and their byproducts can significantly alter hepatocyte function, spread systemically to induce sepsis, and trigger pathogens for infections of the blood, lungs, wound, or bladder (Figure 24-3). Substantial evidence indicates that these events are linked to the development of multisystem organ failure syndrome.

Prevention of these events is relatively straightforward. Adequate resuscitation ensures mesenteric blood flow. Enteral nutrition in general and glutamine in particular have a tropic effect on the enterocytes that preserves mucosal integrity.

Immune Consequences

Patients who have sustained serious burn injuries demonstrate marked decreases in their immune status and ability to resist infection. To date, almost every measure of immune function has been used to document this decline in immunologic status. With immunosuppression from massive tissue injury, necrotic tissue, and bacterial translocation, infection is the major cause of death in patients who survive beyond the initial resuscitation period.[9,31] Immunosuppression results from a combination of excess stimulation/utilization and endogenous inhibitors.

Neutrophils are essential for prevention and control of bacterial infections. Decreased neutrophil function after burn injury is a major cause of infectious complications in these patients. Specific deficits in neutrophil chemotaxis,[41] phagocytosis, and intracellular bacterial killing have been documented.[2,29,40] The mechanism for the latter appears to result from a decreased ability to utilize the oxidant-dependent microbial killing system.[4]

Other aspects of immune function are decreased as well. Cell-mediated immunity, as measured by skin testing, is often impaired. This deficiency is related to decreased lymphocyte activation and suppressive mediators in the serum of burn patients.[18,40] Mechanistic studies have suggested that the decrease in helper T-cell function partly results from decreased synthesis of interleukin-2.[22] Other studies have shown a decrease in immunoglobulin synthesis as well.[37]

QUANTIFICATION OF BURN SEVERITY

Mortality and morbidity can be reasonably well predicted by the depth and size of the burn, the presence of inhalation injury, and the patient's age (Figure 24-4).

Depth of Injury

The depth of the thermal injury varies from inconsequential injuries of the superficial epidermis to deep injuries involving muscle and bone. The depth of injury determines the homeostatic response and the necessary treatment. Lay descriptions of burns are related to the viability of the remaining skin. In general, these are anatomically based (Figure 24-5 and Table 24-1).

First-degree burns involve only the superficial epidermis. The skin is red, dry, and hypersensitive. The epidermal barrier remains intact. Therefore the metabolic response and risk of infection are not present. No treatment except analgesia is necessary.

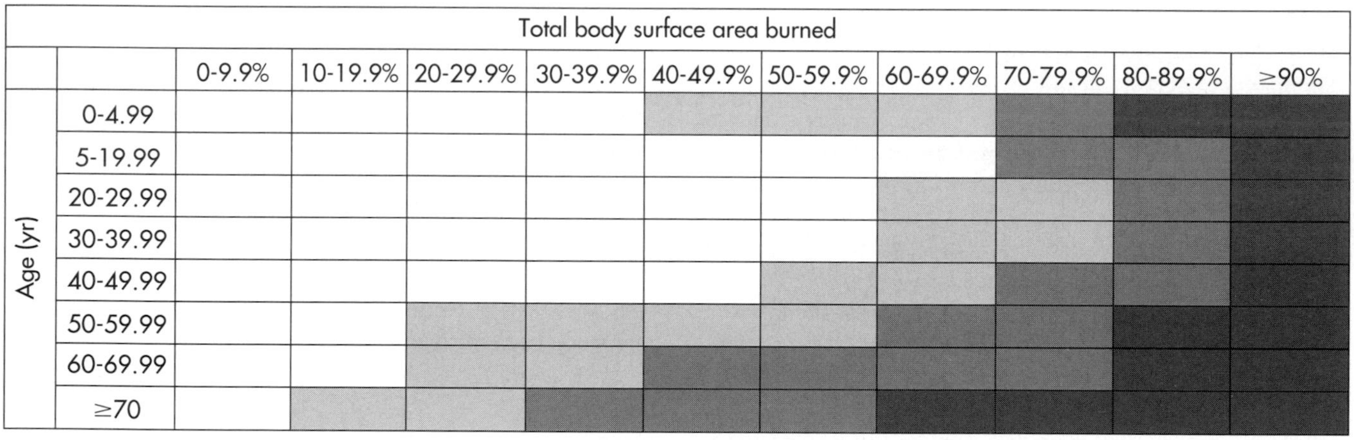

	Total body surface area burned									
Age (yr)		0-9.9%	10-19.9%	20-29.9%	30-39.9%	40-49.9%	50-59.9%	60-69.9%	70-79.9%	80-89.9%	≥90%
0-4.99											
5-19.99											
20-29.99											
30-39.99											
40-49.99											
50-59.99											
60-69.99											
≥70											

Figure 24-4. Survival rates after burn injury. Darker squares indicate increasing mortality.

Table 24-1.
Signs and Symptoms of Burn Injury

	BURN DEPTH (DEGREE)		
	FIRST	**SECOND**	**THIRD**
Cause	Flash Sunburn	Hot liquids	Flame Grease
Appearance	Red Slight swelling	Red Edematous	White/brown Contracted
Surface	Dry	Wet	Dry
Sensation	Painful	Very painful	Anesthetize

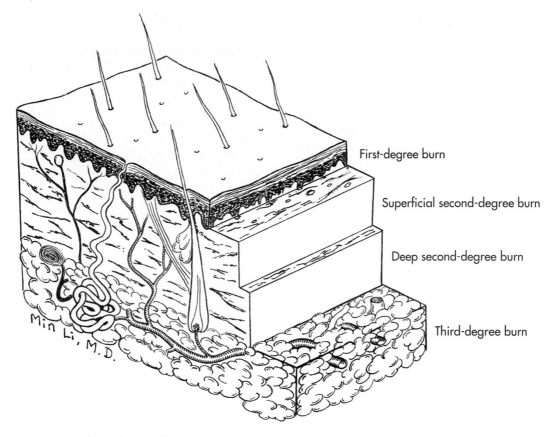

Figure 24-5. Depth of burn injury is related to skin level that is injured. First-degree burns are localized to epidermis. In second-degree burns, epidermis and some of dermis are injured. In third-degree burns, both these skin layers are completely destroyed.

In *second-degree burns* the epidermis is destroyed and part of the dermis is injured. The skin is edematous, red, wet, and painful, and blistering usually occurs. Because the epidermal barrier is lost, treatment is necessary to prevent infection during the healing process. Healing is by epidermal proliferation and migration from epidermal reservoirs in skin appendages. A hypermetabolic response is common, although limited to the time necessary to heal the wound.

Third-degree burns (full-thickness skin loss) differ most importantly from more superficial injuries because surgical intervention is necessary. The tissue is pale, contracted, insensate, and leathery. Deeper injuries, involving the underlying muscle, bone, or other structures, are sometimes described as *fourth-degree burns.* Alternately, these can be described as deep full-thickness injuries involving these structures.

Extent of Injury

A well-established relationship exists between the size of a burn and the rate of survival. The size of the burn is usually described as percentage of the total body surface area (% TBSA) that is injured. As noted, burn size, patient age, and inhalation injury are the three most important factors in predicting survival.

Several methods are available for calculating % TBSA. The most accurate is the use of BSA charts. The simplest is the "rule of nines" (Figure 24-6), which provides an approximate and

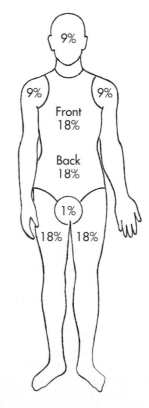

Figure 24-6. "Rule of nines" used for predicting survival rate in burn patients.

quick estimate of burn size. The body is divided into regions and each region described as a multiple of nine, with arms and head 9%, legs 18%, and torso 36%. The relative amount of each area is multiplied by its body percentage and the results summed. It is sometimes useful to remember that the patient's palm is 1% of the body.

Other factors affect mortality and morbidity from a burn injury, especially the patient's age, concomitant injuries, and preexisting medical problems. In general, a direct inverse relationship exists between age and survival for burns of any size. Thus, although the mortality from a burn greater than 40% TBSA in a 20-year-old patient is 8%, the mortality in a patient over age 70 is 94%. Children less than 1 year old also have lower survival rates with large burns. These effects partly result from preexisting medical conditions, such as cardiac, pulmonary, renal, or hepatic dysfunction. When present in younger individuals, these problems further decrease survival. Finally, concomitant injuries increase the degree of injury and physiologic stress. The result is increased complications, delayed recovery, and decreased survival rates.

INHALATION INJURY

Inhalation injury is the most serious complication of thermal injury. Several studies have documented a significant negative effect on survival.[36,39] Inhalation injury has three potential components: (1) carbon monoxide (CO) intoxication, (2) upper airway swelling, and (3) acute respiratory failure. Each of these may occur alone or in combination and may vary in severity from inconsequential to life-threatening.

Inhalation injury is usually evident by a characteristic history and physical examination (Box 24-2). Patients are typically injured in an enclosed space, such as a house or motor vehicle. They may be coughing up carbonaceous sputum. Physical stigmata include facial burns, singed nasal hair, and soot in the pharynx. New-onset hoarseness may indicate vocal cord swelling and the need for immediate airway visualization.

Carbon Monoxide
CO is a colorless, odorless gas that can form during combustion. CO binds to hemoglobin 200 times more avidly than oxygen, thereby limiting the ability to transport oxygen. The toxicity of CO is directly related to the percentage of hemoglobin it saturates (Table 24-2). Less than 15% to 20% saturation results in few sequelae; more than 50% is associated with severe neurotoxicity, central nervous system damage, and death. This phase of inhalation injury occurs in the first minutes to several hours after injury.

Treatment is based on the ability of higher oxygen concentrations to increase the rate that CO is diffused. A 100% oxygen concentration increases the rate of CO diffusion from 4 hours to 45 minutes. Although hyperbaric oxygen is useful in treating patients with isolated CO intoxication, its use complicates the care of those with skin injury. Patients should be referred to a hyperbaric facility only if the institution also has a burn center.

Box 24-2. Indicators of Inhalation Injury
Burned in closed space
Burned in motor vehicle accident
Face burns
Singed nasal hairs
Carbonaceous sputum
Carbonaceous particles in larynx

Table 24-2.
Signs and Symptoms of Carbon Monoxide Toxicity

CARBOXYHEMOGLOBIN (%)	SIGNS/ SYMPTOMS
0-10	None
10-30	Headache
30-50	Headache, nausea, dizziness, tachycardia
50-60	Central nervous system dysfunction, coma
60+	Death

Airway Swelling
Upper airway swelling is the most common form of inhalation injury. It results from dissipation of heat energy into the tissues of the pharynx, larynx, and vocal cords. The result is airway obstruction. This process begins several hours after injury and lasts for 2 to 4 days as tissue edema wanes. The diagnosis is made by direct visualization of the upper airway.

If swelling, erythema, or soot is present, the patient should undergo endotracheal intubation. The airway should be visualized again at 48 hours and daily thereafter to assess airway edema. Extubation is safe when the soft tissue swelling has decreased. If the patient can breathe or talk with the endotracheal tube occluded and the cuff deflated, airway swelling has usually subsided.

Respiratory Failure
Acute respiratory failure can occur hours to days after burn injury. This process is a chemical pneumonitis caused by toxic products of combustion. Generalized tissue edema and a systemic and local inflammatory response, as occurs after a major burn, can worsen the process. Poorer survival rates in patients with concomitant skin and pulmonary injuries are well documented.

Patients with acute respiratory failure should be treated using positive end-expiratory pressure (PEEP), low inspired-oxygen fraction, frequent suctioning, and other supportive measures. A detailed description of such treatment is beyond the scope of this chapter.

OPERATIONS

NONSURGICAL TREATMENT

The initial treatment of a burn wound is to remove all necrotic tissue, ruptured blisters, and debris, I believe removal of blisters simplifies care and may be beneficial, although this is somewhat controversial. Only blisters less than 1 cm in diameter or those on the soles of feet are left intact. The wound is washed with soap and tap water, then covered with a topical antimicrobial dressing. Topical antibiotics are used to decrease microbial growth and prevent invasive infection. Clinical studies have documented that systemic antibiotics do not achieve this result. The patient should then have daily dressing changes until healing or surgical intervention.

In the past, most practitioners performed twice-daily dressings. Recently, many patients have been dressed daily with a significant decrease in cost, nursing time, and pain. This strategy is ideal for children with superficial scald burns. Clear criteria have not been established for patients unresponsive to this treatment but would include those with infection or persistent eschar. During these dressings the wound should gently washed with pathogen-free tap water and mild soap. The previously applied topical antibiotics should be completely removed. Fibrinous exudate and loosely adherent eschar should be removed with a wet washcloth or scissors. Extensive bedside debridements are very painful and are not indicated. In most patients the wound should then be covered with antibiotic cream and gauze (Figure 24-7).

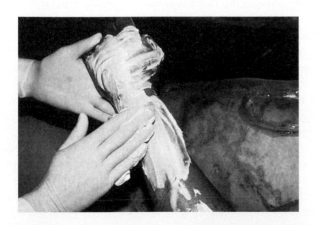

Figure 24-7. Burn wound care should be performed once or twice daily. Wound should be cleaned thoroughly to remove nonadherent skin, exudate, and debris. Light coating of antimicrobial ointment (e.g., silver sulfadiazine) is then applied and wound covered with gauze dressing.

The most frequently used antibiotic is *silver sulfadiazine* (Silvadene). It has the benefits of broad-spectrum antimicrobial coverage and few complications. The 1% incidence of leukopenia does not appear to have functional consequences.

Two other topical antimicrobials often used are mafenide (Sulfamylon) and silver nitrate. *Mafenide* can penetrate tissue and eschar, making it especially valuable in treating infected wounds or eschar. It has significant disadvantages, however, including pain on application, poor antifungal activity, and metabolic acidosis from its inhibition of carbonic anhydrase. *Silver nitrate* is used as a 0.5% soak. Its antibacterial activity is less than the that of preceding agents. Silver nitrate stains tissue and surrounding objects and induces a hypochloremic alkalosis as the silver ions precipitate chloride.

In general, when a patient's wounds are not healing at a rate sufficient to expect closure within 2 to 3 weeks, surgery should be considered.

In small, superficial, or previously debrided wounds an occlusive dressing is an excellent alternative dressing. The dressing can be kept in place for several days, decreasing pain and nursing costs.

Fluid Resuscitation

The local and systemic inflammatory response described earlier results in the loss of fluid from the intravascular space into the extracellular space. The resulting hypovolemia is proportional to the burn's extent (% TBSA burned). This has led to the development of formulas to guide treatment.

The *Parkland formula,* using lactated Ringer's solution (Ringer's lactate) as the primary resuscitation fluid, has become the standard method for resuscitating burn-injured patients. During the initial 24 hours after injury the patient receives 4 ml/kg/% TBSA burn of Ringer's lactate. Half this total is given in the first 8 hours after injury and the remaining half in the subsequent 16 hours (Table 24-3). This fluid is best administered through large-bore peripheral intravenous (IV) lines.

During this period of endothelial leak and fluid administration, significant loss of intravascular protein occurs. To maintain dynamic forces between the intravascular and extracellular spaces, this oncotic protein is replenished by administering 0.5 ml c/kg/% TBSA of 5% albumin when the endothelial integrity is restored, usually 24 hours after injury. This latter phase of resuscitation is only necessary in patients with large burns, greater than 30% TBSA. After the initial resuscitation, further albumin administration is not necessary.

In uncomplicated cases the adequacy of resuscitation is documented by the restoration of urine output greater than 30 to 50 ml/hr (0.5 to 1 ml/kg/hr in children). Lesser responses require intervention. Greater urine output suggests excessive resuscitation, which may be associated with increased tissue edema.

Clinical studies have found that the Parkland formula overestimates fluid needs for adults with moderate-sized burns (15% to 40% TBSA). This fact should remind the practitioner that a resuscitation formula is a guide, not a protocol. Fluid administration should be adjusted based on the individual

Table 24-3.
Fluid Resuscitation in Burn Patient

FORMULA	EXAMPLE*
• Ringer's lactate: 4 ml/kg/% TBSA burned	• 4 ml × 100 kg × 65% TBSA = 26,000 ml
• Give ½ in first 8 hours after injury.	• Give 13 L Ringer's lactate in next 4 hours: 3250 ml/hr.
• Give ¼ over each of next two 8-hour periods.	• Give 13 L Ringer's lactate over next 16 hours: 800 ml/hr.
• Begin 0.5 ml/kg/% TBSA of 5% albumin in Ringer's lactate 24 hours after injury, over 8 hours.	• Adjust fluid administration to maintain urine output of 30-60 ml/hr.
	• Give 400 ml/hr of Ringer's lactate with 5% albumin for 8 hours.

*100-kg male with 65% total body surface area (TBSA) burn who arrives 4 hours after injury.

Box 24-3.
Causes of Failed Fluid Resuscitation in Burn Patient

Inaccurate estimate of burn size
Undiagnosed inhalation injury
Concomitant traumatic injury
Cardiac dysfunction
Refractory shock
Mathematic miscalculation

---

patient's response. Failure to respond to the calculated resuscitation may be caused by any of several factors (Box 24-3).

In addition, characteristic myocardial dysfunction is mediated by the inflammatory cytokine TNF after major burn injury.[11,17] These patients do not respond to fluid resuscitation alone and require inotropic support for optimal treatment. When the patient does not respond to fluid resuscitation as expected, has preexisting or burn-induced cardiac dysfunction, is elderly, or has serious pulmonary injury that complicates treatment, invasive monitoring that includes pulmonary artery catheters can be extremely useful.

A variety of alternate resuscitation fluids and associated agents have been recommended. These include hypertonic saline (3% NaCl), hypertonic saline dextran (7.5% NaCl in 6% dextran 70), and deferoxamine and ascorbic acid as free radical scavengers. Although the use of each of these is supported by experimental evidence, no clinical evidence supports their widespread use in burn patients. One comparative trial even found that renal failure increased fourfold and mortality twofold with hypertonic saline resuscitation.[23]

When survival from a burn injury is virtually impossible, practitioners should strongly consider not beginning fluid resuscitation. Elderly patients with large burns will not survive. If resuscitated, they will survive for days to weeks before eventually dying of sepsis and organ failure. Many of these patients are alert and communicative early after injury. In general, these patients and their families appreciate frank discussions about survival. When resuscitation is not performed, the patient should be kept warm, pain free, and with their family.

Administration of large volumes of fluid can result in significant secondary morbidity. Practitioners should remember that excessive fluid administration results in generalized tissue edema, which can be as detrimental to survival as inadequate resuscitation. Examples include the following:
1. Pulmonary edema superimposed on existing inhalation injury
2. Tissue swelling within full-thickness burns, resulting in an increased need for escharotomies
3. Development of ileus due to bowel edema
4. Hyponatremia

Administration of large volumes of Ringer's lactate can result in metabolic alkalosis as the lactate is metabolized.

ESCHAROTOMY. During resuscitation it is important to remember that full-thickness extremity burns, particularly circumferential injuries, can prevent swelling of the underlying tissue. The result is elevated tissue pressures and impairment of tissue perfusion. In addition, inflexible eschar and underlying tissue edema can prevent chest wall motion and thus limit ventilation.

Surgical division of these constricting eschars (escharotomy) is performed to maintain distal extremity blood flow. Because the eschar is insensate, this procedure can be performed in most patients at the bedside using sedation and analgesics. Both sharp division and electrocautery are effective. Escharotomies should be performed on the midlateral or medial aspects of limbs and digits to prevent joint exposure. The eschar should be divided completely to viable underlying tissue and should separate the entire length to release the obstruction fully.

In addition to escharotomies, *fasciotomies* may be needed in patients with large burns and generalized massive tissue edema, crush injuries, or electrical burns.

GROWTH HORMONE. Various agents have been used in association with fluid resuscitation., The intervention that shows the most promise is administration of human growth hormone. Both wound healing and survival are improved in small trials.[25] The cost/benefit ratio of this treatment will be determined in future randomized trials.

Nutritional Support

Burn injury and the resulting inflammatory and cytokine responses induce a marked increase in metabolic rate. The result is a great increase in energy expenditures, twofold to threefold above normal. These patients require intensive nutritional support or will develop a severe catabolic state. The immunologic and wound healing responses to burn injury require amino acids for protein synthesis and adequate calories. These need to be provided early in the postinjury period.

The preferred method for delivering nutrition is via the gastrointestinal (GI) tract. When a patient or experimental animal does not receive alimentary feedings, the intestinal villae atrophy. This increases the likelihood of bacterial translocation from within the lumen of the gut into the portal circulation. Deitch et al[10] and other authors have documented this process in animals and associated it with systemic sepsis and the eventual development of multisystem organ failure.

This process is prevented by GI, not IV, feedings. Nutritional support is begun within 18 hours of admission through a Dobbhoff feeding tube. Attempts are made to slide the tube's tip past the pylorus by using stimulatory agents such as metoclopramide or erythromycin. Alternately, the tube is manipulated under fluoroscopy. Although gastric feedings are safe in most patients, placing the tip more distally prevents aspiration of gastric feedings during anesthesia and allows the patient to be fed continuously, without holding feedings before and during repetitive debridement and grafting sessions.

The patient's caloric requirements can be estimated using either the Curreri formula (25 kcal/kg + 40 kcal/% TBSA) or twice the Harris-Benedict estimate. Because these estimates can be very inaccurate, however, most practitioners measure *resting energy expenditure* (REE) by indirect calorimetry and then provide 20% more than this figure. REE should be measured on admission and weekly thereafter. Clinical measurements of protein requirements for these patients suggest that they require a nonprotein kilocalorie/nitrogen ratio of 100:1 and at least 2 g of protein/kg/day. In most patients, effectiveness of nutritional support is documented by quantitation of acute-phase protein concentration.

Outpatient Burn Care

Many patients with minor burn injuries can be cared for as outpatients. In general, those considered to have "minor" burns by the criteria of the American Burn Association (ABA) can be safely treated in this manner (Box 24-4). Several additional criteria should be met before initiating this treat-

---

Box 24-4.
American Burn Association Burn Center Referral Criteria

- Second-degree and third-degree burns of more than 10% total body surface are (TBSA) in patients under 10 or over 50 years old
- Second-degree and third-degree burns of more than 20% TBSA in all other age groups
- Second-degree and third-degree burns with serious threat of functional or cosmetic impairment that involve face, hands, feet, genitalia, perineum, and major joints
- Third-degree burns of more than 5% TBSA in any age group
- Electrical burns, including lightning injury
- Chemical burns with serious threat of functional or cosmetic impairment
- Inhalation injury
- Circumferential burns of extremity and chest
- Transfer of burned children to hospital with qualified personnel and equipment

From Demuth MWE, Dimick AR, Gillespie RW, et al: *Advanced burn life support course manual*, 1994, American Burn Association.

---

ment plan. The patient or family must be mentally capable of caring for the wound, and the home environment should be stable and supportive. The patient should have no significant comorbidity and should agree with the decision for outpatient management.

The possibility of *child abuse* must be excluded. Abuse should be considered in any child or elderly burn patient when the mechanism of injury is suspect. The best indicator of abuse is a history that does not fit the patient or injury, such as an 8-month-old child or bedridden elderly person with leg contractures turning on the hot water and getting in the bathtub without supervision. Symmetric injuries can result from "dipping" a child in hot water and should be investigated (Figure 24-8).

At the initial visit the wound is thoroughly cleaned. The patient or family member is then instructed in twice-daily silver sulfadiazine (Silvadene) dressing. Prescriptions are given for Silvadene, gauze, and analgesics. Nutrition and signs of infection are thoroughly discussed. The first follow-up visit should be within 48 to 72 hours, when success of outpatient care can be assessed before the patient develops irreversible problems. Healing progress is then assessed at regular intervals, depending on the patient's healing rate and success at dressing care.

When the wound has healed, use of moisturizer and sunscreen is stressed. All patients are instructed in range of motion (ROM) exercises, and the need for therapy is determined on subsequent visits. Return-to-work issues are addressed as the wound heals and are resolved on an individual basis. A late follow-up visit at 3 to 4 months is arranged for all patients,

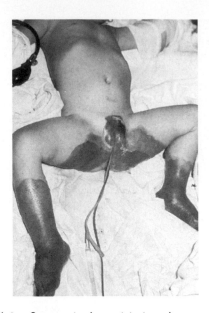

Figure 24-8. Symmetric burn injuries that resulted from "dipping" in hot water during child abuse. (From Demuth MWE, Dimick AR, Gillespie RW, et al: *Advanced burn life support course manual,* 1994, American Burn Association.)

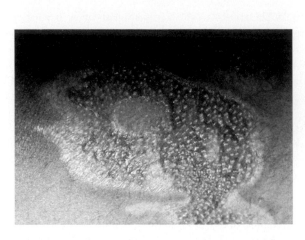

Figure 24-9. Partial-thickness wound healing by reepithelialization 8 days after injury. Note migration of epidermal cells into wound from margins and outgrowth of cells (seen as white dots) within wound.

except those with the most superficial injuries, to assess return of normal motion and degree of scarring.

Some patients with limited areas of full-thickness injury (less than 5% TBSA) can be cared for as outpatients. Patient screening is essential for success. After surgery the patient returns home with a protective dressing or splint and appropriate pain medicine. The graft is checked in the clinic 3 to 5 days later, and postoperative care then follows the usual protocols. Ambulation without weight bearing is allowed in patients with burned lower extremities.

Burn Wound Healing

Wound healing in the burn patient is complicated by the systemic response to injury and the presence of dead tissue. Small burns heal the same as other injuries. Partial-thickness injuries heal by reepithelialization and full-thickness injuries by contraction or surgery. The systemic inflammatory response that occurs in large injuries can persist within the wound and slow healing. Hypermetabolism may remove nutritional precursors from the wound. Necrotic tissue is easily infected because the epidermal barrier is destroyed and the patient is immunosuppressed. In general, the treatment for these problems is straightforward, as follows[33]:

1. Debridement of necrotic tissue
2. Topical antibiotic dressings to limit infection
3. Aggressive nutritional support
4. Aggressive attempts at wound closure

Partial-thickness burns heal by reepithelialization (Figure 24-9). Skin appendages, hair follicles, apocrine glands, and sebaceous glands are lined with epidermal cells. In response to epidermal damage and loss of contact inhibition, these cells replicate and migrate outward to resurface the wound. In most patients, reepithelialization occurs in days to a few

weeks, regenerates a normal epidermis, and results in little or no scar.

Full-thickness burns require surgical treatment. In most patients, split-thickness skin grafting is the procedure of choice. In special circumstances, small areas of full-thickness burn can be allowed to heal by contraction, including burns measuring 2 to 3 cm in diameter in noncritical areas not overlying joints and those 1 cm in diameter in critical areas. Although these wounds are at greater risk for contracture and hypertrophic scar, in many patients this results in an acceptable outcome without the need for surgery.

SURGICAL TREATMENT

Surgical care of burn wounds should be used when the injury is full thickness or is unlikely to heal within 3 weeks. After this time the risks of hypertrophic scar and contracture formation increase, outweighing the morbidity and costs of surgery. When the depth of injury is uncertain, a 7- to 10-day delay before initiating surgical intervention is reasonable. The sooner definitive care is begun, however, the more rapidly the patient will be ready to return to preinjury functioning. In unusual situations, such as small full-thickness burns of the trunk or in the lower extremities of paraplegic patients, a prolonged period of local wound care is reasonable.

Before the 1970s, most full-thickness burn injuries were treated expectantly. When proteolytic enzymes in the wound induced separation of the eschar, the wound was considered suitable for grafting. This usually resulted in a prolonged illness with infection.

The introduction of early debridement, using the principle of tangential excision, radically changed the operative care of the burn wound. This technique applies the standard surgical principle of removing all necrotic tissue from any wound. The result is shortened hospitalizations, earlier rehabilitation, and decreased expense.

Debridement

After the decision to care for the wound surgically has been made, the procedure should proceed expeditiously. In general, debridement should begin when the patient is stable after resuscitation, approximately 48 hours after injury. Because the risk of wound infection increases after 6 to 7 days, debridement should be completed before this time.

Tangential excision is debridement of graduated amounts of dead tissue until the level of viable tissue is reached. This usually can be determined by punctate hemorrhages in the wound bed. The advantages of this technique are accurate removal of necrotic tissue and preservation of as much subcutaneous tissue as possible. The disadvantage is blood loss.

In patients with deep burns or massive burn injuries, excision to fascia is an alternative. In these cases the viability of the subcutaneous fat is questionable. Fascial excision can be performed with electrocautery, decreasing blood loss. The disadvantages are contour irregularities and decreased mobility.

Whatever the method of debridement, it is essential that it be continued until only viable tissue remains. Bacteremia typically occurs after debridement. Patients should receive perioperative antibiotics and be monitored for clinical signs of sepsis during the first 12 hours after debridement.

Grafting

The second phase of surgical treatment is wound closure. Although wound closure usually involves some type of skin grafting, care should be individualized using standard reconstructive principles. Occasionally, small burns can be excised and closed primarily. This is gives an excellent result but is seldom possible.

The most frequent method and gold standard of wound closure is autologous split-thickness skin grafting. Two important surgical decisions must be made in regard to grafting.

AESTHETIC OUTCOME. First, if the expected survival and functional outcomes from the burn are good, the aesthetic outcome of the treatment options should be included in the surgical decision making. This consideration is important, since *mesh grafting* traditionally was used in burn wound closure except for the hand and face, which were treated with sheet grafts. Meshed grafts have a better "take rate" and achieve closure effectively. The resulting "cobblestone" appearance, however, is unsightly and very difficult to reconstruct.

In patients with small to moderate-sized burns, in children, and in patients concerned about the aesthetic result, the surgeon should strongly consider *sheet grafting*. Patients with major burns and those with insufficient donor sites or wounds that have previously failed grafting are better treated by mesh grafting. In the elderly patient the increased metabolic demands of a large donor site and lack of concern about aesthetic

outcome make mesh grafting a better option. Although full-thickness grafts can be used to close small burns, donor site availability limits this option.

DONOR SITE. The second surgical decision is selection of the donor site. When possible, donor sites should be chosen after discussion with the patient. Taking grafts from the body region that was burned or from areas usually covered by clothing or hair decreases the scarred areas and improves the long-term result. Comparative studies of back and thigh donor sites in children documented less donor site scarring in the back.[20] This region should be considered rather than the anterior thigh, the major advantage of which is easy access for the surgeon.

Various methods of dressing donor sites can be used. I most often use an occlusive dressing, since it decreases pain and simplifies the need for future wound care.

Splinting

Before surgery, joint mobility is maintained by encouraging the patients to use burned areas. After grafting, patients are kept immobile until the grafts have adhered. This is achieved by the use of splints. When available, prefabricated, low-temperature, thermoplastic material splints are extremely useful. They can be reused after the first dressing change, can be washed, and are more durable then plaster splints.

In general, splints are used to prevent motion and therefore graft loss. The splints should be designed to place joints at maximal stretch. Specific recommendations for positions include the following:

Axilla at 90 degrees, horizontal with bedside troughs, or in airplane splint

Elbow fully extended

Wrist slightly extended (10 degrees)

Metacarpal joints of fingers flexed and interphalangeal joints fully extended

Thumb in 40 to 50 degrees of abduction with interphalangeal joint extended

Small Burn Injury

A practicing plastic surgeon can successfully treat most uncomplicated small burn injuries. These include burns of the hand or face, which are difficult for other surgeons to treat. As noted, many patients with small injuries, less than 5% TBSA, can be cared for as outpatients.

Before entering the operating room (OR), the patient should be thoroughly informed about the planned procedure, the expected need for therapy and scar management, planned donor sites, and the possibility of blood transfusions. Donor sites ideally are planned before arrival in the OR. Likewise, if low-temperature thermoplastic material splints will be used, they can be fabricated before surgery.

Because large areas of the patient may be exposed during the procedure, it is important to adjust the room temperature and continuously monitor core temperature. If the patient's temperature decreases by more than 2° F, the OR should be warmed and as much of the patient covered as possible.

After induction of anesthesia the patient is positioned to allow easy access to the burn and donor sites. Although position changes are sometimes necessary when the back is used as a donor site, distal upper and lower extremity burns can be treated with the patient in a prone position. The surgeon checks for easy access before beginning the procedure. If both donor and recipient sites are not readily accessible, a position change is planned during the procedure. Open wounds are prepared with the sponge side of a prep brush and donor sites with standard preparation.

Burn debridements can induce significant blood loss, so the surgeon should use various strategies to limit bleeding. A tourniquet can be used during debridement of extremity burns, but the limb is not exsanguinated before the tourniquet is inflated. This allows mild but identifiable bleeding when the debridement reaches the level of viable tissue. The injection of epinephrine (Ringer's lactate with 2 ml 1:1000 epinephrine per liter) into the subcutaneous tissue beneath the burn decreases bleeding.

Thorough regional debridement is followed by wound treatment with topical thrombin and coverage with phenylephrine-soaked sponges (14 mg phenylephrine per liter Ringer's lactate). This limits the total blood loss by minimiz-ing the bleeding from each region as debridement proceeds. Topical thrombin is used to control hemorrhage from large or difficult wounds. Because the clot that results from its use must be removed before grafting, and because rebleeding frequently occurs, I do not use thrombin during treatment of small burn.

Figure 24-10 demonstrates debridement and grafting of a hand burn. Both Goulian and Watson knives are used to remove the burn eschar tangentially. Debridement should proceed until all injured tissue is removed. This can be recognized by punctate bleeding and a normal tissue appearance. Tissue with a reddish brown color is injured and should be removed. Hemostasis is obtained with electrocautery and phenylephrine-soaked sponges. Depending on the anesthesiologist's experience with burn debridement, the surgeon should remain aware of the patient's temperature, urine output, and ongoing blood loss. Grafts can be stapled or sutured into position.

My preference when treating children or applying small grafts in adults is to suture grafts in position with a running absorbable suture, such as 4-0 or 5-0 Monocryl. The increase in operative time is well balanced by the increase in patient comfort. The donor site is dressed with Biobrane. The dressing is changed 4 days after surgery, and therapy is initiated (see later discussion).

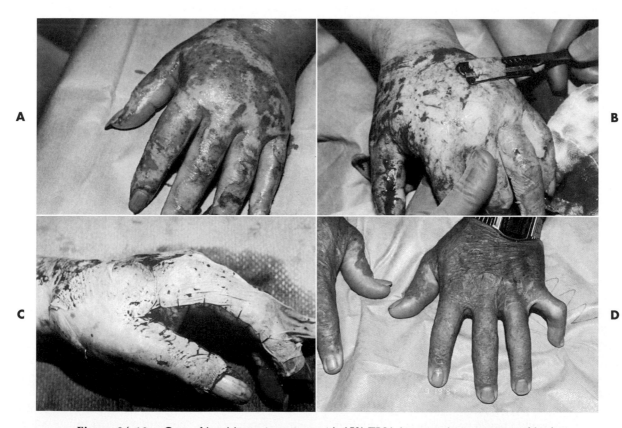

Figure 24-10. Care of hand burns in patient with 15% TBSA burn involving portions of both upper extremities and chest. **A,** Three days after injury, hand is prepped with tourniquet inflated but without exsanguinating arm. **B,** Tangential excision is used to remove full-thickness eschar. Note punctate bleeding sites and intact subcutaneous veins in uninjured subcutaneous fat. **C,** Unmeshed skin graft was harvested from anterolateral thigh and stapled into position. After surgery, patient was splinted for 3 days, then began regimen of hand therapy and pressure garment scar management. **D,** Fourteen months later, at time of release of little finger contracture.

Alternatives to Autograft

In patients with large partial-thickness burns, or when autograft is insufficient to close the wound after debridement, the surgeon should consider closing the wound with a biologic dressing. The advantages include decreased pain, prevention of infection and water loss, and faster reepithelialization.

The most frequently used biologic dressing is *human cadaver allograft*. Although somewhat limited in availability, many organ donors also donate skin, which is available through skin banks throughout the United States. Porcine xenograft (freeze dried) was used in the past, but is now seldom available.

The allograft "takes" similar to a skin graft and is then rejected through cell-mediated immunity 10 to 14 days later. In patients with massive burns who are immunosuppressed, allograft may remain intact for weeks. This strategy is valuable in maintaining wound bed integrity until donor sites have healed and are ready for reharvesting.

Approximately 20 years ago, researchers developed the technology to culture epidermal cells in the laboratory. *Cultured epidermal autografts and allografts* (CEAs) were then used to treat burn wounds. The results of this treatment and the role of this technique in the care of burn patients have been controversial. All agree, however, that CEAs are extremely fragile and sensitive to infection, antimicrobial agents, shear forces, and dressing changes. The limited data also suggest that CEAs do not increase survival or decrease costs.[34]

Allogeneic grafts are not a useful treatment for full-thickness wounds. Although keratinocytes do not usually express HLA DR antigens, allogeneic cells do stimulate rejection. Therefore, it takes 3 to 4 weeks to grow sufficient cells from a tissue biopsy to resurface a significant burn wound. During this time many wounds become infected, prolonging the period before CEAs can be used to close the wound.

After successful engraftment the resulting epidermis remains fragile and frequently blisters, apparently from slow development or abnormal anchoring of these complexes; some components of this structure are synthesized by dermal fibroblasts. This may partially explain why results of epidermal grafting are much better when the cells are used as a composite graft.

At present, most practitioners believe that CEAs are of uncertain value and should be reserved for treatment of massive burn injuries. Anecdotally, CEAs appear to decrease the incidence of hypertrophic scar but are associated with significant contraction problems.

Many surgeons now use CEAs in conjunction with a bioengineered dermis or allograft from which the epidermis is removed.[8] The U.S. Food and Drug Administration (FDA) has approved three bioengineered skin analogs. These products provide temporary wound coverage, improve the success of epidermal cell grafting, and allow the use of thinner autografts, which promote donor site healing. They may decrease contracture formation and improve appearance. In general they are expensive, however, and the cost/benefit ratio of these products is uncertain.

POSTOPERATIVE CARE

After surgical wound closure, supportive care continues, including fluid balance, nutrition, and infection surveillance. No ideal time exists to perform the first dressing change. If performed early, the graft may not be adherent, and its take may be compromised. This is particularly true when it is difficult to replace the bolster protecting the grafted area. Hematomas and seromas can be drained, however, and dislodged or misplaced grafts can be successfully repositioned in the first 2 days after placement. Early graft infection can sometimes be effectively treated with topical antimicrobials.

I individualize the timing of the first dressing change. Sheet-grafted areas that can be easily redressed, such as in the upper extremity, are inspected at 48 hours. If present, problems are corrected, and the dressing is not changed for an additional 2 days. Wounds at risk for infection are inspected at 3 days, and a daily Silvadene dressing is used to treat signs of infection. Most other graft sites are changed at 4 days. Areas that are difficult to protect from mechanical forces, such as with both anterior and posterior surface burns on the buttocks, are sometimes kept dressed for longer periods.

When graft take is stable, usually at 4 days after surgery, therapy is begun. Box 24-5 lists the goals of therapy. In general, active and passive ROM exercises are used to retain motion. Splinting is used when the patient is not moving to retain position. The positioning guidelines are the same as those for the immediate postoperative period. Because burn injury stimulates intense wound contraction, early and aggressive use of these modalities is essential to maintain function. When the grafts are secure, most patients are measured for pressure garments.

Scar Management

The most significant factor limiting recovery from survivable burn injuries is formation of *hypertrophic scar* (HTS).

HTS is a dermal fibrosis characterized by excessive collagen synthesis and wound contraction. The result is thick, prominent scars and contracture formation. The pathophysiology is

---

Box 24-5.
Goals of Therapy for Burn Patients

1. Correct, prevent, or minimize deformity.
2. Protect weak muscles from overstretching.
3. Provide a functional position.
4. Assist in maintaining range of motion.
5. Protect exposed tendons and joints.
6. Provide immobilization across joints after grafting.
7. Minimize scarring with pressure garment therapy.
8. Develop functional skills to facilitate independence in activities of daily living.
9. Facilitate community reentry through group activities, patient and family education, and community-based activities.

not completely understood but appears to result from an excessive healing response in the wound and a change in the nature of the cells within the wound. I and others have documented increases in the transforming growth factor beta (TGF-β) in burn HTS.[14,16]

HTS is more common in children, in dark or colored skin, and in areas of stretch or motion. It is different from other types of dermal fibrosis, such as keloid.

Treatment of HTS includes prevention by early wound closure, nonsurgical scar management, and surgical treatment (see Chapter 29).

Nonsurgical scar management is an important adjunct in controlling HTS. Pressure garments have long been used to limit the intensity of HTS formation. The garments are custom-fitted to provide about 25 mm of pressure and are worn at all times. The mechanism of action is thought to be a combination of pressure-induced remodeling and hypoxia-induced tissue atrophy. Anecdotal experience strongly supports the use these devices, although a recent prospective, randomized study found no benefit.[6]

When silicone sheeting is placed with worsening of HTS, the result is improved appearance, decreased redness, and less itching.[1] Silicone sheeting is applied for 12 hours a day and can be used with pressure garments.

Small HTS can be treated with corticosteroid injections. Steroid-induced suppression of macrophage release of growth factors (e.g., TGF-β) is proposed as a mechanism of action. The technique is painful, is not more effective then the previous methods, and can only be used in limited areas.

Heterotopic Ossification

Heterotopic bone formation is a serious but unusual complication of burn injury. It is characterized by deposition of bone in pericapsular tissues of joints, particularly the elbow. The pathogenesis is unknown. Associations with burn size, nonhealing wounds, superimposed trauma, and immobility have been reported, but some cases do not fulfill any of these criteria.

The first sign of heterotopic ossification (HO) typically is increased pain with joint motion, usually during passive ROM exercise. As HO progresses, joint motion decreases with a "bone end feel" at the limitations of motion. The diagnosis is confirmed by radiographs.

The clinical incidence of HO at burn centers is approximately 2%. When elbow and shoulder radiographs are acquired from many burn patients, 16% to 23% demonstrate HO. This difference suggests that symptoms, not radiographs, should be used to make the diagnosis.

Treatment protocols have been derived empirically. Aggressive therapy is withheld and only active ROM used. Surgical removal of the abnormal bone is delayed until the ossification process has stabilized and the overlying skin has fully healed. In the past, removal was delayed until the bone was mature and quiescent. Recent reports have suggested that this length of delay may not be necessary.

At surgery the abnormal bone should be completely excised. The result obtained in the OR is the best outcome the surgeon can expect.

Pain Control

The pain associated with burn injuries is a significant problem.[24] The acute injury is painful, the treatments are painful, and both continue for a lengthy recovery period. In partial-thickness burns the nerve endings are damaged but continue to generate pain impulses. The release of mediators (e.g., histamine, prostaglandins, bradykinin) within the injured tissue has been proposed as a mechanism. Full-thickness burns are anesthetizing but are surrounded by sensate tissue, which can hurt. After debridement these injuries add to the patient's pain.

The need for daily dressings and physiotherapy and the frequency of repetitive surgeries add to the problem by increasing the patient's anxiety. Therefore the surgeon treating these patients must recognize the need for analgesics and then administer them in effective doses.

Opioids are the most important modality for treating burn patients. Scheduled narcotic dosing is necessary early in these patients' hospital course. In seriously ill patients the drug can be administered intravenously. Intramuscular injections have variable absorption during periods of hemodynamic instability and may not be effective.

Patient-controlled analgesia (PCA) is an excellent method for treating more stable patients. *Morphine* (MS Contin) is another alternative. Additional dosing should be administered before wound care, painful therapy, or other procedures.

OUTCOMES

Successful recovery from a thermal burn injury requires a commitment by the patient and the healthcare system. Comprehensive rehabilitation programs attempt to correct the patient's biologic, psychologic, and social dysfunctions caused by injury. The goal is to enable the patient to regain maximum independence. Rehabilitation is receiving renewed interest as health care reforms mandate that outcomes, assessment, and documentation reflect quality of care.

SURVIVAL

Survival rates after thermal burns have improved dramatically during the last 25 years. In 1971, 50% of the patients admitted with a 40% or greater TBSA died; in 1990, 50% of the patients admitted with a 50% or greater TBSA routinely survived. Survival rates have increased by almost 1% every year because of improvements in resuscitation, the treatment of inhalation injuries, and other advances in critical care. The ability to treat the wound has also improved because of the following:

1. Earlier eschar excisions with aggressive wound treatment
2. Better ability to control infection, including improved antibiotics

3. Improved grafting techniques
4. Use of biologic dressings, which facilitates earlier coverage of large wounds

Even small burns can be lethal in elderly patients, and large burns are fatal. Patients over 50 years of age who sustain a 25% or greater TBSA have a 50% mortality rate. In contrast, patients under 5 years of age with a 50% or greater TBSA have only a 12.5% mortality rate. Elderly patients admitted with an inhalation injury in association with a 30% TBSA burn almost never survive. Aged patients sustain a higher incidence of inhalation injury as a result of slower reactions, reduced mobility, and sensory impairment that affects vision, smell, and hearing.

PSYCHOSOCIAL OUTCOMES

The family greatly influences the patient's recovery and must always be considered as part of the treatment plan. The quality of a patient's family support is the most important factor influencing a patient's postburn adjustment. Patients who receive more social support have a more positive body image, greater self-esteem, and less depression.

In addition to family support, other support systems can be extremely helpful. Burn survivor groups have formed in most metropolitan areas and greatly facilitate physical and emotional recovery.

Body Image

Many burn patients develop altered perceptions of and decreased satisfaction with their body image.[40] Fear of social rejection or ridicule because of the change in their appearance is a frequent response to visible scars. Concern about public acceptance makes burn patients more vulnerable to depression.

The treating surgeon must be aware of possible depression and other psychosocial issues so that proper counseling can be offered to the patient and family during hospitalization and after discharge. Interventions with the patient and family, both cognitive and emotional, can resolve these issues and facilitate appropriate burn adjustment.

Posttraumatic Stress Disorder

Posttraumatic stress disorder (PTSD) is a common result of a serious burn injury. This can be masked, however, by depression, self-image problems, self-blame behavior (typical in burn-injured adults), and burn-induced pain. The hospital staff should be aware of the following symptoms of PTSD:

Insomnia
Daytime flashbacks
Nightmares
Irritability
Heightened anger
Diminished concentration
Low self-esteem
Apprehension around source of injury
Emotional detachment from family and friends
Inability to relate to others
Less involvement with activities

PTSD is treated successfully with pharmacotherapy and psychotherapy.

Long-term Results

Empiric data regarding long-term sequelae of burn injury indicate that many burn survivors do achieve a quality of life that is satisfying to them. Judging from external criteria, many also appear to be well-adjusted individuals.

Good psychologic adjustment after burn injury is indicated by employment status. Burn patients who return to work have higher self-esteem, less behavioral avoidance, and greater attention to goals.

Return to Work

A 1986 study cited hand burns, grafting, and percentage of TBSA burned as the most significant variables influencing return to work after injury, whereas a 1989 study cited the degree of burn, hand burns, victim's age (those under 45 have a higher return-to-work rate), and type of work done before injury. The length of time a patient is off work, their burn size and their preinjury employment are the best predictors of eventual return to work.[43] Other variables increasing a patient's probability of being employed after burn injury include the following:

1. Being white
2. Not blaming oneself
3. Receiving workers' compensation (because of increased availability of acute care and rehabilitation services)
4. Being employed before injury

This 1995 study reported that a patient employed before the burn injury is 171 times more likely to return to work than one not employed before injury.[43]

On average, burn patients with a mean TBSA of 5% returned to work within 1 month, those with TBSA of 10% within 1 to 6 months, patients with TBSA of 20% within 6 months to 1 year, and those with TBSA of 35% more than 1 year later.[43] The patient's length of hospital stay (LOS) also predicted return to work. Patients with an LOS less than 10 days returned to work in 2 months and those with an LOS of 30 days returned in 6 to 12 months.

The successful return of patients to the workplace is influenced by health insurance companies' ability to fund work-hardening and other rehabilitation programs. Patients without these resources may have more difficulty regaining the physical strength their jobs require. Patients in professions that require dexterity or strength usually need more time than atypical office workers. Employers can facilitate a patient's return to work by initially offering light-duty work or a change to part-time status. Because scar and contracture may result in permanent changes in function, patients with hand burns often change jobs.[21,32]

Interdisciplinary involvement, such as counseling, group therapy, and both occupational and physical therapy, is important in maximizing a patient's clinical outcome. Interventions designed to aid adjustment, work-hardening and other rehabilitation services, and marital/family therapy are also important.

REFERENCES

1. Ahn ST, Monafo WW, Mustoe TA: Topical silicone gel: a new treatment for hypertrophic scars, *Surgery* 106:781-786, 1989.

2. Alexander JW, Meakins JL: A physiological basis for the development of opportunistic infections in man, *Ann Surg* 176:273-287, 1972.

3. Becker RA, Vaughan GM, Goodwin CW Jr, et al: Plasma norepinephrine, epinephrine, and thyroid hormone interactions in severely burned patients, *Arch Surg* 115:439-443, 1980.

4. Bjerknes R, Vindenes H, Laerum OD: Altered neutrophil functions in patients with large burns, *Blood Cells* 16:127-143, 1990.

5. Bucky LP, Vedder NB, Hong HZ, et al: Reduction of burn injury by inhibiting CD18-mediated leukocyte adherence in rabbits, *Plast Reconstr Surg* 93:1473-1480, 1994.

6. Chang P, Laubenthal KN, Lewis RW II, et al: Prospective, randomized study of the efficacy of pressure garment therapy in patients with burns, *J Burn Care Rehabil* 16:473-475, 1995.

7. Crum RL, Dominic W, Hansbrough JF, et al: Cardiovascular and neurohumoral responses following burn injury, *Arch Surg* 125:1065-1069, 1990.

8. Cuono CB, Langdon R., Birchall N, et al: Composite autologous-allogenic skin replacement: development and clinical application, *Plast Reconstr Surg* 80:626-637, 1987.

9. Curreri PW, Luterman A, Braun DW, et al: Burn injury: analysis of survival and hospitalization time for 937 patients, *Ann Surg* 192:472, 1972.

10. Deitch EA, Rutan R, Waymack JP: Trauma, shock and gut translocation, *New Horiz* 4:289-299, 1996.

11. DeMeules JE, Pigula FA, Mueller M, et al: Tumor necrosis factor and cardiac function, *J Trauma* 32:686-692, 1992.

12. Demling RH, LaLonde C: Early post-burn lipid peroxidation: effect of ibuprofen and allopurinol, *Surgery* 107:85-93, 1990.

13. Friedl HP, Till GO, Ward PA: Roles of histamine, complement and xanthine oxidase in thermal injury of skin, *Am J Pathol* 1:203-217, 1989.

14. Garner WL, Rittenberg T, Ehrlich HP, et al: Hypertrophic scar fibroblasts accelerate collagen gel contraction, *Wound Rep Reg* 3:185-191, 1995.

15. Garner WL, Rodriguez JL, Miller C, et al: Acute skin injury releases neutrophil chemoattractants, *Surgery* 116:42-48, 1994.

16. Ghahary A, Shen YJ, Scott PG, Tredget EE: Immunolocalization of TGF-beta 1 in human hypertrophic scar and normal dermal tissues, *Cytokine* 7:184-190, 1995.

17. Giroir BP, Horton JW, White DJ, et al: Inhibition of tumor necrosis factor prevents myocardial dysfunction during burn shock, *Am J Physiol* 267:H118-H124, 1994.

18. Gough DB, Jordan A, Collins K, et al: Suppressor T-cell levels are unreliable indicators of the impaired immune response following thermal injury, *J Trauma* 32:677-682, 1992.

19. Grayson LS, Hansbrough JF, Zapata-Sirvent RL, et al: Quantitation of cytokine levels in skin graft donor site wound fluid, *Burns* 19:401-405, 1993.

20. Greenhalgh DG, Barthel, PP, Warden GD: Comparison of back versus thigh donor sites in pediatric patients with burns, *J Burn Care Rehabil* 14:21-25, 1993.

21. Heinberg LJ, Fauerbach JA, Spence RJ, et al: Psychologic factors involved in the decision to undergo reconstructive surgery after burn injury, *J Burn Care Rehabil* 18:374-380, 1997.

22. Horgan AF, Mendez MV, O'Riordain DS, et al: Altered gene transcription after burn injury results in depressed T-lymphocyte activation, *Ann Surg* 220:342-352, 1994.

23. Huang PP, Stucky FS, Dimick AR, et al: Hypertonic sodium resuscitation is associated with renal failure and death, *Ann Surg* 221:543-547, 1995.

24. Kinsella J, Booth MG: Pain relief in burns: James Laing Memorial Essay 1990, *Burns* 17:391-395, 1991.

25. Knox J, Demling R, Wilmore D, et al: Increased survival after major thermal injury: the effect of growth hormone therapy in adults, *J Trauma* 39:526-532, 1995.

26. Ljunghusen O, Berg S, Hed J, et al: Transient endotoxemia during burn wound revision causes leukocyte B2 integrin up-regulation and cytokine release, *Inflammation* 19:457-468, 1995.

27. Mallonee S, Istre GR, Rosenberg M: Surveillance and prevention of residential-fire injuries, *N Engl J Med* 335:27-31, 1996.

28. Mileski W, Borgstrom D, Lightfoot E, et al: Inhibition of leukocyte-endothelial adherence following thermal injury, *J Surg Res* 52:334-339, 1992.

29. Nelson RD, Hasslen SR, Ahrenholz DH, et al: Mechanisms of loss of human neutrophil chemotaxis following thermal injury, *J Burn Care Rehabil* 8:496-502, 1987.

30. Nwariaku FE, Sikkes PJ, Lightfoot E Jr, et al: Inhibition of selectin- and integrin-mediated inflammatory response after burn injury, *J Surg Res* 63:355-358, 1996.

31. Pruitt BA, Tumbuschi WT, Mason AD, et al: Mortality in 1,100 consecutive burns treated at a burn unit, *Ann Surg* 159:396, 1964.

32. Riis A, Anderson M, Pederson MB, et al: Long-term psychosocial adjustment in patients with severe burn injury: a follow-up study, *Burns* 18:121-126, 1992.

33. Robson MC, Burns BF, Smith DJ: Acute management of the burned patient, *Plast Reconstr Surg* 89:1155-1168, 1992.

34. Rue LW, Cioffi WG, McManus WF, Pruitt BA Jr: Wound closure and outcome in extensively burned patients treated with cultured autologous keratinocytes, *J Trauma* 34:662-668, 1993.

35. Sharar S, Winn R, Murry C: A CD18 monoclonal antibody increases incidence and severity of subcutaneous abscess formation after high-dose *Staphylococcus aureus* injection in rabbits, *Surgery* 10:213, 1991.

36. Smith DL, Cairns BA, Ramadan F, et al: Effect of inhalation injury, burn size, and age on mortality: a study of 1447 consecutive burn patients, *J Trauma* 37:655-659, 1994.

37. Teodorczyk-Injeyan JA, Sparkes BG, Mills GB: Impairment of T cell activation in burn patients: a possible mechanism of thermal injury–induced immunosuppression, *Clin Exp Immunol* 65:570-581, 1986.

38. Till GO, Guilds LS, Mahrougi M, et al: Role of xanthine oxidase in thermal injury of skin, *Am J Pathol* 135:195-202, 1989.

39. Tredget EE, Shankowsky HA, Taerum TV, et al: The role of inhalation injury in burn trauma: a Canadian experience, *Ann Surg* 212:720-727, 1990.

40. Ward H, Moss R, Darko D, et al: Prevalence of post-burn depression following burn injury, *J Burn Care Rehabil* 8:294-298, 1987.

41. Warden GD, Mason AD, Pruitt BA Jr: Evaluation of leukocyte chemotaxis in vitro in thermally injured patients, *J Clin Invest* 54:1001-1004, 1974.

42. Wolfe JHN, Wu AVO, O'Connor NE, et al: Anergy, immunosuppressive serum, and impaired lymphocyte blastogenesis in burn patients, *Arch Surg* 117:1266-1271, 1982.

43. Wrigley M, Trotman K, Dimick A, et al: Factors relating to return to work after burn injury, *J Burn Care Rehabil* 16:445-450, 1995.

CHAPTER

Electrical Injuries

Robert L. McCauley
Juan P. Barret

INTRODUCTION

Electrical injuries occur worldwide and constitute 5% to 10% of all occupational fatalities.[26,46] Ore and Cassini[39] reported an annual estimated mortality rate of 2.7 per 100,000 workers for electrical injuries, with construction workers four times more likely to be electrocuted at work than those in all other industries combined.

Although the percentage of patients admitted to burn units with electrical injuries is low, the high morbidity rates can have a significant impact on these patients' functional rehabilitation. Hussmann et al[25] noted that although electrical injuries constituted only 6.5% of total admissions to their burn unit, 73% of these patients developed significant long-term neurologic deficits. The limb amputation rate remains at 45% to 71%. Not surprisingly, therefore, only 5.3% of patients with high-voltage (more than 1000 V) electrical injuries return to their jobs.[24,48]

INDICATIONS

ETIOLOGY

An analysis of human factors contributing to electrocutions has shown that carelessness is a major contributor.[37]

Death from electrocutions may result from *ventricular fibrillation,* as seen with a low-voltage (less than 1000 V) alternating current, or from *respiratory arrest* secondary to tetanic contractions of respiratory muscles, as seen with high-voltage injuries. High-voltage injuries may also cause death from damage to the brain's respiratory control center.

Muscular contractions that tend to tetany occur with currents of 8 to 12 milliamperes (mA) or greater. Such contractions may prevent victims from releasing their hold on electrical conductors, thereby prolonging the time of exposure and increasing tissue damage. Muscular injury, joint dislocations, and fractures can result from high-voltage electrical trauma. In addition, currents of 25 mA may produce ventricular fibrillation and cardiac arrest. Although cardiac muscle damage is not always evident, the electromechanical dissociation can be devastating. Without direct myocardial damage, life-threatening arrhythmias (dysrhythmias) may not recur. Currents of 100 mA can cross the brain and may produce loss of consciousness, whereas convulsions and suppression of the respiratory and circulatory centers occur with currents of 200 to 1200 mA.[32]

Grube et al[19] documented that 48% of patients who sustained electrical injuries greater than 380 V lost consciousness; 28% of these patients required cardiopulmonary resuscitation (CPR) before admission, and 9% died.

Low-voltage electrical injuries typically involve accidents with household appliances, whereas high-voltage injuries tend to be industrial accidents.[26,37,46]

PATHOPHYSIOLOGY

Our understanding of the pathophysiology of electrical injuries continues to evolve. Factors that determine the type and extent of electrical injuries include voltage, type of current, duration of contact, skin resistance, and current flow.

Since electrical injuries can produce a spectrum of soft tissue injuries, clinicians have divided these injuries into two categories based on the projected amounts of soft tissue, vascular, muscular and nerve damage: (1) high-voltage injuries (greater than 1000 V) and (2) low-voltage injuries (less than 1000 V). Low-voltage injuries occurring in the home are usually from 120-V, 60-cycle current and result in cutaneous burns with or without soft tissue injury.[19] High-voltage electrical injuries, however, are characterized by varying degrees of cutaneous thermal damage combined with extensive destruction of deeper layers.

Historically, the mechanism for damage was believed to be the conversion of electrical energy into heat, the *joule effect.* High-voltage electrical injuries may be characterized by extensive burns, soft tissue coagulation, rhabdomyolysis, and peripheral nerve injury.[50] The amount of heat produced is determined by *Ohm's law,* which states that the amount of current traveling through tissue is determined by the voltage divided by resistance ($V = 1/R$). Heat production, the joule effect (J), is expressed by the following equation:

$$J = I^2RT$$

where I is the amount of current, R is the resistance, and T is the time of contact. From this relationship, tissue resistance is directly proportional to the amount of heat imparted to a particular tissue type.

Skin has the highest resistance of all tissues. The amount of skin resistance is not consistent and varies as a function of thickness and moisture. The resistance of dry skin is 100 to 1000 times higher than that of moist skin. Wet skin allows a greater proportion of current to flow through the body, thereby increasing the risk of internal damage. Once skin resistance is breached, current flow increases.

Tissue temperature rises when heat production exceeds dissipation into the surrounding environment. It is believed that a rise in temperature to 50° C (122° F) will produce irreversible damage. Further temperature increases can result in coagulation necrosis and charring.

Ten Dais[50] emphasizes that the amount of heat generated by an equal current in an extremity is a function of resistance, as well as the magnitude and time of the current flow. Since resistance is inversely proportional to the extremity's diameter, in locations with small diameters (e.g., joints), heat production may be higher than in locations with large muscle bellies. Resistance of various tissue types occurs in the following order of decreasing resistance: bone, cartilage, tendon lung, skin, muscle, blood, and nerves. Consequently, heat production within an extremity is not uniform.

Sances et al[48] found that although nerves and arteries are excellent conductors, muscles carry the highest percentage of current because of the larger cross-sectional area. The bone, heated secondarily, has prolonged dissipation of heat, which explains why the highest temperatures occur in muscle areas adjacent to bone.

Although heat production plays a major role is the pathogenesis of electrical damage, Lee et al[30,31] clearly demonstrated another nonthermal component to this problem. Their experimental data suggest that muscle and nerve cell membrane rupture by *electroporation* may play a significant role, even in the absence of significant heat production.[7] This is clinically evident with elevated levels of arachidonic acid and large releases of myoglobin, which indicate intracellular damage, as seen in patients with electrical trauma.

Although heat production and cell membrane rupture may explain the spectrum of clinical manifestations of electrical trauma, management of its consequences continues to be less than optimal.

The most common types of electrical burns may be classified into two types: arc injuries and thermoelectrical burns. *Arc injuries* can occur in electrical accidents as well as in lightning accidents. Typically, as one approaches an electrical conductor, if the distance is short enough, the air becomes ionized and breaks down. Consequently, current jumps in an arclike manner. The arc is composed of ionized air particles. The particles between the current and the contact consumes much of the electrical energy, resulting in a rapid voltage drop. If the victim forms part of the arcing process, the current is transformed into heat, thereby producing a thermal injury.[52]

Pure *electrothermal burns* are produced from direct contact with an electrical conductor. The flow of current through the skin and subsequent heating can cause significant tissue damage. In high-voltage injuries the inability to release the conductor produces prolonged current flow with significant heating. A combination of the joule effect and electroporation produces soft tissue, vascular, muscular, and nerve damage.

ASSESSMENT AND INITIAL THERAPY

Although the detailed resuscitation of patients with high-voltage electrical trauma is beyond the scope of this chapter, evaluation of the airway, breathing, and circulation are crucial in the initial assessment of all patients. Associated injuries, particularly in high-voltage electrical trauma, require documentation. Significant head injuries, fractures, dislocations, spinal cord injuries, and intraabdominal injuries have been reported with high-voltage electrical trauma.[47]

Resuscitation and initial assessment of all injuries is crucial for survival and rehabilitation of these patients. Muscle damage may be severe and worsened by the edema from the inflammatory mediators released by the damaged tissues. If a compartment syndrome develops within a muscle group, fasciotomies are necessary to prevent necrosis.

Myoglobin is released from the damaged muscles and normally is cleared by the kidneys. When massive amounts of myoglobin are released, however, *acute renal failure* may result from the deposition of myoglobin in the renal tubules. Patients with electrical injury who develop acute renal failure may have a mortality rate are as high as 50%.[20] Consequently, alkalinization of the urine along with a high urine output is crucial to prevent renal failure.

Controversy surrounds whether or not the tissue damage in electrical injuries is progressive. Initial studies by Robson et al[45] suggested that progressive tissue necrosis does occur, primarily through the increased production of arachidonic acid and metabolites. More specifically, elevated levels of the potent vasoconstrictor *thromboxane,* which causes thrombosis in the microvasculature, are believed to enhance tissue necrosis. This group also suggested that prostaglandin inhibitors may be useful in the prevention of late tissue injury.

In a primate model using angiographic studies, microscopy, and nerve conduction studies, however, Zelt et al[55] analyzed the pathophysiology of electrical trauma and concluded that progressive tissue necrosis does *not* occur in electrical trauma.

The initial damage is less extensive than the damage documented 48 to 72 hours later. Consequently, "second-look" procedures have become routine to determine the extent of electrical injury. Although electroporation of muscular, neural, and endothelial cells may be responsible for the extension of tissue necrosis, the inability to assess accurately the extent of initial tissue damage may be the reason for "progressive tissue necrosis."

Although various tests have been used to examine muscle viability, their effect on management of these patients has been limited. Quinby et al[43] suggested using frozen and permanent sections for histologic examination to determine muscle viability. Similarly, xenon-131 and technetium-99m, stannous pyrophosphate scintigraphy has been useful in the evaluation of skeletal muscle ischemia.[11,24] Unfortunately, because of their expense, time-consuming nature, and increased sensitivity in the evaluation of ischemic muscle, these tests have not gained widespread use in the management of these patients.

OPERATIONS

The spectrum of anatomic manifestations from electrical trauma is quite varied. The management of these acute wounds has progressed over time, with the emphasis changing from a conservative approach to wound closure, then to a more aggressive doctrine of improving the functional and aesthetic outcome of these patients.

HEAD INJURIES

Scalp and Skull

Injuries to the head and face regions are frequently an entry or contact point in high-voltage electrical injuries. The damage may range from loss of pericranium to loss of the inner table with underlying brain injury.[12]

Conservative approaches to this problem are of historic interest only. More dated approaches to calvarial injuries promoted the use of dressing changes over exposed bone. The skull could be removed later as a sequestrum before skin grafting.[11] Unfortunately, the risk of infectious complications, such as osteomyelitis, meningitis, and epidural abscesses, precludes the use of this treatment modality.

More aggressive approaches have been advocated, such as excision of devitalized outer-table bone before coverage of the wound with skin grafts or flaps. In most clinical situations, full-thickness calvarial injuries may not appear different than injuries limited to the outer table. Such an approach is risky, however, and may leave the brain devoid of bony protection.

In such patients, I prefer early coverage of exposed calvarial bone with either a rotation or a transposition scalp flap without debridement. If local tissue is not available, vascularized coverage of the exposed skull may be accomplished using a free tissue transfer. With the underlying devitalized bone serving as a bone graft, early definitive coverage can be obtained with minimal complications (Figure 25-1).[22,33] Continued follow-up for these patients is crucial to optimize long-term management.

If skin grafts are used to cover the donor site for a scalp flap, reconstruction of the alopecia segment may require serial excision or soft tissue expansion. The use of tissue expanders in the reconstruction of scalp defects secondary to burn injuries has become a safe and reliable method for the reconstruction of extensive areas of alopecia.[34,36]

Subsequent evaluation of devitalized bone beneath the scalp flap is crucial. If the injury is a full-thickness calvarial injury, bony resorption may occur without adequate regeneration of new bone beneath the scalp flap (Figure 25-2). Calvarial reconstruction then becomes an important issue to provide protection for the brain. The methods for reconstruction depend on the defect's size, the available donor tissue, and the patient's age. Reconstruction of large cranial defects can be challenging. Although the sources of autologous grafts are numerous, har-

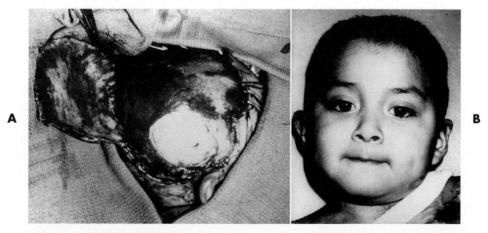

Figure 25-1. **A,** Four-year-old girl sustained 45% total body surface area (TBSA) burn after wandering into transformer box at housing complex. She had full-thickness calvarial injury and open linear skull fracture with epidural air and cerebrospinal fluid leak in right parietooccipital area. Defect measured 6 × 8 cm. Within 24 hours after transfer to hospital, large transposition scalp flap was used to provide watertight seal, with split-thickness skin graft covering pericranium from donor flap site. **B,** One month after healing, with no signs of infectious complication. Scalp flap remained 100% viable.

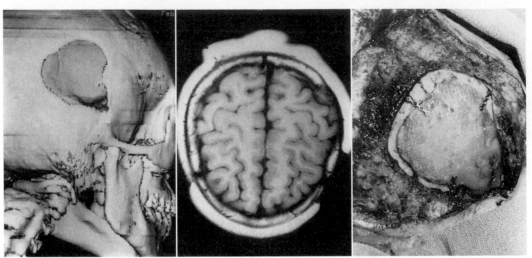

Figure 25-2. A, Computed tomography (CT) scan of 10-year-old female who sustained electrical trauma skull with resulting linear skull fracture. Area was covered with vascularized scalp flap. Six years later, incomplete bone regeneration was noted over skull. **B,** CT scan shows failure of complete bone regeneration. **C,** Closure of full-thickness defect with polymethylmethacrylate and coverage with scalp flap.

vesting of cranial bone grafts has proved to be a reliable sources of cortical bone for calvarial reconstruction.[4,5,41,56]

Cranial bone grafts may be frozen autologous grafts or fresh calvarial autografts. Although frozen autologous cranial bone can be of benefit, many surgeons believe that these grafts are complicated by increased resorption rates and infection. Clearly, fresh autologous cranial bone is superior. Both in situ and ex vivo methods are available for harvesting calvarial bone grafts to cover large defects.

IN SITU GRAFTS. Split calvarial bone grafts taken in situ have the advantage of avoiding a craniotomy. The parietal region is the site of choice because of bone thickness.[41] Grafts are not harvested any closer than 2 cm from the sagittal suture in an attempt to avoid injury to the sagittal sinus. The technique, although well described, is designed for small defects with a width of 3 cm or less.[56] Complications include graft irregularities, thin bone, dural exposure, and dural tears.

EX VIVO GRAFTS. Ex vivo split calvarial bone grafts require a full-thickness craniotomy and subsequent separation of the inner and outer tables. The advantages of this procedure are as follows[5]:

1. Large amounts of bone may be harvested.
2. Thin skulls become reliable donor sites.
3. Any part of the skull may be chosen as a donor site.
4. The graft is technically easier to split.

The disadvantages of this technique include longer operat-

ing room time, risk of dural tears, and conversion of one into two free grafts. Despite these potential problems, many authors have come to rely on the low complication rate and large amounts of bone available for harvesting using the ex vivo technique.

Full-thickness craniotomy has been advocated as a safe method for harvesting cranial bone, particularly in children as young as 1 year of age.[4]

POLYMETHYLACRYLATE. Acrylic resins became available in 1937 and were first used medically in 1940.[2] Calvarial reconstruction using polymethylmethacrylate (PMMA) is a useful alternative to split calvarial bone grafts in adolescent and adult patients with vascularized coverage over a full-thickness calvarial defect. Although potential complications of this type of cranioplasty include infection, plate failure, and poor aesthetic results, many surgeons continue to use this technique. With the use of preoperative and postoperative antibiotics and antibiotic-impregnated PMMA, the infection rate of 5% for PMMA cranioplasty is equivalent to that of fresh autologous cranial bone grafts[5] (Figure 25-2, *C*).

Lip and Oral Commissure

Although burn-related injury is the leading cause of accidental death in the home for children under 14 years of age, low-voltage electrical burns represent less than 4% of all burn injuries in children.[27] Gifford et al[17] reported that most low-voltage electrical injuries in children are around the mouth. These injuries occur most often from biting on an electrical

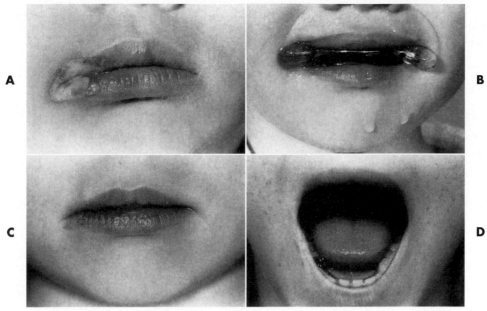

Figure 25-3. **A,** Two-year-old child with burn of right commissure. **B,** Application of custom-made splint bonded to first maxillary primary molars within 2½ weeks after injury. Child wore splint for 4 months. **C** and **D,** Functional and aesthetic outcome 4 years later.

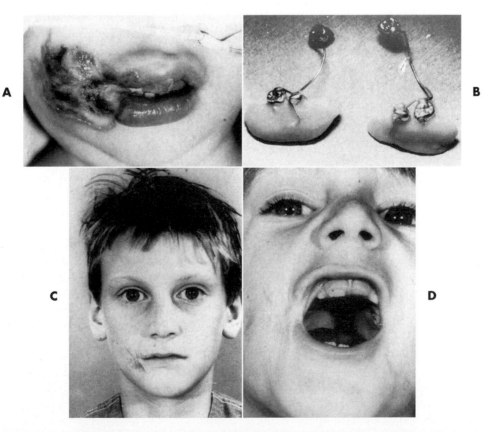

Figure 25-4. **A,** Four-year-old child with extensive electrical burn involving right upper lip, lower lip, and commissure with extension into cheek. **B,** Appearance of earlier splints attached to maxillary teeth. **C** and **D,** Aesthetic and functional outcome 6 years later.

cord or sucking on a wall socket. The most frequently affected site is the upper and lower lip with the connecting commissure, followed by the tongue and the alveolus. The wounds can be extensive, with thermal injury to the surrounding cheek regions.

Initial management of these injuries has progressed from surgical treatment in the early 1970s to a more conservative nonsurgical approach to prevent scar contractures, which can lead to microstomia or commissural asymmetry. Custom-made splints are important in the prevention of such contractures (Figure 25-3). Compliance can be a problem, however, and may affect the final outcome. The use of intraoral splints bonded to the maxillary primary molars (and the central incisors if possible) is a useful method to ensure compliance. Such splints do not inhibit speech or eating but remain in place for the time needed for wound maturation. Once the healing process is complete, the splints are removed from the mouth as an outpatient procedure (Figure 25-4).

The aesthetic outcome in patients using this conservative approach is generally good, even in the most severe cases. If microstomia or commissural asymmetry develops, however, surgical correction is indicated.

Reconstruction of a contracted commissure requires precise measurements and positioning. The development of skin and mucosal flaps allows identification of the scarred orbicularis oris muscle and subsequent repositioning of the muscle laterally, with or without reconstruction of the modiolus and coverage with intraoral mucosal flaps. The use of tongue flaps has fallen into disfavor because the tongue's anterior surface bears little resemblance to the lip. Donelan[15] has achieved excellent results, however, using a ventral tongue flap for commissure reconstruction.

EXTREMITY INJURIES

The extremities frequently exhibit the disastrous effects of electrical trauma in high-voltage injuries. Although variable, amputation rates generally remain high regardless of early attempts at debridement and decompression.[25,47] Although Mann et al[35] documented a decrease in amputation rate from 45% to 10% with immediate selective decompression of the upper extremity in high-voltage electrical injuries, most authors report significantly higher amputation rates after decompression.

Most surgeons approach high-voltage electrical injuries to the extremities with decompression, as clinically indicated, and multiple procedures to remove devitalized tissue, including nerves, tendons, muscles, and arteries. Successful attempts at debridement with preservation of blood flow are frequently characterized by extensive muscle loss and peripheral nerve damage. In children, even low-voltage electrical injuries to the hand can produce significant damage requiring early debridement and wound coverage to maximize functional outcome.

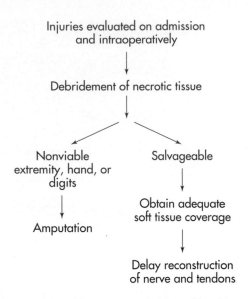

Figure 25-5. Management of electrical hand burns.

High-voltage electrical injuries involve the hand in most cases. The initial clinical presentation largely determines the ultimate outcome in the extremity.[1,35] Contracted, charred extremities without distal pulses usually result in amputation despite early, aggressive management. Viable extremities that maintain blood flow may require the release of the carpal tunnel, as well as additional surgical interventions for muscle debridement to maximize functional outcome.

Achauer et al[1] documented a 40% amputation rate in the upper extremity for patients with high-voltage injuries. Patients undergoing staged reconstruction, however, had greatly improved hand function.

Patients may have an insensate, nonfunctional upper extremity. A thorough examination of motor function with neurosensory mapping is crucial to reconstruction in such patients. Although documentation of peripheral neuropathies of the upper extremity after electrical trauma is incomplete, studies show that the median nerve and then the ulnar nerve are injured most often.[18]

I follow the general principles outlined by Achauer for staged reconstruction of the upper extremity (Figure 25-5). Good soft tissue coverage is also important if nerve grafts will be used to restore sensation. The success of nerve grafts in these patients depends on the quality of the graft bed and the overlying soft tissue coverage. Arteriography is necessary as a preliminary study if free tissue transfer is contemplated to provide better coverage.[44] If arteriography shows a single vessel supplying the hand, local flaps for coverage may be the safest approach, since the remaining vessel perfusing the hand is not only damaged but also extremely sensitive to vasospasm (Figure 25-6). In addition to local flaps, many free tissue transfers have been described to achieve soft tissue coverage for both upper and lower extremity injuries.

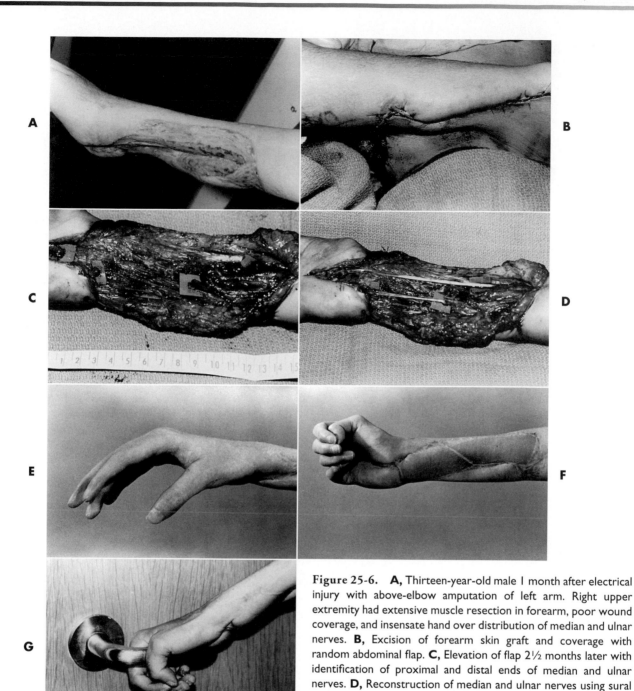

Figure 25-6. **A,** Thirteen-year-old male 1 month after electrical injury with above-elbow amputation of left arm. Right upper extremity had extensive muscle resection in forearm, poor wound coverage, and insensate hand over distribution of median and ulnar nerves. **B,** Excision of forearm skin graft and coverage with random abdominal flap. **C,** Elevation of flap 2½ months later with identification of proximal and distal ends of median and ulnar nerves. **D,** Reconstruction of median and ulnar nerves using sural nerve grafts. **E to G,** Functional outcome at 1 year.

Continued

Adequate soft tissue coverage is the first step in the reconstruction of the extremity damaged by high-voltage electricity. Later, flap elevation and identification of the proximal and distal ends of the upper extremity nerves can be done. Because the normal anatomy is completely destroyed in the area of electrical trauma, surgical knowledge of the course of the median and ulnar nerves proximal and distal to the area of injury is crucial in identification of the nerve ends. Sural nerve grafts harvested from one or both lower extremities can reestablish neuronal continuity using an epineural repair, with good results.

In a series of eight patients, McCauley et al[44] performed median and ulnar nerve grafts in seven extremities after high-voltage electrical injury. Soft tissue coverage was required in five extremities before nerve grafting. All patients were delayed referrals, and time from injury to reconstruction was 14 months. Two patients underwent reconstruction of the median nerve alone, and five had reconstruction of both the median and the ulnar nerves. The mean length of the sural nerve grafts were 9 to 10 cm. All patients developed protective sensation within a few months.

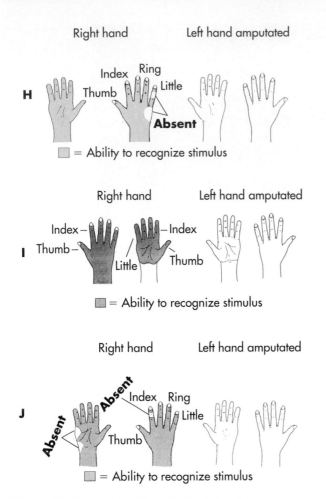

Figure 25-6, cont'd. H to J, Analysis of touch responses at 2 years: **H,** temperature; **I,** light touch; **J,** sharp and dull sensations.

OUTCOMES

Electrical burns are unique; the low incidence of hospital admission is offset by the high short-term and long-term morbidity rates. Interestingly, a large percentage of patients with low-voltage electrical burns do not require hospital admission, and up to 40% of these burns may represent oral injuries.[57] Amputation rates are low when extremities are involved and appear to be limited to digits in children.

High-voltage electrical injuries are devastating, however, and full-thickness burns are complicated by deeper destruction of tissues that involves muscle and neurovascular structures. Most clinical series document high amputation rates even with early escharotomy and fasciotomy. The neurologic sequelae of these injuries remain significant, with less than 6% of adult patients returning to their jobs. Despite increased knowledge about the pathophysiology of these lesions, morbidity rates for those patients remain excessively high.

HEAD INJURIES

Scalp and Skull

When the head is the site of contact in high-voltage electrical injuries, large areas of scalp necrosis may occur. The presence of denuded calvarium with damage to the outer table presents a management challenge to reconstructive surgeons.

Historically, wound closure was only attempted after sequestration was complete.[3,53] Reports indicate that the sequestration process may be accelerated with the drilling of burr holes through the calvarium.[13,28]

Current management of these defects has evolved to the point where removal of devitalized bone or development of granulation tissue is not necessary to achieve early wound closure. At present, early closure of full-thickness calvarial injuries, even with cerebrospinal fluid leaks, can be safely obtained without excision of devitalized skull using local scalp flaps or free tissue transfers. Wang et al[51] evaluated 24 patients using this approach with uniform success.

Several authors have addressed the fate of devitalized bone beneath a vascularized scalp flap. Although it is believed that the underlying necrotic bone regenerates under the protection of a scalp flap, this is not uniformly seen. Most published reports fail to report adequate follow-up to assess the completeness of subsequent calvarial regeneration after such an injury.[42,49,53,54]

Neck

Little data exist on reconstruction of the neck after high-voltage electrical trauma. Because of the vital structures within the neck, however, early debridement is advocated to assess the extent of damage.

Palao et al[40] reported the use of deltoid-pectoral flaps in four patients with electrical trauma to the neck to achieve early wound closure. Two of the patients also had exposed mandibles. Use of these flaps for wound closure was uniformly successful.

The use of free tissue transfers may be required if defects in the head and neck region occur in a pattern that precludes the use of local flaps for wound closure.[21]

Lips and Oral Commissure

Electrical burns to the mouth are relatively common in young children.[6,8,14,38] These injuries classically result from biting on the electrical cords of house appliances. Males usually outnumber females by a 2:1 ratio.

Components of both an arc burn and a contact burn may be present. *Arc burns* result from electrolyte-containing saliva bridging the polarity gap of the wires. An arc or flash develops and can produce temperatures as high as 3000° C. *Contact burns* occur as the current travels across a pathway of least resistance from the mouth to the ground.[8] Significant hemorrhage from the labial artery may occur after eschar separation; it is easily controlled with pressure.

Controversy surrounds the optimal method for management of these patients. Protocols have ranged from the conservative approach of no surgery and no splints to the aggressive approach of early commissuroplasty. A third option is nonsurgical management with splints. The goal of each treatment regimen is to maintain or restore function and to minimize scarring in the shortest possible time.

NO SURGERY OR SPLINTS. Canady et al[8] retrospectively evaluated 24 patients with oral commissure burns who were treated conservatively without splinting or early surgery at the University of Iowa. Early surgical intervention was not indicated because the extent of soft tissue injury could not be precisely defined. Patients were allowed to heal their wounds without splinting of the commissure.

To soften the resulting scars, massage, triamcinolone (Kenalog) cream, and vitamin E were used. Prolonged use of splints was thought to cause excessive scarring, which could complicate later reconstruction. Although the timing and type of reconstructive procedure varied, the authors concluded that conservative surgical management after scar maturation resulted in successful functional and aesthetic outcomes.[8]

Barone et al[6] retrospectively evaluated 29 patients with perioral electrical burns. Patients were divided into three groups based on treatment modalities and were evaluated for aesthetic and functional outcome. The parameters judged were lip length, scar, vermilion quality, and lip roll. Group 1 patients were managed without surgery and without splints. Group 2 patients were treated with extraoral splints only. Group 3 patients underwent commissuroplasty. Although the timing of commissuroplasty was not clearly defined, these authors believed that splinting alone provided the best overall results.

Neale et al[38] reviewed 116 children with perioral electrical burns and also advocated the use of splints until scar maturation occurred. Once wounds were completely healed, commissuroplasty was considered.

EARLY COMMISSUROPLASTY. Earlier studies by de La Plaza et al[14] of 58 children who sustained electrical burns to the mouth revealed better overall results with aggressive early surgical management. They concluded that surgery allows early resolution of the problem by excision of devitalized tissue, with shorter hospital stays and fewer operations to achieve a satisfactory final result.[1] Unfortunately, such results have not been reproduced by other authors.[6,8,38]

NONSURGICAL MANAGEMENT WITH SPLINTS. The use of dynamic splinting to prevent microstomia has gained in popularity.[29] Most authors believe that better functional restoration and overall aesthetic results are obtained through nonsurgical management of these patients using splints. The primary drawback of this type of treatment is noncompliance.

The use of custom-fitted intraoral splints bonded to the maxillary primary molars (and if possible, central incisors) serves as an effective method that not only splints the wound until maturation occurs but also eliminates compliance issues. Within 2 weeks after injury, dental impressions are made in the operating room, and in a few days the appliance is fixed to the maxillary teeth. This method allows the patient to eat and talk during the healing process.

My results to date with intraoral splints have been uniformly satisfactory.

DELAYED RECONSTRUCTION OF COMMISSURE. Once contraction of the commissure occurs, surgical intervention is the only alternative to correct microstomia or commissural asymmetry. Careful preoperative planning for repositioning of the commissure is crucial to achieve a satisfactory outcome.

Several investigators propose excision of the burn scar with lateral advancement of the orbicularis oris muscle, readvancement of the modiolus labii, and reestablishment of vermilion continuity.[42] Various types of mucosal flaps have been described to reestablish a normal appearance, but to date, no particular technique has been associated with uniform success.

Although reconstruction of all layers of the commissure, including vermilion continuity, is crucial to optimize outcome, large contracted defects with extension into the cheek may not always produce satisfactory outcomes because of the extent of scarring. These patients may also have significant intraoral scarring, which may prevent normal intraoral excursion.

The use of tongue flaps for intraoral contractures represents an alternative method for coverage of intraoral contractures. Donelan[15] has used the ventral tongue flap for extraoral reconstruction of the oral commissure in children with electrical burns with good results.

Individual methods of reconstruction are based on sound principles. Results of commissure reconstruction, however, are not uniformly satisfactory.

EXTREMITY INJURIES

Although the amputation rate in patients with high-voltage electrical injuries is reported as 45% to 73%, it can be as high to 90% when the hand and forearm are considered individually. Total return of function in upper extremities is only about 6%, with partial return up to 53%. No functional return is documented at 28%.[16]

Providing vascularized tissue to the injured area has been advocated as a method to improve outcome in electrical injuries to the upper extremity. Cho et al[10] used a free innervated dorsalis pedis tendocutaneous flap in composite hand reconstruction. Long-term follow-up showed that two-point discrimination of the transferred flaps averaged 25 mm. Recovery rates for range of motion of the metacarpophalangeal joints ranged from 83% to 99%.

Excellent sensory recovery has also been achieved with vascularized ipsilateral ulnar nerve transfers with the flexor carpi ulnaris muscle as a carrier. In patients with extensive loss of skin and subcutaneous tissues, large free flaps, such as the combined scapular/parascapular flap, have provided successful tendon gliding under the flap and excellent nerve recovery in all patients treated. Chick et al[9] performed by immediate coverage of high-voltage electrical injuries, with a 62.5% recovery of 10 mm of two-point discrimination in all digital nerves involved. Persistent peripheral nerve pathologies, however, occur in 48% of all patients.[23]

Data relative to the outcome of the nonamputated lower extremity affected by electrical trauma is scarce. Various types of flap coverage for the foot and lower leg areas have been advocated. The radial artery forearm flap and the scapular flap are popular for forefoot reconstruction. Muscle flaps (e.g., gracilis, rectus abdominis) have been used for heel defects. Earlier studies documented the use of the cross-leg flap in lower extremity reconstruction.

The outcome for lower extremities with high-voltage injuries remains poor; 40% require amputations. More than 60% of affected lower limbs develop persistent dysesthesias, insensate parts, or motor palsies.

REFERENCES

1. Achauer B, Applebaum R, Vanderkam VM: Electrical burn injury to the upper extremity, *Br J Plast Surg* 47:331-340, 1994.

2. Albertstone CD, Benzel CC: Polymethylmethacrylate cranioplasty. In Rengachary SS, Benzel EC, editors: *Calvarial and dural reconstruction,* Park Ridge, Ill, 1998, American Association of Neurological Surgeons.

3. Bagozzi IC: Reparative procedures in large losses of scalp and bone of the skull caused by severe electrical lesions, *Br J Plast Surg* 8:49-54, 1955.

4. Barone CM, Jimenez DF: Split calvarial grafts in young children, *J Craniofac Surg* 8:43-47, 1997.

5. Barone CM, Jimenez DF, Boschert MT: Cranioplasty using autologous bone. In Rengachary SS, Benzel EC, editors: *Calvarial and dural reconstruction,* Park Ridge, Ill, 1998, American Association of Neurological Surgeons.

6. Barone CM, Hulnick SJ, de Linde LG, et al: Evaluation of treatment modalities in perioral electrical burns, *J Burn Care* 15:335-340, 1994.

7. Block TA, Aarsvold, Matthews KL, et al: Nonthermal-mediated muscle injury and necrosis in electrical trauma, *J Burn Care Rehabil* 16:581-588, 1995.

8. Canady TW, Thompson SA, Bardach J: Oral commissure burns in children, *Plast Reconstr Surg* 97:738-744, 1996.

9. Chick LR, Lister GD, Sowder L: Early free-flap coverage of electrical and thermal burns, *Plast Reconstr Surg* 89:1013-1019, 1992.

10. Cho BC, Lee JH, Weinzweig N, Baik BS: Use of the free innervated dorsalis pedis tendocutaneous flap in composite hand reconstruction, *Ann Plast Surg* 40:268-276, 1998.

11. Clayton JM, Hayes PC, Hammel J, et al: Xenon-133 determination of muscle blood flow in electrical injury, *J Trauma* 17:283-297, 1977.

12. Curtin JW, Lathans WD, Greely PN, et al: Catastrophic loss of scalp and contiguous structures, *Plast Reconstr Surg* 32:1-11, 1963.

13. Dale RH: Electrical accidents, *Br J Plast Surg* 7:44-66, 1954.

14. De La Plaza R, Quetglas A, Rodriguez E: Treatment of electrical burns of the mouth. In *Burns, including thermal injury,* 10:49-60, 1983.

15. Donelan MB: Reconstruction of electrical burns of the oral commissure with a ventral tongue flap, *Plast Reconstr Surg* 95:1155-1164, 1995.

16. Engrav LH, Gottlieb JR, Walkinshaw MD, et al: Outcome and treatment of electrical injury with immediate median and ulnar nerve palsy at the wrist: a retrospective review and a survey of members of the American Burn Association, *Ann Plast Surg* 25:166-168, 1990.

17. Gifford GH, Marty AT, Collum MA: The management of electrical mouth burns in children, *Pediatrics* 47:113-119, 1971.

18. Grube BJ, Heimbach DM: Acute and delayed neurological sequelae of electrical injury. In Lee RC, Cravalho EG, Burke JF, editors: *Electrical trauma: pathophysiology, and clinical management,* New York, 1992, Cambridge University Press.

19. Grube BJ, Heimbach DM, Engrav LD, et al: Neurologic consequences of electrical burns, *J Trauma* 30:254-258, 1990.

20. Gupta KL, Kunar R, Sekha MS, et al: Myoglobin acute renal failure following electrical injury, *Ren Fail* 13:23-25, 1991.

21. Hardesty RA, Jones NF, Swartz WM, et al: Microsurgery for macro defects, *Am J Surg* 154:399-405, 1987.

22. Hartford CE: Presentation of devitalized calvarium following high voltage electrical injury: case reports, *J Trauma* 29:391-394, 1989.

23. Huberal MA, Gurer S, Akman N, Basgoze O: Persistent peripheral nerve pathologies in patients with electric burns, *J Burn Care Rehabil* 17:147-149, 1996.

24. Hunt JL, Lewis S, Parkey R, et al: The use of technetium-99m stannous pyrophosphate scintigraphy to identify muscle damage in acute electric burns, *J Trauma* 19:409-413, 1979.

25. Hussmann J, Kucan JO, Russel JC, et al: Electrical injuries: morbidity, outcome and treatment rationale, *Burns* 21:530-535, 1995.

26. Janicak CA: Occupational fatalities caused by contact with overhead power lines in the construction industry, *J Occup Environ Med* 34:328-332, 1997.

27. Keusch CF, Gifford GH, Eriksson E: Pediatric electrical burns. In Res RC, Cravalho EG, Burke JF, editors: *Electrical trauma: pathophysiology, manifestations and clinical management,* New York, 1992, Cambridge University Press.

28. Kraugh LV, Erich JB: Treatment of electrical injuries, *Am J Surg* 101:419, 1961.

29. Leake, JE, Curtin JW: Electrical burns of the mouth in children, *Clin Plast Surg* 11:669-683, 1994.

30. Lee RC, Kolodney MS: Electrical injury mechanisms: dynamics of the thermal response, *Plast Reconstr Surg* 80:663-671, 1987.

31. Lee RC, Gzylor DC, Brett D, Israel DA: Role of cell membrane rupture in the pathogenesis of electrical trauma, *J Surg Res* 44:709-719, 1988.

32. Less V, Frame JD: Electrical burns. In JD Settler, editor: *Principles and practice of burn management,* New York, 1996, Churchill Livingstone.

33. Luce EA, Hoopes JE: Electrical burn to the scalp and skull: case report, *Plast Reconstr Surg* 54:359-363, 1974.

34. Manders EK, Schenden, Furrer, JA et al: Soft tissue expansion: concepts and complications, *Plast Reconstr Surg* 74:493-497, 1948.

35. Mann R, Gbran N, Engrav L, Heimbach D: Is immediate decompression of high voltage electrical injuries to the upper extremity always necessary? *J Trauma* 40:584-589, 1996.

36. McCauley RL, Oliphant JR, Robson MC: Tissue expansion in the correction of burn alopecia: classification and methods of correction, *Ann Plast Surg* 25:103-115, 1990.

37. Mellen PF, Weedn VW, Kao G: Electrocution: a review of 155 cases with emphasis on human factors, *J Forensic Sci* 37:1016-1022, 1992.

38. Neale HW, Billmire DA, Gregory RO: Management of perioral burn scarring in the child and adolescent, *Ann Plast Surg* 15:212-217, 1985.

39. Ore T, Cassini V: Electrical fatalities among U.S. construction workers, *J Occup Environ Med* 38:587-592, 1996.

40. Palao RG, Gomez PG, Casaudoume CP, et al: Use of flaps in the treatment of burns in the acute phase, *Int Soc Burn Inj* 10:17, 1998.

41. Pensler J, McCarthy JG: The calvarial donor site: an anatomic study in cadavers, *Plast Reconstr Surg* 75:648-651, 1995.

42. Pensler JM, Rosenthal A: Reconstruction of the oral commissure after electrical burn, *J Burn Care Rehabil* 11:50-53, 1990.

43. Quinby WC Jr, Bunke JF, Trelstad RL, et al: The use of microscopy as a guide to primary excision of high tension electrical burns, *J Trauma* 18:423-429, 1978.

44. Roberts L, Meyers R, Pierre E, McCauley RL: Sensory analysis of nerve grafting in children with electrical burns of the upper extremity, *Proc Am Burn Assoc* 28:13, 1996.

45. Robson MC, Murphy RC, Heggers JP: A new explanation for the progressive tissue loss in electrical injuries, *Plast Reconstr Surg* 73:431-437, 1984.

46. Rossignol M, Pinesault M: Classification of fatal occupational electrocutions, *Can J Public Health* 85:322-325, 1994.

47. Rouse RG, Dimick AR: Treatment of electrical injury compared to burn injury, *J Trauma* 18:43-47, 1978.

48. Sances A, Mykel Bust JB, et al: Experimental electrical injury studies, *J Trauma* 21:589, 1981.

49. Shen Z: Reconstruction of refractory defect of scalp and skull using microsurgical free flap transfer microsurgery, 15:633-638, 1994.

50. Ten Dais HJ: Acute electrical burns, *Semin Neurol* 15:381-386, 1995.

51. Wang KW, Miller G, Zapata-Sirvent RL, et al: Regeneration of full-layer necrosed skull after high tension electrical injury. In *Burns, including thermal injuries* 12(3):206-211, 1986.

52. Worthen EF: Surgical management of electrical burns of the scalp and skull: past and present, *Clin Plast Surg* 9:161-165, 1982.

53. Worthen EF: Regeneration of the skull following a deep electrical burn, *Plast Reconstr Surg* 48:1-13, 1971.

54. Wright HR, Drake DB, Gear AJL, et al: Industrial high-voltage electrical burn of the skull, a preventable injury, *J Emerg Med* 3:345-349, 1996.

55. Zelt RG, Daniel RK, Ballard PA, et al: High voltage electrical injury: chronic wound evolution, *Plast Reconstr Surg* 82:1027-1039, 1988.

56. Zins JE, Weinzweig N, Hahn J: A simple fail-safe method for the harvesting of cranial bone, *Plast Reconstr Surg* 96:1447, 1995.

57. Zubair M, Besner GE: Pediatric electrical burns: management strategies, *Burns* 23:413-420, 1997.

CHAPTER

Chemical Burns

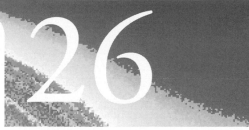

Philip Edelman

Chemical burns constitute a diverse group of injuries with varying pathology. Thus the definition of a chemical burn is elusive. Acute inflammation of the skin from allergic phenomena or contact dermatitis may be difficult to distinguish from a chemical burn, but each may occur acutely after chemical exposure.[25] For a broad and inclusive definition, chemical burns are inflammatory or corrosive reactions of the integument caused by some chemical property of the agent other than its inherent thermal energy. Extremes of pH, oxidative potentials, cellular poisoning, and other factors may cause the "burn."

Jelenko[24] described the nature of chemical burns, their severity, and their prognosis in 1974; many of his observations remain valid today. These agents do not cause a thermal injury; rather, they act in various ways to coagulate, saponify, poison, and oxidize proteins and related tissues. Lewis[29] noted that chemical burns were underestimated more frequently than thermal injuries and suggested that greater morbidity was associated with chemical injuries.

Some chemicals may generate significant heat on contact with the water in the skin. The heat of hydration is substantial for materials such as concentrated sulfuric acid. Therefore chemical burns may include a thermal component when the chemical reacts exothermally with tissue components.

Although chemicals with extremes of hydrogen ion concentration (or activity) are generally corrosive, one cannot assume that neutral materials are harmless. For example, various epoxy catalysts cause skin injury despite near-neutral pH.

The treatment of chemical burns may differ from that of thermal burns because of the following factors[11]:
1. Estimation of severity may be elusive.
2. Systemic toxicity may ensue from the absorption of chemical(s).
3. Ocular and inhalation injuries may occur from splashes and inhalation.
4. Antidotes may be needed.

Most importantly, systemic effects may follow skin burns. Neligan[33] reported the systemic absorption of metals from a burn wound induced by an 88° C (190.4° F) solution with nickel and cobalt salts.

Factors that affect the severity of a chemical burn include the following:
1. Concentration of the chemical
2. Duration of skin contact
3. Manner of skin contact (e.g., under occlusive garment)
4. Prior condition of the skin
5. Lipid solubility of the chemical
6. Inherent toxicity of the compound

This chapter focuses on the tissue effects that result when chemicals cause burns, as well as the potential systemic effects. A discussion of gastrointestinal (GI) or ocular chemical injuries is beyond the scope of this chapter.

This chapter first addresses decontamination and safety in relation to chemical burns, then discusses specific substances. The alphabetic listing of chemicals, with antidotes as appropriate, constitutes the "Indications, Operations, and Outcomes" for this chapter. Chapters 24, 25, and 29 discuss plastic surgical principles and reconstruction for burn injuries.

DECONTAMINATION

Rescuers and health care providers can decrease the duration of the victim's contact with the offending agent by properly decontaminating the patient. The importance of this critical factor cannot be overstated. Many patients are treated in the field by paramedics or may be treated in an emergency department, but patients often are not decontaminated before hospital admission.

All patients with chemical contamination must be decontaminated as early as possible. Although extended washing and flushing of the skin may not always be possible before transport, some attempt at decontamination should be made. This may simply involve the removal of contaminated garments and a brief showering. The duration of showering needed to cleanse the skin has not been specified, so best judgment should be used. Certainly, patients who are outdoors in very cold environments should not be showered for more than 1 or 2 minutes because hypothermia may occur without heated water. Some patients with serious injuries require immediate transport, and treatment may not be available with decontamination equipment; however, contaminated clothing should be removed.

Oils and related agents has been used to increase the back diffusion of chemicals from the skin. Although agents such as mineral oil may remove some additional phenol from the skin after a soap-and-water wash, the clinical benefit is unclear.[8,35] As a general recommendation, contaminated skin should be washed for at least 5 and preferably 15 minutes with water (and mild soap if available) after removal of contaminated clothing. The eyes should also be irrigated with appropriate eyewash solutions whenever ocular contamination is possible, especially by alkali.

Several proprietary materials are sold as special neutralizing agents for chemical burns, but no studies support their routine use. Special solutions should be considered a secondary measure.

Although some chemicals (e.g., sodium metal) are water reactive, such skin contamination is rare; the theoretic presence of a water-reactive compound should not deter one from flushing contaminated skin with copious volumes of water. Even with a water-reactive agent, a stream of water with a high flow rate will remove the generated heat. The one caveat is that some chemicals react with water to form more toxic substances. For example, aluminum phosphide powder reacts with water to form phosphine, a highly toxic gas used for fumigation.

Early and thorough irrigation is especially necessary for alkali burns.[41]

Safety of Personnel

Decontamination is not only beneficial for the patient, but also a mandatory preventive measure to protect all subsequent health care providers who will treat the patient. Although most reports of health care workers secondarily exposed to chemicals from patients suggest mild effects, some workers have incurred significant injury.

Health care workers, paramedics, and others who may be in contact with contaminated patients should have proper training and resources to select the appropriate methods of protection. Specifically, the recommended gloves and air-filtration cartridge-canister masks should be available. Consultation with a certified industrial hygienist or the nearest Occupational Safety and Health Administration (OSHA) consultation office should provide useful guidance in this area. Regular training is mandatory for the proper use and selection of these devices.

ALKALIS (LYE, SODIUM AND POTASSIUM HYDROXIDE)

Lye is used in janitorial applications, electroplating, drain cleaners (Figure 26-1), oven cleaners (Figure 26-2), detergent manufacture, and many other applications. As with many other strong alkalis, lye in contact with the skin feels slippery, because saponification of the fat in the skin with the strong

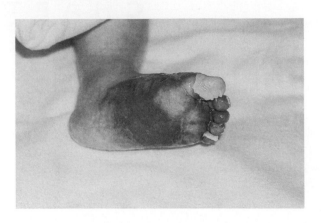

Figure 26-1. Child's foot about 4 hours after being placed in tub of water with residual alkaline drain cleaner.

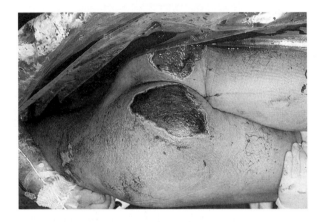

Figure 26-2. Deep burns of buttock in male who was sprayed with jellylike substance and left semiconscious in parking lot. Substance was later identified as an alkaline oven cleaner.

base forms a soap. Burn injuries from lye are typically liquefaction necrosis with deep penetration of the tissues.

Several patients who have fallen into lye vats incurred lethal injuries. Death resulted from sepsis, and myocutaneous gangrene developed in one patient, with incalculably high creatine kinase (CK) values. Two patients' white blood cell counts dropped to about 1000 cells/ml, only to rebound a day later. At that time, most of the cells were mature, suggesting that the lye injury caused a temporary margination of the neutrophils in the peripheral tissues.

Other patients have survived falls into a lye pit, and a recent report demonstrates the difficulties associated with determination of chemical burn wound severity.[18] Aggressive techniques led to this patient's recovery after an 85% total body surface area (TBSA) burn.

Other industrial accidents have resulted in death with a spray of lye.[28]

The superficial layers of skin may be dissolved and may "float" off with showering. With severe injuries the subcutaneous tissues may have a doughy and crepitant sensation on palpation. Again, these findings suggest deep saponification of the integument and underlying adipose tissues. Injuries to the GI tract and ocular tissues are infamous and severe; if survived, they may lead to long-term problems and complications. Appropriate consultations should be obtained if the lungs, GI tract, or eyes are affected.

Antidotes and Recommendations

No antidotes are applicable for alkalis such as lye. Supportive care is usually sufficient but may not overcome severe caustic injuries. No analysis of biologic fluids for lye has clinical value.

Washing the skin with sodium acetate caused a more rapid return of subcutaneous pH toward normal in animal models.[42] The relevance to human outcomes is uncertain.

AMMONIA

Burns of the skin from ammonia are usually a result of prolonged contact. A strong alkali base, ammonia is capable of causing severe injuries to the skin, eyes, and GI tract, with liquefaction necrosis. Concurrent inhalation of ammonia gas is life threatening because the respiratory tract may be severely compromised.[2,27]

Ammonia is among the most devastating chemicals to injure the eye. Because of its small molecular size, its relatively low apparent charge, and its strong alkalinity, ammonia is able to diffuse readily through the tissues and exert severe injury to the eye.

The effects on the respiratory tract depend on victims' ability to remove themselves from exposure. Prolonged inhalation may occur when a victim is unable to escape a cloud of ammonia gas. The immediate effects on the eye, resulting in severe lacrimation and lid closure or blindness, may contribute to the victim's inability to reach breathable air.

Because of ammonia's high water solubility, its irritating effects are usually limited to the upper airway. It rapidly produces a cough and choking sensation, which, along with its distinct odor, make its presence immediately known. Generally, as with other highly water-soluble gases, ammonia does not reach the lower airways in sufficient concentration to result in injury. When victims are unable to extricate themselves from exposure, however, severe pneumonia or bronchiolitis may result.

When ammonia inhalation has likely occurred, careful evaluation of the upper airway for stridor, hoarseness, or obstruction should be a high priority. Evaluation for pulmonary parenchymal injury should also be undertaken, especially in patients with prolonged inhalation or who demonstrate serious upper airway injury.

Antidotes and Recommendations

No antidotes exist for ammonia exposure. Involvement of the integument should be treated with copious irrigation and standard burn treatment. Involvement of the eyes, even with exposure only to gases or vapors, mandates prolonged and repeated irrigation and immediate ophthalmologic consultation.

The absorption of ammonia is not of systemic importance. Obtaining blood ammonia concentrations for patient exposures has no benefit.

ARYLAMINES

Aniline and its derivatives fall into the arylamine class. Many of these chemicals are used as chemical intermediates and in pharmaceutical manufacturing, dyes, and other laboratory uses. Several of these chemicals can cause burns, which generally are superficial. Burns are often violet to brown in color and are not painful.

Many of these compounds, however, including aniline, may cause severe systemic toxicity with absorption. Methemoglobinemia may develop, with shortness of breath, tachycardia, tachypnea, and cyanosis. Hepatic injury may also occur; an early elevation of serum hepatic transaminases may result.

Symptomatic patients or those with a methemoglobin level greater than 30% require treatment. Patients with anemia, heart disease, or other conditions that might be affected by decreased oxygenation may also need therapy. Blood samples for methemoglobin must be analyzed within an hour because the value may change in vitro.

Many of these compounds are formulated with other solvents, which may contribute to the corrosive nature and the systemic toxicity.[36]

Antidotes and Recommendations

Methylene blue may be needed for the treatment of methemoglobinemia, and 1 to 2 mg/kg of body weight is the usual intravenous (IV) dose in adults. The antidotal effect is rapid and peaks in about 30 minutes. Excessive doses may paradoxically cause methemoglobinemia and hemolysis.

Methylene blue may be ineffective in patients with glucose-6-phosphate dehydrogenase (G6PD) deficiency because of the lack of available NADPH necessary for its effectiveness. Additional doses may be needed. Further evaluation by a toxicologist or through a poison control center is advisable.

BLEACH SOLUTIONS (SODIUM OR CALCIUM HYPOCHLORITE)

Household bleaches are an aqueous solution of sodium or calcium hypochlorite, usually of about 5% concentration. Industrial applications of this solution may use much higher concentrations. Hypochlorite solutions are used as bleach in laundry operations, as chemical reagents, and for disinfection. When used as a disinfectant, bleach is legally controlled as a pesticide (germicide).

Hypochlorite solutions are strong oxidizers. They must be stabilized by adjustment of the pH and are generally maintained at a pH greater than 10 by the addition of sodium hydroxide. Therefore bleach solutions may cause injury to the integument and mucous membranes because of their alkalinity (Figure 26-3). Oral ingestion of small quantities, however, is usually not a problem. Prolonged contact with skin may cause full-thickness burns.

The potential release of toxic gases from bleach solution is a frequent concern. At the range of pH for these products,

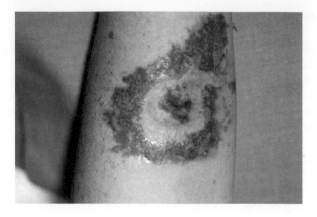

Figure 26-3. Burn from alkaline hypochlorite solution (bleach) associated with prolonged skin contact under kitchen glove.

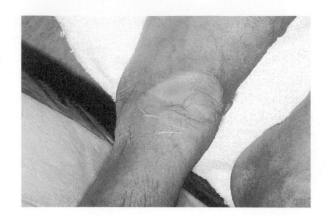

Figure 26-4. Initial appearance of chromic acid burn with typical yellow discoloration.

chlorine gas will not form spontaneously. If acid is added to the solution, however, altering the pH, chlorine gas may escape. This occurs when an acid cleaning agent is mixed with bleach. Also, ammonia is often mixed with bleach, producing *chloramine,* not chlorine.

Both chlorine and chloramine are irritants to the respiratory tract. Both are sufficiently water soluble and irritating to warrant adequate warnings of their presence. Some people continue to work in such potentially hazardous environments, risking respiratory tract injury. Usually this is limited to the upper and middle airways. With sufficiently heavy exposure, however, laryngeal edema occurs and may progress to pneumonitis.

Exposure to chlorine or chloramine is unlikely to cause skin burns. Isolated burns while using bleach solutions suggest direct and prolonged contact with the liquid. In these patients, and without a history of improperly mixed solutions, inhalation injury would not be expected. Regardless of the scenario, the patient with airborne exposure is usually aware of ocular or respiratory tract irritation.

Antidotes and Recommendations

No specific antidotes are available for exposure to bleach or its potential formed gases. Treatment is symptomatic and supportive.

With mild to moderate exposure to these gases, hoarseness, upper airway edema, and chemical bronchitis are the likely outcomes. With severe exposure, pulmonary edema may occur over hours.

CEMENT

Cement used today contains lye and, when wet, has a pH greater than 12. Skin in contact with wet cement for a prolonged time will develop severe burns (see section on lye).[7,9,15,19]

Professional cement workers use kneepads to protect themselves from this injury. Dabblers in cement work often

are not aware of the dangers, however, and may develop injuries.

CHLORATES

Chlorates are substances composed of chlorine-oxygen molecules that have high reactivity and oxidizing potential. Chlorates react exothermally and produce oxygen.

Chlorate cylinders ("candles") are used as a substitute for compressed-gas oxygen cylinders on aircraft. Chlorate canisters were recently implicated in a major airline accident in Florida. When activated to generate oxygen, these canisters become extremely hot, so they must be shielded from flammable materials and to prevent skin contact. Most burns occur as a result of contact with the canister.

If chlorates directly contact the skin, they can generate substantial heat, causing a thermal injury. When removing residual chlorates, caregivers must realize that heat may be generated, with possible ignition from the liberated oxygen.

The absorption of chlorates may result in methemoglobinemia (see section on arylamines) and intravascular hemolysis. With inhalation, the patient should be observed for injuries to the respiratory tract. Methemoglobin levels and serial hemoglobin and hematocrit readings are needed to detect hemolysis.

CHROMIC ACID

This strong acid and oxidizing agent is used in electroplating and as a laboratory reagent. Burns from chromic acid are generally severe compared with those from other acids at a corresponding pH. Burn injuries typically have an initial yellow-orange appearance (Figures 26-4 and 26-5), changing over 12 hours to a white, coagulative necrosis with a thin, erythematous border. These are usually deep burns.

Absorption of chrome ions may result in acute cardiac, hepatic, and renal toxicity.[39] Some authors advocate the use of

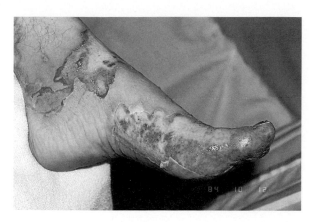

Figure 26-5. Burns from concentrated chromic acid sustained at chrome-plating shop.

chelating agents for the chrome, but this seems unnecessary and probably is ineffective. With chronic exposure, chrome is a human carcinogen.

Antidotes and Recommendations

No specific antidotes exist for chrome burns. Chelating agents are not recommended. Cardiac, renal, or hepatic toxicity must be evaluated and treated as necessary. Supportive measures should be used as appropriate.

A few case reports suggested early burn wound excision to prevent absorption of chrome, but these are too limited to make a recommendation.[26]

DIMETHYLFORMAMIDE

Dimethylformamide (DMF) is frequently used as a solvent in the plastics industry. This liquid has significant hepatotoxicity.

Skin contact with DMF may result in a thick, white, bullous lesion and may occur in individuals who have used this chemical in the past. The cause of the skin change is unclear. Typically, after being exposed for several hours, the fingertips are affected, and the patient develops a painless area of thickened white tissue that resembles "waterlogged" skin. If excised, the underlying tissue is erythematous but otherwise undamaged.

Observation of these lesions is adequate without intervention. They generally resolve within a few days, with no skin loss.

Antidotes and Recommendations

No specific antidotes for DMF exposure or toxicity are available. Hepatotoxicity has not been seen with less extensive skin injuries. Patients generally can be managed on an outpatient basis without difficulty.

Often, patients with skin injuries also had chronic dermal exposure, and particular attention to liver function is warranted. Serial liver function studies over several days should be documented.

ETHYLENE OXIDE (EtO)

Ethylene oxide (EtO) is a gas used as an ethylating agent in chemical reactions. It is also a common gas-sterilizing agent in biomedical applications. For gas sterilization, it is often diluted with an inert gas, with resulting EtO concentrations of about 12%. EtO has caused minor burns of the skin with bullous formation and erythema. Retained EtO in medical products was associated with at least one injury.[2]

EtO can also be inhaled and cause pulmonary irritation at higher concentrations. EtO can cause lymphocytosis and hepatocellular injury, neither of which has been a clinical problem. EtO is considered a human carcinogen, based primarily on animal data but also some human epidemiologic studies. EtO has caused peripheral neuropathy in some patients. The neuropathy and cancer outcomes should be considered effects of chronic exposures.

Routine wound care and supportive measures should be employed.

Antidotes and Recommendations

No specific antidote exists for EtO. Biologic monitoring for presence of the gas is not feasible or clinically useful.

Tests of deoxyribonucleic acid (DNA) effects, unscheduled DNA synthesis, and sister chromatid exchange have not been useful in the monitoring of chronically exposed patients. These tests also would not be useful in the acute setting.

FORMALDEHYDE

Formaldehyde is a widely used chemical in many industrial processes. It is used as a disinfectant, as a tissue fixative, and in other laboratory operations. It may be used in insulating materials and as embalming fluid and is contained in the formulation of resins and plastics. Solutions of 47% formaldehyde are called *formalin*.

Formaldehyde is recognized as a probable human carcinogen.

Burns generally require only flushing and observation. More severe injuries may occur, however, if formaldehyde contacts the eyes or GI tract. Inhalation of formaldehyde gas or vapor may result in significant respiratory distress and asthma. If ingestion is suspected, GI consultation should be obtained, with ophthalmologic consultation for ocular contact.

Significant absorption of formaldehyde from the integument may occur. This generally does not result in systemic toxicity but a mild metabolic acidosis may occur.

Antidotes and Recommendations

No specific antidote is required with formaldehyde. Supportive care is adequate. Some potential biologic markers of exposure may be available, but none would be clinically useful in the acute setting.

FORMIC ACID

Formic acid is used in laboratories and in geologic studies to dissolve certain rocks. It causes a brown discoloration of the skin with fine blistering.

Formic acid has caused substantial metabolic acidemia. This is out of proportion to the amount of acid potentially absorbed and suggests a direct metabolic effect of the formate ion.

Antidotes and Recommendations

No specific antidote is available at this time. Correction of acid-base balance may become necessary with formic acidemia.

HALOGENATED HYDROCARBONS

The halogenated hydrocarbons are those containing chlorine, bromine, iodine, or fluorine. The *chlorinated hydrocarbons* are the most widely used group within this class. They have a variety of industrial applications, including as solvents, paint strippers, carburetor cleaners, and spot removers. They are found in many products as solvents for glues, adhesives, coatings, and as antispatter agents in welding.

The toxic effects of *carbon tetrachloride* on the liver are well known. Used for many years in dry cleaning, carbon tetrachloride was replaced by *trichloroethylene,* which was subsequently found to be toxic to the liver, kidney, and central nervous system (CNS). Trichloroethylene occasionally causes burns with skin contact.[4] Currently, *perchloroethylene* is used for dry cleaning in the United States.

As with the hydrocarbons or petroleum distillates, the chlorinated hydrocarbons can cause profound narcosis. Their tissue penetration and kinetics vary considerably. The degree of metabolism in the liver and subsequent excretion by the kidneys also are variable. The more volatile members of this group may have substantial excretion through exhalation.

Some halogenated hydrocarbons are considered carcinogenic. These substances have the potential for causing serious skin burns, and all of them cause significant defatting of the skin, especially with chronic exposure. Unique within this group is the corrosive *dichloromethane,* or *methylene chloride;* in addition to causing dermal burns (Figure 26-6), it also is metabolized to carbon monoxide in the body. Patients with chemical burns and elevated (and especially increasing) carboxyhemoglobin (COHb) levels should be suspected of having absorbed methylene chloride. COHb levels of 20% have been reported. It is unlikely that the COHb alone would account for the degree of altered mental status, but the COHb certainly would be one factor altering CNS function.

The halogenated hydrocarbons sensitize the myocardium and predispose to dysrhythmias. Hypoxemia and sympathomimetic amines must be avoided. Dysrhythmias should be treated accordingly, with particular attention to oxygen status.

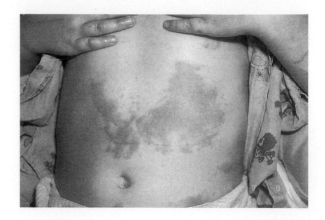

Figure 26-6. Burns from methylene chloride (dichloromethane) in child who found can of the solvent in alley behind her home. Absorption can lead to dysrhythmia, narcosis, and production of carboxyhemoglobin from metabolism of methylene chloride.

Antidotes and Recommendations

No specific antidotes are available for the chlorinated hydrocarbons. If carboxyhemoglobinemia develops from dichloromethane, however, supplemental oxygen should be used. The role of hyperbaric oxygen in dichloromethane-induced elevation of COHb has not been evaluated. As noted, sympathomimetic amines are avoided because they have a synergistic effect with halogenated hydrocarbons in promoting dysrhythmias.

Although no specific antidotes exist for the potential hepatotoxic effects of the halogenated hydrocarbons, the mechanism is most likely the production of free radicals during the metabolism of some of these compounds. Based on analogy with other chemicals that cause free radical hepatocellular injury, *N*-acetylcysteine may be of some benefit. This has not been sufficiently studied, however, to make any recommendations at this time.

HYDROCHLORIC ACID

Unlike its sister halogen acid, hydrofluoric acid (see next section), hydrochloric acid causes immediate symptoms of burning and discomfort and a typical acid burn with coagulative necrosis. Hydrochloric acid burns occur less often than other acid injuries, however; hydrochloric acid is less aggressive in causing burns, and other agents are used more often and in settings more likely to cause skin contact.

No systemic toxicity follows absorption of hydrochloric acid. Immediate irrigation and routine burn treatment are appropriate.

As with other acid and corrosive substances, hydrochloric acid may cause serious injuries to the ocular tissues. Injuries to the upper GI tract can occur, but this usually follows the ingestion of highly concentrated acid. Recognizing that the stomach contains hydrochloric acid with a pH of about 2, small amounts of this acid understandably have little effect on the stomach and esophagus. Clearly, concentration is an important factor. Further, the upper respiratory and GI tracts are subject to injury.

Antidotes and Recommendations

No antidotes are required for hydrochloric acid. Any absorbed hydrogen chloride is handled by the body with its usual homeostatic mechanisms. No useful biologic monitoring exists for hydrochloric acid exposure.

HYDROFLUORIC ACID

Hydrofluoric acid (HFA) is a highly corrosive material to all human tissues; injury results from the fluoride ion more than the hydrogen ion. Although frequently stated to be a strong acid, HFA is much weaker than hydrochloric acid; HFA's dissociation constant (K_d) is about 10^3 less.[16] This likely accounts for a greater proportion of HFA remaining in an uncharged state, allowing for more dermal penetration.

Applications

Hydrofluoric acid is used in a variety of chemical processes, including as a catalyst to increase the octane ratings in gasoline during the refining process and for product recovery in oil wells. Because of its extreme electronegativity, HFA is used in metallurgy and in electroplating.

The avidity of the fluoride ion for calcium, magnesium, and other metals has significant industrial and biologic ramifications. Thus HFA is used in a variety of applications to remove calcium scaling and rust (e.g., from boilers) and to brighten aluminum. It may be used to clean air-conditioning coils and other equipment that tend to collect metal deposits from water. HFA is used in laundries to remove rust from fabric.

Because it etches glass, HFA is used to frost glass and to etch thin glass layers in the production of computer chips. It is also used in dental laboratories, janitorial services, and chemical laboratories.

Systemic Effects

Hydrofluoric acid may be concentrated to a maximum of 70% in water. Solutions above about 50% may generate a significant mist ("fuming acid"), especially in moist air.

Serious systemic effects resulting from hypocalcemia and hypomagnesemia may follow skin burns and absorption,[6,20,31] including lethal dysrhythmias.[32] Severe local burns may result from HFA contact with any tissue. The systemic effects are life threatening and generally caused by severe depletion of available ionic calcium. Available magnesium may also be decreased. Burns greater than 5% TBSA should be considered life threatening.

Treatment Considerations and Modalities

Because of the absence of controlled human studies, the best therapy for HFA burns under various conditions has not been determined.[30] Animal studies vary with respect to concentration of acid, duration of exposure, method of treatment, and measurement of effect.

INITIAL THERAPY AND TOPICAL AGENTS. For more than 50 years, standard practice has been to apply a chemical agent to the exposed tissue to decrease the bioavailability of the fluoride ion. This has been accomplished using a variety of modalities. Both magnesium and calcium salts have been applied to the integument because these divalent metals bind with fluoride.[10] Quaternary ammonium salts are also able to bind with fluoride.

Pain out of proportion to the apparent visible injury is common and is a hallmark of dilute HFA burns. Therefore, since the physical effects may be delayed, all suspected exposures to HFA should be treated expectantly. Initial thorough irrigation of the tissue is mandatory. Application of topical agents may be done without concern of side effects.

Although topical agents may be effective immediately after skin contamination, the presence or persistence of pain after topical treatment of 30 minutes suggests that more aggressive, invasive techniques are needed. Other indications for possible invasive therapy include a delay in skin decontamination, severe pain, or contact with solutions greater than 40% HFA.

CALCIUM GLUCONATE. If a commercially available preparation of calcium gluconate is not available, a solution of magnesium sulfate (Epsom salts) in water may be used for topical application with HFA exposure. Calcium gluconate solution is often mixed with a water-soluble gel (e.g., examination lubricant) and applied to the affected skin.

When topical therapy fails, injection with 10% calcium gluconate is the preferred treatment. Approximately 0.5 ml solution/cm^2 tissue is injected intradermally and subdermally. For the digits, no more than 0.5 ml of 10% calcium gluconate per phalanx is injected. *(Never use calcium chloride; it is corrosive to tissue.)* Extreme swelling of the digits may preclude local infiltration because of vascular compromise from further introduction of fluid.

NAIL BEDS AND SUBJACENT TISSUES. The majority of HFA burns involve the hands (Figure 26-7), and many of these involve the nail bed (Figure 26-8). The acid is able to penetrate

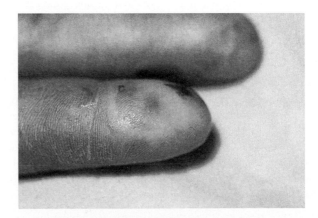

Figure 26-7. Hydrofluoric acid burns to digits from concentrated solution 1 hour before presentation. Patient noted pain within minutes of contact.

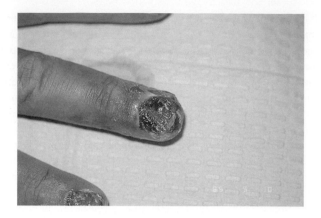

Figure 26-8. Hydrofluoric acid (HFA) burn of digits in metal worker about 36 hours after injury. Burn was from 60% HFA concentration with about 5 minutes of contact.

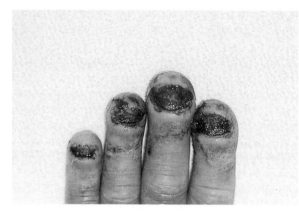

Figure 26-9. Involvement of all digits and subungual tissues 10 hours after injury in male worker using 30% hydrofluoric acid as cleaning agent. He did not use glove protection.

around and under the fingernail at locations that are not fully protected by a continuous layer of stratum corneum. Despite diffuse exposure to the hands, the fingernails and fingertips are often the tissues affected most (Figure 26-9). This creates a problem, since the presence of the nail precludes local infiltration into these tissues.

Erythema or discoloration of the nail bed requires removal of the nail under local anesthesia (Figure 26-10). This predilection for the nails probably reflects the importance of the lipid barriers of the skin in protecting from HFA burns.[34]

HFA can also cause significant injury to the subjacent tissues. Severe nonsuppurative *tenosynovitis* has been reported, and injuries to the nerves may cause protracted pain syndromes in rare cases. *Osteolysis* may occur where osseous structures are not protected by intervening tissues; the hands are particularly susceptible. Baseline radiographs of the tissues may be useful for detection of early changes of osteolysis.

EXTREMITIES. Intraarterial infusion of calcium gluconate is an alternative treatment for burns of the extremities. Neither prospective nor case-control studies have been reported using intraarterial calcium gluconate with any other method of treatment. However, intraarterial infusion appears safe and effective. Removal of the fingernail may not be necessary with intraarterial infusion. This may have a profound effect on a worker's ability to return to work earlier.

In the upper extremity the brachial artery is cannulated, and 3 g of calcium gluconate in 300 ml of 5% dextrose in water (D5W) is infused over 4 hours; this may be repeated several times over a 12-hour period. No human or animal data describe the best dosage, timing, or total dose of calcium gluconate. Other authors have suggested using magnesium sulfate and calcium chloride.

In the lower extremity, 5 g of calcium gluconate in 500 ml of D5W is used in the femoral artery. Again, the dosage is arbitrary but apparently was effective in most patients. With extravasation of fluid, calcium gluconate is less irritating than calcium chloride salts.

DMSO AND MAGNESIUM SULFATE. Other treatment alternatives have included the use of calcium salts in dimethyl sulfoxide (DMSO), primarily used in pediatric patients. Bordelon et al[6] reported an infant in whom various calcium preparations were used, including DMSO; the child had cardiac arrest before finally recovering. DMSO can cause other skin damage, can carry injurious materials into the skin and circulation, and can cause systemic reactions; thus it is not preferred.

Although IV administration of calcium gluconate is useful for the treatment of systemic hypocalcemia, it is not sufficient for local effects because the tissue concentrations of calcium will not reach the burned area. Reporting on an animal study, Williams et al[40] reported efficacy of high-dose (160-mg/kg) IV magnesium sulfate in rats. Cox and Osgood[14] reported on the use of IV magnesium sulfate on a rabbit ear model with HFA burns and suggested that this IV preparation was efficacious. Henry and Hla[22] reported the use of IV infusion into the upper extremity in a single case as a method analogous to a Bier block (instead of lidocaine, calcium gluconate was used).

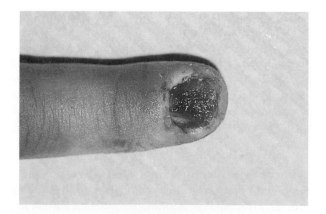

Figure 26-10. Hydrofluoric acid (HFA) burn of digit after nail was removed to relieve pain and decontaminate tissues. Concentration of HFA was 20% with prolonged exposure of 1 hour.

PROPHYLAXIS. The systemic effects of HFA burns are primarily caused by the severe decrease in available (ionizable) calcium and magnesium. Tetany, cardiac dysrhythmias, and negative inotropic effects leading to hypoperfusion and electromechanical dissociation have been well documented. In patients with normal renal function, the additional calcium load provided as therapy will not cause a problem and will be rapidly excreted.

If patients develop dysrhythmias from hypocalcemia induced by HFA, they are refractory to treatment. Early prophylactic provision of systemic calcium to patients with HFA burns from greater than 5% TBSA is critical in some cases. Patients meeting this criterion should have continuous cardiac monitoring for the evaluation of prolonged QTc intervals associated with hypocalcemia. Serial (about every 2 hours) serum calcium (ionizable) levels should be obtained. Magnesium should similarly be evaluated and replaced as needed.

Immediate excision of the burned tissue has been attempted to decrease the further absorption of the fluoride ion.

Ocular and Gastrointestinal Injury
Ocular contamination with HFA requires immediate irrigation. Although these injuries may result in significant ocular damage, people generally are aware of these injuries and irrigate them immediately, diminishing the duration of exposure and the severity of the injury. Ocular instillation of calcium gluconate drops has been suggested but this is based on anecdotal cases and speculation at best.

Similarly, HFA inhalation can cause serious pulmonary edema, airway edema, and upper airway compromise. Although the inhalation of nebulized calcium gluconate has been suggested, this also is not suggested by adequate human or animal data.

The stratum corneum is of critical importance in the protection of the human integument, and therefore the mucosal surfaces of the GI tract are more susceptible to injury. Intentional and accidental HFA ingestions and intentional HFA enemas have been devastating. Immediate GI consultation should be obtained. Full extent of the injury may be delayed, and HFA should not be equated with other acid injuries of the GI tract.

Fluoride Concentration
Urinary fluoride determinations may be useful to confirm HFA exposure and absorption. The concentration of this ion in blood or urine, however, does not provide prognostic or therapeutic information.

Antidotes and Recommendations
As discussed, controversy still surrounds the best topical or injectable preparation for HFA burns of the skin. The reports of human therapy are uncontrolled studies, case reports, and supposition. Animal studies do not provide sufficient information to recommend a specific therapy and even appear contradictory regarding the most efficacious agent and method of delivery. Various treatments have numerous proponents.

Despite this, some treatment is necessary with all HFA injuries other than brief, low-concentration exposures without residual pain. For small areas where injectable calcium gluconate does not appear contraindicated, intradermal and subdermal injection is useful. For multiple digits, periungual and subungual tissues, or severe injuries of the hand or foot, intraarterial calcium gluconate appears to be efficacious without serious adverse effects. The use of calcium gluconate eye drops or eyewash (1%) for eye contamination is largely anectodal.

Patients who have intentionally ingested HFA do poorly. If the patient does not succumb to the immediate toxic effects, severe corrosive effects to the esophagus are the rule.

With inhalation injuries the role of inhaled, nebulized calcium gluconate is again anecdotal. With burns greater than 5% TBSA, ingestions, or enemas, however, calcium gluconate (or another salt) is essential by IV supplementation. Constant cardiac monitoring and serial calcium and magnesium levels are necessary. Aggressive replacement of calcium and magnesium is mandatory.

LIQUID NITROGEN AND OTHER CRYOGENIC AGENTS

Nitrogen is a gas at ambient temperature and pressure. Liquefied gases (e.g., propane, butane, Freon, nitrogen) are cryogenic and can cause severe frostbite (Figure 26-11). Pressurized gases emitted from a narrow orifice generally have a cooling effect and can cause cryogenic injuries. Slow rewarming of the tissues is indicated. Vascular stasis occurs, and the skin slowly demarcates the injured area over several hours.

Most chemicals used in cryogenics are hazardous not only because of the local injury but also because of their ability to expand to a gas and displace oxygen in an area with limited ventilation. Dilutional hypoxia may cause severe CNS injury. Some extremely cold liquefied gases can also liquefy surrounding oxygen, resulting in explosive potential.

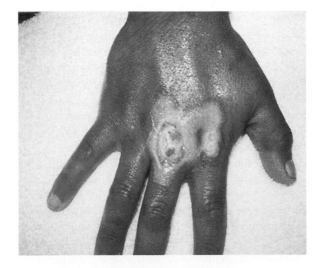

Figure 26-11. Severe "frostbite" from release of halocarbon from pressurized industrial line.

An open flame in the vicinity of halogenated hydrocarbons used as refrigerants may release the various halogen acids and carbonyl compounds (e.g., HFA, hydrochloric acid, phosgene, carbonyl fluoride). These have serious and often delayed pulmonary effects.

Antidotes and Recommendations

No specific antidotes are available. Biologic monitoring for the underlying agent has no clinical value.

METHYL BROMIDE

Methyl bromide is used in some chemical processes and in the past was used as a fire suppressant on aircraft engines. Methyl bromide is also used as a pesticide for structural and agricultural purposes. Although its popularity has declined in recent years for control of termites in buildings, it continues to be used in agricultural settings. For termites the structure is tented, and heated methyl bromide vapors are "shot" into it.

Methyl bromide is highly neurotoxic and has lead to several deaths. Severe CNS effects, coma, seizures, hepatic failure, and death may occur. The presence of coma and seizures carries a high mortality rate; those who recover may have severe neuropsychiatric deficits.

When burns occur from contact with liquid methyl bromide, they are usually superficial with bullous formation but may be deeper.[23] To introduce the vapor into the structure or into the soil for fumigation, it is heated from the liquid phase. Therefore the vapors may initially have thermal energy and thus cause a burn.

Antidotes and Recommendations

No specific antidotes exist for methyl bromide. Neither topical nor systemic agents are of proven value. Because the hepatotoxic nature of methyl bromide is likely related to hepatic transformation to a free radical, however, it has been proposed that N-acetylcysteine may be helpful. This is routinely used in acetaminophen poisoning, where free radical formation causes liver injury. By analogy, other chemical exposures causing hepatotoxicity by this mechanism are thought to benefit from N-acetylcysteine, although no human data are available to determine its efficacy. Consultation with a poison control center regarding N-acetylcysteine dosing may be considered for treatment of liver toxicity.

Seizures, if they occur, are severe, prolonged, and difficult to control. Aggressive, standard antiseizure therapy should be instituted, and general anesthesia may be needed.

No useful specific biologic monitoring is available, but serum and probably cerebrospinal fluid bromide levels are elevated. This analyte is for total *inorganic* bromide and not specifically organic bromide. Therefore a dietary contribution to inorganic bromide is a real factor, and "normal" values up to about 5 mg/dl are reported without methyl bromide exposure. Many laboratories use traditional reference ranges from the era of cold preparations containing bromides, and therefore most ranges for bromide are not relevant for methyl bromide exposure. If a laboratory report indicates that the bromide level is "not toxic," this may have no validity for organic bromide compounds. It is therefore more important to recognize false-negative bromide results than false-positive results when assessing methyl bromide.

With a significant history of exposure to methyl bromide, bromide levels greater than 5 to 10 mg/dl may be significant, and levels of 20 to 30 mg/dl or more may be lethal. Data on inorganic bromide in methyl bromide exposure are insufficient, however, to determine a prognostic or therapeutic value.

NITRIC ACID

Nitric acid is a simple acid with moderate oxidizing capacity. Nitric acid is used in various metallurgical operations, including pickling of steel. As with other acids, nitric acid may be heated for certain reactions or cleaning processes in metallurgy.

Typical of the other simple acids, nitric acid causes a coagulation necrosis. The oxidative effects are not as devastating as with chromic or perchloric acids. Burns may be severe and deep with concentrated solutions. Nitric acid burns are often a yellow color with minor injuries, as though a yellow marking pen was applied to the skin. With severe injuries a deeper burn may develop, but again a yellow hue is present. This coloration occurs as the acid nitrosates the aromatic ring-containing amino acids in the skin, forming a yellow compound. Nitric acid is also corrosive to the ocular and GI tissue, similar to other acids.

When nitric acid reacts with organic or carbonaceous matter, oxides of nitrogen are generated. This may occur when a high-carbon steel is accidentally placed into a nitric acid pickling solution. This orange-red-brown gas forms with smoke and is distinctive.

The oxides of nitrogen are toxic to the lung; reported effects include bronchospasm, airway inflammation, pulmonary edema, and bronchiolitis obliterans. Aggressive pulmonary support may be necessary. After apparent recovery and about 10 to 14 days after exposure, the patient may have a relapse of the asthmalike condition. This recurrence may be worse than the acute pulmonary injury. The mechanism for this late reaction is unknown.

Antidotes and Recommendations

No antidotes are available for nitric acid. Standard burn wound therapy and supportive care are appropriate. For inhalation, aggressive pulmonary care may be needed, and the patient must be aware of the potential late pulmonary sequelae. Laboratory analyses are not specific.

PERCHLORIC ACID

Perchloric acid is used in specialized laboratory processes. It is highly reactive and a very strong oxidizing agent. Perchloric acid can cause severe burns, but few reports exist on the dangers from burns.

Systemic toxicity is not expected. Clearly, perchloric acid would also have severe effects with ingestion or ocular contact.

Antidotes and Recommendations

No antidotes are required for perchloric acid. Supportive care and routine burn treatment are recommended. No relevant laboratory monitoring methods are available.

PETROLEUM DISTILLATES AND OTHER HYDROCARBONS

This group constitutes a variety of organic chemicals (Figure 26-12). Some petroleum distillates are effectively inert, whereas others may cause inflammatory reactions of the integument after prolonged contact. Because some are gases at ambient temperature, they may be liquefied. Liquefied *butane* or *propane* discharging from a narrow orifice may cause frostbite injuries (see section on liquid nitrogen). Materials such as *gasoline* and *kerosene* have sufficient corrosiveness to the skin that contact with the liquid or saturated garments can cause injuries that range from erythema to full-thickness burns[21,37] (Figure 26-13).

For most of these petroleum distillates, removal of the agent from contact with the body is sufficient treatment. Although many of these chemicals have specific additional toxicity with absorption, such effects are usually confined to chronic exposures. The exception is the narcotic effects of the hydrocarbons. This acute CNS effect is dose dependent and occurs with acute or even one-time exposure.

Dermal absorption of solvents usually involves concomitant inhalation of the chemicals as well. With high exposures to some of the petroleum distillates, *pneumonitis* may occur. With accidental ingestions, some organic chemicals may be aspirated (probably a function of their surface tension), which may lead to hydrocarbon pneumonitis, a serious complication.

The solvent *n-hexane* is not only extremely flammable but also causes a peripheral neuropathy with chronic exposure. The same is true of methyl-n-butyl ketone. With chronic exposure, *benzene* is hematotoxic and is known to cause acute myelogenous leukemia in humans. Acute exposures are unlikely to cause these problems, but patients with acute burns from chemicals may also have been poorly supervised and overexposed long before their burn. For this reason, attention to these risks should not be ignored.

Antidotes and Recommendations

No specific antidotes are indicated for petroleum distillates.

Evaluation of CNS status is usually indicated after solvent overexposure. The liver and kidney are also common target organs, and serial hepatic enzyme determinations and renal function testing may also be indicated. With pure hydrocarbons, patient monitoring may be tailored to the specific agent involved. Hydrocarbon mixtures (e.g., gasoline) are more common, however, making monitoring less focused.

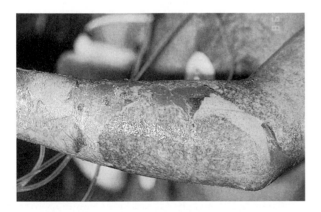

Figure 26-12. Injury from a chlorinated hydrocarbon corrosive used as degreaser. Patient slipped and partially fell into vat.

PHENOLS

Phenol and substituted phenols are capable of causing skin burns (Figure 26-14). Phenols are used as paint strippers, disinfectants, solvents, organic reagents, and concrete cleaners. They have also been used medically to fix tissues, such as the appendiceal stump in an appendectomy, and for chemical

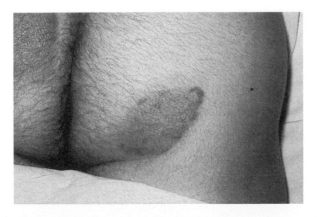

Figure 26-13. Burn of buttocks in worker from sitting in pool of gasoline for 1 hour while eating lunch at a loading dock.

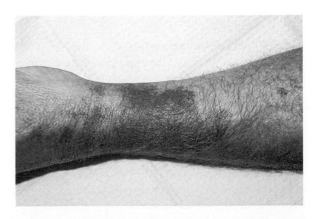

Figure 26-14. Phenol burn after about 2 hours. Superficial skin will desquamate in about 2 days, leaving bright erythematous base. Burns usually are not full thickness but may be anesthetic because of phenol. Phenol is rapidly absorbed and may be apparent on patient's exhaled breath.

"peels." Phenol is a weak acid. *Carbolic acid* (phenol) has been reported to cause gangrene.[1]

Burns from phenol typically evolve over several days. The initial appearance is a reddish brown area; in about 2 days this superficial skin desquamates, leaving an erythematous base. As this heals over several weeks, the remaining skin may be hypopigmented.

Phenol and many of the substituted phenols rapidly penetrate the skin and are absorbed by the bloodstream. Phenol may acutely cause dysrhythmias, hepatocellular injury, and kidney damage. It also has stimulant and narcotic effects on the CNS. Most importantly, some of the substituted phenols (e.g., chlorophenols) are respiratory poisons, inhibiting oxidative phosphorylation. This can result in elevated body temperature, confusion, and seizures. Such patients must avoid aspirin and related salicylates because these can amplify this effect.

Decontamination of the skin should be accomplished as soon as possible. Some studies have addressed the ideal materials for decontamination, whereas others have recommended increased removal of phenol from the skin or a decrease in blood levels. No clinical benefit has been demonstrated from this additional removal.

Antidotes and Recommendations

No specific antidotes exist for phenol(s). Supportive care is needed; dysrhythmias and seizures may occur. After dermal absorption of phenol, the odor may be present on the breath as it is cleared by the lungs.

POVIDONE-IODINE TINCTURE

Burns from povidone-iodine (Betadine) used in surgical preparation have been reported.[13] These have occurred in children, generally on a plastic cooling blanket, such that the solution pools at the child's dependent pressure points. The mechanism has not been determined.

Awareness and prevention are the keys to this problem. Standard burn treatment is adequate. Systemic toxicity has not been a problem.

Antidotes and Recommendations

No antidotes are necessary. Since these injuries are invariably iatrogenic, prevention through education is imperative.

RESINS AND CATALYSTS

Various epoxy resins and related catalysts are corrosive to the skin, despite their near-neutral pH. Many of these contain reactive amine groups, which appear to be responsible for the biologic activity of these compounds.

These chemicals are frequently sensitizers and are independently capable of causing dermatitis or asthma. Acute skin absorption does not appear capable of causing internal or systemic injury, although chronic exposure to some of these agents may be toxic. Little opportunity exists for inhalation of resins because most are viscous liquids with low or intermediate vapor pressures. However, when heated or reacted exothermally, sufficient vapor may evolve, causing dermatitis or pulmonary effects (asthma).

The various catalysts used are small, volatile liquids that are highly reactive and can act as *haptens,* causing allergic reactions. *Isocyanates,* used in urethanes, are typical examples, as are many of the amine catalysts used in epoxy systems. Chronic exposure may lead to bronchospastic conditions.

Antidotes
No antidotes are available.

SULFURIC ACID

Sulfuric acid is a strong acid and oxidizing agent. It is a common agent causing burns in humans. It is used in automobile lead storage batteries, where its ability to cause burns is infamous. Sulfuric acid is also used in many metallurgical operations, electroplating, petroleum refining as a catalyst for higher-octane gasoline, and sulfonation reactions. It may also be a component of drain cleaners. Highly concentrated sulfuric acid with *sulfur trioxide,* or oleum (oil), is viscous.

The burns from concentrated sulfuric acid are potentially devastating. Contact with moisture releases significant heat of hydration. The skin becomes red-brown, then gray. It has a moderately dried, leathery appearance and later rehydrates over 8 to 12 hours, turning gray, mottled, and swollen (Figure 26-15). After about 18 hours, a white coagulate necrosis develops with an erythematous border. Until this time, it is difficult to define the ultimate wound margins.

No systemic toxicity occurs, but inhalation of sulfuric acid "fumes" is highly irritating. Upper and possible lower airway injury may occur. Ocular and GI exposures require appropriate evaluation and consultation.

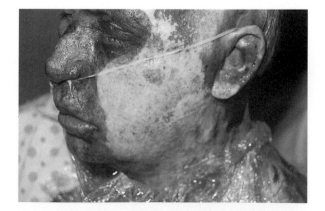

Figure 26-15. Sulfuric acid burns of face in assault case. It takes about 4 to 12 hours for oxidation of tissues to establish coagulation necrosis. Initially, tissues are inflamed, but with central grayish cast.

Antidotes

No specific antidotes are required.

WHITE PHOSPHORUS

White phosphorus is used in munitions, agrochemicals, and flares. It ignites spontaneously in air.

Skin lesions are often hardened, white tissue. It is difficult to see the pieces of white phosphorus embedded in the skin. Because these pieces need to be surgically debrided, a 10% solution of copper sulfate is often used to paint over the area. This turns the white phosphorus blue, enabling removal. Copper sulfate solutions applied over large body surface areas, however, may cause hemolytic anemia,[38] and caution should be used.

Eldad et al[17] concluded that a water flush is as effective as any other method of removal and that copper sulfate is not needed.

Typically, substantial pain relieved with submersion of the affected tissues in water. Also useful for diagnosis, white phosphorus fluoresces under a black light (Figure 26-16). White phosphorus exerts toxic effects on the heart, liver, and kidneys.[3,5]

Antidotes and Recommendations

No specific antidotes are useful. Copper sulfate is not an antidote but aids the ability to see white phosphorus for debridement purposes.

SUMMARY

Chemical burns are a diverse set of injuries requiring special attention not only to the dermal injury, but also to the potential systemic effects from chemical absorption. The extent of chemical burns is often underestimated. They often result in greater morbidity than thermal burns.

Although specific antidotes are not typically available, hydrofluoric acid is a particular exception. Thorough, early decontamination is essential. All other "neutralizing" agents should be considered secondary. When needed, consultation with a toxicologist or poison control center is recommended for systemic effects.

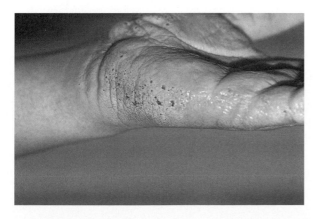

Figure 26-16. Burns from white phosphorus 4 hours after injury in high-school student. Extreme pain resolved with placement of hand in water. Particles fluoresced under ultraviolet light.

REFERENCES

1. Abraham AJ: A case of carbolic acid gangrene of the thumb, *Br J Plast Surg* 25:282-284, 1972.
2. Andersen SR: Ethylene oxide toxicity: a study of tissue reactions to retained ethylene oxide, *J Lab Clin Med* 77:346-356, 1971.
3. Appelbaum J, Ben-Hur N, Shani J: Subcellular morphological changes in the rat kidney after phosphorus burn, *Pathol Eur* 10:145-154, 1975.
4. Balakrishnan C, Leonard MW, Marson D: Trichloroethylene "burn," *J Burn Care Rehabil* 14:461-462, 1993.
5. Ben-Hur N: Phosphorus burns, *Prog Surg* 16:180-181, 1979.
6. Bordelon BM, Saffle JR, Morris SE: Systemic fluoride toxicity in a child with hydrofluoric acid burns: case report, *J Trauma* 34:437-439, 1993.
7. Boyce DE, Dickson WA: Wet cement: a poorly recognized cause of full-thickness skin burns, *Injury* 24:615-617, 1993.
8. Brown VKH, Box VL, Simpson BJ: Decontamination procedures for skin exposed to phenolic substances, *Arch Environ Health* 30:1-6, 1975.
9. Buckley DB: Skin burns due to wet cement, *Contact Dermatitis* 8:407-409, 1982.
10. Burkhart KK, Brent J, Kirk MA, et al: Comparison of topical magnesium and calcium treatment for dermal hydrofluoric acid burns, *Ann Emerg Med* 24:9-13, 1994 (abstract).
11. Cartotto RC, Peters WJ, Neligan PC, et al: Chemical burns, *Can J Surg* 39:205-211, 1996.
12. Close LG, Catlin FI, Cohn AM: Acute and chronic effects of ammonia burns on the respiratory tract, *Arch Otolaryngol* 106:151-158, 1980.
13. Corazza M, Bulciolu G, Spisani L, Virgili A: Chemical burns following irritant contact with povidone-iodine, *Contact Dermatitis* 36:115-116, 1997.
14. Cox RD, Osgood KA: Evaluation of intravenous magnesium sulfate for the treatment of hydrofluoric acid burns, *Clin Toxicol* 32:123-136, 1994.
15. Early SH, Simpson RL: Caustic burns from contact with wet cement, *JAMA* 254:528-529, 1985.
16. Edelman PA: Hydrofluoric acid burns, *Occupational Medicine* 1:89-103, 1986.
17. Eldad A, Wisoki M, Cohen H, et al: Phosphorus burns: evaluation of various modalities for primary treatment, *J Burn Care Rehabil* 16:49-55, 1995.
18. Erdmann D, Hussmann J, Kucan JO: Treatment of a severe alkali burn, *Burns* 22:141-146, 1996.
19. Flowers MW: Burn hazard with cement, *Br Med J* 1:12, 1978.
20. Greco RJ, Hartford CE, Haith LRJ, Patton ML: Hydrofluoric acid–induced hypocalcemia, *J Trauma* 28:1593-1596, 1988.
21. Hansbrough JF, Zapata-Sirvent R, Dominic W, et al: Hydrocarbon contact injuries, *J Trauma* 25:250-252, 1985.

22. Henry JA, Hla KK: Intravenous regional calcium gluconate perfusion for hydrofluoric acid burns, *Clin Toxicol* 30:203-207, 1992.

23. Jarowenko DG, Mancusi-Ungaro HRJ: The care of burns from methyl bromide (case report), *J Burn Care Rehabil* 6:119-123, 1985.

24. Jelenko C: Chemicals that "burn," *J Trauma* 14:65-72, 1974.

25. Kanerva L, Tarvainen K, Pinola A, et al: A single accidental exposure may result in a chemical burn, primary sensitization and allergic contact dermatitis, *Contact Dermatitis* 31:229-235, 1994.

26. Laitung JK, Earley M: The role of surgery in chromic acid burns: our experience with two patients, *Burns* 10:378-380, 1984.

27. Leduc D, Gris P, Lheureux P, et al: Acute and long term respiratory damage following inhalation of ammonia, *Thorax* 47:755-757, 1992.

28. Lee KA, Opeskin K: Fatal alkali burns, *Forensic Sci Int* 72:219-227, 1995.

29. Lewis GK: Chemical burns, *Am J Surg* 98:928-937, 1959.

30. Matsuno K: The treatment of hydrofluoric acid burns, *Occup Med* 46:313-317, 1996.

31. Mayer TG, Gross PL: Fatal systemic fluorosis due to hydrofluoric acid burns, *Ann Emerg Med* 14:149-153, 1985.

32. Mullett T, Zoeller T, Bingham H, et al: Fatal hydrofluoric acid cutaneous exposure with refractory ventricular fibrillation, *J Burn Care Rehabil* 8:216-219, 1987.

33. Neligan PC: Transcutaneous metal absorption following chemical burn injury, *Burns* 22:232-233, 1996.

34. Noonan T, Carter EJ, Edelman PA, Zawacki BE: Epidermal lipids and the natural history of hydrofluoric acid (HF) injury, *Burns* 20:202-206, 1994.

35. Pullin TG, Pinkerton MN, Johnston RV, Kilian DJ: Decontamination of the skin of swine following phenol exposure: a comparison of the relative efficacy of water versus polyethylene glycol/industrial methylated spirits, *Toxicol Appl Pharmacol* 43:199-206, 1978.

36. Raskin W, Canada A: Acute topical exposure to a mixture of benzene, chloracetyl chloride and xylidine, *Vet Hum Toxicol* 23:42-44, 1981.

37. Schneider MS, Mani MM, Masters FW: Gasoline-induced contact burns, *J Burn Care Rehabil* 12:140-143, 1991.

38. Summerlin WT, Walder AI, Moncrief JA: White phosphorus burns and massive hemolysis, *J Trauma* 7:476-484, 1967.

39. Wang XW, Davies JW, Zapata SR, Robinson WA: Chromic acid burns and acute chromium poisoning, *Burns* 11:181-184, 1985.

40. Williams JM, Hammad A, Cottington EC, Harchelroad FC: Intravenous magnesium in the treatment of hydrofluoric acid burns in rats, *Ann Emerg Med* 23:464-469, 1994.

41. Yano K, Hata Y, Matsuka K, et al: Experimental study on alkaline skin injuries: periodic changes in subcutaneous tissue pH and the effects exerted by washing, *Burns* 19:320-323, 1993.

42. Yano K, Hata Y, Matsuka K, et al: Effects of washing with a neutralizing agent on alkaline skin injuries in an experimental model, *Burns* 20:36-39, 1994.

Necrotizing Soft Tissue Infections and Spider Bites

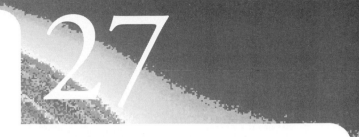

Greg Borschel
Riley Rees

INTRODUCTION

Necrotizing soft tissue infections are particularly dangerous because they often present suddenly and progress rapidly. The areas involved are often diffuse and lack a central area of necrosis typical of localized soft tissue infections. Deeper tissues are usually more infected and devitalized than the overlying tissues. Therefore the diagnosis and treatment is often delayed, leading to higher rates of morbidity and mortality.[15]

Brown recluse and hobo spider bites and the resulting skin necrosis are discussed in the sections on operations and outcomes later in this chapter.

INDICATIONS

ETIOLOGY

The first account of a necrotizing soft tissue infection was in 1883, when Fournier[20] described the rapidly progressive necrotizing infection of the scrotum that is now known as *Fournier's gangrene.* In 1924 Meleney[40] identified what we now term *necrotizing fasciitis.* Brewer and Meleney[7] later recognized the significance of bacterial synergism in necrotizing soft tissue infections. Since then, a number of pathogens, including bacteria, fungi, and protozoa, have been implicated in necrotizing infections.[1,33]

Since these earlier descriptions, different names have been given to the various forms of necrotizing soft tissue infection. Collectively, they can affect the skin, subcutaneous tissue, superficial and deep fascial planes, and muscle. All necrotizing soft tissue infections carry a significant risk of tissue destruction, wound dehiscence,[13] loss of function, sepsis, and death. Although many individual disease entities have been described in the literature, most infections leading to tissue destruction are part of a continuous spectrum of severity. They are therefore managed using a common approach[15,16,21,27] (Figure 27-1).

Early diagnosis and prompt definitive surgical management are required for successful treatment of these conditions. Comorbidities such as diabetes increase both the frequency and the severity of these infections. If no surgery is performed on a patient with a necrotizing soft tissue infection, the mortality rate is high, approaching 100% in some series,[53] despite systemic antibiotic therapy.

PATHOPHYSIOLOGY

Diabetes, wound contamination, devitalized tissue, foreign bodies, immunosuppression, chronic systemic disease, trauma, and burns have been identified as general factors predisposing to necrotizing soft tissue infections.[38] Factors that cause a particular soft tissue infection to progress to tissue loss are not well understood. Anaerobic wound environment, toxic lytic enzymes, bacterial synergy, and vessel thrombosis, however, appear to play a significant role in the transition of a wound from nonnecrotizing to necrotizing soft tissue infection.[36]

The presence of a microaerobic environment, as in ischemic tissue, facilitates the growth of *Clostridium* spores, which allow the proliferation of facultative anaerobes. The facultative anaerobes consume available tissue oxygen, thereby lowering the oxidation-reduction (redox) potential, allowing fastidious anaerobes to grow. The synergism between aerobic and anaerobic bacteria is thought to lead to tissue necrosis through a variety of mechanisms (see following discussion).

Microorganisms produce toxic enzymes that can potentiate local effects and also produce systemic effects. Rapidly progressive streptococcal infections are thought to be accelerated through elaboration of streptokinase and other proteolytic enzymes.[37] In clostridial infections, exotoxins produce multiple effects. Lecithinase, or *alpha toxin,* destroys cell membranes, increases capillary permeability, and causes hemolysis. *Theta toxin* is cardiotoxic and produces tissue necrosis and hemolysis. *Kappa toxin* and *nu toxin* act together as collagenase and hyaluronidase to dissect enzymatically through tissue planes and increase the rate of infection spread.[36] Pseudomonal necrotizing fasciitis has been shown to be mediated in part by a bacterial collagenase.[39]

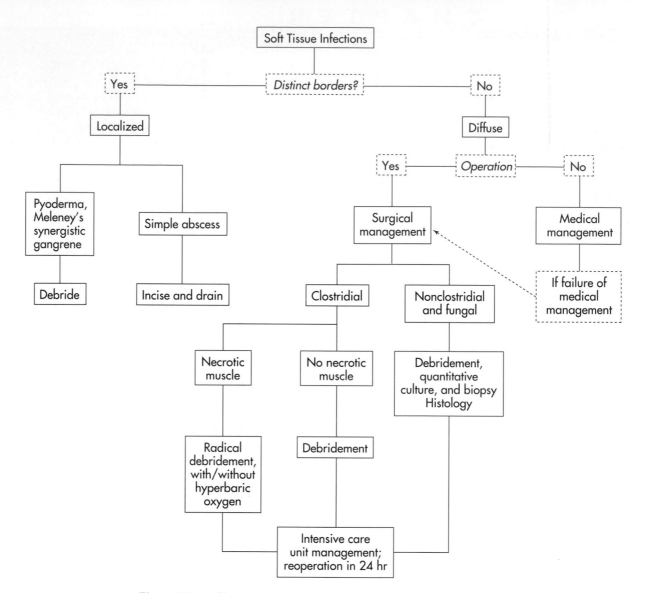

Figure 27-1. Management approach to necrotizing soft tissue infections.

Bacterial Synergism

Synergism may play a role in many necrotizing soft tissue infections because most severe wound infections are polymicrobial. In necrotizing fasciitis, for example, β-hemolytic streptococci synergize with *Staphylococcus aureus* to cause tissue loss. In animal studies, Seal and Kingston[50] found that intradermal injection of β-hemolytic streptococci produced spreading lesions (cellulitis or necrotizing fasciitis) in 12% of patients, whereas injection with *S. aureus* produced spreading lesions in 50%. When the β-hemolytic streptococci were injected with staphylococcal alpha lysin, the rate of spreading infection was 75%.

Other studies demonstrated bacterial synergy between various combinations of organisms, including *Bacteroides* and *Fusobacterium* species, *Bacteroides* and *Escherichia coli*, *Neisseria* and *Bacteroides*, *Streptococcus* and *Bacteroides*, and *Fusobacterium* and *Corynebacterium*.[8,9,28,41]

MELENEY'S SYNERGISTIC GANGRENE

In Meleney's synergistic gangrene, also known as *progressive postoperative gangrene,* and *progressive synergistic bacterial gangrene* tissue loss occurs over several days to weeks, usually after thoracic or abdominal procedures. Most often, this gangrene develops after appendectomy or empyema drainage.[14]

The etiology of Meleney's synergistic gangrene is controversial. No studies conclusively show that it has a characteristic microbiology. Meleney believed that the infection was caused by synergism between microaerophilic staphylococci and streptococci.[7]

Strong evidence indicates, however, that this infection is caused by *Entamoeba histolytica*, a parasite that first enters the intestinal tract and then migrates into surrounding tissues. Microscopic examination of pus on a wet mount can reveal the organisms, as can examination of tissue prepared with a periodic acid–Schiff stain. Evidence also suggests that concomitant bacterial infection can increase the virulence of *E. histolytica*.[33]

Over days to weeks the lesion progresses to a shaggy-edged, purplish ulcer with a granulating base. The wound is severely painful. Multiple fistulous tracts and extensive undermining may be present, requiring extensive debridement. The slow time course and multicolored appearance of the wound distinguish Meleney's synergistic gangrene from other necrotizing soft tissue infections.

Surgical excision of the lesion with concurrent use of metronidazole is the definitive treatment.[14]

CLOSTRIDIAL AND NONCLOSTRIDIAL NECROTIZING INFECTIONS

Clostridial infections differ somewhat from nonclostridial infections in their presentation, diagnosis, and treatment. Diffuse infections caused by streptococci (e.g., necrotizing fasciitis, Fournier's gangrene) initially present with painful areas of erythema. Unlike nonclostridial infections, clostridial infections present with severe pain out of proportion to the findings on physical examination. Both clostridial and nonclostridial infections present with edema extending beyond the boundaries of erythema.

For these reasons, clostridia are generally more virulent than other bacteria producing necrotizing infection. Clostridial infections can produce more severe systemic illness than nonclostridial infections. With progression of clostridial infections, the overlying skin can develop a bronzed appearance with hemorrhagic bullae. Advanced cases of both clostridial and nonclostridial infection progress to skin necrosis and crepitus.[15,38] Gram staining of clostridial infections reveals gram-positive rods without inflammatory cells.

Surgical treatment of microbiologically demonstrated clostridial infections should be more aggressive than for nonclostridial infections. Hyperbaric oxygen is a useful adjunct (see later section).

Regardless of microbial etiology, the following findings usually warrant surgical exploration with possible debridement[15]:
1. Marked edema extending beyond erythema
2. Bulla formation
3. Crepitus
4. Radiologic evidence of gas within tissues
5. Rapidly progressive infection
6. Signs of early shock
7. Failure of medical treatment

In patients with equivocal history and physical examination findings, fine-needle aspiration biopsy or incisional biopsy with frozen section can be used to establish the diagnosis quickly.[38] If frozen section demonstrates necrosis, bacteria, fungal hyphae, or vessel thrombosis, immediate debridement is indicated.[35]

FUNGAL INFECTIONS (CUTANEOUS MUCORMYCOSIS, PHYCOMYCOSIS, ZYGOMYCOSIS)

Fungal infections, often unrecognized, can be severe enough to require operative management. It is easy to underestimate both the importance and the prevalence of fungal infections.

Fungal infections typically occur in diabetic, immunocompromised, neonatal, and elderly patients. Other predisposing conditions include surgery, trauma, burns, hepatic or renal insufficiency, malnutrition, synthetic grafts, intravenous (IV) drug abuse, and use of contaminated elasticized dressing tape. Fungal infections have also occurred in otherwise healthy patients.

Fungi of the class Zygomyces and order Mucorales (genera *Rhizopus, Absidia,* and *Mucor*) are responsible for the majority of necrotizing fungal infections in humans. Affected sites can include the lungs, brain, bowels, heart, kidney, and skin with underlying structures.[1] Unlike infections caused by other organisms, fungal infections are not limited by tissue planes and often invade directly through fascia into underlying muscle and bone.

The initial presentation of cutaneous mucormycosis is variable. Usually the affected area is purple and indurated, and mold may be seen growing at the wound edge. Most cases of cutaneous mucormycosis are superficial and slowly progressing. Some penetrate below fasciae and progress rapidly, however, requiring urgent, aggressive surgical debridement.

Correct diagnosis of necrotizing fungal infections requires histologic specimens. Tissue samples should be taken from the deeper layers of the wound because a simple swab culture of the wound surface is insufficient.[34] Subcutaneous wound biopsy specimens show broad, eosinophilic, nonseptate hyphae. Hematoxylin and eosin staining must be performed carefully, since overstaining of the slide will fail to identify the eosinophilic hyphae. Follow-up fungal cultures can confirm the diagnosis.

Amphotericin B, 0.5 mg/kg/day to a maximum of 50 mg/day, is given to slow the progression of infection before debridement is performed.[55]

OPERATIONS

Even as late as the second half of the twentieth century, debate surrounded the merits of radical debridement versus incision and drainage or medical treatment alone for necrotizing soft tissue infections. In early studies the mortality rate remained high with radical debridement; however, the mortality rate without radical debridement approached 100%.[53]

Current surgical management of necrotizing soft tissue infections is directed at early recognition and aggressive debridement of all infected or devitalized tissue. Any foreign bodies in the wound should be removed. Tissue should be excised until brisk bleeding is encountered from the skin and subcutaneous fat. The wound should be bluntly probed in all directions in search of pockets or subcutaneous extensions of infected tissue.[15] If fascia and muscle are involved, they must be resected until viable tissue is identified.[13] Intraoperative quantitative culture and biopsy specimens should be obtained.

The samples sent during debridement can assist in narrowing the spectrum of antimicrobial coverage. Histologic analysis should be performed using a deep tissue specimen. Preferably, the tissue sample is obtained through intact, sterilized skin a few centimeters from the wound.[15] Subcutaneous wound fluid should be sent for Gram stain and culture. When debridement is complete, a specimen should be sent for quantitative culture and biopsy. If the border between involved and uninvolved tissue is not distinct, frozen sections can be useful in determining the necessary extent of debridement.[38]

The wound should be dressed with silver sulfadiazine (Silvadene) gauze soaked in normal saline. Repeat exploration and debridement should be performed within 24 to 48 hours, and quantitative culture and biopsy should be repeated. The culture results can assist in deciding whether subsequent debridements are necessary.

Clostridial infections may require even more aggressive debridement, and in cases affecting the limbs, amputation may be necessary.[15,52] Unfortunately, the rate of amputation in clostridial infections of the limbs has not been reported.

Initial antimicrobial coverage should include coverage for gram-positive and gram-negative organisms as well as anaerobes. In a nosocomial setting, vancomycin will provide broad gram-positive coverage until sensitivities demonstrate that penicillin analogs will be effective. An aminoglycoside (e.g., gentamicin) or a third-generation cephalosporin can be used to provide excellent gram-negative coverage. Anaerobes can be effectively covered with clindamycin or metronidazole. Amphotericin B can be used if fungal infection is suspected, based on histologic criteria, or if the patient does not improve with antibiotics. Antimicrobial coverage can be narrowed pending culture and sensitivity results.

Postoperative care should initially take place in an intensive care unit. Pulmonary artery pressure measurements, arterial pressure monitoring, and mechanical ventilatory support are indicated immediately postoperatively in many of these patients before resolution of sepsis. If a limb is affected, it should be immobilized and elevated.[55] Early adequate nutrition is essential postoperatively. Creatine kinase (CK) levels should be followed if muscle necrosis is suspected. If CK levels are high or if myoglobinuria is present, repeat exploration is indicated.[38]

Despite the lack of prospective studies, *hyperbaric oxygen* (HBO) therapy is generally thought to be of benefit in clostridial infection.[22] Currently, no clear consensus exists on the effectiveness of HBO in nonclostridial necrotizing infections.[10,24,49] Some authors claim a significant decrease in morbidity and mortality, whereas others demonstrate only a nonsignificant trend toward reduced mortality. A recent study of HBO in perineal necrotizing fasciitis (Fournier's gangrene) showed significantly reduced mortality with HBO.[24]

In most patients with clostridial necrotizing infection, we recommend that HBO be used in conjunction with prompt, aggressive debridement of the wound. Its use in nonclostridial infection has not been validated.

ABDOMINAL WALL INFECTIONS

The management of full-thickness abdominal wall infections deserves special consideration, since the source for infection is often intraperitoneal. Computed tomography (CT) scanning has been recommended to rule out intraabdominal pathology (e.g., perforated viscus).

After debridement of the infected abdominal wall, the exposed viscera should be covered with saline gauze if the wound is less than 6 cm in diameter. Primary closure of these wounds results in dehiscence.[54] When the wound is greater than 6 cm, nonabsorbable mesh provides tension-free initial closure of the wound. After resolution of sepsis, the mesh may be covered with abdominal flaps, which are preferable to skin grafts. Definitive closure of the resulting defect may be performed later using tensor fascia lata or other tissue.[13]

Perineal infections may require other procedures in addition to debridement. Fecal diversion with a colostomy is typically done to avoid fecal wound contamination.[18] Extensive scrotal debridement may require formation of a testicular thigh pouch for gonadal preservation; otherwise, orchiectomy may be indicated.[22] Suprapubic urinary diversion is indicated with extensive penile and perineal debridement and evidence of periurethral abscess.[24] Skin grafts and local advancement flaps are used to provide soft tissue coverage of the resulting defect.

BROWN RECLUSE SPIDER BITES

Entomology

The brown recluse spider *(Loxosceles reclusa)* inhabits homes and other buildings primarily in the southeastern United States, where it is a common cause of necrotic skin bites. With the expansion of interstate travel, brown recluse spiders have colonized the South and the western Midwest.

The *reclusa* is the most prevalent of the 12 species of *Loxosceles*. Members of the genus *Loxosceles* have a dark-brown violin-shaped mark on the dorsal cephalothorax, providing the name "fiddleback" spider. The spider is generally timid, nocturnal, and tends to hide in piles of debris, biting only when disturbed.[19] The spider's ovoid body is about 1 cm long, and mature spiders measure approximately 3 cm from leg tip to leg tip. All *Loxosceles* species have three pairs of eyes on the cephalothorax, which differentiates them from most other spiders, which usually have four pairs (Figure 27-2).

In 1872 Caveness[12] published the first description of skin necrosis secondary to a spider bite. The clinical diagnosis of such bites is based on a history of spider bite and seeing the brown spider. A typical appearance of the lesion is usually confirmatory but often is misleading without supporting evidence, since no diagnostic test is readily available.

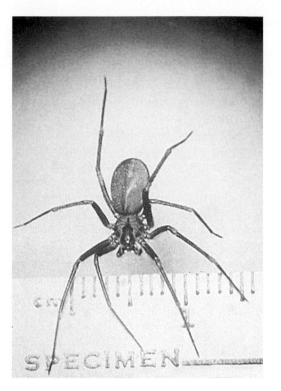

Figure 27-2. Brown recluse spider.

An early bite wound may only have superficial erythema on a large area of purplish discoloration. Later, full-thickness skin necrosis may occur (68%), or an abscess may appear at the bite site. In addition to skin lesions, brown recluse venom induces systemic effects, ranging from fever (12%), generalized myalgia (39%), gastrointestinal upset (39%), and general malaise (45%) to pulmonary, renal, or hematologic disorders (very rare).[23] Collectively, these findings are known as *loxoscelism* or *necrotic arachnidism.*

Pathophysiology

The pathophysiology of the brown recluse spider bite is not fully understood and may have several mechanisms. The venom is directly cytotoxic to endothelial cells but also appears to employ the victim's own immune system to produce neutrophil-mediated tissue necrosis.

The venom contains a protease, hyaluronidase, esterase, sphingomyelinase D, and other compounds. The sphingomyelinase D component appears to act on cell membranes and, when injected intradermally in rabbits, produces skin necrosis.[47] This component, through activating interleukin-8 (IL-8), may be the inciting factor leading to dermatonecrosis in brown recluse spider bites.

Platelet activity is affected by the brown recluse venom. In experimental animals, purified venom produces a persistent thrombocytopenia and a 24-hour decrease in complement levels. Purified venom produces dose-dependent platelet aggregation as well as secretion of serotonin, without platelet lysis or disruption of other platelet granules. Effects of brown recluse venom on platelets may represent the mechanism responsible for the platelet thrombi seen histologically. Leuko-

cytic infiltration is typically seen in tissue sections of animals dying from systemic loxoscelism. The leukocyte aggregates produce an acute shock lung syndrome with interstitial pulmonary edema.[44]

Brown recluse venom is known to potentiate release of granulocyte-macrophage colony-stimulating factor (GM-CSF) and IL-8 within hours of the initial injury. Experimental neutrophil-depleted animals do not form dermatonecrotic lesions, indicating that neutrophil activity is essential in the process leading to tissue necrosis.[42] The venom, by activating endothelial cells, causes release of GM-CSF and IL-8, which in turn stimulates adhesion of neutrophils and release of granules.[51] The invasion of unregulated neutrophils, combined with endothelial injury, leads to cell death, localized vasculitis, and tissue loss.

A small erythematous lesion appears within 6 hours of the spider bite. Slight itching and pain may occur for a short time after injury. Major symptoms do not appear for 12 hours, when the area becomes erythematous and painful; a blister may appear. After 12 to 24 hours, fever, chills, malaise, nausea, vomiting, and restlessness may occur in severe cases. Children are more likely to develop systemic signs than adults.

At about 36 hours a faint macular erythematous rash is frequently seen over the body and extremities. Areas of skin loss usually become apparent during the second day. Blanching surrounds the injection site, followed by splotchy areas of hemorrhage or venous stasis. The exact extent of necrosis, however, is not evident until 6 to 7 days after injury, when a well-outlined eschar begins to form.[19]

Histologic studies show a polymorphonuclear perivasculitis with hemorrhage in the skin and subcutaneous tissues. Later, lesions demonstrate epidermal and arterial wall necrosis, followed by gradual resolution and scarring, with occasional fat necrosis in certain anatomic areas. Rarely an eosinophilic infiltrate forms around vessel walls. Capillary thrombosis with hemorrhage has been seen experimentally. Protein-rich pink fluid may be noted between swollen collagen bundles in the rabbit.[11]

Treatment

Initial medical management of brown recluse bites should include irrigation, application of ice packs, tetanus prophylaxis, and elevation if an extremity is bitten. Erythromycin has been advocated in preventing superinfection, and antihistamines have been used for symptomatic relief.[6]

Controversy continues over the appropriate timing of surgical intervention, as well as the use of various agents to reduce the area of affected tissue.[5] Formerly, treatment included intralesional steroid injection, early wide excision of the evolving lesion, and use of antihistamines and phentolamine.[19] Early excision was performed because it was assumed that removing the residual venom would prevent further tissue necrosis. This is not true, however, and surgery worsens the situation.

It is now accepted that most lesions from brown recluse bites do not progress to significant tissue loss.[4]

Some severe bites, however, develop delayed wound healing; repeatedly reject skin grafts; produce recurrent, pyoderma gangrenosum–like lesions; and may cause deep venous thrombosis.[29-31,43-45,48]

All suspected, early brown recluse bites (less than 24 hours) should be evaluated to determine if the lesion may be caused by an infection or any of several causes of urticaria, cellulitis, or pyoderma. Development of necrotic skin within 24 to 72 hours excludes many possible causes, and thus the coexistence of systemic symptoms becomes important. In an otherwise healthy nondiabetic and immunocompetent adult, this diagnostic decision is usually made within the first 72 hours. The physician and patient can be more comfortable with the prognosis when this potentially unstable period is over and no serious illness is present.

Similarly, the suspected brown recluse bite victim should be tested to see if a hemolytic anemia or thrombocytopenia has developed. If proven or suspected brown recluse bites do not become clinically necrotic within 72 hours, a serious wound-healing problem occurs only rarely.

We recommend administering dapsone, a leukocyte inhibitor used to treat leprosy, for any brown recluse bite. Dapsone has been shown to reduce the need for surgical intervention.[45] Immediate surgical excision produces more complications than using dapsone with or without delayed surgical excision and repair.

Clinical and experimental studies demonstrate that using intralesional steroids as formerly advocated has no benefit.[4] Applying heat to brown recluse bite sites makes lesions much worse. Blisters, necrosis, and ulceration are induced when heat is applied to typical brown recluse bites. Clinically, applying ice or cold packs to bite sites greatly reduces inflammation and slows the evolution of lesions.[29]

Because secondary infections also increase localized skin temperature, erythromycin or cephalosporins should be given, as well as aspirin. Brown recluse bites have a more favorable clinical course if they are treated with ice packs and elevation. Strenuous activity should be avoided. Until definitive diagnostic methods are available, further management of brown recluse spider bites should be guided by response to therapy, cultures, and biopsies.[32]

The use of dapsone carries a small risk of methemoglobinemia, sulfonamide-induced rash, and hemolytic anemia. Therefore patients should have baseline hematologic studies, including hematocrit, before initiation of therapy. Treatment should begin with 50 to 100 mg of dapsone orally a day.[26]

A preliminary study demonstrated that a specific antivenom was as effective as dapsone. The antivenom (not commercially available) used in combination with dapsone did not enhance wound healing or improve outcome.[46]

If the patient is unresponsive to medical therapy, the lesion should be allowed to demarcate. Debridement should then be performed, followed by reconstruction. Usually only a skin graft is required because the necrosis is typically confined to the skin. Frequent follow-up is necessary because the rate of skin graft failure can be high, especially without the use of dapsone.[45]

HOBO SPIDER BITES

The hobo spider, or common aggressive house spider (*Tegenaria agrestis*), arrived in the Pacific Northwest in 1936 from Europe. It can be found indoors from March through December. The hobo spider feeds on insects and other spiders. It is more aggressive than the brown recluse and can be a common cause of spider bite in its range.

The hobo spider measures 10 to 15 mm in length and has a herringbone stripe running longitudinally on the abdomen. The bite, which may be painless, becomes indurated with an erythematous periphery. Sometimes the lesion progresses to an ulcer. About half of all hobo spider bites produce systemic signs of illness similar to brown recluse bites.

Treatment is largely medical (ice packs, elevation, tetanus prophylaxis), and surgical intervention is needed only rarely.[6]

OUTCOMES

Outcomes analysis of necrotizing infections is confusing because of the relative rarity of these infections. Prospective studies are lacking.

Currently, necrotizing soft tissue infections are managed with aggressive surgical debridement. When infections are managed medically, the mortality rate is very high, approaching almost 100% in some series. Even with appropriate surgical management, about half these patients do not survive.[10,24,49,53]

Delay in diagnosis and treatment results in increased mortality. Despite significant advances in critical care, the overall mortality rate has remained unchanged for decades. This finding may be attributed to the increasing number of elderly and immunocompromised patients with severe infections.

Most necrotizing soft tissue infections ultimately require serial surgical debridement.[10] Limb involvement, especially if circumferential, frequently results in amputation.

Additional outcome data are needed to assess better the costs and functional results of various treatments. A prospective study with adequate statistical power would be helpful, to define conclusively, for example, the role of HBO therapy in treatment of these infections.

SPIDER BITES

In 1974 Auer and Hershey[2] reported a series comparing nonoperative treatment of brown recluse bites, delayed excision of bite sites, and early excision of bite sites at 3 to 10 days. They concluded that early excision of bite sites produced the best result.

In 1983 Wasserman and Anderson[56] advocated conservative wound care and no initial antibiotics. They believed that most victims of brown recluse bites do not have necrotic wounds or secondary infections. The authors did not think that excision was indicated for most brown recluse bites.

A later prospective study compared the outcomes of patients treated with dapsone and late surgical intervention versus early surgical intervention. Patients who underwent a 2-week course of oral dapsone had fewer complications and faster wound healing than patients treated with early excision.[45] The early-excision group developed a number of complications, including delayed wound healing longer than 1 month, postoperative abscess formation, painful incisional scar requiring flap reconstruction, and postoperative ulnar nerve entrapment requiring neurolysis. Eight of 14 patients in the early-excision group experienced complications in wound healing. In the dapsone-treated delayed-excision group, only one of 17 patients required a skin graft, and patient acceptance was much higher. The dapsone group also healed with less aesthetically objectional scarring.

Brown recluse spider bites of the upper extremity can cause severe functional deficits. In one series of patients with bites to the hand, 20% had chronic hand dysfunction.[17] The most common cause of long-term hand dysfunction was chronic pain, which occurred in 16% of patients with upper extremity bites. Recurrence of pain was associated with delayed wound healing, including skin graft failure, secondary to a persistent inflammatory response. In this series, 15% of skin grafts failed. Further complications included single cases of pyoderma gangrenosum and ulnar nerve entrapment. Complications were much more common when patients were treated with early lesion excision and intralesional steroids.

These studies demonstrate that the outcome with dapsone and delayed excision is better than with early excision. Some clinicians are reluctant to use dapsone, however, citing its potential for adverse reactions, including nausea, vomiting, headache, methemoglobinemia, and hemolytic anemia, all of which are rare.[3,25,26]

REFERENCES

1. Adam RD, Hunter G, Ditomasso J, et al: Mucormycosis: emerging prominence of cutaneous infections, *Clin Infect Dis* 19:67-76, 1994.
2. Auer A, Hershey F: Surgery for necrotic bites of the brown spider, *Arch Surg* 108:612-618, 1974.
3. Berger R: Management of brown recluse spider bite, *JAMA* 251(7):889, 1984.
4. Berger RS: The unremarkable brown recluse spider bite, *JAMA* 225(9):1109-1111, 1973.
5. Berstein B, Ehrlich F: Brown recluse spider bites, *J Emerg Med* 4:457-462, 1986.
6. Blackman J: Spider bites, *J Am Board Fam Pract* 8:288-294, 1995.
7. Brewer GE, Meleney FL: Progressive gangrenous infection of the skin and subcutaneous tissues following operation for acute perforative appendicitis: a study in symbiosis, *Ann Surg* 84:438, 1926.
8. Brook I: Pathogenicity of capsulate and noncapsulate members of *Bacteroides fragilis* and *B. melaninogenicus* groups in mixed infection with *Escherichia coli* and *Streptococcus pyogenes, J Med Microbiol* 27:191-198, 1988.
9. Brook I: Encapsulated anaerobic bacteria in synergistic infections, *Microbiol Rev* 50:452-457, 1986.
10. Brown DR et al: A multicenter review of the treatment of major truncal necrotizing infections with and without hyperbaric oxygen therapy, *Am J Surg* 167:485-489, 1994.
11. Butz WC, Stacy LD, Heryfor NN: Arachnidism in rabbits: necrotic lesions due to the brown recluse spider, *Arch Pathol* 91:97-100, 1971.
12. Caveness WA: Insect bite, complicated with fever, *Nashville J Med Surg NS* 10:333, 1872.
13. Chassin JL: Operations for necrotizing infections of abdominal wall and infected abdominal wound dehiscence. In *Operative strategy in general surgery,* ed 2, New York, 1994, Springer-Verlag.
14. Davson J, Jones DM, Turner L: Diagnosis of Meleney's synergistic gangrene, *Br J Surg* 75:267-271, 1988.
15. Dellinger EP: Necrotizing soft tissue infections. In Davis JM, Shires GT, editors: *Principles and management of surgical infections,* Philadelphia, 1991, Lippincott.
16. Dellinger EP: Severe necrotizing soft tissue infections: multiple disease entities requiring a common approach, *JAMA* 246:1717, 1981.
17. DeLozier J, Reaves L, King L, Rees R: Brown recluse spider bites of the upper extremity, *South Med J* 81:181-184, 1988.
18. Dunn DL: Infection. In Greenfield LG et al, editors: *Surgery: scientific principles and practice,* ed 2, New York, 1997, Lippincott-Raven.
19. Fardon DW et al: The treatment of brown spider bite, *Plast Reconstr Surg* 40:482-488, 1967.
20. Fournier JA: Gangrene foudrayante de la verge, *Med Pratique (Paris)* 4:589, 1883.
21. Freischlag JA, Ajalat G, Busuttil RW: Treatment of necrotizing soft tissue infections: the need for a new approach, *Am J Surg* 149:751, 1985.
22. Hart GB, Lamb RC, Strauss MB: Gas gangrene, *J Trauma* 23:991-1000, 1983.
23. Hershey F, Aulenbacher C: Surgical treatment of brown spider bites, *Ann Surg* 170:300-308, 1969.
24. Hollabaugh RS et al: Fournier's gangrene: therapeutic impact of hyperbaric oxygen, *Plast Reconstr Surg* 101:94-100, 1998.
25. Ingber A et al: Morbidity of brown recluse spider bites, *Acta Derm Venereol (Stockh)* 71:337-340, 1991.
26. Iserson K: Methemoglobinemia from dapsone therapy for a suspected brown spider bite, *J Emerg Med* 3:285-288, 1985.
27. Kaiser RE, Cerra FB: Progressive necrotizing surgical infections: a unified approach, *J Trauma* 21:349, 1981.
28. Kelly MJ: The quantitative and histological demonstration of pathologic synergy between *Escherichia coli* and *Bacteroides fragilis* in guinea pig wounds, *J Med Microbiol* 11:513-523, 1978.
29. King LE Jr, Rees RS: Brown recluse spider bites: keep cool, *JAMA* 254:2895-2896, 1985.

30. King LE Jr, Rees R: Dapsone treatment of a brown recluse spider bite, *JAMA* 250:648, 1983.

31. King LE Jr, Rees R: Management of brown recluse spider bite, *JAMA* 251:889-890, 1984.

32. King LE Jr, Rees R: Treatment of brown recluse spider bites, *J Am Acad Dermatol* 14:691-692, 1986 (letter).

33. Kingston D, Seal DV: Current hypotheses on synergistic microbial gangrene, *Br J Surg* 77:260-264, 1990.

34. Lehrer RI et al: Mucormycosis, *Ann Intern Med* 93:93-108, 1980.

35. Lewis RT: Necrotizing soft-tissue infections, *Infect Dis Clin North Am* 6:693, 1992.

36. Lewis RT: Soft tissue infection. In Meakins JL, editor: *Surgical infections: diagnosis and treatment,* New York, 1994, Scientific American.

37. McCafferty EL: Suppurative fasciitis as the essential feature of hemolytic streptococcus gangrene, *Surgery* 24:438, 1948.

38. McHenry CR, Malangoni MA: Necrotizing soft tissue infections. In Fry DE, editor: *Surgical infections,* New York, 1995, Fry.

39. Meade JW, Muller CB: Necrotizing infections of subcutaneous tissue and fascia, *Ann Surg* 168:274, 1968.

40. Meleney FL: Hemolytic streptococcus gangrene, *Arch Surg* 9:317, 1924.

41. Onderdonk AB, Kasper DL, Mansheim BJ, et al: Experimental animal models of anaerobic infections, *Rev Infect Dis* 1:291-301, 1979.

42. Patel K, Modur V, Zimmerman G, et al: The necrotic venom of the brown recluse spider induces dysregulated endothelial cell-dependent neutrophil activation: differential induction of GM-CSF, IL-8, and E-selectin expression, *J Clin Invest* 94:631-642, 1994.

43. Rees R, Fields J, King LE Jr: Do brown recluse spider bites induce pyoderma gangrenosum? *South Med J* 78:283-287, 1985.

44. Rees R, O'Leary P, King L: The pathogenesis of systemic loxoscelism following brown recluse spider bites, *J Surg Res* 35:1-10, 1983.

45. Rees RS et al: Brown recluse spider bites: a comparison of early surgical excision versus dapsone and delayed surgical excision, *Ann Surg* 202:659-663, 1985.

46. Rees RS et al: The diagnosis and treatment of brown recluse spider bites, *Ann Emerg Med* 16:945-949, 1987.

47. Rees RS et al: Interaction of brown recluse spider venom on cell membranes: the inciting mechanism? *J Invest Dermatol* 83:270-275, 1984.

48. Rees RS et al: Management of the brown recluse spider bite, *Plast Reconstr Surg* 68:768-773, 1981.

49. Riseman JA et al: Hyperbaric oxygen therapy for necrotizing fasciitis reduces mortality and the need for debridements, *Surgery* 108:847-850, 1990.

50. Seal DV, Kingston D: Streptococcal necrotizing faciitis: development of an animal model to study its pathogenesis, *Br J Exp Pathol* 69:813-831, 1988.

51. Smith CW, Micks DW: The role of polymorphonuclear leukocytes in the lesion caused by the venom of the brown spider, *Lab Invest* 22:90-93, 1970.

52. Smith DJ et al: Drug injection injuries of the upper extremity, *Ann Plast Surg* 22:19-24, 1989.

53. Stone HH, Martin JD: Synergistic necrotizing cellulitis, *Ann Surg* 175:702-711, 1972.

54. Stone HH et al: Management of acute full-thickness losses of the abdominal wall, *Ann Surg* 193:612, 1981.

55. Vainrub B et al: Wound zygomycosis (mucormycosis) in otherwise healthy adults, *Am J Med* 84:546-548, 1988.

56. Wasserman G, Anderson P: Loxoscelism and necrotic arachnidism, *Clin Toxicol* 21:451-472, 1983.

CHAPTER

Radiation Effects

Gregory R. D. Evans

INTRODUCTION

Radiation therapy is being used with increasing frequency for both definitive and adjunctive treatment of cancer and other disease etiologies. Definitive irradiation may allow functional preservation of structures that otherwise would be excised. Adjunctive therapy after surgical resection of the primary lesion treats regional lymph nodes and sites of primary extension in patients with a high risk for microscopic involvement.[56] When used with surgical excision, the amount of resection and subsequent deformity from extirpation may be minimized.

Despite the apparent benefits of radiotherapy, the resultant chronic changes may be lifelong and cumulative. Reconstruction of complex wounds after adjuvant radiation therapy requires a change in the approach to the patient. These chronic changes and the need for well-vascularized, undamaged tissue have complicated the reconstructive purview for the plastic surgeon.

INDICATIONS

With the discovery of x-rays by Wilhelm Konrad Roentgen in 1895, ionizing radiation became a diagnostic tool and a therapeutic modality. The goals of ionizing radiation, alone or with surgical extirpation, are local regional tumor control and functional preservation. High doses of irradiation can be delivered with specialized techniques to minimize late complications. Radiation portals precisely outline tissues at risk and exclude uninvolved regions by applying individualized treatment blocks. Verification films and computed tomography (CT) assist with the development of individualized treatment plans.[56]

Despite success in current technology, changes occur from radiation, as first exemplified by the development of acute radiation dermatitis[13] and soon after by a cutaneous malignancy of the dorsal hand.[28] The daily dose of radiation is one of the most important factors in the development of radiation

sequelae. To avoid such sequelae, variations in dosing should not exceed 10% over the portal being treated. Body contour can account for variations in dose, necessitating the use of filters for dosing consistency and equality.

TECHNIQUES

Traditionally the absorbed dose of radiation has been described in units called *rads,* but contemporary designation uses the term *gray* (Gy).[56] The equivalent units of energy for this dosing are as follows:

$$1 \text{ joule/kg} = 1 \text{ Gy} = 100 \text{ rads}$$
$$1 \text{ rad} = 0.01 \text{ Gy} = 1 \text{ cGy}$$

The therapeutic doses for carcinoma depend on tissue toxicity but normally range from 45 to 80 Gy.[12]

Ionizing radiation is classified as particulate or electromagnetic.[56] *Particulate radiation* is created by high-energy subatomic particles, such as electrons, protons, neutrons, and helium (alpha) particles. *Electromagnetic radiation* is composed of waves of electrical and magnetic energy transmitted as discrete photons. They are usually from a naturally occurring photon source that collides with a metal target, yielding a shower of electromagnetic energy.

DELIVERY

Radiation may be delivered by external beam therapy (e.g., linear accelerators, cobalt[60] [^{60}Co] units) or by brachytherapy, with radioactive isotopes applied close to the lesion. *External beam therapy* is prescribed with daily fractions (200 cGy/day) over a 5- to 6-week course. In contrast, *brachytherapy* allows a continuous application of radiation to the tumor bed.

Ionizing irradiation is administered from specialized machines that emit gamma rays from housed isotopes (e.g., ^{60}Co) or from generated x-rays 1000 times more potent than those used for diagnostic purposes. Different photon energies allow more selective administration of treatment to the tumor while sparing superficial structures.

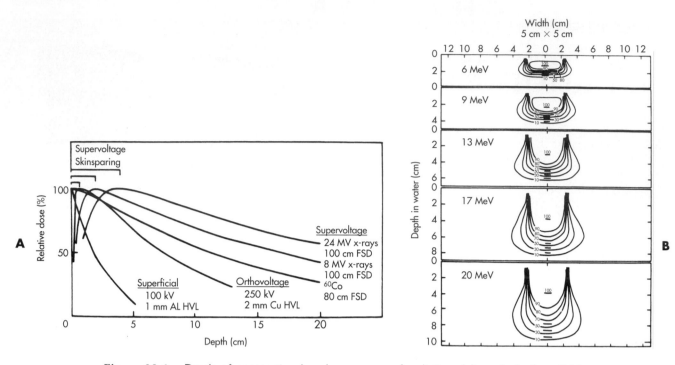

Figure 28-1. Depth of penetration based on energy of radiation delivered. **A,** Superficial, orthovoltage, and supervoltage irradiation. *FSD,* Focal skin distance. **B,** Penetration depth and width with different megaelectron volt doses.

Electron beam energy allows precise localization of the radiation to superficial lesions while sparing underlying critical structures. *Proton beam therapy* (radiosurgery) has limited application and is primarily used to deposit large amounts of radiation to a well-defined volume of tumor while sparing intervening tissues. Since precision is based on millimeters, pretherapy mapping is critical.

Finally, *neutron irradiation* is reserved for patients with a history of aggressive therapy or with large tumor burdens. The *radiation biologic effectiveness* (RBE) describes the relative efficiency of different radiation beams in terms of a dose ratio to produce the same level of cellular damage. When comparing particulate energy, the RBE is greatest with neutron therapy.[33]

As with any form of energy, radiation from an external source loses energy as it enters the skin. The depth at which the maximum radiation dose (D_{max}) is delivered is determined in part by the energy of the radiation (Figure 28-1). *Superficial irradiation* penetrates only a short distance and has similar dosing to diagnostic irradiation (10 to 125 kiloelectron volts, or keV). *Orthovoltage irradiation,* (125 to 400 keV) penetrates more deeply but is currently of historic value only because of its complications (osteonecrosis).[56] *Supervoltage irradiation* (greater than 400 keV) penetrates the deepest and has been employed in the treatment of deep-seeded tumors (e.g., in pelvis) while sparing superficial structures such as the skin.

Brachytherapy

Brachytherapy involves the placement of radioactive isotopes within the tumor bed (Figure 28-2). Radiation is delivered to the tumor bed over a predetermined number of minutes or hours based on the isotope selected and its radioactive properties (e.g., depth of penetration, degradation) (Figure

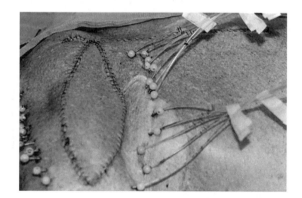

Figure 28-2. Placement of brachytherapy catheters after resection of recurrent malignant fibrohistiocytoma and reconstruction with transverse rectus abdominis myocutaneous (TRAM) rotational flap to groin in 45-year-old male.

28-3). Advantages include reduction in overall treatment time and sparing of uninvolved tissue.

Brachytherapy catheters are placed at surgery, usually after tumor extirpation and before wound coverage. The catheters must be placed such that the threading of the isotopes can be easily performed. Catheters with significant bends will impede the delivery of isotopes. This may preclude the use of brachytherapy catheters in certain anatomic locations. Because radiation is localized within 3 cm of the catheters, considerably less normal tissue damage occurs.

Tissue hypoxia from previous surgery and therapy greatly reduces the sensitivity of radiotherapy, and brachytherapy can increase the efficacy of radiation delivery.[56] Because of potential wound complications, catheters are not threaded

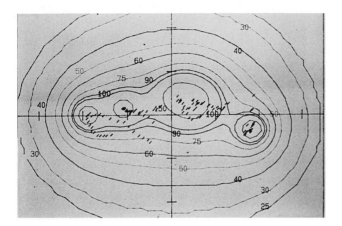

Figure 28-3. Delivery dose versus distance from isotopes placed for brachytherapy.

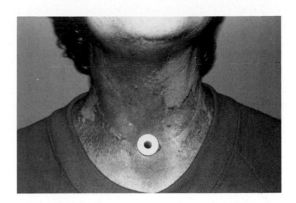

Figure 28-4. Acute radiation changes demonstrated by erythema and inflammation in 44-year-old woman after undergoing 6 weeks of radiation therapy (50 Gy) following total pharyngolaryngectomy and reconstruction with free jejunal transfer.

with isotopes until postoperative day 5. Brachytherapy catheters can be placed in a variety of locations, including intracavitary positioning for uterine or vaginal tumors and within bile ducts, bronchi, or the esophagus (intraluminal brachytherapy). The catheters can be easily removed after therapy is concluded.

Plesiotherapy involves the treatment of superficial lesions with a mold containing a radioactive source. Its use is usually reserved for the palate, nasopharynx, nasal septum, and eyes.

Radiation Dose

External beam irradiation remains the most widely available treatment approach to cancer therapy. The concept of *fractionating irradiation* allows treatment of the cancer while not exceeding the tolerance of the surrounding normal tissue, thus providing adequate time for repair. In general the larger the daily dose of irradiation, the lower is the total dose that can be administered because of normal tissue tolerance.[56]

Unfortunately, the dose necessary for tumor irradiation is indexed to the tumor volume. Consequently the larger the irradiation dose, the more tumor cells are killed. Thus a balance must be struck between tumor cells killed and total dose administered, which is limited by radiation effects on normal tissue. Standard treatment regimens attempt to exploit the differences in cell kinetics between tumor cell populations and the normal tissue. Delivery fractions of conventional radiation normally involve 180 to 200 cGy over 24-hour intervals. A total dose of 50 to 70 Gy is usually achieved over 6 to 7 weeks.

Altered fractionation defines an external beam radiation schedule outside the realm of conventional treatment. This includes *hyperfractionation,* used to treat rapidly growing tumors and local disease that cannot be surgically resected. Radiation is delivered by two small daily doses separated by 6-hour intervals.

Accelerated fractionation defines a radiation treatment schedule that delivers the same daily and total dose as conventional regimens but over a shorter period (e.g., a boost dose after conventional fractionation). *Hypofractionation* is generally applied to palliative treatment of advanced tumors (e.g., spinal cord compression) or definitive treatment of malignant mela-

noma. Large daily doses are administered, restricting the total dose.

RADIATION INJURY

The nature of tissue injury from ionizing radiation is thought to be caused by the following two discrete mechanisms:

1. Deoxyribonucleic acid (DNA) disruption, which can cause a lethal injury if genes critical to routine cellular processes are affected. More often, however, cell death occurs from the disruption of normal cell division. In general, cells are most sensitive to radiation in the G2-M phase and most resistant in the last S phase.[74]
2. Generation of oxygen free-radicals, which has a direct toxic effect on the cell, culminating in cell death. Consequently, radiosensitivity is partly based on the oxygen tension in the tumor.

The effect of radiotherapy on the molecular structure appears to be an all-or-none phenomenon. The extent of energy absorption by normal structures depends on the absolute number and the energy level of the ionizing particles.

The *alpha/beta ratio* is a function of tissue radiosensitivity and is based on acute and late reacting tissues. Acute reacting tissues demonstrate the effects of irradiation during the course of treatment, usually by an inflammatory response. Late radiation effects most frequently present as scar tissue. Thus the alpha/beta ratio specifically relates to the radiobiologic repair of normal tissues.

Acute Effects

Acute radiation effects occur during or immediately after the course of radiation therapy. They are characterized by an inflammatory response in rapidly proliferating tissues, such as the skin and mucosal surfaces. Most patients manifest these changes by erythema and hyperpigmentation of the skin (Figure 28-4).

Because of their rapidly dividing nature, keratinocytes are sensitive to ionizing radiation. This early erythematous reaction is believed to be related to activation of proteolytic enzymes, resulting in an increase in capillary permeability and local inflammatory response.[7,48,66] The main erythematous reaction may appear approximately 8 days after a single dose and peak at a set time frame later. Because of the fractionation, the erythematous reactions from each dose overlap. Mucosal surfaces may exhibit mucositis or cystitis limited to the portal of therapy. Dry desquamation occurs at moderate doses and moist desquamation at higher doses.[42]

The acute response usually resolves within 1 month after cessation of radiation therapy.

Late Effects

Late radiation effects can occur in any tissue. No association exists between the intensity of the acute reaction and the late radiation effects. Factors that appear important in the development of chronic changes, however, are total dose and fractionation.

Tissue fibrosis appears to be the most common histologic effect of late radiation changes. Alopecia and xerostomia may also occur. Late radiation changes produce an irregular epidermis, with areas of atrophy alternating with variable hyperplasia. Pigmentary changes may be seen, with thickening and fibrosis of the skin and subcutaneous tissues (Figure 28-5). These pigmentary changes are believed to result from the increased transfer of melanin from the melanocytes to kerati-

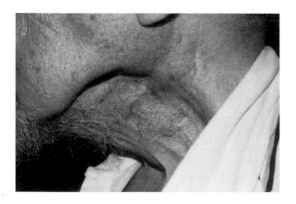

Figure 28-5. Chronic radiation changes demonstrated by pigmentation, atrophy, alopecia, and woody and fibrotic skin in 72-year-old male with prior irradiation and neck dissection.

nocytes through melanosomes.[7,56] Further epidermal melanocytes may be deposited in the dermis and engulfed by macrophages, resulting in pigmentary changes.

The histopathology of chronic irradiated tissue reveals hyalinization and swelling of collagen bundles. Many of the changes seen are thought to be caused by a decrease in the proliferative ability of fibroblasts for wound healing.[7,38,66] Telangiectasia, sebaceous and sweat gland dysfunction, necrosis, and the potential for tumorigenesis are present.

Tolerance Dose

A National Cancer Institute (NCI) task force has determined the tolerance dose (TD) of tissues and organs as a function of the likelihood of a treatment-related complication in 5 years using conventional fractionation. Thus the minimal TD is defined as that dose that will create a complication in 5% of the patients at 5 years for that specific tissue (TD 5/5). As the dose increases, the TD ratio also increases. For example, the dose causing 50% complications at 5 years is expressed as TD 50/5.[9,56]

SKIN. The organ that most reveals the effects of radiation therapy is the skin. The clinical endpoint for complications is defined as skin necrosis and telangiectasia. For a 100-cm² radiation field, the TD 5/5 is equivalent to 55 Gy. The complication rate increases to 50% when 70 Gy is used. This TD frequently limits the ability to deliver the desired tumor-killing energy.[9,44,56]

MUSCLE. Muscle is more difficult to assess. Using clinical myositis as the endpoint, however, the TD 1/5 is considered to be 50 Gy.[9,56]

BONE. The effects of irradiation on bone have been based on location. The humoral and femoral heads have a TD 5/5 of 52 Gy and a TD 50/5 of 65 Gy based on necrosis and fracture.

The endpoint for osteonecrosis of the mandible and temporomandibular joint is difficult to determine. The degree of trismus related to radiation has not been fully evaluated. The risk for osteoradionecrosis of the mandible depends on the tumor location, dental status, radiation technique, and total dose (Figure 28-6). Assuming excellent dental care, external

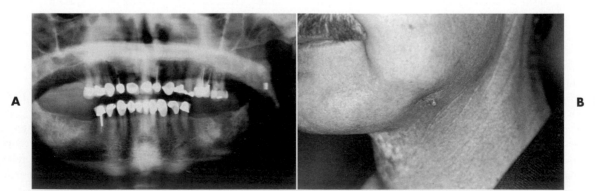

Figure 28-6. Previous squamous cell carcinoma of floor of mouth in 43-year-old male was treated with surgical resection and radiotherapy. Several years later, patient had osteoradionecrosis of right mandible: **A,** radiographic view; **B,** clinical presentation of chronic draining sinus tract.

beam irradiation, and no initial bony involvement, the TD 5/5 is considered to be 65 Gy when one third or less of the mandible is irradiated and 60 Gy when larger radiation portals are used.[9,56,67]

Pathologic fractures are determined to be the endpoint of radiation complications related to the ribs. The data are based on experience with chest wall irradiation after breast cancer. If tangential irradiation is delivered to one third or less of the rib cage, the TD 2/5 was 45 Gy, TD 8/5 was 58 Gy, and TD 20/5 was 65 Gy.

Growth arrest occurs only in patients with incomplete bone maturation and is ultimately based on the patient's age and degree of maturation. Although bone hypoplasia has been reported with doses as small as 12 Gy, the most significant risk is with doses greater than 35 Gy. This risk is increased in patients less than 2 years old who receive radiation therapy.[46,56]

All components of bone are affected by radiation therapy. Epiphyseal plate irradiation has the greatest effect on growth in endochondral bones. Arrested chondrogenesis occurs, with reduced chondroblasts and disorderly maturation. Radiation affects periosteal activity, causing errors in bone formation and remodeling.

NERVES. Peripheral nerves are somewhat radioresistant. Doses for a TD 5/5 appear to be 60 Gy for treatment of the brachial plexus and cauda equina.

BLOOD VESSELS. Radiation changes for blood vessels have not been well categorized by the NCI task force.[76] These are outlined in clinical studies discussed later.

Malignant Change

Since radiation effects cellular DNA, the risk of late malignant changes is present. Intermediate doses (2 to 10 Gy) seem to be more tumorigenic, but it is difficult to calculate the risk of this tumorigenesis. Previous studies demonstrated that the incidence of malignant cutaneous lesions in patients who have undergone irradiation is increased, especially in sun-exposed areas.[7,26] Basal and squamous cell carcinomas are typically seen within chronic dermatitis. Sarcomas induced by irradiation, although less common, are highly malignant with poor long-term outcomes.

The latency periods between the conclusion of radiotherapy and tumor presentation may be quite long.

OPERATIONS

The mechanism of wound healing is a complex process that involves cellular migration, proliferation, and differentiation, as well as a variety of growth factors used to accelerate the dermal and epidermal processes. Radiation adversely affects soft tissue by modifying the normal environment.

The dermis is the tissue principally responsible for wound healing and most influenced by late radiation ef-

fects. With a full dose of irradiation, endothelial, mesenchymal, and epithelial cells have severely impaired proliferative capacity.[2,59]

Decreasing the number of blood vessels impairs tissue oxygen delivery and the normal angiogenic response to wounding. The various responses in the vasculature lead to wound ischemia and delayed wound healing. Fibroblasts cultured from irradiated wounds have decreased ability to attach to the substrate and form colonies and also have significantly longer cell lines.

One year after radiation therapy, impaired lymphatic drainage is thought to be related to transient changes in the connective tissue associated with the evolution of late radiation effects. Thus the usually efficient regeneration of lymphatics is impaired.[58] To add to this difficulty, radiation impairs normal polymorphonuclear antibacterial function, leaving irradiated tissue more susceptible to infection.[59] Also, a general release of polypeptide growth factors appears to occur from irradiated cells in vitro, but the clinical applicability of this phenomenon is not yet fully appreciated.[75]

Further understanding of these factors is necessary, as well as the development of ways to reduce perioperative wound complications after surgical resection and adjuvant radiation.

HYPERBARIC OXYGEN

The use of hyperbaric oxygen (HBO) in the management of poor wound healing and radiation necrosis was introduced in the mid-1980s.[45] In the normal wound, a steep oxygen gradient exists between the normal and damaged tissue. The mechanism whereby hyperbaric oxygen is able to revascularize irradiated tissue is thought to occur through the creation of steep oxygen gradients naturally present in noncompromised wounds. These oxygen gradients allow the body to recognize irradiated tissue as being a true wound, and the chemotactic and biochemical messenger response proceeds as in normal tissue angiogenesis.

Clinically, HBO may or may not be effective in complicated wounds. The use of well-vascularized tissues (e.g., free fibula for osteoradionecrosis of the mandible) may provide wound healing in a one-step, more cost-effective manner. The use of HBO for children with radiation-induced bone and soft tissue complications appear safe and results in few significant adverse effects.[4]

THERAPEUTIC GOALS AND CHARACTERISTICS

With the efficacy of combined therapy in the treatment of malignancies, the approach to the patient undergoing surgical reconstruction has become more complex. The goal of reconstructive cancer surgery is maintenance or enhancement of the quality of life, as measured by resultant function and cosmesis. In addition, the availability of reconstructive techniques combined with radiotherapy allows resection of large tumors that otherwise would be unresectable. The reconstructive technique chosen should have the following optimal characteristics[34]:

1. Reliability
2. Expediency
3. Good functional results and cosmesis

Reliability is perhaps the most important factor in any type of oncologic reconstruction. A failed reconstruction that prolongs hospitalization time and increases cost does not improve the quality of life. Furthermore, prolonged reconstruction is time taken away from family or additional adjuvant therapy.[34]

Expediency must also be considered, and in most cases a one-stage reconstruction should be employed. Patients seldom benefit from multistage procedures that take several months to complete, delaying adjuvant therapy and interfering with valuable family time.[34]

The type and grade of the tumor as well as the patient's psychologic makeup determine the reconstructive method that will provide the best function and contour.

EVALUATION AND COMPLICATIONS

The key to patient evaluation and surgical planning is to avoid the potential complications that may arise from irradiated tissue. Radiation changes appear to be lifelong and cumulative. The longer the interval between radiation exposure and surgery, the greater is the tendency for complications to occur.

When evaluating a patient, the physician must estimate degree of tissue damage using the history and radiation dosing. Although no direct correlation exists, the higher the radiation dose, the more likely a complication will occur. Examination of the skin may reveal atrophy, pigmentary changes, and alopecia. The skin may feel woody, firm, and leathery with indications of deep fibrosis. Skin with this appearance must be approached with care. Meticulous handling of the tissues, avoidance of tension, and strict sterile technique are mandatory for successful wound closure.

When adherence to these guidelines are not possible, alternative well-vascularized tissue must be considered. We believe that free tissue transfers or pedicle flaps outside the field of irradiation must be employed if any doubt exists regarding tissue viability. The placement of viable healthy tissue increases wound healing factors impaired by radiotherapy. Surgery or an underlying connective tissue disease may accelerate or result in an excessive expression of late radiation effects without affecting the basic radiobiologic process occurring in the epidermis.[73]

It is still unclear how other medical conditions, such as collagen vascular disease, diabetes, and neurologic disease, affect the long-term outcomes of radiotherapy.

POSTOPERATIVE THERAPY

Postoperative radiation has the advantage of promptly resecting the disease to relieve symptoms associated with the tumor, allowing surgery in nonirradiated tissue and reducing the potential for metastatic spread. Disadvantages of postoperative radiation therapy include (1) the increased dose required to encompass the entire surgical bed plus margins and (2) the hypoxic effects of scarring. A further concern is the potential for repopulating the tumor bed in the hiatus between surgery and radiotherapy.

Radiotherapy is usually begun 3 to 4 weeks after wound healing. A single dose of 18 Gy has been demonstrated to reduce wound strength at 90 days to levels 30% to 50% lower than in nonirradiated wounds. When a healing wound was irradiated within 5 days of surgery, the effects on wound healing were the same as preirradiation of the skin. If perioperative irradiation was delayed for 12 days after the incision, the healing rate was slowed only slightly, and wound strength ultimately equaled that of nonirradiated skin.[56]

PREOPERATIVE THERAPY

Preoperative irradiation is administered at a lower total dose to a smaller field that includes a 5-cm to 7-cm margin around the tumor and draining lymphatics. The advantage of preoperative radiation therapy includes possible tumor necrosis and regression, allowing easier surgical resection.

Problems with preoperative irradiation are the potential for wound complications and the delay in surgical extirpation of a tumor. The rate of wound complications for sarcoma ranges from 6% to 37%.[70] Factors that increase this wound morbidity include age, tumor location, blood loss, and prolonged wound healing. In an attempt to decrease these wound complications, standard surgical practice has been to wait 1 week for each week of radiotherapy before surgical resection. Closure of these wounds with well-vascularized tissue from free tissue transfer or pedicled flaps also may decrease these potential wound problems.

BRACHYTHERAPY

Wound healing issues involving brachytherapy are unique (see earlier discussion). The volume of tissue is not significant because brachytherapy administers well-localized radiation.

Wound healing complications associated with brachytherapy have primarily been associated with the interval between surgery and insertion of the radioactive source. Placement of isotopes before the fifth postoperative day has been associated with increased complications. The judicious use of well-vascularized tissue has decreased these problems.[69]

HEAD AND NECK

Treatment of head and neck tumors typically employs radiotherapy. Larson et al[50,51] demonstrated at least one significant complication involving bone or soft tissue in 40% to 70% of these patients, depending on the site of primary disease. Judicious use of preoperative antibiotics is important for the patient undergoing head and neck surgery, since atrophy of the salivary glands from radiotherapy may alter the antibacterial and lubricating action of saliva.

External and intraoral incisions must be designed with full knowledge that wound dehiscence may cause exposure of tissue. The altered tissue response to desiccation or bacterial contamination may result in a catastrophic event.[12] Thus incisions should be designed to protect the carotid vessels. In both human and animal experiments, disruption of its vasa vasorum places a carotid vessel in an extremely vulnerable position to exposure and intraoperative manipulation. Premature atherosclerosis and fibrosis of the adventitia have also occurred.[36]

Irradiation and neck dissection can also adversely affect the internal jugular vein. Fisher et al[27] noted clotted internal jugular vasculature on the CT scans of two patients who underwent surgical neck dissection after radiotherapy. While evaluating ultrasound scans of patients who had undergone modified neck dissection after radiotherapy, Docherty et al[14] noted that the flow pattern in the internal jugular vein was normal in only 18% (Figure 28-7).

Primary closure of intraoral defects must be done with caution because fistula formation often occurs. Tissue ischemia and edge necrosis from excessive tension are the most common causes of fistula formation. Further, local infection may lead to suture line dehiscence. If fistula formation occurs, adequate debridement and drainage are the first attempts at closure. HBO treatment may also be of some benefit, but in our experience the success at spontaneous closure in an irradiated field is variable.

Although occurring infrequently, osteoradionecrosis of the mandible is another problem. HBO therapy may be of some assistance. In our practice the resection and replacement of the bone with a well-vascularized, free bone transfer is the best treatment for this difficult problem.

Free tissue transfer has become an important part of the primary and secondary treatment of head and neck malignancies. The external carotid artery and internal jugular

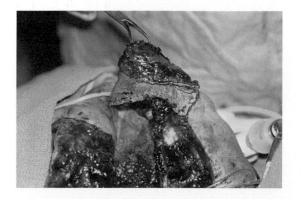

Figure 28-7. Recurrent squamous cell carcinoma of floor of mouth in 52-year-old female was initially treated with radiotherapy, and patient underwent surgical resection for recurrence. Reconstruction with radial forearm free flap became cyanotic on postoperative day 5; internal jugular vein had thrombosed.

vein in an end-to-side anastomosis are the vessels most frequently used, providing a robust blood supply. The vessels must be assessed before attempting the transfer. If the vessels are thrombosed, the opposite neck should be considered. This may require vein grafts; in our practice the saphenous vein is most often used. All necrotic tissue must be replaced with well-vascularized tissue outside the irradiated field. The flaps should be designed to fill the three-dimensional defect created.

The intraoral defect and the lumen must be closed carefully. Absorbable sutures in a simple or vertical mattress fashion are used to avoid necrosis of the flap edges. Free tissue transfers must be carefully monitored. The use of a skin paddle placed intraorally allows for Doppler monitoring of the flap. Alternately, if the skin paddle is placed externally, the muscle or fascial lining of the flap can be sutured to the native mucosa. This can be allowed to epithelialize or can be skin grafted to complete an adequate internal lining (Figure 28-8).

CHEST WALL AND LOWER BACK

Resection of chest wall lesions in previously irradiated fields also requires the transfer of well-vascularized tissue if tension or skin ischemia is a consideration. Radionecrosis or ulceration of the chest wall after radiotherapy may range from small lesions not compromising pulmonary function to large lesions requiring resection and with possible life-threatening consequences. With current technology and adjustment of radiation portals, radionecrosis has decreased in incidence.[11,30,77]

Frequently the lesion appears as an inverted cone, with the cutaneous component representing a much larger defect. As with any ulcerative lesion, the potential for recurrent tumor must be evaluated.

In the primary or secondary reconstructive setting the latissimus dorsi, pectoralis major, rectus abdominis muscle, or the omentum can provide the necessary tissue for adequate wound healing (Figure 28-9). Occasionally the latissimus dorsi or the pectoralis major muscle may be included in the radiation portal. The surgeon must carefully evaluate the pedicle before flap transfer and should consider avoiding the use of flaps in previously irradiated fields.[3] Polymethylmethacrylate or other autogenous substances for rib reconstruction must be used cautiously in these patients. Simple closure of the skin over such a reconstruction may not allow adequate vascular cover. Placement of a flap over this autogenous material may prevent future complications.

Although lower back wounds are rarely suitable for split-thickness skin grafts, such grafts are certainly an option when repairing smaller wounds. The success of skin grafts is unpredictable, however, especially in irradiated tissue. The effects of shearing may compromise long-term protection and durability.[18] The use of local skin and fasciocutaneous flaps to the back is limited by radiation-induced constraints on the vascular pedicle and the unpredictability of their random components. Thoracolumbar fascial extensions of the latissimus dorsi

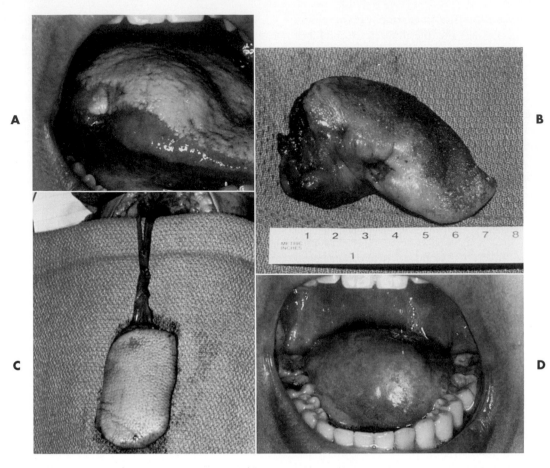

Figure 28-8. **A,** Squamous cell carcinoma of right buccal tongue in 21-year-old oriental female. **B,** Tongue after surgical resection. **C,** Reconstruction with radial forearm free flap. **D,** Eight months and after radiation therapy, flap is well healed with native tongue.

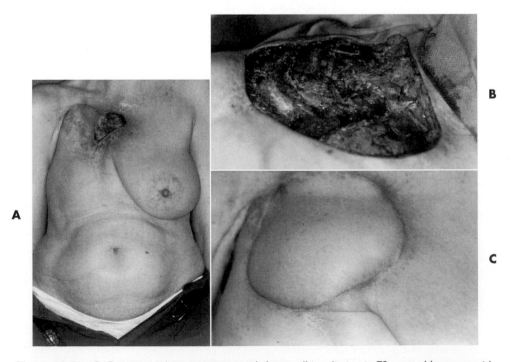

Figure 28-9. **A,** Previous right mastectomy and chest wall irradiation in 72-year-old woman with ulcerative chest lesion. **B,** Defect after surgical resection. **C,** Healing wound 2 months after reconstruction with rotational TRAM flap.

muscle, gluteus maximus muscle rotation, and paraspinous muscle have been used individually or in combination.

The transverse rectus abdominis myocutaneous (TRAM) flap has been described for back reconstruction. This flap has been transposed through the retropubic space of Retzius and is brought out near the defect next to the ischial tuberosity. A superiorly or inferiorly based pedicle can be used in the reconstruction. Flap size may be restricted by the ability to close the donor site, and the "reach" may be limited by the liver on the right.

Omentum has also been used for lower back closures. Frequently the omentum is used when tumor resection involves entering the peritoneal cavity. It can conform to multiple geometric configurations in the retroperitoneal cavity and can cover wounds up to 600 cm in size. Laparotomy is required, however, and the potential exists for fat necrosis and delayed abdominal hernia. Despite these limitations, the omentum does provide the surgeon with vascularized tissue for repairing wounds frequently compromised by the factors previously discussed.

Finally, free tissue transfer offers the advantage of well-vascularized distant tissue for stable reconstruction. The paucity of free flap recipient vessels and the need for close monitoring have convinced us to use local tissue for coverage when possible (Figure 28-10).

A systematic approach is needed to repair chest wall and lower back wounds in the irradiated patient. Multiple methods may be necessary to repair one wound in the same patient. Preoperatively the surgical team must devise more than one reconstructive plan in the event the resected area is larger than anticipated or potential recipient vessels are inadequate. All options should be available to the surgeon, and each wound must be treated individually with the most appropriate techniques available.[18]

ABDOMEN AND PERINEUM

With the frequency of visceral tumors, the abdomen and perineum are exposed to a variety of treatments for tumor control. Ulcerations are not as common as other manifestations of radiation exposure, including enteritis, proctitis, and cystitis. Radiation injury to the rectal wall eventually causes connective tissue fibrosis and obliterative endarteritis, with subsequent local tissue ischemia.[5,31,60]

The severity of radiation-induced damage to the intestinal tract is progressive, and the prognosis depends on subsequent surgical exploration and intestinal fistulas.[43] The omental pedicle "hammock" has been used in an attempt to prevent radiation-induced enteropathy. The exclusion of bowel by this technique may allow the application of larger doses of irradiation, thus avoiding complications.[10]

A variety of factors must be considered in perineal reconstruction. The high concentration of enteric organisms demands watertight closure with well-vascularized tissue. Failure to deliver this vascularized tissue can lead to wound infection and breakdown. Urinary and fecal diversion may be necessary to avoid wound contamination. Alternatively, pharmacologic management of excretory frequency may be required.

In assessing the defect after surgical excision, the physician must consider the nature and quantity of soft tissue, bone, and special structures, such as the pelvic floor and anal sphincter. Skin, subcutaneous tissue, and muscle can be imported using a variety of flaps. The amount of skin required to close a defect is usually self-evident. For defects not requiring skin replacement, the muscle, subcutaneous fat, and deepithelialized skin from the flap can be used to obliterate dead space.

Further treatment of perineal defects requires tissue that can

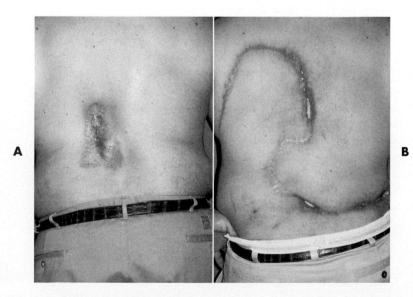

Figure 28-10. **A,** Recurrent malignant fibrohistiocytoma of lower back in 43-year-old male, who previously received radiotherapy and chemotherapy. **B,** Six months after reconstruction with two large rotational musculocutaneous flaps.

bear weight and prevent herniation of the pelvic contents. The deepithelialized dermal layer of myocutaneous flaps is ideal for this purpose. Small gaps in bone, after a partial pubic symphyseal resection, for example, can be bridged with the deepithelialized skin paddle. If the flap is insufficient for structural support, placement of synthetic mesh may allow added stability. If a superficial ulcer is present, potential communications with the intestines, bladder, and vagina should be found.

After adequate debridement of radiated tissue, a variety of muscle and myocutaneous flaps have been employed for reconstruction. The gracilis muscle provides well-vascularized tissue, but the distal one third of the skin paddle is frequently unreliable. The maximum size of the skin paddle from a gracilis myocutaneous flap is approximately 20 × 8 cm.

Occasionally the gracilis muscle is thin and has insufficient bulk to fill large defects. Use of bilateral muscles, however, may allow reconstruction of a neovagina, for example, and may correct tissue deficits. If tissue is still lacking, a TRAM flap may be more suitable. The rectus abdominis is an excellent myocutaneous flap for pelvic reconstruction. The rotation of this flap may be based on the inferior epigastric vessels, which occasionally are compromised in pelvic surgery. Also, placement of colostomies and ileal conduits frequently precludes use of the rectus muscle.

Another flap is the posterior thigh, a substantial axial skin flap based on the descending branch of the inferior gluteal artery. It can provide excellent cutaneous rotation but is frequently insufficient to fill dead space.

The rectus femoris muscle and the tensor fascia lata for groin and suprapubic defects can also be used. The tensor fascia lata is a popular flap, receiving its dominant blood supply from a terminal branch of the lateral circumflex femoral artery.[19] The flap's large size (20 × 40 cm) allows for either internal or external coverage. Its fascial component can be used to assist with reconstruction of the pelvic floor defect; in our experience, however, the tensor fascia lata has not been large enough to allow for stable coverage of the bony defect.

The rectus femoris muscle is frequently limited by its arch of rotation, and thus only lower abdominal defects seem appropriate for closure with this flap.[19] The rectus femoris also receives its dominant blood supply from the lateral circumflex femoral artery. The rectus femoris can be raised in a similar manner as the tensor fascia lata, and the combination of these flaps provides soft tissue coverage of most of the pelvic floor defects and synthetic mesh, if used. The undersurface of the rectus femoris contains a thick fascial layer, further adding to the support of the defect.

The omentum is a readily accessible vascularized tissue that can fill dead space. Omentum is probably the ideal coverage, but previous surgery and adjuvant therapy often limit its use. Fixation of the omentum to the sacrum and posterior pelvis provides the necessary inner layer of vascularized tissue if mesh is used.

Traditional methods for pelvic floor reconstruction involve soft tissue repair with either local tissue advancement or muscle flap transfer. These methods work if the bony integrity is intact, which allows for anchorage to the pelvic ring and structural support of the pelvic floor.

In cases that include bony resection, we prefer to use prosthetic mesh for the reestablishment of pelvic floor and bony support. Anchoring this mesh posteriorly to the sacrum, coccyx, and posterior iliac wing provides stable points of fixation.[19] Several sheets of mesh can be used and joined to recreate the contour of the pelvic floor. The mesh is pliable and can be rotated on itself anteriorly, with anchorage to the costal margins for reconstruction of the entire anterior abdominal wall and pelvic floor, if necessary. The mesh can be laterally secured by suture fixation to the abdominal fascia. This fixation seals in the abdominal contents to prevent hernia formation (in effect, an internal "diaper").

We have not employed Dexon or Vicryl absorbable mesh because we believe the absorption will eventually lead to recurrent hernia formation. Use of nonabsorbable mesh also may result in complications, however, and adequate soft tissue coverage by one of the options outlined is necessary for limiting potential morbidity.

Although used infrequently, free tissue transfer can provide both internal and external coverage. Recipient vessels include the internal and external iliac vessels and their tributaries. In our experience, sufficient rotational muscle options are available. Reconstruction of the pelvic floor after bone and soft tissue resection necessitates a combination of proven techniques, with the goal of stable pelvic reconstruction. Adjuvant therapy does not appear to limit this reconstructive approach.

The organization and judicious use of these techniques permit the safe resection of tumors involving the pelvic bone, which historically were fraught with unacceptable patient morbidity[19] (Figure 28-11).

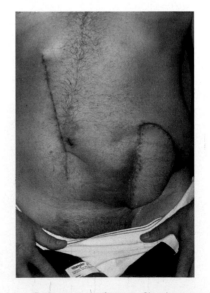

Figure 28-11. Recurrent malignant fibrohistiocytoma of left groin in 45-year-old male after initial resection and radiation therapy. Reconstruction was with rotational TRAM flap.

EXTREMITIES

The advent of neoadjuvant therapy changed the surgical approach to the patient with extremity cancer. Amputation was no longer the rule, which altered the reconstructive purview from stump coverage to durable, functional extremity salvage. To ensure this salvage, the integrity of bone, blood vessels, and nerves is vital, either by preservation or reconstruction.[8,17,39,55,65,68]

Defects of the extremity vary widely, and the strategy for reconstruction needs to be tailored to each defect. It is important within this strategy first to consider skeletal stability. Satisfactory reconstruction of osseous defects in the extremity requires restoration of stability and length while maintaining mobility. To accomplish these goals, the following methods are available:

1. *Bone shortening* may be considered if the defect is limited. This is rarely an option in upper extremity tumors.
2. *Conventional bone grafting* is also an option for segmental defects of limited length (less than 6 cm) but requires stable soft tissue coverage and a well-vascularized bed. This method should be avoided in irradiated tissues.
3. *Cadaveric allografts* can be used for large defects that may involve joint surfaces, and they heal similar to conventional bone grafts (creeping substitution). Because of their large volume and possible low-grade immune activity, cadaveric allografts may require up to 1 year for healing and are more prone to complications.
4. *Resection and arthroplasty* may result in a functional extremity when tumors are close to the ends of long bones.
5. *Vascularized bone transfer* provides a useful alternative to some of these techniques or may be used in conjunction with them to enhance successful bone healing. Vascularized bone provides healing even in compromised tissue beds and reduces the volume of bone to heal by creeping substitution, speeding stable bony union and functional recovery. A variety of donor sites have been described for vascularized bone transfer. Generally, the most useful of these for the extremity is the fibula. Up to 25 cm of bone may be easily

obtained, and the thick cortex allows reliable fixation with plates and screws. In cases requiring soft tissue, a skin paddle may be harvested with the bone as a reliable composite.

Soft tissue coverage to the extremities can be provided by a variety of local and distant muscle flaps. Again, the theory is to provide the transfer of well-vascularized muscle.

Local tissue options include the use of the major muscles in the thigh, including the rectus femoris, vastus lateralis, and vastus medialis. Frequently the gracilis muscle is too small for significant coverage, but it is appropriate for exposed vessels or vital structures. Loss of mobility must be considered when using these muscles. The gastrocnemius and soleus muscles are options for proximal lower leg reconstruction. The muscle chosen should be outside the field of irradiation, and the surgeon must assess the pedicle's viability.

Distant tissue flaps include the latissimus dorsi, the rectus abdominis, and the radial forearm free flap. If reconstruction of the hand or foot requires well-vascularized fascia, use of the temporalis or dorsalis pedis is an option. The surgeon must consider performing the microsurgical anastomosis outside the field of irradiation. This may require the use of vein grafts. Alternatively, large-caliber vessels in an end-to-side anastomosis may be employed.

Reconstruction of the extremity involves a complex set of functional and anatomic structures that require attention during tumor resection. The surgeon must address each potential defect in the restoration of function and improvement in quality of life (Figure 28-12).

OUTCOMES

It is difficult to quantitate the surgical effects of radiotherapy. Although the focus is frequently on complications, radiotherapy has many benefits. This section defines some of these surgical and therapeutic outcomes by region.

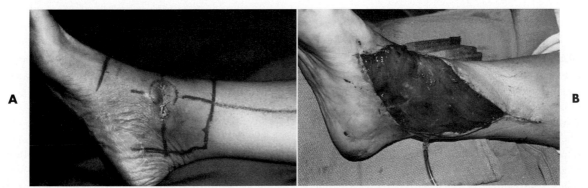

A   **B**

Figure 28-12. A, Sarcoma of right dorsal foot in 42-year-old woman. Patient received radiotherapy after attempted initial excision. **B,** Further surgical excision was required, and defect was reconstructed with rectus abdominis free tissue transfer and skin grafting.

HEAD AND NECK

The inclusion of radiotherapy in treatment of the head and neck has provided better local and regional control of malignancies. Placement of free tissue transfer into the head and neck appears to be well tolerated with this adjuvant regimen.[12] Outcomes of radiotherapy, however, have not always been positive.

Recent clinical reports indicate that patients receiving radiotherapy that includes the auditory system are likely to develop an irradiation-induced hearing loss. These changes appear to occur in the inner ear as well as the auditory nerve and brain stem with fractionated doses of 2 to 2.5 Gy and total doses of 50 Gy.[1]

Previous radical radiotherapy has been demonstrated to predispose a patient strongly to postlaryngectomy fistula. Further, these fistulas tend to survive longer and are more likely to require surgical repair.[54] Irradiation causes subendothelial proliferation and atherosclerotic changes. Occasionally these changes may lead to carotid artery "blow out."[32] Revascularization for radiation-induced arterial disease can be performed, but prosthetic grafts should be used with caution.[62] The effects of irradiation on tissue and the vasculature are progressive and lifelong. Vessel dissection must be performed with care. Vessel compliance is decreased, and suture material must be placed gently because the vessel wall may tear.

Evaluation of free tissue transfer in the head and neck revealed no increase in flap loss when using irradiated vessels.[6] Several additional reports have confirmed the safety of postoperative adjuvant radiotherapy after reconstruction with various types of free tissue transfer.[35] Vascularized skin, muscle, and bone tolerate ionizing radiation better than the nonreconstructed "ischemic" and fibrotic tissue resulting from primary closure.

Free jejunal transfers have been noted to withstand 45 to 60 Gy without acute or chronic problems.[47] In a series of 93 reconstructions in our institution, the jejunal transfer appeared to tolerate irradiation, and the stricture rate was 15%.[63] The most common reason for strictures in many of these series was recurrent disease.[12] With judicious use, free tissue transfers seem to tolerate preoperative and postoperative radiotherapy.

CHEST WALL AND LOWER BACK

The treatment of chest wall and lower back tumors and of complications from radiation is a challenging problem. The cellular and noncellular changes combined with the progressive nature of the radiation damage frequently require modifications in wound closure.

The outcomes of using irradiated versus nonirradiated muscle in chest wall reconstruction has recently been evaluated.[3] One hundred consecutive, previously irradiated wounds closed with muscle or musculocutaneous flaps were analyzed.

These 100 patients has 151 muscles transposed for coverage; 43 had the muscle transposed from the primary field of radiation, and 57 patients had closure with nonirradiated muscle. Patients who had radiated transposed muscles had a complication rate of 32%, with the entire muscle dying in 14%. The subgroup who had nonirradiated muscle had a complication rate of 19.3%, with no muscle dying completely. The authors recommended using nonirradiated muscle for closure of irradiated wounds.

In the patient with chest wall irradiation, surgical considerations must include possible pulmonary complications. A lymphocytic alveolitis develops in both lung fields after unilateral thoracic irradiation, suggesting a generalized lymphocyte-mediated hypersensitivity reaction.[64]

HBO as an adjunctive treatment for delayed radiation injury of the chest wall may have some benefit when combined with appropriate debridement of necrotic tissue and bone.[25]

BREAST

Radiotherapy for small breast malignancies combined with lumpectomy appears to result in the same local control and survival as modified radical mastectomy.[75] This treatment modality is now a routine procedure. Despite success, however, complications have occurred.

Skin telangiectasia in patients with conservative cancer treatment can be minimized by higher total radiation doses, longer schedules, and lower fraction sizes.[15] To minimize late responses to radiation, interval variations have been tested; a radiation interval of 4 hours resulted in the same late reactions as an 8-hour interval.[61] Other studies have shown that sucralfate cream protects the skin during electron beam therapy.[53] Topical agents must compensate for variations in portal delivery, however, and their use should not be encouraged.

Lumpectomy and radiation therapy can alter the aesthetic outcome for some women, with problems in treatment of recurrent disease. Radiotherapy combined with lumpectomy may cause significant deformity in small breasts; modified radical mastectomy may be more appropriate for these patients.

In women who have undergone mastectomy and desire reconstruction, options become more difficult. With implant reconstruction, capsular contracture (Baker III and IV) and complication rates for breast implants appear to be a significant in patients who receive adjuvant radiotherapy. These complications are unrelated to implant type or interval between implant placement and radiotherapy. Placement of implants before or after irradiation had no effect on outcome. Autogenous tissue does not seem to offer a protective environment for the implant.

With the current emphasis on cost containment, "simpler" reconstructive techniques will be promoted. Surgeons must be cautious with the irradiated patient. Multiple complications can easily exceed the potential for cost control.[24] Reconstruction with autogenous tissue appears to have better results. In a review of 19 patients who had TRAM breast reconstruction and received postoperative irradiation, all women reported excellent results with good locoregional control.[41]

When approaching a woman with previous chest wall irradiation, the surgeon must take care in developing the breast flaps. Necrosis and tissue loss should be expected, and the need for a large TRAM skin paddle may be necessary. Use of the latissimus dorsi muscle may be in question because the previous irradiation may have compromised the thoracodorsal pedicle. Free tissue transfer is more difficult in previously irradiated patients. Frequently the previously irradiated vessels are small and fibrotic. Careful evaluation must be performed before flap transfer.

To determine whether the ipsilateral internal mammary arteries can be used as a viable blood supply for a pedicle TRAM flap, we used ultrasound probes to detect patent internal mammary vessels in patients with previous chest wall irradiation. Despite known clinical and pathologic effects in blood vessels after radiotherapy, we were unable to demonstrate a statistical difference in vessel diameter or peak systolic velocity using sonographic evaluation of the internal mammary artery. Also, we noted no significant differences between patients with a documented dose of radiation to the internal mammary region using specific radiation portals and patients treated with tangential radiation portals. We identified significant increases in blood flow in the irradiated side, however, compared with documented radiation portals to the internal mammary chain. Therefore the indirect measurements indicate that the ipsilateral muscle may not need to be eliminated as a possible source for TRAM reconstruction, although more clinical data are needed.[23]

ABDOMEN AND PERINEUM

The fundamental principles of management of radiation-related wounds apply to the pelvis and perineum. The optimum reconstruction of the pelvis requires the introduction of fresh, well-vascularized tissue as well as wide debridement of necrotic tissue in chronic wounds. Pelvic fractures have been reported after the administration of irradiation.[37]

The combination of irradiation and radical pelvic surgery is associated with significant morbidity and mortality. Radical hysterectomy after full-dose pelvic irradiation is associated with a high fistula rate, high operative mortality, and decreased survival rate compared with primary radical hysterectomy. Radical hysterectomy should not be recommended after full-dose irradiation.[52]

EXTREMITIES

Radiotherapy has achieved better local control of extremity sarcomas, fostering the expansion of limb-sparing therapeutic options. Radiation treatment portals precisely outline tissues at risk and attempt to exclude uninvolved regions from radiation effects with individualized treatment blocks.

Adjuvant therapy did not increase the complication rate of free tissue transfers for limb salvage to the lower extremity (25% with and 31% without adjuvant therapy). For comparison, we examined the complication rates in patients who had surgery with adjuvant therapy but without free tissue transfer for reconstruction. Of 663 cases performed between 1960 and 1992, 158 had complications (24%). Surgery alone was performed in 25% of the patients, and adjuvant therapy was employed in the other 75%. Wide local excision was performed in 70% of the patients, which could be closed by skin grafting or primary closure, and amputation was done in 11%.[20]

Although comparison to our free tissue transfers could not be done because the defect types are not alike, we would hypothesize that the larger defects may have fared much worse with primary closure alone. The timing of adjuvant therapy did not influence the microvascular transfer, and similarly, the transfer did not affect the timing of therapy. We would hypothesize that higher doses of irradiation may be employed because of the well-vascularized microvascular closure, which offers a more stable wound. Combined with this adjuvant therapy, we believe microvascular transfer allows for more frequent limb salvage.[20]

The radiosensitivity of nerve reconstruction in a previously irradiated field and postoperative irradiation of nerve grafts have also been evaluated.[16,22] Rats received isografts into the posterior tibial nerve, then postoperative irradiation according to clinical parameters for 3, 5, 7, and 9 weeks (2-Gy/day fractions) for a total dose of 46, 66, 86, and 106 Gy. Walking-track analysis was performed monthly, and the rats were evaluated for 8 months. Functional parameters were not significantly different between the irradiated rats and the nonirradiated controls. Histomorphologic parameters did demonstrate a statistically lower number of axons/mm^2 and nerve fiber density in the distal nerve segments of irradiated nerves.[21]

Rats were further examined for potential functional changes with grafting nerves into a posterior tibial defect after the administration of irradiation. Similar doses were applied in a fractionated regimen of 2 Gy/day for 3, 5, 7, and 9 weeks. Placement of the isograft was performed after waiting 6 weeks, allowing some chronic changes to occur. After 8 months, again, functional parameters were not significantly different between the irradiated rats and nonirradiated controls. Histomorphologic parameters, however, were different in the distal nerve segment, again for axon number/mm^2.

It thus appears that acute nerve grafting can be performed in an irradiated bed and that the functional outcome may not be affected by postoperative irradiation[16,22] (Figure 28-13).

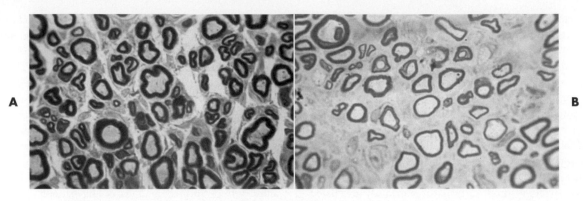

Figure 28-13.   Histomorphology of **A,** distal nerve used as control, and **B,** distal nerve irradiated with 106 Gy. Note fewer number of axons, thinning of myelin, and fibrosis in irradiated segment.

SKIN

Recently the effects of radiation therapy on skin grafts have been evaluated. Ulceration and wound breakdown in the rat were noted as the irradiation dose increased, after waiting 4 weeks between applying the skin graft and administering a single dose of irradiation. Skin grafting thus does not appear to be a reliable, durable cover for wounds.[72]

FUTURE TRENDS

Surgical abilities have advanced such that surgeons can successfully transfer tissue, pedicled or free, from a nonirradiated location to the injured tissue. As demonstrated, this well-vascularized tissue has allowed healing in wounds traditionally difficult to close. Surgeons must remember, however, that successful reconstruction is based not only on tissue transfer survival but also on functional outcome.

With today's managed care environment, cost containment and procedural justification are as important as successful tissue transfer. What are the economic considerations with radiotherapy versus surgical extirpation? Does surgery, radiation, or a combination yield the best results in restoring quality of life?

Patients treated with external beam radiotherapy alone had excellent results in understandable speech (tumor grade T1, 94%; T4, 88%). Neck dissection had no impact on the functional outcomes evaluated. Functional results did not deteriorate and remained stable with prolonged follow-up of more than 5 years. Many results were even superior to surgical resection.[57]

Further studies have demonstrated that good to excellent functional outcomes in speech and swallowing were preserved in 18 of 20 patients with squamous cell carcinoma of the head and neck treated with radiotherapy alone.[40]

Future trends in health care will demand outcome evaluations for surgeries performed. Local and regional control will continue to be vital in the establishment of surgical techniques, but long-term functional assessments and quality of life values will have to be measured as well. It is in these latter areas that determination of cost-effective techniques is difficult.

SUMMARY

The field of plastic surgery is rapidly changing. Most of the focus today is on one-stage immediate reconstruction, which has permitted more extensive ablation and superior reconstructive outcomes. Such procedures demand close patient monitoring and a team approach. With the increasing use of radiotherapy, careful perioperative planning has allowed for an improved quality of life through functional and cosmetic restoration.

REFERENCES

1.   Anteunis LJC, Wanders SL, Hendriks JJT, et al: A prospective longitudinal study on radiation-induced hearing loss, *Am J Surg* 168:408-411, 1994.

2.   Ariyan S, Marfuggi RA, Harder G, Goodie MM: An experimental model to determine the effects of adjuvant therapy on the incidence of postoperative wound infection. I. Evaluating preoperative radiation therapy, *Plast Reconstr Surg* 65:328-337, 1980.

3.   Arnold PG, Lovich SF, Pairolero PC: Muscle flaps in irradiated wounds: an account of 100 consecutive cases, *Plast Reconstr Surg* 93:324-327, 1994.

4.   Ashamalla HL, Thom SR, Goldwein JW: Hyperbaric oxygen therapy for the treatment of radiation-induced sequelae in children, *Cancer* 77:2407-2412, 1996.

5.   Babb RR: Radiation proctitis: a review, *Am J Gastroenterol* 91:1309-1311, 1996.

6.   Bengtson BP, Schusterman MA, Baldwin BJ, et al: Influence of prior radiotherapy on the development of postoperative complications and success of free tissue transfers in head and neck cancer reconstruction, *Am J Surg* 166:326-330, 1993.

7. Bernstein EF, Sullivan FJ, Mitchell JB, et al: Biology of chronic radiation effect on tissues and wound healing, *Clin Plast Surg* 20:435-453, 1993.

8. Brennan MF: Management of extremity soft-tissue sarcoma, *Am J Surg* 158:71, 1989.

9. Brenner DJ: Dose, volume and time-control predictions in radiotherapy, *Int J Radiat Oncol Biol Phys* 26:171-179, 1993.

10. Choi HJ, Lee HS: Effect of omental pedicle hammock in protection against radiation-induced enteropathy in patients with rectal cancer, *Dis Colon Rectum* 38:276-280, 1995.

11. Clay RP, Arnold PG: Management of intrathoracic defects, *Clin Plast Surg* 20:551-557, 1993.

12. Coleman JJ: Management of radiation-induced soft-tissue injury to the head and neck, *Clin Plast Surg* 20:491-505, 1993.

13. Daniel J: The x-rays, *New Sci* 3:562, 1896.

14. Docherty JG, Carter R, Sheldon CD, et al: Relative effect of surgery and radiotherapy on the internal jugular vein following functional neck dissection, *Head Neck,* November-December 1993, pp 553-556.

15. Dodwell DJ, Povall J, Gerrard G, et al: Skin telangiectasia: the influence of radiation dose delivery parameters in the conservative management of early breast cancer, *Clin Oncol* 7:248-250, 1995.

16. Evans GRD, Goldberg D: Principles of extremity reconstruction. In Schusterman MA, editor: *Microsurgical reconstruction of the cancer patient,* Philadelphia, 1997, Lippincott-Raven.

17. Evans GRD, Miller MJ: Upper extremity reconstruction. In Schusterman MA, editor: *Microsurgical reconstruction of the cancer patient,* Philadelphia, 1997, Lippincott-Raven.

18. Evans GRD, Reece GP: Lower back reconstruction: an approach to wound closure in the cancer patient, *Plast Reconstr Surg* 96:635-642, 1995.

19. Evans GRD, Goldberg DP, Ames FC: Complex abdominal-perineal reconstruction: options after pelvic bone resection, *Plast Reconstr Surg* 98:735-739, 1996.

20. Evans GRD, Black JJ, Robb GL, et al: Adjuvant therapy: the effects on microvascular lower extremity reconstruction, *Ann Plast Surg* 39:141-144, 1997.

21. Evans GRD, Brandt K, Ang KK, et al: Peripheral nerve regeneration: the effects of postoperative irradiation, *Plast Reconstr Surg* 100:375-380, 1997.

22. Evans GRD, Brandt K, Saval T, et al: Preoperative irradiation: the effect on peripheral nerve regeneration. Presented at the Plastic Surgery Research Council 42nd Annual Meeting, Galveston, Tex, 1997.

23. Evans GRD, David CL, Loyer LM, et al: The long-term effects of internal mammary chain irradiation and its role in the vascular supply of the pedicle TRAM flap breast reconstruction, *Ann Plast Surg* 35:342-348, 1995.

24. Evans GRD, Schusterman MA, Kroll SS, et al: Reconstruction and the radiated breast: is there a role for implants? *Plast Reconstr Surg* 96:1111-1118, 1995.

25. Feldmeier JJ, Heimbach RD, Davolt DA, et al: Hyperbaric oxygen as an adjunctive treatment for delayed radiation injury of the chest wall: a retrospective review of twenty-three cases, *Undersea Hyperbaric Med* 22:383-393, 1995.

26. Fineberg S, Rosen PP: Cutaneous angiosarcoma and atypical vascular lesions of the skin and breast after radiation therapy for breast carcinoma, *Am J Clin Pathol* 102:757-763, 1994.

27. Fisher CB, Mattox DE, Zinreich JS: Patency of the internal jugular vein after functional neck dissection, *Laryngoscope* 98:923-927, 1988.

28. Frieben EA: Cancroid des rechten Handrückens nach langdauernder Einwirkung von Roentgenstrahlen, *Forstchr Roentgenstr* 6:106, 1902.

29. Goldwein JW, Meadows A: Influence of radiation on growth in pediatric patients, *Clin Plast Surg* 20:455-464, 1993.

30. Granick MS, Larson DL, Solomon MP: Radiation-related wounds of the chest wall, *Clin Plast Surg* 20:559-571, 1993.

31. Granick MS, Solomon MP, Larson DL: Management of radiation-associated pelvic wounds, *Clin Plast Surg* 20:581-587, 1993.

32. Gupta S: Radiation induced carotid artery blow out: a case report, *Acta Chir Belg* 94:299-300, 1994 (letter).

33. Hall EJ: LET and RBE. In *Radiobiology for the radiologist,* ed 2, Hagerstown, Md, 1978, Harper & Row.

34. Hanna DC: Present and future trends in reconstructive surgery for head and neck cancer patients, *Laryngoscope* 88(suppl 8):96, 1978.

35. Hayden R: Tolerance of gastric mucosal flap to postop irradiation, *Laryngoscope* 101:462, 1991.

36. Haywood RH: Arteriosclerosis induced by radiation, *Surg Clin North Am* 52:359, 1972.

37. Henry AP, Lachman E, Tunkel RS, Nagler W: Pelvic insufficiency fractures after irradiation: diagnosis, management and rehabilitation, *Arch Phys Med Rehabil* 77:414-416, 1996.

38. Hicks GL: Coronary artery operation in radiation-associated atherosclerosis: long-term follow-up, *Ann Thorac Surg* 52:670-674, 1992.

39. Hidalgo DA, Carrasquillo IM: The treatment of lower extremity sarcomas with wide excision, radiotherapy, and free-flap reconstruction, *Plast Reconstr Surg* 89:96-101, 1992.

40. Horwitz EM, Frazier AJ, Martinez AA, et al: Excellent functional outcome in patients with squamous cell carcinoma of the base of the tongue treated with external irradiation and interstitial iodine 125 boost, *Cancer* 78:948-957, 1996.

41. Hunt KK, Baldwin BJ, Singletary SE, et al: Postoperative radiotherapy does not interfere with TRAM flap viability or cosmetic results in patients with high risk breast cancer. Presented at the Society of Surgical Oncology, Boston, 1995.

42. Jacob RFK. Management of xerostomia in the irradiated patient, *Clin Plast Surg* 20:507-516, 1993.

43. Jahnson S, Westerborn O, Gerdin B: Prognosis of surgically treated radiation-induced damage to the intestine, *Eur J Surg Oncol* 18:487-493, 1992.

44. Janjan NA: Radiation effects on the eye, *Clin Plast Surg* 20:535-549, 1993.

45. Kindwall EP: Hyperbaric oxygen's effect on radiation necrosis, *Clin Plast Surg* 20:473-483, 1993.

46. Kroll SS, Woo SY, Santin A, et al: Long-term effects of radiotherapy administered in childhood for the treatment of malignant diseases, *Ann Surg Oncol* 1:473-479, 1994.

47. Kulungowski M, Coleman JJ: The effect of postoperative radiotherapy on the jejunal free autograft, American Society of Plastic and Reconstructive Surgeons Annual Scientific Meeting, 1991, Seattle.

48. Kureshi SA, Hofman FM, Schneider JH, et al: Cytokine expression in radiation-induced delayed cerebral injury, *Neurosurgery* 35:822-830, 1994.

49. Lanciano R, Corn B, Martin E, et al: Perioperative morbidity of intracavitary gynecologic brachytherapy, *Int J Radiat Oncol Biol Phys* 29:969-974, 1994.

50. Larson DL: Long-term effects of radiation therapy in the head and neck, *Clin Plast Surg* 20:485-490, 1993.

51. Larson DL, Lindberg RD, Lane E, Goepfert H: Major complications of radiotherapy in cancer of the oral cavity and oropharynx, *Am J Surg* 146:531-536, 1983.

52. Magrina JF: Complications of irradiation and radical surgery for gynecologic malignancies, *Obstet Gynecol Surv* 48:571-575, 1993.

53. Maiche A, Isokangas OP, Gröhn P: Skin protection by sucralfate cream during electron beam therapy, *Acta Oncol* 33:201-203, 1994.

54. McCombe AW, Jones AS: Radiotherapy and complications of laryngectomy, *J Laryngol Otol* 107:130-132, 1993.

55. McDonald DJ, Capanna R, Gherlinzoni F, et al: Influence of chemotherapy on perioperative complications in limb salvage surgery for bone tumors, *Cancer* 65:1509-1516, 1990.

56. Miller MJ, Janjan NA: Treatment of injuries from radiation therapy. In Kroll SS, editor: *Reconstructive plastic surgery for cancer,* St Louis, 1996, Mosby.

57. Moore GJ, Parsons JT, Mendenhall WM: Quality of life outcomes after primary radiotherapy for squamous cell carcinoma of the base of the tongue, *Int J Radiat Oncol Biol Phys* 36:351-354, 1996.

58. Mortimer PS, Simmonds RH, Rezvani M, et al: Time-related changes in lymphatic clearance in pig skin after a single dose of 18 Gy of X rays, *Br J Radiol* 64:1140-1146, 1991.

59. Mustoe TA, Porras-Reyes BH: Modulation of wound healing response in chromic irradiated tissues, *Clin Plast Surg* 20:465-472, 1993.

60. Nussbaum ML, Campana TJ, Weese JL: Radiation-induced intestinal injury, *Clin Plast Surg* 20:573-580, 1993.

61. Nyman J, Turesson I: Does the interval between fractions matter in the range of 4-8 h in radiotherapy? A study of acute and late human skin reactions, *Radiother Oncol* 34:171-178, 1995.

62. Phillips GR, Peer RM, Upson JF, Ricotta JJ: Late complications of revascularization for radiation-induced arterial disease, *J Vasc Surg* 16:921-925, 1992.

63. Reece GP, Schusterman MA, Miller MJ, et al: Morbidity and functional outcome after pharyngoesophageal reconstruction using free jejunal transfer, *Plast Reconstr Surg* 96:1307-1316, 1995.

64. Roberts CM, Foulcher E, Zaunders JJ, et al: Radiation pneumonitis: a possible lymphocyte-mediated hypersensitivity reaction, *Ann Intern Med* 118:696-700, 1993.

65. Rosenberg SA, Glatstein EJ: Acute and long-term effects on limb function of combined modality limb sparing therapy for extremity soft tissue sarcoma, *Int J Radiat Oncol Biol Phys* 21:1493-1499, 1991.

66. Rudolph R, Vandeberg J, Schneider JA, et al: Slowed growth of cultured fibroblasts from human radiation wounds, *Plast Reconstr Surg* 82:669-675, 1988.

67. Sanger JR, Matloub HS, Yousif NJ, Larson DL: Management of osteoradionecrosis of the mandible, *Clin Plast Surg* 20:517-530, 1993.

68. Shiu MH, Castro EB, Hajdu SI, Fortner JG: Surgical treatment of 297 soft tissue sarcomas of the lower extremity, *Ann Surg* 182:597-602, 1975.

69. Shiu MH, Turnbull AD, Nori D, et al: Control of locally advanced extremity soft tissue sarcomas by function saving resection and brachytherapy, *Cancer* 53:1385-1392, 1984.

70. Skibber JM, Lotze MT, et al: Limb sparing surgery for soft tissue sarcomas: wound related morbidity in patients undergoing wide local excision, *Surgery* 102:447-452, 1987.

71. Stinson SF, DeLaney TF, Greenberg J, et al: Reconstruction after excision of soft tissue sarcomas of the limbs and trunk, *Br J Surg* 75:774-778, 1988.

72. Tadjalli H, Evans GRD, Gürlek A, Ang KK: Skin graft survivability following external beam irradiation. Presented at the Plastic Surgery Research Council 42nd Annual Meeting, Galveston, Tex, 1997.

73. Taylor JMG, Mendenhall WM, Parsons JJ, Lavey RS: The influence of dose and time on wound complications following post-radiation neck dissection, *Int J Radiat Oncol Biol Phys* 23:41-46, 1992.

74. Terasima R, Tolmach LJ: X-ray sensitivity and DNA synthesis in synchronous populations of HeLa cells, *Science* 140:490-492, 1963.

75. Veronesi U, et al: Comparing radical mastectomy with quadrantectomy, axillary dissection and radiotherapy in patients with small cancers of the breast, *N Engl J Med* 305:6, 1984.

76. Witte L, Fuks Z, Haimovitz-Friedman A, et al: Effects of irradiation on the release of growth factors from cultured bovine, porcine and human endothelial cells, *Cancer Res* 9:279, 1989.

77. Zinzani PL, Gherlinzoni F, Piovaccari G, et al: Cardiac injury as late toxicity of mediastinal radiation therapy for Hodgkin's disease patients, *Haematologica* 81:132-137, 1996.

CHAPTER

Burn Reconstruction

Bruce M. Achauer
Victoria M. VanderKam

After acute thermal injury the burn survivor may be faced with impaired function and disfiguring scars. The goals of reconstructive surgery are to maximize function and minimize disfigurement. The effective surgeon must listen to and work with the patient to determine what treatment and when to do it. Although the surgeon may continue to seek improvement, the patient decides when reconstruction must end.

Successful burn reconstruction requires using good judgment and establishing priorities. The surgical reconstruction must be integrated into the patient's overall rehabilitation. A holistic approach to reconstruction ensures that the patient is not only functionally and aesthetically corrected, but also socially and psychologically healed.

Priorities for surgical procedures fall into three categories for the burn patient: (1) urgent, (2) essential, and (3) desirable. *Urgent procedures* are required in the acute phase to preserve function. Examples of acute needs are exposed ear cartilage, exposed cornea, or severely injured hands. *Essential procedures* are required to regain function. For example, contractures may decrease range of motion or interfere with activities of daily living. *Desirable procedures,* as typically envisioned by patients, are attempts to restore a more normal appearance. Examples include restoration of the nose or correction of scar alopecia.

The following discussion of burn reconstruction is organized anatomically, from head to toe, and includes indications and preferred operations, within each anatomic area covered.

SCALP

Indications
The primary indication for scalp reconstruction after a burn is scar alopecia or an unstable scar.

Classification
Minor defect: up to 5% of scalp surface area involved
Moderate defect: 7% to 70% of scalp involved
Extensive defect: greater than 70% involved

Operations
MINOR DEFECT. Immediate treatment is done by early skin grafting, with reconstruction performed later. The skin graft is excised by a staged procedure. Advancement and rotation of adjacent scalp flaps fill the defect.

MODERATE DEFECT. This defect cannot be effectively treated by excision. Tissue expansion is the treatment of choice. This allows the area to be reconstructed with like tissue and with no donor defect. A skin graft is placed during the acute phase. Placement of tissue expanders or flap advancement at the time of injury is risky and not recommended.

Once healing is complete, normal adjacent skin is expanded to replace the skin grafts. Guidelines for tissue expansion include the following:

1. Plan for more tissue than is needed.
2. Plan incision carefully, avoiding scar tissue.
3. Use EMLA Cream (lidocaine and prilocaine) over the needle entry site to ensure maximum patient comfort.
4. Rapid expansion is usually unnecessary; weekly injections are sufficient.

EXTENSIVE DEFECT. Defects in this range may be too large to be corrected with tissue expansion. Skin grafting or scalp flaps are required. Orticochea[26] described a scalp reconstruction using three flaps, each with its own vascular pedicle. Jurkewicz and Hill[23] also describe flaps to cover large defects.

Extensive injuries involving full-thickness or deeper skull defects represent a difficult situation. Immediate reconstruction is required as a lifesaving measure. Free tissue transfer may be required. The most common source of tissue is the omentum or the latissimus dorsi myocutaneous flap.

FACE

Indications
The primary indication for facial reconstruction after burns is improvement of scars.

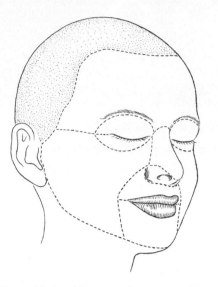

Figure 29-1. Classic aesthetic units of face.

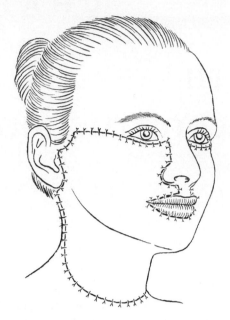

Figure 29-2. Large full-thickness skin graft can cover entire face as single aesthetic unit. Tissue from neck and chest areas can be used for this graft. (Redrawn from Feldman JJ: In Serafin D, Georgiade NG, editors: *Pediatric plastic Surgery*, St Louis, 1984, Mosby.)

Operations

Aesthetic units, described by Gonzales-Ulloa[20] in 1956, are the primary consideration that governs all grafting of the face (Figure 29-1). The following two factors are important so that skin grafts conform to these aesthetic units:

1. Normal skin may need to be excised to follow aesthetic units. This is a difficult decision for the surgeon. The sacrifice of normal skin in a burn patient must be weighed carefully and discussed with the patient.
2. Grafts should be made larger than the aesthetic unit. With healing, contraction occurs, altering the original plan. The oversized graft helps resolve this problem.

Successful facial reconstruction requires vision. The surgeon should look at the face and ask the following:

What is missing?

What is out of place?

What features call attention to the injured area?

What tissue and techniques are available for reconstruction?

Photography is recommended and is helpful for preoperative planning. Many current concepts from aesthetic surgery are applicable to burn patients, including facelift techniques to excise preauricular scars, contouring of the face with lipectomy, and chin augmentation to improve the chin position and profile.

In addition to full-thickness skin grafts (FTSGs), flaps may be used for facial reconstruction. Flaps have the advantage of providing quality skin texture and color match. Grafts fall short in both these areas. The major objection to flaps is that they mask facial expression and obscure normal angles and contours of the face.

Almaguer et al[6] compared outcomes of grafts versus flaps on the face. Split-thickness skin grafts (STSGs) from below the clavicle resulted in poor color match in 50% of patients. FTSGs from above the clavicles had good color and texture in 98%, whereas those from below the clavicle demonstrated poor color matches in 55%. Eleven of 12 patients with flap reconstruction had excellent color and texture.

The *forehead* is best resurfaced with a single high-quality STSG. Preferred donor sites are the scalp or supraclavicular area. With bony destruction, flap reconstruction is indicated. Free flap reconstruction may be needed as an urgent procedure during the acute phase with a deep burn of the forehead. The parascapular flap is preferred.

Cheeks are most often reconstructed with flaps. Tissue expansion provides an excellent alternative for cheek reconstruction. After tissue expansion, adjacent local tissue can be advanced to reconstruct the cheek.

Some promising concepts regarding facial reconstruction have been proposed. Feldman[19] describes the one-unit approach, which uses one large FTSG to cover the face as an aesthetic unit (Figure 29-2). Angrigiani[7] uses a very large scapular flap with two pedicles to cover the entire face. Despite the thickness of this flap, some difficult cases have had excellent results (Figure 29-3). Rose[30] uses carefully sculpted free flaps to restore missing contours. Hemifacial defects can be reconstructed with a patterned free scapular flap (Figure 29-4). Rose[29] also details the vascular supply of this flap (Figure 29-5).

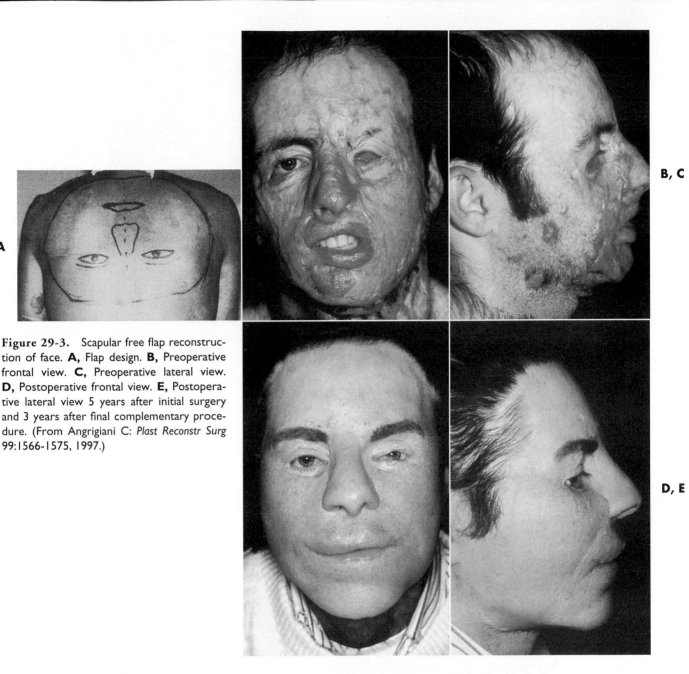

Figure 29-3. Scapular free flap reconstruction of face. **A,** Flap design. **B,** Preoperative frontal view. **C,** Preoperative lateral view. **D,** Postoperative frontal view. **E,** Postoperative lateral view 5 years after initial surgery and 3 years after final complementary procedure. (From Angrigiani C: *Plast Reconstr Surg* 99:1566-1575, 1997.)

NECK

Indications
Severe contracture, drooling, dental deterioration, folliculitis, significant deformity and obstacle for intubation for general anesthesia are reasons to reconstruct the neck.

Classification
Mild defect: scar band which involve less than ⅓ of the anterior surface of the neck.
Moderate defect: more than one third but less than two thirds of the anterior surface involved.
Severe defect: greater than two thirds of the anterior surface of the neck.
Extensive defect: a mentosternal adhesion.

Operations
MILD DEFECT. Mild scar bands can generally be corrected surgically by the use of local flaps or Z-plasties. Vertical scars of the neck are likely to produce a contracture. If the vertical scar is converted to a transverse orientation, the problem can be obviated.

MODERATE DEFECT. Moderate contractures cannot be adequately corrected with local flaps. Tissue expansion is the first consideration (Figure 29-6). The unscarred, lateral aspects of the neck are expanded. Skin grafting is avoided if possible. Limitations of tissue expansion are the lack of hard tissue immediately underneath so that some of the expansion is lost. Also, the transposed skin tends to contract as the neck angle does not oppose shrinkage. Tissue expansion can be effective if

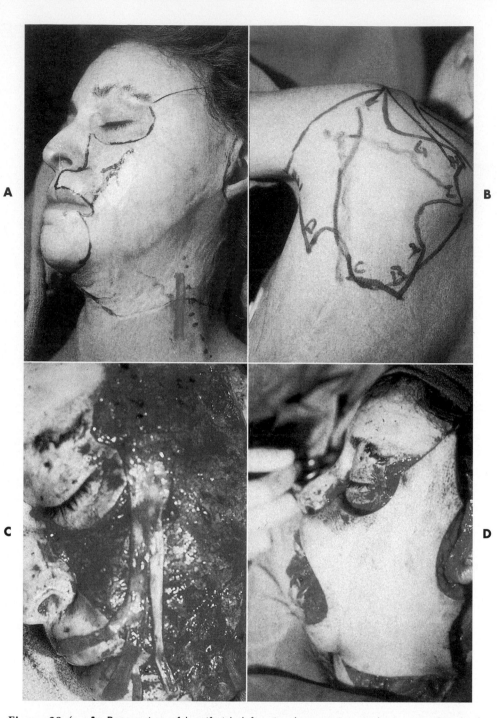

Figure 29-4. **A,** Preparation of hemifacial defect involves tracing aesthetic unit, the cheek. **B,** Prepatterned scapular flap corresponding to hemifacial unit. **C,** "Triple-tail" fascia lata sling. **D,** Flap ready for inset. (From Rose EH: *Aesthetic facial restoration,* Baltimore, 1998, Lippincott, and Williams & Wilkins.

the lateral neck skin can be stretched and brought medially. Be aware that tissue expansion may compress the trachea, internal jugular vein and carotid arteries but is almost always very safe.

SEVERE DEFECT. Severe contractures require that skin be imported in the form of a skin graft or flap. Local flaps are not adequate.

EXTENSIVE DEFECT. Extensive (mentosternal adhesion) contractures require an extensive surgical release and skin grafts. Release of the neck contracture is complicated. Induction of anesthesia may be difficult. Intubation may in fact be impossible. Fiberoptic endoscopes provide an excellent alternative to standard intubation and have in fact prevented many emergency release and tracheostomies. Always be prepared for

A　　　　　　　　**B**　　　　　　　　**C**

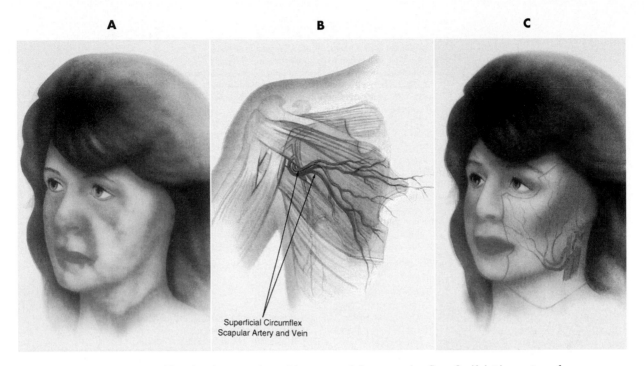

Superficial Circumflex
Scapular Artery and Vein

Figure 29-5. Hemifacial restoration with patterned free scapular flap. **A,** Keloid scarring of entire lateral cheek and neck. **B,** Design of patterned scapular flap. **C,** Inset of flap into left hemisphere of face. (From Rose EH: *Aesthetic facial restoration,* Philadelphia, 1998, Lippincott-Raven.)

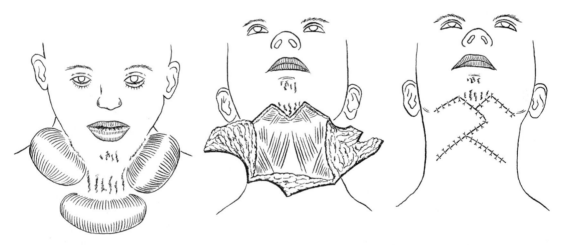

Figure 29-6. Tissue expanders are helpful for moderate neck deformities with insufficient skin for advancement flaps. Unscarred tissue on lateral aspect of neck is expanded, then brought into area of contracture.

an emergency release to facilitate an endotracheal intubation or tracheotomy.

The importance of an extensive, complete release cannot be overemphasized. The most common error is to do an inadequate release. All contracture bands no matter the depth (strap muscles) or the width (at least to midlateral neck) must be released. When the skin graft is placed there is a tendency for recurrent contracture. In order to obtain maximum improvement the release should be done extensively. After thorough release and careful hemostasis a sheet of split thickness skin grafts (non-meshed) is placed. If seams are necessary they

should be oriented transversely. A pressure dressing is applied. Foam rubber sponges are cut to match the shape of the graft. This is held in place with staples. The dressing provides gentle, even pressure, allows room for drainage, is readily available and convenient to use. The neck is immobilized for several days. A four poster neck brace works well for this purpose. Nasogastric feeding is usually required for several days to provide immobility of the mouth. A custom made splint is applied 10-14 days after surgery. Waymack et al[35] noted an 89% recurrences rate without splinting compared to a 17% rate when a splint was employed.

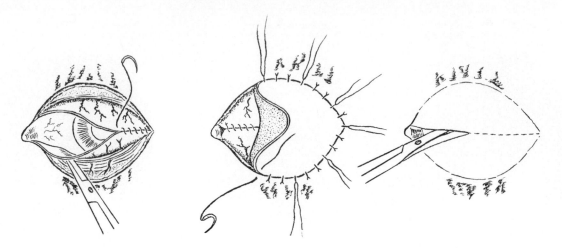

Figure 29-7. Mobilization of conjunctiva and skin flap coverage. Even thin and transparent conjunctiva will support skin graft.

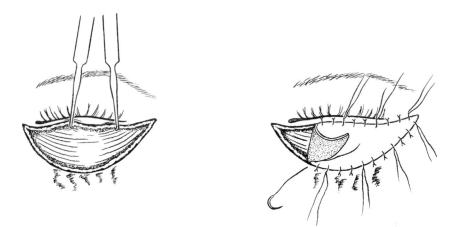

Figure 29-8. Surgical correction of lower lid ectropion. Release is extended beyond medial and lateral canthus. Full-thickness skin graft is most often used.

EYELIDS

Indications

Exposed cornea, ectropion (of the upper and lower eyelids), and medial and lateral canthal contractures are the major indications for burn reconstruction of the eyelids.

Operations

TISSUE LOSS. If the eyelids are destroyed, the conjunctiva can be mobilized and covered with skin grafts (Figure 29-7).

EXPOSED CORNEA. Tarsorrhaphy is *not* recommended for an exposed cornea. The procedure has limitations and results in loss of eyelid tissue.

ECTROPION. Ectropion is a persistent problem around the eyes despite preventive measures such as custom-made conformers and splints. In the early postburn period the patient may have chronic eye irritation and corneal damage. The area is treated with topical ointment and eye shields.

Any extrinsic causes of ectropion must be eliminated before focusing on the eyelid itself. The face, neck, and forehead must be examined for contractures that may be transmitting forces to the eyelid, leading to a secondary ectropion. Once all extrinsic causes have been corrected, residual ectropion is managed by eyelid correction.

Even a small abnormality of the eyelid may cause problems. For example, a patient may have no apparent ectropion on examination in an upright position but may have difficulty closing the eye while sleeping, opening the mouth, or looking upward.

CONTRACTURES. Flaps are of little use in reconstruction of eyelid contractures. Skin grafts are the treatment of choice. First, a thorough, wide, overcorrecting release is required. The releasing incision on the lower eyelid is placed as close to the eyelashes as possible while preserving tissue to allow for suturing (Figure 29-8). The releases should extend beyond the medial and lateral canthal areas.

Debate has surrounded which type of skin graft is ideal.

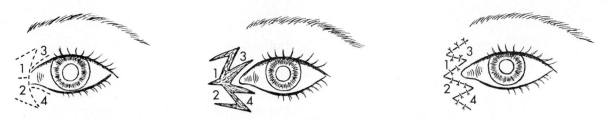

Figure 29-9. Medial epicanthal scar bands released and repaired using series of Z-plasties. (Redrawn from Converse JM: *Surg Clin North Am* 47:323, 1967.)

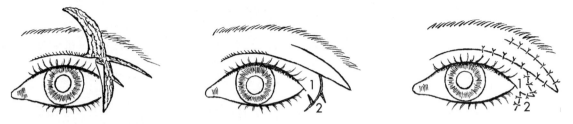

Figure 29-10. Lateral epicanthal scar bands corrected by local transposition flap. (Redrawn from Tajima S, Aoyage F: *J Br Plast Surg* 30:200-201, 1977.)

Most agree that good-quality full-thickness skin such as postauricular tissue is best for the lower eyelid. Thick STSGs are frequently used for the upper eyelids. The upper eyelid is a more mobile unit and therefore suitable to this type of graft.

The lateral incision of the lower eyelid must extend beyond the lateral and medial canthi. If this is not done, a downcast, sad look will result. Sloan et al[31] recommend that this incision be elevated 15 degrees above the horizontal and extended 15 mm beyond the canthus.

Appropriate timing of the reconstruction is important. Both upper and lower lids should *not* be done at the same sitting, since it is difficult to produce the needed overcorrection when simultaneously operating on both eyelids. Also, because the release should extend beyond both the medial and the lateral canthi areas, operating on both upper and lower lids is not practical.

Web deformities of the medial canthus may be corrected with Z-plasties or local flaps (Figure 29-9).[15] If scarred tissue is incorporated into the correction, a Y-V plasty should be considered. In this correction the tips of the flaps are not elevated and transposed, thus allowing scar tissue to be used.

Vertical contracture of the medial canthus may also occur. This type of contracture is similar to that seen with trauma or congenital anomalies. Lateral canthal scar bands may occur and are corrected with a local transposition flap (Figure 29-10).[34]

EYEBROWS

Indications

Eyebrows may be destroyed in deep facial burns. Attention to the eyebrows is considered after all functional and appearance problems have been solved. For some patients, tattooing or makeup may be sufficient. Surgical correction is not indicated for every patient but may benefit a patient with extensive facial scarring.

Operations

Techniques for reconstruction include (1) free scalp composite grafts, (2) micrografts, and (3) island flaps based on the superficial temporal artery and vein.

Scalp *composite grafts* are the preferred method for eyebrow reconstruction. Attention to detail is required, and hair orientation is critical to a desirable result (Figure 29-11).[11] The outline of the opposite eyebrow (if present) is copied, although the normal side cannot be mimicked exactly.

When harvesting the graft, the surgeon chooses an area of the scalp where the angle of the hair follicle exiting the skin is similar to the angle of the remaining or the opposite eyebrow. Incisions are made parallel to the hair follicle to avoid damaging the follicle. Small grafts present less risk of graft failure; grafts are placed in a scar bed where "take" is less predictable. The surgeon should consider grafting in stages or using several small pieces to customize the angles of the eyebrow.

Clodius and Smahel[14] recommend inducing an artificial catagen phase by epilating the donor site 6 to 10 days before grafting. Their theory is that during the catagen phase the bulb of the hair is high in the dermis and therefore less susceptible to injury during surgical transfer.

Micrografts of hair follicles to the eyelid may also be considered.[9]

Pensler et al[27] found that complications of eyebrow reconstruction, including partial graft loss and malalignment, were much less common in free scalp grafts than in vascularized flaps. Patients with composite grafts had 90% acceptable results versus 38% in patients with the island pedicle technique.

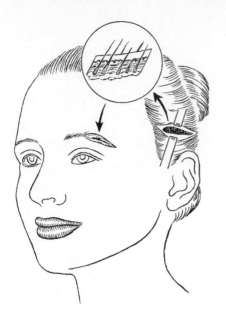

Figure 29-11. Graft reconstruction of eyebrow. Hair follicles must mimic direction of eyebrow on opposite side and must have same shape. Reconstructed side should be smaller than other side. (Redrawn from Brent B: *Plast Reconstr Surg* 55: 312-317, 1975.)

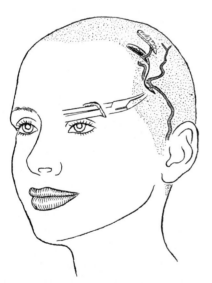

Figure 29-12. Island pedicle flap based on superficial temporal artery.

The vascularized *island pedicle flap* is reserved for patients with heavy hair density in the remaining eyebrow or for failed composite grafts. An island flap is based on the superficial temporal artery, which is identified with a Doppler stethoscope. A pattern is made and placed over the artery. The vascular pedicle is tunneled under the skin to the eyebrow (Figure 29-12). A large tunnel is necessary, and usually an excellent, bushy eyebrow results.

EARS

Indications
Involvement of the ears is common in facial burns (90%). Defects may range from partial loss to total loss of the external ear. Patient selection requires communication regarding priorities and expectations. Alternatives to reconstruction are using a prosthetic ear or wearing the hair long.

Classification
Mild defect: loss of helix and upper part of auricle without extensive scarring

Moderate defect: concha nearly normal, although may be adherent to side of head; upper half of ear missing; antihelix and its posterior crura also missing

Severe: remnant of concha; external ear orifice normal or stenosed; local soft tissues scarred.

This classification provides a framework for discussing the injury and determining treatment.

Operations
Reconstructive techniques vary with the extent of injury.

TOTAL ABSENCE OF AURICLE. The vascularized temporoparietal flap provides the tissue necessary to reconstruct the ear with a cartilage graft. Although infrequently done, this technique is successful. Some of the problems of congenital ear loss are not encountered with the burn patient; for example, the concha is intact, and the ear location is not in doubt.

An alternate approach is an osteointegrated prosthesis.[36]

SUBTOTAL ABSENCE OF HELICAL RIM. Helical defects may be either partial or complete. A partial defect may be treated with the adjacent ear tissue. The Antia procedure is effective for restoring the helical rim (Figure 29-13).[8] Local flap reconstruction is preferred if possible[18] (Figure 29-14). These procedures are usually completed as one-stage, uncomplicated operations and provide major improvement.

When the entire helix is missing, a tubed skin flap may be used (Figure 29-15).

EAR LOBE DEFORMITY. Ear lobe deformities usually are easily corrected. Adherence of the ear lobe to the adjacent neck skin is the most common deformity, and Z-plasty or local flaps are generally sufficient for correction (Figure 29-16).

If the ear lobe is absent, it may be reconstructed using a variety of local flaps.[5,10,24,33] The most common flap is a vertical or horizontal extension from the ear lobe that is folded on itself to create a detached ear lobe.

MEATAL STENOSIS. A stenotic external auditory meatus may result from a scar contracture. Splinting may be used as a preventive measure and may eliminate the need for surgical correction. If surgical release is necessary, local flaps are considered first. If flaps are insufficient, skin grafts are required. After grafting the patient wears a conformer in the ear canal for 4 to 6 months to prevent recurrence.

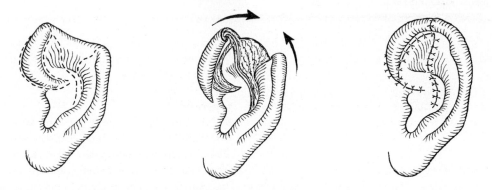

Figure 29-13. Antia procedure to restore helical rim. Smaller ear does result. (Redrawn from Antia NH, Buch VI: *Plast Reconstr Surg* 39:472-477, 1967.)

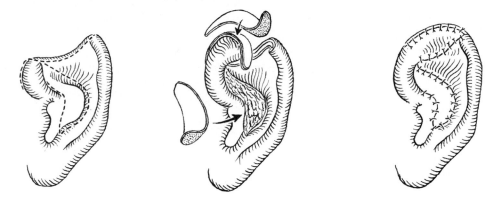

Figure 29-14. Local flap reconstruction of burned ear. Conchal cartilage and overlying skin are usually preserved and have reliable pedicle anteriorly. After alignment in new position with donor defect, flap is sutured in place and donor defect covered with skin graft.

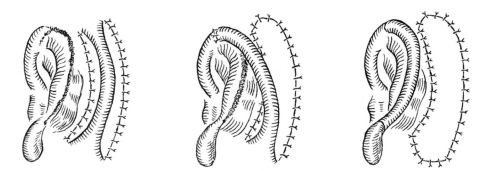

Figure 29-15. Reconstruction with long, thin cervical tube pedicle when helical rim entirely destroyed.

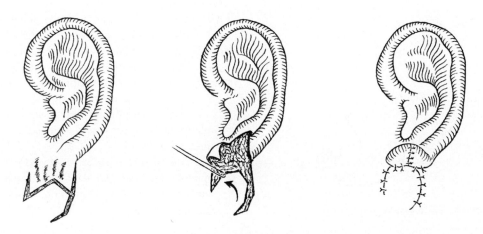

Figure 29-16. Simple local flap to reconstruct ear lobe and break up scar line.

NOSE

Indications
Nasal ectropion, extensive tissue loss and nostril stenosis are typical indications for nasal reconstruction.

Classification
Burn scar deformity: without major tissue loss

Nasal ectropion: classic nasal burn deformity resulting from loss of alar rim substance. As the scar heals and matures, a scar contracture pulls the tip of the nose up, everting the nostrils; the lower lateral cartilages are rotated externally.

Subtotal tissue loss: more than tip involved but not entire nose

Extensive tissue loss: virtually all soft tissue of nose destroyed or deformed

Nostril stenosis: unusual deformity distinct from others. With

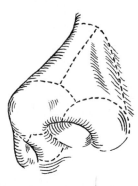

Figure 29-17. Aesthetic units of nose are guidelines for reconstruction. Plastic surgeon may not want to repair entire tip and entire nose, but should include at least a subunit when resurfacing with skin graft or other reconstruction. (Redrawn from Burget GC, Menick FJ: *Plast Reconstr Surg* 76: 239, 1985.)

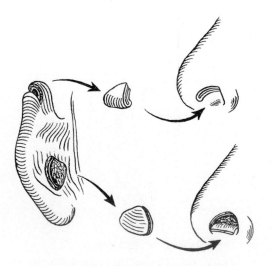

Figure 29-18. Composite graft to nose.

minimal tissue loss and scar contracture, the nostrils can close almost totally.

Operations
SCAR. Burn scar deformity without major tissue loss involves deformities such as hypertrophic scars, scar bands, discoloration, hyperpigmentation, hypopigmentation, and asymmetry. The major corrections required are scar revision and resurfacing skin grafts. The preferred procedure is use of adjacent tissue. Again, aesthetic units are the major reconstructive guidelines (Figure 29-17).[12]

ECTROPION. Nasal ectropion is best treated with composite grafts (Figure 29-18) or turn-down flaps with an FTSG. These simple techniques are very effective.

SUBTOTAL DEFECT. Subtotal tissue loss requires that tissue be imported. Flaps are usually required, but total reconstruction is unnecessary. Local scar flaps are useful.

EXTENSIVE DEFECT. The borderline between subtotal and extensive tissue loss is not well defined and must be determined by each reconstructive surgeon. A more precise way to make this judgment is needed. Resurfacing the nose is one reconstructive option (Figure 29-19).

Total nose reconstruction may be necessary. Forehead flaps are the first choice but may not be available in the burn patient. Traditional tube pedicles can be created in a variety of locations and transferred to the nose.[3]

NOSTRIL STENOSIS. This rare complication of burn injury is not difficult to correct surgically. Repair is done with release and skin grafting (Figure 29-20).[1] Splints must be worn for a minimum of 6 months after surgery to prevent recurrence.

LIP AND MOUTH

Indications
Indications for lip and mouth reconstruction include oral commissure contractures, microstomia, ectropion, and obliterated lip features.

Operations
Oral commissure burns are typically unilateral, which complicates reconstruction because the surgeon must match the normal side. The oral commissure is an important anatomic feature and thus must be restored with as much accuracy as possible. The following principles are important:

1. Wait for scar maturation, which may require more than 1 year. Dental appliances may help with scar control. At maturation the scar is softer; the softer the scar, the better the correction.
2. The commissure must be in a location symmetric with its opposite member. Accurate measurement will determine and ensure the proper position. Some overcorrection is generally advisable.

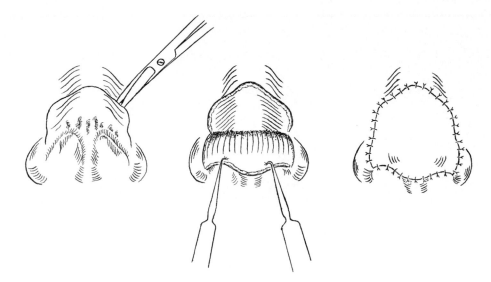

Figure 29-19. Resurfacing of nose with full-thickness skin graft.

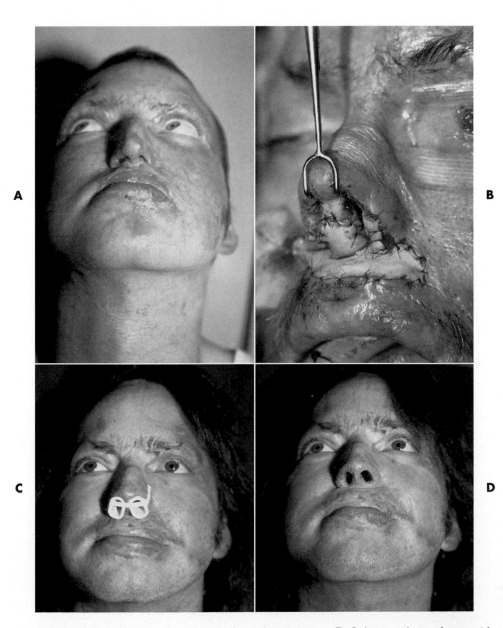

Figure 29-20. **A,** Contracture of upper lip and nostril area. **B,** Release and resurfacing with full-thickness skin grafts on lip, columella, and ala. **C,** Controlling scar tissue with splint. **D,** Postoperative result. (From Achauer BM: *Burn reconstruction,* New York, 1991, Thieme.)

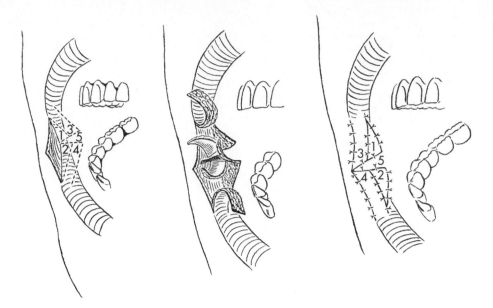

Figure 29-21. Mucosal flaps for commissure and lip reconstruction. Triangular section of scar tissue has been moved, leaving oral mucosa intact. Dotted lines show three flaps created on oral mucosa: triangular flap for lateral margin of commissure and other two flaps for vermilion of upper and lower lips. After flaps are advanced to new position, excision of dog ears may be required. (Redrawn from Converse JM: In Kazanjian VH, Converse JM, editors: *The surgical treatment of facial injuries,* Baltimore, 1959, Williams & Wilkins.)

3. The oral commissure has a unique, definite shape; it is *not* triangular. The lateral margin has a small vertical component. By reconstructing this area, the result is more natural in appearance.
4. Use like tissue for repair, that is, vermilion for vermilion and skin for skin.

Converse[16] described a mucosal flap that has served well for decades. A release is performed to the desired point, as determined by measuring the normal side. A vertical flap of mucosa reconstructs the vertical part of the commissure, and two other mucosal flaps reconstruct the upper and lower lips (Figure 29-21).

The lateral margin of the oral commissure is determined by measuring from the midline to the uninvolved side. Typically this point is just below the pupil or the end of the nasolabial fold. A slight overcorrection is desirable with extensive scarring.

AXILLA

Indications
Axillary reconstruction usually involves a scar contracture resulting in decreased mobility and function.

Classification
Scar band of either anterior or posterior axillary fold, with apex scarred
Scar bands of both anterior and posterior axillary folds
Entire axilla scarred
Scars of adjacent areas

Operations
Scar bands of either the anterior or the posterior axillary fold are a common problem. Skin grafts should be avoided. One preferred method of release and correction is with the inner arm fascial-intermuscular flap. Typically, unburned tissue is present in the inner aspect of the arm. This skin is suitable for an axillary release. The fascia is included, and limited release can be obtained.[1]

Another method is multiple Z-plasties (Figure 29-22).[1] A Z-plasty with scarring at the base will jeopardize circulation. Tip necrosis is often seen. This flap is most successful if it does not incorporate any burned tissue.

MINOR DEFECT. For minor contractures a better choice is the Y-V–plasty (Figure 29-23).[1] The triangular flap is not separated from its subjacent tissue. Using this technique, even scar tissue can be advanced without sequelae. The Y-V–plasty is also technically simpler than the Z-plasty. This procedure provides a modest release.

MODERATE DEFECT. Moderate contracture of the axilla may be corrected with a latissimus dorsi fasciocutaneous flap[4] (Figure 29-24). This narrow flap is designed to conform to the shape of the axilla. The origin of the flap allows it to be rotated and to reach the anterior axillae. The flap may have burn scar. If the scar tissue is limited to the base, the flap may be successfully transferred. This procedure is our treatment of choice and offers the following advantages over STSGs:
1. Decreased postoperative immobilization
2. Reduced postoperative therapy

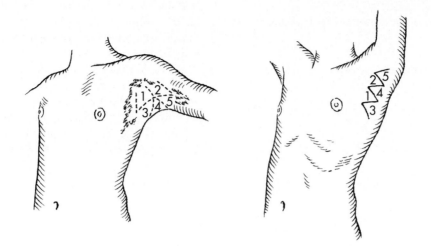

Figure 29-22. Double opposing Z-plasty for axillary release, typically with scar band on anterior axillary fold. Flaps should be unscarred. Scar tissue will not survive being elevated, undermined, or transposed. (Redrawn from Achauer BM: *Burn reconstruction,* New York, 1991, Thieme.)

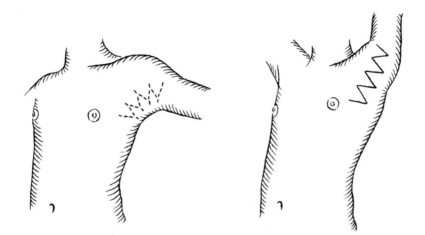

Figure 29-23. Y-V–plasty release of axillary contractures, excellent for small defects. Some flaps may involve scar tissue if they are not undermined or transposed. Y-plasty increases in size from end of scar to center of axilla and decreases at other end. Triangular flaps are then advanced into defect made by leg of Y. Each tip is secured with half-buried mattress suture, with one or two sutures in each side of triangle. (Redrawn from Achauer BM: *Burn reconstruction,* New York, 1991, Thieme.)

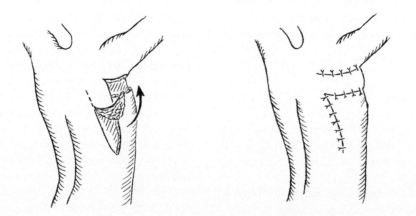

Figure 29-24. Fasciocutaneous flap for axillary contracture release has proved extremely useful. Its base superiorly overlies lateral margin of latissimus dorsi muscle. Flap has excellent thickness to resurface axilla. (Redrawn from Achauer BM: *Burn reconstruction,* New York, 1991, Thieme.)

3. Decreased hospitalization
4. Less likelihood of repeat operations for scar contracture release

SEVERE DEFECT. Severe contractures produce a large defect after release, and STSGs are required.

UPPER EXTREMITY

Indications

Claw deformity (complete or incomplete) and palmar contracture are major indications for burn reconstruction of the hand. Web space deformities include adduction contractures and syndactylism. Hypertrophic scar and contracture bands, amputation deformity, and nail bed deformity are other indications. Elbow defects include flexion contracture, extensive tissue loss from deep burns, and heterotopic ossification.

As with all burn deformities, prevention reduces the incidence of these complications. The indications for surgery are determined by the presence and severity of these defects. A claw deformity that does not interfere with hand function or appearance may not require surgery. Occasional palm contractures are mild enough that they can be left untreated. Web space deformities can be tolerated if they are mild.

With the deformities just mentioned, however, their presence is almost always an indication for surgery. Even a small claw deformity usually persists to become a major deformity in regard to function and appearance. Any tightness of the palm interferes with appearance, function, and comfort. Web space deformity can be corrected, producing normal web spaces that are more comfortable, functional, and normal appearing.

Before treating scar bands and contractures, the importance of repair should be discussed with the patient. The patient should decide whether elimination of the specific symptoms warrants undergoing a surgical procedure. Many burn patients have had many procedures and are not willing to undergo more without significant benefit.

The surgeon must consider timing when planning these operations. It is important to delay surgery until after the immature scar stage if possible. Surgery on immature scars is not recommended; the recurrence rate is high, and the deformity is not usually corrected fully. Occasionally the surgeon must operate before scar maturation to provide the patient with a functional state.

Operations

Hand reconstruction involves local flaps and STSGs or FTSGs. Local flaps can be used even in the presence of scar tissue or skin grafts. In web space deformities, for example, the procedure described can be done regardless of scarring in the area, since the flaps are not moved from their attachment to the underlying soft tissue.

When a Z-plasty is indicated in a burn patient, the surgeon performs only half the procedure. That is, one local transposition flap of unburned tissue is used to break up a straight-line contracture, and the reciprocal triangular flap is a burn scar and thus is not developed because it will be transposed. If lifted, it would be detached from its underlying tissue. Even though some small scar flaps will survive, they are not reliable and can usually be avoided.

Thick STSGs often give the best functional result with minimal contracture. FTSGs are useful for this as well. FTSGs are the first choice for grafts of the palm.

With a paucity of grafts or a problem with donor sites because of a scarcity or propensity to hypertrophic scarring, an alternative is a dermis graft. A thin graft can be used over a freeze-dried cadaver dermis (Alloderm) or other dermal substrate (Integra, Dermagraft TC). This technique provides the benefit of a thick dermis without the complications of a donor site.

CLAW DEFORMITY. The most common hand reconstruction is for claw deformity. The imbalance of forces after a dorsal hand burn result in a claw deformity. This deformity occurs when efforts to prevent it in the early stage fail. With severe deformity, the proximal interphalangeal (PIP) joint is largely destroyed. Fusion of the PIP joint allows more balance, a better-positioned hand, and relief of many problems.

The second most common procedure for the burn claw deformity is release of the dorsum with a thick STSG or an FTSG.

CONTRACTURES. Palmar contractures typically occur in children who have grasped hot objects or in persons with seizure disorders. Grafting is done when possible. The incidence of late contracture is high. After scar maturation, the deformity is excised and the area resurfaced, preferably with an FTSG.

Extra care is taken with hemostasis and immobilization postoperatively. Prolonged splinting is usually needed.

WEB SPACE DEFORMITY. The most common defect requiring correction at our burn center is the web space deformity. Despite early grafting, excellent therapy, and compliance with a treatment plan, web space contractures do occur. Z-plasty has proved to be a reliable and straightforward technique (Figure 29-25).[1]

AMPUTATION DEFORMITY. Typically, burn amputation deformities are not repaired. A major exception is amputation after an electrical injury (see Chapter 25). Typical amputation deformities involve distal and interphalangeal joints and possibly middle phalanges. Toes as well as fingers are usually involved. The most common reconstructive procedure involves deepening the web space to produce a longer digit.

Pollicization is indicated for severe deformity (Figure 29-26).[25] The thumb amputation deformity associated with electrical injury can be corrected with toe-to-thumb transfer (Figure 29-27).

NAIL BED DEFORMITY. These deformities can be reconstructed if necessary. The loss of the eponychial fold can be symptomatic in workers who rely on their hands in their

A **B** **C**

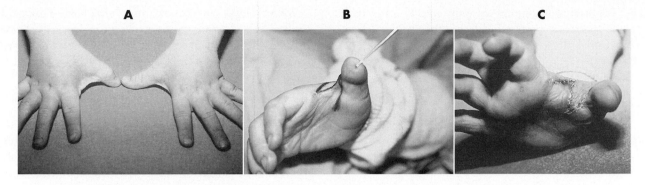

Figure 29-25. **A,** Contracture of first web space. **B,** Z-plasty flaps outlined. **C,** Definitive correction of contracture with transposition flaps. (From Achauer BM: *Burn reconstruction,* New York, 1991, Thieme.)

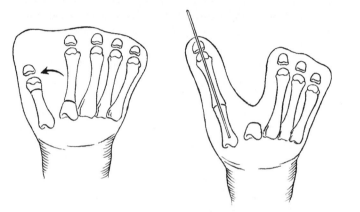

Figure 29-26. When performing pollicization for burn scar deformity, advancement may improve functional result. Normally, thumb reconstruction is made shorter than opposing phalanges. If multiple fingers have been amputated, however, a longer thumb may be useful. By manipulating bone cuts, transposed unit can be lengthened. (Redrawn from May JW Jr, Donelan MB, Toth BA: *J Hand Surg* 9A:484-489, 1984.)

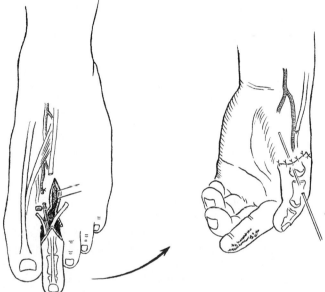

Figure 29-27. Electrical burn injury may result in amputation of thumb as well as loss of flexor tendons and neurovascular bundles. Great toe may be transferred to replace thumb.

job. Bilateral, triangular flaps have been quite useful (Figure 29-28).[2] This procedure produces a more stable nail fold over time.

OTHER DEFECTS. *Flexion contractures* occur at the wrist and elbow. These are typically released by extensive, 180-degree release through the joint's axis of rotation.

Heterotopic ossification is a rare but complicated problem that may occur in the elbow.[22]

LOWER EXTREMITY

Indications

Contractures, functional or anatomic deficiencies, and soft tissue defects are the major indications for reconstructive surgery of lower extremity structures.

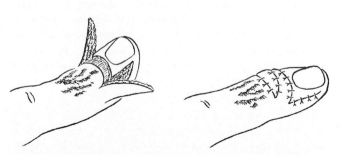

Figure 29-28. Bilateral, proximally based flaps transposed in single-stage procedure are most effective for correction of postburn nail bed deformity. (Redrawn from Achauer BM, Welk RA: *Plast Reconstr Surg* 85:937-941, 1990.)

KNEE. Popliteal contractures include medial or lateral bands and posterior popliteal defects. Soft tissue defects include exposed deep structures and unstable scars of the anterior knee.

LEG. Exposed deep structures and unstable scars are indications for burn reconstruction.

ANKLE. Achilles tendon contractures and soft tissue defects are typical ankle deformities indicating surgery.

FOOT. Indications for foot reconstruction after burns include the following:
1. Hammer toe deformity
2. Metatarsophalangeal extension
3. Phalangeal contracture
4. Web space deformity
5. Soft tissue defect

Operations
KNEE AND LEG

Popliteal Contractures: Medial or Lateral Bands. Local skin flaps should be used whenever possible. Skin flaps are preferred to grafts so that postoperative therapy and splinting are minimized. The surgeon should avoid using burned tissue when creating these flaps, since it results in a less reliable reconstruction. Postoperative immobilization with plaster is recommended.

Posterior Popliteal Contractures. If the entire popliteal area is involved, a more extensive release is indicated. Excision is done from one axis of rotation of the joint through the other to allow complete release. A deep scar is usually present and must be released to complete the correction. An STSG is placed and immobilized with a foam sponge to provide a gentle, effective "stent" dressing.

The extremity is immobilized for 5 to 7 days with a splint or cast. Once the graft has taken well, therapy is initiated. This includes daily stretching exercises and splinting at night for 3 to 6 months.

Soft Tissue Defects: Exposed Deep Structures. Flaps are usually required when an extensive deformity is present. Natural choices for the knee include the medial or lateral gastrocnemius muscle or musculocutaneous flaps. Fasciocutaneous flaps and free flaps may also be advantageous, although these are not typically used for thermal burns.

Unstable Scars. An unstable scar of the anterior knee is the primary reconstructive problem after a burn to the knee. Coverage with a skin graft may be too thin, leading to unstable correction. When a partial-thickness burn has healed without grafting, a poorly vascularized scar may result.

Minor trauma can lead to chronic breakdown. This may be resolved by *overgrafting* with a medium to thick STSG or even an FTSG. The epithelium is excised. Any available dermis is saved. A good-quality graft is added, thereby increasing the thickness of dermis.

ANKLE

Achilles Tendon Contracture. This is a ubiquitous problem in extensively burned patients with lower extremity involvement. Because patients with very large burns are often unable to stretch the Achilles tendon, prophylactic splinting should be used. The splints must not put pressure on the leg because this may lead to necrosis.

Surgical correction usually involves importing distant tissue as a free flap. Ramakrishnan et al[28] used fasciocutaneous flaps as an alternative, with excellent success rates. The inferiorly based flap was created over the heel or Achilles area, deepithelialized, and turned over. This resulted in adequate padding for the deep wound. The exposed surfaces were skin grafted.

We have no experience with distally based flaps and prefer a temporoparietal fascial flap.

Soft Tissue Defects. Deep soft tissue defects of the ankle may require imported tissue. Free flaps are the first choice, with the cross-leg musculocutaneous flap as a possible alternative.

FOOT. The common deformities in the foot listed earlier should be surgically repaired if symptomatic, particularly in children. The usual reconstruction is by release with STSGs. The position is held with Kirschner wires with or without a cast. Some type of splinting device is usually warranted. In some patients, splinting may be accomplished with firm shoes. A shoe insert may be required. Consultation with a therapist is indicated.

In the past, patients with skin grafts of the feet were hospitalized and kept on bedrest for several days with feet elevated. In acute burn therapy, pressure wraps such as the Unna boot, plaster casts, or Coban provide appropriate pressure, eliminating the need for bedrest. With these types of dressings, skin graft procedures of the feet can also be managed on an outpatient basis.

Web Space Deformity. This defect is corrected using a technique similar to that used for the hand. Repair of web space deformity in the foot, however, is not as crucial as in the hand. The surgeon should choose a simple procedure and repair only major deformities.

Amputation Tissue Defects. These deformities are common in patients with large burns. Toes are often lost, and generally no treatment is required. This can be an inconvenience, however, if the patient has also lost fingers or thumbs. The microvascular transfer may be considered.

ABDOMEN

Indications

Unstable or unattractive abdominal scars may cause a functional deficit or anatomic deformity. Usually, however, scar deformities of the abdomen have relatively low priority if other burn scars exist. On the other hand, abdominal scars may be the only deformities and may result in significant functional limitations for the patient.

Operations

SMALL DEFECT. Small defects may be managed with primary excision and closure.

MODERATE DEFECT. Moderate defects are managed with staged serial excision. Problematic scar bands can be released and reconstructed with local flaps and STSGs. Skin grafts are a quick solution but often leave an irregular contour.

LARGE DEFECT. Extensive hypertrophic scarring may become a major problem. Although skin grafts can be used to cover excision of scars, they may cause scarring at the donor site.

Some patients benefit from extensive tissue expansion (Figure 29-29). Children tolerate extensive tissue expansion well. Large areas of scar can be replaced by local tissue. Tissue expansion provides the best approach for like-for-like tissue replacement.

BREAST

Indications

Scarring, deformity, and asymmetry are major indications for breast reconstruction.

The most common breast burns result from scald injuries after hot liquid is poured on the chest and abdomen of a young girl. The surgeon must be extremely conservative in debriding the nipple area. The first priority is to not alter the breast bud. This is left in place so that the breast will develop. Typically the breast is distorted as it develops.

Follow-up should continue through puberty. After scar maturity, and puberty, reconstructive surgery can be planned.

Operations

Surgical intervention can range from a release, typically done in the inframammary fold, to extensive excision of an unyielding scar. STSGs are then used, allowing the breast to take its typical shape (Figure 29-30). Usually the nipple retains patent ducts, with a good chance of successful nursing. A four-flap nipple procedure is done to lengthen the nipple (Figure 29-31). This does not disturb the duct but does leave a raw area around the nipple. An FTSG over these areas simulates the areola. The final result can be enhanced by tattooing of the nipple and areola.

Breast reconstruction with implants or with flaps, such as the latissimus dorsi myocutaneous flap or the transverse rectus abdominis myocutaneous (TRAM) flap, are options but are rarely indicated.

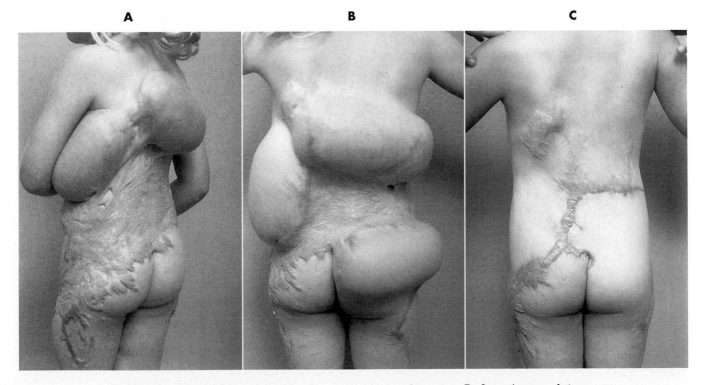

A   **B**   **C**

Figure 29-29.   A, Tissue expansion for extensive truncal scarring. **B,** Second stage of tissue expansion. **C,** Postoperative result.

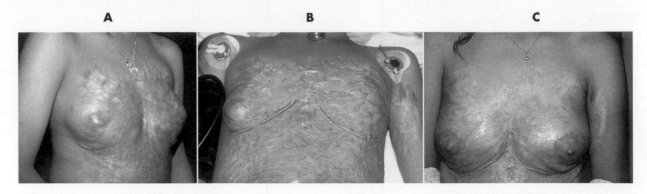

Figure 29-30. **A,** Extensive scarring of chest restricting breast tissue. **B,** Surgical preparation. **C,** After release and skin grafting, with nipple reconstruction.

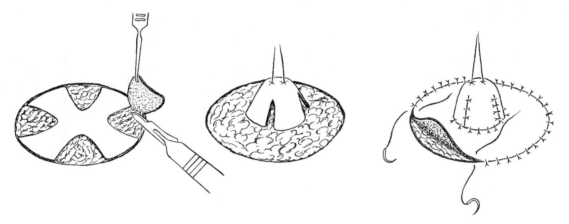

Figure 29-31. Nipple reconstruction with four-flap technique.

PERINEAL AREA

Indications

Contractures represent a net loss of functional tissue in the perineal region.

Operations

As with any area of the body that has symptomatic scars, perineal scars are amenable to excision and direct closure (Figure 29-32). Transposition flaps may also be used.

Perineal burns can lead to sexual dysfunction, it and psychologic care can ease the resulting anxiety. A sympathetic nurse may also be helpful. Adolescent females are reticent to discuss this with a male physician or most adults. Functional problems can almost always be improved with appropriate surgical and psychologic care.

GENITALIA

Indications

Contractures and partial or complete loss of the external genitalia are the major indications for burn reconstruction of the genitalia.

Loss of genitalia rarely occurs with thermal burns but is seen with electrical burns. Penile reconstruction may be required (see Chapter 35). Unfortunately, these patients have many other injuries, and the first or second choice for reconstruction may not be available. The surgeon may need to plan a unique reconstruction using an individualized approach.

Operations

Scar contracture may lead to functional loss, such as difficulty with sex or urination. Release of scar contracture with skin grafting is indicated, but this is rarely done.

Total penile reconstruction may be indicated for total loss of the genitalia. The neurosensory radial forearm flap is preferred.[13] The limiting factor of this procedure is scarring of the forearms.

OUTCOMES

Doctor et al[17] examined the outcomes of 91 patients after severe burn injury, collecting longitudinal data over 1 year. Their study used a prospective design and a widely used generic measure of health status, the *sickness impact profile* (SIP). The SIP provides a measure of sickness-related dysfunction. This is measured on an interval scale and is therefore a quantitative measure of dysfunction.

Survivors of severe burns have stable and relatively good health status compared with other patient populations (Table 29-1). Over time, however, their health status is inferior to that

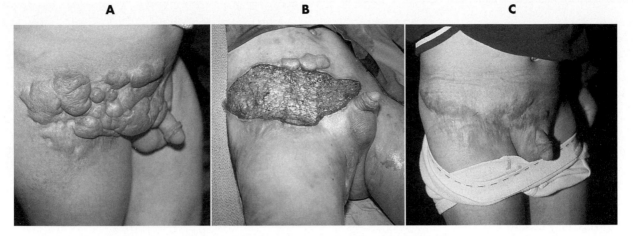

Figure 29-32. **A,** Extensive scarring of inguinal area. **B,** Intraoperative view showing extent of excision. **C,** After excision and direct closure.

Table 29-1.
Health Outcomes Measured by Sickness Impact Profile (SIP) for Survivors of Major Burn Injuries Compared with Other Patient Populations

PATIENT POPULATION	SIP SCORE (% OVERALL DYSFUNCTION)
SIP SCORES <CI .95*	
General population: preinjury	2.5
General population	3.3
Ulcerative colitis	5.2
ESRD: posttransplantation	5.5
Myocardial infarction (no arrest)	6.9
SIP SCORES WITHIN CI .95	
Cataract: before surgery	7.5
Coronary artery disease	7.5
Angina pectoris: NYHA class I	8.3
Crohn's disease	8.6
Hearing-impaired elderly	9.2
Major burn injury survivors: 1 month after injury	9.3
Lower extremity fracture	9.8
Cardiac arrest survivors	10.3
Female patients who have undergone CABG	10.3
Congestive heart failure	10.4
Elderly outpatients	11.4
SIP SCORES >CI .95	
Continuous peritoneal dialysis	13.7
Total hip arthroplasty	14.2

Continued

Table 29-1.
Health Outcomes Measured by Sickness Impact Profile (SIP) for Survivors of Major Burn Injuries Compared with Other Patient Populations—cont'd

PATIENT POPULATION	SIP SCORE (% OVERALL DYSFUNCTION)
SIP SCORES >CI .95—CONT'D	
End-stage arthritis	14.9
Rheumatoid arthritis	15.6
Head injury	15.7
Angina pectoris: NYHA class II	16.1
Chronic lung disease	16.2
Parkinson's disease	16.8
Recurrent syncope	16.8
HIV positive	17.4
Chronic pain	17.7
Hemodialysis	18.0
HIV disease: stages 3 and 4	18.8
Low back pain	20.8
ARC and AIDS	21.0
Multiple sclerosis outpatients	21.1
Angina pectoris: NYHA class III	22.3
Osteoarthritis of knee and hip	23.3
Liver transplantation candidates	23.4
Hospitalization for combined medical and psychiatric problems	23.8
Chronic low back pain	23.8
Stroke (cerebrovascular accident)	25.4
Heart transplantation candidates	31.7
Amyotrophic lateral sclerosis	32.3
Nursing home residents	40.4

Modified from Doctor JN, Patterson DR, Mann R: *J Burn Care Rehabil* 18:490-495, 1997.
ESRD, End-stage renal disease; *NYHA class,* New York Heart Association classification; *CABG,* coronary artery bypass grafting; *HIV,* human immunodeficiency virus; *ARC,* AIDS-related complex; *AIDS,* acquired immunodeficiency syndrome.
*CI .95, 95% confidence interval for major burn injury survivors.

of the general population. Vocational and psychosocial functioning are the most troublesome for the burn survivor (Table 29-2).[17]

Staley et al[32] have defined functional outcomes for burn patients, emphasizing the importance of measuring function. Helvig et al[21] have developed quality indicators for burn outcomes as a project of the American Burn Association Committee on Organization and Delivery of Burn Care. We hope that these efforts will result in future documentation of outcomes in the burn population.

The literature lacks studies on the effects of reconstruction. This would be an interesting area for future research.

Table 29-2.
Sickness-related Dysfunction across 12 Categories of Everyday Living Measured by Sickness Impact Profile (SIP) 1 Month after Burn Injury

CATEGORY	SIP (+/− SEM)
PHYSICAL SUBSCALE	
Ambulation	8.1 (1.5)
Mobility	5.2 (1.1)
Body care/movement	4.0 (0.8)
PSYCHOSOCIAL SUBSCALE	
Communication	5.4 (1.2)
Alertness behavior	10.2 (2.2)
Emotional behavior	12.8 (1.7)
Social interaction	10.9 (1.6)
INDEPENDENT SUBSCALE	
Sleep and rest	10.4 (1.6)
Eating	4.3 (3.4)
Work	25.4 (3.4)
Home management	14.2 (2.1)
Recreation	17.7 (2.0)

Modified from Doctor JN, Patterson DR, Mann R. *J Burn Care Rehabil* 18:492, 1997.

REFERENCES

1. Achauer BM: *Burn reconstruction,* New York, 1991, Thieme.
2. Achauer BM, Welk RA: One stage reconstruction of the postburn nail-fold contracture, *Plast Reconstr Surg* 85:937-941, 1990.
3. Achauer BM, Daly B, Martinez S: The role of pedicled flaps in burned nose reconstruction, *Eur J Plast Surg* 18:314-315, 1995.
4. Achauer BM, Spenler CW, Gold ME: Reconstruction of axillary burn contractures with the latissimus dorsi fasciocutaneous flap, *J Trauma* 28:211-213, 1988.
5. Alanis SZ: A new method for earlobe reconstruction, *Plast Reconstr Surg* 45:254-257, 1970.
6. Almaguer E, Dillon BT, Parry SW: Facial resurfacing at Shriners Burns Institute: a 16 year experience in young burned patients, *J Trauma* 25:1081-1082, 1985.
7. Angrigiani C: Total face reconstruction with one free flap, *Plast Reconstr Surg* 99:1566-1575, 1997.
8. Antia NH, Buch VI: Chondrocutaneous advancement flap for the marginal defect of the ear, *Plast Reconstr Surg* 39:472-477, 1967.
9. Barrera A: Micrograft and minigraft megasession hair transplantation results after a single session, *Plast Reconstr Surg* 110:1524-1530, 1997.
10. Brent B: Earlobe construction with an auriculo-mastoid flap, *Plast Reconstr Surg* 57:389-391, 1976.
11. Brent B: Reconstruction of the ear, eyebrow and sideburn in the burned patient, *Plast Reconstr Surg* 55:312-317, 1975.
12. Burget GC, Menick FJ: The subunit principal in nasal reconstruction, *Plast Reconstr Surg* 76:239, 1985.
13. Chang T, Hwang W: Forearm flaps in one stage reconstruction of the penis, *Plast Reconstr Surg* 74:251-258, 1984.
14. Clodius F, Smahel J: Resurfacing denuded areas of the beard with full-thickness scalp grafts, *Br J Plast Surg* 32:295-299, 1979.
15. Converse JM: Burn deformities of the face and neck, *Surg Clin North Am* 47:323, 1967.
16. Converse JM: Technique of elongation of the oral fissure and restoration of the angle of the mouth. In Kazanjian VH, Converse JM, editors: *The surgical treatment of facial injuries,* Baltimore, 1959, Williams & Wilkins.
17. Doctor JN, Patterson DR, Mann R: Health outcome for burn survivors, *J Bone Care Rehabil* 18:490-495, 1997.
18. Donelan MB: Conchal transposition flap for postburn ear deformities, *Plast Reconstr Surg* 83:641-654, 1989.
19. Feldman JJ: Reconstruction of the burned face in children. In Serafin D, Georgiade NG, editors: *Pediatric plastic surgery,* St Louis, 1984, Mosby.
20. Gonzales-Ulloa M: Restoration of the face covering by means of selected skin in regional aesthetic units, *Br J Plast Surg* 9:212-221, 1956.
21. Helvig EI, Upright J, Bartleson BJ: The development of outcome statements for burn care, *Semin Periop Nurs* 6:197-200, 1997.
22. Hoffer MN, Brody G, Ferlic F: Excision of heterotopic ossification about elbows in patients with thermal injury, *J Trauma* 18:667-670, 1978.
23. Jurkiewicz MJ, Hill HL: Open wound of the scalp: an account of methods of repair, *J Trauma* 21:769-778, 1981.
24. Kazanjian VH: Deformities of the external ear. In Kazanjian VH, Converse JM, editors: *The surgical treatment of facial injuries,* Baltimore, 1949, Williams & Wilkins.
25. May JW Jr, Donelan MB, Toth BA: Thumb reconstruction in the burned hand by advancement pollicization of the second ray remnant, *J Hand Surg* 9A:484-489, 1984.
26. Orticochea M: New three-flap scalp reconstruction techniques, *Br J Plast Surg* 24:184-188, 1971.
27. Pensler JM, Dillon B, Perry SW: Reconstruction of the eyebrow in the pediatric burn patient, *Plast Reconstr Surg* 76:434-439, 1985.
28. Ramakrishnan KM, Ch M, Jayaramoan V, et al: Deepithelialized turnover flaps in burns, *Plast Reconstr Surg* 82:262-266, 1988.
29. Rose EH: *Aesthetic facial restoration,* Philadelphia, 1998, Lippincott-Raven.
30. Rose EH: Aesthetic restoration of the severely disfigured face in burn victims: comprehensive strategies, *Plast Reconstr Surg* 96:1573-1585, 1995.

31. Sloan DF, Huang TT, Larson DL, Lewis SR: Reconstruction of eyelids and eyebrows in burned patients, *Plast Reconstr Surg* 58:340-346, 1976.

32. Staley M, Richard R, Warden GD, et al: Functional outcomes for the patient with burn injuries, *J Burn Care Rehabil* 17:362-368, 1996.

33. Subba-Rao YV, Ventkateswara-Roa P: A quick technique for ear lobe reconstruction, *Plast Reconstr Surg* 41:13-16, 1968.

34. Tajima S, Aoyage F: Correcting post-traumatic lateral epicanthal folds, *J Br Plast Surg* 30:200-201, 1977.

35. Waymack JP, Law E, Park R, et al: Acute upper airway obstruction in the postburn period, *Arch Surg* 120:1042-1044, 1985.

36. Wolfaardt JF, Coss P, Levesque R: Craniofacial osseointegration: technique for bar and acrylic resin substructure construction for auricular prostheses, *J Prosthet Dent* 76:603-607, 1996.

Pressure Sores

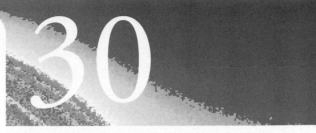

John S. Mancoll
Linda G. Phillips

INTRODUCTION

Pressure sores result from a complex process of tissue destruction, and a thorough knowledge of this pathophysiology is essential for their successful treatment. As with many multifaceted disease processes, a multidisciplinary approach to treatment is required. The team includes physicians from various fields (plastic surgeons, general surgeons, internal medicine specialists, endocrinologists, neurologists), nurses, nutritionists, and mental health experts. Plastic surgeons are uniquely suited to lead this team of medical specialists.

INDICATIONS

DEFINITION AND ETIOLOGY

The terms *pressure sores, decubitus ulcers,* and *bedsores* have been used synonymously to refer to the tissue ulceration typically seen in debilitated patients. The term *decubitus* comes from the Latin *decumbere,* "to lie down." Although this term may be appropriate for bedridden patients, it does not correctly describe the ulcers in mobile patients (e.g., ischial ulcers in wheelchair-bound patients).[4] The common physiologic process in all patients with decubitus ulcers is unrelieved pressure, and thus *pressure sore* is the best descriptive term.

In addition to unrelieved pressure, factors contributing to the formation of pressure sores include the following:

1. Altered sensory perception
2. Incontinence
3. Exposure to moisture
4. Altered activity and mobility
5. Friction and shear forces
6. Poor nutrition

Individually, any one of these factors does not lead to ulcer formation, but the combination with unrelieved pressure may result in irreversible tissue injury.

EPIDEMIOLOGY

The incidence of pressure sore formation is highly variable and depends on patient population evaluated. Over the last 25 years, several studies have determined the incidence of pressure sores in various settings. The Fourth National Pressure Ulcer Prevalence Survey (NPUPS) found an incidence of 1.4% to 36.4%, with a mean of 10.8%, in the acute care setting.[3] Most ulcers were stage I or II. All studies cited the association with other medical problems, including cardiovascular disease (41%), acute neurologic disease (27%), and orthopedic injury (15%).[11,38,59]

In chronic care facilities the incidence rises sharply. Reports vary from as low as 3.5% to as high as 50% in some series.[67,68] The more significant ulcerations, however, tend to occur in acute care patients; the primary disease process may overshadow other concerns, and pressure sores may be allowed to progress unnoticed for longer periods. In addition to medical problems, age is an associated factor. In 1997 the Fourth NPUPS found that 63% of patients with ulcers were more than 70 years old.[3]

The incidence in patients with spinal cord injuries has decreased greatly with the advent of rehabilitation centers and overall awareness of the problem. Initial reports after World War II measured pressure sores in up to 85% of veterans in the Veterans Administration (VA) system.[11] In 1983 Stal et al[77] cited a 20% incidence in paraplegic patients and 26% in quadriplegic patients.

The most common locations involving pressure sores in paraplegic patients are the ischial, trochanteric, and sacral regions. In the acute care setting, supine patients who are predominantly bedridden have a slightly different distribution. Of the 6603 ulcer reported in the NPUPS in 1997, 36% were sacral, 30% heel, and 6% ischial, trochanteric, or malleolar[3] (Table 30-1).

INFORMED CONSENT

Treating patients with pressure sores involves more than managing with a nonhealed wound. Treatment options are largely

Table 30-1.
Pressure Sore Staging

STAGE	DESCRIPTION
I	Skin intact but reddened for more than 1 hour after relief of pressure
II	Blister or other break in dermis with or without infection
III	Subcutaneous destruction into muscle with or without infection
IV	Involvement of bone or joint with or without infection

Modified from Barczak C, Barnett R, Child E, et al: *Adv Wound Care* 10(4):19, 1997.

determined by the patient's and family's ability to comply with the regimen. Thus the patient must be both mentally and physically prepared for surgery.

Proper informed consent of these patients must include information about the overall disease process, the mechanism of injury, and the prevention of pressure sores. They must realize that this is a lifelong disease process and that they must be committed for therapy to be successful. They should be informed about the high recurrence rates associated with both surgical and nonsurgical approaches. Other aspects of informed consent mainly explain the potential complications of treatment (see Outcomes section).

PATHOPHYSIOLOGY

Since the most successful treatment of pressure sores is prevention, all practitioners must have an adequate understanding of the pathophysiology. Although initial theories regarding pressure sore development by Charcot (1879), Leyden (1874), and Munro (1940) all stressed the importance of neurologic impairment, we now know that pressure is the single most important etiologic factor.[7,70] The compression of soft tissues results in ischemia and, if unrelieved, will progress and cause necrosis and ulceration. In susceptible patients this sequence of events may be accelerated because of other endogenous sources, such as infection, malnutrition, diabetes, or altered neurologic states.

Pressure

Pressure is the most important feature in the formation of ulcers.[16] Of all pressure sores, 96% occur below the level of the umbilicus.[57] For most patients the wounds develop in either the supine or the seated position. Not surprisingly, therefore, up to 75% of all pressure sores are located around the pelvic girdle.[3]

In 1930 Landis[51] used a microinjection system to determine that capillary blood pressure in a single capillary ranged from 12 mm Hg on the venous end to 32 mm Hg on the arterial end. If the external compressive force exceeds capillary bed pressure, capillary perfusion is impaired and ischemia will ensue.

This effect is not instantaneous, however, or everyone would have pressure sores. An inverse relationship exists between the amount of pressure and the length of time required to cause ulceration. Early studies by Kosiak et al[49] demonstrated that 70 mm Hg applied over 2 hours was sufficient to cause pathologic changes in dogs. Similarly, Daniel et al[18] also demonstrated ischemic changes in a paraplegic pig model. He showed that 500 mm Hg applied for 2 hours or 100 mm Hg for 10 hours was sufficient to cause muscle necrosis. Interestingly, it was not until 600 mm Hg was applied for 11 hours that ulceration of the skin could be seen. These results not only confirmed the relationship between pressure and time, but also demonstrated that the initial pathologic changes occurred in the muscle overlying the bone. They also showed that muscle is more susceptible than skin to ischemia, as evidenced by the increased time necessary to see skin changes.[67]

In their classic 1965 study, Lindan et al[57] used a compressible bed of springs and nails to measure the external distribution of contact pressure in patients in the supine and seated positions (Figure 30-1 and 30-2). They found that in the supine position the maximal recorded pressures were 40 to 60 mm Hg near the heels, buttocks, and sacrum. In the sitting position the pressures were greatest near the ischial tuberosities, with measurements up to 100 mm Hg.

Husain[45] studied the effects of pressure versus time to determine which had the greater impact on ulcer formation. He believed that low pressures maintained for long periods induced more tissue damage than high pressures for short periods. Kosiak et al[49] investigated dogs subjected to constant pressure for varying times. They noted an inverse parabolic relationship between the amount of pressure and duration of exposure (Figure 30-3). Dinsdale[21] confirmed these results in a pig model but also demonstrated minimal tissue injury if pressure could be relieved for as briefly as 5 minutes. This reversal was seen even with pressures as high as 450 mm Hg. Le[52] et al demonstrate characteristic pressure gradient highest directly over the bony prominence, tapering in all directions radiating from the bony prominence. The result is a conical shaped wound, which is typical of pressure sores. This is consistent with previous findings showing the most tissue destruction directly overlying the bony prominence but still extending to the surrounding tissue. Round off the bone versus not cutting it out, as shown in this figure (Figure 30-5).

Infection

Pressure sore formation is the culmination of many different factors combining to cause tissue destruction. As previously mentioned, Daniel et al[18] demonstrated a resistance to ulceration of the skin in studies in which only pressure and time was altered. In the clinical setting, skin involvement occurs with nearly all pressure sores. Clearly, some other factor must be significantly involved.

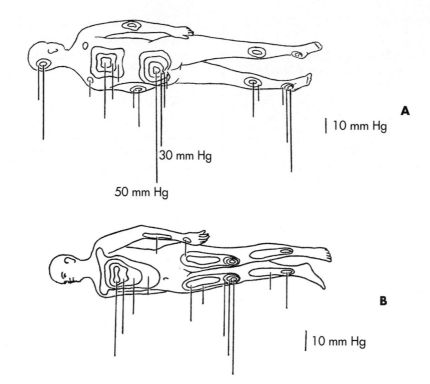

Figure 30-1. Pressure distribution in **A,** supine, and **B,** prone positions.

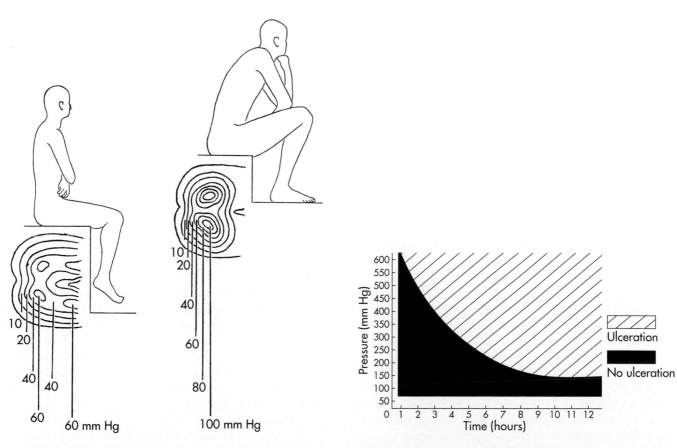

Figure 30-2. Pressure distribution in sitting positions.

Figure 30-3. Inverse relationship between time and pressure in formation of pressure sores. (Modified from Kosiak M et al: *Arch Phys Med Rehabil* 39:623, 1958.)

Box 30-1.
Results of Bacterial Growth in Control Wounds and Wounds Subjected to Pressure

Incisions inoculated with 5×10^7 *Staphylococcus aureus*

Pressure limbs: Control limbs:
3×10^8 1×10^5

Pressure: 1 psi/hr

From Robson MC and Krizek TJ: In Frederick S, Brody GS: *Symposium on neurologic aspects of plastic surgery*, St Louis, 1978, Mosby.

Some propose that the rapid rate of skin breakdown in a pressure sore suggests a bacterial process. The accelerated rate at which necrosis can occur in a pressure sore may be the result of the collagenolytic activity known to accompany bacterial infections. Compressed skin has less resistance to bacterial invasion.[39]

In 1942 Groth[33] demonstrated that bacteria would accumulate in areas of increased pressure. He simultaneously injected rabbits with bacteria while applying external pressure to the gluteal region. This resulted in localized collections of bacteria in the compressed sites.

Robson and Krizek[73] quantified the effect of pressure on bacterial count. They showed that surgical incisions created in areas of applied pressure and inoculated with known concentrations of organisms allowed for a 100-fold greater bacterial growth than in areas not subjected to pressure (Box 30-1). The proposed mechanisms include impaired lymphatic function, ischemia, denervation, and impaired immune function.[70]

Edema
The role of edema in promoting the infectious process seen in pressure sores must not be overlooked. Compressed, denervated skin is known to become edematous by several processes. Landis[51] demonstrated the pressure needed to overcome end capillary pressure in the skin. Once external pressures exceed 12 mm Hg, the veins become engorged, and total tissue pressure increases. As this process continues, end arterial pressure increases; at this point, plasma extravasation occurs, leading to edema formation. Also, the tissues are denervated, which compounds this process. This leads to loss of sympathetic tone in the blood vessels, which causes vasodilation and increased engorgement of the vessels and greater edema.

Denervation indirectly contributes to lymphatic edema. In their study of hemiplegic patients, Exton-Smith and Crockett[25] noted edema 2 weeks after injury in 16% of the patients, persisting up to 6 months. They postulated that this was the result of injury to the lymphatic pump, which depends on skeletal muscle to function.

Edema formation in pressure sore patients also results from inflammatory mediators released in response to the trauma of compression. The normal homeostasis between prostaglandins $F_{2\alpha}$ and PGE_2 is disrupted in favor of PGE_2. This leads to increased leakage through the cell membranes and ultimately increased interstitial fluid accumulation. As interstitial plasma concentrations rise, the concentration of sebum is diluted. Sebum has been shown to be important in the defense against both streptococcal and staphylococcal infections.[70]

Shear
Vertical shear, or *shearing,* is a factor often overlooked by health care professionals when treating patients with pressure sores. Every time a patient is dragged up to the head of the bed and then allowed to slump down again, the area of the body in contact with the bed is subject to shear forces. Vertical shearing might contribute more to pressure sore formation than compression. When a patient slides against the sheets, the skin and subcutaneous tissue tend to adhere to the sheets, whereas the underlying fascia, muscle, and bone tend to follow the pull of gravity. The perforating blood vessels are stretched, may avulse, and may ultimately lead to tissue ischemia.

Using computed tomographic (CT) analysis of patients, Conner and Clack[10] were able to demonstrate that vertical shear forces result when a patient is in the supine position. The patient's weight against the underlying surface causes morphologic changes in the tissues, resulting in tension and strain on the tissues. These strains are most obvious near bony prominences. The authors further studied the effects of various air and foam mattresses on this phenomenon and determined that an air mattress with 3 inches of foam was most effective at eliminating the effects of vertical shear.

PREOPERATIVE CARE

The treatment of pressure sores is one of the most challenging areas in plastic surgery today. Recurrence rates as high as 95% have been reported. Preparing a patient and the family for long-term management requires a team approach. Consultation with medical personnel from internal medicine, endocrinology, neurology, urology, nutrition, physical and occupational therapy, and psychiatry, as well as with a wound care nurse specialist, is essential.[77] All components of the patient's overall care must be optimized before surgery. Specific contributing factors must be corrected to facilitate successful wound closure.

Nutrition
The patient's nutritional condition must be reviewed. Patients may be malnourished because of the primary disease or the inability to obtain adequate nutritional support. Daily calorie counts should be started as soon as the patient is hospitalized to determine daily caloric intake. Assuming no other stress factors, 25 to 35 cal/kg of nonprotein calories should be delivered daily. Daily protein requirements are 1.5 to 3.0 g/kg depending on the ulcer's size and the patient's starting protein and albumin levels.

As a marker for impaired healing, hypoalbuminemia is controversial. Early reports by Howe et al[40] demonstrated decreased incisional strength in animals. In 1987 Felcher and Schwartz[26] failed to demonstrate impaired healing in analbuminemic rats. Robson et al[76] demonstrated normal healing potential in clinical trails as long as serum albumin was maintained above 2.0 g/dl. It is difficult to be protein depleted without also lacking other minerals and trace elements critical to pathways necessary for proper healing.

Vitamin C is essential for proper collagen production. The role of vitamin C in hydroxylation of proline and lysine for proper collagen stranding is well documented.[60] Other essential vitamins include vitamin A. The exact role of vitamins is not completely known but involves cell differentiation and epithelialization. Vitamins can increase cell-mediated immunity, contribute to the early inflammatory response seen in wound healing, and may contribute to angiogenesis.[55]

Trace elements are also critical for wounds to heal properly. Zinc is specifically involved with epithelialization and fibroblast proliferation through its effects on metalloenzymes (e.g., RNA polymerase, DNA polymerase and transcriptase.) Zinc also contributes to many aspects of the immune response, including phagocytosis, cellular and humoral immunity, and bactericidal activity. Ferrous iron is needed for hydroxylation of lysine and proline; copper is needed for lysyl oxidase; and both are needed for normal collagen metabolism. Blood levels should be assessed and supplemented as part of the patient's nutritional care. The amount needed daily of these elements will vary. No study has demonstrated that supraphysiologic levels will accelerate wound healing beyond normal.[28,37,55,81]

If the patient is unable to take an adequate amount of daily nutrition, supplemental means should be used. Tube feedings, either continuous or at night, can deliver the necessary additional calories needed for wound repair. It may also be important to deliver these supplements in a low-residue form, since fecal incontinence and soiling of these wounds are significant problems in many patients. If enteral feeding is not possible, parenteral hyperalimentation should be used. Catheter-related problems must be monitored daily, including infection, catheter malposition, and local extravasation.

Treatment of Infection

Concomitant infections may occur in patients with pressure sores. Indwelling bladder catheters or self-catheterization programs can result in urinary sepsis in one third of patients with paraplegia. If left untreated, urinary infections can be a constant source of bacteremia. As previously shown by Groth[33] and others, ischemic tissues surrounding pressure areas are particularly susceptible to seeding, and any infection must be controlled.

Patients with high spinal cord lesions are also susceptible to developing pulmonary infections because of poor diaphragmatic function. A program of pulmonary toilet is recommended preoperatively and postoperatively and includes positioning, side-to-side rolling, deep breathing and coughing, chest physical therapy, and bronchodilators.

Osteomyelitis is another infection seen in patients with pressure sores. The incidence has been reported to be as high as 23% in spinal cord–injured patients with pressure sores. The workup for suspected osteomyelitis includes complete blood count, erythrocyte sedimentation rate, and plain radiographs.[56] This combination of studies has a sensitivity of 73% and a specificity of 96%. Although other diagnostic methods are available, including technetium 99m, CT, and magnetic resonance imaging (MRI) scanning, these studies can be costly and may expose the patient to radiation risks (Figure 30-4).

When preoperative studies are negative but osteomyelitis is still suspected, a needle core biopsy can be performed at the bedside. Bone biopsy can be considered the gold standard for diagnosing osteomyelitis but can have a significant false-positive rate if not carefully performed, since bacterial contamination is common in these wounds. The accuracy of the biopsy can be increased if adequate debridement is first performed and if careful adherence to sterile technique is maintained.

The use of antibiotics should include topical antimicrobial agents as well as systemic therapy. Before initiation of antibiotic therapy, wound biopsies should be sent for quantitative culture. The accuracy rates for tissue biopsies range from 90% to 100%. Swabbing of the wound is discouraged, however, because the specimen may only represent surface contaminants and thus may not be as reliable. The reported accuracy rate for swabbing is 65% to 98%.[72,78]

Appropriate antibiotics should include coverage of gram-positive, gram-negative, and anaerobic organisms. The most common organisms cultured from pressure sores include common skin flora (staphylococci, streptococci, corynebacteria) and enteric organisms *(Proteus, Escherichia coli, Pseudomonas)*. Chronic suppressive therapy may be needed to deal with persistent urinary infections.

Relief of Pressure

The initial goal is to avoid progression of the sore by relieving the source of pressure. Wound healing will not occur in the presence of ischemia or infection.

A simple program of turning the patient allows for recirculation in the affected areas. As previously stated, the deleterious effects of pressure can be negated by relieving it for as briefly as 5 minutes every 2 hours. In addition, a variety of mattress systems are designed to relieve pressure, including foam, static flotation, alternating-air, low-air-loss, and air-fluidized beds.[9] The purpose of these beds is to distribute the patient's weight more evenly to minimize pressure in any one area.

The Clinitron bed is designed with medical-grade optical beads fluidized with a constant flow of warm air.[69] The Clinitron bed is most effective at reducing external pressures when the patient is supine. It has disadvantages, however, including a weight of 1700 to 2000 pounds, which may be too bulky or heavy for patients treated at home. The bed is known to cause electrolyte and water losses, especially in elderly patients, which may lead to hallucinations and disorientation. Also, if any padding (pillow, foam wedge, bolster) is placed under the patient, pressures are redistributed and end capillary pressure may be exceeded. In patients with compromised breathing, pulmonary toilet may be impaired. The Clinitron bed does not negate the need for good wound care; it only helps relieve the pressure that caused the problem.

Management of Spasm

Spasticity is common in patients with spinal cord injuries. Loss of supraspinal inhibitory pathways is believed to be the mechanism of spasm in these patients. The incidence of spasm varies with the level of injury. The more proximal the lesion, the higher is the incidence of spasm: almost 100% in cervical, 75% in thoracic, and 50% in thoracolumbar regions. If spasm is not eliminated before any surgical procedure, the pressure sore will inevitably recur.

Medications are available to reduce spasm (Table 30-2). Our choice is diazepam (Valium), 10 mg every 4 to 6 hours or in combination with baclofen (Lioresal). Baclofen is usually started at 5 mg every 6 hours and may be increased to as much as 20 mg every 6 hours. Also available is Dantrolene (Dantrium), 25 mg every 12 hours. Physicians should use caution with these drugs because hepatic toxicity has been reported, and serum transaminases should be monitored. If patients do not respond to medical therapy, surgical intervention may be indicated.

The surgical management of spasm includes peripheral nerve blocks, epidural stimulators, baclofen pumps, and rhizotomy. *Rhizotomy* can be surgical or medical using subarachnoid blocks with phenol (phenol rhizotomy). Since clinical improvement can occur up to 18 months after injury, surgical rhizotomy is not performed during this period. In addition, some spinal cord lesions are not complete, and rhizotomy must be used with care to avoid exacerbating the injury.

Table 30-2.
Medications Used to Treat Spasm

DRUG	USUAL DOSE (mg)	RANGE (mg)	FREQUENCY
Diazepam (Valium)	10	5-20	Every 4-6 hours
Baclofen (Lioresal)	5	5-20	Four times a day
Dantrolene (Dantrium)	25	25-100	Every day to four times a day

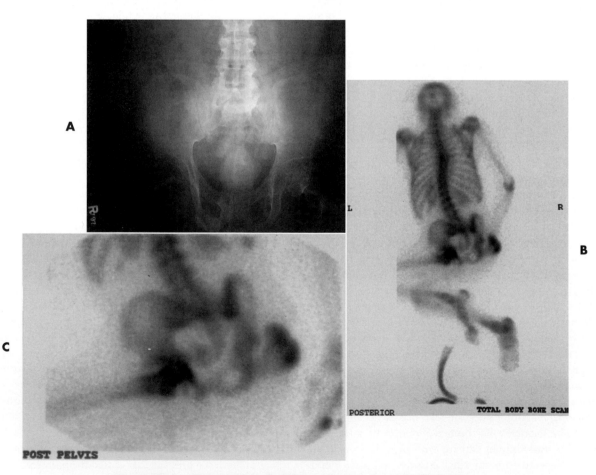

Figure 30-4. Osteomyelitis. **A,** Pelvic radiograph. **B** and **C,** Bone scans.

Contracture Therapy

Joint contractures may occur in patients with longstanding denervation. Unless an aggressive program of physical therapy is initiated early, these patients will have a significant problem. Contractures are caused by tightening of both muscles and joint capsules. Because the hip flexors are so strong, contractures are common in this region, contributing to the formation of trochanteric, knee, and ankle ulcers.[35]

Every attempt should be made to treat significant hip and knee contractures before surgery. If they persist, the pressure sores will recur. If the patient is placed in an alternative position, the pressure is only redistributed, putting a different area at risk for breakdown.

If physical therapy is unsuccessful at relieving the contractures, tenotomies are performed. In mobile, wheelchair-bound patients, releasing the hip contractures can lead to a flail extremity, which may interfere with transferring.

NONSURGICAL TREATMENT

The ultimate treatment of pressure ulcers is not necessarily surgical correction. It is always prudent to attempt ulcer closure without surgical means. Proper preoperative assessment and preparation usually allow the ulcers to be observed. If the ulcer appears to be healing significantly during this time, continuation of nonsurgical treatment is indicated.

Some patients may never be candidates for surgical correction because of significant medical problems. In these patients, avoidance of unrelieved pressure, control of infection (local and remote), control of incontinence, and improved nutrition may lead to successful ulcer closure or at least may allow for a stable wound that does not progress.

In some patients, ulcer closure may be accelerated by the use of topical agents other than antibiotics. In two separate studies, Robson et al[74-76] demonstrated improved healing in ulcers treated with recombinant human platelet-derived growth factor BB and basic fibroblast growth factor. Although use of protein growth factors has been shown to improve wound healing, their widespread use has been limited to date. As the cost and accessibility of these agents improves, they may provide an option not available to most patients today.

Many practitioners believe that nonsurgical treatment can offer adequate treatment for these difficult problems, given the high recurrence rates associated with surgery. In part this philosophy can be attributed to the creation of wound care specialists and the associated industry. Many wound care products have recently become available for the nonsurgical treatment of pressure sores. As a result, many health care professionals are now choosing to treat these ulcers by themselves rather than consult a reconstructive surgeon.

Isenberg et al[46] reviewed the practice patterns of health care professionals whose patients required treatment for pressure sores. A surgeon was consulted in less than 25% of the cases. The study demonstrated that 82% of the patients' ulcers either showed no change or increased in size during the hospitalization. This study underscores the importance of surgical input in the proper care of pressure sores. Even if nonsurgical treat-

ment is chosen, the reconstructive surgeon's expertise in guiding this form of therapy is critical.

OPERATIONS

Surgical management of pressure sores is based on the following three principles (Figure 30-5):
1. Excisional debridement of the ulcer, its bursa, and any heterotopic calcification
2. Partial or complete ostectomy to reduce the bony prominence
3. Wound closure with healthy tissue that is durable and can provide adequate padding over the bony prominence

DEBRIDEMENT

In general, debridement of pressure sores should be accomplished in the operating room, where adequate light, assistance, and ability to control bleeding can be obtained. Limited bedside debridement may be useful to facilitate local wound care preoperatively. This usually means unroofing the eschar or opening the cutaneous window to allow adequate exposure for dressing changes.

The surgical treatment of pressure sores starts with debridement of the ulcer. The patient is placed on the operating table in a position that gives the surgeon maximal exposure. Positioning should also allow the surgeon to appreciate the maximum volume of the wound while debriding the ulcer. If the wound is closed in this position, tension on the suture line will not increase, regardless of the patient's postoperative positioning. By following this simple guideline, the surgeon may avoid one of the most common reasons for early postoperative dehiscence: suture line tension.

The ulcer's true boundaries may be difficult to determine. A dilute 1% solution of methylene blue can be placed in the wound to stain the bursa. The wound is then irrigated with

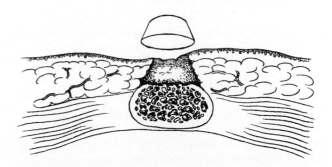

Figure 30-5. Typical configuration of pressure ulcer. Proper technique involves removing conical shaped bursa. The remaining defect is filled with adjacent, healthy viable tissue, as needed. When bone is involved only partial bony excision is necessary.

hydrogen peroxide to remove the excess dye.[48] This helps to define the cavity and provides a visual guide for excision.

In some patients, cellulitis or other adjacent infection is present, and surgical closure in a single procedure is not advisable. In these patients, specimens must be sent for culture to assist in postoperative antibiotic coverage and in selection of the most effective topical antimicrobial agent. This might also include bone biopsies to rule out bone involvement.

The wound can be lightly packed with Kerlex gauze soaked in saline or a topical agent. Silver sulfadiazine, mafenide, Betadine, and Dakin's solution are frequently used agents.[62] Although all these agents are bactericidal, they are also toxic to fibroblasts and macrophages. Only a buffered Dakin's solution at 0.025% is both bactericidal and nontoxic to cells involved in wound healing. Dressings are changed every 6 to 8 hours. The mechanical debridement associated with dressing changes may be responsible for decreasing the bacterial count as much as the solution employed.

OSTECTOMY

Removal of the bony prominence is an integral part of the surgical treatment of pressure sores. Radical ostectomy, however, should be avoided. Excision of exposed bone and infected bone is necessary to close the wound, but overaggressive bony excision will lead to additional problems, including excessive bleeding, skeletal instability, and redistribution of pressure points to adjacent areas.[84]

Ischial ulcers represent a unique problem, and some authors have advocated total ischiectomies. Although the recurrence rate decreased from 38% to 3%, ischiectomy was also associated with formation of a contralateral ischial ulcer in almost a third of the patients. Bilateral ischiectomy has also been proposed, but redistributed pressure has caused perineal ulceration, which can be complicated by the formation of urethral fistulas.[2] To minimize the creation of new problems, Vasconez et al[83-85] recommend removing a minimal amount of ischium in the debridement of ischial pressure ulcers (see Figure 30-5).

PRESSURE SORE CLOSURE

The operative procedure chosen should be customized to the patient as well as the ulcer. When planning a surgical strategy the surgeon should consider subsequent surgical procedures as well as the present surgery.

The choice of skin flaps versus musculocutaneous flaps depends on not only the location, size, and depth of the ulcer, but also the previous surgeries. Primary closure may be appealing, but the surgeon should remember that these ulcers represent an absence of tissue and that primary closure almost always leaves a subcutaneous "dead space." In addition, adjacent tissues are usually less compliant than would be necessary for a tensionless, primary closure.

Skin grafting of pressure sores may be possible with superficial ulceration, but this tends to provide unstable coverage, and the success rate is only 30%.[13] Therefore wound closure usually requires rotation of local skin, fasciocutaneous, or musculocutaneous flaps.

The theoretic superiority of musculocutaneous flaps over skin flaps in the closure of infected wounds has been demonstrated in animal and clinical studies.[6,14,15] The advantages of musculocutaneous flaps for coverage of pressure sores include the following:

1. Excellent blood supply
2. Provision of bulky padding
3. Ability to readvance or rerotate flaps to treat recurrences
4. Proven effectiveness in treating infected wounds

The disadvantages are also significant in that muscle (1) is the tissue most sensitive to external pressure, (2) may be atrophic in elderly patients and in those with spinal cord injuries, and (3) may lead to a functional deformity in ambulatory patients.

The advantages of fasciocutaneous flaps are as follows[88]:

1. Adequate blood supply
2. Durable coverage
3. Minimal potential for a functional deformity
4. Better reconstruction of the normal anatomic arrangement over bony prominences

The disadvantages include the limited bulk for the treatment of large ulcers.

Several common locations of pressure sores require specific considerations.

Ischial Pressure Sores

The ischial pressure sore occurs in seated patients. These patients tend to have a high recurrence rate, at least partly because they typically return to the seated position after the acute perioperative period. Figure 30-6 demonstrates the pertinent anatomy of this region. Conway and Griffith[12] reported on the treatment of 1000 ischial pressure sores. Regardless of the type of treatment (nonoperative or operative), the recurrence rate was 75% to 77%.

In most cases, placing the patient in the jackknifed flexed position during surgery is best for accurately determining the ulcer's size. Flap design should allow coverage of the ulcer but not prevent the use of other, secondary flaps for pressure sore recurrence. Additional consideration when designing a flap to close ulcers in this region include (1) size and depth of the ulcer, (2) quality and pliability of the surrounding skin, and (3) presence of previous surgical scars. Although the simplest surgical technique, excision with wound closure is also the least successful, given the significant tension usually associated with primary closure in this area.

Local random flaps, such as the medial or laterally based posterior thigh flap, can be used successfully to treat some superficial ulcers. The major limitations with these simple flaps include the need for skin grafting at the donor site and the inability to use secondary flaps from this region if the perforating vessels have been transected. These flaps may also lack the

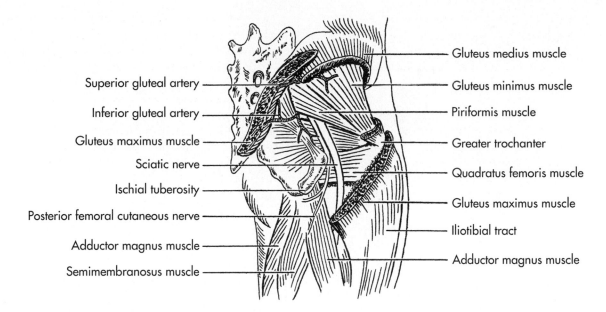

Figure 30-6. Pertinent anatomy of pelvic region.

necessary bulk to close the wound, so additional muscle or musculocutaneous flaps may be needed.[80]

Many different flaps can be used for ulcers in the ischial region (Figure 30-7).[43,44,79] The inferior gluteal musculocutaneous flap, based on the inferior gluteal artery, uses only the lower half of the gluteus maximus muscle. This rotation flap has many advantages because it does not eliminate later use of the posterior thigh flap. Also, it is less likely to interfere with stair climbing in ambulatory patients, since the insertion into the femur may be preserved. The superiorly based gluteal flap may also be used. In designing this flap, the surgeon must not place the incisions over the bony prominences when the patient is seated.

The biceps femoris, semimembranosus, and semitendinosus musculocutaneous flaps, with their overlying medial posterior thigh skin, are excellent flaps when moderate to large ischial ulcers need to be closed[42,50] (Figure 30-8). The advantage of these flaps is the ability to bring well-padded tissue into the wound and to readvance them if necessary. This is possible because of the segmental blood supply in this region from the femoral artery. These flaps are most reliably designed as V-Y advancement flaps.

Occasionally a turnover flap may be designed, but great care must be taken not to devascularize its distal aspect. This can occur while trying to achieve adequate muscle mobilization to reach the ischial ulcer. Closure of the donor site can usually be done with primary closure, but occasionally skin grafts are needed.

Tobin et al[82] describe modifications of the posterior thigh flap. Instead of "islandizing" the skin paddle, they leave a medial or lateral skin bridge to maximize the skin's blood supply. If the skin impedes mobilization, it can always be released (Figure 30-9).

The tensor fascia lata (TFL) flap can occasionally be used to close ischial ulcers.[58] Unfortunately, the distal aspect of the TFL flap is needed to reach the ischial region and is usually too thin to offer adequate padding for this type of ulcer.

Sacral Pressure Sores

Sacral pressure sores occur in supine patients. Ulcers in this area can be treated with a variety of procedures, ranging from simple primary closure to free flaps. As with ulcers in other regions, primary closure usually results in a short-term solution with significant recurrence rates. Superficial ulcers can be treated with skin grafts, but because of the unstable nature and constant pressure in the sacral region, 70% will recur. The most frequently employed flaps for closure of sacral defects are musculocutaneous or fasciocutaneous flaps (see Figure 30-12, **A** and **B**).

One of the first fasciocutaneous flaps was a rotational flap described by Conway and Griffith.[12] In their series of 34 patients, only 16% developed a recurrence. The most common musculocutaneous flaps are based on the gluteus maximus muscle. Depending on the size of the ulcer, previous surgeries, and ambulation of the patient, many options are available. The gluteal flap can be based superiorly or inferiorly; part or all of a muscle or both muscles may be used; the flap can be constructed of muscle or muscle and skin; and it may be rotated, advanced, or turned over[30,61,71] (Figure 30-10).

Other available flaps include the transverse and vertical lumbosacral flap, which is based on lumbar perforating vessels[36] (Figure 30-11).

Although many flaps are available for the treatment of sacral ulcers, the underlying problem facing these spinal cord–injured patients is lack of protective sensation. In an effort to restore protective sensation, tissue expansion of sensate skin[23] more cranially on the back has been described, as well as various techniques for placing small sensate "buttons" from intercostal origins.[17,19,20,53] Although this concept is appealing, the associated complications have limited the usefulness of these techniques.[8]

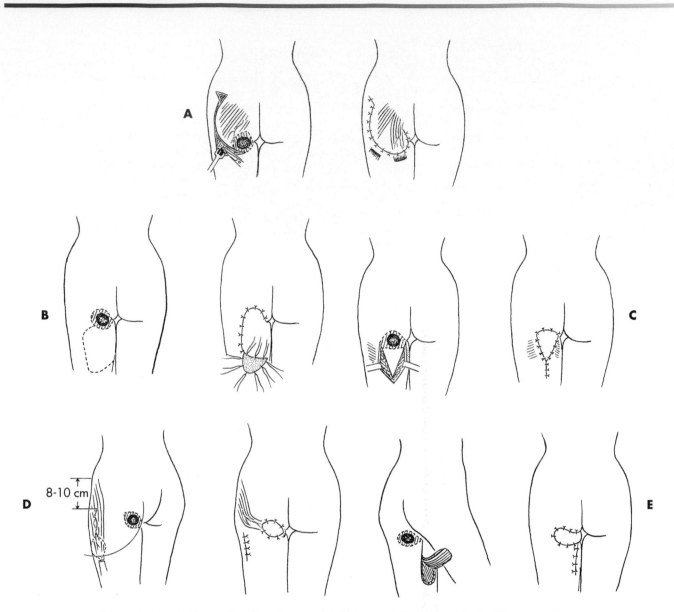

Figure 30-7. Different flaps for closure of ischial wound (not to scale). **A,** Gluteus maximus superiorly based rotation flap. **B,** Posterior thigh advancement flap and skin graft of donor site. **C,** Posterior thigh V-Y advancement flap. **D,** Tensor lata flap. **E,** Medial thigh rotation flap.

Trochanteric Pressure Sores

Trochanteric ulcers develop in patients who lay in the lateral decubitus position for too long. The problem may be accentuated in patients with significant hip flexion contractures. As with ulcers in other sites, treatment with primary closure and skin grafting will lead to recurrence.

The flap used most often for treatment of trochanteric ulcers is the TFL musculocutaneous flap.[64,65,79] This highly reliable flap is based on the perforating vessels from the TFL muscle. The pivot point of the flap is 8 cm (about 3 inches) below the anterosuperior iliac spine. Its potential length in some patients also makes it useful for the treatment of ischial and sacral ulcers (Figure 30-12).

The surgeon must use caution because the TFL flap's distal aspect is mostly a thin fascial sheet and its available bulk is limited. Sensation from the nerve roots of L1, L2, and L3 by the lateral femoral cutaneous nerve makes this a potentially sensate flap in patients with spinal cord injury below L3. This may apply to more than 60% of meningomyelocele patients.[20]

OTHER CONSIDERATIONS

In patients with multiple pressure sores or who have undergone multiple previous procedures, no local options may remain. In the extreme cases it may be necessary to consider total thigh flaps, amputation, hemipelvectomy, or hemicorporectomy to obtain enough soft tissue to close the ulcer (Figure 30-13). The impairment of body image may be significant for these patients.

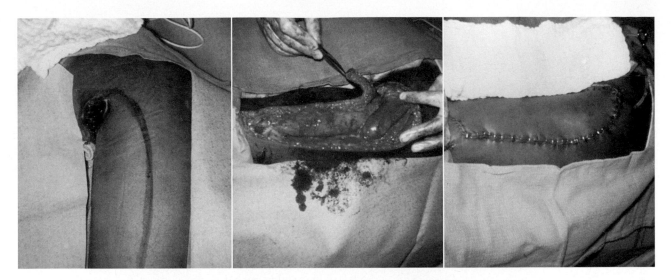

Figure 30-8. Posterior thigh–based flap.

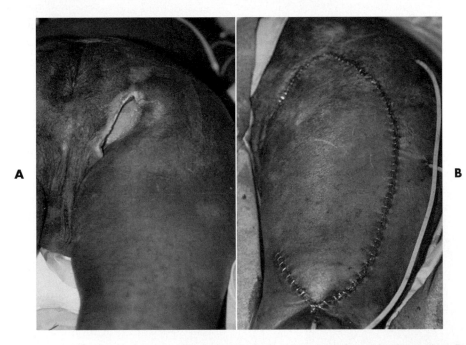

Figure 30-9. **A,** Preulcer excision. **B,** After debridement of ischeal ulcer and advancement flap.

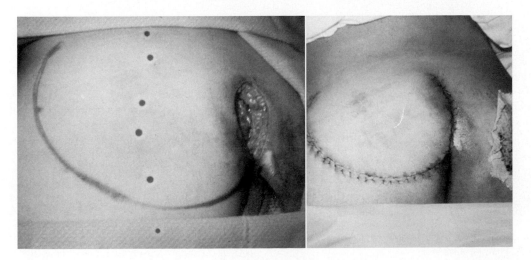

Figure 30-10. Superiorly based gluteal rotation flap.

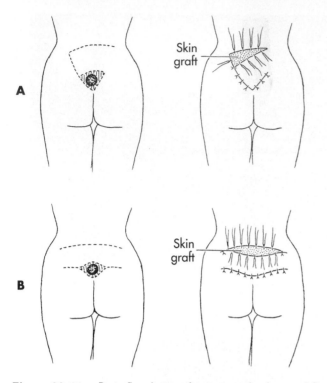

Figure 30-11. Basic flap design of transverse lumbosacral flap. **A,** Rotation; **B,** pedicle.

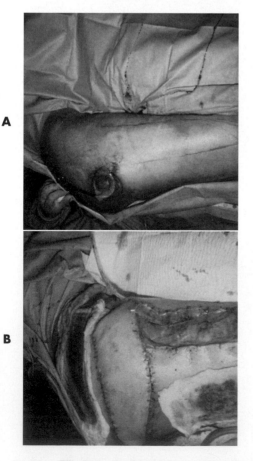

Figure 30-12. TFL flaps. **A,** Preoperative view of patient in lateral position. **B,** Postoperative view.

POSTOPERATIVE CARE

The postoperative care of these patients is usually a continuation of the preoperative care. Nutritional, medical (spasm, diabetes, hypertension), psychologic, and rehabilitative care should be continued and only altered so as not to interfere with the acute postoperative recovery period. Careful nursing care is critical to postoperative success. Pressure is avoided on the operative site (1) by positioning the patients so that they are not lying on the surgical site or (2) by using special mattresses. As previously described, the Clinitron bed may be helpful, but its improper use can cause excessive pressure.

Positioning should be done so as not to transfer excessive pressure to a different location. This can be avoided by turning the patient every 2 hours. An absorptive nonocclusive dressing should be used on the wound to keep it clean and dry. Every effort should be made to avoid macerating the wound. Overuse of topical ointments can cause maceration. The control of urine and stool is important and should have been addressed preoperatively. Drains are usually placed intraoperatively for both removal of serous drainage and to aid in opposition of the flaps to the wound bed. The drains are left in place until the collagen deposition in the wound is sufficient, usually 14 days.

The surgery usually induces significant bacteremia, and patients generally continue receiving antibiotics during the perioperative period. Since most pressure sore cultures are polymicrobial, broad-spectrum antibiotics are used. These may be altered as preoperative culture sensitivities become available.

After surgery, patients generally do not need to stay in the hospital. After 2 or 3 days, patients usually are stable and can be safely transferred to an intermediate-level care facility. For many patients, this may be their nursing home or a rehabilitation center. The patients are kept in the postoperative position, with no pressure allowed to the surgical site for 2 to 3 weeks. At this point in wound healing, most patients have progressed enough to bear weight on the affected site. This process is usually started at 15- to 30-minute intervals, progressing up to 2 hours by 6 weeks.

OUTCOMES

In addition to the acute complications related to treating pressure sores (e.g., hemorrhagic, pulmonary, cardiac, infectious), long-term complications include recurrence and carcinoma.

RECURRENCE

The most common complication associated with pressure sores is their extremely high recurrence rate, as high as 95% in some

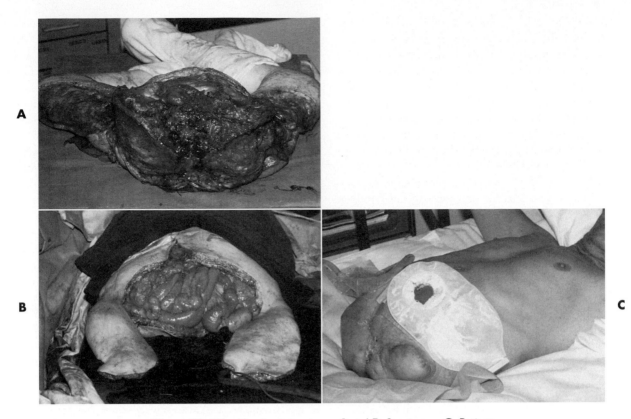

Figure 30-13. Hemicorporectomy. **A** and **B,** Specimens. **C,** Patient.

series.[12,22,24,32,46] Prevention of recurrence requires at least the patient's or caregiver's cooperation and motivation. Any breakdown in this support and care system will result in recurrent ulceration.

The reasons for the high rates of recurrence are multifactorial but include the following:

1. The underlying medical problems that originally contributed to ulcer formation usually persist, such as spinal cord injury or altered mentation in elderly patients.
2. The labor-intensive nursing care issues (e.g., turning, local wound care, avoidance of urine and fecal contamination) may not have changed from the preoperative setting.
3. Diabetes, smoking, and cardiovascular disease are associated with increased rates of recurrence.[66]

Unless the predisposing factors can be modified (e.g., change behavior, eliminate spasm, release contractures), no reason exists to provide surgical treatment to an otherwise clean wound.

CARCINOMA

In 1828 Marjolin described a tumor originating in a chronic wound. Dupuytren subsequently identified the lesion as a malignancy.

The term *Marjolin's ulcer* is used to describe carcinoma arising in a chronic wound. The most common cell type is squamous cell carcinoma. Unlike most other tumors of this type, these malignancies tend to be more aggressive and have a poorer overall survival, with 2-year mortality rate varying from 66% to 80%.[34,63] The metastatic rate in these lesions is 61%, compared with a rate of 34% for Marjolin's ulcers arising in burn scars. The time until development of Marjolin's ulcers is also reduced. Although the usual time to appearance is 25 years, compared with 30 years in burn-related carcinomas, this time span can be as short as 3 years.

Because of the aggressive nature of Marjolin's ulcers, wide surgical excision to clear margins is recommended. Prophylactic lymph node dissection is not recommended, but therapeutic node dissection is indicated in patients with clinically involved nodes. Adjuvant radiation and chemotherapy may be indicated for unresectable tumors or if the patient refuses surgery.

ECONOMIC FACTORS

The cost of treating pressure sores is staggering. One study estimated that $836 million was spent in 1992 to treat the almost 34,000 inpatients who developed pressure sores.[47] Numerous studies have examined resource utilization associated with pressure sore treatment, citing costs ranging from $20,000 to $50,000 per patient.* Therefore great incentives exist to treat these lesions as effectively as possible but at the lowest price.

---

*References 1, 3, 5, 27, 29, 31, 54.

The obvious approach to reducing costs is prevention. Hu et al[41] examined the cost of preventing pressures sores in patients identified as being at high risk in the acute care setting. The cost in labor and materials would be $15.13 to $43.00 per day, depending on the patient population.[66,86] These costs included nursing time to turn and position the patient, foam or pressure mattresses, and sheepskin or other pressure-relieving boots. These figures contrast sharply with caring for a pressure sore in a chronic care facility, where the total daily cost ranged from $0.35 to $10.83 per day.[54,87]

Another factor that affects costs is the pressure sore's extent. Stage II and IV ulcers can cost almost twice as much to treat as a stage I or II ulcer. Therefore ulcers must be identified early, with initiation of aggressive treatment and prevention programs.

PSYCHOLOGIC FACTORS

A pressure sore often develops in a paraplegic patient during times of stress. The presence of a pressure sore in a patient with no problem for years is a major adverse psychologic event. It may represent a failure to the patient in the ability to attend to personal needs. A new ulcer may also affect the caregivers, who also may feel some responsibility for the problem.

Although no specific article addresses the psychologic effect that closure of a pressure sore may have on the patient, ulcer development clearly implies a larger problem. Psychosocial consultation and a therapist's involvement can help the patient and family work through the underlying problem.

SUMMARY

The proper treatment and care of patients with pressure sores are mandatory. Plastic surgeons confront no other disease process that carries such high recurrence rates, economic strains, and emotional concerns. All surgeons who care for these patients must understand the disease process and all available treatment options. With this knowledge, plastic surgeons can lead the team of health care professionals dedicated to preventing and treating pressure sores.

REFERENCES

1. Allman RM: Outcomes in prospective studies and clinical trials, *Adv Wound Care* 8:28-61, 1995.
2. Arregui J et al: Long-term evaluation of ischiectomy in the treatment of pressure ulcers, *Plast Reconstr Surg* 36:583, 1965.
3. Barczak C, Barnett R, Childs E, et al: Fourth National Pressure Ulcer Prevalence Survey, *Adv Wound Care* 10(4):18-26, 1997.
4. Bergstrom N, Bennett A, Carlson CE, et al: *Pressure ulcer treatment: a critical practice guideline,* AHCPR Pub No 95-0653, Rockville, MD, 1994, U.S. Department of Health and Human Services, Public Health Service, Agency for Health Care Policy and Research.
5. Bolton LL, Rijswijk L, Shaffer FA, et al: Quality wound care equals cost-effective wound care: a clinical model, *Adv Wound Care* 10(4):33-38, 1997.
6. Bruck JC, Buttemeyer R, Grabosch A, et al: More arguments in favor of myocutaneous flaps for the treatment of pelvic pressure sores, *Ann Plast Surg* 26:85, 1991.
7. Charcot JM: Note sur la Fomation rapide dúne eschare a la Fesse du cote paralyse dans l'hemiplesie recente de cause cerebrale, *Arch Physiol Norm Path Paris* 1:308, 1868.
8. Cochran JH, Edstrom LE, Dibbell DG: Usefulness of the innervated tensor fascia lata flap in paraplegic patients, *Ann Plast Surg* 7:286, 1981.
9. Colin D, Loyant R, Abraham P, et al: Changes in sacral transcutaneous oxygen tension in the evaluation of different mattresses in the prevention of pressure ulcers, *Adv Wound Care* 9(1):25-28, 1996.
10. Conner LM, Clack JW: In vivo (CT scan) comparison of vertical shear in human tissue caused by various support surfaces, *Decubitus* 6:20-28, 1993.
11. Controller, Department of Medicine and Surgery: *Mortality report in spinal cord injury,* 1958, Washington, DC, Reports and Statistics Service, Veterans Administration.
12. Conway H, Griffith BH: Plastic surgery for closure of decubitus ulcers in patients with paraplegia: based on experience with 1,000 cases, *Am J Surg* 91:946, 1956.
13. Conway H et al: The plastic surgical closure of decubitus ulcers in patients with paraplegia, *Surg Gynecol Obstet* 85:321, 1947.
14. Daniel RK, Faibisoff B: Muscle coverage of pressure points—the role of myocutaneous flaps, *Ann Plast Surg* 8:446, 1982.
15. Daniel RK, Hall EJ, MacLeod MK: Pressure sores—a reappraisal, *Ann Plast Surg* 3:53, 1979.
16. Daniel RK, Priest DL, Wheatley DC: Etiologic factors in pressure sores: an experimental model, *Arch Phys Med Rehabil* 62:492, 1981.
17. Daniel RK, Terzis JK, Cunningham DM: Sensory skin flaps for coverage of pressure sores in paraplegic patients: preliminary report, *Plast Reconstr Surg* 58:3, 1976.
18. Daniel RK, Wheatley DC, Priest DL: Pressure sores and paraplegia: an experimental model, *Ann Plast Surg* 15:15, 1985.
19. Dibbell DG: Use of long island flap to bring sensation of the sacral area in young paraplegics, *Plast Reconstr Surg* 54:220, 1974.
20. Dibbell DG, McCraw JB, Edstrom LE: Providing useful and protective sensibility to the sitting area in patients with myelomeningocele, *Plast Reconstr Surg* 64:796, 1979.
21. Dinsdale SM: Decubitus ulcers: role of pressure and friction in causation, *Arch Phys Med Rehabil* 55:147, 1974.
22. Disa JJ, Carlton JM, Goldberg NH: Efficacy of operative cure in pressure sore patients, *Plast Reconstr Surg* 89:272, 1992.
23. Esposito G, Di Caprio G, Ziccardi P, et al: Tissue expansion in the treatment of pressure ulcers, *Plast Reconstr Surg* 87:501, 1991.

24. Evans G, Dufresne CR, Manson PN: Surgical correction of pressure ulcers in an urban center: is it efficacious? *Adv Wound Care* 7(1):40, 1994.

25. Exton-Smith AN, Crockett DJ: Nature of edema in paralyzed limbs of hemiplegic patients, *Br Med J* 2:1280, 1957.

26. Felcher A, Schwartz J, Schechter C, et al: Wound healing in normal and analbuminemic (NAR) rats, *J Surg Res* 43:546-549, 1987.

27. Ferrell B: Outcomes in quality improvement activities, *Adv Wound Care* 8(4):28-65, 1995.

28. Flanigan KH: Nutritional aspects of wound healing, *Adv Wound Care* 10(5):48-52, 1997.

29. Frantz R, Bergquist S, Specht J: The cost of treating pressure ulcers following implementation of a research-based skin care protocol in a long-term care facility, *Adv Wound Care* 8:36-45, 1995.

30. Ger R: The surgical management of decubitus ulcers by muscle transposition, *Surgery* 69:106, 1971.

31. Goldberg N: Outcomes in surgical intervention, *Adv Wound Care* 8:28-69, 1995.

32. Griffith BH, Schultz R: The prevention and surgical treatment of recurrent decubitus ulcers in patients with paraplegia, *Plast Reconstr Surg* 27:248, 1961.

33. Groth KE: Klinische Beobachtungen und experimentelle Studien uber die Enstelung des Dekubitis, *Acta Chir Scand* 87(suppl 76):198, 1942 (English summary).

34. Grotting JC, Bunkis J, Vascoez LO: Pressure sore carcinoma, *Ann Plast Surg* 18:527, 1987.

35. Haher JN, Haher TR, Devlin VJ, et al: The release of flexion contractures as a prerequisite for the treatment of pressure sores in multiple sclerosis: a report of ten cases, *Ann Plast Surg* 11:846, 1983.

36. Hill HL, Brown RG, Burkiewicz MJ: The transverse lumbosacral back flap, *Plast Reconstr Surg* 62:177, 1978.

37. Himes D: Nutritional supplements in the treatment of pressure ulcers: practical perspectives, *Adv Wound Care* 10(1):30-31, 1997.

38. Hoffman R, Pase M, VanLeuwen DM: Use and perceived effectiveness of pressure ulcer treatments in extended care facilities, *Adv Wound Care* 9(4):43-47, 1996.

39. Howe CW: Experimental wound sepsis from transient bacteremia, *Surg Gynecol Obstet* 126:1066, 1968.

40. Howe E, Briggs H, Shea R, et al: Effect of complete and partial starvation on the rate of fibroplasia in the healing wound, *Arch Surg* 27:846, 1933.

41. Hu T, Stotts NA, Fogarty TE: Cost analysis for guideline implementation in prevention and early treatment of pressure ulcers, *Decubitus* 6:42-46, 1993.

42. Hurteau JE, Bostwick J, Nahai F, et al: V-Y advancement of hamstring musculocutaneous flap for coverage of ischial pressure sores, *Plast Reconstr Surg* 68:539, 1981.

43. Hurwitz DJ, Walton RL: Closure of chronic wounds of the perineal and sacral regions using the gluteal thigh flap, *Ann Plast Surg* 8:375, 1982.

44. Hurwitz DJ, Swartz WM, Mathes SJ: The gluteal thigh flap: a reliable , sensate flap for the closure of buttock and perineal wounds, *Plast Reconstr Surg* 68:521, 1981.

45. Husain T: An experimental study of some pressure effects on tissues with reference to the bedsore problem, *J Pathol Bacteriol* 66:347, 1953.

46. Isenberg JS, Ozuner G, Restifo RJ: The natural history of pressure sores in a community hospital environment, *Ann Plast Surg* 35:361, 1995.

47. Isik F, Engrav L, Rand R, et al: Reducing the period of immobilization following pressure sore surgery: a prospective, randomized trail, 100:350, 1997.

48. Jones NF, Wexler MR: Delineation of the pressure sore bursa using methylene blue and hydrogen peroxide, *Plast Reconstr Surg,* 68:798, 1981.

49. Kosiak M et al: Evaluation of pressure as a factor on the prediction of ischial ulcers, *Arch Phys Med Rehabil* 39:623, 1958.

50. Kroll SS, Hamilton S: Multiple and repetitive uses of the extended hamstring V-Y myocutaneous flap, *Plast Reconstr Surg* 84:296, 1989.

51. Landis EM: Micro-injection studies of capillary blood pressure in human skin, *Heart* 15:209, 1930.

52. Le KM, Madsen BL, Barth PW, et al: An in-depth look at pressure sores using monolithic silicon pressure sensors, *Plast Reconstr Surg* 74:745, 1984.

53. Lesavoy M, Dubrow TJ, Korn N, et al: "Sensible" flap coverage of pressure sores in patients with meningomyelocele, *Plast Reconstr Surg* 85:390, 1990.

54. Leshem OA, Skelskey C: Pressure ulcers: quality management, prevalence, and severity in a long-term care setting, *Adv Wound Care* 7(2):50, 1994.

55. Levenson SM, Demetriou AA: Metabolic factors. In Cohen IK, Diegelmann RF, Lindblad WJ: *Wound healing,* Philadelphia, 1992, Saunders.

56. Lewis VL, Bailey MH, Pulawski G, et al: The diagnosis of osteomyelitis in patients with pressure sores, *Plast Reconstr Surg* 81:229, 1988.

57. Lindan O, Greenway RM, Piazza JM: Pressure distribution of the surface of the human body. I. Evaluation of lying and sitting positions using a bed of springs and nails, *Arch Phys Med Rehabil* 6:378, 1965.

58. Little JW, Lyons JR: The gluteus medius–tensor fascia lata flap, *Plast Reconstr Surg* 71:366, 1982.

59. Meehan M: National Pressure Ulcer Prevalence Survey, *Adv Wound Care* 7(3):27, 1994.

60. Miller TA, editor: *Physiologic basis of modern surgical care,* St Louis, 1988, Mosby.

61. Minami RT, Mills R, Pardoe R: Gluteus maximus myocutaneous flaps for repair of pressure sores, *Plast Reconstr Surg* 60:242, 1977.

62. Morgan JE: Topical therapy of pressure ulcers, *Surg Gynecol Obstet* 141:945, 1975.

63. Mustoe T, Upton J, Marcellino V, et al: Carcinoma in chronic pressure sores: a fulminant disease process, *Plast Reconstr Surg* 77:116, 1986.

64. Nahai F, Hill HL, Hector TR: Experiences with the tensor fascia lata flap, *Plast Reconstr Surg* 63:788, 1979.

65. Nahai F, et al: The tensor fascia lata musculocutaneous flap, *Ann Plast Surg* 6:788, 1979.

66. Niazi ZB, Salzberg A, Byrne DW: Recurrence of initial pressure ulcer in persons with spinal cord injuries, *Adv Wound Care* 10(3):38-42, 1997.

67. Nola GT, Vistnes LM: Differential response of skin and muscle in the experimental production of pressures sore, *Plast Reconstr Surg* 66:728, 1980.

68. Oot-giromini BA: Pressure ulcer: prevalence, incidence and associated risk factors in the community, *Adv Wound Care* 6(5):24, 1993.

69. Parish LC, Witkowski JA: Clinitron therapy and the decubitus ulcer: preliminary dermatologic studies, *Int J Dermatol* 19:517, 1980.

70. Phillips LG, Robson MC: Pathobiology and treatment of pressure ulcerations. In Jurkiewicz MJ, Krizek TJ, Mathes SJ, Ariyan S, editors: *Plastic surgery: principles and practice,* St Louis, 1991, Mosby.

71. Ramirez OM, Hurwitz DJ, Futrell JW: The expansive gluteus maximus flap, *Plast Reconstr Surg* 74:757, 1984.

72. Robson MC, Heggers JP: Bacterial quantification of open wounds, *Milit Med* 134:19, 1969.

73. Robson MC, Krizek TJ: The role of infection in chronic pressure ulcerations. In Frederick S, Brody GS: *Symposium on neurologic aspects of plastic surgery,* St Louis, 1978, Mosby.

74. Robson MC, Phillips LG, Lawrence WT, et al: The safety and effect of topically applied recombinant basic fibroblast growth factor on the healing of chronic pressure sores, *Ann Surg* 216:401, 1992.

75. Robson MC, Phillips LG, Thomason A, et al: Recombinant human platelet-derived growth factor-BB for the treatment of chronic pressure ulcers, *Ann Plast Surg* 29:193, 1992.

76. Robson MC, Phillips LG, Thomason A, et al: Platelet-derived growth factor-3B for the treatment of chronic pressure ulcers, *Lancet* 339:23, 1992.

77. Stal S, Serer A, Donovan W, et al: The perioperative management of the patient with pressure sores, *Ann Plast Surg* 11:347, 1983.

78. Stotts NA: Determination of bacterial burden in wounds, *Adv Wound Care* 8(4):28-46, 1995.

79. Teflon M: The tensor fascia lata: variation on a theme, *Plast Reconstr Surg* 63:59, 1981.

80. Teflon M, Nihau F, Bostick J: Gluteus maximus island musculocutaneous flap for closure of sacral and ischial ulcers, *Plast Reconstr Surg* 68:533, 1981.

81. Thomas D: Specific nutritional factors in wound healing, *Adv Wound Care* 10(4):40-43, 1997.

82. Tobin GR, Brown GL, Deer JAW, et al: V-Y advancement flaps: reusable flaps for pressure ulcer repair, *Clin Plast Surg* 17:727, 1990.

83. Vasconez LO, McCraw, JB: The use of muscle in plastic and reconstructive surgery. In Krizek TJ, Hoopes J, editors: *Symposium on application of basic science to plastic surgery,* St Louis, 1976, Mosby.

84. Vasconez LO, Bostwick J, McCraw J: Coverage of exposed bone by muscle transposition and skin grafting, *Plast Reconstr Surg* 53:526, 1974.

85. Vasconez LO, Schneider WJ, Jurkiewicz MJ: Pressure sores. In *Current problems in plastic surgery,* Chicago, 1977, Year Book.

86. Xakellis GC, Frantz RA: The cost-effectiveness of interventions for preventing pressure ulcers, *J Am Board Fam Pract* 9(2):79-85, 1996.

87. Xakellis GC, Frantz R, Lewis A: Cost of pressure ulcer prevention in long-term care, *J Am Geriatr Soc* 43:496-501, 1995.

88. Yamamoto Y, Ohura T, Shintomi Y, et al: Superiority of the fasciocutaneous flap in reconstruction of sacral pressure sores, *Ann Plast Surg* 30:116, 1993.

Lymphedema of the Extremity

Dominic F. Heffel
Timothy A. Miller

INTRODUCTION

Throughout the world, approximately 100 to 250 million persons have lymphedema.[29] This disease is characterized by the abnormal accumulation of protein-rich interstitial fluid within the skin and subcutaneous tissue; the deep muscle compartments are spared.

No medical or surgical cure exists for lymphedema. The goals of therapy are as follows:

1. Reduction of fluid accumulation and production
2. Reduction of associated complications
3. Improvement of limb function and appearance

INDICATIONS

ETIOLOGY AND CLASSIFICATION

The diagnosis can be made after a complete history and physical examination. Typically the fluid accumulation occurs within a *unilateral* extremity. The gradual development of a soft pitting edema, beginning distally and ascending proximally over months, is the usual presentation. The increase in limb diameter and weight often causes patients to complain of fatigue in the involved extremity. Over time, inflammatory changes occur within the subcutaneous tissue, and the involved limb becomes indurated and develops a nonpitting edema.

Systemic disorders (e.g., cardiac failure, hepatic failure) cause *bilateral* edema and can generally be excluded on this basis.[1] Lymphedema does occur rarely in the midline, but bilateral crossover drainage mitigates this occurrence.

Historically, lymphedema has been defined as a deficiency in the lymphatic system. A deficiency in lymph flow exists in the presence of normal capillary flow, thus generating fluid collection within the extremity's interstitium.

The etiology of the lymph flow abnormality has led to a traditional classification scheme that categorizes lymphedema as primary or secondary. In "primary lymphedema" the disease is believed to be genetically determined. The genetic expression of this disease, however, can occur at birth *(Milroy's disease)*, puberty *(lymphedema praecox)*, or midlife *(lymphedema tarda)*. In "secondary lymphedema" the disease is believed to be caused by a known inciting event, such as infection or surgical ablation.

Authors' Paradigm

We believe that the conceptualization of this disease requires revision. We propose a new paradigm based on the principle that lymphedema represents a spectrum of disease. The disease may be manifested in its most severe form as lymphedema occurring at birth and in its mildest form as a subclinical process unknown to both the patient and the health care provider. This latter underlying lymphatic abnormality does not appear clinically because of a compensatory mechanism.

All patients who experience an inciting event (e.g., lymph node dissection, trauma, infection, irradiation, malignancy) do not develop lymphedema. An individual's ability to compensate for lymphatic destruction may explain this. Within a large population with functionally abnormal lymphatics, a subgroup may compensate extremely well for any insult to the lymphatic system (Figure 31-1). Within that same population, other subgroups may compensate satisfactorily, marginally, or not at all. Patients incapable of compensating for any increase in transcapillary lymph flow would manifest the disease very early (at or near birth). Patients with *marginal compensation* would manifest the disease later in life, depending on the number of lymphatic insults; those with *satisfactory compensation* may not manifest lymphedema at all.

Therefore lymphedema should not be classified as primary or secondary. Based on our paradigm, the current classification of lymphedema is misleading.

SURGICAL GUIDELINES

The traditional classification of lymphedema does not aid the surgeon because it does not guide surgical management. At this time, regardless of etiology, long term follow-up studies demonstrate that, with a probable exception, only one operation for the lymphedematous extremity provides lasting improvement:

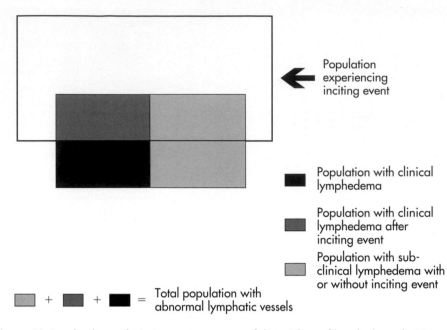

Figure 31-1. A scheme depicting a new concept of the etiology of lymphedema. Inciting events include trauma, ablative surgery, infection, and irradiation. Shaded rectangles represent different populations, and their sum is total population with abnormal lymphatic vessels. *Darkest rectangle,* population who develop lymphedema separately from inciting event and early in life. *Intermediate-gray rectangle,* population who develop lymphedema after inciting event or cumulative events *(marginal compensator). Light-gray rectangles,* populations who have abnormal lymphatic vessels but do not manifest disease, either because they do not experience inciting event or because they can compensate *(satisfactory compensator)* for inciting event.

staged subcutaneous tissue excision. This statement does not preclude the development of a better operation; it only reflects, unfortunately, the status of surgical science at this time.

The exception may be microsurgical attempts to "short-circuit" the normal lymph-to-venous flow. In select patients, procedures designed to circumvent an isolated lymphatic obstruction have shown early promise. Because of the requirement for a patent distal lymph vessel, the microsurgical procedures must be performed before the sequelae of lymphedema become manifest; this interval is not known. Also, venous disease is a contraindication to lymphovenous bypass. Another limitation occurs when the patient has lymphedema from incomplete development of lymphatic vessels.

Again, long-term follow-up is limited, and existing data are not completely convincing.

When conservative therapy fails to control the swelling, the surgeon must make the decision on the next course of action. Surgery is indicated in about 10% of all patients with lymphedema,[11] although some lymphologists argue against any surgery.[8]

When surgery is pursued, it is a continuum of therapy and is generally performed to improve limb function and appearance through the reduction of limb weight and size. Profound limb swelling produces discomfort and fatigue and reduces mobility. Abnormal limb appearance also produces psychologic handicaps.[37] The plastic surgeon can palliate these problems (Box 31-1).

> **Box 31-1.**
> **Lymphedema: Indications for Surgery**
>
> Failed conservative therapy
>   Impaired extremity function
>   Gross extremity size and weight
> Recurrent lymphangitis: more than three episodes of infection per year
> Severe skin changes

Surgery is also pursued as a preventive measure to decrease the incidence of lymphangitis and cellulitis.

Risks and Complications

The patient must understand that surgery is not curative and does not obviate the need for continued medical therapy. Informed consent depends on the choice of procedure. Many procedures exist, but firm, quantitative, long-term data on outcome are sparse. When skin and subcutaneous tissue are removed, the patient can expect decreased sensation over the area of tissue excision and a surgical scar.

Additional risks of excisional procedures include nerve damage (sural, peroneal, ulnar) and skin flap necrosis. Within a series of 82 patients, no inadvertent nerve damage occurred. Three cases of skin flap necrosis healed well by secondary intention, based on personal observation.

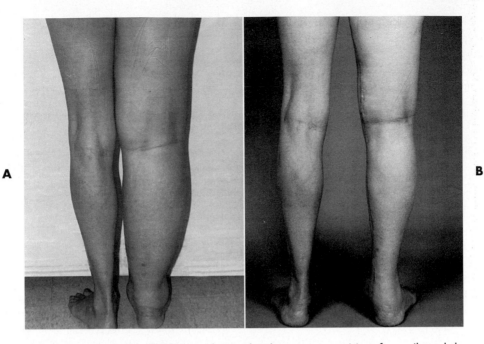

Figure 31-2. Three-year follow-up of staged subcutaneous excision for unilateral lower extremity lymphedema. **A,** Before surgery. **B,** After surgery. Note maintenance of extremity contour.

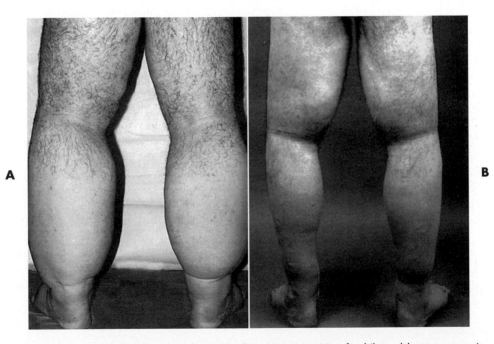

Figure 31-3. Six-year follow-up of staged subcutaneous excision for bilateral lower extremity lymphedema. **A,** Before surgery. **B,** After surgery. Note return and maintenance of extremity contour.

Mortality is estimated at less than 0.5% when superficial lymphangiectomy is performed.[31]

POSTOPERATIVE EDEMA. With long-term attenuation of extremity swelling, surgical results are not predictable. When performed on the lower extremities, surgery does not worsen the disease. Some patients may experience dramatic long-term relief from extremity swelling (Figures 31-2 and 31-3). Con-versely, some patients may experience poor improvement and develop swelling equivalent to preoperative levels within a few years. The degree of postoperative edema depends greatly on the patient's compliance with a postoperative medical and physical therapy regimen.

These outcomes should not be surprising because the surgery is not curative and at best is palliative. The patient will always experience symptoms of lymphedema.

LYMPHANGITIS. The risks depend on the continuing enlargement despite medical management, with further impairment of limb function and the potential for recurrent infection. Recurrent lymphangitis occurs in about 25% of patients with lymphedema. Lymphangitis and cellulitis further accelerate the rate of subcutaneous fibrosis and consequent lymphatic obstruction, aggravating the disease. As swelling increases, so do the complications of hyperkeratosis, papillomatosis, induration, lichenification, and lymphorrhea.

LYMPHANGIOSARCOMA. Lymphedema-induced lymphangiosarcoma does occur, although rarely. The incidence of postmastectomy lymphangiosarcoma is 0.07% to 0.45%, and the average interval between mastectomy with lymphedema and presentation with lymphangiosarcoma is 10 years. Lymphangiosarcoma is rapidly progressive and always fatal. Median survival after diagnosis is about 19 months.[14] No evidence indicates that surgery for lymphedema decreases the incidence of lymphangiosarcoma.

ALTERNATIVE THERAPY

Conservative therapy is used first and is the mainstay of treatment for lymphedema.[18,24] In this chronic disease, conservative therapy and surgery must be regarded as a continuum of treatment. Surgery, since it is not curative, must be followed by a conservative therapy regimen (Box 31-2).

Some treatment modalities have not been verified by randomized, controlled prospective studies.[3] Also, unreasonable success is often claimed. Unfortunately the choice of method is often based on anecdotal observations or investigator bias, not science. This unscientific method of selection is replete throughout the surgical literature.

Recently, however, research for pharmaceutical manipulation of lymphedema has shown therapeutic effect in randomized, double-blind, placebo-controlled prospective trials.[30] *Coumarin* (5,6-benzo-[α]-pyrone) reduces lymphedema in both animals and humans.[5] (Coumarin has no anticoagulant activity.) This drug is thought to function by increasing (1) the number of macrophages at the site of edema and (2) the rate of macrophage-mediated proteolysis. Thus another route for the removal of excess protein is theoretically created.

Micronized diosmin (Daflon), a flavonoid compound, has had some success in the treatment of ulcers caused by chronic venous insufficiency and has shown some promise in initial trials on patients with lymphedema. Micronized diosmin decreases capillary permeability and white blood cell margination and increases venous tone and lymphokinetic activity. These properties are thought to account for the beneficial effects noted in a small study of patients with lymphedema.[30]

ABNORMAL ANATOMY

Traditionally, lymphedema has been categorized by its abnormal anatomy seen on lymphangiography (i.e., lymphatic aplasia, hypoplasia, hyperplasia with incompetent valves) or by the anatomy related to a specific insult (e.g., obstructive lymphedema secondary to surgical ablation).[1,18] In patients who develop lymphedema without a specific insult, 77% will show a hypoplastic pattern and 15% an aplastic pattern on lymphangiography. Aplasia and agenesis represent an extreme form, and lymphangiograms reveal absence of lymphatic vessels. The remaining 8% of those patients who develop congenital lymphedema demonstrate a hyperplastic pattern, characterized by valvular incompetence and dilated, tortuous lymphatic vessels.

Damage or removal of regional lymph nodes as a result of surgery, trauma, radiation, tumor invasion, infection (e.g., filariasis, tuberculosis, lymphogranuloma, actinomycosis, cat-scratch fever), or inflammation (e.g., chronic lymphangitis, chronic venous disease with ulceration, snakebite, insect bite) is the most common factor causing lymphedema. In women, upper extremity lymphedema is a well-recognized complication of radical mastectomy, axillary dissection, and radiation. One year after surgery, moderate lymphedema was present in 5.2% and severe lymphedema in 3.4% of 58 women in one retrospective study.[19] Another study employing strict definition criteria and volume displacement measurements reported a postmastectomy lymphedema incidence of 7.6%.[12]

PATHOPHYSIOLOGY

Within the extremities, lymphedema is confined to the subcutaneous compartment, apparently sparing the deep muscle compartments. The accumulation of protein-rich lymphatic fluid results when fluid formation exceeds lymphatic transport capacity. Normal lymphatics have a substantial reserve capacity and may increase their flow rate tenfold. An increase in the rate of interstitial fluid formation by itself does not produce lymphedema. Therefore lymphatic dysfunction must be a prerequisite for the diagnosis of lymphedema.

Box 31-2.
Lymphedema: Components of Conservative Therapy

Benzopyrones and related flavonoids: optional
Diuretics: judicious use, as during acute water gain
Elastic compression combined with exercise
External pneumatic compression: contraindicated in presence of infection, neoplastic/metastatic disease, chemotherapy/radiation, and arterial insufficiency of involved extremity
Heat: optional
Limb elevation
Massage
Skin maintenance
Treatment of infection
Weight loss

Early in the course of lymphedema, the accumulation of protein-rich interstitial fluid results in only a soft, pitting edema. Over time, decreased macrophage function and increasing amounts of protein-rich fluid result in a chronic inflammatory state and consequent fibrosis. This fibrosis in the subcutaneous tissue converts the edema to the nonpitting variety. The degree of subcutaneous fibrosis correlates with the difficulty encountered with conservative management. Moreover, the accumulation of protein-rich fluid combined with lymphatic stasis predisposes to recurrent episodes of lymphangitis. The combination of fluid stasis, inflammation, fibrosis, and infection inevitably leads to progression of the disease as the existing lymphatic vessels are further destroyed or their function is compromised by scarring.

OPERATIONS

Many surgical procedures of varying theoretic persuasion have offered the potential to relieve the symptoms of lymphedema (Table 31-1). Most of the multiple surgical procedures are not substantiated by long-term follow-up studies that document lasting effectiveness. For an incurable disease that will last a lifetime, the surgical procedure of choice should have documented effectiveness beyond 3 years.

The multitude of operations proposed suggests a general lack of satisfaction with any one procedure, and randomized, prospective studies comparing procedures are not available. We believe the only consistently successful operation, especially within the lower extremity, is the staged subcutaneous

Table 31-1.
Operations for Lymphedema

PROCEDURE	DESCRIPTION/COMMENTS
Lymphangioplasty	Implantation of various materials into subcutaneous compartment to facilitate lymph drainage No demonstrated long-term benefit
Lymphovenous anastomosis	Anastomosis between lymph vessel and vein/node Shows promise in select cases Technically difficult and operator dependent
Lympholymphatic anastomosis	Autologous, nondiseased lymph vessels are transposed/transplanted into affected extremity Shows promise in select cases Technically difficult and operator dependent
Enteromesenteric bridge	Ileal segment denuded of mucosa and apposed to transected iliac or inguinal lymph nodes Requires celiotomy and bowel anastomosis Limited to proximal obstructive lymphedema No demonstrated long-term benefit
Omental transposition	Omentum transposed into lymphedematous extremity Celiotomy required High complication rate Tissue excision part of operation No demonstrated long-term benefit
Buried dermal flap	Excisional procedure No documented evidence of dermal flap drainage into deep lymphatic system
Total subcutaneous tissue and skin excision	Excisional procedure Poor cosmetic result
Staged subcutaneous tissue excision	Excisional procedure Not operator dependent Low complication rate Good long-term results Best surgical option at this time

tissue excision described later. This operation is not ideal but appears to be the best choice among procedures available at this time.

HISTORY

When describing surgical approaches, two differing types appear: excisional and physiologic. *Excisional procedures* remove various amounts of the diseased subcutaneous tissue and excess skin. If the skin is severely affected with the complications of longstanding lymphedema, it is also excised rather than preserved as skin flaps.

Physiologic procedures attempt to create de novo lymphatic connections between the subcutaneous tissue and the unaffected compartments. Attempts to construct these new connections have used the interposition of native tissue and artificial material. More recently, microsurgery has been used to short-circuit the normal lymphatic-to-venous pathways.

Charles described a surgical technique for the treatment of scrotal edema in 1901. The *Charles procedure,* however, has become an eponym for an operation in which the involved lower extremity is debulked and the limb covered with skin grafts from the surgical specimen. In this operation the end cosmetic result is often worse than the initial presentation, with many complications. When split-thickness skin grafts are used to resurface the extremity, the results may be catastrophic.

Lymphangioplasty was first proposed by Handley in 1908. Silk threads were placed subcutaneously with the hope that fibrous channels would form around the foreign body and transport lymph from the extremity by capillary action. Long strips of nylon have also been proposed to function is a similar manner. Follow-up studies of the lymphangioplasty procedure demonstrated no long-term benefit. The mean duration of effect in one study was 13 months, and the authors advocated the procedure only for those patients with limited life expectancy.[32]

In 1912 Kondoleon attempted to drain the abnormal subcutaneous compartment into the uninvolved deep compartment by excising strips of underlying muscle fascia. This strategy was also unsuccessful because of scar formation and fascial regeneration. In 1918 Sistrunk[33] described his experiences with this procedure, as have others.[18]

In 1962 Thompson[35] attempted to drain the subcutaneous compartment into the deep subfascial area with a buried dermal flap. This procedure involved significant subcutaneous tissue excision and was performed in stages. Follow-up lymphangiograms failed to demonstrate lymphatic connections between the apposed tissues, suggesting that the excisional component of the procedure (removal of subcutaneous tissue and skin) was responsible for the extremity reduction.

Pedicle flap procedures juxtapose lymphatic-rich flaps and lymphedematous tissue to induce lymphatic communication and provide drainage for the lymphedematous tissue. To date, skin, omentum, and small bowel have been used as pedicle flaps. Theoretically these procedures seem appealing, but the

juxtaposition of omentum or small bowel to lymphedematous tissue has a major drawback: celiotomy is required. The patient is then predisposed to hernia development, adhesion formation, and bowel obstruction or strangulation. All these complications have been documented. We have operated on three patients to repair hernias secondary to omental transposition surgery.

The theory that lymphatic connections would be established between transposed omentum and lymphedematous tissue seems untenable. Omentum is covered by a mesothelial layer that prevents its adherence to tissue. When omentum is transposed to the chest to cover mediastinal structures, it *slides* rather than adheres. The same situation occurs when the omentum is transposed for treatment of hemifacial atrophy. The omentum becomes surrounded by a bursalike sac and remains mobile within the sac. The formation of new lymphatic connections is difficult to imagine under this condition.

After long-term evaluation of *omental transposition,* Goldsmith[10] claimed sustained extremity reduction and decreased incidence of lymphangitis. However, no objective data defined the extent of size reduction, the complication rate was high because the peritoneal cavity was violated, and the data did not clarify how many patients had been followed beyond 3 years. Goldsmith acknowledged that the lymphedema surgical literature was replete with investigator bias and added that he would recommend a Thompson procedure or a staged subcutaneous excision.

Hurst et al[13] followed eight patients who underwent an *enteromesenteric bridge procedure* for 2½ to 7 years. Again, this procedure required a celiotomy and bowel reanastomosis. It was physically limited to patients with proximal lymphatic obstruction at the level of the iliac or lower aortic nodes. Of the patients treated, 25% failed to improve and underwent an excisional procedure. In five patients followed beyond 3 years, the authors noted clinical improvement but provided no objective data.

Microsurgical procedures designed to reestablish lymphatic drainage to an affected extremity can be divided into two operative categories: (1) lymph nodal–venous shunts, or lymphovenous shunts, and (2) lympholymphatic shunts. Lymph nodal-venous and lymphovenous shunts were first reported in the early 1960s. Lympholymphatic shunts were developed in the late 1970s and show promise as a means of constructing artificial collateral vessels in selected patients. To date, long-term follow-up is not reliably available.

One study indicated persistence of lymphovenous anastomoses on follow-up lymphoscintigrams, but the clinical significance of this persistence was uncertain without concurrent data on limb size.[38] Another study compared microsurgical procedures to combined microsurgical-excisional procedures, suggesting that the combination approach may be superior to microsurgery alone.[27] A third study presented long-term follow-up data (greater than 5 years) on lymphovenous and lymphatic capsule–venous anastomoses.[4] Although the data seemed promising, some of the accompanying photographs appeared qualitatively inferior to those of our preferred procedure.

PATIENT PREPARATION

All patients are placed on bedrest, and the extremity is elevated. Although this step can be started at home, the patient is usually admitted to the hospital 1 to 3 days preoperatively, and the lower extremity is elevated using a modified Thomas orthopedic splint suspended from an overhead frame. The rate of edema resolution is proportional to the chronicity of the condition and the amount of subcutaneous fibrosis. The extremity is washed daily in the hospital.

Other than a single preoperative prophylactic dose, antibiotics are not routinely used. An overt or smoldering infection is an obvious contraindication to surgery.

SURGICAL OPTIONS

With the exception of the microsurgical procedures, all the operations described here remove excess lymphedematous tissue to improve function and cosmesis and reduce complications. Some procedures, such as the buried dermal flap, have physiologic and excisional components.

Microsurgery

Although theoretically attractive, the microsurgical procedures are more technically demanding and operator dependent than the common excisional procedures. Microsurgical approaches have the same drawback as surgery, a patent distal lymphatic vessel, which may be absent in longstanding chronic lymphedema or congenital lymphedema. Furthermore, lymphovenous anastomosis is contraindicated in the patient with venous hypertension.

Microlymphaticovenous surgery is described in detail elsewhere.[25] Briefly, patent blue dye is injected into the web spaces of the involved extremity to facilitate vessel identification. Exploration is carried out concurrently on the dorsum of the wrist/ankle and the anteromedial aspect of the midarm/thigh. Superficial veins and patent lymphatics are localized. No definitive number of anastomoses are required, but as many lymphatics and superficial veins as possible are marked. End-to-end anastomoses are created between suitable vessels with interrupted 11-0 nylon under an operating microscope. If a suitable number of veins are not present, end-to-side anastomoses are performed. If microanastomoses are possible only at the wrist/ankle, a proximal excisional procedure may be performed.

For regional lymphatic blockage, *lymphatic grafting* has been proposed.[2] Lymphatic vessels are harvested from the ventromedial bundle of the normal thigh after patent blue injection. Dye is not injected into the lymphedematous extremity. In the abnormal extremity, lymphatic vessels are identified under the microscope.

Magnification up to 40 times is used to create three to five tension-free anastomoses with 11-0 suture. For postmastectomy lymphedemas, grafts are used to bypass blockade in the axilla, and the anastomoses are created between ascending arm lymphatics and lymphatic vessels in the neck. A suction catheter tube can function as a guide through the subcutaneous tissue between incisions.

In lower extremity unilateral edema the lymphatic graft remains attached to the groin lymph nodes. The free distal end is pulled over the symphysis pubis and anastomosed to lymph vessels in the lymphedematous limb.

Total Skin and Subcutaneous Tissue Excision

This operation, typically referred to as the *Charles procedure,* has been described in detail by McKee and Edgerton.[20] In the lower extremity, all the skin and subcutaneous tissues are excised from the tibial tuberosity to the malleoli (except for tissue overlying the calcaneal tendon). Tapering of tissue at the proximal and distal margins is performed to prevent a step deformity. The defect is closed with a split-thickness skin graft (STSG) or a full-thickness skin graft (FTSG) from the resected specimen or with an STSG from an uninvolved donor site.

Coverage with an STSG is technically easier and gives a satisfactory initial appearance. These grafts, however, are easily injured, ulcerate frequently, scar extensively, become hyperpigmented, and may develop a severe hyperkeratotic, weeping chronic dermatitis. The end result is almost always much worse than the original problem. We strongly oppose the use of STSG resurfacing after subcutaneous excision.[22]

Coverage with an FTSG is technically more demanding but produces a more durable graft site. Nevertheless, regions of graft breakdown and substantial scar formation can also occur with FTSGs.

Long-term follow-up studies (greater than 20 years) have documented the effectiveness of Charles procedure in reducing extremity size, which is not surprising.[7] Conceptually, this procedure is closely related to staged subcutaneous tissue excision; cosmetically, no comparison exists. This procedure should be performed only in the patient with extremely severe skin changes.

Buried Dermal Flap

The buried–dermal flap operation involves the following:
1. A portion of the lymphedematous subcutaneous tissue is resected beneath flaps.
2. A flap edge is deepithelialized.
3. The resulting dermal flap is buried into the underlying muscle compartment.

Thompson[36] presents more detail on the operation. The *Thompson procedure* is based on three hypotheses, as follows:
1. The buried dermis permits the formation of lymphatic connections between the subdermal lymphatic plexus of the flap and the deep lymphatics of the muscle compartment.
2. Muscle contraction increases the lymphatic flow rate through the subdermal plexus.
3. The buried flap provides a physical barrier against deep fascia regeneration.

Although the operative success of the Thompson procedure is attributed to the formation of lymphatic connections between the flap and the muscle compartment, postoperative lymphangiography has failed to demonstrate any lymphatic anastomosis.[6,16] Radiolabeled albumin (RIHSA) clearance studies have demonstrated postoperative improvement in the rate of lymphatic isotope clearance. Comparable improvement in RIHSA clearance was noted after skin and subcutaneous excision alone, however, suggesting the tissue excision may account for postoperative improvement.

Staged Subcutaneous Excision Underneath Flaps

This approach provides the most reasonable surgical treatment for the symptoms of lymphedema. Within the lower extremity, 80% of the lymphatic fluid is carried by the superficial lymphatic system, which explains why surgical therapy should be directed at this compartment.[9] The theory underlying staged subcutaneous excision is removal of diseased lymphatics and lymphedematous tissue with preservation of the dermal lymphatic plexus, thus altering the relative ratio between lymph-producing tissue and functioning lymphatics.

Staged subcutaneous excision offers reliable long-term improvement and minimizes postoperative complications. It produces results comparable to those of the Thompson procedure but has a lower complication rate. Improvement is directly related to (1) the amount of skin and subcutaneous tissue removed, (2) postoperative care, and (3) patient compliance with the postoperative regimen. The surgical procedure is offered to patients as a means of managing their lymphedema and not as a cure.

During the operation, as much subcutaneous tissue and skin as possible are removed while attempting to maintain a viable skin flap and achieve primary skin closure. An experience with 652 cases over 40 years demonstrated the safety and efficacy of this approach.[31]

The following section describes our preferred surgical approach for this operation.

TECHNIQUE: STAGED EXCISION

Staged subcutaneous tissue excision is done in two stages, with at least 90 days between procedures. The medial side of the extremity is usually completed first and involves the largest amount of tissue resection. A pneumatic tourniquet is placed as proximally as possible before surgery.

Lower Extremity

A medial incision is made in the leg approximately 1 cm posterior to the tibial border and extended proximally into the thigh. Flaps about 1.5 cm thick are elevated anteriorly and posteriorly to the midsagittal plane of the calf. The dissection is less extensive in the thigh and ankle. All subcutaneous tissue underneath the flap is removed.

After excising the subcutaneous fat from the periosteum of the tibia, the deep fascia is incised, permitting an easy plane of dissection to develop. The sural nerve is identified and preserved. All the attached subcutaneous fat and deep fascia along the medial aspect of the calf are removed (Figure 31-4). The dissection is kept superficial to the deep fascia at the knee

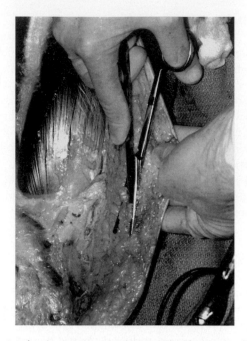

Figure 31-4. Intraoperative photograph of staged subcutaneous excision of lower extremity lymphedema. Fascia over gastrocnemius muscle is removed. Field is bloodless because of pneumatic tourniquet.

and ankle. Flaps in the ankle are rarely longer than 6 cm. The redundant skin is excised after removal of the subcutaneous fat.

A suction catheter is placed in the dependent portion of the posterior flap and is left in place for 5 days. Interrupted and continuous 4-0 nylon is employed for skin closure. No subcutaneous or dermal sutures are placed.

The second stage is performed on the lateral aspect of the limb 3 months later. The operation is essentially identical, except that the deep fascia is not removed. Great care is taken to avoid damaging the peroneal nerve.[21]

Upper Extremity

A medial incision is made from the distal ulna across the medial epicondyle of the humerus to the posterior medial upper arm. Flaps approximately 1 cm thick are elevated to the midsagittal aspect of the forearm, and the dissection is tapered distally and proximally. The edematous subcutaneous tissue is removed, but the deep fascia is spared. The ulnar nerve is identified in the region of the medial epicondyle and preserved. The redundant skin is excised. If necessary, the tourniquet can be removed, the area prepped, and the operation continued into the axilla.

A suction catheter is placed, and the skin is closed with 4-0 nylon suture. No subcutaneous or dermal sutures are used.

DIAGNOSTIC AND POSTOPERATIVE TESTING

In most patients the diagnosis of lymphedema can be made from the history and physical examination.[1] Laboratory studies are obtained to distinguish other sources of edema. Venous studies are helpful if a component of venous insufficiency is suspected.

A variety of imaging techniques may be used in the differential diagnosis and in the assessment of the results of therapy. *Lymphoscintigraphy* using radiocolloids has been successful in delineating the anatomy of lymph vessels and evaluating the kinetics of lymph flow. *Computed tomography* (CT) and *magnetic resonance imaging* (MRI) may be useful early in the diagnosis of lymphedema to rule out malignancy. In some centers, CT evaluation of lymph node number and size is supplanting lymphoscintigraphy as the diagnostic modality of choice.[28]

Although frequently used in the past, *lymphangiography* has been largely abandoned. One report suggests that lymphangiography may significantly worsen lymphedema and predispose the patient to complications such as pulmonary infarction, central nervous system events, and death.[26] We oppose lymphangiography.

Since the vast majority of cases can be diagnosed by history and physical examination, one could argue that no indication exists for a diagnostic test. A diagnostic test should be employed only when it will benefit patient management. A preoperative lymphoscintigram or lymphangiogram cannot guide surgical management if an excisional procedure is contemplated. If a microsurgical procedure is considered, the best assessment of lymphatic vessel status is through surgery and injection of patent blue dye or by direct visualization under an operating microscope, not by lymphangiography or lymphoscintigraphy.

POSTOPERATIVE CARE

Lower Extremity
The extremity is immobilized with a posterior splint and gauze dressing and kept elevated. The suction catheter is usually removed on the fifth postoperative day. Sutures are usually removed on the eighth day. The patient is measured for an elastic stocking, and dependency of the leg is begun on the ninth day. Ambulation is started on the eleventh postoperative day, but only with the leg tightly wrapped.

Upper Extremity
The arm is immobilized and elevated for 5 days.[23] The suction catheter can often be removed after the third day. Otherwise, the postoperative management is similar to that described for the lower extremity.

SECONDARY PROCEDURES

Suction curettage has been reported as a useful adjunct to the surgical management of primary and secondary lymphedema. This method cannot be used to treat extremity lymphedema of any significant magnitude without a concomitant resection of the expanded skin envelope. Excisional procedures continue to be the mainstay of surgical treatment.

OUTCOMES

We have performed staged subcutaneous tissue excision on more than 100 patients. Recently, 32 patients with lower extremity lymphedema underwent long-term follow-up (shortest, 3 years; longest, 27 years), with chart reviews, interviews, questionnaires, and photographs. Substantial sustained improvement was seen in at least 75% of the patients, as evidenced by significant reduction in extremity size, functional recovery, and decreased incidence or absence of cellulitis. Except for partial wound separation in one patient and three cases of ischemic flap necrosis (which healed by secondary intention), patients had no significant complications. Although many experienced decreased sensation at the incision site, this was not a source of complaint. None of these patients had inadvertent nerve injury or any alteration in hand or foot sensation. Some recurrence of swelling occurred in all patients.

The surgical results for postmastectomy lymphedema are much less predictable. In patients with massive swelling, postoperative improvement is usually significant, and function can often be restored. In 10 of 14 patients, postoperative arm volume was reduced by 250 to 1200 ml.[23] In the remaining four patients, arm swelling continued to progress despite initial surgical reduction. Three of these patients had a progressive increase in hand edema after surgery. Long-term data are not available in this series.

The success of staged subcutaneous excision differs between the upper and lower extremities. Foot swelling is not aggravated. The cause of hand swelling is unclear at this time but may result from the surgery or disease progression. Regardless, we do *not* believe that staged subcutaneous excision is indicated in patients with moderate postmastectomy arm swelling. A greater degree of conservatism should be reserved for the upper extremity.

Some authors employing a microsurgical approach have noted a reduction in hand swelling after reconstruction.[27] Interestingly, in some series, microsurgery has been relatively more successful in the upper extremity compared with the lower extremity. To conclude that one operation is indicated in the upper extremity and another in the lower extremity would be premature at this time.

Data on economic outcomes after surgery for lymphedema are nonexistent. Apparently, however, lymphedema is a chronic disease that can debilitate the patient in its more severe forms. This debilitation can manifest as recurrent infections, pain, functional impairment from increased extremity size and decreased joint mobility, musculoskeletal problems secondary to limb weight, psychosocial distress caused by cosmetic issues, and difficulty carrying out activities of daily living.[3] If the incidence of these problems can be decreased through a multidisciplinary approach, the economic cost of this disease can be reduced as well. Patients who undergo effective treatment decrease in-hospital stays and medication use and can obtain employment.

Again, no procedure cures lymphedema, and some edema inevitably follows any procedure. Compared with all available methods of surgical management, staged subcutaneous excision beneath skin flaps is the most reliable, consistently beneficial, and uncomplicated means of surgically managing the symptoms of lymphedema at this time. This opinion is based on the comparable ease of the operation, the minimal postoperative complications, and the results on long-term follow-up.

The continuing debate on the best surgical approach to lymphedema underscores the need for intensified research. Rather than an evolution of methods, the surgical literature represents a trial-and-error approach. As mentioned, one significant problem is the lack of randomized, controlled prospective studies, except for pharmaceutical trials. Furthermore, no well-defined standards exist with which to compare the various surgical procedures.

A useful preoperative or postoperative evaluation should not be undertaken early in the day, after the patient has been sleeping supine, but late in the afternoon, after the patient has been upright for several hours. Fluid displacement (volumetric measurement) likely provides the most objective assessment of results. Circumferential measurements are difficult to compare and standardize. A small variation in where and when the measurement is done can account for significant variations.

SUMMARY

No cure exists for lymphedema because the basic pathophysiology is not completely understood. Why do some people who experience an inciting event (e.g., axillary node dissection) develop lymphedema, whereas the majority do not? After traumatic amputation of an extremity and reimplantation, why do some patients *not* develop lymphedema? Why do patients undergoing a free flap operation *not* develop lymphedema? In these latter two situations, all lymphatic vessels are transected, including collateral vessels, but no lymphedema develops.

Theoretically, those who develop lymphedema seem incapable of either lymphatic generation or lymphatic regeneration. Alternately, development of lymphedema may be related to the abnormal handling of extravascular protein. An intrinsic abnormality in the macrophage may explain the beneficial effects of the coumarin derivatives, which increase proteolysis. Evidence suggests the presence of growth factors specific for the lymphatic system[15,17] and a capability for lymphatic regeneration.[34]

After lymphatic compromise, is there a lack of lymphatic vessel repair, a response to a growth factor, or *lack* of a growth factor? We must conclude some abnormality in an individual's genetic makeup permits that person to develop lymphedema. This defect, however, remains unknown.

REFERENCES

1. Ashby ER, Miller TA: Lymphedema and tumors of the lymphatics. In Moore WS, editor: *Vascular surgery: a comprehensive review,* ed 4, Philadelphia, 1993, Saunders.
2. Baumeister RG, Siuda S: Treatment of lymphedemas by microsurgical lymphatic grafting: what is proved? *Plast Reconstr Surg* 85:64, 1990.
3. Brennan MJ, DePompolo RW, Garden F: Focused review: post-mastectomy lymphedema, *Arch Phys Med Rehabil* 77:S74, 1996.
4. Campisi C, Boccardo F, Alitta P, Tacchella M: Derivative lymphatic microsurgery: indications, techniques, and results, *Microsurgery* 16:463, 1995.
5. Casley-Smith JR, Morgan RG, Piller NB: Treatment of lymphedema of the arms and legs with 5,6-benzo-[α]-pyrone. *N Engl J Med* 329:1158, 1993.
6. Chilvers AS, Kinmonth JB: Operation for lymphedema of the lower limbs: a study of the results in 108 operations using vascularized dermal flaps, *J Cardiovasc Surg* 16:115, 1975.
7. Dellon AL, Hoopes JE: The Charles procedure for primary lymphedema: long-term clinical results, *Plast Reconstr Surg* 60:589, 1977.
8. Foldi E, Foldi M, Clodius L: The lymphedema chaos: a lancet, *Ann Plast Surg* 22:505, 1989.
9. Gloviczki P: Physiologic changes in lymphatic dysfunction. In White RA, Hollier LH, editors: *Vascular surgery: basic science and clinical correlations,* Philadelphia, 1994, Lippincott.
10. Goldsmith HS: Long-term evaluation of omental transposition for chronic lymphedema, *Ann Surg* 180:847, 1974.
11. Hafez HM, Wolfe JHN: Basic data underlying clinical decision making: lymphedema, *Ann Vasc Surg* 10:88, 1996.
12. Hoe AL, Iven D, Royle GT, Taylor I: Incidence of arm swelling following axillary clearance for breast cancer, *Br J Surg* 79:261, 1992.
13. Hurst PAE, Stewart G, Kinmonth JB, Browse NL: Long-term results of the enteromesenteric bridge operation in the treatment of primary lymphoedema, *Br J Surg* 72:272, 1985.
14. Janse AJ, van Coevorden F, Peterse H, et al: Lymphedema-induced lymphangiosarcoma, *Eur J Surg Oncol* 21:155, 1995.
15. Jeltsch M, Kaipainen A, Joukov V, et al: Hyperplasia of lymphatic vessels in VEGF-C transgenic mice, *Science* 276:1423, 1997.
16. Kinmonth JB, Hurst PA, Edwards JM, Rutt DL: Relief of lymph obstruction by use of a bridge of mesentery and ileum, *Br J Surg* 65:829, 1978.
17. Kukk E, Lymboussaki A, Taira S, et al: VEGF-C receptor binding and pattern of expression with VEGFR-3 suggests a role in lymphatic vascular development, *Development* 122(12):3829, 1996.
18. Manson PN, Watts D: Lymphedema. In Cameron JL, editor: *Current surgical therapy,* ed 5, St Louis, 1995, Mosby.
19. Markowski J, Wilcox JP, Helm PA: Lymphedema incidence after specific post-mastectomy therapy, *Arch Phys Med Rehabil* 62:449, 1981.

20. McKee DM, Edgerton MT Jr: The surgical treatment of lymphedema of the lower extremities, *Plast Reconstr Surg* 23:480, 1959.

21. Miller TA: How I do it: surgical management of lymphedema of the extremity, *Ann Plast Surg* 1:184, 1978.

22. Miller TA: Charles procedure for lymphedema: a warning, *Am J Surg* 139:290, 1980.

23. Miller TA: Surgical approach to lymphedema of the arm after mastectomy, *Am J Surg* 148:152, 1984.

24. Mortimer PS: Therapy approaches for lymphedema, *Angiology* 48:87, 1997.

25. O'Brien BM: Microlymphatic surgery. In O'Brien BM, Morrison WA: *Reconstructive microsurgery,* Edinburgh, 1987, Churchill Livingstone.

26. O'Brien BM, Das SK, Franklin JD, Morrison WA: Effect of lymphangiography on lymphedema, *Plast Reconstr Surg* 68:922, 1981.

27. O'Brien BM, Mellow CG, Khazanchi RK, et al: Long-term results after microlymphaticovenous anastomoses for the treatment of obstructive lymphedema, *Plast Reconstr Surg* 85:562, 1990.

28. O'Donnell TF, Bry JDL: Diagnosis and management of lymphedema. In Haimovici H, editor: *Haimovici's Vascular surgery,* ed 4, Cambridge, Mass, 1996, Blackwell Science.

29. Olszewski W: The enigma of lymphedema: a search for answers, *Lymphology* 24:100, 1991 (editorial).

30. Pecking AP, Fevrier B, Wargon C, Pillion G: Efficacy of Daflon 500 mg in the treatment of lymphedema (secondary to conventional therapy of breast cancer), *Angiology* 48:93, 1997.

31. Servelle M: Surgical treatment of lymphedema: a report on 652 cases, *Surgery* 101:485, 1987.

32. Silver D, Puckett CL: Lymphangioplasty: a ten-year evaluation, *Surgery* 80:748, 1976.

33. Sistrunk WE: Further experiences with the Kondoleon operation for elephantiasis, *JAMA* 71:800, 1918.

34. Slavin SA, Upton J, Kaplan WD, Van den Abbeele AD: An investigation of lymphatic function following free tissue transfer, *Plast Reconstr Surg* 99:730, 1997.

35. Thompson N: Surgical treatment of chronic lymphedema of the lower limb with preliminary report of new operation, *BMJ* 2:1566, 1962.

36. Thompson N: Surgical treatment of chronic lymphedema of the extremities, *Surg Clin North Am* 47:445, 1967.

37. Tobin MB, Lacey HJ, Meyer L, Mortimer PS: The psychological morbidity of breast cancer–related arm swelling, *Cancer* 72:3248, 1993.

38. Weiss M, Baumeister RG, Tatsch K, Hahn K: Lymphoscintigraphy for noninvasive long-term follow-up of functional outcome in patients with autologous lymph vessel transplantation, *Nuklearmedizin* 35:236, 1996.

Lower Extremity Reconstruction

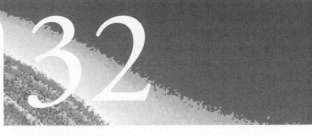

Randy Sherman
Michael Law

INTRODUCTION

Lower extremity reconstruction with limb salvage is a relatively new endeavor, unlike many other subspecialties within the field of plastic and reconstructive surgery. Medical historians can trace the roots of craniomaxillofacial, aesthetic, and hand surgery back at least a century and even centuries in some cases, such as nasal reconstruction. The basic functions of the lower extremity help explain plastic surgery's late arrival to this area. Well-performed amputations and well-rehabilitated amputees set a functional benchmark that was easily achieved with proportionally low morbidity. Until recently, surgeons could not reconstruct most lower extremity wounds and have outcomes meeting or exceeding those of amputation and prosthesis.

Less than 30 years have elapsed since the inception and development of vascularized tissue transfer for treatment of lower extremity injuries. Over that time, options have expanded for the coverage of open wounds and treatment or prevention of osteomyelitis, a problem previously solved by amputation. Surgeons have managed injuries caused by trauma, infection, peripheral vascular disease, diabetes, arthritis, cancer, and congenital anomalies. Coverage of open fractures, osteomyelitic defects, exposed total joint replacements, endoprostheses, and allografts have provided great challenges for the reconstructive surgeon.

Most recently, surgeons have tempered their zeal for limb salvage. With the experience of both spectacular successes and catastrophic failures, they have narrowed the indications for reconstruction, choosing only those candidates who would truly benefit from an improved functional outcome.

This chapter first reviews the anatomy of the lower extremity and its function involving gait, load bearing, and stance. Injuries are classified according to tissue and location, and specific reconstructive options are discussed for each part of the lower limb. Adjunctive considerations include the treatment of osteomyelitis, diabetes, and ulcers; nerve repair; amputation alternatives; and associated outcomes.

INDICATIONS

FUNCTIONAL ANATOMY AND DYSFUNCTION

Functionally the lower extremity serves two basic purposes: (1) static support of the trunk in the upright position and (2) ambulation. Its osseous and soft tissue components are specifically integrated to provide weight-bearing and locomotion capabilities. These stress tolerating forces and gravitational forces greatly exceed those loaded on the upper extremity. Although one lower limb constitutes approximately one sixth of total body weight, during one-legged stance the force exerted on the standing hip joint is about two and one-half times body weight. This phenomenon occurs partly because the thigh abductors pull forcibly across the joint to stabilize the pelvis. If the thigh abductors are weak, the pelvis dips greatly during the stance phase and creates a lurching gait referred to as Trendelenberg gait.

On ambulation the hip is loaded with the equivalent of three times body weight, and during running or stair climbing the load borne by the hip joint as each leg strikes the ground increases to about five times body weight. A similar relationship exists at the ankle because of the muscles pulling across this joint to balance the tibia on the talus. Under the stress of such massive, repetitive loading, dysfunction of lower extremity muscle groups may lead to progressive degenerative arthritis.[27]

Knowledge of lower extremity anatomy therefore must be integrated with an understanding of how the actions of the involved anatomic structures translate into static support of the trunk and locomotion. Attention to functional anatomy underscores the anatomic relationships that are clinically important in lower extremity reconstruction.

Hip Joint

The lower limb functions as a lever arm with joints, allowing coordinated bipedal locomotion. The skeleton of the lower limb consists of a stable girdle, the pelvis, and a mobile lever arm comprising the femur, tibia, and foot bones. The two hip bones (os coxae) are joined anteriorly at the pubic symphysis and posteriorly by the sacrum, the inferior extension of the

Table 32-1.
Muscle Groups Affecting Hip Motion

MOTION AT HIP JOINT	MUSCLES (PRIMARY, SECONDARY)
Thigh flexion	**Iliacus/psoas major**
	Rectus femoris
	Tensor fascia lata
	Pectineus
	Sartorius
	Adductor longus/brevis
	Adductor magnus (anterior part)
	Gluteus minimus
Thigh extension	**Gluteus maximus**
	Adductor magnus (sciatic part)
	Biceps femoris
	Semitendinosus/ semimembranosus
Thigh abduction	**Gluteus medius**
	Gluteus minimus
	Tensor fascia lata
	Sartorius
Thigh adduction	**ANTERIOR GROUP**
	Adductor magnus (obturator part)
	Adductor longus/brevis
	Pectineus
	Gracilis
	POSTERIOR GROUP
	Gluteus maximus
	Biceps femoris (long head)
	Obturator externus
	Quadratus femoris
	Semitendinosus/ semimembranosus
Internal rotation	**Tensor fascia lata**
	Pectineus
	Gluteus minimus (anterior part)
	Adductor longus
	Adductor brevis
	Adductor magnus
	Iliacus/psoas major
External rotation	**Gluteus maximus**
	Piriformis
	Obturator internus/gemelli
	Obturator externus
	Quadratus femoris
	Gluteus medius (posterior part)
	Sartorius

vertebral column. This construct forms a stable arch that transmits the body's weight from the trunk to the lower extremities. The hip joint provides a ball-and-socket articulation with the trunk that is capable of motion in three dimensions. In contrast to the shoulder girdle of the upper limb, the pelvic girdle is extremely stable because of its deep articulation and strong capsular, ligamentous, and muscular attachments.

Functionally the configuration of the hip joint provides stability by sacrificing range of motion, unlike the shallower and more mobile glenohumeral joint. Motion at the hip consists of flexion/extension, abduction/adduction, and internal/external rotation. The muscles responsible for these actions not only control hip motion but also serve to stabilize the pelvis, with considerable overlap in their individual actions (Table 32-1).

Thigh

Structurally the thigh consists of the femur and its associated muscles, which either insert on or arise from it and produce motion at the hip and knee joints. The femur is surrounded as far distally as the supracondylar area by these thick muscle groups, and thus traumatic exposures of the supracondylar femur are relatively unusual. The thigh muscles reside in three fascial compartments. Although some functional overlap occurs, each muscle has major actions on the hip and knee joint and receives innervation from a particular nerve. The anterior compartment contains hip flexors/knee extensors, the medial compartment has thigh adductors/flexors, and the posterior compartment contains hip extensors/knee flexors (Table 32-2).

Blood flow to the muscle groups is provided by the femoral artery for the anterior compartment, the profunda femoris and obturator arteries for the medial compartment, and branches of the profunda femoris artery for the posterior compartment.

Knee

The knee is the largest joint in the body and consists of three articular surfaces: the two articulations of the medial and lateral femoral condyles with the medial and lateral aspects of the tibial plateau and the patellofemoral articulation. The knee joint is stabilized by the external medial and lateral collateral ligaments and the intraarticular anterior and posterior cruciate ligaments, as well as by a thick capsule that fuses posteriorly with periarticular ligaments. Functional motion at the knee consists mainly of flexion and extension and, to a lesser degree, internal and external rotation.

Active knee extension is produced solely by the quadriceps, which consists of the rectus femoris and three vasti muscles. The major thigh extensor, the gluteus maximus muscle, and the major foot plantar flexors, the gastrocnemius and soleus muscles, indirectly contribute to knee extension in the weight-bearing extremity. Since the knee may not flex in the loaded limb (with the foot fixed) without concomitant thigh flexion and ankle dorsiflexion, the muscles, which oppose these two actions, help to maintain the knee in an extended position. This allows a relatively normal (although slower) gait on level

Table 32-2.
Muscle Groups and Motor Nerves of Thigh

COMPARTMENT	MOTOR NERVE	MUSCLES
Anterior	Femoral (L2-4)	Quadriceps femoris Sartorius Iliacus/psoas Pectineus
Medial	Obturator (L2-4)	Gracilis Adductor longus Adductor brevis Adductor magnus Obturator externus
Posterior	Sciatic (L4-S3)	Biceps femoris Semitendinosus Semimembranosus Adductor magnus (portion)

L, Lumbar; *S*, sacral.

ground in a patient with femoral nerve palsy and a nonfunctioning quadriceps.

Knee flexion is produced by the hamstrings (biceps femoris, semitendinosus, semimembranosus) and the gracilis and sartorius muscles, all of which span the knee joint and insert on the proximal tibia or fibula. The semitendinosus, sartorius, and gracilis share a common insertion on the tibia just medial and inferior to the tibial tuberosity, the pes anserinus. Two calf muscles, the gastrocnemius and popliteus, may also contribute to knee flexion because they arise posteriorly above the joint and insert below.

The knee flexors and extensors also produce internal and external rotation of the knee. The flexors all pass to the medial side of the joint and are therefore internal rotators, as is the popliteus, which passes from the posterior aspect of the lateral femoral condyle to the anteromedial aspect of the proximal tibia. The biceps femoris, which passes laterally to insert on the anterior aspect of the fibular head, is an external rotator of the knee. The greatest range of rotational motion at the knee, approximately 40 degrees, occurs with the knee flexed.

Neurovascular structures pass posterior to the knee joint and are fairly well protected by overlying soft tissues. The anterior, medial, and lateral aspects of the joint are almost immediately subcutaneous, as is the patella, and thus orthopedic approaches to the knee generally proceed from the anterior aspect. For this reason, soft tissue coverage is often required in this region with treatment of complex injuries and exposure of orthopedic hardware.

Lower Leg

The lower leg skeleton, comprising the larger tibia and lesser fibula, transmits the muscle groups that produce motion of the ankle, foot, and toes. The four fascial compartments in the lower leg contain muscles of similar or related function (Table 32-3).

The sciatic nerve divides above the knee into the tibial and common peroneal nerves; the common peroneal then divides below the knee into the deep and superficial peroneal nerves. These three terminal motor branches supply the separate muscle groups of the anterior, lateral, and superficial and deep posterior compartments. Within the sciatic nerve the separation into tibial and peroneal fascicles occurs proximally, and thus partial lacerations, crush injuries, and traction injuries may produce deficits manifested predominantly in one of the two terminal motor branches.

Anterior compartment muscles dorsiflex the foot at the ankle joint, extend the toes, and produce inversion of the foot at the subtalar and transverse tarsal joints. Superficial posterior compartment muscles plantar flex the foot at the ankle joint, and the gastrocnemius also assists in knee flexion as it arises above the knee from the femoral condyles. Deep posterior compartment muscles plantar flex the toes and ankle, and the tibialis posterior also inverts the foot. Lateral compartment muscles plantar flex the foot and evert the foot at the subtalar and transverse tarsal joints. The transverse arch of the foot is supported medially by the tibialis anterior and posterior muscles and long toe flexors and laterally by the peronei muscles.

The bellies of the lower leg muscles reside predominantly in the upper and middle thirds of the leg and are mainly tendinous in the lower third. The muscle groups are arranged around the posteromedial, posterior, and lateral aspects of the tibia and fibula, whereas the anteromedial aspect of the tibia remains immediately subcutaneous throughout the lower leg's

Table 32-3.
Fascial Compartments of Lower Leg

COMPARTMENT	MUSCLES	MOTOR NERVE	ARTERY
Anterior	Tibialis anterior Extensor digitorum longus Extensor hallucis longus Peroneus tertius	Deep peroneal	Tibialis anterior
Lateral	Peroneus longus Peroneus brevis	Superficial peroneal	Peroneal (branches)
Superficial posterior	Gastrocnemius Plantaris Soleus	Tibialis	Tibialis posterior
Deep posterior	Popliteus Flexor digitorum longus Flexor hallucis longus Tibialis posterior	Tibialis	Tibialis posterior

length. Therefore the tibia is frequently exposed in open fractures, particularly in the distal third, where the investing soft tissue envelope is the thinnest.

Ankle Joint

The articulation of the tibia and fibula with the talus forms a hinge joint capable of flexion (plantar flexion) and extension (dorsiflexion). The articulation of the distal tibia and fibula is fibrous with little inherent motion and is referred to as a *mortise joint,* which is stabilized by a system of fused periarticular ligaments termed the *syndesmosis.* Although the tibia bears approximately 80% to 90% of a load (at the ankle) placed on the leg, stability of the ankle mortise also is necessary to prevent degenerative changes in the ankle joint. Normal range of motion is from 15 to 20 degrees of dorsiflexion through 45 to 50 degrees of plantar flexion, although normal gait requires only 5 to 10 degrees of plantar flexion. Rotational motion between the lower leg and foot is provided below the ankle level by the subtalar and transverse tarsal joints.

Foot

The function of the foot is twofold: (1) to support the body's weight and (2) to serve as a lever to propel the body forward in ambulation. Because its osseous anatomy consists of a series of mobile small bones rather than a single large one, the foot is pliable and can adapt itself to uneven surfaces. It is thus a segmented lever, which allows the long flexors and short muscles of the foot to exert their influence on the forefoot, the site of push-off for forward gait. This greatly assists the propulsive action of the gastrocnemius and soleus muscles.

A segmented structure such as the lever of the foot is only able to tolerate loading effectively if it is arranged as an arch. The foot is thus arranged as three interrelated arches: (1) trans-

verse, (2) medial longitudinal, and (3) lateral longitudinal. The transverse arch consists of the cuboid and cuneiform bones, with the intermediate and lateral cuneiforms serving as "keystones." The medial and lateral arches are formed by the articulations of the subtalar bones with the metatarsals. These arches are supported by the tendons of the tibialis muscles, the long flexors, and the peronei muscles, as well as by the inherent shape of the bones and the dense plantar ligaments and fascia.

Foot inversion and eversion occur at the subtalar joint, the articulation of the talus and calcaneus. This joint is especially important in accommodating uneven terrain and absorbing forces that would otherwise be transmitted directly to the ankle joint. *Chopart's joint* is the midtarsal joint that allows some independence of motion between the forefoot and hindfoot. The tarsal-metatarsal articulation is referred to as *Lisfranc's joint* and is often a site of overlooked dislocations, particularly in the neuropathic foot.

The sole of the foot is a specialized structure designed to tolerate extremes of direct pressure and shear stress. The skin is quite thick and is densely bound to the underlying plantar fascia by numerous fibrous bands. The cutaneous innervation of the sole is a major consideration in reconstruction, since protective sensation is required to prevent further soft tissue damage and to allow effective gait. The majority of the sole is innervated by the following terminal sensory branches of the tibial nerve (fourth lumbar to first sacral, L4-S1):

1. Medial plantar nerve (L4-5), which supplies the medial forefoot
2. Lateral plantar nerve (S1-2), which supplies the lateral forefoot
3. Medial calcaneal branches (S1-2), which supply the skin immediately below the calcaneus

The inferior distribution of the saphenous nerve (L3-4), a terminal branch of the femoral nerve, includes the skin of the medial arch. The inferior distribution of the sural nerve (S1-2) includes the skin of the lateral arch and the lateral aspect of the heel.

The intrinsic muscles of the foot are essentially analogous to those of the hand, with short flexors and extensors, lumbricals, and interossei present. In the foot, stability is provided at the expense of mobility, and the ranges of motion of the foot and ankle are therefore much less than those of the wrist and hand.

OSSEOUS ANATOMY AND HEALING

An understanding of blood supply to the long bones is critical to appreciate the necessity of thorough bony debridement of comminuted fractures. Diaphyseal fragments bereft of firmly adherent, vascularized soft tissue attachments inevitably form a nonvital sequestrum, which then serves as a nidus for ongoing osteomyelitis. Likewise, osseous infections must be widely debrided to produce the well-perfused, sterile environment required for osseous union.

The tibia has a blood supply typical of long bones and is an excellent experimental and clinical model of bone healing. The cross-sectional anatomy of long bones consists of the following:

1. Outer fibrous periosteum, a thick cortical layer that provides structural stability
2. Inner endosteum, which lies on the inner surface of the cortex
3. Central medullary canal

The tibia receives its blood supply from three sources: a primary nutrient artery, proximal and distal metaphyseal vessels, and the periosteum. The nutrient artery is a branch of the posterior tibial artery that penetrates the cortex and arborizes within the medullary canal to supply the inner two thirds of the cortex from its endosteal surface. The metaphyseal vessels enter the tibia at the proximal and distal metaphyses, penetrating the cortex and forming arcades with the longitudinally oriented endosteal vessels.

The periosteal vessels arise from all the primary blood vessels of the lower leg. These vessels are oriented perpendicular to the long axis of the tibia and normally supply the outer one third of the cortex. This vascular arrangement becomes clinically significant with displaced fractures, in which the longitudinally oriented endosteal blood supply is, by definition, disrupted. The outer periosteal circulation becomes the sole blood supply of displaced diaphyseal fragments, and fragments that have little or no soft tissue attachment are therefore avascular and must be debrided.

Osseous healing thus requires a good blood supply and rigid stabilization of fracture fragments. Rhinelander[46] has demonstrated clinically that although the endosteal circulation remains dominant in nondisplaced fractures, the periosteal circulation is the primary blood supply for healing bone in displaced fractures. Pluripotent mesenchymal cells, which appear to arise from the periosteum, enter the fracture sites and differentiate into cell lines capable of forming callus, bridging the osseous defect, and then laying down new cortical bone.

Some evidence indicates that overlying soft tissue, particularly muscle, may provide blood supply to a fracture site, although this issue remains controversial. Also, muscle flaps may be more effective than random skin flaps or fasciocutaneous flaps in promoting clearance of bacterial contamination of wounds.[10,44] Clearly, however, normal bone healing will not occur without vascularized soft tissue coverage.

GAIT

Lower extremity reconstruction aims to provide a patient with a functional limb capable of effective gait, and gait analysis is a means of objectively assessing lower limb function. *Gait analysis* consists of measuring objectively quantifiable parameters that can be compared with normative data and with repeated measurements in the same patient over time. Typical parameters include gait velocity, step and stride length, cadence (steps per minute), and single stance time. Because local muscle units are frequently used for wound coverage in lower limb reconstruction, gait analysis may also be used to delineate the overall effect on lower limb function when a given muscle (or muscle group) is mobilized and therefore defunctionalized.

The term *gait* refers to the cyclic series of lower extremity movements that results in forward locomotion. It is generally divided into stance and swing phases. The *swing phase* is initiated by the push-off action of the toes and forefoot and concludes with heel strike. The *stance phase* therefore lasts from heel strike to push-off. In normal gait, the swing phase occupies about one-third the cycle and stance the remaining two-thirds; both feet are thus simultaneously in the stance phase one-third the time. *Stride* refers to the distance between heel strikes of the same foot, and *step length* refers to the distance between heel strikes of opposite feet.

Single support refers to the period when one leg is in contact with the ground; *double support* is the period when both feet contact the ground simultaneously. As the speed of gait and the time spent in the swing phase increase, the period of double support decreases from approximately 20% of the cycle in normal walking. Running involves no period of double support but instead a period of "double swing" in which neither foot contacts the ground.

The stance phase consists of contact (heel strike), loading, midstance and terminal stance, and preswing. At contact the knee is extended and the foot dorsiflexed to prevent foot slap. As the foot is loaded, the ankle plantar flexes, which is resisted by the anterior compartment muscles that draw the tibia forward. In *midstance* the body advances over the stationary foot as the ankle rocks from plantar flexion to dorsiflexion, and in *terminal stance* the heel rises as the calf muscles contract and the weight is shifted to the forefoot. In *preswing* the knee flexes passively and hip flexors begin to contract to propel the entire lower extremity forward. The ankle is maximally plantar flexed.

The swing phase is divided into initial swing, midswing, and terminal swing. During *initial swing* the hip flexors fire to bring the lower extremity forward from its trailing position behind the body. The knee passively flexes and the ankle dorsiflexors fire, both of which assist in toe clearance. At *midswing,* toe clearance is critical as the ankle dorsiflexors bring the foot up to a neutral position. The opposite limb is at midstance. In *terminal swing* the hip extensors fire to slow down and stop hip flexion, and the quadriceps extends the knee in preparation for heel strike.[27]

Normal gait thus requires the coordinated action of opposing muscle groups. If a given muscle group is dysfunctional, predictable patterns of gait abnormalities occur. These relationships must be considered in planning reconstructive surgery of the lower extremities. For example, during the swing phase, inadequate passive knee flexion or excessive ankle plantar flexion will result in toe drag. In such patients, "vaulting" by the opposite extremity may be required to clear the toes. During loading a weakened quadriceps mechanism may result in buckling and instability of the knees, which can be partially compensated for by increased tension in the hip extensors.

WOUND CLASSIFICATION

The two primary considerations in wound evaluation of the lower extremity are *location* and *tissue-based assessment* of the wound. Wound location affects both functional issues and the ability to use local tissues in reconstruction. A full-thickness wound of the midthigh 6 cm in diameter may be managed with a skin graft or local skin flap, whereas the same wound over the distal tibia or the calcaneus may require free tissue transfer for coverage.

The surgeon also must determine the individual components missing in the defect to develop a rational plan for reconstruction. This affects the decision to use local versus remote tissue as well.

Wound Location
Each region of the lower extremity possesses unique anatomic and functional characteristics that must be evaluated. It is useful to categorize the thigh, lower leg, and foot into separate anatomic units when planning reconstruction, as follows:
1. The thigh is divided into the hip and proximal/lateral thigh, midthigh, and supracondylar knee.
2. The lower leg is also divided into thirds corresponding to the changing relationship of the tibia with its surrounding soft tissues: the proximal one-third, middle one-third, and distal one-third.
3. The foot is divided into (a) the Achilles and malleolar area (proximal non-weight-bearing foot), (b) the heel and proximal plantar area (proximal weight-bearing foot), (c) the distal plantar area, and (d) the dorsum.

Tissue-based Wound Assessment
SKIN AND MUSCLE. The most common posttraumatic tissue loss is skin and subcutaneous tissue. Proximal cutaneous defects may be effectively managed by skin grafting or local skin or composite flaps, but wounds of the distal tibia, ankle,

and foot often present a greater challenge because of limited soft tissue coverage over osseous structures.

The loss of muscle tissue presents problems of both soft tissue coverage and functional deficits. Muscle loss may be (1) posttraumatic, as in patients with comminuted fractures; (2) ischemic, following compartment syndrome or prolonged hypoperfusion; (3) postablative, as with resection of lower extremity sarcomas; or (4) associated with debridement of infectious processes, such as osteomyelitis and necrotizing fasciitis.

BONE AND JOINTS. Osseous defects are most often posttraumatic, associated with high-energy injury mechanisms such as pedestrian–motor vehicle accidents and motorcycle accidents (Table 32-4). These mechanisms frequently produce open, comminuted fractures that require debridement of nonviable bone. Osteomyelitis, usually accompanied by osteonecrosis and sequestrum, demands extensive osseous debridement. The nature, location, and length of an osseous defect will determine the need for bone grafting, bone lengthening, or vascularized bone transfer or for amputation if the defect is deemed unreconstructable (Table 32-5).

Joint exposure is also an important consideration. When the normally closed, sterile joint environment is compromised, chronic infection and rapid articular destruction may result. Open joint injuries should be closed immediately with local flaps when possible.[45] Chronically contaminated open joints require debridement of exposed, infected synovium and granulation tissue before wound closure.

BLOOD VESSELS AND NERVES. Vascular injuries and neurologic deficits must be thoroughly assessed in developing a plan for lower extremity reconstruction. In the trauma patient, neurovascular injuries usually accompany massive lower extremity injury, and the vascular and neurologic status of the involved limb may be the final determinant of reconstructability. These patients must also be carefully monitored for the presence of compartment syndrome, which is reported to

---

Table 32-4.
Force Imparted to Different Tibial Fracture Mechanisms

INJURY TYPE	DISSIPATED ENERGY (FOOT-POUNDS)
Fall from curb	100
Ski injury	300-500
High-velocity gunshot wound	2000
Automobile bumper collision	100,000

Data from Chapman M: *Instr Course Lect* 31:75-87, 1982.

occur in 9% of open tibial fractures[5] and, if treated late, may result in an unsalvageable extremity.

Irreversible neurologic deficits may require special consideration, such as a peroneal nerve palsy resulting in footdrop, or may obviate the usefulness of reconstruction, as in the patient with an insensate foot. In patients with open tibial fractures an associated vascular injury (Gustilo type IIIc) greatly increases the probability of ultimate amputation. McNutt et al[36] have reported amputation in six of 17 (35%) IIIc tibial fracture patients undergoing tibial artery vascular repair for distal ischemia, despite a patent vascular reconstruction at the time of amputation in three patients. No extremities were salvaged in patients with two or more of the following findings:

Involvement of three or more fascial compartments

Two or more injured tibial and peroneal vessels

Failed vascular reconstruction

Cadaveric foot at initial examination

Severe muscle crush or muscle tissue loss

Table 32-5.
Gustilo Classification of Open Tibial Fractures

GRADE	DESCRIPTION
I	Skin opening of 1 cm or less, quite clean Most likely from inside to outside Minimal muscle contusion Simple transverse or short oblique fractures
II	Laceration more than 1 cm long, with extensive soft tissue damage, flaps, or avulsion Minimal to moderate crushing component Simple transverse or short oblique fractures with minimal comminution
III	Extensive soft tissue damage, including muscles, skin, and neurovascular structures Often a high-velocity injury with severe crushing component
IIIA	Extensive soft tissue laceration with adequate bone coverage Segmental fractures, gunshot injuries
IIIB	Extensive soft tissue injury with periosteal stripping and bone exposure Usually associated with massive contamination
IIIC	Vascular injury requiring repair

Data from Gustilo R: *J Orthop Trauma* 2:54-55, 1988.

Chronic peripheral vascular disease may also impact the reconstructive plan. The patient with peripheral vascular disease must be carefully evaluated because occlusive lesions may compromise the circulation of potential muscle or myocutaneous flaps. In the patient with an occlusive lesion proximal to a wound that requires free tissue transfer for coverage, preliminary peripheral vascular reconstruction may permit successful subsequent microsurgical reconstruction.[7,12] Revascularization may also prevent ulceration or wound breakdown and may change a plan for amputation to a more distal, functional level.

DIABETES. Diabetic patients requiring lower extremity reconstruction present additional concerns. In addition to frequently compromised arterial inflow, diabetes is associated with an obliterative microangiopathy that may result in chronic tissue ischemia. Diabetic wounds are often colonized with resistant bacteria, are prone to osteomyelitis, and demonstrate abnormal wound healing. The peripheral neuropathy associated with diabetes eventually leads to a poorly sensate or insensate foot, which may result in a spectrum of foot deformities, including chronic metatarsophalangeal joint dislocation, transverse and longitudinal arch collapse, and eventually the end-stage Charcot's foot.

Lower extremity reconstruction must be individualized in these patients. The surgeon must balance the possibility of achieving a closed and stable wound with the probability that the patient will be able to use the reconstructed limb for effective, long-term ambulation.

DEVICES. The presence of exposed orthopedic hardware may alter the soft tissue coverage requirements, as may the need to obliterate a "dead space" after debridement or elective resection of osseous structures. For example, total knee prostheses typically require vascularized coverage after drainage of infection and may be temporarily explanted while the infectious process is allowed to resolve.

PATIENT ASSESSMENT

History

Patient assessment begins with a history of the primary event or disease process leading to the development of a lower extremity wound. Previous operations, including fracture management, vascular procedures, debridement of infection, and prior reconstructive surgery, must be explored in detail. When possible, operative reports should be obtained, particularly in the case of prior vascular or reconstructive surgery. If recent infections are reported, bacteriology reports must be obtained as well as documentation of recent antibiotic therapy.

Associated conditions that may complicate wound healing and the patient's metabolic state must be identified. These include systemic processes such as diabetes, renal failure, collagen vascular disease, and steroid dependency. A smoking history should be obtained and a smoking cessation program initiated if possible. Regional disease processes that may affect limb vascularity also must be identified, such as peripheral vascular disease or a history of deep venous thrombosis.

Because lower extremity reconstruction aims to restore function, current and previous ambulatory capacity should be reviewed. In most patients a subjective assessment of gait suffices, although formal gait analysis may be obtained if more objective data are required. The patient's type of employment and current job status are documented, as well as personal goals for return to activity, employment, and avocation.

Physical Examination

Examination includes an assessment, as previously described, of the location and composite nature of the lower extremity wound. In addition, a careful vascular examination should be performed, including evaluation of distal pulses and capillary refill and inspection for signs of chronic ischemia or venous insufficiency. Absence of distal pulses should initiate a more detailed evaluation for peripheral vascular occlusive disease, such as arterial duplex examination, magnetic resonance angiography, or conventional angiography.

Doppler examination may be a useful adjunct in some patients but can be misleading, particularly in diabetic patients with arterial calcinosis. Doppler examination does provide a means for performing a lower extremity "Allen's test" by assessing Doppler signals in one end artery as another end artery is compressed. For example, an audible signal over the dorsalis pedis artery that can be obliterated by manual occlusion of the tibialis posterior artery at the ankle implies reversal of flow in the dorsalis pedis, most likely from an occlusive lesion of the anterior tibial artery proximally.

Digital pressures in the toes and transcutaneous oxygen tension measurements may also provide useful information regarding distal perfusion and likelihood of wound healing.

Careful neurologic assessment is required, and any muscle group weakness or motor nerve deficit is noted. Motor deficits may require external splinting or an arthrodesis in some cases. A detailed evaluation of cutaneous sensibility must be performed, particularly for the foot's weight-bearing surface. Insensate feet quite frequently develop neuropathic ulcers and degenerative changes, and the prognosis for long-term salvage of the distal lower extremity in this setting is poor.

Joint motion should also be carefully assessed, since restriction caused by prior trauma, infection, or surgery may adversely affect the functional status of the involved extremity. The presence of sinus tracts may indicate chronic underlying joint or bone infection. Radiographs and relevant studies (e.g., computed tomography, and bone scintigraphy) must be reviewed to determine the exact nature of osseous defects and associated orthopedic hardware. An understanding of nomenclature associated with internal and external fixation devices is important for effective communication with orthopedic surgeons involved in the care of these patients, particularly in planning intraoperative access to sites potentially obstructed by devices.

OPERATIONS

LOCATION-BASED WOUND RECONSTRUCTION

Thigh

HIP AND PROXIMAL/LATERAL THIGH. Hip and proximal/lateral thigh wounds usually result from complications in the management of hip fractures or from pressure necrosis over the greater trochanter. Hip wounds therefore often require vascularized coverage of exposed orthopedic hardware or obliteration of dead space after explantation of infected prostheses. Local lower extremity muscle or myocutaneous flap options include the tensor fascia lata, vastus lateralis, and rectus femoris flaps, all of which are based on the lateral circumflex femoral artery.

The *tensor fascia lata (TFL) flap* does not have much inherent muscle bulk but does allow a long inferior fascial extension to be elevated to just above the knee. If the distal portion is delayed, a larger skin paddle may be raised with the flap, which remains innervated if the iliohypogastric (twelfth thoracic, T12) and lateral femoral cutaneous (L2-3) nerves are preserved. A complication of TFL elevation may be lateral destabilization of the knee in some patients.

The *vastus lateralis muscle flap* provides a larger bulk of muscle and can provide a skin paddle overlying its proximal half.[15] This flap has the functional advantage of producinglittle or no effect on ambulation when mobilized and can reach most of the inferior and posterior pelvis. It is useful for large soft tissue defects and is often employed to fill the dead space created by a Girdlestone resection of the femoral head.

The *rectus femoris muscle flap* is easily mobilized and has a fairly wide arc of rotation. It can be elevated with a small skin paddle, which allows primary closure of the donor site. The rectus femoris flap does not provide as much bulk as the vastus lateralis flap and is associated with some loss of strength in knee extension.

An excellent alternative for closure of large hip defects, particularly after explantation of an infected hip prosthesis, is the *extended deep inferior epigastric (EDIE) flap* (Figure 32-1). The EDIE flap is essentially a vertical rectus abdominis myocutaneous flap, elevated with a random cutaneous extension adjacent to the paraumbilical perforators.[53] A portion or all of the large cutaneous paddle may be deepithelialized for use in filling extensive soft tissue defects. Its arc of rotation may extend as far inferiorly as the knee. This versatile flap should be considered when local lower extremity muscle flaps are unavailable, are inadequate in size, or are thought to be unreliable because of vascular disease or prior radiation.[17,59]

When the nature of the wound or of potential donor sites precludes the use of pedicled flaps, free tissue transfer is indicated. The *latissimus dorsi free flap* is an obvious first choice because it provides the maximum possible soft tissue coverage and a donor site that is anatomically remote from the wound. A potential problem with microsurgical tissue transfer to this area is the availability of easily accessible, reliable recipient vessels.

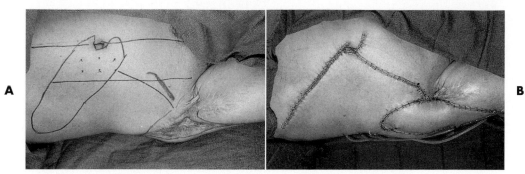

Figure 32-1. A, Unstable scar over infected right total hip replacement, with outline for extended deep inferior epigastric (EDIE) flap. **B,** After transposition, complete resurfacing of right hip with obliteration of deep dead space using rectus abdominis component.

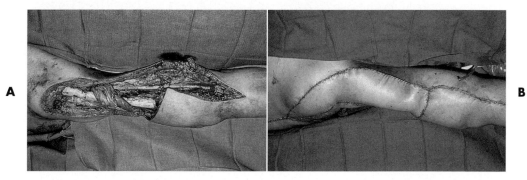

Figure 32-2. A, Midthigh defect with long exposure of femoral diaphysis. **B,** EDIE flap, also known as extended rectus abdominis myocutaneous flap, used for extensive coverage of lateral midshaft defect.

MIDTHIGH. Wounds of the midthigh can often be closed with skin grafts or local fasciocutaneous flaps because the femur is protected by a thick envelope of soft tissue. Exposure of a femoral fracture or orthopedic hardware, however, requires well-vascularized muscle flap coverage. The TFL, vastus lateralis, and rectus femoris flaps may all be useful for midthigh wounds if the lateral circumflex femoral pedicle is intact.

The *gracilis flap,* based on the medial circumflex femoral artery, is available for coverage on the medial aspect of the thigh. Although it does not provide much muscle bulk, the gracilis can be "unfurled" by careful longitudinal dissection of intramuscular septa to cover broad defects.

The *vastus medialis muscle flap* is supplied by perforators from the profunda femoris proximally and the superficial femoral artery distally and cannot be rotated on a vascular pedicle. It may be mobilized on its perforators, however, and transposed medially for coverage of the femur. When left attached proximally, the vastus medialis flap may be used for reconstruction of the patellar tendon and restoration of knee extension.[2,55]

The rectus abdominis muscle and more specifically the EDIE flap are useful in patients with extensive soft tissue loss (Figure 32-2). When recurrent infection of an underlying fracture requires wide soft tissue debridement, free tissue transfer may be the best management option. As opposed to the hip area, adequately sized and easily accessible vessels for inflow and outflow are usually available in the thigh.

SUPRACONDYLAR KNEE. The femur flares distally into medial and lateral condyles, and the soft tissue envelope surrounding it tapers accordingly. This area is at or beyond the limit of the arc of rotation for the previously described rotation flaps. For coverage of exposed fractures and hardware at this level, an *extended medial gastrocnemius muscle or myocutaneous flap* is useful. This flap incorporates a random fasciocutaneous extension of the usual gastrocnemius skin paddle and can effectively cover wounds at and just proximal to the level of the femoral condyles. In general the skin paddle of the medial gastrocnemius flap is reliable up to 10 cm above the medial malleolus. Delayed coverage with a more distal portion may allow incorporation of a skin paddle that extends within 5 cm of the malleolus.

Lower Leg

PROXIMAL-THIRD TIBIA. Proximal tibial defects may usually be covered with a *medial or lateral gastrocnemius muscle or myocutaneous flap* or a combination of the two (Figure 32-3). These muscles have a dominant proximal vascular pedicle, the medial and lateral sural arteries, respectively, and when completely "islandized" on their pedicles, they may reach most wounds adjacent to the knee. These flaps are extremely

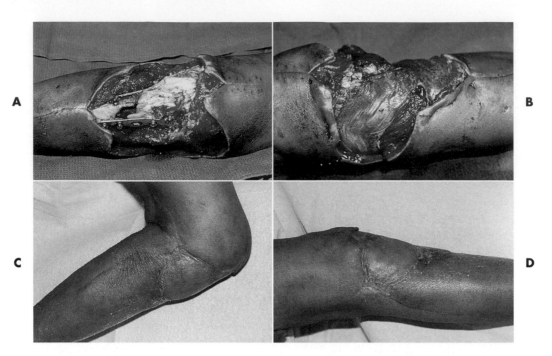

Figure 32-3. **A,** Comminuted tibial plateau fracture with large, overlying soft tissue defect. **B,** Coverage using both medial and lateral gastrocnemius muscle flaps. **C,** Successful closure with maximal knee flexion. **D,** Successful closure with maximal knee flexion and knee extension.

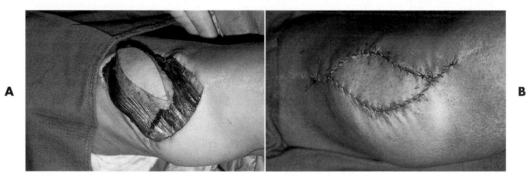

Figure 32-4. **A,** Gastrocnemius muscle flap harvested with overlying skin paddle. **B,** Flap inset demonstrates superior contour of myocutaneous construct.

reliable, are easily elevated, and pose no functional deficiency if one muscle is mobilized. Perpendicular scoring of the fascial envelope of the gastrocnemius muscle, particularly on its undersurface, adds length and width to the muscle belly. If both muscles are elevated as flaps, many patients will demonstrate weakness in ankle plantar flexion.

If the *soleus muscle flap* is used along with the medial or lateral gastrocnemius flap for an extensive defect of the proximal to middle tibia, a minimal to moderate functional defect results if one head of the gastrocnemius remains in situ. A cutaneous paddle can easily be raised with the muscle, which may obviate the need for skin grafting in some patients (Figure 32-4).

Other local muscle flaps have been described, such as a bipedicled tibialis anterior transposition flap, but none has gained wide clinical use because of questionable reliability. A wide variety of fasciocutaneous flaps have been reported, based on superficial perforating vessels from the deep arterial system, such as the saphenous artery and sural artery flaps. These flaps are less reliable than muscle flaps, may create unfavorable donor defects, and have a relatively high rate of complications.[22]

Proximal-third tibial and knee defects that cannot be closed using gastrocnemius flaps generally require free tissue transfer, most often of a rectus abdominis or latissimus dorsi muscle flap with skin graft. Extremely large defects may require transfer of a free EDIE flap, which may allow recontouring of wounds with large skin and subcutaneous tissue defects. A combined latissimus dorsi–serratus anterior flap can be transferred on a common pedicle.

MIDDLE-THIRD TIBIA. The *soleus flap* can be raised only as a muscle flap and is the primary coverage for middle-third tibial defects (Figure 32-5). As with the gastrocnemius flap, the

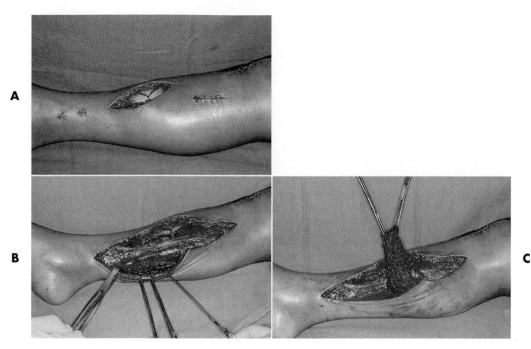

Figure 32-5. **A,** Typical type IIIB middle-third tibial fracture. **B,** Soleus muscle identified at its confluence with Achilles tendon. **C,** Soleus muscle dissected free and rotated.

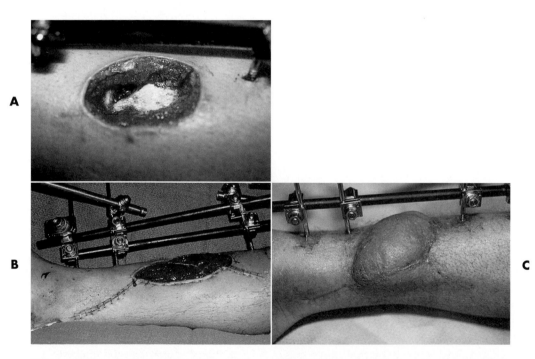

Figure 32-6. **A,** Composite middle-third type IIIB tibial fracture. **B,** Soleus muscle completely covers defect. **C,** Several weeks after soleus transposition with overlying skin graft.

soleus flap is reliable and easily raised (Figure 32-6). Its bipennate morphology allows the soleus to be split into a larger medial flap and much smaller lateral hemisoleus flap.[54] We have found no advantage, however, to bisecting the soleus in most situations.

The soleus muscle has a dominant proximal vascular supply from branches of the popliteal artery and a secondary distal supply from branches of the tibialis posterior artery. A reversed soleus flap has been described based on the inferior circulation for coverage of lower tibial and heel defects,[56] but its reliability is questionable.

As mentioned, large defects may require a combination of a soleus and medial or lateral gastrocnemius flap. In these patients it is usually more appropriate to choose free tissue transfer using either the rectus abdominis or the latissimus dorsi muscle.

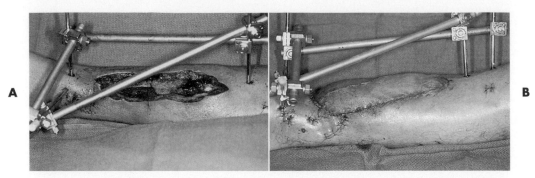

Figure 32-7. **A,** Middle-third and distal-third type IIIB tibial fracture with external fixator in place. **B,** Immediately after surgery, with transfer of rectus abdominis muscle and overlying skin graft.

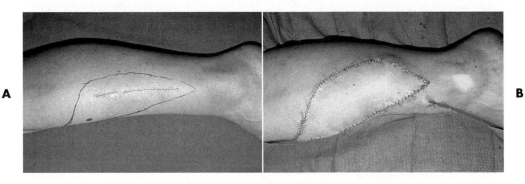

Figure 32-8. **A,** Proposed composite excision of malignant fibrous histiocytoma (MFH). **B,** After resection and reconstruction using parascapular fasciocutaneous flap.

LOWER-THIRD TIBIA. Distally based fasciocutaneous flaps may be adequate for small wounds of the distal third of the lower leg, but most wounds involving significant tibial exposure and essentially all open tibial fractures require coverage by free tissue transfer. This is particularly true in patients with osteomyelitis. Again, the rectus abdominis and latissimus dorsi free flaps are most often employed for large three-dimensional defects, especially when segmental tibial defects must be filled before formal osseous reconstruction (Figure 32-7). The gracilis flap is also readily available, reliable, and useful for smaller, narrower defects. Although less often used, the scapular or parascapular fasciocutaneous free flaps are as effective (Figure 32-8).

The widespread application of early wound closure by free tissue transfer for comminuted, open distal-third tibial fractures has resulted in a dramatic decrease in the incidence of osteomyelitis and subsequent amputation.

If thinner soft tissue coverage is required for recontouring of defects in the lower-third tibial area, the radial forearm and temporoparietal fascia free flaps are easily raised and reliable. The fasciocutaneous flaps described previously for smaller defects are essentially distally based, reverse-flow flaps that are perfused by septocutaneous perforators from the tibial or peroneal vessels. Great care must be taken to preserve the tenuous inflow to these flaps during elevation, and flap length should not greatly exceed the width.

Foot

Hidalgo and Shaw[23] have developed a classification system for foot injuries that quantifies soft tissue deficits, as well as associated osseous injuries, as follows:

Type I injuries: limited soft tissue loss only

Type II injuries: major soft tissue deficits with or without distal amputation

Type III injuries: major soft tissue loss and accompanying open fracture(s) of the ankle, calcaneus, or bimalleolar area

The foot is divided anatomically into the following four areas for reconstruction:

1. Achilles tendon and malleolar area
2. Heel and midplantar area
3. Distal plantar area and forefoot
4. Dorsum

As with all extremity injuries, the surgeon must consider the nature of the injury, the specific anatomic area involved, and the relative and absolute contraindications before formulating a plan for reconstruction. Although cutaneous sensibility is not as absolute prerequisite for adequate weight bearing on the reconstructed foot,[33] complete loss of plantar sensation after tibial nerve avulsion is a strong contraindication to foot salvage in patients with type III injuries.

ACHILLES TENDON AND MALLEOLAR AREA. Type I wounds of the proximal non-weight-bearing area of the foot

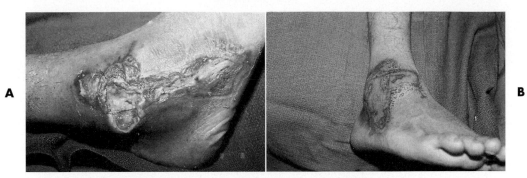

Figure 32-9. A, Unstable scar over lateral malleolus with exposed bone. **B,** Closure using temporoparietal fascial flap with skin graft adds minimal bulk.

may be reconstructed with local fasciocutaneous flaps and muscle flaps. Plantar flaps generally are not useful for this area because of a limited arc of rotation and problems associated with disrupting the plantar surface as a donor site.[23]

The *lateral calcaneal artery flap* is based on the terminal branch of the peroneal artery and may be useful for limited Achilles tendon area coverage.[18,60] It has the advantage of providing sensate coverage (sural nerve) and can be designed with a flap length of up to 14 cm if delayed.

The *dorsalis pedis flap* may also be mobilized sufficiently to reach malleolar and distal Achilles tendon area defects and provides sensate coverage. Flap elevation is tedious, however, and potential donor site morbidity makes this flap a secondary option in hindfoot reconstruction.

Several muscle flaps can be elevated for Achilles tendon and malleolar area coverage, although most are limited both in size and in their arc of rotation. The *extensor digitorum brevis flap* is the most useful of the local muscle rotation flaps and is based on the lateral tarsal–dorsalis pedis arterial pedicle.[28,29] The muscle belly averages 5 × 6 cm in size and effectively covers one malleolar area. It is somewhat easier to elevate than the dorsalis pedis flap and has less associated donor site morbidity.

Type II and III defects of this area generally require free tissue transfer for coverage. The *temporoparietal fascia (TPF) free flap* (with split-thickness skin graft)[6] and *radial forearm free flap* may provide thin coverage for large Achilles tendon or malleolar area exposures and allow for tendon gliding on the undersurface (Figure 32-9). These flaps can be elevated simultaneously with dissection of the recipient vessels, usually the tibialis posterior system. The TPF flap has the potential advantage of a less conspicuous donor site.

Wounds that need more extensive soft tissue replacement may require a thicker fasciocutaneous flap, such as the parascapular or lateral arm flap.

Large type III wounds of the hindfoot, particularly those with exposed joints or fractures, require free muscle transfer for coverage. Successful treatment of these injuries demands adequate osseous debridement and stabilization (Figure 32-10). The gracilis muscle is especially well suited for this area because it is long and narrow, can be "unfurled" by dissection of intramuscular septa to provide thin coverage, and can even be split transversely and transferred as two separate free flaps, using a minor distal pedicle to revascularize the distal half

of the muscle (Figure 32-11). The rectus abdominis and latissimus dorsi muscles are also reliable and readily available.

HEEL AND MIDPLANTAR AREA. A wide array of plantar flaps have been described for coverage of the proximal weight-bearing areas.[40,47,48] Conceptually these flaps attempt to provide sensate coverage using like tissue from the non-weight-bearing midsole area. Such flaps may include the abductor hallucis or flexor digitorum brevis muscles and one or both plantar arteries and may be dissected in a deep subfascial, fascial, or superficial plane.

Shaw and Hidalgo[49,50] have reported a comprehensive anatomic and clinical evaluation of a medially based instep flap perfused by a vascular plexus superficial to the plantar fascia. The plantar nerves are mobilized with the flap, providing sensate, glabrous coverage of wounds up to 7 cm in diameter.

As with the Achilles tendon and malleolar area defects, only relatively small, type I wounds can be reliably closed using local tissue. More extensive defects require free tissue transfer (Figure 32-12). With the weight-bearing surface of the foot, free muscle flaps covered with split-thickness skin grafts may be more stable and functional than fasciocutaneous flaps. Although such flaps are initially insensate, neurotization along vascular channels with subtotal return of various sensory modalities has been widely reported in free tissue transfer. Some degree of proprioception may return.

May et al[32] reported on nine patients who underwent this reconstruction for wounds of the weight-bearing heel or sole. Plantar wound breakdown or ulceration occurred in only one patient over an average follow-up of 19 months. This complication was thought to result from the muscle being inset under too little tension to keep the flap from folding on itself when subjected to pressure.

DISTAL PLANTAR AREA AND FOREFOOT. Most wounds of the distal plantar area require free tissue transfer for coverage (Figure 32-13). Plantar flaps cannot be sufficiently mobilized distally because of a tethering effect by the plantar nerves that innervate them. Sensate toe flaps have been described, but the associated donor defect is unfavorable. As for the proximal weight-bearing foot, free muscle flaps with split-thickness skin grafts appear to provide the most stable, durable coverage.

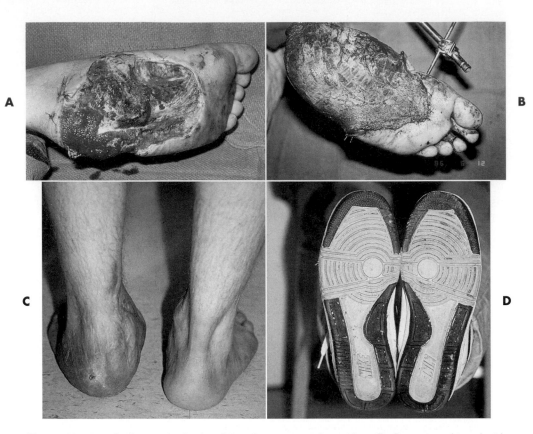

Figure 32-10. **A,** Composite heel avulsion after motorcycle accident. **B,** Coverage achieved with latissimus dorsi muscle flap. **C,** Eight months after wound closure, patient is ambulatory with stable, closed wound. **D,** Satisfactory shoe fit after reconstruction.

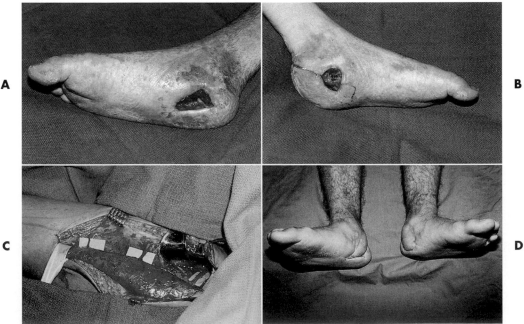

Figure 32-11. **A,** Calcaneal osteomyelitis of right foot after four-story fall. **B,** Similar wound on left foot. **C,** Gracilis muscle demonstrates major and both minor pedicles. This one donor muscle was split to fill both recipient defects. **D,** Successful closure of wounds 1 year after transfer. Patient ambulates without assistance.

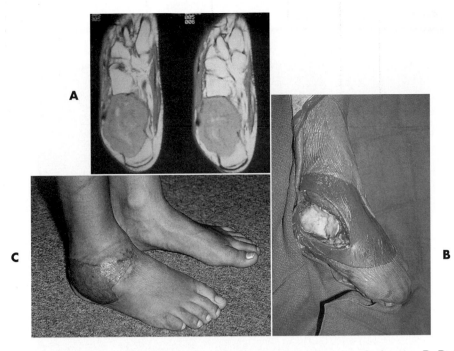

Figure 32-12. **A,** Computed tomography scan showing giant cell tumor of calcaneus. **B,** Defect temporarily filled with methylmethacrylate before rectus abdominis muscle transfer and split-thickness skin graft. **C,** Eighteen months after initial resection, flap has been elevated, methylmethacrylate removed, and bone graft placed and subsequently incorporated.

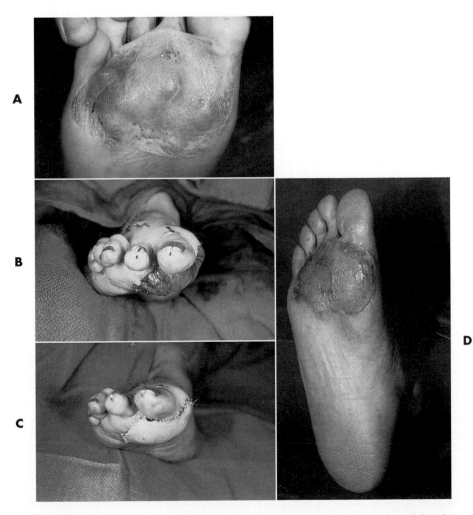

Figure 32-13. **A,** Plantar forefoot 5 years after resection of melanoma followed by skin graft over metatarsophalangeal joints. Patient was unable to ambulate on this area and underwent recurrent skin graft breakdown. **B,** Partial latissimus dorsi muscle flap used for plantar reconstruction, with thoracodorsal pedicle threaded through intermetatarsal space and anastomosed to dorsalis pedis vessels. **C,** Full-thickness skin graft applied over latissimus dorsi flap. **D,** Four years after reconstruction, patient is fully ambulatory with stable, closed wound.

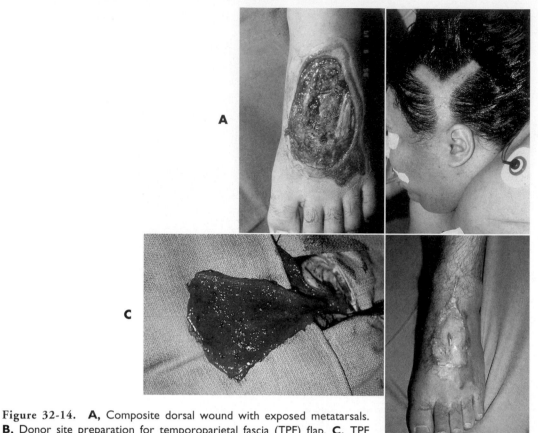

Figure 32-14. A, Composite dorsal wound with exposed metatarsals. **B,** Donor site preparation for temporoparietal fascia (TPF) flap. **C,** TPF flap isolated on superficial temporal vessels. **D,** Closed wound with TPF flap and skin graft adds no bulk.

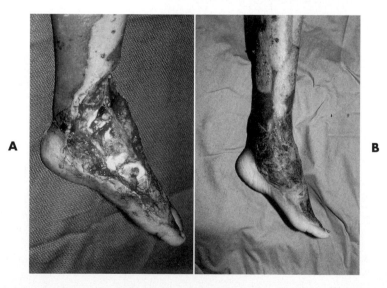

Figure 32-15. A, Dorsal avulsion of all soft tissues with tangential metatarsal fractures in 5-year-old boy. **B,** Latissimus dorsi muscle with split-thickness skin graft provides stable coverage with surprisingly minimal bulk.

DORSUM. Soft tissue wounds of the dorsum with intact paratenon may be closed with split-thickness skin grafts, but direct exposure of tendon or bone requires vascularized coverage. Fascial free flaps (e.g., TPF) provide thin coverage and permit tendon gliding below the reconstruction (Figure 32-14). For deeper wounds in the adult, thin fasciocutaneous flaps (e.g., radial forearm, parascapular) provide a more aesthetic reconstruction than muscle flaps with skin grafts. For severe injuries associated with open fractures (type III), however, coverage with a muscle free flap may be prudent.

Surprisingly, in young children the latissimus dorsi muscle is nearly ideal for reconstructing these subtypes (Figure 32-15).

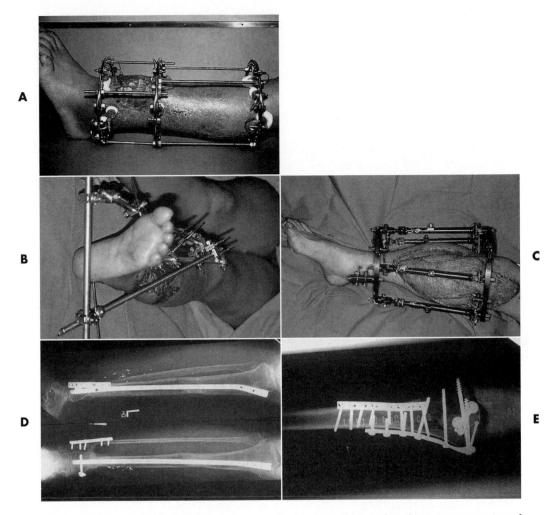

Figure 32-16. **A,** Ilizarov device in place, usually employed for bone lengthening or correction of malunion. **B,** A-O unilateral half-frame external fixator, used more often than any other device for tibial fractures. **C,** Ace-Fisher hybrid device for external fixation, often used for comminuted intraarticular fractures. **D,** Radiograph of interlocking intramedullary (IM) nail after reduction of tibial shaft fracture. **E,** Radiograph of buttress plates used for tibial plateau fracture.

SPECIAL RECONSTRUCTIVE CONSIDERATIONS

Neuropathic Ulcers

The diabetic lower extremity undergoes the combined insults of sensory denervation (peripheral neuropathy) and impaired peripheral circulation. Diabetes also adversely affects immune function. The combination of these factors predisposes to foot ulceration, which may be refractory to local measures and prone to infection with multiple organisms. Underlying osteomyelitis is present in the vast majority of diabetic foot ulcers, including those without exposed bone.[42]

After adequate wound debridement, including involved bone, and initiation of culture-guided antibiotic therapy, the mainstay of treatment for these difficult wounds is relief of pressure on the prominent weight-bearing surfaces. Total contact casting has been adopted from the treatment of leprosy patients and attempts to increase the sole's weight-bearing surface area. This method has been shown to be highly effective in the management of diabetic foot wounds in properly selected patients, with 82% of ulcers healed over 6

weeks in one report.[51] Metatarsal head resection is another effective means of eliminating pressure and promoting healing of plantar wounds localized in that area.[19]

For diabetic patients with more complex foot wounds, local flaps should be avoided because of the associated lower extremity neurologic and vascular impairments. The decision involves amputation versus free tissue transfer, and must be individualized for each patient. This depends on (1) available proximal inflow, (2) necessity for further debridement, and (3) the patient's functional status and personal needs and goals. Free tissue transfer may permit limb salvage in diabetic patients with severe foot wounds provided that adequate inflow is available and preliminary thorough debridement is performed.[3,26]

Orthopedic Hardware

Because most lower extremity reconstruction is undertaken in conjunction with orthopedic trauma or its sequelae, the surgeon must have a working knowledge of fixator devices. Bone-stabilizing hardware may be applied as either internal or external fixation (Figure 32-16).

Plates and screws are primarily used in femoral shaft and epicondylar fractures. Blade plates are typically employed for distal femur and intracondylar injuries. Plating of the tibia and fibula is much more limited and plays an important role in plateau fractures, also known as proximal tibial interarticular fractures. Small plates are often used to stabilize the distal fibula in patients with plafond fractures or distal tibial intraarticular injuries. More recently, intramedullary nailing, either reamed or unreamed, has become the preferred method of tibial diaphyseal reduction.

Several external fixator options are available for type III tibial fractures and osteomyelitis-related defects after debridement. The A-O half-frame is by far the most popular and adaptable. With extension bars, it can be used to allow access to circumferential wounds. The device does not permit fine wire placement for comminuted intraarticular fractures.

Other devices include the Ace-Fisher, the EBI, and the Ilizarov. Insertion of the Ilizarov device is complex and labor intensive but adds the mechanical ability to undertake bone transport for closure of osseous defects. Knowledge of these devices and their orthopedic nomenclature will help the plastic surgeon understand and apply the reconstructive algorithm.

Osseous Reconfiguration

The reconstruction of osseous deficiencies is a challenging facet of lower extremity reconstruction that has evolved considerably in the recent past. Skeletal reconstruction focuses on the restoration of bone length and stability and the prevention or elimination of osteomyelitis. Options for restoring strength and stability include nonvascularized bone autografts and allografts, vascularized bone transfer, and distraction osteogenesis. As with other aspects of lower extremity reconstruction, the surgeon must individualize decision making and consider the nature of the injury, functional requirements, and associated soft tissue injury.

The use of autologous bone to restore bone continuity is the gold standard of osseous reconfiguration. The most frequently used donor site is the iliac crest, an excellent source of cortical and cancellous bone. The success of this technique depends on an adequately debrided, sterile wound and vascularized coverage of the grafted area. Early prophylactic bone grafting of high-energy tibial fractures greatly reduces the time to union.[4,8,9]

With a colonized or severely infected fracture site, external skeletal stabilization, wide debridement, and vascularized coverage followed by delayed (4 to 8 weeks) autogenous bone grafting have provided the most reliable form of treatment. Gustilo[20] noted that a delay of at least 6 weeks results in accelerated fracture healing, which may relate to time required for complete clearance of bacterial contamination and resolution of inflammatory changes. Segmental tibial defects as long as 14 cm have been successfully reconstituted using this technique, employing both iliac crests as donor sites.[11] Although allograft bone is readily available, this material consists of acellular corticocancellous bone only, and its use is not widely recommended for this indication.

Taylor[52] popularized the *free fibula graft,* initially describing reconstruction of tibial defects up to 12.5 cm. The treatment of defects more than twice that length has subsequently been reported. Proponents of vascularized bone transfer claim the following advantages[38,58]:

1. Reduced time to osseous union
2. Shorter period of immobilization compared with conventional bone grafting
3. Option for incorporating soft tissue elements with the fibular diaphysis

Potential disadvantages include the following[61]:

1. Donor site morbidity associated with elevation of the free fibula flap
2. Risk of nonunion at the proximal or distal tibial interface
3. Lower inherent strength of the fibula, which may lead to fatigue fracture

Bone lengthening by the *Ilizarov method of distraction osteogenesis*[24] has been widely investigated in the lower extremity, particularly for segmental tibial defects.[13,43] Osseous transport and consolidation for tibial defects as long as 18 cm have been reported. The primary disadvantage of the Ilizarov method is the prolonged period of immobilization and non-weight-bearing status required to achieve lengthening. In one series of 11 patients (10 tibias, one femur) the average defect bridged was 6.7 cm (range 2 to 18 cm), and the average duration of treatment was 13 months (range 8½ to 22 months).[41]

Osteomyelitis

The single greatest obstacle to the successful treatment of open fractures of the lower extremity is the prevention or eradication of posttraumatic osteomyelitis. In 1970 Ger and Efron[16] enumerated the following factors associated with persistent infection after open fractures:

1. Retention of devitalized or infected bone (sequestrum)
2. Presence of dysvascular or infected soft tissues
3. Dead space in the surgical site
4. Inadequate soft tissue coverage

The authors advocated aggressive debridement of all pathologic tissue and the obliteration of dead space. Other investigators later reported success with these principles, combined with muscle flap coverage and delayed osseous reconstruction.[8,9,21]

These principles have now become axiomatic in the management of severe lower extremity trauma and posttraumatic osteomyelitis. The ability to perform free tissue transfer for coverage of complex lower extremity wounds has significantly expanded the possibilities for limb salvage in these patients.[34,35]

Nerve Repair and Functional Reconstruction

Peripheral nerve injuries associated with lower extremity trauma may cause significant disability and may even preclude the usefulness of reconstruction. Open wounds, missile wounds, and displaced fractures are potential mechanisms of nerve laceration, and motor nerve deficits may be associated with these injuries.

Sharp lacerations require immediate repair. For injuries with extensive tearing and contusion, however, repair is usually delayed for 2 to 3 weeks to permit a more accurate assessment of the true extent of injury. Blunt trauma or blast injuries most often produce nerve contusions. These patients may benefit from an initial period of close observation for spontaneous recovery, with exploration reserved for those who show no improvement over 3 to 4 months.

The prognosis for recovery of nerve function after repair in the lower extremity varies anatomically. Prognosis depends on the distance from the injury to the motor end plate or sensory end organ, and these distances tend to be longer for the lower than the upper extremity. Functional recovery depends on the clinical significance of the functional loss associated with a given nerve injury. Careful assessment of peripheral nerve function must be performed in all patients undergoing lower extremity reconstruction, since their level of function should influence the treatment plan.

Femoral nerve palsy results in an inability to complete the last 15 degrees of knee extension, mainly due to paralysis of the vastus medialis. This permits adequate ambulation on flat ground but marked disability with uphill walking and stair climbing, which require powerful knee extension. The sensory deficit is limited to a small area medial and superior to the patella. Most patients with femoral nerve repair can be expected to recover some function. Exploration is recommended for all patients with traumatic, complete femoral nerve palsy.

Sciatic nerve injuries are most often associated with posterior hip dislocations, posterior acetabular fractures, and operations on the femoral head. Prognosis for recovery of function varies, with return of function more likely in the tibial than the peroneal nerve distribution. Repair of lesions at the buttock level often allows partial return of plantar flexion and may provide protective plantar sensation. Patients with high sciatic lesions, however, are frequently plagued with severe vasomotor and trophic changes.[1] Peroneal nerve division with muscle function usually does not return. Delayed repairs carry a poor prognosis, and thus all sciatic nerve injuries should be explored early.

Tibial nerve injuries are extremely disabling because the terminal sensory branches (medial and lateral plantar nerves, medial calcaneal branches) provide plantar sensibility. Plantar sensation is crucial for proper weight bearing and ambulation and to prevent neuropathic bone and joint injury. In addition, most sympathetic innervation to the foot is from the tibial nerve, and thus severe vasomotor and trophic changes may be associated with tibial nerve palsy, further predisposing the affected extremity to ulceration.

The insensate sole is widely considered to be an absolute contraindication to distal lower extremity reconstruction. Using free muscle transfer, however, much of the sole or in some patients the entire sole may be recontoured, with effective, long-term weight bearing and ambulation. Proximal tibial nerve lesions are complicated by loss of plantar flexion, foot inversion, and toe flexion, which is disabling for activities requiring forceful push-off, such as running and stair climbing.

The most important objective in tibial nerve repair is restoration of plantar sensation, because an anesthetized sole inevitably develops chronic ulceration and eventually requires amputation. Partial return of sensory and motor function can be expected in most patients undergoing tibial nerve repair. The best results are obtained with sharp lacerations in young patients undergoing early exploration. Sole hyperesthesia may be a problematic complication in many patients undergoing tibial nerve repair.

The *common peroneal nerve* is the most frequently injured peripheral nerve of the lower extremity because of its superficial position proximally at the fibular neck. Postoperative results are the poorest of all lower extremity peripheral nerves. The peroneal nerve is also subject to traction injuries, in which it is tethered between the sciatic notch and fibular neck, and such injuries carry the worst prognosis for return of function. The functional loss involves ankle dorsiflexion, foot eversion, and toe extension and produces footdrop and a tendency toward equinovarus deformity. The sensory deficit along the lateral margin of the foot (sural nerve) is not significant. Ankle dorsiflexion and a normal gait may be restored in children and in patients with sharp, distal lacerations undergoing early repair. Less encouraging results can be expected with increasing patient age and delay of nerve repair.

Patients with permanent footdrop caused by peroneal nerve injury can be managed by splinting or tendon transfer. Millesi[37] reported useful recovery in the majority of 23 patients undergoing tibialis posterior tendon transfer for footdrop. In general an ankle-foot orthosis is preferable to ankle fusion.

AMPUTATION

Despite aggressive treatment of open fractures and osseous infections of the lower extremity, some patients inevitably require amputation for unsalvageable situations. In determining an appropriate level for amputation, the surgeon must consider (1) the extent of debridement necessary to allow primary healing and (2) the optimal site for prosthetic fitting.

The ultimate goal is to provide the patient with the most expeditious pathway to bipedal ambulation using some form of prosthesis. This requires a stump that can tolerate total contact and partial end bearing, which is achievable from the forefoot to the supracondylar region. In general, the more distal the amputation, the greater is the likelihood of effective weight bearing and ambulation.

When retained, viable portions of the lower extremity are dysfunctional. A midfoot amputation in a patient with an insensate plantar surface will eventually lead to recurrent ulceration and more proximal amputation. Similarly, a below-knee amputation in a patient with a knee joint contracture will preclude effective use of a prosthesis.[39]

Toes may be amputated at essentially any level, with extension to ray amputation of associated metatarsals if indicated. Such amputations permit essentially normal walking in most patients. When possible, preservation of the great toe is preferable to transmetatarsal amputation of the entire forefoot, since the former generally requires no special orthotic shoe inserts. Transmetatarsal amputation requires a shoe filler but also permits walking without a prosthesis.

A variety of tarsal and intertarsal level amputations have been described. These include Lisfranc's (midfoot, or tarsometatarsal) and Chopart's (hindfoot, or intertarsal) disarticulations, which may be performed when soft tissue is insufficient for coverage of a short transmetatarsal amputation. Orthotic inserts may be adapted to any level of amputation. In some patients these amputations may be more functional than ankle disarticulation (Syme's amputation), but muscle imbalance may lead to equinovarus deformity. A more extensive shoe filler is required, and heel cord lengthening with tendon transfer may be required later to correct the equinovarus.[25]

Syme's amputation refers to tibiotalar disarticulation, and the goal is to retain the proprioceptive heel pad. The patient is able to walk without a prosthesis. Walking may be improved using a prosthesis, which coapts a shoe to the stump and diffuses end weight bearing, with lower energy consumption than for a below-knee amputation.[57] A bulbous stump can be avoided by removing the medial and lateral malleoli. Heel pad migration can be averted by anchoring the plantar aponeurosis to the distal tibia and fibula.

A modification of Syme's technique is *Pirogoff's calcaneotibial arthrodesis,* which may better maintain heel pad position and provide a more aesthetic stump.

All ankle-level amputations are functionally superior to those performed at a more proximal level.[25]

Preservation of a functional knee joint is invaluable in lower extremity rehabilitation. Every effort must be made to salvage an unreconstructable foot or lower leg at the below-knee level. Above-knee amputations result in much higher energy demands for ambulation, and above-knee prostheses are more difficult to use. The general recommendation is to retain as long a stump as feasible, providing as much strength, leverage, and proprioception as possible.

Below-knee amputations that progress to primary healing rarely require late revision. Stumps that measure more than 5 cm from the medial joint line may be effectively fitted with a prosthesis. Thus every effort must be made to salvage this length of tibia, including local muscle rotation flap coverage and even free tissue transfer.

OUTCOMES

MacKenzie et al[31] examined physical impairment and functional outcomes after severe lower extremity fracture in 444 patients; 85% were interviewed at 6 months, and 68% returned for a clinical assessment. Disability was measured using the sickness impact profile (SIP). The overall SIP score denoted a moderate level of dysfunction or disability. The most notable of the subscores was the return to work. Analysis showed that 48% of those working before injury had returned to work at 6 months. Limitations of this study were the

6-month period, the wide age range (18 to 64 years), and injury variables. For example, some patients had open wounds, and some had more than one fracture site. Further study will be enhanced by limiting the number of variables in the study groups.

Dillingham et al[14] studied the incidence, length of stay, and rehabilitation of traumatic amputee patients. Their Maryland hospital database suggests a decline in incidence of amputation from 1979 to 1993. The authors reported a low rate of transfer to inpatient rehabilitation service. This epidemiologic study demonstrated increasingly shorter acute care hospital stays and low rates of discharge to inpatient rehabilitation. These findings highlight the need to determine their impact on the long-term outcomes of amputee patients.

MacKenzie et al[30] developed the functional capacity index, which is the first step toward a measure of expected functional outcome. This promises to become a valuable tool for the evaluation of outcomes across a wide range of injury types.

REFERENCES

1. Aldea P, Shaw W: Lower extremity nerve injuries, *Clin Plast Surg* 13:691-699, 1986.
2. Arnold P, Prunes-Carillo F: Vastus medialis muscle flap for functional closure of the exposed knee joint, *Plast Reconstr Surg* 68:69-72, 1981.
3. Banis J, Richardson D, Derr J, Acland R: Microsurgical adjuncts in salvage of the ischemic and diabetic lower extremity, *Clin Plast Surg* 19:881-893, 1992.
4. Blick S, Brumback R, Lakatos R, et al: Early prophylactic bone grafting of high energy tibial fractures, *Clin Orthop* 240:21-41, 1989.
5. Blick S, Brumback R, Poka A, et al: Compartment syndrome in open tibial fractures, *J Bone Joint Surg* 68A:1349-1353, 1986.
6. Brent B, Upton J, Acland R, et al: Experience with the temporoparietal free flap, *Plast Reconstr Surg* 76:177-188, 1985.
7. Briggs S, Banis J, Kaebnic H: Distal revascularization and microsurgical free tissue transfer: an alternative to amputation in ischemic lesions of the lower extremity, *J Vasc Surg* 2:806-811, 1985.
8. Byrd H, Cierny G, Tebbetts J: The management of open tibial fractures with associated soft tissue loss: external pin fixation with early flap coverage, *Plast Reconstr Surg* 68:73-79, 1981.
9. Byrd H, Spicer T, Cierney GI: Management of open tibia fractures, *Plast Reconstr Surg* 76:719-728, 1985.
10. Chang N, Mathes S: Comparison of the effect of bacterial inoculation in musculocutaneous and random pattern flaps, *Plast Reconstr Surg* 70:1-10, 1982.
11. Christian E, Bosse M, Robb G: Reconstruction of large diaphyseal defects, without free fibular transfer, in grade IIIb tibial fractures, *J Bone Joint Surg* 71A:994-1003, 1989.
12. Colen L: Limb salvage in the patient with severe peripheral vascular disease: the role of microsurgical free tissue transfer, *Plast Reconstr Surg* 79:389-395, 1987.
13. Dagher F, Roukoz S: Compound tibial fractures with bone loss treated by the Ilizarov technique, *J Bone Joint Surg* 73B:316-321, 1991.

14. Dillingham TR, Pezzin LE, MacKenzie EJ: Incidence, acute care length of stay, and discharge to rehabilitation of traumatic amputee patients: an epidemiologic study, *Arch Phys Med Rehabil* 79:279-287, 1998.

15. Dowden R, McCraw J: The vastus lateralis muscle flap: technique and applications, *Ann Plast Surg* 4:396-404, 1980.

16. Ger R, Efron G: New operative approach in the treatment of chronic osteomyelitis of the tibial diaphysis: a preliminary report, *Clin Orthop* 70:165-169, 1970.

17. Gottleib M, Chandrasekhar B, Terz J, Sherman R: Clinical applications of the extended deep inferior epigastric flap, *Plast Reconstr Surg* 78:782-787, 1986.

18. Grabb W, Argenta L: The lateral calcaneal artery skin flap (the lateral calcaneal artery, lesser saphenous vein, and sural nerve skin flap), *Plast Reconstr Surg* 68:723-730, 1981.

19. Griffiths G, Wieman T: Metatarsal head resection for diabetic foot ulcers, *Arch Surg* 125:832-835, 1990.

20. Gustilo R: Bone grafting in open fractures, *J Orthop Trauma* 2:54-55, 1988.

21. Gustilo R, Anderson J: Prevention of infection in the treatment of one thousand and twenty-five open fractures of long bones, *J Bone Joint Surg* 58A:453-458, 1976.

22. Hallock G: Complications of 100 consecutive fasciocutaneous flaps, *Plast Reconstr Surg* 88:264-268, 1991.

23. Hidalgo D, Shaw W: Reconstruction of foot injuries, *Clin Plast Surg* 13:663-680, 1986.

24. Ilizarov G: Pseudoarthroses and defects of long tubular bones. In Ilizarov G, editor: *Transosseous osteosynthesis,* New York, 1992, Springer-Verlag.

25. Keblish P: Amputation alternatives in the lower limb, stressing combined management of the traumatized extremity, *Clin Plast Surg* 13:595-618, 1986.

26. Lai C, Lin S, Chou C, et al: Limb salvage of infected diabetic foot ulcers with microsurgical free muscle transfer, *Ann Plast Surg* 26:212-220, 1991.

27. LaMont J: Functional anatomy of the lower limb, *Clin Plast Surg* 13:571-579, 1986.

28. Landi A, Soragni O, Monteleone M: The extensor digitorum brevis muscle island flap for soft-tissue loss around the ankle, *Plast Reconstr Surg* 75:892-897, 1985.

29. Leitner D, Gordon L, Buncke H: The extensor digitorum brevis as a muscle island flap, *Plast Reconstr Surg* 76:777-780, 1985.

30. MacKenzie EJ, Damiano A, Miller T, Luchter S: The development of the functional capacity index, *J Trauma* 41:799-807, 1998.

31. MacKenzie EJ, Cushing BM, Jurkowvich, et al: Physical impairment and functional outcomes six months after severe lower extremity fractures, *J Trauma* 34:528-539, 1993.

32. May JJ, Halls M, Simon S: Free microvascular muscle flap with skin graft reconstruction of extensive defects of the foot: a clinical and gait analysis study, *Plast Reconstr Surg* 75:627-639, 1985.

33. May JW Jr, Rohrich R: Foot reconstruction using free microvascular muscle flaps with skin grafts, *Clin Plast Surg* 13:681-689, 1986.

34. May JW Jr, Gallico GG, Jupiter JB, Savage R: Free latissimus dorsi muscle flap with skin graft for treatment of traumatic chronic bony wounds, *Plast Reconstr Surg* 73:641-649, 1984.

35. May JW Jr, Jupiter J, Gallico GG, et al: Treatment of chronic traumatic bone wounds—microvascular free tissue transfer: a thirteen-year experience in 96 patients, *Ann Surg* 214:241-250, 1991.

36. McNutt R, Seabrook G, Schmitt D, et al: Blunt tibial artery trauma: predicting the irretrievable extremity, *J Trauma* 29:1624-1627, 1989.

37. Millesi H: Nerve grafts: indications, techniques, and prognosis. In Omer G, Spinner M, editors: *Management of peripheral nerve problems,* Philadelphia, 1980, Saunders.

38. Moore J, Weiland A: Free vascularized bone and muscle flaps for osteomyelitis, *Orthopedics* 9:819-824, 1986.

39. Moore W: General principles of amputation level selection. In Moore W, Malone J, editors: *Lower extremity amputation,* Philadelphia, 1989, Saunders.

40. Morrison W, Crabb D, O'Brian B: The instep of the foot as a fasciocutaneous island and a free flap for heel defects, *Plast Reconstr Surg* 72:56-63, 1983.

41. Naggar L, Chevalley F, Blanc C, Livio J-J: Treatment of large bone defects with the Ilizarov technique, *J Trauma* 34:390-393, 1993.

42. Newman L, Waller J, Palestro C, et al: Unsuspected osteomyelitis in diabetic foot ulcers: diagnosis and monitoring by leukocyte scanning with indium 111 in oxyquinoline, *JAMA* 266:1246-1251, 1991.

43. Paley D, Catagni M, Argnani F, et al: Ilizarov treatment of tibial nonunions with bone loss, *Clin Orthop* 241:146-165, 1989.

44. Pappas C, Goldich G, Cundy K, Wong W: Skin flaps versus muscle flaps: coping with infection in the presence of a foreign body, *Plast Surg Forum* 3:133-135, 1980.

45. Patzakis M, Dorr L, Ivler D, et al: The early management of open joint injuries, *J Bone Joint Surg* 57A:1065-1071, 1975.

46. Rhinelander F: Tibial blood supply in relation to fracture healing, *Clin Orthop* 105:34-81, 1974.

47. Rieffel R, McCarthy J: Coverage of heel and sole defects: a new subfascial arterialized flap, *Plast Reconstr Surg* 66:250-260, 1980.

48. Shanahan R, Gingras R: Medial plantar sensory flap for coverage of heel defects, *Plast Reconstr Surg* 64:295-298, 1979.

49. Shaw W, Hidalgo D: Anatomic basis of plantar flap design, *Plast Reconstr Surg* 78:627-636, 1986.

50. Shaw W, Hidalgo D: Anatomic basis of plantar flap design: clinical applications, *Plast Reconstr Surg* 78:637-649, 1986.

51. Sinacore D, Mueller M, Diamond J, et al: Diabetic plantar ulcers treated by total contact casting, *Phys Ther* 67:1543-1549, 1987.

52. Taylor G: The current status of free vascularized bone grafts, *Clin Plast Surg* 10:185-209, 1983.

53. Taylor G, Corlett R, Boyd J: The extended deep inferior epigastric flap: a clinical technique, *Plast Reconstr Surg* 72:751-765, 1983.

54. Tobin G: Hemisoleus and reversed hemisoleus flaps, *Plast Reconstr Surg* 76:87-96, 1985.

55. Tobin G: Vastus medialis myocutaneous and myocutaneous-tendinous composite flaps, *Plast Reconstr Surg* 75:677-684, 1985.

56. Townsend P: An inferiorly based soleus muscle flap, *Br J Plast Surg* 31:210-213, 1978.

57. Waters R, Perry J, Antonelli D, Hislop H: Energy cost of walking amputees: the influence of level of amputation, *J Bone Joint Surg* 58A:42-46, 1976.

58. Weiland A, Moore J, Daniel R: The efficacy of free tissue transfer in the treatment of osteomyelitis, *J Bone Joint Surg* 66A:181-193, 1984.

59. Wellisz T, Sherman R, Nichter L, et al: The extended deep inferior epigastric flap for lower extremity reconstruction, *Ann Plast Surg* 30:405-410, 1993.

60. Yanai A, Park S, Iwao T, Nakamura N: Reconstruction of a skin defect of the posterior heel by a lateral calcaneal flap, *Plast Reconstr Surg* 75:642-646, 1985.

61. Youdas J, Wood M, Cahalan T, Chao E: A quantitative analysis of donor site morbidity after vascularized fibula transfer, *J Orthop Res* 6:621-629, 1988.

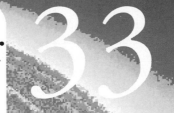
Diabetes and Lower Extremity Reconstruction

Lawrence B. Colen

INDICATIONS

It has been estimated that 1.5 million Americans, 15% of all diabetic patients, have foot wounds during their lifetime. In addition, 20% of all diabetic patients admitted to hospitals are admitted for foot problems.[1]

Of the many complications affecting patients with diabetes mellitus, none is more devastating, both psychologically and economically, than gangrene of the extremity and its attendant risk of major limb amputation. Diabetic patients account for approximately 50% of all lower extremity amputations for nontraumatic indications. More than 56,000 major amputations due to diabetes were reported in 1987 in the United States.[2] Patients who have undergone such an amputation have a 50% incidence of contralateral limb disease and a 30% to 40% incidence of contralateral amputation within 2 to 3 years of the primary procedure.[3]

The cost of managing "the diabetic foot" in the United States is enormous. An estimated 5% to 6% of the U.S. population is diabetic, and the annual cost of their health care exceeds $20 billion, of which more than $1.5 billion is directly related to the amputations that result from foot infections.[4] The actual health care dollars spent may be insignificant compared with the lost productivity of these patients and the psychologic impact of their limb loss. In one study, 77% of patients undergoing major lower extremity amputations were candidates for a prosthesis, and only 90% of below-knee amputees with prostheses could be successfully rehabilitated.[5]

The pathophysiology of diabetic foot ulceration is multifactorial. The interaction of diffuse sensorimotor neuropathy, abnormalities in capillary blood flow secondary to hemorheologic disturbances, diabetic patients' increased propensity for infection, and infrapopliteal arterial occlusive disease in the lower extremity best describes the pathogenesis. The "mal perforans" is the usual mode of patient presentation, although cellulitis, with or without plantar abscess formation, may occur in a significant number. Osteomyelitis, Charcot deformities, Achilles tendon contractures, and the sequelae of generalized atherosclerosis may further complicate the management of these patients.

The trend in management of the diabetic patient with foot disease has shifted during the past two decades from primary below-knee amputation to limb-salvage techniques using a multispecialty approach. Although indications for primary amputation exist (e.g., systemic sepsis, major tissue loss, significant comorbid factors, poor patient compliance, nonreconstructible peripheral vascular disease), the goal in the management of these patients is to preserve limb length and thus bipedal ambulation. The reasons for this are relatively straightforward.

Many of these patients experience disabling increases in energy expenditure of ambulation with a below-knee or above-knee amputation. Individuals with concurrent heart disease or prior stroke may never be able to ambulate with a prosthesis. The oxygen consumption of an amputee walking with an above-knee prosthesis is 2.3 times that of an age- and disease-matched control patient.[6] Above-knee prosthesis walking requires 63% of maximum aerobic capacity at 45% of the control patient's gait velocity. This data is derived from the more favorable 30% to 66% of amputees who are successfully rehabilitated to prosthesis walking (30% for above-knee and 66% for below-knee levels). Even patients with hindfoot amputations such as the Syme's require 33% more oxygen consumption per unit distance at two-thirds the control patient's velocity.

Patients who do not successfully ambulate with a prosthesis fall into one of several categories. They either fail rehabilitative efforts or are unable to be fitted with a prosthesis because of dementia, stroke, or debilitation. Crutch walking without a prosthesis demands even more energy expenditure and usually results in tachycardia and a wheelchair-dependent patient. The incidence of contralateral foot disease increases rapidly after limb amputation.[3,7] Ambulation with bilateral prostheses is even less likely than with a unilateral prosthesis; only 30% of those with mixed amputations achieve satisfactory rehabilitation.[6]

During the past 15 years, new information on the etiology of diabetic foot disease and major advances in plastic, vascular, orthopedic, and podiatric surgical specialties have set the stage for improved limb salvage in this difficult group of patients. Foot revascularization using autogenous venous conduits has become commonplace. With successful revascularization, surgeons can perform soft tissue repair, tendon transfers, and bony fusions when indicated.

The hypothesis that aggressively closing diabetic foot wounds decreases the incidence of life-threatening or limb-threatening infections seems well founded. Patients with chronic ulceration are treated with broad-spectrum antibiotics until wound cultures are finalized. Surgical debridement, drainage of localized infections, and local wound care with topical antibacterials may be followed with appropriate wound closure procedures. Strict attention to diabetes control and nutritional support is mandatory.

During the same hospitalization, appropriate management of relevant peripheral vascular, orthopedic, and podiatric problems is undertaken. This approach has resulted in major lower limb amputation rates of less than 3% during the past 15 years. Frequent multidisciplinary follow-up must be strict to maintain these results. This includes massive efforts at patient education and a dedicated "diabetic foot team." Patients must inspect their feet daily and minimize callosities with the use of pumice stones and routine podiatric care. Custom-molded orthotic devices may be necessary after the loss of the transverse and longitudinal arches of the foot from either Charcot changes or reconstructive surgery.

PATHOPHYSIOLOGY

The etiology of foot ulceration in the diabetic patient is quite complex. Evolving knowledge about the pathophysiology of diabetes mellitus continues to define the processes that interact and ultimately lead to foot wounds. The interplay among diffuse peripheral neuropathy, peripheral vascular disease, hemorheologic abnormalities, immune system impairment, and the effects of advanced glycosylation end products on the Achilles tendon (biomechanics) must be understood and properly managed to treat these patients successfully.

Neuropathy

Peripheral neuropathy involving motor, sensory, and autonomic pathways is the fundamental abnormality that sets the stage for plantar ulceration in the diabetic patient. Although the understanding of diabetic peripheral neuropathy has advanced significantly during the past two decades, a reliable "cure" is not yet available.[8] No single "form" of diabetic neuropathy may exist, and the complex etiology may differ from patient to patient. Autoimmune and microvascular mechanisms have recently been implicated for the segmental demyelination that is found on nerve biopsy. Endoneural edema and slow axoplasmic flow significantly contribute to the nerve dysfunction that has been termed *diabetic peripheral neuropathy.*

The incidence of carpal tunnel syndrome in diabetic patients is greater than that seen in nondiabetic controls. Considerable evidence has been accumulated to suggest that peripheral nerve compression, in concert with the underlying metabolic dysfunction, may be responsible for neuropathic symptoms in some patients. The "double-crush hypothesis"

implies that each insult to a nerve is additive and that the nerve abnormalities and symptoms are a result of this.[9]

As previously stated, diabetic nerves are characterized by endoneural edema. Peripheral nerve compression secondary to a bony foramen, a muscular band, or a bony or ligamentous tunnel (i.e., tarsal, carpal, or cubital) may therefore occur more easily in these patients.[10,11] It therefore may be appropriate to select diabetic patients carefully for peripheral nerve releases to help restore nerve function.[12]

Nerve dysfunction in the diabetic patient involves motor, sensory, and autonomic pathways. Intrinsic muscle weakness within the foot leads to the loss of both the transverse and the longitudinal arches. The derangement in the normal toe flexor/extensor balance leads to pes cavus deformity, toe extensor subluxation, and plantar metatarsal head prominence. These Charcot changes have a direct effect on skin breakdown and ulcer formation. Infection soon follows because both pressure and denervation have been shown to contribute to increased bacterial localization and replication.[13,14]

The inability to perceive pain or pressure as a result of sensory abnormalities plays a major role in the chronic wounds on the diabetic foot's plantar surface. Autonomic dysfunction results in both anhidrosis and hyperkeratosis. Calluses develop over insensate pressure areas and further increase the forces that act on the plantar skin. Small hemorrhages and fissures develop, ultimately with the classic "mal perforans" ulcer.

Vascular Disease

For decades, surgeons were taught that ischemic ulcers could occur in the diabetic patient with normal pedal pulses. The theory was that microvascular disease and small-vessel endothelial proliferation were the primary reasons for ulceration in the diabetic foot.[15] The original work published by Goldenberg et al[16] 40 years ago propagated these misconceptions. Several better designed anatomic studies contradicted Goldenberg's work and elucidated the nature of the blood flow problems in the diabetic limb.[17,18] Both diabetic and nondiabetic patients were found to have similar degrees of intimal hyperplasia.

More recent functional studies have also helped to clarify these issues. Arteriolar reactivity and arteriolar resistance measurements performed during arterial bypass grafting were no different in diabetic and nondiabetic patients.[19] Transcutaneous oxygen measurements performed on the foot also did not differ in diabetic and nondiabetic patients with peripheral arterial disease.[20] In fact, later studies have shown that diabetic patients with neuropathy have increased transcutaneous oxygen measurements adjacent to their foot ulcers compared with nondiabetic patients or diabetic patients without neuropathy.[21]

Peripheral vascular disease may play a role in the persistence of ulceration in the diabetic foot in some patients but is clearly not the primary etiologic concern. Thickened capillary basement membranes and abnormal functioning of these structures have been confirmed in diabetic muscle but not in skin.[22] The incidence of peripheral vascular disease is no greater in the diabetic than the nondiabetic patient, although its onset may be earlier in diabetic patients and may favor the infrapopliteal vessels over the iliofemoral system.[23] Many diabetic patients have disease within the tibioperoneal trunk, with the pedal circulation unaffected. This "pedal sparing" is an important concept and is responsible for the excellent results with bypass graft surgery of the ankle or foot dorsum.[24] Adequate arterial inflow allows successful wound closure in these patients.

Hemorheology

Although our concepts of "small-vessel disease" in diabetic patients have been radically altered, how do we explain that nutritive blood flow is *not* normal in many of these individuals? Diabetic patients exhibit alterations in blood flow secondary to elevations in blood viscosity and abnormalities in erythrocyte deformability.[25] Of the many factors responsible for elevated blood viscosity, platelet aggregation, erythrocyte aggregation, and increased fibrinogen levels are well documented in diabetic patients and account for most changes. Altered viscosity is further exacerbated by the serum protein shifts that result from the increased capillary permeability.[26] A pattern of increasing blood viscosity can develop. As increases in viscosity occur, blood flow slows, predisposing to further development of platelet aggregates and rouleaux forms. Since insulin quickly reverses some of these viscosity changes, not all of them result from the nonenzymatic glycosylation of the erythrocyte or platelet cell membrane.[27]

Reduced erythrocyte deformability has been shown to occur even in juvenile-onset diabetes, in contrast to the plasma protein abnormalities seen in the adult. The inability of the red blood cell (RBC) to deform in a "parachute-like" manner impairs its ability to enter the smallest of capillary beds, thus significantly impacting the perfusion within microcirculatory beds. RBC deformability has been shown to depend directly on adenosine triphosphate (ATP) metabolism.[28] With increases in intracellular ATP, the rigid cell membranes become more pliable, resulting in improved perfusion within capillaries.[29] Pentoxyfylline is a methylxanthine derivative that increases intraerythrocyte ATP levels and thus offers a clinically promising therapy for diabetic patients with lower extremity wound healing problems.[30-33]

The energy required to disrupt circulating RBC aggregates and to deform rigid erythrocytes has the indirect effect of altering local vessel pressures and shear forces. This leads to greater serum albumin leakage, the development of advanced glycosylation end products, and subsequent stiffening of the capillary walls. Erythrocyte membrane changes result in elevated large-vessel resistance to flow and atherosclerosis.[34]

In addition to pentoxyfylline, other therapeutic interventions include the intake of fish oils (omega-3 fatty acids), aspirin ingestion, smoking cessation, and tight glucose control. Fish oils contain eicosapentanoic acid and have been shown to act as competitive substrates for cyclooxygenase in prostaglandin biochemistry. The result is a decrease in the vasoconstrictive and proaggregatory effects of thromboxane and less endothelial proliferation.[35,36]

Immunology

Both cell-mediated and humoral-mediated types of immune system dysfunction are seen in the diabetic patient. The trivial fissure that occurs on the plantar surface of the diabetic foot provides an entry port for bacteria. The functional deformities of polymorphonuclear neutrophil leukocytes (PMNs) in these patients facilitate the resultant foot infections. In the diabetic patient these cells have been shown to have decreased adherence to the blood vessel wall, decreased chemotaxis, decreased phagocytosis, decreased diapedesis, and abnormal bactericidal activity.[37,38]

No consensus seems to exist in the literature regarding the etiology of this problem. Some studies show that these deficiencies may be reversed by normalizing serum glucose levels or overcoming ketoacidosis, whereas others show the effects to be independent of glucose regulation.[39,40] Whereas the ingestion of opsonized particles complexed with lipopolysaccharide is similar in normal patients and normoglycemic diabetic patients, diabetic PMNs show slow migration that is unaffected by blood glucose levels.[41] Some evidence indicates that the defect may be a function of serum abnormalities rather than a primary defect of the PMN.[42] In addition, staphylococcal killing is reduced in diabetic PMNs, independent of blood glucose levels.[43]

Abnormalities of the lymphocyte and of cell-mediated immunity have been described as well. Impairments in blast transformation, skin test reactions, granuloma formation, and intracellular killing have been quite reproducible.[44] T-cell response is delayed and monocyte phagocytosis hampered. This may partly explain the susceptibility of diabetic patients to fungal infections.[45]

The loss of metabolic control in the diabetic patient may influence the development of sepsis in a separate manner. High serum glucose levels favor the growth of gram-positive organisms and actually inhibit growth of gram-negative organisms in vitro.[46] Clinically, a retrospective study of 214 patients with septicemia showed that 81% of those with serum glucose levels less than 110 mg/dl had cultures that grew gram-negative organisms, whereas 82% of patients with serum glucose levels greater than 130 mg/dl had cultures with gram-positive organisms.[47]

Biomechanics

About 35% of diabetic patients develop significant peripheral neuropathy, many of whom have abnormalities of gait. The most severe manifestation of this neuropathic condition is the Charcot foot. The most widely accepted explanation for these degenerative changes is neurotraumatic; that is, joint collapse results from accumulated damage caused by insensitivity to pain, although small-fiber functions may be preserved.[48]

CHARCOT FOOT. The destructive changes that occur in the Charcot foot cause a collapse of the medial longitudinal arch, which alters the biomechanics of gait. The normal calcaneal pitch is distorted, which in turn causes severe strains to the ligaments that bind the metatarsal, cuneiform, navicular, and other small bones that form the foot's long arch.[49] These degenerative changes further alter the gait, resulting in abnormal weight-bearing stress and foot collapse. Unfortunately, ulceration, infection, gangrene, and limb loss are frequent outcomes if the process is not arrested in its early stages.

ACHILLES TENDON. The Achilles tendon is the most important tendon affecting foot function. In patients with diabetic neuropathy, an extremely tight Achilles tendon combined with sensory deprivation contributes to abnormal gait patterns that eventually result in soft tissue ulceration and Charcot joint collapse. Diabetic patients with midfoot and forefoot ulcerations typically have concomitant equinus deformity related to shortening of the Achilles tendon complex.[50] This restriction in ankle motion in the diabetic has the following two consequences:

1. At first, excessive pressures are borne by the plantar forefoot structures during all phases of gait.
2. Over time, loss of dorsiflexion at the ankle because of Achilles tendon shortening is compensated for by increased mobility in Lisfranc's joint, a normally nonmobile region of the foot. This "unweights" the forefoot during gait, but the midfoot begins to bear the excessive forces.

As such, Achilles tendon contracture must be considered as one of the etiologic factors in the formation of the Charcot foot as well as the "mal perforans" ulcers seen in the forefoot and midfoot. Abnormalities within the Achilles tendons of diabetic subjects have been well documented and may be related to excessive collagen cross-linking due to nonenzymatic glycosylation.[50] The results of these studies provide a scientific justification for treatment of the diabetic foot by Achilles tendon lengthening instead of casting, shoes with extra depth, and other methods that have limited success.[51]

OPERATIONS

The therapeutic approach to the management of foot disease associated with diabetes and vascular disease involves three major components: (1) a thorough preoperative evaluation and

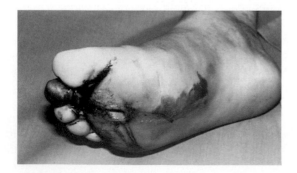

Figure 33-1. Foot with plantar abscess originating from a second metatarsal head ulcer.

preparation, (2) a well-executed surgical and medical program, and (3) a closely supervised postoperative routine. Before surgery, testing should be directed toward the complete diagnosis of the problem while optimizing the patient's medical status. This often includes tests that assess neurologic function, bony abnormalities, gait disturbances, and peripheral vascular status, as well as provide information about the contralateral extremity.

If the patient has an acute infection, basic surgical principles should be followed. Bedrest, elevation of the extremity, and broad-spectrum antibiotic coverage may need to be supplemented with serial surgical debridement. Plantar space abscess may be a subtle finding in some patients and a limb- or life-threatening concern, so prompt diagnosis and treatment are mandatory (Figure 33-1). Aspiration of the plantar space with a 19-gauge needle is often helpful. If necessary, magnetic resonance imaging (MRI) can diagnose necrotizing infections quite well. The liberal use of topical antimicrobials and subcutaneous heparin help to eradicate infection while providing prophylaxis against deep venous thrombosis. The role of hyperbaric oxygen (HBO) remains controversial, although most would consider adjuvant HBO therapy in the treatment of anaerobic infections.[52]

PREOPERATIVE EVALUATION

Once acute infection has been properly managed, the assessment of diabetic patients with lower extremity disease should focus on five distinct areas: (1) systemic disease, (2) radiologic abnormalities, (3) peripheral vascular status, (4) neurologic status, and (5) gait disturbances.

Systemic Evaluation
Many of these patients have concomitant coronary, cerebrovascular, pulmonary, and renal disease. Nephropathy is often accompanied by proteinuria, which contributes to low serum albumin levels and thus promotes poor wound healing. Every effort should be made to optimize the patient's status systemically before beginning a surgical reconstruction. The preoperative involvement of endocrinology, cardiology, nephrology, pulmonary medicine, and anesthesia is often required to attain these goals. Thallium stress testing is necessary to help determine cardiac risk in some patients.[53] Perioperative cardiac monitoring should be considered as well.

Poor glucose control, characterized by high serum hemoglobin A_{1c} levels, must be corrected to improve the associated hemorheologic and immunologic abnormalities. This may be rapidly accomplished by the careful administration of continuous intravenous (IV) insulin and supplemental crystalloid. Endocrine consultation is necessary for most patients because concurrent infection will increase insulin requirements.

Radiologic Analysis
Plain bone radiographs should be obtained before any surgical intervention on the foot is planned. Bone spurs, bony promi-

nences, malunion, nonunion, Charcot deformities, and other abnormalities may be readily identified. The information obtained is extremely useful in the formulation of the operative plan, since almost all wound closures on the diabetic foot are accompanied by an osseous procedure. High-resolution, three-dimensional imaging techniques may provide additional information on abnormal bony anatomy that should be corrected with an osteotomy, ostectomy, or arthrodesis (Figure 33-2).

In the diabetic patient the diagnosis of osteomyelitis can usually be made with plain roentgenograms, although most patients will have additional studies. Osteomyelitis occurs from the direct extension of the pressure ulcer through the soft tissues and into the bone, which shows cortical irregularities on plain films. After plain-film evaluation, most patients have nuclear scans, which are misleading and unnecessary. These studies are often "positive" at the level of the ankle, midfoot, and forefoot in patients with diabetes mellitus who have *no* associated foot ulceration. The neuroarthropathy in these patients usually results in false-positive scans.

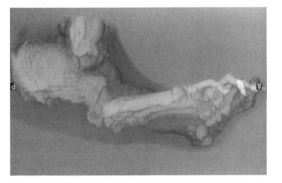

Figure 33-2. 3-D CT scan of the foot assists the surgeon in understanding the exact nature of the bony abnormalities that can lead to plantar ulceration.

My group is currently evaluating the use of Ceretec scans (technetium-labeled white blood cell studies). We believe, however, that MRI is the current study of choice unless prior surgical intervention with placement of hardware prohibits its use. Reports have documented that MRI has a much higher sensitivity and specificity than any other radiologic assessment for the detection of bone infections.[54]

Regardless of the radiologic method used to diagnose osteomyelitis, a bone biopsy is mandatory before the decision is made to use long-term IV antibiotic therapy. Even MRI has false-positive results (Figure 33-3). The study shows the presence of edema within the marrow space quite well. This finding is correlated with infection but is not always accompanied by it. MRI does help us decide which patients to biopsy. A patient with a positive study will undergo bone biopsy, whereas a patient that has a negative study will usually be spared the procedure.

The biopsy may be accomplished through a separate approach (e.g., dorsally with a plantar ulcer) or, more often, directly through the wound at the time of reconstruction. If performed through the wound bed, the surgeon should disregard culture data and assess only the histologic data because the wound will often contaminate the specimen. Medullary tissue should be harvested with a previously unused curette and submitted to the laboratory for processing.

If the diagnosis of osteomyelitis is made on biopsy and the procedure included removal of the entire involved bone (phalanx, metatarsal, tarsal), perioperative antibiotics are sufficient. If parts of the involved bone are left in situ, as with metatarsal head resection, the physician should consider a 6-week antibiotic regimen to treat the portions of bone remaining.

Vascular Evaluation

Improved understanding of the prevalence and nature of the vascular disease in diabetic patients has led to a more aggressive

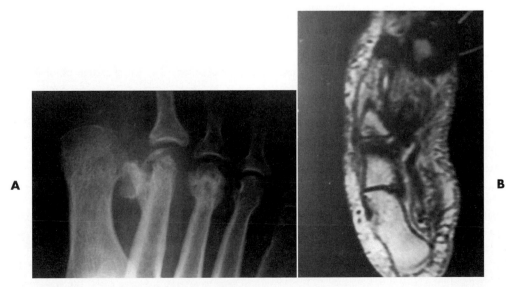

Figure 33-3. **A,** X-ray of forefoot with changes in the second and third metatarsal heads consistent with osteomyelitis. **B,** MRI shows changes in the same location that are consistent with osteomyelitis *(upper right).* Bone biopsy was negative.

approach to limb salvage. The presence of chronic foot ulceration in patients with palpable pedal pulses was thought to be secondary to the widespread occlusion of smaller vessels in the foot. Over the past three decades, many studies have dispelled this myth.[22,55,56] The role of peripheral vascular disease in the etiology of diabetic foot ulceration should not be minimized but rather put into proper perspective.

The vast majority of diabetic foot wounds are neuropathic in origin, with peripheral vascular components acting to exacerbate these lesions. Diabetic patients tend to develop peripheral vascular disease at younger ages than their nondiabetic counterparts. In addition, the vessels below the inguinal ligament tend to be involved more than those of the aortoiliac system. The success or failure of soft tissue repair in the diabetic foot is directly related to the blood supply of the lower extremity. Vascular evaluation is therefore essential.[57,58]

Vascular studies begin with a careful physical examination for atrophic skin changes associated with the chronic ischemia and indurated skin discoloration that accompany longstanding venous insufficiency. Palpation of pedal pulses offers a "qualitative" assessment of blood flow, but a more "quantitative" assessment may be obtained by measuring ankle-brachial indices and Doppler waveforms.[57,58] Ankle-brachial indices exceeding 0.7 are believed to be acceptable for soft tissue reconstruction without procedures directed toward improving the blood flow. These ratios are often falsely elevated in diabetic patients, however, and may give a misleading picture of the circulation. Toe pressures greater than 30 to 50 mm Hg are more indicative of healing, and their measurement should be a routine part of the vascular laboratory investigation of these patients.

Occasionally, additional tests of skin perfusion may be required before proceeding with soft tissue repair. Some patients improve only marginally with vascular bypass surgery, whereas others may not be considered good candidates for bypass procedures because of poor vascular "runoff" anatomy. In these patients, I obtain transcutaneous oxygen determinations as a measure of skin blood flow. In studies performed on patients with foot ulceration, nearly all wounds healed spontaneously with transcutaneous oxygen tensions of at least 25 mm Hg.

Directional Doppler flow studies are extremely important in planning the reconstructive procedures necessary to effect prompt wound closure. This is particularly true when the ankle-brachial indices are falsely elevated. The normal Doppler waveform is triphasic, with two forward-flow components and one reverse-flow component. As stenoses or occlusions occur, the waveforms deteriorate to biphasic, monophasic, and aphasic patterns (Figure 33-4).

Every effort should be made to improve blood flow in the affected extremity before scheduling foot reconstruction, especially when microvascular procedures are necessary to obtain limb salvage. Our recent studies indicate that patients with triphasic, biphasic, and even "good" monophasic flow can have a successful microvascular flap transfer without the need for "preoperative" vascular intervention. Controversy surrounds patients with monophasic patterns of flow. Provided the upstroke of the analog trace is brisk and the width of the

complex is narrow, successful free flap transfer is possible. On review of our patients who have undergone combined distal bypass surgery and free tissue transfer, we have found that the bypass procedure, at best, restored "good" monophasic blood flow to the extremity rather than biphasic or triphasic patterns.

If free tissue transfer is the only procedure that will adequately close the foot wound, Duplex scanning of the extremity is required. This study combines real-time B-mode ultrasound imaging with pulsed Doppler recordings and can be used to delineate both the arterial and the venous anatomy of the extremity. Within the arterial tree, the study can identify areas of adequate arterial diameter and areas of localized atherosclerosis. Venous valve competency and vein patency and size can be similarly evaluated. This permits preoperative selection of possible targets for free tissue transfer. When regional fasciocutaneous flaps are available as donor tissue, a duplex scan is invaluable in the mapping of flaps based on the leg's perforating vessels.[59]

Angiography is still considered the gold standard for delineating the vascular anatomy of the lower extremity. Duplex ultrasonography, however, may offer more information than the angiogram when soft tissue reconstruction is being planned. All patients undergoing distal bypass procedures will have a standard angiogram ordered by their vascular surgeon. New digital subtraction techniques decrease the amount of contrast that is required to obtain a high-quality study. Isotonic dye should be used in this patient population, and careful attention to the patients' hydration status is important to prevent the procedure's renal complications. In special circumstances (e.g., patients with contrast allergy or declining renal function), magnetic resonance angiography (MRA) can offer extremely detailed information without the need for iodine contrast material.

Since the etiology of these patients' foot wounds is primarily neuropathic, vascular surgeons should use a more liberal approach. Vascular interventions (e.g., bypass procedures, transluminal angioplasties) should be performed regardless of their expected long-term patency rates. The goal should be to obtain

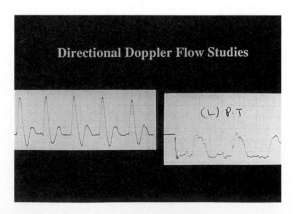

Figure 33-4. The normal Doppler waveform (*left*) is triphasic. Distal to arterial stenoses (*right*) the waveform is dampened. The amplitude is decreased and the waveform complex becomes widened and monophasic.

a healed wound and to correct the biomechanical abnormalities that led to the chronic ulceration. This may only require patency of the procedure for months rather than years.

Before performing any soft tissue repair, the plastic surgeon should completely evaluate the pedal circulation with a 9-MHz, hand-held Doppler device. The posterior tibial and dorsalis pedis arteries should be examined both with and without compression of the other vessel to help determine direction of blood flow. The dorsal and plantar circulations may be distinctly separate, without the usual communications between them. This will greatly affect the reconstructive plan.

Neurologic Evaluation

A careful clinical evaluation of the sensory and motor deficits in diabetic patients should be completed before any reconstructive procedure. When partial sensory loss is limited to the area of ulceration, the surgeon can develop a reconstructive plan that transfers sensate tissue at the time of soft tissue reconstruction (Figure 33-5).

Nerve conduction studies usually show evidence of a diffuse, symmetric polyneuropathy and are not always useful in planning the reconstruction. Such studies are appropriate, however, when a superimposed peripheral nerve compression is suspected. Nerve conduction may be decreased across areas of anatomic narrowing. These sites of compression should be addressed during the soft tissue procedure.

Patients with a clinically positive Tinel's sign are candidates for additional evaluation with nerve conduction studies. Percussion of the posterior tibial nerve in the region of the tarsal tunnel usually elicits Tinel's sign if considerable nerve compression has occurred in that area. The same applies to the peroneal nerve in the proximal calf (region of fibular head). The physician should be careful, however, because some

patients have a positive Tinel's sign all along the course of a specific nerve, from the infragluteal crease to the ankle. These patients usually have longstanding diabetes mellitus and significant sensorimotor disturbances, and nerve release does not seem to be beneficial. In properly selected patients, however, improved pedal sensibility after nerve decompression may help prevent recurrent ulceration and should therefore be given careful consideration.

Gait Analysis

Abnormalities of gait can be detected in most candidates for soft tissue repair. Midfoot and forefoot ulceration is often accompanied by shortening of the Achilles tendon, with increased weight-bearing pressures over these regions during ambulation. Patients with prior transmetatarsal amputations and recurrent forefoot ulceration are another group with biomechanical disturbances causing their wounds. These problems are usually related to equinus deformity and varus abnormalities. Soft tissue repair should be accompanied by Achilles tendon lengthening and tibialis anterior tendon transfer. Finally, patients with chronic heel ulceration often bear excessive weight on this area during gait. This may be a result of a prior, excessive Achilles tendon–lengthening procedure or a previously undetected Achilles tendon injury. Reconstruction should include some method of shortening and strengthening this important musculotendinous unit.

Preoperative evaluation of gait should include a measure of ankle dorsiflexion and computer gait analysis. When determining equinus deformity, the leg must be held in complete extension in an effort to keep the gastrocnemius muscles at their full resting length. Computer gait analysis uses probes that record pressures on the sole during all phases of gait. Areas of excessive compression during weight bearing can be displayed graphically and help plan the biomechanical components of the planned reconstruction (Figure 33-6). Changes that occur with tendon transfer or tendon-lengthening procedures may also be documented with this technique.

ANATOMY

Inherent in any reconstructive procedure is a sound understanding of the regional vascular anatomy. The cutaneous vascular territories of the foot communicate significantly with neighboring territories, but some generalizations may be made.

The dorsalis pedis artery and its branches supply the dorsum of the foot and ankle as well as the malleoli and the first web space (Figure 33-7).[60] Some communication, however, occurs with the medial plantar artery in the instep region. The peroneal artery contributes to the circulation around the lateral malleolus as well as the lateral ankle and hindfoot (Figure 33-8).[60]

On the sole, the calcaneal branches of the posterior tibial and peroneal arteries coalesce to supply the heel pad and overlying skin (Figure 33-9).[60] The medial plantar artery supplies the instep region, whereas perforators arising from the lateral plantar artery supply the more lateral portions of the plantar

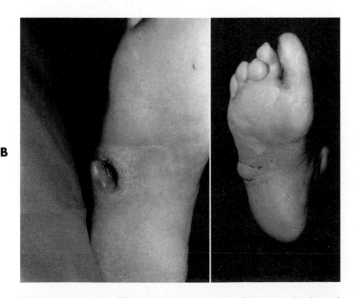

, B

Figure 33-5. A, This patient had sensory loss over the lateral plantar nerve distribution with resultant neurotrophic ulceration. **B,** A neurovascular island flap from the lateral side of the great toe (medial plantar nerve distribution) was used to close the wound and provide protective sensation.

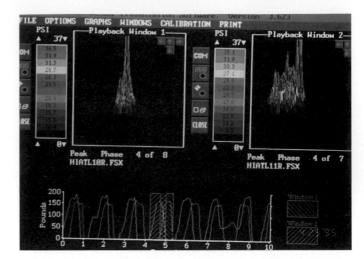

Figure 33-6. This computer gait analysis shows how the distribution of pressure on the plantar surface of the foot has moved from the instep *(left)* to the heel *(right)* during the same phase of gait after an Achilles' tendon lengthening procedure.

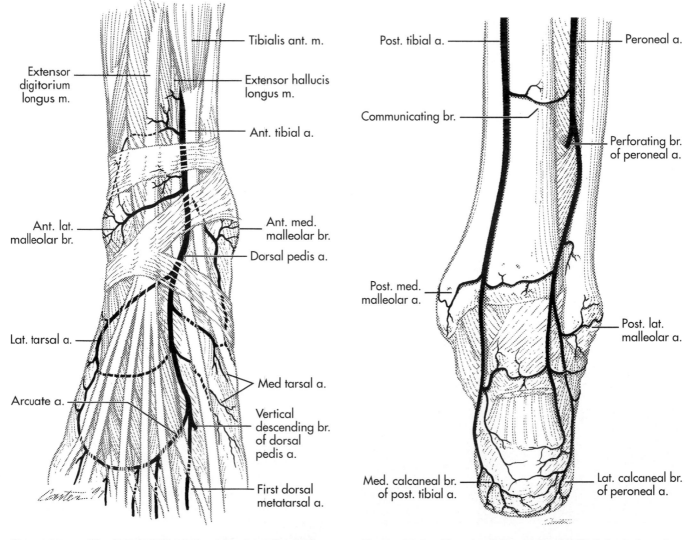

Figure 33-7. The dorsalis pedis artery and its branches perfuse the foot dorsum and communicate with the plantar circulation (posterior tibial artery and its branches) via the vertical descending branch of the dorsalis pedis artery. From Jurkiewicz MJ, Culbertson JH, editors: *Operative techniques in plastic and reconstructive surgery,* Philadelphia, 1997, WB Saunders.

Figure 33-8. The circulation to the hindfoot is via branches of the peroneal artery and the posterior tibial artery. From Jurkiewicz MJ, Culbertson JH, editors: *Operative techniques in plastic and reconstructive surgery,* Philadelphia, 1997, WB Saunders.

surface[61] (see Figure 33-9). In the forefoot the plantar common metatarsal and individual digital arteries provide the blood flow to the plantar skin and toes (Figure 33-10).[62] The dorsal and plantar circulations are closely associated in this region because of the communication through the vertical descending branch of the dorsalis pedis artery (Figure 33-11).[62]

In general the dorsal and instep circulation parallels that of the leg, with a network of vessels that course just superficial to the deep fascia.[61,63] The plantar surface is primarily composed of perforating vessels that course through and around the thick plantar fascia to arborize within the subcutaneous tissues.[61]

Details of the vascular anatomy as it applies to specific soft tissue reconstructive procedures are outlined later. The "normal" intercommunications between the peroneal artery, dorsalis pedis artery, and posterior tibial artery do not always exist in the diabetic patient. Thorough preoperative evaluation with the hand-held Doppler device, as described earlier, helps to ensure a safe reconstructive procedure.

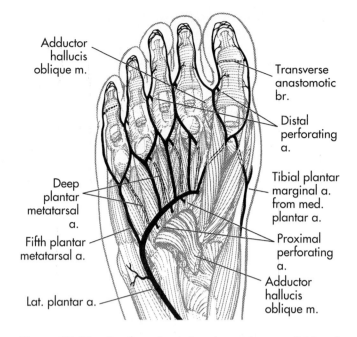

Figure 33-10. Forefoot circulation shows the superficial and deep plantar metatarsal arteries arising from the plantar arch (lateral plantar artery) that give rise to the digital vessels. From Jurkiewicz MJ, Culbertson JH, editors: *Operative techniques in plastic and reconstructive surgery,* Philadelphia, 1997, WB Saunders.

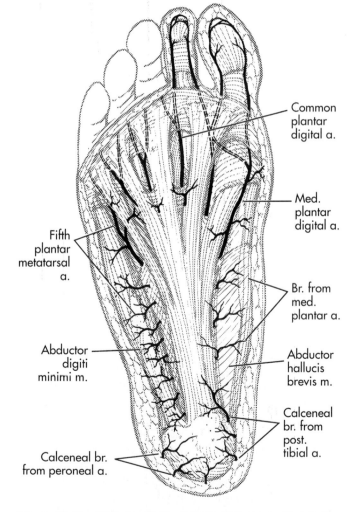

Figure 33-9. Perfusion to the plantar soft tissues is through the posterior tibial artery and its medial and lateral plantar branches. The heel pad derives its circulation from the medial calcaneal artery (from the posterior tibial artery) and the lateral calcaneal artery (from the peroneal artery). From Jurkiewicz MJ, Culbertson JH, editors: *Operative techniques in plastic and reconstructive surgery,* Philadelphia, 1997, WB Saunders.

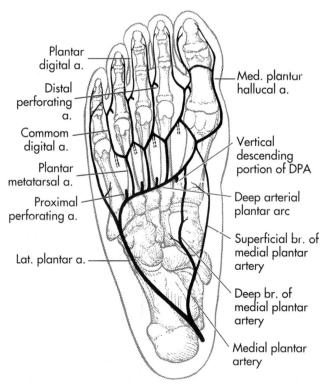

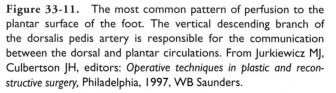

Figure 33-11. The most common pattern of perfusion to the plantar surface of the foot. The vertical descending branch of the dorsalis pedis artery is responsible for the communication between the dorsal and plantar circulations. From Jurkiewicz MJ, Culbertson JH, editors: *Operative techniques in plastic and reconstructive surgery,* Philadelphia, 1997, WB Saunders.

SURGICAL TECHNIQUES

The plantar skin is a unique weight-bearing structure in which the glabrous epidermis and underlying dermis are much thicker than in other areas of the body (up to 3.5 mm in depth). The vertically oriented fascial septa resist the shear forces of ambulation while enclosing the subcutaneous fat into discrete units that act as shock absorbers during ambulation. Skin on the dorsal surface and overlying the Achilles tendon is much thinner and more mobile. Reconstructive procedures for the plantar surface are often suboptimal for these other regions. In general, skin grafting techniques may be employed for shallow wounds on non-weight-bearing surfaces with a well-vascularized base. Split-thickness skin grafts (STSGs) placed on the plantar surface have a 50% incidence of breakdown, requiring further reconstructive procedures.

The surgical plan should provide stable wound closure using the simplest techniques available. The surgeon must consider the possibility of future ulceration; thus the "reconstructive ladder" concept applies here as it does with the neuropathic pressure sores seen in the paraplegic patient. As such, skin grafts, local flaps, limited amputations, midfoot amputations, regional flaps, and free tissue transfer procedures must be within the reconstructive surgeon's armamentarium. Limited toe or ray amputations or more extensive transmetatarsal or Lisfranc's procedures may provide the best functional result in many patients with forefoot wounds rather than complex microvascular reconstructions. Despite the increasing number and reliability of flaps, both pedicled and free, patient characteristics often influence the choice for wound closure.

Recently, use of vacuum assisted closure techniques has greatly simplified some wound closure procedures, especially in debilitated patients who might otherwise have been candidates for amputation. It has some inherent risks, however, since these patients must be monitored closely for intercurrent infection.

Most of the local flaps available for plantar foot reconstruction depend on antegrade blood flow within the posterior tibial artery and its medial and lateral plantar branches. The sural artery, lateral calcaneal artery, and lateral supramalleolar flaps are exceptions to this "rule" because their circulation is derived from the peroneal artery, the best preserved of the tibial vessels in the diabetic population.[23] These procedures are of limited use, however, distal to the heel region. Therefore patients with plantar foot wounds and accompanying peripheral vascular disease within the posterior tibial artery and its plantar branches are usually poor candidates for local flap reconstructions. This is especially true for patients who have had revascularization procedures using bypass grafts to either the distal anterior tibial–dorsalis pedis artery or the distal peroneal vessels. Flow in the plantar vessels is usually retrograde and unable to support this type of flap transfer. In such patients, wound closure may require free tissue transfer techniques with end-to-side arterial anastomoses performed either directly to the bypass graft or to the most suitable vessel, as outlined by preoperative noninvasive vascular studies (e.g., duplex scanning).

When wounds are large or local flaps are unavailable or unsafe, free tissue transfer techniques must be employed.

A recent review of lower extremity bypass combined with free flap reconstruction identified several groups of patients who would benefit from this aggressive approach (see later discussion).

The bony and tendinous abnormalities previously outlined must be addressed to prevent recurrent ulceration. This usually mandates orthopedic or podiatric consultation. The reconstructive plastic surgeon should have the assistance of either an orthopedic or a podiatric surgeon who is interested and proficient in surgery for diabetic biomechanical abnormalities. Tendon lengthening, tendon transfer, ostectomy, osteotomy, ankle fusion, or midfoot fusion may be the essential procedure to ensure a complication-free future for these patients. As in surgery of the hand and upper extremity, surgeons frequently use a tourniquet throughout the flap dissection portion of the procedure. Patients with tenuous circulation and those who have been revascularized with either angioplasty or bypass grafts are exceptions to this rule.

It is helpful to separate the foot and ankle into four distinct regions when outlining the options available for wound closure: (1) ankle and foot dorsum, (2) plantar forefoot, (3) plantar midfoot, and (4) plantar hindfoot.

Ankle and Foot Dorsum

The superficial wounds resulting from minor trauma, burns, or poorly fitting shoes may be successfully closed with STSGs in most patients. Exposed tendons devoid of paratenon or bone devoid of periosteum usually require flap techniques; both local and free flap procedures may be applicable. In many patients, excision of dorsal extensor tendons permits successful STSGs for closure of an otherwise complex dorsal foot wound.

Many of these patients have hyperextension deformities of the metatarsophalangeal joints (hammer toes) and benefit secondarily from tendon excision (Figure 33-12). Thin free flap transfers are best to reconstruct more extensive tissue loss with accompanying malleolar exposure and major ankle tendon exposure, such as the tibialis anterior or peroneus tendons (Figure 33-13).

Useful local flaps include the extensor digitorum brevis muscle flap, the sural neurocutaneous flap, and the lateral supramalleolar flap. The sural flap may be employed for coverage of anterior ankle wounds but is primarily useful in hindfoot repair (see later discussion).

EXTENSOR DIGITORUM BREVIS MUSCLE FLAP. Although often not considered, this flap is extremely useful for coverage in the perimalleolar area and foot dorsum. The pedicled island flap may be based on three different blood supplies. The lateral tarsal artery permits limited rotation to the medial and lateral foot dorsum and to the perimalleolar region. Sacrifice of the anterior tibial–dorsalis pedis axis is avoided. If the muscle is elevated on the anterior tibial artery, any site on the leg may be reached with the flap. Distally based flaps may also be used for coverage over the distal foot dorsum. In these cases the blood supply is from the perforating branch of the dorsalis pedis artery between the first and second metatarsal bases.

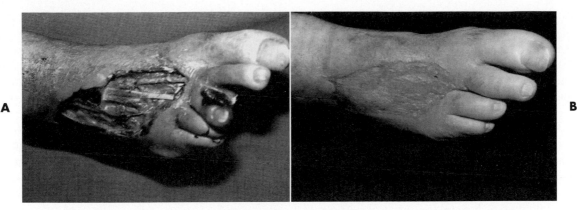

Figure 33-12. **A,** Necrotizing infection with dorsal tendon exposure. **B,** Following tendon excision, local wound care, and split thickness skin grafting.

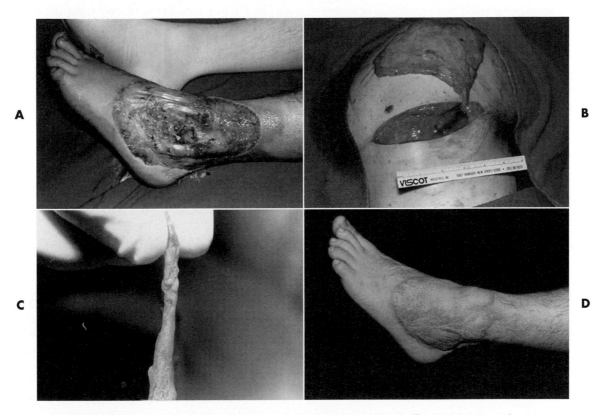

Figure 33-13. **A,** Lateral leg/ankle/foot wound after debridement. **B,** The dorsal thoracic fascia is an excellent source of "thin" flap tissue for resurfacing this area. **C,** This fascial flap is no more than 2 to 4 mm in thickness. **D,** Following flap transfer and split thickness skin grafting.

Through a curvilinear dorsal foot incision, retraction of the extensor digitorum longus tendons and preservation of the dorsal foot sensory nerves expose the muscle flap. Sequential division of the distal tendons permits lateral retraction of the muscle and isolation of the lateral tarsal artery branch of the dorsalis pedis artery. The proximal muscle may then be released from its calcaneal attachments. The lateral tarsal artery will supply the muscle but will continue laterally, along the muscle's undersurface, to anastomose with the peroneal artery (see Figure 33-10). Ligation of this connection is necessary. At this point the flap may be transposed. If additional pedicle length is necessary, ligation of the medial tarsal artery and dorsalis pedis artery should be considered.

Plantar Forefoot

The area from the midshaft of the metatarsals distally is referred to as the *forefoot.* More than 50% of ulcerations typically occur in this part of the foot because Charcot arthropathy usually manifests first in this region. Excessive distribution of weight to the forefoot during ambulation occurs in the presence of Achilles tendon shortening. Soft tissue reconstruction should be combined with Achilles tendon lengthening if preoperative computer gait assessment confirms these findings.

Toe ulceration complicated by underlying osteomyelitis is best managed by amputation of the affected phalanx. This avoids the need for prolonged IV antibiotic administration. Dorsal or plantar flaps of uninvolved skin can usually assist in preservation of length while obtaining stable wound closure.

Because peripheral vascular disease often accompanies these wounds, a thorough evaluation of the affected limb in the vascular laboratory is mandatory before undertaking any surgical procedure. If the infectious process involves both the phalanx and its associated metatarsal, the surgeon should consider ray amputation. Because the proximal portions of the affected metatarsal are left in situ, a 6-week course of antibiotics is indicated. Patients often do well with two ray resections in the same foot. If three or more ray amputations are necessary, the surgeon should proceed to formal transmetatarsal amputation, since this is a much more biomechanically stable procedure than the alternative.

All bony tissue removed must be sent for careful histologic analysis. Every effort must be made to differentiate osteitis from osteomyelitis. In *osteitis* the changes are reactive in nature, secondary to the nearby ulcerative process. In *osteomyelitis,* invasive infection with an associated leukocytic response is seen within the marrow of the affected bone.

Metatarsal head ulceration is the most frequent sequela of Charcot forefoot arthropathy. Toe fillet flaps,[64] neurovascular island flaps from the lateral side of the great toe,[65,66] and plantar V-Y fasciocutaneous flaps[61] are three useful procedures for the surgical closure of these wounds. They may be performed rapidly and safely in patients with adequate arterial inflow and should be accompanied by resecting the underlying bony prominence and off-loading the forefoot by lengthening the Achilles tendon.

Recurrent ulceration after transmetatarsal amputation often requires more proximal amputation techniques when local flap procedures are no longer of value. These problems can be avoided, however, by reducing the stresses of weight bearing on the forefoot with lengthening of the Achilles tendon.

TOE FILLET FLAP. The fillet of an adjacent toe based on its plantar digital vessels (see Figure 33-10) permits closure of wounds up to 3 cm in diameter. Depending on the wound, the toe flap may be dissected as an island flap or simply transposed into the defect after its bony framework and germinal matrix are resected (Figure 33-14).

The nail bed and underlying distal phalanx are resected, leaving the plantar pad intact. A midlateral incision to bone allows subperiosteal resection of the remaining phalanges. By retaining one or two neurovascular bundles, the soft tissue flap may be transposed into a nearby plantar defect without risk.

NEUROVASCULAR ISLAND FLAP. The flap is centered over the area of the Doppler pulse of the fibular neurovascular bundle of the great toe. Dissection of the flap is begun distally at the level of the phalangeal periosteum. Proceeding more proximally, the neurovascular pedicle in the first web space is identified and preserved. Additional dissection provides greater freedom in flap transposition.

Small wounds of 2 to 3 cm may be closed with this technique. Depending on the size of the flap elevated, the donor site will either close directly or require a small STSG (Figure 33-15).

V-Y PLANTAR FLAP. This flap may be raised either singly or in pairs to reconstruct defects up to 4 to 5 cm in diameter. This is my first choice for flap repair of the forefoot region. Perfusion is based on the numerous perforating vessels on the foot's planar surface (Figure 33-16). The V-Y flap is incised circumferentially and must include the underlying plantar fascia with the skin and subcutaneous fat incision. The release of this fascia allows the soft tissues to stretch and advance into the wound (Figure 33-17).

If necessary, additional advancement may be accomplished by the careful release of the vertical attachments of the plantar fascia to the underlying metatarsals. Wounds too large to be closed with one flap may be reconstructed with two opposing flaps without difficulty.

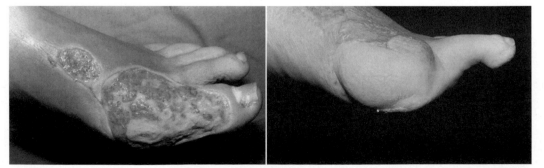

A **B**

Figure 33-14. **A,** Exposure of the capsule of the metatarsal-phalangeal joint of the great toe.
B, Following great toe fillet flap based on the plantar neurovascular structures.

FOREFOOT AMPUTATIONS. Reconstructive surgeons managing patients with foot ulceration should be well versed in the options available for forefoot amputation, since these procedures are often the simplest alternative in providing stable healing and bipedal ambulation. Transmetatarsal amputation is indicated once three or more rays have been deleted. This is usually accomplished by using a plantar flap of skin, subcutaneous tissue, and fascia to advance over the metatarsal stumps. With significant plantar ulceration, however, dorsal soft tissues may be needed for this purpose. The key is to preserve as much soft tissue as possible (both dorsal and plantar) to maintain length and help suture lines free of tension. More proximal applications of the transmetatarsal amputation may be necessary in selected patients (Figure 33-18).

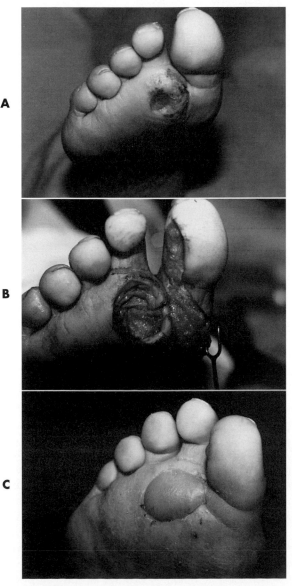

A

B

C

Figure 33-15. **A,** Second metatarsal head ulceration. **B,** Debrided wound and a neurovascular island flap based on the lateral side of the great toe. **C,** Three months after flap transfer. The donor site was closed primarily.

The surgeon should be careful to avoid injury to the vertical descending branch of the dorsalis pedis artery (see Figure 33-11). This vessel courses between the first and second metatarsal bases and is at risk of injury with nearby bony resection. In patients with significant stenoses in the posterior tibial artery, the vertical descending branch of the dorsalis pedis artery may be the only blood supply to the plantar forefoot.

Plantar Midfoot

The *midfoot* is defined as the region between the proximal tarsal row and the midshaft of the metatarsals. It comprises the medial non-weight-bearing arch as well as the more lateral weight-bearing structures. Ulceration in this region is usually secondary to severe Charcot deformities, which must be addressed at wound closure to prevent recurrent ulceration.

Historically, reconstruction of the midfoot has been the most challenging of all regions of the foot. The complexity of repairs in this region accounts for the high incidence of below knee amputations that are performed for these problems. With strict adherence to an organized approach to wound management in the midfoot, however, the need for major amputation has been less than 5% in our patients versus the greater than 80% previously reported.[67]

As discussed earlier, deformity at Lisfranc's joint (tarsometatarsal junction) occurs when a shortened gastrocnemius-soleus complex alters normal ankle motion. The inability to dorsiflex fully at the ankle puts undo strain across Lisfranc's joint during gait. Over time, this inability to dorsiflex the ankle contributes to increased motion (dorsiflexion) at the midfoot level, with breakdown of Lisfranc's joint and resultant midfoot deformity. Soft tissue ulceration is inevitable.

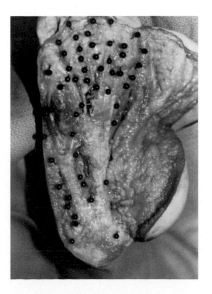

Figure 33-16. After colored latex is injected into the posterior tibial artery in this "fresh" cadaver specimen, the small tacks show the location of the numerous perforating vessels that communicate with the subdermal plexus of vessels on the plantar surface of the foot.

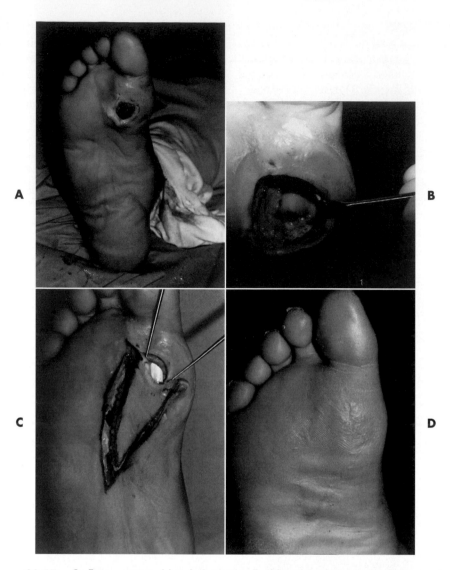

Figure 33-17. **A,** First metatarsal head ulceration. **B,** After debridement, the flexor tendon is retracted medially to expose the fibular sesamoid bone. **C,** After excision of the fibular sesamoid, the V-Y flap is advanced by incising through the skin, subcutaneous fat, and the plantar fascia. **D,** Three years after wound closure and Achilles' tendon lengthening.

If the wounds are superficial and the arch is preserved, skin grafting may be an acceptable solution. This, however, is rarely the case. Based on the anatomic studies used to develop the toe flap, neurovascular island flap, and the V-Y plantar flap procedures discussed for forefoot repair, similar techniques may be used for small wounds of the midfoot (Figure 33-19). The toe island flap will need to be more extensively dissected on its dominant circulation (either the dorsal or the plantar metatarsal artery) in order for the flap to reach wounds of the midfoot. If the dorsal circulation is dominant, division of the transverse metatarsal ligament is necessary for safe flap transposition.

When wounds exceed 4 to 6 cm, options for repair include either midfoot amputation or free flap reconstruction to ensure ample soft tissue for a tension-free repair.[57,68] Microvascular free tissue transfer is particularly useful for the reconstruction of the guillotine midfoot amputation because it permits maximal salvage of tissues, leading to a functional midfoot amputation (Figure 33-20). Details for these procedures are discussed with hindfoot repair.

MIDFOOT AMPUTATIONS. Midfoot amputation may be the preferred "repair" because the procedure is simple and may be performed relatively rapidly without the significant morbidity associated with more complex reconstructions. If patients are appropriately chosen and the procedure is executed properly, the surgeon may be able to salvage a limb that provides a stable platform for ambulation without increasing the energy expenditure involved.

The two most common procedures are Lisfranc's amputation (previously discussed) and Chopart's amputation. Lisfranc's amputation involves removal of all metatarsal remnants. Chopart's procedure requires an intertarsal resection and is therefore a more proximal amputation. Both procedures

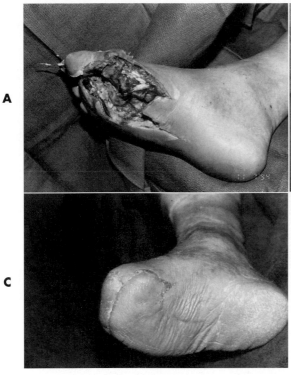

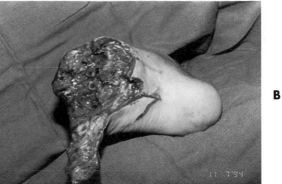

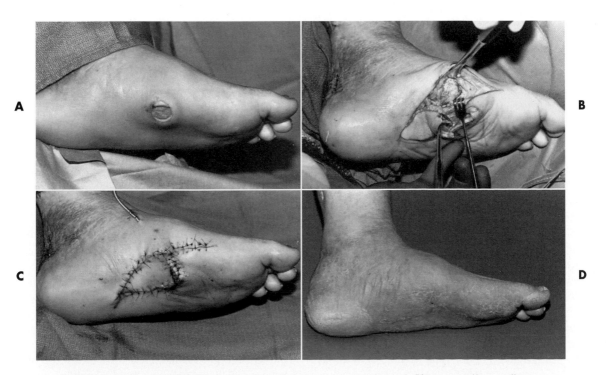

Figure 33-18. **A,** Infectious complications following forefoot surgery led to soft tissue necrosis. **B,** This patient had significant peripheral vascular disease. Following femoral-popliteal bypass grafting, a forefoot "fillet" procedure was performed to generate a laterally based flap to close the debrided wound. **C,** Six weeks after wound closure and concomitant Achilles' tendon lengthening.

Figure 33-19. **A,** Midfoot ulceration secondary to neuropathy and Charcot midfoot collapse. **B,** A V-Y flap has been elevated. A distal extension of the incision is made to provide adequate access to the underlying bony prominence. **C,** After ostectomy of the medial cuneiform/navicular the flap may be advanced and the wound closed. **D,** Two months after surgical closure.

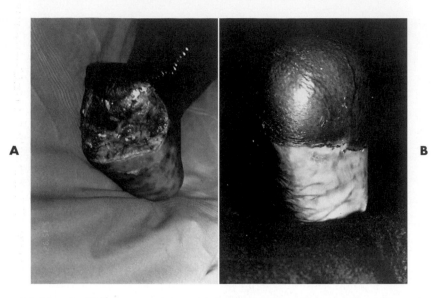

Figure 33-20. **A,** Midfoot amputation with loss of additional plantar skin. This patient was recently revascularized to the dorsalis pedis artery. **B,** After serratus anterior free flap transfer and split thickness skin grafting. The arterial anastomosis was performed to the bypass graft.

affect the patient's ability to dorsiflex and evert the involved foot, since they may jeopardize the insertions of the peroneus and tibialis anterior tendons. Lengthening of the Achilles tendon and repositioning of the tibialis anterior tendon more laterally on the foot dorsum greatly assist the reconstruction.[69]

Plantar Hindfoot

The *hindfoot* extends from the insertion of the Achilles tendon to the level of the proximal tarsal row. It is the second most frequently involved area of ulceration in diabetic patients. The thick, durable heel pad and its associated fibrous septations contrast with the thin, pliable soft tissue coverage that overlies the Achilles tendon and posterior heel.

Soft tissue reconstruction in this area must consider both the form and the function of the tissue deficiency. The plantar heel pad bears more than 50% of the patient's weight during the early phases of gait, so recurrent ulceration after reconstruction is quite common. The surgeon should treat problems in this region similar to ischial pressure sores in the paraplegic patient. The present reconstruction must not interfere with possible future reconstructions.

Unlike in other regions of the foot, numerous local flaps may be useful in the management of hindfoot wounds. The intrinsic foot muscle flaps and the instep island flap are based on antegrade blood flow through the posterior tibial artery and its medial and lateral plantar branches. Extremities that derive their vascular supply from the anterior tibial–dorsalis pedis system (because of atherosclerosis within the posterior tibial system or recent arterial bypass grafting to the distal anterior tibial–dorsalis pedis vessels) are not good candidates for these simpler repairs.

Three intrinsic foot muscles of the plantar area have been used for proximal rotation and coverage of the plantar heel: the abductor hallucis muscle, the flexor digitorum brevis muscle, and the abductor digiti minimi. The abductor digiti minimi muscle is rarely useful; its small size and arc of rotation significantly impair its ability to assist in wound repair.

The lateral calcaneal artery flap, based on terminal branches of the peroneal artery, was a useful procedure for posterior hindfoot coverage.[70] It has largely been replaced with the *sural neurocutaneous flap*, however, since the donor site is more acceptable. Also, flap size and arc of rotation of the sural flap are superior.

ABDUCTOR HALLUCIS MUSCLE FLAP. This small flap may be used by itself or with the flexor digitorum brevis muscle flap to close wounds of the plantar heel. The abductor hallucis muscle is elevated through a medial foot incision by dividing the tendon distally and separating the lateral border of the muscle from the medial head of the nearby flexor hallucis brevis muscle. The blood supply enters the muscle proximally through branches of the medial plantar artery, which may be included in the flap to increase its arc of rotation.[71]

FLEXOR DIGITORUM BREVIS MUSCLE FLAP. Although small, this muscle is significantly larger than the abductor hallucis and can be useful for wounds 3 to 5 cm in diameter. Its blood supply is derived from branches of the medial and lateral plantar vessels, with the latter being dominant.

Exposure of the muscle and its overlying plantar fascia is obtained through a midline plantar foot incision. After division of the distal four tendons, the muscle may be dissected in a retrograde manner off the underlying quadratus plantae muscle. The surgeon should be able to elevate the muscle flap and its associated plantar fascia without division of the medial or lateral plantar vessels if plantar heel pad coverage is required (Figure 33-21). Including the plantar fascia increases the flap's volume.

To increase this flap's arc of rotation (for coverage of the heel's posterior, non-weight-bearing portion), ligation of the

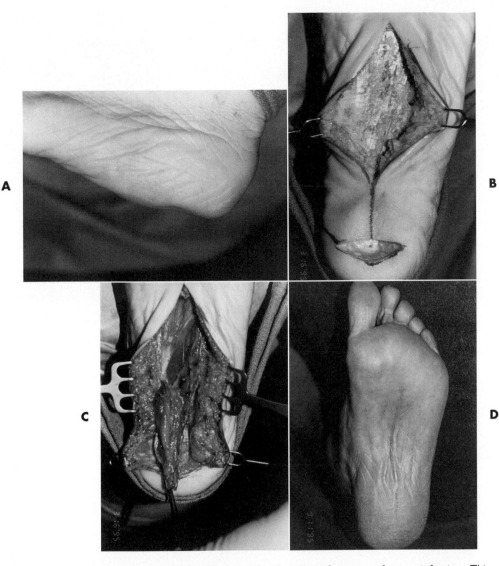

Figure 33-21. A, Loss of plantar heel pad subcutaneous soft tissues after an infection. This patient has heel pain when walking. **B,** The approach to the flexor digitorum brevis muscle is through a midplantar approach. The plantar fascia is left attached to the muscle and elevated with it to increase the "bulk" of the transfer. **C,** The muscle flap is elevated, beginning distally, and "turned over" into the soft tissue defect. Proximal medial and lateral plantar branches coursing into the muscle are preserved. **D,** Six months post op, the contour of the heel pad is improved and the patient is pain free.

lateral plantar artery distally and dissection of the flap based on this vessel can be accomplished well into the tarsal tunnel. Division of the abductor hallucis muscle's origin will "unroof" the tarsal tunnel and greatly simplify the dissection.[72]

MEDIAL PLANTAR ARTERY FLAP. This flap is useful for heel pad reconstruction if no significant Charcot midfoot collapse is present. To ensure durability of the instep donor site, it must not be a weight-bearing surface. Instep collapse is a relative contraindication to this procedure. This flap should not be routinely used for heel repairs since future collapse of the midfoot may occur and initiate ulceration through the skin-grafted donor site.

The course of the medial plantar artery should be mapped preoperatively with the Doppler probe. The flap dimensions should not exceed the boundaries of the non-weight-bearing instep. After tourniquet inflation, the distal extent of the flap is incised through the plantar fascia so that the medial plantar neurovascular pedicle may be isolated in the cleft between the abductor hallucis and flexor digitorum brevis muscles. The pedicle must be elevated with the overlying soft tissues. Arterial branches to the muscles are ligated, while an interfascicular dissection of the medial plantar nerve preserves the fascicles to the medial toes and provides fascicular continuity to the flap.

Because most patients requiring this procedure have significant neuropathy, transecting the nerve at the time of plantar artery ligation may be more appropriate. Dissection of the pedicle should continue until it is seen emerging from the distal

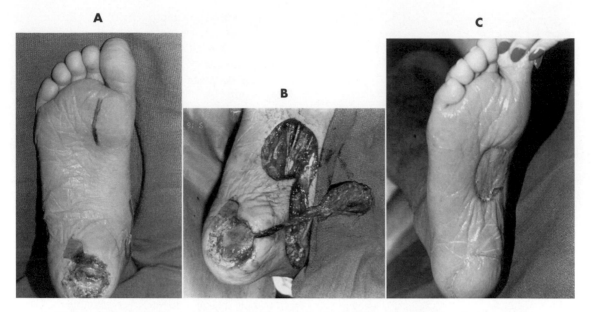

Figure 33-22. A, Neurotrophic ulceration of the heel. Note the well-formed plantar arch. **B,** The instep flap is elevated as an "island" based on the medial plantar artery. **C,** Six months after flap inset and skin grafting to the donor site.

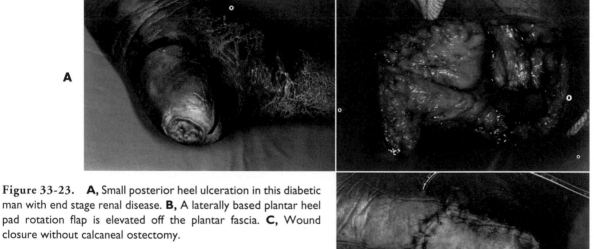

Figure 33-23. A, Small posterior heel ulceration in this diabetic man with end stage renal disease. **B,** A laterally based plantar heel pad rotation flap is elevated off the plantar fascia. **C,** Wound closure without calcaneal ostectomy.

extent of the tarsal tunnel. If additional length is required, the abductor hallucis muscle's origin should be divided to release the tarsal tunnel (Figure 33-22).[73]

HEEL PAD ROTATION WITH OR WITHOUT CALCA-NECTOMY. Small wounds of the posterior heel may be reconstructed using a suprafascial flap of heel pad tissue based either medially or laterally.[63] To ensure a tension-free closure

and to avoid the need for a skin graft to the donor area, adjuvant calcanectomy should be considered.

Flap elevation is performed superficial to the plantar fascia. The blood supply enters the soft tissues through vessels that course around the medial and lateral aspects of the origin of the thick plantar fascia. Medially based flaps require division of the lateral vessels, and vice versa (Figure 33-23). Generous calcanectomy may provide enough soft tissue excess to close

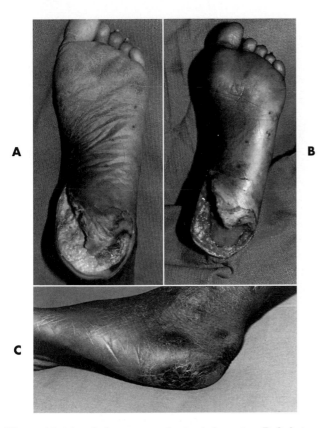

Figure 33-24. **A,** Large posterior heel ulceration. **B,** Soft tissue debridement is accompanied by release of the proximal plantar midfoot soft tissues off the plantar fascia and generous calcanectomy. **C,** Eight months after surgery. This patient has a soft heel lift placed in her shoe.

larger wounds without resorting to more complex procedures. This technique is especially useful in patients with significant comorbid factors that render them poor candidates for free flap reconstruction (Figure 33-24).

LATERAL SUPRAMALLEOLAR FLAP. This flap has been most useful in the coverage of bony defects that accompany loss of soft tissue over the lateral malleolus. The flap should be distally based because the blood supply is derived from the perforating branch of the peroneal artery as it pierces the interosseous membrane 5 cm proximal to the tip of the lateral malleolus (see Figure 33-8). Cutaneous vessels then course upward, anterior to the fibula, and anastomose with the vascular network that accompanies the superficial peroneal nerve.

The perforating branch of the peroneal artery may be located with the hand-held Doppler probe. The base of the flap should be centered at this point. Flap width includes the tissue between the fibula and the tibia. The length should be adequate to reach the lateral malleolus (6 to 8 cm).[74] I generally elevate the tissue as a fascial flap, turn it over like the page of a book, and skin graft its surface. When done in this way, the donor site may be closed directly.

The skin incision is made so that skin flaps may be elevated off the underlying deep fascia. The fascia is then incised along its anterior margin and progressively reflected until the perforating branch is seen. Branches of the superficial peroneal nerve course within the fascia and must be divided to permit safe elevation and rotation. Final release of the flap requires incision through the posterior margin and release of its attachments to the septum that separates the anterior and lateral muscular compartments (Figure 33-25).

SURAL FLAP. The blood supply to this flap is derived from the small arteries that accompany the sural nerve along its course in the posterior aspect of the distal two thirds of the lower leg. In most patients this is a "vascular network," although occasionally a well-defined median superficial sural artery may accompany the nerve. Numerous anastomoses exist between this "network" and the peroneal artery; the most important is the most distal anastomosis, located approximately 5 cm cephalad to the lateral malleolar region. This location is usually audible with the Doppler probe, which may be useful in mapping the flap preoperatively. The flap should not be outlined cephalad to the junction of the two heads of the gastrocnemius muscle because the nerve and its accompanying arteries are subfascial as they course to the popliteal fossa. The pedicle consists of a 2-cm-wide strip of subcutaneous tissue and fascia containing the sural nerve, its associated arteries, and the lesser saphenous vein.

The sural flap is outlined over the raphe between the two heads of the gastrocnemius muscle. A line is drawn from the flap's inferior edge to the pivot point for the pedicle, approximately 5 cm from the lateral malleolus. Flap elevation is begun along its cephalic portion. Through this incision, the sural nerve and the lesser saphenous vein are identified and ligated so that they may be elevated along with the overlying soft tissue. The pedicle is created by elevating two skin flaps off the subcutaneous fascial pedicle. The flap and pedicle may then be separated from the underlying muscle layers by dividing small arteries that arise from the peroneal artery.

The flap's arc of rotation allows coverage of the heel and anterior ankle. The donor site may be closed primarily if small or with STSGs if larger (Figure 33-26).[75]

FREE FLAP RECONSTRUCTION. Free tissue transfer may be the only alternative to amputation in patients with wounds greater than 6 cm in size, those without posterior tibial arterial flow, or those with revascularization to the distal anterior tibial–dorsalis pedis artery through long saphenous vein grafts. Patients who require both distal bypass grafting and free tissue transfer procedures for limb salvage are a unique group (see later discussion).

Although many neurosensory free flap donor sites have been described, they have little usefulness in the diabetic patient with significant peripheral neuropathy. Free flap donor sites should be located in the upper torso or upper extremity to minimize the incidence of atherosclerosis in the donor vessels. Because of its proximity to the wound margin, the posterior tibial artery is the preferred recipient vessel. If the recipient artery is either a dorsally placed bypass graft or the anterior tibial vessel, a long donor pedicle becomes essential. Therefore

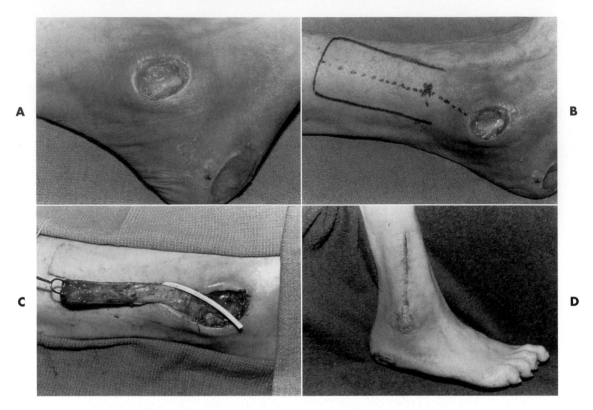

Figure 33-25. **A,** Chronic lateral malleolar ulcer. **B,** The lateral supramalleolar artery may be easily heard with the hand-held Doppler probe and its course traced on the extremity. **C,** After elevation of skin flaps, the underlying fascia may be elevated based on the lateral supramalleolar artery and then "turned over" to cover the debrided wound. **D,** Three months after flap transfer and split thickness skin grafting.

the serratus anterior muscle is usually a first choice for donor tissue. Venous outflow is through the deep system, which should be thoroughly mapped preoperatively using a duplex imaging system (Figure 33-27).

HINDFOOT AMPUTATION. The *Syme's amputation* has a definite role in the reconstruction of the diabetic foot. The procedure involves using the heel pad as the soft tissue cover over the distal end of the tibia and fibula. Amputation is performed through the distal tibia and fibula at the level of the medial and lateral malleoli. "Filleting" of the heel pad must be performed at the level of the calcaneal and talar periosteum so that "button holing" of the thin soft tissues just distal to the ankle is avoided.

Incisional closure should avoid tension. This usually means that the remaining medial and lateral "dog ears" are revised at a second procedure. Significant wounds of the plantar heel require the foot dorsum as a flap, which is turned down to provide closure over the bone ends.

Although beneficial in most patients, Syme's amputation may be most helpful for patients who have already undergone contralateral below-knee amputations. Redundancy of the soft tissues at the stump is a typical consequence of the procedure and usually mandates revision.

Combined Distal Bypass Vascular Surgery and Free Flap Reconstruction

Improved techniques for lower extremity bypass surgery usually result in successful limb salvage despite initially severe ischemia. Venous bypass grafts to the distal tibial and pedal arteries have particularly benefited diabetic patients primarily with infrapopliteal occlusive disease. Despite these advances, some patients have such extensive tissue loss that primary healing cannot be anticipated, even after successful arterial reconstruction. These large wounds are accompanied by large segments of exposed bone and tendon and are often on the foot's weight-bearing plantar surface.

Distal leg arterial reconstruction and microvascular free tissue transfer offer possible limb salvage for patients with extensive ischemic tissue loss who would normally require amputation. Combining these two techniques should be reserved for patients whose only alternative is limb loss. Wounds of the forefoot are easily managed by partial foot amputation. In general, the best candidates for this combined approach are those with extensive wounds of the midfoot and hindfoot who would predictably not achieve ambulation after a primary amputation. This includes patients with a previous contralateral amputation or diabetic patients with a high likelihood of subsequent contralateral

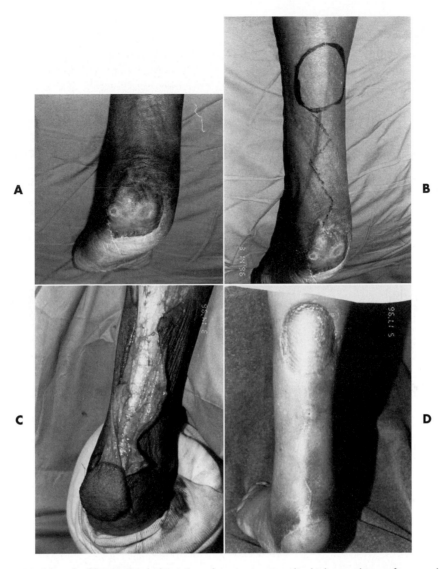

Figure 33-26. **A,** Chronic heel ulceration after numerous split thickness skin graft procedures. **B,** The sural flap is outlined over the course of the sural nerve and the lesser saphenous vein. The arc of rotation is approximately 5 cm above the lateral malleolus. **C,** The flap is elevated with a 2 cm width of deep fascia containing the sural nerve and lesser saphenous vein. **D,** Two months after flap transfer. A split thickness skin graft was placed on the flap donor site.

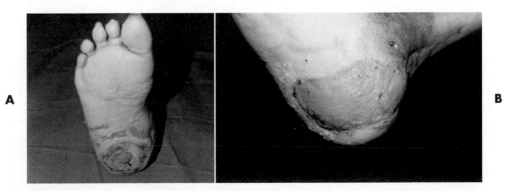

Figure 33-27. **A,** Chronic osteomyelitis of the calcaneous after multiple attempts at debridement and local flap repair. **B,** Successful outcome after generous calcanectomy to remove areas of devitalized bone and coverage using a serratus anterior free flap and skin graft.

amputation. Five groups who may fit these criteria include patients with the following:

1. Diabetic neurotrophic ulcers
2. Posttraumatic infected ulcers (Figure 33-28)
3. Postoperative wound complications (Figure 33-29)
4. Open midfoot amputations (Figure 33-20)
5. Ischemic wounds in extremities without "target" vessels to bypass ("nutrient" flaps)

Successful limb salvage has been reported in patients with "nutrient flaps," although my experience is that a successful revascularization procedure must accompany the free flap reconstruction or poor flap incorporation into the defect occurs with eventual amputation.[76]

Poor candidates for combined revascularization and free tissue transfer include high-risk patients, noncompliant pa-

tients, nonambulatory patients, and patients with small forefoot ulcers.

A variety of free flap donor sites have been described, but muscle flaps harvested from the subscapular vascular axis may be most useful. The donor vessels are usually free from atherosclerotic deposits, and both long and short vascular pedicles may be obtained. If the recipient artery is severely calcified, a Carrel patch for the thoracodorsal artery can be made from its connection with the subscapular or circumflex scapular artery to facilitate a wide anastomosis (see Figure 33-30). Combined muscle flaps (serratus anterior and latissimus dorsi) on one vascular pedicle may also be used.

Free tissue transfer may be delayed after arterial reconstruction or performed during the same procedure. The optimal

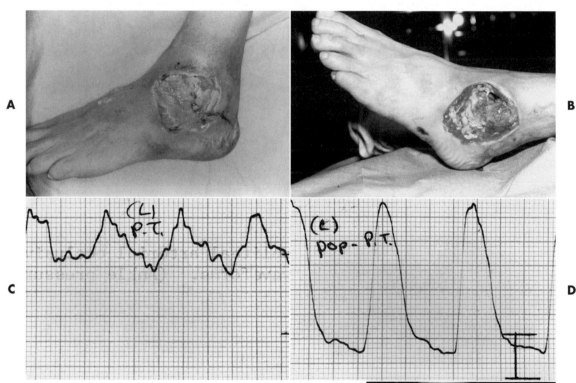

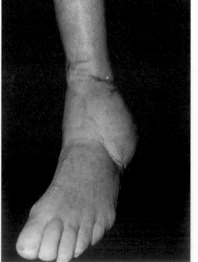

Figure 33-28. **A,** Posttraumatic wound over the lateral ankle. **B,** After judicious debridement of obviously devitalized tissues. This patient has significant peripheral vascular disease; hence, definitive debridement should follow revascularization surgery. **C,** The analog Doppler waveforms in the posterior tibial artery are monophasic. **D,** After popliteal artery angioplasty and popliteal-posterior tibial artery bypass grafting, the Doppler waveforms are markedly improved. **E,** The wound is closed with a serratus anterior free flap and split thickness skin graft. The arterial anastomosis is to the vein bypass graft.

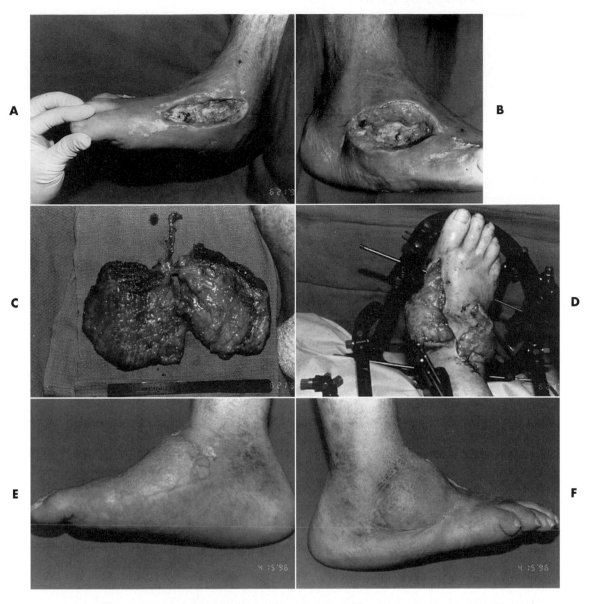

Figure 33-29. **A,** Medial foot wound. This patient had Charcot midfoot reconstruction and required internal fixation. Postoperative infection lead to breakdown of the incisions and exposure of the hardware. **B,** Lateral foot wound. **C,** A combined serratus anterior and latissimus dorsi muscle flap is harvested based on a single pedicle (the thoracodorsal artery). **D,** The internal fixation devices are removed and external fixation applied at the time of flap transfer and inset into the separate foot wounds. **E,** Medial foot reconstruction 10 months postoperative. **F,** Lateral foot repair 10 months postoperative.

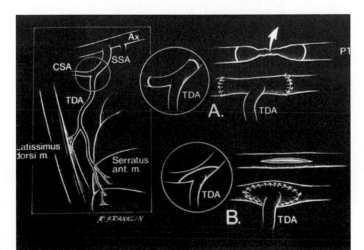

Figure 33-30. There are many options available to the reconstructive microsurgeon when the subscapular vascular axis is chosen as the donor site for free tissue transfer. The thoracodorsal artery may be harvested with either the serratus anterior muscle and/or the latissimus dorsi muscle with a segment of subscapular artery/circumflex scapular artery *(upper right)* or with a Carrel patch *(lower right)* to simplify flap transfer in patients with significant atherosclerosis in their recipient vessels.

timing depends on several factors. If durability of the arterial reconstruction is questionable, the free flap transfer should be delayed. For patients with significant infection or necrosis, debridement rather than wound closure should accompany revascularization.

For some patients, however, simultaneous procedures may be the best approach, especially if the soft tissue defect encompasses the course of the arterial bypass graft. Simultaneous revascularization and free tissue transfer may hasten rehabilitation, decrease hospital length of stay, and reduce cost. This approach is appropriate for patients with optimal arterial reconstructions and limited infection or soft tissue necrosis.

POSTOPERATIVE CARE

All patients are maintained on non-weight-bearing status for 3 to 4 weeks after procedures that place suture lines on the foot's plantar surface. This is essential to ensure normal healing. The use of strict bedrest and wheelchairs after reconstruction varies with the procedure performed. Local flaps generally require a day of extremity elevation, skin grafts 3 to 5 days, and free flaps up to 2 weeks. Control of pedal edema is important and may be accomplished with bedrest and elevation or careful use of elastic wraps once the patient is permitted to place the limb in a dependent position. During the bedrest phase, low-molecular-weight heparin may significantly reduce the incidence of deep venous thrombosis.

Postoperative antibiotic use is dictated by the findings at surgery. Patients with no acute infection and a negative bone biopsy should receive 5 days of broad-spectrum antibiotics. Patients with acute infection require a 2-week course of culture-specific antibiotics. These drug regimens are usually started intravenously in the hospital and continued orally after discharge. Patients with biopsy-proven osteomyelitis may be more problematic. If the debridement procedure completely removes the offending bone, a 2-week course of antibiotic therapy is recommended.

The L'Nard splint has been a very useful tool in keeping the posterior heel off the surface of the bed (to prevent posterior heel ulceration) while providing immobilization of the foot and ankle. It is lightweight and therefore beneficial when the patient begins non-weight-bearing ambulation with crutches or a walker. The Cam walker boot is often used to protect foot repairs and tendon transfers or lengthenings when the patient becomes weight bearing. A heavy device (similar to a cast), it comfortably and effectively immobilizes the foot and ankle while allowing for adjustment of the degree of equinus required at the ankle level.

Sutures are generally removed just before the patient begins weight-bearing ambulation at 3 to 4 weeks. Sutures often incite callus formation on the plantar surface. When a callus is thoroughly debrided, "new" areas of small ulceration are often found. I manage these small areas with Regranex gel (becaplermin) and find that they rapidly contract and epithelialize provided the foot has been corrected biomechanically.

Follow-up at the diabetic limb clinic is frequent and performed in a multidisciplinary manner involving plastic surgery, vascular surgery, endocrinology, orthopedic surgery, podiatry, and orthotics. Experienced nursing personnel adept at all aspects of wound assessment and care contribute as well. As discussed next, this approach is as important as any other intervention in the prevention of recurrent wounds.

OUTCOMES

Data have only recently become available regarding the outcomes from a closely supervised multidisciplinary approach to the management of the diabetic foot. Review of the literature suggests that limb salvage is improved when certain management schemes are followed. Because of the many variables within the few studies published, it is difficult to determine exactly which variables account for the improved outcomes. For example, reports that deal with surgical interventions compare groups of patients who have undergone certain procedures with "controls." The improved outcomes after surgery are attributed to the procedure itself, although the frequent follow-up that accompanies the postoperative care may be important as well.

Several groups have reported their experience using a multidisciplinary approach within a diabetic foot clinic. A study from the University of Louisville compared two groups of patients. One group developed ulcers while receiving prophylactic care at a multidisciplinary clinic (group I), and the other, identical group was referred to the clinic after ulceration had already occurred (group II). The sites and sizes of the lesions were no different between the two groups. Despite the similarities between the two groups, group I patients had a significantly better prognosis than those in group II. The conclusions reached supported the contention that the establishment of a dedicated diabetic foot care clinic and regular patient review can reduce the morbidity associated with diabetic foot ulceration. New ulceration is detected sooner, and leads to more effective management to attain limb preservation.[77]

The role of early, aggressive revascularization surgery in the long-term outcome of diabetic foot management is addressed in several recent studies as well. Researchers from the University of California, San Francisco, have shown that a multidisciplinary wound care program that includes vascular surgery and adjuvant HBO therapy can provide limb salvage that is both cost-effective and durable. In 63% of patients, their wounds healed and remained so during the 5 years of follow-up.[78]

The vascular surgery section at New England Deaconess Hospital similarly showed the beneficial effects of revascularization surgery in diabetic foot management, comparing outcomes of patients during two different intervals. The "modern" approach included distal bypass arterial grafting and led to improved care, as evidenced by the following:

1. Decrease in major and minor amputation rates
2. Reduced hospital length of stay
3. Reduced cost for care

Despite this, however, reimbursement through Medicare remained insufficient, with an average loss of $7480 per admission.[79]

Many studies have specifically examined frequent multidisciplinary wound care and its effect on the healing of diabetic foot ulceration. They repeatedly show that foot wounds will heal when pressure points are "off loaded" and wound management is done properly at frequent intervals.[80-82] Recurrent ulceration results from the difficulty in maintaining "off loading" with orthotic devices alone.

One series compared the outcomes of patients who had wound closure surgery (flap repairs) with those who underwent identical procedures but combined with the removal of bony prominences, repair of Charcot midfoot deformities, and Achilles tendon lengthening. The first group of patients underwent surgery from 1983 to 1990 and the second from 1990 to 1997. All patients were followed a minimum of 2 years, with average follow-up of 5 years. All patients were fitted with footwear appropriate to the procedures performed. When wounds were closed without attention to correction of the biomechanical abnormalities, ulcer recurrence rates were 25%. With the addition of the procedures mentioned, recurrence dropped to 2%.[83]

Finally, a recent study evaluated long-term outcomes in 52 patients who required both arterial revascularization surgery and free tissue transfer procedures to obtain limb salvage; 54 limbs required 60 free flap procedures. Follow-up averaged 48 months, at which time 52% of patients had died. Cardiac events were the main cause of mortality, and patients with diabetes more than 10 years correlated with a higher risk of mortality at follow-up. Early limb salvage rates were 95%, with late preservation in 91% of extremities. Perioperative myocardial infarction occurred in 24% of patients. Operative mortality rates were 5% per patient and 1.3% per procedure. Postreconstructive function was rated as good in 35%, intermediate in 50% and poor in 15% of patients. This was related to wound location and status of the contralateral extremity. Based on this data, a selective approach to the management of these problems is advocated.[84]

REFERENCES

1. Palumbo PJ, Melton LJ III: Peripheral vascular disease and diabetes. In *Diabetes in America: diabetes data compiled in 1984,* NIH pub 85-1468, Washington, DC, 1985, US Government Printing Office.
2. Lower extremity amputations. In *Diabetes surveillance, 1980-1987,* Atlanta, 1990, Centers for Disease Control and Prevention.
3. Kucan J, Robson M: Diabetic foot infections: fate of the contralateral foot, *Plast Reconstr Surg* 77:439, 1986.
4. Apelquist J et al: Long-term costs for foot ulcers in diabetic patients in a multidisciplinary setting, *Foot Ankle Int* 16:388, 1995.
5. Couch NP et al: Natural history of the leg amputee, *Am J Surg* 133:469, 1977.
6. Waters R, Perry J, Antonelli D, et al: Energy cost of walking of amputees: the influence of the level of amputation, *J Bone Joint Surg* 8A:42, 1986.
7. Goldner MG: The fate of the second leg in the diabetic amputee, *Diabetes* 9:100, 1960.
8. Cameron N, Leonard M, Roos I: The effects of sorbinil on peripheral nerve conduction velocity, polyol concentrations, and morphology in the streptozotocin-diabetic rat, *Diabetologica* 29:168, 1986.
9. Upton A, McComas A: The double crush in nerve entrapment syndromes, *Lancet* 2:359, 1973.
10. Sammarco G, Chalk D, Feibel J: Tarsal tunnel syndrome and additional nerve lesions in the same limb, *Foot Ankle* 14:71, 1993.
11. Morain W, Dellon A, Mackinnon S, Colen L: Current concepts in plastic surgery for the diabetic, *Adv Plast Reconstr Surg* 4:1, 1987.
12. Dellon A: A cause for optimism in diabetic neuropathy, *Ann Plast Surg* 20:103, 1988.
13. Robson M: Difficult wounds: pressure ulcerations and leg ulcers, *Clin Plast Surg* 6:537, 1979.
14. Groth K: Clinical observations and experimental studies on the pathogenesis of decubitus ulcers, *Acta Chir Scand Suppl* 87:206, 1942.
15. Tooke J: Microcirculation and diabetes, *Br Med Bull* 45:206, 1989.
16. Goldenberg S, Alex M, Joshi R, et al: Nonatheromatous peripheral vascular disease of the lower extremity, *Diabetes* 8:261, 1959.
17. Strandness D, Priest R, Gibbons G: Combined clinical and pathological study of diabetic and nondiabetic peripheral arterial disease, *Diabetes* 13:366, 1964.
18. Conrad M: Large and small artery occlusion in diabetics and nondiabetics with severe vascular disease, *Circulation* 36:83, 1967.
19. Bower H, Kaiser G, Willman V: Blood flow in the diabetic leg, *Circulation* 43:391, 1971.
20. Wyss C, Matsen F, Simmons C, et al: Transcutaneous oxygen tension measurements on limbs of diabetic and nondiabetic patients with peripheral vascular disease, *Surgery* 95:339, 1984.
21. Gaylorde P, Fonseca V, Llewellyn G, et al: Transcutaneous oxygen tension in legs and feet of diabetic patients, *Diabetes* 37:714, 1988.
22. LoGerfo F, Coffman J: Vascular and microvascular disease of the foot in diabetes, *N Engl J Med* 311:1615, 1984.
23. Haimovici H: Patterns of arteriosclerotic lesions of the lower extremity, *Arch Surg* 95:918, 1967.
24. Donaldson MC, Mannick JA, Whittemore AD: Femoral-distal bypass with in situ greater saphenous vein, *Ann Surg* 213:457, 1991.
25. Macmillan D: The effect of diabetes on blood flow properties, *Diabetes* 32 (suppl 2):56, 1983.

26. Rand P, Lacomb E: Hemodilution and blood viscosity, *J Clin Invest* 43:2214, 1964.

27. Vague P, Juhan I: Red cell deformability, platelet aggregation and insulin action, *Diabetes* 32 (suppl 2):88, 1983.

28. Weed R, Labelle P, Meirill E: Metabolic dependence of red cell deformability, *J Clin Invest* 48:795, 1969.

29. Nakao M, Nakao T, Yamoro S: Adenosine triphosphate and maintenance of shape of red cells, *Nature* 187:945, 1960.

30. Ehrly A: The effect of pentoxyfylline on the deformability of erythrocytes and on the muscular oxygen pressure in patients with chronic arterial disease, *J Med* 10:331, 1979.

31. Armstrong M, Kunar D, Cummings C: Effect of pentoxyfylline on myocutaneous flap viability in pigs, *Otolaryngol Head Neck Surg* 109:668, 1993.

32. Schwartz R, Logan N, Johnson P: Pentoxyfylline increases extremity blood flow in diabetic atherosclerotic patients, *Arch Surg* 124:434, 1989.

33. Porter J, Cutter B, Lee B: Pentoxyfylline efficacy in the treatment of intermittent claudication: multicenter controlled, double-blind trial with objective assessment of chronic occlusive arterial disease patients, *Am Heart J* 104:66, 1982.

34. Brownlee M, Vlassara H, Cerami A: Non-enzymatic glycosylation and the pathogenesis of diabetic complications, *Ann Intern Med* 101:527, 1984.

35. Singer P, Berger I, Luck K, et al: Long-term effect of mackerel diet on blood pressure, serum lipids and thromboxane formation in patients with mild essential hypertension, *Atherosclerosis* 62:259, 1986.

36. Fox P, DiCorleto PE: Fish oils inhibit endothelial cell production of platelet-derived growth factor–like protein, *Science* 241:453, 1988.

37. Ainsworth SK, Allison F: Studies on the pathogenesis of acute inflammation. IX. The influence of hyperosmolality secondary to hyperglycemia upon the acute inflammatory response induced by thermal injury to ear chambers of rabbits, *J Clin Invest* 282:123, 1970.

38. Brayton RG, Stokes PE, Schwarz MS, et al: Effect of alcohol and various diseases on leukocyte mobilization, phagocytosis and intracellular bacterial killing, *N Engl J Med* 49:433, 1970.

39. Bagdale JD, Stewart M, Walters E: Impaired granulocyte adherence: a reversible defect in host defense in patients with poorly controlled diabetes, *Diabetes* 27:677, 1978.

40. Mowat AG, Baum J: Chemotaxis of polymorphonuclear leukocytes from patients with diabetes mellitus, *N Engl J Med* 234:621, 1971.

41. Kjersen H, Hilsted J, Madsbad S, et al: Polymorphonuclear leukocyte dysfunction during short-term metabolic changes from normo- to hypoglycemia in type I (insulin-dependent) diabetic patients, *Infection* 4:215, 1988.

42. Bagdale JD, Root R, Bulger JR: Impaired leukocyte function in patients with poorly controlled diabetes, *Diabetes* 23:9, 1974.

43. Richardson R: Immunity in diabetes: influence of diabetes on the development of anti-bacterial properties in the blood, *J Clin Invest* 12:1143, 1943.

44. Plouffe JF, Silva J, Fekety FR, et al: Cell-mediated immunity in diabetes mellitus, *Infect Immun* 21:425, 1978.

45. Kahn CR, Weir GC, editors: *Joslin Diabetes,* ed 12, Malvern, Pa, 1985, Lea & Feiberger.

46. Robson MC, Heggers JP: Effect of hyperglycemia on survival of bacteria, *Surg Forum* 20:56, 1969.

47. Robson MC, Heggers JP: Variables in host resistance pertaining to septicemia. I. Blood glucose level, *J Am Geriatr Soc* 17:991, 1969.

48. Stevens MJ, Edmond ME, Foster AVM, Watkins PJ: Selective neuropathy and preserved vascular response in the diabetic foot, *Diabetologia* 35:148, 1992.

49. Hoeldtke RD, Cavanaugh ST: Treatment of orthostatic hypotension with dihydroergotamine and caffeine, *Ann Intern Med* 105:168, 1996.

50. Grant WP, Sullivan RS, Vinik AI, et al: Electron microscopic investigation of the effects of diabetes mellitus on the Achilles tendon, *J Foot Ankle Surg* 36:1, 1997.

51. Lin SS, Lee TH, Wapners KL: Plantar forefoot ulceration with equinus deformity of the ankle in diabetic patients: the effect of tendo-Achilles lengthening and total contact casting, *Orthopedics* 19:465, 1996.

52. Cianci P: Adjunctive HBO therapy in the treatment of the diabetic foot, *Wounds* 4:158, 1992.

53. Mangano DT, London MJ, Tubau JF, et al: Dipyridamole thallium-201 scintigraphy as a preoperative screening test: a reexamination of its predictive potential, *Circulation* 84:493, 1991.

54. Yuh W, Corson J, Baraniewski H, et al: Osteomyelitis of the foot in diabetic patients, *Am J Radiol* 152:795, 1989.

55. Wyss CR, Matsen FA, Simmons CW, et al: Transcutaneous oxygen tension measurements on limbs of diabetic and nondiabetic patients with peripheral vascular disease, *Surgery* 95:339, 1984.

56. Krahenbuhl B, Mossaz A: On vascular non-disease of the foot in diabetes, *N Engl J Med* 312:1190, 1985 (letter).

57. Colen L: Limb salvage in the patient with severe peripheral vascular disease: the role of microsurgical free tissue transfer, *Plast Reconstr Surg* 79:389, 1987.

58. Colen L, Munsen A: Preoperative assessment of the peripheral vascular disease patient for free tissue transfer, *J Reconstr Microsurg* 4:1, 1987.

59. Miller J, Potparic Z, Colen LB, et al: The accuracy of duplex ultrasonography in the planning of skin flaps in the lower extremity, *Plast Reconstr Surg* 95:1221, 1995.

60. Cormack GC, Lamberty BGH: *The arterial anatomy of skin flaps,* Edinburgh, 1986, Churchill Livingstone.

61. Colen LB, Replogle SL, Mathes SJ: The V-Y plantar flap for reconstruction of the forefoot, *Plast Reconstr Surg* 81:220, 1988.

62. Sarrafian SK: *Anatomy of the foot and ankle,* Philadelphia, 1993, Lippincott.

63. Shaw WW, Hidalgo DA: Anatomic basis of plantar flap design, *Plast Reconstr Surg* 78:637, 1986.

64. Morain WD: Island toe flaps in neurotrophic ulcers of the foot and ankle, *Ann Plast Surg* 13:1, 1984.

65. Colen LB, Buncke HJ: Neurovascular island flaps from the plantar vessels and nerves for foot reconstruction, *Ann Plast Surg* 12:327, 1984.

66. Buncke HJ, Colen LB: An island flap from the first web space of the foot to cover plantar ulcers, *Br J Plast Surg* 33:242, 1980.

67. Weiman T, Griffiths GD, Polk HC Jr: Management of diabetic midfoot ulcers, *Ann Surg* 215:627, 1992.

68. Oishi S, Levin S, Pederson W: Microsurgical management of extremity wounds in diabetics with peripheral vascular disease, *Plast Reconstr Surg* 92:485, 1993.

69. Roach J, Macfarlane D: Pioneer amputators for a new age, *Contemp Surg* 35:44, 1989.

70. Grabb W, Argenta L: The lateral calcaneal artery skin flap (the lateral calcaneal artery, lesser saphenous vein and sural nerve skin flap), *Plast Reconstr Surg* 68:723, 1981.

71. Ger R: The management of chronic ulcers of the foot by muscle transposition and skin grafting, *Br J Plast Surg* 29:199, 1976.

72. Hartrampf C, Scheflan M, Bostwick J: The flexor digitorum brevis muscle island pedicle flap: a new dimension in heel reconstruction, *Plast Reconstr Surg* 66:264, 1980.

73. Morrison WA, Crabb DM, O'Brien BM, et al: The instep of the foot as a fasciocutaneous island and as a free flap for heel defects, *Plast Reconstr Surg* 72:56, 1983.

74. Masquelet AC, Beveridge J, Romana MC, Gerber C: The lateral supramalleolar flap, *Plast Reconstr Surg* 81:74, 1988.

75. Griffiths GD, Wieman TJ: Meticulous attention to foot care improves the prognosis in diabetic ulceration of the foot, *Surg Gynecol Obstet* 174:49, 1992.

76. Cianci P, Hunt T: Long-term results of aggressive management of diabetic foot ulcers suggest significant cost effectiveness, *Wound Repair Regen* 5:141, 1997.

77. Gibbons GW, Marcaccio EJ, Burgess AM, et al: Improved quality of diabetic foot care, 1984 vs. 1990: reduced length of stay and costs, insufficient reimbursement, *Arch Surg* 128:576, 1993.

78. Boulton AJ, Meneses P, Ennis WJ: Diabetic foot ulcers: a framework for prevention and care, *Wound Repair Regen* 7:7, 1999.

79. Edmonds ME, Blundell MP, Morris ME, et al: Improved survival of the diabetic foot: the role of a specialized foot clinic, *Q J Med* 60:763, 1986.

80. Sibbald RG, Kensholme A, Carter L: Special foot clinics for patients with diabetes, *J Wound Care* 5:238, 1996.

81. Colen LB: Unpublished data.

82. Colen LB, Reus WF, Sasmor MT: Long-term follow-up of patients undergoing vascular bypass procedures and free tissue transfer for limb salvage, *Plast Reconstr Surg* (submitted).

CHAPTER 34

Lower Extremity Tumors and Reconstruction

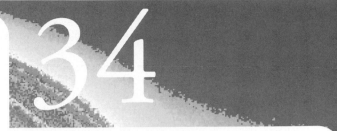

Bernadette H. Wang
Frank J. Frassica
Bernard Chang

INDICATIONS

The most common locations of bone and soft tissue sarcomas are in the lower extremities. Each year in the United States, about 5000 soft tissue sarcomas are diagnosed, less than 1% of the 1.3 million new cancer cases.[4] These sarcomas account for the majority of the neoplastic extremity defects seen by the reconstructive surgeon. The most common histologic types include liposarcoma, malignant fibrous histiocytoma, fibrosarcoma, synovial sarcoma, and rhabdomyosarcoma. Despite differences in tumor biology of each sarcoma, they all pose similar problems of clinical management in terms of resection and reconstruction.[28]

Local recurrence is common after inadequate excision. Sarcomas tend not only to invade the structure of origin, but also to expand centripetally with microinvasion. This effectively compresses normal muscle and fascia at the periphery and produces a pseudocapsule at the margins of the lesion. Because sarcomas demonstrate invasive properties, the pseudocapsule and local neural, vascular, and bony structures may be penetrated by the tumor.

Primary soft tissue sarcomas may be *intracompartmental* (arising within a major anatomic compartment) or *extracompartmental* (within but spreading outside the compartment). The site of the primary lesion in part dictates the potential spread of satellite lesions. In general, major fascial planes serve as a barrier to local invasion of sarcoma. An intracompartmental primary sarcoma can easily spread to any tissue within the anatomic compartment, and satellite lesions typically arise close to the primary lesion. An extracompartmental lesion can spread easily along the fascial planes and exposes all neighboring structures to potential tumor seeding. Subcutaneous lesions usually spread to subcutaneous tissue surrounding the primary sarcoma and also have a greater likelihood of lymphatic involvement.[14,29]

Amputation and disarticulation have traditionally provided local control for soft tissue sarcomas of the lower extremity. This aggressive resection, however, must be weighed against permanent loss of an extremity and still carries the risk of treatment failure secondary to distant metastases.[28] Improvements in diagnostic imaging, advances in adjuvant therapy, and the evolution of microsurgical techniques now make limb-sparing surgery possible in 90% of patients with extremity tumors.[10] Importantly, limb-sparing surgery has not compromised survival or local recurrence rates.[18,26] Furthermore, limb preservation offers potential functional, aesthetic, and psychologic benefits to the patient.

Reconstruction of complex wounds of the lower extremity after tumor extirpation requires a multidisciplinary approach. Specialists in surgical oncology, reconstructive surgery, radiation therapy, chemotherapy, and rehabilitation must coordinate their efforts to improve the patient's overall and disease-free survival and provide optimal functional and aesthetic outcomes.

CLINICAL PRESENTATION

Patients with lower extremity tumors generally present with a slowing enlarging mass. Patients may or may not have pain. Occasionally, patients give a history of sudden onset of a painful mass when hemorrhage into a previously unnoticed lesion occurs. Neurovascular symptoms are rare unless the tumor is located in an area where neurovascular structures can become compressed as the lesion expands, such as the popliteal fossa or femoral triangle. Systemic symptoms also are rare, although a few patients may have fever, malaise, or anemia.

PREOPERATIVE PLANNING

Preoperative planning in the management of lower extremity malignancies is crucial to optimal oncologic and functional outcomes. Radiographic imaging studies not only localize and delineate the extent of the primary tumor (intracompartmental, extracompartmental, or subcutaneous regions), but also show the anatomic relationships among the primary lesion and adjacent bone, blood vessels, and nerves. Biopsy is essential for diagnosis and histologic grading. The need for preoperative and postoperative adjuvant radiation and chemotherapy must be addressed. A structured rehabilitation program and orthoses and assistive devices should be considered preoperatively.

Imaging

Anatomic localization of the tumor must be accomplished before biopsy is undertaken. Routine radiographs usually are obtained but have limited benefit. Magnetic resonance imaging (MRI) provides the most valuable information in assessment of tumor location.[20] Proximity to vascular structures is easily demonstrated, but neural structures other than the sciatic nerve are more difficult to visualize on the MR scan. Satellite lesions can occasionally be seen. The tumor's pseudocapsule often enhances with intravenous contrast.

Technetium bone scans were used more often before the advent of MRI. Cortical bone involvement and periosteal reactions can be defined better with MRI than bone scanning. Angiography may be necessary when computed tomography (CT) and radionuclide imaging do not adequately delineate the lesion's blood supply.

Biopsy

Biopsy for diagnosis and histologic grading is performed only after anatomic localization of the lesion. Ideally the oncologic surgeon should perform the biopsy because placement of the biopsy incision is critical to the definitive surgical resection. Traditionally the incisional biopsy is performed through a longitudinal incision that will not compromise complete excision of the biopsy tract at definitive resection. Strict hemostasis must be achieved because tumor cells may be disbursed along tissue planes within the field of the biopsy hematoma.

INFORMED CONSENT

Informed consent should include the usual surgical risks, including bleeding, infection, scarring, poor wound healing, numbness, and repeat operations, in addition to the risks associated with the location and degree of tumor invasion. These additional risks may include motor nerve injury, vascular injury, flap or tissue loss, and possible amputation if an extremity is involved.

OPERATIONS

Amputation was the primary treatment for extremity sarcomas in the middle of the twentieth century because of their high propensity to infiltrate along tissue planes and spread to tissues far beyond the visible primary lesion. At that time, recurrence rates for limited or even wide excisions ranged from 50% to 90%, whereas local recurrence rates after amputation ranged from 8% to 15%.[10]

In 1958 Bowden and Booher[3] described a limb-sparing surgical approach to extremity sarcomas that addressed local tumor spread. They advocated removing the entire muscle groups surrounding the primary lesion, from origin to insertion. This resulted in a reasonable local recurrence rate of 17% for tumors in the middle of muscle groups, but failure rates were much higher when the primary lesion was near the groin or popliteal fossa.

The addition of radiation and chemotherapy and refinements in their delivery have made wide excision, not compartmental resection, the surgical treatment of choice. At present, local failure rates range from 5% to 20% when wide excision is combined with adjuvant therapy. Amputation is still necessary in certain cases, but its use is now reserved for multicentric or locally recurrent disease.

EXCISION

Marginal excision is the removal of the tumor and pseudocapsule by shelling it from the surrounding tissue. This leaves microscopic tumor and results in local recurrence. Thus marginal excision is not considered therapeutic in the treatment of malignant lower extremity tumors.

Wide local excision is the removal of the tumor with a cuff of normal tissue, usually at least 2 to 5 cm in size, and includes the biopsy tract. *Radical excision* is the complete removal of the major anatomic compartment in which the tumor arises. Wide local excision with adjuvant therapy has local recurrence rates comparable to those of radical compartmental excision. Therefore wide excision is the surgical treatment of choice today.

RECONSTRUCTION

Adequate soft tissue reconstruction is critical to the success of limb preservation in lower extremity tumors. The type of reconstruction is determined by the tumor's size and location, as well as by the adjacent structures that need to be sacrificed with the resection. The surgeon usually can establish the skin, soft tissue, and bony requirements early in the resection. If the oncologic margins are not predictable, delayed reconstruction is advised.

Primary Closure or Skin Grafts

A wide local excision that removes significant muscle bulk through longitudinal incisions can sometimes be closed primarily if subcutaneous dissection preserves the lateral and medial skin flaps. Wide elliptic excisions, radiation changes, or vascularly compromised skin flaps, however, will not allow primary closure with a reproducible degree of success.

Subcutaneous sarcomas treated by wide local excision with underlying fascia and muscle as a deep margin can sometimes be treated with a split-thickness skin graft. When these lesions occur around joints, however, simple skin grafting can compromise joint function. The reconstructive surgeon often confronts wounds for which primary closure with skin grafting is not an option.

Local Flaps

Local flaps using nonirradiated autologous tissues can obliterate dead space after tumor extirpation and provide reliable, expedient wound closure. Local muscle flaps, however, usually provide only limited tissue. Furthermore, blood supply to local flaps may be compromised by preoperative radiation or the tumor resection. In addition, a local muscle flap may lead to some loss of function in an already compromised limb. Also, the risks of spreading the primary tumor theoretically increase with dissection in regional tissue planes.

Free Tissue Transfer

In recent years, advances in free vascularized tissue transfer have offered a broad range of options for reconstruction. Transfer of healthy, well-vascularized, nonirradiated soft tissue can obliterate large dead spaces without skin flap tension and can protect the underlying blood vessels, nerves, and bones. Furthermore, free flaps can withstand adjuvant therapy and the mechanical forces associated with limb use.

In general the principles of free flap reconstruction for lower extremity tumors follow those used in lower extremity trauma (see Chapter 32). Free flaps are indicated for coverage of the following.

1. Neurovascular structures, especially if irradiated
2. Bone stripped of periosteum
3. Allografts or prostheses that cannot be effectively covered by local tissue

In many of these cases, local flaps either cannot reach or cannot cover the entire defect. Furthermore, the blood supply to these local flaps may be sacrificed by tumor resection or compromised by radiation therapy. Depending on design, failure of these local flaps can even result in a higher level of amputation.

Cordeiro et al[9] demonstrated that free tissue transfer for lower extremity reconstruction after oncologic resection has a high success rate that is similar to other free flap applications. They also showed that free flaps permit uninterrupted adjuvant therapy and enhance the efficacy of limb salvage surgery.

Because adjuvant therapy has become an integral part of lower extremity tumor management, use of free flaps must not delay or preclude the use of radiation or chemotherapy. In a study by Evans et al[12] the timing of adjuvant therapy did not influence microvascular transfer, and vice versa. The authors hypothesized that higher doses of irradiation may be used because of the well-vascularized closure, which offered a more stable wound.

In general, postoperative chemotherapy or external radiation therapy can begin once wound healing has progressed to a substantial degree, usually about 3 to 4 weeks after surgery. It has also been demonstrated that free flaps can safely tolerate postoperative brachytherapy, often starting 1 week postoperatively[17,23] (Figure 34-1).

Surgical details, including incisions, design of skin flaps, exposure, and preservation of recipient site vessels, must be planned with the oncologic surgeon. Selection of the free flap donor site is determined primarily by the extent of the defect and the tissue types needed in reconstruction. Defects after resection of lower extremity tumors are often large. Those requiring only soft tissue replacement can generally be covered by a rectus abdominis or latissimus dorsi muscle flap (Figure 34-2). Bony defects can be reconstructed with prostheses and allografts in conjunction with a soft tissue free flap. Alternatively, long bony defects with small soft tissue requirements may be reconstructed with free fibula flaps.

The choice of recipient site vessels is determined primarily by the defect's location and extent. Microvascular anastomoses should be performed outside the immediate zone of resection if possible. Irradiated vessels can be used with caution, but the surgeon should consider using distant vessels, possibly with vein grafts. Free flaps to the distal thigh can easily be anastomosed to the proximal superficial femoral vessels. Anastomoses to the popliteal vessels pose more awkward exposure and positioning problems. In the lower leg the posterial tibial artery and vein are usually the best-caliber vessels.

OUTCOMES

RECURRENCE

Recurrence rates vary with the surgical approach. After marginal resection of gross tumor, the rate of local recurrence is 80% to 90%. After wide excision with margins of at least 2 to 5 cm, the recurrence rate is 20% to 40%.[10] Even after amputation the rate of local recurrence is 5% to 20%.[13] When irradiation is combined with negative surgical margins, the local failure rate drops below 5%.

Despite optimal, limb-sparing multimodality treatment, local recurrence occurs in 10% to 20% of patients with primary extremity sarcoma.[1,5-8,11,15] An early prospective trial from the National Cancer Institute randomized patients with extremity sarcoma to receive either limb-salvage surgery with radiation therapy or amputation. Both groups received postoperative chemotherapy with doxorubicin, cyclophosphamide, and methotrexate. With a follow-up longer than 9 years, five of 27 patients who underwent limb-sparing surgery developed local recurrence, compared with one of 17 patients who had amputations ($p = 0.22$).[26]

Other studies also demonstrated no statistically significant differences in recurrence rates after limb-salvage surgery combined with adjuvant therapy versus amputation.[18] In their

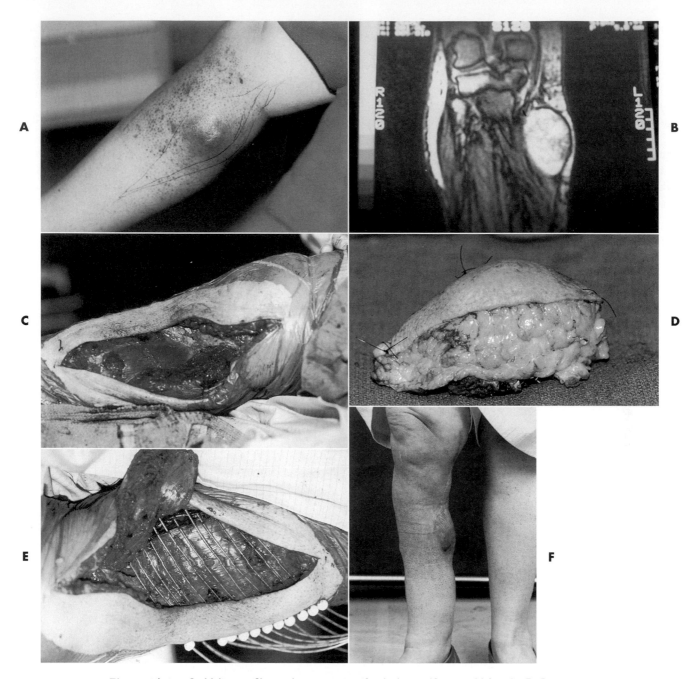

Figure 34-1. A, Malignant fibrous histiocytoma of right leg in 62-year-old female. **B,** Preoperative MRI scan. **C,** Defect after wide resection. **D,** Specimen. **E,** Tube placement for brachytherapy. **F,** Six months after medial gastrocnemius muscle rotation flap and split-thickness skin flap.

series of 911 patients treated for primary extremity sarcoma, Lewis et al[19] found that local recurrence was strongly associated with the development of subsequent metastasis and tumor mortality.

FUNCTIONAL OUTCOME

The patient can have a functional, pain-free limb after limb-salvage surgery for lower extremity tumors. A comprehensive rehabilitation program, however, is critical to the

successful outcome. Restoring and maintaining the integrity of the involved extremity reduce perioperative morbidity and facilitate early return to function.

Few studies specifically address the functional outcome of limb salvage in patients with lower extremity tumors. Weinberg et al[32] analyzed 26 patients who underwent limb-sparing procedures for tumors around the knee. Their functional evaluations revealed good function in the group as a whole. Evans et al[12] reported on 22 patients who underwent limb-sparing surgery and free flap reconstruction. All these patients could ambulate postoperatively except one, who had

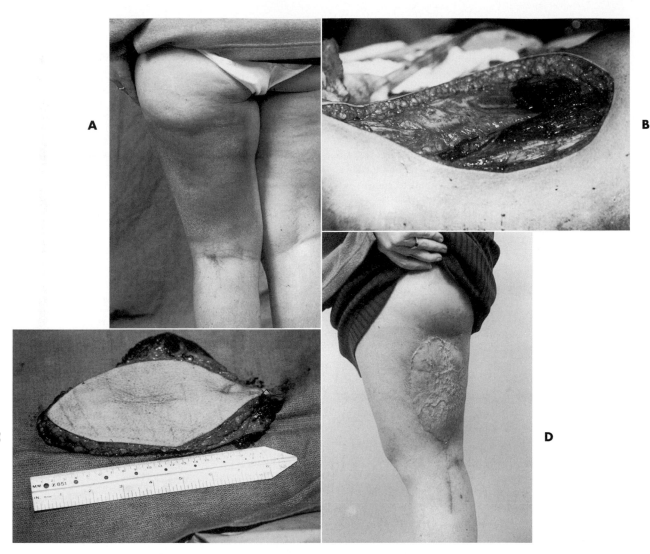

Figure 34-2. **A,** Liposarcoma of left posterior thigh in 38-year-old female. **B,** Defect after resection. **C,** Specimen. **D,** Eight months after latissimus dorsi free flap and split-thickness skin flap.

a local recurrence. In a series from Heiner et al,[16] nine of 10 patients who had limb-sparing surgery returned to their preoperative jobs.

COMPLICATIONS

Although local control and survival after limb-salvage surgery are comparable to those after primary amputation, wound healing complications can be more problematic in limb-sparing procedures. Achieving a stable wound is important because postoperative wound complications are associated with a poorer functional outcome.[2] Furthermore, postoperative wound healing complications may lead to subsequent amputation. In a study of 73 patients who had limb-sparing surgery for osteosarcoma of the femur, 10 patients underwent amputation after developing a local wound complication.[30]

Oncologic surgeons have long been aware of the increased likelihood of wound healing problems after resection of large, malignant extremity tumors because of the large dissection required, the resultant dead space, and the compromised circulation of remaining skin flaps. Peat et al[24] reported a 16% wound healing complication rate in 137 patients treated with local or primary direct wound closure. They identified preoperative irradiation and specimen resection diameter as risk factors for wound complications. Furthermore, patients with thigh sarcomas were at higher risk if ligation of the profunda femoris artery was necessary. With local or primary wound closure, infection rates as high as 10% to 15% have been reported.[27]

Despite improving local control, adjuvant therapy has been well documented to delay wound healing and increase the complication rate in patients treated with local or primary closure.[12] McDonald et al[21] reported an 8% increase in wound complications for patients treated with chemotherapy after limb-salvage surgery for bone tumors. Ormsby et al[22] reported increased wound complication rates of 48% and 14% in patients with soft tissue sarcomas treated with wide excision, primary closure, and brachytherapy starting either before or after postoperative day 5, respectively.

Lower extremity reconstruction using a well-vascularized flap from a distant site offers a more stable wound and tends to have less wound healing complications. Thus the need for adjuvant therapy often influences the selection of free tissue transfer as the method of reconstruction.

Cordeiro et al[9] reported only one of 57 patients with prolonged wound healing after free flap reconstruction of lower extremity sarcomas treated with limb-salvage surgery and adjuvant therapy. Evans et al[12] showed that adjuvant therapy did not increase the complication rate for free tissue transfer in the lower extremity. In addition, Hildalgo and Carrasquillo[17] and Panchal et al[23] demonstrated that brachytherapy can be delivered in the early postoperative period after free flap reconstruction without an increase in wound breakdown.

These series and others demonstrate that free flaps enhance the efficacy of limb-salvage surgery and provide reliable reconstruction for extremity tumors, with greater than 95% flap success rates.[16]

QUALITY OF LIFE

Although most health indices used in outcome-oriented clinical research focus on physical function, an evolving part of outcome analysis focuses on quality-of-life assessments. Unfortunately, quality of life is difficult to define and even more difficult to assess using standardized methods. The measure of quality of life is a dynamic process that requires periodic evaluations of psychosocial, economic, and global well-being factors.

Long-term effects, such as repeated hospitalizations, time lost from work, increased interpersonal stress, and financial burdens, can have a significant impact on an individual's quality of life over time. Future long-term outcome studies that assess quality-of-life issues may better elucidate the patient's overall experience.

Yasko et al[33] summarized the majority of the studies that analyzed quality-of-life issues in patients with extremity tumors. Weddington et al[31] evaluated 35 patients treated for extremity sarcoma by either limb-sparing surgery or amputation. Their assessment included comprehensive quality-of-life measures using the cognitive capacity screening examination, the Hopkins symptom check list, the Beck depression inventory, the profile of mood states scale, the Karnofsky performance scale, global adjustment to illness scale, and the schedule for affective disorders. Both the patients who underwent amputation and those who had limb-salvage surgery scored similarly with respect to mood, cognition, body image, global physical functioning, global adjustment to illness, and lifetime prevalence for psychiatric disorders.

Posma et al[25] evaluated 33-patients who underwent either amputation or limb-salvage surgery for extremity bone sarcomas. Quality-of-life assessments included self-report questionnaires, interviews, and visual analog scales for psychoneurotic and somatic distress, activities of daily living, self-esteem, and adjustment to illness. Amputees reported more problems with self-esteem and socialization, whereas limb-salvage patients cited more physical complaints.

REFERENCES

1. Barr LC, Stotter AT, A'Hern RP: Influence of local recurrence on survival: a controversy reviewed from the perspective of soft tissue sarcoma, *Br J Surg* 78:648-650, 1991.

2. Bell RS, O'Sullivan B, Davis A, et al: Functional outcome in patients treated with surgery and irradiation for soft tissue tumors, *J Surg Oncol* 48:224, 1991.

3. Bowden L, Booher RJ: The principles and techniques of resection of soft parts for sarcoma, *Surgery* 44:963-977, 1958.

4. Brennan MF: Management of extremity soft-tissue sarcoma, *Am J Surg* 158:71-78, 1989.

5. Brennan MF, Casper ES, Harrison LB, et al: The role of multimodality therapy in soft-tissue sarcoma, *Ann Surg* 214:328-336, 1991.

6. Brennan MF, Hilaris B, Shiu MH, et al: Local recurrence in adult soft tissue sarcoma: a randomized trial of brachytherapy, *Arch Surg* 122:1289-1293, 1987.

7. Choong PF, Gustafson P, Willen H, et al: Prognosis following locally recurrent soft-tissue sarcoma: a staging system based on primary and recurrent tumour characteristics, *Int J Cancer* 60:33-37, 1995.

8. Collin CF, Friedrich C, Godbold J, et al: Prognostic factors for local recurrence and survival in patients with localized extremity soft tissue sarcoma, *Semin Surg Oncol* 4:30-37, 1988.

9. Cordeiro PG, Neves RI, Hidalgo DA: The role of free tissue transfer following oncologic resection in the lower extremity, *Ann Plast Surg* 33:9-16, 1994.

10. Drake DB: Reconstruction for limb-sparing procedures in soft-tissue sarcomas of the extremities, *Clin Plast Surg* 22:123-128, 1995.

11. Emrich LJ, Ruka W, Driscoll DL, et al: The effect of local recurrence on survival time in adult high-grade soft tissue sarcoma, *J Clin Epidemiol* 42:105-110, 1989.

12. Evans GR, Black JJ, Robb GL, et al: Adjuvant therapy: the effects on microvascular lower extremity reconstruction, *Ann Plast Surg* 39:141-144, 1997.

13. Fine G, Ohorodnik JM, Horn RC Jr, et al: Soft tissue sarcomas: their clinical behavior and course and influencing factors. In *Seventh National Cancer Center Conference proceedings*, Philadelphia, 1973, Lippincott.

14. Frassica FJ, Thompson RC: Evaluation, diagnosis, and classification of benign soft-tissue tumors, *J Bone Joint Surg* 78A:126-140, 1996.

15. Gustafson P, Dreinhofer KE, Rydholm A: Metastasis-free survival after local recurrence of soft-tissue sarcoma, *J Bone Joint Surg* 75A:658-660, 1993.

16. Heiner J, Rao V, Mott W: Immediate free tissue transfer for distal musculoskeletal neoplasms, *Ann Plast Surg* 30:140-146, 1993.

17. Hidalgo DA, Carrasquillo IM: The treatment of lower extremity sarcomas with wide excision, radiotherapy and free flap reconstruction, *Plast Reconstr Surg* 89:96-101, 1992.

18. Karakousis CP, Emrich LF, Rao U, et al: Feasibility of limb salvage and survival in soft tissue sarcomas, *Cancer* 57:484-491, 1986.

19. Lewis JJ, Leung D, Heslin M, et al: Association of local recurrence with subsequent survival in extremity soft tissue sarcoma, *J Clin Oncol* 15:646-652, 1997.

20. Ma LD, Frassica FJ, McCarthy EF, et al: Benign and malignant musculoskeletal masses: MR imaging differentiation with rim-to-center differential enhancement ratios, *Radiology* 202:739-744, 1997.

21. McDonald DJ, Capanna R, Gherlinzoni F, et al: Influence of chemotherapy on perioperative complications in limb salvage surgery for bone tumors, *Cancer* 65:1509-1516, 1990.

22. Ormsby MV, Hilaris BS, Nori D, et al: Wound complications of adjuvant radiation therapy in patients with soft-tissue sarcomas, *Ann Surg* 210:93-99, 1989.

23. Panchal JI, Agrawal RK, McLean NR, et al: Early postoperative brachytherapy following free flap reconstruction, *Br J Plast Surg* 46:511-515, 1993.

24. Peat BG, Bell RS, Davis A, et al: Wound-healing complications after soft-tissue sarcoma surgery, *Plast Reconstr Surg* 93:980-987, 1994.

25. Postma A, Kingma A, De Ruiter J, et al: Quality of life in bone tumor patients comparing limb salvage and amputation of the lower extremity, *J Surg Oncol* 51:47-51, 1992.

26. Rosenberg SA, Tepper J, Glatstein E, et al: The treatment of soft-tissue sarcoma of the extremities, *Ann Surg* 196:305-315, 1982.

27. Saddegh MK, Bauer HCF: Wound complication in surgery of soft tissue sarcoma: analysis of 103 consecutive patients managed without adjuvant therapy, *Clin Orthop* 289:247-253, 1993.

28. Shiu MH, Castro EB, Hajdu SI, et al: Surgical treatment of 297 soft-tissue sarcomas of the lower extremity, *Ann Surg* 182:597-602, 1975.

29. Sim FH, Frassica FJ, Frassica DA: Soft-tissue tumors: diagnosis, evaluation, and management, *J Am Acad Orthop Surg* 2:202-211, 1994.

30. Simon MA, Aschliman MA, Thomas N, et al: Limb-salvage treatment versus amputation for osteosarcoma of the distal end of the femur, *J Bone Joint Surg* 68A:1331, 1986.

31. Weddington WW JR, Segraves KB, Simon MA: Psychological outcome of extremity sarcoma survivors undergoing amputation of limb salvage, *J Clin Oncol* 3:1393-1399, 1985.

32. Weinberg H, Kenan S, Lewis M, et al: The role of microvascular surgery in limb-sparing procedures for malignant tumors of the knee, *Plast Reconstr Surg* 92:692-698, 1993.

33. Yasko AW, Reece GP, Gillis TA, et al: Limb-salvage strategies to optimize quality of life: the MD Anderson Cancer Center experience, *CA* 47:226-238, 1997.

Reconstruction of Genitourinary Anomalies

Charles E. Horton
Charles E. Horton, Jr.

Plastic surgical reconstruction is appropriate for many genital deformities, both congenital and acquired. This chapter reviews the most frequently encountered genitourinary anomalies, including hypospadias, epispadias, Peyronie's disease, lymphedema, and vaginal agenesis. We also discuss conditions that may be appropriate for elective reconstruction, such as phalloplasty after trauma or in gender dysphoria.

HYPOSPADIAS

Hypospadias is a congenital anomaly of the penis and urethra that affects approximately one in 350 males. In hypospadias the urethra does not develop completely and opens on the underside of the penis, in the scrotum, or occasionally in the perineum. Interestingly, reports suggest that both the incidence and the severity of hypospadias may be increasing.[11] The more severe variants of hypospadias are usually associated with *chordee,* or a downward curvature of the penile shaft. The prepuce is usually abnormally developed as well, with a dorsal hood of foreskin covering the top of the glans but absent ventrally.

Hypospadias may affect both urinary and sexual functioning of the penis. When the urethral meatus opens ventrally, micturition is affected, and the urinary stream is directed downward rather than straight ahead, making it difficult for these males to stand while voiding. In general, hypospadias is not associated with internal anomalies of the urinary tract, with no increased risk of urinary tract infections. Sexual intercourse may be difficult because of the small size and downward curvature of some hypospadiac penises. In severe cases, fertility can be impaired.

Fortunately, about two thirds of all hypospadias cases constitute minor variants of the condition, with the urethral meatus opening on the distal shaft or glans. Functional impairment is minimal in these patients; however, because of the unique psychosexual aspects of the penis, issues related to body image, self esteem, and psychologic development are significant considerations.[1]

Given the high success and low morbidity of modern surgical techniques, we strongly believe that all but the most trivial cases of hypospadias should be repaired. When successfully completed between age 6 and 18 months, hypospadias surgery gives a boy the opportunity to grow and develop normally with no knowledge of ever having had a genital abnormality.

Operations

The first recorded hypospadias surgery consisted of penile amputation distal to the existing meatus (Heliodorus and Antyllus, AD 100 to 200). In the 1800s a plethora of multistaged procedures were devised for severe hypospadias. Because of the potential for catastrophic complications, mild and moderate hypospadias cases were not even addressed. In general the first-stage operation was designed to straighten the penis, with later stages planned to transfer skin and complete the urethroplasty. Such a series of procedures required years to complete, and as mentioned, complications occurred frequently and were severe. The modern age of hypospadias surgery began in the late 1950s with the advent of reliable, single-stage procedures for simultaneous correction of hypospadias and chordee.

Literally hundreds of different operations have been described for hypospadias repair, and the surgeon cannot become familiar with all of them. Often, multiple techniques are equally successful for repair of any given form of hypospadias. Correction of all forms of hypospadias can be achieved using a variation of the following six recommended techniques[7]:
1. Meatal advancement and glansplasty (MAGPI)
2. Urethral advancement
3. Tubularized incised plate (TIP) urethroplasty
4. Flip-flap urethroplasty
5. Full-thickness graft urethroplasty
6. Preputial flap urethroplasty

MEATAL ADVANCEMENT AND GLANSPLASTY. The MAGPI procedure is useful only for true glanular hypospadias (Figure 35-1, *A*). Although it has the advantage of simplicity, in our experience, when the MAGPI technique is inappropriately used for a subcoronal meatus, the result is often a retrusive and unacceptable meatal position.

The MAGPI technique involves a vertical incision of the transverse mucosal bar just distal to the hypospadiac meatus. This incision is closed transversely, thus advancing the dorsal lip of the meatal mucosa out toward the tip of the glans. Glansplasty is achieved by midline approximation of lateral glanular wings, which first are freed from the corporal tunica.

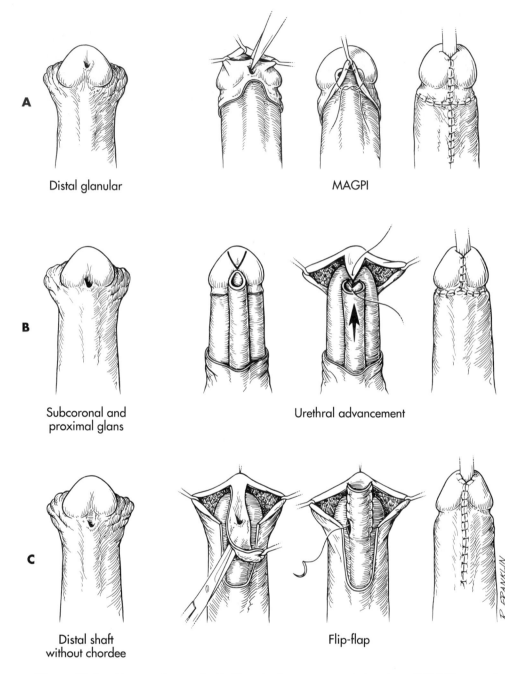

Figure 35-1. Hypospadias repair. **A,** Meatal advancement and glansplasty (MAGPI) procedure. **B,** Urethral advancement. **C,** Flip-flap urethroplasty. *Continued*

Closure of the glans flaps effectively moves the urethral meatus out toward the glans tip. It is important to close the glans securely in two layers to support the urethra. Excessive preputial skin is resected.

Because the MAGPI procedure is relatively easy, it lends itself to overuse. It achieves no effective urethral lengthening and does not correct any element of chordee; it simply transfers the position of the meatus and wraps glans tissue behind it.

URETHRAL ADVANCEMENT. For subcoronal or distal shaft hypospadias, in which a well-formed urethra and corpus spongiosum are present distally, urethral advancement is an effective method of treatment (Figure 35-1, *B*). The penis is degloved with a circumcising incision. The urethra and corpus spongiosum are mobilized proximally, well down into the penoscrotal level. This generally affords sufficient mobility so that the urethra and corpus spongiosum can be advanced out to the tip of the penis.

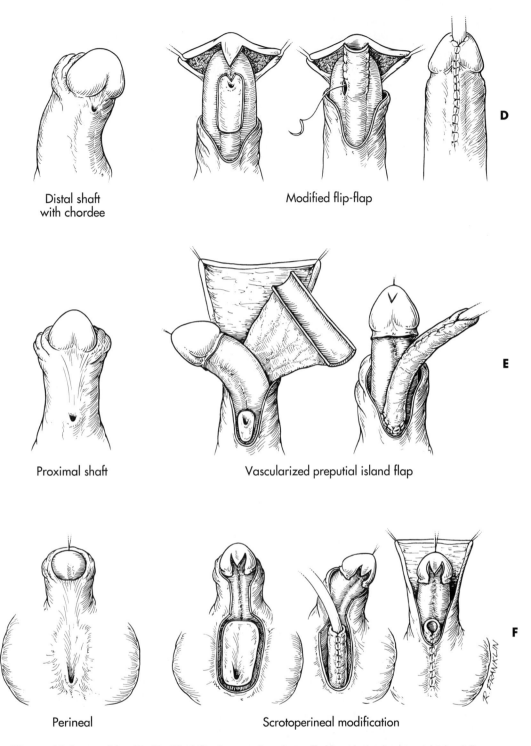

Distal shaft
with chordee

Modified flip-flap

D

Proximal shaft

Vascularized preputial island flap

E

Perineal

Scrotoperineal modification

F

Figure 35-1, cont'd. **D,** Modified flip-flap urethroplasty. **E,** Vascularized preputial island flap. **F,** Scrotoperineal modification.

This technique takes advantage of the urethra's elasticity. The glans is split in the midline, and lateral glans wings are mobilized and closed over the urethra. To avoid the development of meatal stenosis, a triangular flap of glans tissue is inserted into the circular meatal opening. Alternately, a tunnel can be made in the glans, a core of tissue excised, and the urethra advanced through the center of the glans. The advanced meatus is sutured to the glans skin at the tip.

Because this operation avoids urethral reconstruction, no fistula formation should occur. Excess tension on the advanced urethra can cause chordee and must be avoided.

TUBULARIZED INCISED PLATE URETHROPLASTY. In distal shaft and midshaft hypospadias, when the urethral groove is wide and deep, the TIP repair, reported by Snodgrass[13] in 1995, is a useful technique. It represents a modification of the standard Thiersch-Duplay urethroplasty and simply tubularizes the urethral plate in situ.

To address the concern of inadequate urethral width, a longitudinal incision is made through the midline epithelium of the urethral plate, extending from the hypospadiac meatus out to the end of the glans. This incision allows the urethral plate to hinge and be tubularized over a no. 8 or 10 French urethral stent without tension. A deepithelialized subcutaneous flap of dorsal prepuce is mobilized and rotated ventrally to cover the urethroplasty. Finally, glans wings are closed over the urethroplasty in the midline.

In our experience the TIP repair produces a normal-appearing, vertically oriented slit similar to urethral meatus.

FLIP-FLAP URETHROPLASTY. If there is no chordee and the meatal opening is adequate, and if the urethral plate is flat and narrow and does not seem to lend itself to tubularization, we recommend a flip-flap repair (Figure 35-1, *C* and *D*). Parallel incisions on each side of the lateral plate out to the tip of the glans form the dorsal urethral wall. The meatal-based flip-flap of ventral shaft skin makes up the ventral wall. After extension of the meatus onto the tip of the glans, lateral glans wings are approximated over the flip-flap urethroplasty.

PREPUTIAL SKIN FLAPS. If the meatus is too proximal for either a TIP or a flip-flap technique and in all patients with significant chordee, a neourethra must be made using either vascularized preputial flaps or free preputial skin grafts (Figure 35-1, *E*). After degloving the penis and excision of all dysgenetic spongiosal tissue tethering the penis and causing chordee, a meatotomy is made in the existing urethral meatus. When the distal hypospadiac urethra is thin and hypoplastic, the urethra should be mobilized proximally back to good-quality tissue surrounded by spongiosum.

If a free skin graft repair is chosen, in an uncircumcised patient the skin for the neourethra is harvested from the prepuce. The graft is tubularized over an appropriately sized stent, usually no. 10, and a tongue-and-groove anastomosis to the hypospadiac meatus is made using a 7-0 Polydioxanone suture. The neourethra is anchored to the tunica along its course to the glans. Lateral glans flaps are once again used to cover the distal urethra and place the meatus at the tip of the glans. Well-vascularized subcutaneous tissue mobilized from the dorsal prepuce is rotated ventrally and closed as a separate layer over the graft.

As an alternative to splitting the glans, the neourethra can be tunneled and brought out of a central cored area of glans and united with a V-shaped flap of glans at the tip.

An equally acceptable technique for proximal hypospadias entails use of a vascularized preputial flap for urethroplasty. A carefully planned flap can be raised successfully on a dartos pedicle and can be tubularized and transposed to the ventral portion of the penis, where it is anasatomosed as described for the free skin graft neourethra. Torsion of the penis and devascularization of the dorsal penile shaft skin are potential complications unique to this procedure.

A useful variation of the preputial island flap is the *onlay technique,* which preserves the existing urethral plate. The vascularized preputial island flap is sutured onto the urethral plate as a patch, thereby avoiding a circumferential anastomo-sis and decreasing the risk for development of stenosis. With this method if there is chordee, dorsal plication of the tunica albuginea is used to straighten the penis. The onlay flap, compared with tubed flaps or grafts, may decrease the incidence of urethral strictures or meatal stenosis.

In reoperative cases, preputial skin may not be available. Many alternatives have been advocated for these complex situations. In the search for reliable, hairless material, full-thickness extra genital skin, bladder, and oral mucosa have all been used. We have found full-thickness hairless skin harvested from the inguinal area to be the tissue of choice. Bladder mucosal harvesting incurs the risks of cystotomy and is subject to epithelial proliferation at the meatus. More recently, buccal mucosa grafts have been used with favorable results.[2]

SCROTOPERINEAL MODIFICATION. In scrotal and perineal cases, a slight modification is occasionally useful (Figure 35-1, *F*). The proximal urethra may be constructed using the hairless midline scrotal skin that usually surrounds the hypospadiac meatus. A Thiersch type of incision is made, and the scrotal skin is tubed to the base of the penis, converting the perineal hypospadiac meatus to a proximal shaft position. The scrotal skin tube is then anastomosed to either a free skin graft or a vascularized preputial island flap to complete the repair.

SKIN COVERAGE. After a neourethral reconstruction, the final step in hypospadias repair is achieving ventral skin coverage. Most hypospadias repairs require the transfer of the remaining dorsal prepuce to the ventral surface of the penis. Although a variety of methods have been described, we prefer to split the dorsal preputial skin in the midline and redistribute the halves to the ventral surface (Byars flaps). The flaps are approximated in the midline to simulate the median raphe or in a gentle "5" shape. In the absence of preputial skin an appropriate amount of shaft skin can be transferred ventrally from the dorsum of the penis. The dorsal donor site is then covered by a full-thickness skin graft.

Postoperative Care

After all hypospadias surgery, consistent postoperative care is imperative for a good result. Most hypospadias surgeries are now done on an outpatient basis. The penis is dressed in a transparent, semipermeable, bolstered adhesive dressing, which allows for inspection of the flaps, maintenance of shape, and minimization of edema.

Urinary diversion is used in all patients except when the MAGPI or a urethral advancement operation is used. Young boys who are not toilet trained simply have a silicone stent passed through the repair and up into the bladder to serve as a "drippy tube" to drain into a double diaper. For older patients, we recommend a no. 10 or 12 silicone tube placed through the urethra 2 to 3 cm (1 inch) proximal to the urethroplasty. The patient then voids through the stent. We rarely employ suprapubic diversion. Catheters are usually left in place for 5 to 7 days.

Outcomes

The success rate of primary one-stage surgery for hypospadias is approximately 90%. With modern surgery the glans will grow normally, with predictable sexual activity. The appearance of the penis is within normal limits, with minimal visible scarring.

EPISPADIAS

Epispadias is a severe congenital anomaly of the penis that usually occurs in combination with bladder exstrophy. Although it is often considered the counterpart of hypospadias, with the urethral opening on the dorsal aspect of the penis rather than on the ventral aspect, epispadias tends to be a more serious defect than hypospadias and can be much more challenging to correct surgically. Fortunately, epispadias occurs rarely, one in 30,000 males.

Epispadias is part of a spectrum representing incomplete development of various components of the dorsal aspect of the penis and bladder. Most often, epispadias occurs as one part of the bladder-exstrophy-epispadias complex. It can also occur, however, as an isolated penile defect with no bladder abnormality.

Epispadias is classified as *glanular, penile,* or *penopubic,* depending on the location of the urethral opening. In complete epispadias seen with bladder exstrophy, the anterior urethral cleft extends through the urinary sphincter mechanism, resulting in total urinary incontinence.

The care of these patients is complex; they require bladder neck reconstruction to achieve continence and penile reconstruction for the epispadias.

The anatomy of epispadias includes a penis that is usually short, wide, and stubby with an abnormally flat and cleft glans. The crural attachments of the penis to the pubic bones are widely separated because there is lateral diastasis and outward rotation of the pubic bones. The rectus muscles, which insert on divergent pelvic bones, are also laterally displaced; often a midline fascial defect is present. The corporal bodies remain separate throughout the length of the epispadiac penis. The prominent urethral groove opens dorsally. In severe cases the ejaculatory ducts may be exposed.

With the exstrophy-epispadias complex, the anterior urethral cleft extends to the exstrophic bladder, where the trigone, urethral orifices, and posterior bladder wall are exposed. Typically the patient has profound dorsal curvature of the penis caused by shortening of the urethral plate and underlying disgenetic tissue. The prepuce is redundant ventrally and deficient dorsally.

Operations

The essential elements of successful repair of epispadias include the following:

1. Penile lengthening
2. Correction of dorsal chordee
3. Urethroplasty
4. Penile skin coverage

YOUNG TECHNIQUE. Traditionally the mainstay of primary epispadias repair has been the *modified Young urethroplasty.* This technique relies on the Thiersch-Duplay concept of creating a longitudinal mucosal strip in the shape of a tube to form the neourethra.

The Young urethroplasty requires that sufficient penile skin exist, both to construct the new urethra and to cover the penile shaft. Often, tissue is insufficient to accomplish both adequately. In addition, the Young technique does not provide good exposure to the base of the corpora bodies, where the corpora are attached to the pubic bones. To provide true lengthening of the penis, the corpora must be partially detached from the pubic bones.

For these reasons, we use the Young repair only for distal, mild forms of epispadias.

CANTWELL-RANSLEY TECHNIQUE. Our preferred method for primary epispadias repair is an adaptation of the Cantwell-Ransley technique.[4] We often have found it helpful to stimulate the size of these very small penises preoperatively by administering testosterone enanthate at a dosage of 3 mg/kg intramuscularly 5 weeks and 2 weeks before surgery.

The repair begins with a ventral circumcising incision, degloving the shaft down to the base. The urethral plate is outlined with lateral incisions. The urethral plate is subsequently tubularized; if adequate width for tubularization without tension is a concern, the epithelium of the urethral plate can be incised to allow it to hinge. Typically in epispadias, the end of the urethral plate has a dorsal orientation that must be advanced by making a vertical incision in the midline at the tip of the urethral plate and closing it horizontally in a Heineke-Mikulicz fashion. During degloving of the ventral skin, care should be taken to preserve the central mesentery of vascular tissue, which runs dorsally and provides blood supply to the urethral plate.

The urethral plate is approached and mobilized from below. The urethral plate can be mobilized off the underlying corporal bodies, maintaining its vascularity. After the urethral plate has been elevated from the corporal bodies, an artificial erection is obtained and usually demonstrates significant dorsal curvature. In this case, corporotomy incisions through the dorsal tunica are made in the area of maximal curvature. A small dermal graft can be placed into the resulting tunica defect to augment the length of the dorsal corporal bodies. This may require immobilization of the neurovascular bundles.

Occasionally the urethral plate must be divided and a full-thickness graft or flap used to build a larger urethra. The urethral plate is then tubularized over a silicone catheter. The tubularized neourethra is routed ventrally, and the corpora are closed together above it. The glans is then closed. The shaft of the penis is covered with skin, usually available from the unrolled ventral prepuce, which is split in the midline and rotated dorsally. The urethral stent is left in place as a "drippy" catheter for 10 to 12 days.

The advantage of this repair is that it usually allows for preservation of the urethral plate while providing exposure to underlying corporal bodies for correction of the dorsal chordee inherent in epispadias. Rerouting of the reconstructed urethra to its more normal position on the underside of the corporal bodies helps in correcting curvature.

SECONDARY EPISPADIAS: W-FLAP TECHNIQUE. Because of the difficulties inherent with primary epispadias repair, many older patients require additional surgery after puberty. Typically the main issue is persistent debilitating dorsal chordee, along with overall inadequate penile length. This is usually attributed to persistent chordee that restricts growth of the dorsal tunica albuginea. These secondary epispadias cases must be approached with systematic and comprehensive dissection that completely releases and straightens the penis, allowing it to dangle in a dependent manner.[15]

Our approach begins with a W-shaped incision to produce bilateral, superiorly based groin flaps, with the apex of each flap extending below the penoscrotal junction on each side. These W flaps are carefully elevated with abundant subcutaneous tissue attached. In the midline of the incision, unsightly penopubic and lower abdominal scarring, often from previous surgeries, may be excised. The W flaps serve the following purposes:

1. They provide excellent exposure to the base of the penis, where dissection must be done to achieve adequate penile lengthening.
2. When closed in the midline, they normalize the appearance of the escutcheon by transposing the laterally and inferiorly displaced hair-bearing skin to a more normal position.
3. They add healthy skin at the base of the penis, where skin is often deficient.

Additional exposure of the corporal bodies is accomplished through a dorsal midline skin excision extended distally to meet a standard circumcising incision just proximal to the coronal sulcus. Multiple artificial erections are administered during this dissection. After mobilization of the skin, persistent dorsal chordee usually results from tethering due to inadequate urethral length, which causes a "bowstring" effect. In this case the urethra is divided distally and mobilized off the underlying corporal bodies. This provides exposure to allow removal of underlying disgenetic tissues and scar tissues, which also may contribute to chordee.

After transection of the urethra, if artificial erection demonstrates persistent chordee, a dermal graft is used to augment the length of the dorsal tunica albuginea of each corporal body. A transverse corporotomy incision is made through the tunica albuginea, and a small elliptic-shaped dermal graft is harvested from a hairless area of groin skin and placed into the tunica

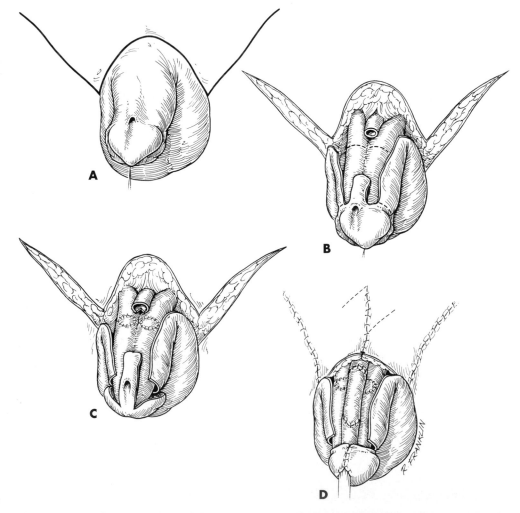

Figure 35-2. Epispadias repair. **A,** Preoperative view. **B,** W-shaped flaps for exposure excision of dorsal skin scar. **C,** Chordee still demonstrated, indicating tunica is short on dorsal surface. Incisions are made in tunica and dermal grafts used to repair it. **D,** W-flaps advanced superiorly to add skin. Full-thickness graft used to build urethra. Penile skin defect covered with reverse Byars flaps.

defect. In our experience, placement of dorsal dermal grafts has resulted in complete correction of chordee and dangling of the shaft in virtually all patients with secondary epispadias. Additional dissection in the penopubic area to mobilize the corporal bodies partly off the pubic bones can result in additional penile length.

After the penis has been completely released and straightened, attention turns to performing a urethroplasty. We usually construct the neourethra using a full-thickness skin graft or flap. Ideally the penile repair is covered by local skin flaps. Reverse Byars flaps can be made by dividing the ventral prepuce in the midline and rotating the skin to the dorsum of the penis. The **W** groin flaps arc closed by rotating them together in the midline. A small suction drain is left under these flaps for 48 hours. A urethral catheter is placed through the repair and left in position for 2 weeks (Figures 35-2 and 35-3).

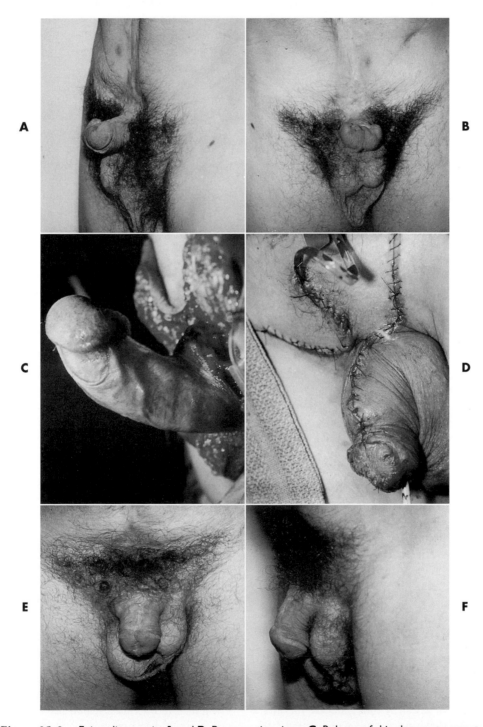

Figure 35-3. Epispadias repair. **A** and **B,** Preoperative views. **C,** Release of skin does not correct chordee. **D,** W-flaps closed, with dermal grafts to tunica and skin closure. **E** and **F,** Postoperative views.

Outcomes

One-stage repair of epispadias is successful in about 90% of all cases. Patients with more severe anomalies can have postoperative complications of fistula, stenosis, and urinary stream spraying. Previous operations have caused severe functional and cosmetic deficits. These problems can be corrected with urethroplasty, skin shifting, and dermal grafts to correct tunica disproportion.

Data on the incidence of complications and functional and aesthetic deficits are scarce. Outcomes studies in these areas would be valuable.

PEYRONIE'S DISEASE

Peyronie's disease is a connective tissue disorder of the penis affecting an estimated 1% of the adult male population. It is primarily seen in the 40- to 60-year-old age group, although we have seen it develop in younger as well as older individuals. The hallmarks of Peyronie's disease include painful erections, penile curvature during erection, and a firm palpable nodule or inelastic plaque on the penile shaft. This condition was first reported in 1743 by François de la Peyronie, who described a patient who "had Rosary beads of scar tissue causing an upward curvature of the penis during erection."

Approximately 10% of patients with Peyronie's disease also have Dupuytren's contracture of the palmar fascia. This has led to speculation that Peyronie's disease may be one component of an overall autoimmune or connective tissue type of disorder. More recent speculation regarding the etiology of Peyronie's disease has centered on the effects of acute or repetitive trauma, which may result simply from normal sexual functioning. Even minimal repetitive trauma to the erect penis during normal sexual intercourse can result in microvascular injury at the dorsal attachment of the intracorporal septum and tunica albuginea. This may lead to fibroblast activation with fibrin deposition, inflammation, and subsequent plaque formation. Most frequently the plaque is on the dorsal midline of the penis. Patients typically complain of curvature either upward or to the left side and only rarely to the right.

After the initial onset of symptoms the natural history of this condition typically progresses through a 1- to 2-year inflammatory phase, during which the penile plaque and degree of curvature may worsen. Eventually, however, the plaque tends to stabilize, and any pain often abates. Once a Peyronie's plaque has become established, no medication is effective in eradicating it.

Vitamin E therapy may help patients during the inflammatory phase of the condition. In our patients, Potaba (aminobenzoate potassium) has been ineffective. Erectile dysfunction with Peyronie's disease occurs in approximately 15% of patients.

Evaluation of patients with Peyronie's disease includes a thorough medical and sexual history, along with physical examination. Polaroid photographs demonstrating the curvature can be helpful. All patients undergo a penile Doppler ultrasound evaluation with a pharmacologic erection using intracavernous injection of vasoactive substances. The penile ultrasound study demonstrates penile vascular anatomy and allows identification of individuals who may have preexisting venoocclusive disorders. It also demonstrates the patient's capacity to maintain and sustain a rigid erection and accurately delineates the area of maximum penile shaft curvature.

In men with mild Peyronie's disease who remain sexually functional, we discourage surgery. In patients who are sexually disabled by their Peyronie's disease, however, we consider three surgical options. Most men with Peyronie's disease are not impotent, and we suggest placement of a penile prosthesis only in those 15% of patients who have complete erectile impotence along with their Peyronie's disease. In men with adequate erectile ability, we consider either a plication procedure or a procedure consisting of excision of the Peyronie's plaque and reconstruction of the corporal bodies with a dermal graft.

A plication procedure is a good option in a man who has only minimal penile curvature (approximately 30 to 45 degrees) and a reasonably long erect penis. If the plaque is extensive and the amount of curvature greater than 45 degrees, however, plication procedures do not yield optimal results. In these patients we have found excision of the plaque along with dermal graft reconstruction of the corporal bodies to be a better technique. Overall, we do more dermal graft than plication procedures.[3]

Our technique of penile plication involves a circumcising incision with degloving of the penile shaft down to the base (Figure 35-4). An artificial erection is then obtained, and the area of maximum curvature is marked. The tunica albuginea opposite the area of maximum curvature is identified. An ellipse is excised from each corporal body, typically measuring 2 mm in width and 0.5 to 1 cm in length. The resulting tunica defects are closed primarily. The artificial erection is then repeated, and if necessary, additional ellipses can be excised until complete straightening has been achieved. This procedure has the disadvantage of slightly shortening the penis.

The dermal graft procedure also involves a circumcising skin incision and complete degloving of the penile shaft down to the base. Incisions are then made through Buck's fascia covering the lateral aspect of each corpus. Circumferential emissary penile veins are usually identified in this plane under Buck's fascia and are divided and ligated. Buck's fascia, containing the dorsal neurovascular structures, is then elevated off the underlying tunica albuginea. Mobilization of Buck's fascia is aided using magnification, and meticulous care is taken to avoid injury to the dorsal neurovascular structures.

After Buck's fascia has been mobilized, the tunica plaque or inelastic ridge is palpated and the circumference of the pathology marked. The bulk of the diseased tunica albuginea is then excised. This usually results in an elliptic tunica defect. Additional relaxing incisions must be extended laterally on each side of this tunica defect to allow the penile shaft to lengthen further and expand. After removal of the plaque and creation of the relaxing incisions, the resulting tunica defect is always two to four times larger than the plaque initially removed. The defect is measured, placing the penis on stretch,

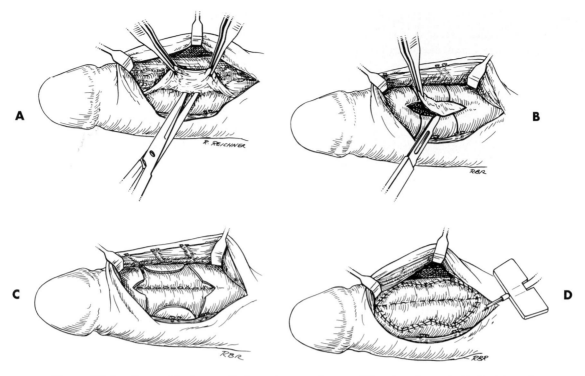

Figure 35-4. Peyronie's disease. **A,** Lateral approach to mobilize dorsal vessels. **B,** Excision of central part of plaque. **C,** Relaxing incision to prevent straight-line contractures of graft-tunica edges. **D,** Dermal graft sutured to repair large tunica defect.

and the size of the dermal graft to be used in the reconstruction is determined.

A dermal graft is then harvested from a hairless area in the lateral groin and defatted. It is sutured to the defect while the penis is placed on stretch. The midline of the dermal graft is attached to the intracorporal septum and to each side of the corporal defect. This lends stability to the graft. A repeat artificial erection is then performed and should demonstrate a straight penis. If a straight penis has not been achieved, more dermal graft should be added to the repair. The penis should be straight at the conclusion of the tunica repair (Figure 35-5).

Postoperative Care

Erections are discouraged during the first 6 postoperative weeks. Sexual activity is restrained in the following 6 weeks to allow the dermal graft to become securely attached. After 12 weeks the patient is counseled that normal erections may still result in some discomfort but will no longer be harmful to the healing phase. The patient's sexual partner is often asked to massage the area with lubricating oil. Both the patient and his partner need to understand that recovery after surgery is gradual and progressive, and it may be up to 6 months before the penis is completely pain free.

Outcomes and Prostheses

In our experience the dermal graft procedure for Peyronie's disease is successful in restoring a straight penis with spontaneous erections satisfactory for intercourse in 85% of patients. A 10% to 15% incidence of erectile insufficiency is seen after dermal graft repairs. Such impotence may be related to the

development of a "venous leak phenomenon." In other patients, postoperative impotence may be psychogenic. Venoocclusive disorder is more likely in older patients and in those who have had resection of extensive Peyronie's plaques.

Degenerative processes such as Peyronie's disease and impotence are seen frequently in our practice. The penile prosthesis is an accepted, well-tolerated remedy when all else fails in the impotent patient. Psychologic counseling, testing, and new medications should always be tried before surgery. Excision of the diseased tunica with dermal graft reconstruction is our treatment of choice. In the few patients who have had this surgery and remain impotent, we recommend placement of a penile prosthesis.

Every patient with Peyronie's disease should have consultation with a sex therapist. We have found this to be helpful in the small percentage of patients who complain of impotence postoperatively, and most have not required placement of a prosthesis.

To alleviate the problems caused by inelasticity of the tunica albuginea, we first use dermal grafting to replace the inelastic scarred tunica. Because most men with Peyronie's disease are not impotent, excision of the plaque with dermal grafting is preferred for initial treatment, as opposed to placement of a penile prosthesis, because the former preserves the patient's ability to have spontaneous erections. Organic impotence may occur with Peyronie's disease, however, and can be corrected by a combination of dermal graft and placement of a prosthesis at the initial surgery.

As noted, approximately 10% to 15% of patients who have the dermal graft procedure for Peyronie's disease will not have

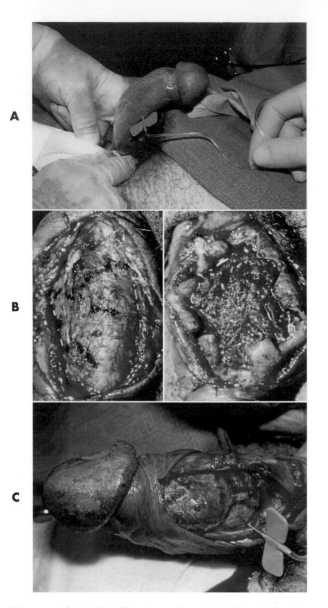

Figure 35-5. A, Chordee of typical Peyronie's disease. **B,** Exposure of tunica after mobilizing dorsal vessels and nerves. *Left,* Excision of central portion of plaque. *Right,* After relaxing lateral incisions. Note enlarged defect. **C,** Dermal graft repair. Artificial erection used to demonstrate correction of chordee.

spontaneous erections that are satisfactory for intercourse, probably because of combined psychologic and physical factors. In these patients, it is a straightforward procedure to implant a penile prosthesis as a second operation. Two types of prostheses are available, and both should be discussed with the patient. One type consists of a permanently stiff rod that keeps the penis firm at all times. The other type of prosthesis may be inflated with a saline pump and deflated when erection is not desired. Both techniques are reliable and worth consideration.

When Peyronie's disease causes severe curvature so that intercourse is physically impossible, surgery with dermal graft repair of the diseased tunica has been successful in a high percentage of patients. This is our treatment of choice, reported first in 1971. It has been used successfully on thousands of patients worldwide.

LYMPHEDEMA

Genital lymphedema can be a difficult challenge for both patient and physician. Lymphedema results from retention of lymphatic fluid in subcutaneous tissues as a result of lymphatic obstruction. In the United States, most cases of genital lymphedema are primary and idiopathic. Congenital lymphedema is known as *Milroy's disease,* whereas edema developing after the onset of puberty is termed *lymphedema praecox.* In developing nations, inflammatory causes such as filariasis predominate. Other secondary causes of penoscrotal lymphedema include postsurgical or postirradiation destruction of the normal lymphatic circulation.[10]

Anatomic considerations reveal there are two systems for lymphatic drainage from the genitalia. The superficial lymphatic network derives from the prepuce and dartols layer of the penile shaft down to Buck's fascia. These superficial lymphatics coalesce and drain into the superficial inguinal lymph nodes. A separate and deeper network of lymphatics drains the urethra, corpus spongiosum, and glans. Generally, genital lymphedema involves only the tissues drained by the superficial system. Therefore no cuff of skin proximal to the coronal sulcus must remain after resection of pathologic edematous skin, or lymphedema will recur in this retained skin. Lymphatics of the scrotum drain laterally into the inguinal nodes from the median raphe. The posterior scrotum has separate lymphatic drainage and may not be involved, even with massive lymphatic enlargement.

Obstruction of lymph flow is the underlying pathology. The histology of chronic lymphedema reveals marked dermal fibrosis and ectasia of the lymphatics in small blood vessels. The gross morphology reveals significant hypertrophy of the skin, which may vary from 2 to 4 cm in thickness. Affected areas may become covered with flat wartlike or nodular excrescences. Edematous skin may become chronically infected because of stasis of protein-rich fluid, which can act as a culture medium for bacteria.

Operations

Our technique for correction of chronic genital lymphedema involves excision of the lymphedematous skin and subcutaneous tissues, along with split-thickness skin graft resurfacing of the underlying genital structures. Surgery is initiated with the patient in a low lithotomy position using Allen stirrups. A Foley catheter is placed through the urethra. Broad-spectrum antibiotic agents are administered preoperatively.

A circumferential incision is made through the distal penile skin immediately adjacent to the coronal sulcus. A longitudinal incision is made down the median raphe of the penile skin, extending through the scrotum toward the perineal body. A circumscribing incision is made around the skin at the edges of the scrotum. The involved skin and subcutaneous tissue is then excised. This dissection is done at the level of Buck's fascia on the penis and down to the tunica vaginalis testis within the scrotum. The spermatic cords and testes are sutured together in the midline.

A split-thickness skin graft measuring approximately ¹⁵⁄₁₀₀₀ of an inch is harvested from each thigh. The scrotal grafts that will cover the testes are then meshed at a ratio of 1.5:1; the grafts for the penile shaft are not meshed. The skin grafts are secured with a combination of 4-0 chromic sutures and interrupted silk stay sutures, which are left long. The skin grafts are covered with Xeroform gauze and a moist cotton dressing, which is placed firmly over the graft sites and secured in place with the lengthy sutures previously placed. The bolster dressing is left in place for 5 or 6 days.

Outcomes

Skin grafts do very well in the genital area, and it is rare not to have 100% take. Postoperatively the patient is instructed to apply vitamin E oil to aid in cleaning and moisturizing the new skin grafts. Flap coverage is not desirable or necessary.

Data on complications rate, functional outcomes, and costs are good areas for future research.

PHALLIC RECONSTRUCTION

Subtotal Techniques

Subtotal phallic reconstruction includes a variety of techniques used to improve the size, function, and appearance of existing penile tissues. It most often is indicated in the setting of trauma, but many types of injury, such as circumcision accidents or severe hypospadias/epispadias (e.g., slough of glans or a corporal body), are appropriate for subtotal phallic reconstruction. Some congenital conditions, such as micropenis or concealed penis, also can be improved with these methods.[6]

When the penis has been damaged and erectile capability persists in the stump, it is often best to optimize the residual penile tissues rather than proceed to total free flap phallic reconstruction. Even in apparently hopeless cases, gratifying results can often be achieved using a combination of the following techniques.

For lengthening the penile stump, the first priority is to release all elements of the existing scar contracture. Scarring and shortness of skin often inhibit extension of the corporal bodies. A circumferential incision is made at the distal end of the penis through the existing shaft skin, and the corporal bodies are degloved down to their base. This often exposes an impressive length of corporal tissue that previously was tethered by the skin scar contracture. Denuded penile shaft tissue must be covered with skin grafts. Full-thickness skin grafts are preferable to split-thickness grafts because they are more durable, develop some sensation, and provide a better cosmetic appearance.

Specific incisions can provide relief for a longitudinally oriented skin contracture extending from the suprapubic area to the penile shaft. A large Z-plasty can "break up" the longitudinal tethering pull of the scar and advance healthy skin onto the shaft. W flaps in the suprapubic skin may also be used. Both these incisions afford excellent exposure to the base of the corporal bodies. If deeper scar tissue surrounds the corpora, it should be excised.

Division of the suspensory ligament may be considered if additional length is desired. The suspensory ligament is aggressively divided in the midline, with care taken to cut it immediately adjacent to the periosteum of the symphysis pubis to avoid injury to dorsal neurovascular structures of the penis. The ligament can usually be detached for about 4 cm (1½ inches). To prevent reattachment, a "spacer" is sutured between the dorsum of the corporal bodies and the base of the pubis. We have used a solid Silastic implant for this purpose, similar to the material used for chin implants.

Augmentation of penile girth is sometimes desired. The circumference of the penile shaft can be reliably increased using a fat-dermal composite graft. The defatted dermal graft is applied as a sheet and wrapped around the shaft, extending from the base to the coronal sulcus in the plane between the skin, with dartos layer above and Buck's fascia below. A large elliptic dermal graft approximately 16 × 8 cm in size is harvested from either the lateral lower abdominal wall skin or the gluteal crease. Before harvesting, the epidermis is removed. Approximately 5 to 10 mm of subcutaneous fat is preserved under the dermal layer. The apex at either end of the graft is spatulated for about 4 cm, which allows it to be wrapped around the shaft at the base and the coronal sulcus. Ventrally the edges of the graft are sutured to Buck's fascia on each lateral edge of the corpus spongiosum.

Many patients also have a prominent suprapubic panniculus, which may engulf and conceal stumps of the corporal bodies. In these cases, the subcutaneous adipose tissue in the suprapubic area is excised down to the anterior rectus fascia. A lipectomy can extend from the umbilicus down to the base of the corpora and laterally between the two spermatic cords.

Other patients may have significant webbing at the penoscrotal junction that may engulf the ventral aspect of the penile shaft. This can obscure the penoscrotal angle and make the penis appear short. A Z-plasty at the penoscrotal junction, with the central limb oriented along the median raphe, serves to recess the scrotum, thus restoring the normal penoscrotal angle.

When the glans has been lost, creation of an artificial coronal sulcus and neoglans provides a visual and palpable step from the shaft skin, which can greatly improve the appearance of the penis. The cap of skin at the penile tip representing the glans is partially undermined, and the proximal edges are furled underneath using chromic mattress sutures tied over small external cotton bolsters circumferentially. The distal edge of the proximal shaft skin (or graft) is advanced under the edge of the furled glans cap for approximately 0.5 cm. This initially leaves a raw distal edge of skin that curves inward as a result of primary healing to create an elevated sulcus. A normal, darker glans color can be simulated by tattooing the tip with appropriate pigment. Multiple treatments may be necessary to achieve optimal appearance.

OUTCOMES. In patients with short penile stumps, exploration of the existing tissue is usually warranted. Many cases are corrected to avoid future extensive reconstruction. Increases in length have been measurable and functional results appreciated in many patients. In those who still desire a larger and longer penis, total phallic microvascular reconstruction can be considered.

Total Phalloplasty

Total phallic reconstruction is best approached by a multidisciplinary team composed of plastic surgeons and urologists. The evolution of phallic reconstruction has paralleled the technical advances in plastic surgery and reconstructive urology. Phallic reconstruction is indicated for total penile destruction after trauma, circumcision accidents, ablative cancer surgery, gender reassignment, and burns. Congenital deformities, such as penile agenesis, micropenis, intersex abnormalities, cloacal exstrophy, and severe hypospadias, may also produce candidates for total phallic reconstruction.[8,14]

The goals of ideal phalloplasty surgery are as follows:

1. Reproducible procedure
2. One-stage operation
3. Cosmetically acceptable phallus
4. Tactile and erogenous sensibility of neophallus
5. Competent urethra to allow voiding while standing
6. Adequate stiffness to allow for sexual intercourse
7. Psychologic adjustment of patient
8. Psychologic adjustment of sexual partner

Unfortunately, no operation or combination of procedures has yet achieved all these goals, but great progress has been made in recent years. The advent of microsurgery has enabled phallic reconstruction to evolve to its present state of the art.[11] The creation of a neophallus has evolved from nonsensate local tube pedicle flaps requiring multiple stages, to myocutaneous flaps, then to free flaps with a defined vascular pedicle that is transferred from its donor to recipient site by microscopically reconnecting its arteriovenous and nerve pedicle.

Several free flaps are available for phallic reconstruction. The most frequently used flap is the *forearm fasciocutaneous free flap* (Figure 35-6). This flap is usually based on the radial artery and its venae comitantes, with skin perfusion occurring through antebrachial fascial perforator vessels and the subdermal plexus. This flap is relatively hairless in most patients on its ulnar border, which allows for construction of a relatively hairless neourethra. If hair is present, epilation is done postoperatively.

This flap is not difficult to raise and does not usually result in any appreciable functional deficit. The donor site defect is covered with a split-thickness graft and is always a cosmetic blemish. The cephalic and basilic veins are usually included to enhance venous drainage. The medial and lateral antebrachial cutaneous nerves of the arm are preserved and coapted to the dorsal nerves of the penis or the pudendal nerves to provide both tactile and erogenous sensation to the neophallus. The dermatome specific to these nerves is in the distal forearm, and thus the optimum sensation is in the glans region of the neophallus when the flap is raised. We anastomose the radial artery to the inferior epigastric artery, the venae comitantes to the inferior epigastric vein, and the cephalic and basilic veins to branches of the saphenous vein.

The urethra is formed by creating a tube from the hairless central portion of the forearm flap. This tube is then enclosed within the phallus, which is formed from the remaining skin of the forearm flap. The neourethra is then anastomosed to the

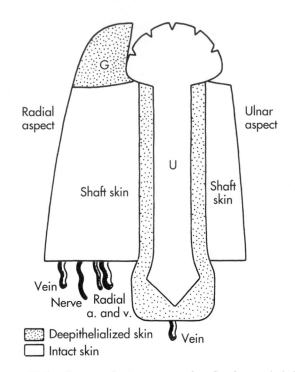

Figure 35-6. Forearm fasciocutaneous free flap for total phallic reconstruction. *G*, Glans flap; *U*, urethra.

native urethra. To prevent a fistula, the urethra-neourethra anastomosis is multilayered and covered with well-vascularized skin or a muscle flap where indicated. The usual muscle used for this flap coverage in transsexual surgery is the rectus abdominis or gracilis. A stricture is further minimized by making the urethral anastomosis oblique and "trumpeting" the proximal neourethra.

On the forearm donor site, great care is taken to preserve the paratenon of the tendons, which provides a reliable bed for a skin graft. The cosmetic appearance of the donor site is greatly improved by using a thick skin graft to resurface the forearm rather than a thin split-thickness graft. The thicker graft allows some hair growth and provides more normal texture and appearance (Figure 35-7).

Outcomes

The ability to achieve adequate rigidity for sexual intercourse is one of the most problematic challenges remaining in total phallic reconstruction.[11] Penile prostheses have a very high failure rate because of extrusion, infection, and inadequate rigidity. The ability to achieve tactile and erogenous sensation reliably in a neophallus has provided the protective mechanism that helps to prevent extrusion of a prosthesis.

Because of this protective sensation and further refinement of surgical techniques, successful insertion of a penile implant is now being reported more frequently. Implant insertion should be delayed until nerve sensation occurs, usually about a year after initial surgery. Since erogenous sensation is present in most patients with a reconstructed neophallus, they can also potentially have normal orgasms.

A sensate, aesthetically desirable total penis can now be reconstructed. This major surgery is indicated when local tissue

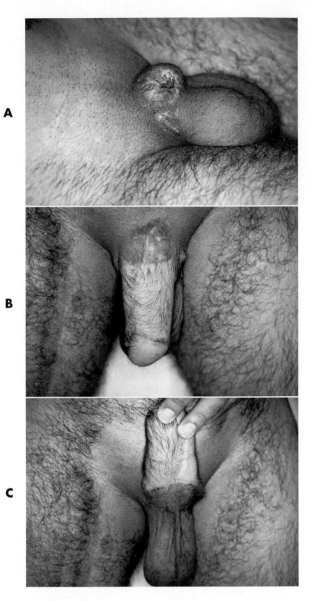

Figure 35-7. Penile reconstruction. **A,** Preoperative view. **B** and **C,** Postoperative views.

rearrangement is inadequate. The success rate for total phallic reconstruction with erogenous sensation approaches 100%.

VAGINAL RECONSTRUCTION

Vaginal reconstruction is considered in the following settings:

1. Females born without a vagina (Mayer-Rokitansky-Küster-Hauser syndrome), most with no uterus but with normal ovaries
2. At adult females' request after extirpative surgery for neoplasm
3. Gender dysphoria for male-to-female transsexual pseudohermaphrodite

In the past, reconstruction of the vagina was usually accomplished by dissecting a tunnel in the perineum (above the rectum and below the bladder) to the peritoneal reflection.

The cavity was then resurfaced with a split-thickness graft (McIndoe procedure).[9] The patient was required to wear a stent for many years postoperatively to prevent stenosis and keep the canal open and adequate. Many patients were helped with this technique, but stenosis and rectal and bladder fistulas were common.

Bowel has also been used for vaginal reconstruction, and a vascularized bowel segment of ileum or colon has successfully been substituted for the lining of the new vaginal canal.[5] Potential disadvantages of bowel for vaginal reconstruction include excess mucus secretion and the tendency for bowel mucosa to be traumatized by normal sexual intercourse. Also, harvesting of the bowel segment requires laparotomy and intraabdominal surgery.

We advocate the use of full-thickness skin grafts for vaginal reconstruction.[12] The new channel is made as described for the McIndoe technique. Full thickness grafts are harvested from a hairless area in the lateral groin. Two grafts are usually required (one on each side) for the channel to be deep and wide. Foam rubber is carved into a stent and covered with a sterile condom. The grafts are sutured together around the condom-covered mold, leaving one end of the tube open. This graft is placed in the new vaginal canal, and the open end is sutured to the vaginal perineal skin.

The stent is removed in 1 week, with new dressings as necessary for 2 to 3 weeks postoperatively. We then ask the patient to obtain various sizes of candles. Condoms are used to cover the appropriately sized candle, which is used in the new vagina for 3 months. At that time the graft should be well healed and will not constrict or shrink. This is a tremendous advantage over the previously used split-thickness graft technique. Also, the donor site of the full-thickness graft can be closed in a linear fashion, and the resulting scar is minimal.

Outcomes

Vaginal reconstruction is usually successful, with few anticipated complications. To avoid pressure on a urethral catheter postoperatively, we usually recommend a suprapubic diversion of urine. Earlier vaginal reconstruction is possible in younger patients because full-thickness grafts will grow with the body, will remain supple and soft, and unlike split-thickness grafts, do not require prolonged stenting.

REFERENCES

1. Berg R, Berg G: Penile malformation, gender identity, and sexual orientation, *Acta Psychiatr Scand* 68:154, 1983.
2. Dessanti A, Rigamont W, Merullus V, et al: Autologous buccal mucosa grafts for hypospadias repair: initial report, *J Urol* 147:1081, 1992.
3. Devine CJ Jr, Horton CE: Peyronie's disease, *Clin Plast Surg* 15(3):405-410, 1988.
4. Gerrhart JP, Leeward MP, Burgess JR, Jeffs RO: The Cantwell-Ransley technique for repair of epispadias, *J Urol* 148:851, 1992.

5. Hendren WH, Atala A: Use of bowel for vaginal reconstruction, *J Urol* 152:752, 1994.

6. Horton CE, Horton CE Jr: Subtotal phallic reconstruction, *Pediatr Urol* 18:3, 1995.

7. Horton CE Jr, Horton CE: Congenital genitourinary anomalies. In Benz ML, editor: *Pediatric plastic surgery,* East Norwalk, Conn, 1998, Appleton & Lange.

8. Jordan GH, Alter GJ, Gilbert DA, Horton CE: Penile prosthesis implantation in total phalloplasty, *J Urol* 152:410, 1994.

9. McIndoe DH: An operation for cure of congenital absence of the vagina, *Br J Obstet Gynecol* 45:490, 1938.

10. Morey AF, Meng MV, McAninch J: Skin graft reconstruction and lymphedema, *Urology* 50:423, 1997.

11. Penlozzi L, Erickson J, Jackson R: Hypospadias trends in two U.S. surveillance systems, *Pediatrics* 100(5):831-834, 1977.

12. Sadove RC, Horton CE: Utilizing full-thickness skin grafts for vaginal reconstruction, *Clin Plast Surg* 15(3):443, 1988.

13. Snodgrass W: Tubularized incised plate hypospadias repair: results at a multicenter experience, *J Urol* 156:839, 1995.

14. Trengove-Jones G, Alter GJ: Total phallic reconstruction, *Pediatr Urol* 18:4-6, 1995.

15. Vortsman B, Horton C, Winslow B: Repair of secondary genital deformities of epispadias-exstrophy, *Clin Plast Surg,* 15(3): 381-392, 1988.

Chest Wall Reconstruction

36

Alan E. Seyfer

INDICATIONS

The major indications for chest wall reconstruction include the following:

1. Restoration of chest wall components after tumor ablation
2. Closure of defects associated with infection or dehiscence of the pleural space or parietes
3. Obliteration of empyemic cavities
4. Repair of congenital defects, such as pectus excavatum ("hollowed breast"), pectus carinatum ("keeled breast"), and Poland's syndrome (anomaly).

Reconstruction involves many factors. The plastic surgeon may be consulted by the surgeon who intends to remove a segment of chest wall or requires assistance because of an open wound or cavity in the chest itself. Obliteration of an open chest wound can (1) ameliorate pulmonary dynamics, (2) provide primary healing, and (3) prevent many long-term complications.

The most important principle in chest wall reconstruction may be provision of durable, well-vascularized coverage for wounds. A well-vascularized cover also has oncologic implications and may provide excellent serviceability if radiotherapy is planned.

With congenital lesions, operative indications may involve the correction of pulmonary dynamics secondary to a severe pectus excavatum deformity. Likewise, cosmetic implications may be important in such patients, as well as in those with Poland's anomaly.

Chest wall restoration is a major procedure, often undertaken in the patient who is at risk for potentially life-threatening problems. An accurate preoperative assessment is critical to detect and treat correctable problems. The assessment of risk is important in the preoperative assessment as well as in providing informed consent to patients and their families.

Many patients who undergo chest wall reconstruction fall into higher risk categories. The Dripps–American Association of Anesthesiology (DAAA) classification may be helpful, and its validity has been confirmed (Table 36-1). The DAAA classification continues to be a useful means of stratifying patients according to operative risk. Functionally, the risk factors associated with a major chest wall reconstruction can be divided into cardiovascular, pulmonary, and nutritional factors.

CARDIOVASCULAR EVALUATION

Overall, the cardiac risk associated with chest wall reconstruction is similar to that of noncardiac procedures. A history of cardiac disability, however, such as a recent myocardial infarction or poorly controlled congestive heart failure, remains a contraindication to elective chest wall procedures. In emergent cases, consultation with the patient's cardiologist and assessment according to Goldman criteria may be appropriate to assess the level of risk (Table 36-2).

In patients who have had chest wall infections, multiple coronary risk factors may be present and may merit special attention. These patients must be aggressively screened to assess the degree of cardiac disability. The use of invasive and noninvasive methods, such as electrocardiography and multigated acquisition scans, may be helpful. Patients with coronary disease may require angiography. Higher Goldman scores correlate with serious cardiac events and death in patients undergoing cardiac procedures.

PULMONARY EVALUATION

A history of pulmonary dysfunction merits preoperative spirometry and routine preoperative pulmonary function testing. These tests may include chest roentgenograms, measurement of arterial (room air) blood gases, and spirometry before and after bronchodilation. The routine chest film may unmask interstitial or pulmonary disease. It may also be useful as an indirect estimate of thoracic volume, inspiratory effort, and rib osteopenia.

Resting blood gas measurements may be helpful in predicting pulmonary risk by estimating ventilation, or carbon dioxide partial pressure (P_{CO_2}). A resting P_{CO_2} above 50 mm Hg remains a relative contraindication to surgery because of the need for prolonged postoperative ventilation. Spirometry continues to be a relatively simple yet informative method of

Table 36-1.
Dripps–American Association of Anesthesiology Classification of Anesthetic Risk

CLASS	DESCRIPTION
I	Pathologic process is localized and not conducive to systemic disturbance.
II	Mild to moderate systemic disturbance is caused by either condition to be treated to other pathophysiologic processes.
III	Rather severe systemic disturbance or pathology is present, even though degree of disability may be uncertain.
IV	Severe systemic disorder is already life-threatening and is not always correctable by procedure.
V	Patient is moribund with little chance of survival but undergoes repeated operations.
Emergent	Any of above classes, patient is in poorer physical condition because emergency operation is necessary.

Modified from Azarow, K, Molloy M, Seyfer AE, Graeber G: *Surg Clin North Am* 69:899-910, 1989.

Table 36-2.
Goldman Cardiac Risk Index

FINDING	POINTS
S3 gallop of jugular venous distention	11
Transmural or subendocardial myocardial infarction in past 6 months	10
More than five premature ventricular contractions documented at any time	7
Premature atrial contractions or other than sinus rhythm on last preoperative electrocardiogram	7
Age >70 years	5
Emergency operation	4
Intrathoracic, intraabdominal, or aortic surgery	3
Evidence of aortic valvular stenosis	3
Poor general medical status*	3

POINTS	GROUP	RISK
0-5	I	None
6-12	II	Minimal
13-25	III	Moderate
>25	IV	Great

Modified from Goldman L: *Ann Intern Med* 98:504-513, 1983.
*Oxygen pressure <60 mm Hg; carbon dioxide pressure >50 mm Hg; serum K^+, 3 mEq/L; HCO_3^- >20 mEq/L; urea nitrogen >50 mg/dl; creatinine >3 mg/dl; elevated aspartate transferase or signs of liver disease; any condition for which patient is chronically bedridden.

Table 36-3.
Assessment of Pulmonary Resectability

FEV₁ × FVC*	PATIENT IMPLICATIONS
>2500	Will tolerate resection of one lobe
>3500	Will tolerate pneumonectomy
<2500	Will have postoperative pulmonary dysfunction even if no pulmonary tissue is resected

Modified from Azarow K, Molloy M, Seyfer AE, Graeber G: *Surg Clin North Am* 69:899-910, 1989.
*Forced expiratory volume at 1 second times forced vital capacity.

Table 36-4.
Assessment for Risk of Postoperative Respiratory Complications

CLASS	DESCRIPTION
0	No dyspnea
I	Dyspnea when walking up incline
II	Dyspnea when walking at own pace on level surface
III	Needs to rest after three blocks
IV	Needs to rest after two blocks

Modified from Azarow K, Molloy M, Seyfer AE, Graeber G: *Surg Clin North Am* 69:899-910, 1989.

assessing pulmonary risk. Forced vital capacity (FVC) and forced expiratory volume (flow) at 1 second (FEV_1) are useful, along with their product, $FVC \times FEV_1$, and can be helpful in estimating the patient's ability to tolerate the removal of all or part of one lung (Table 36-3).

One simple test is walking the patient down the hallway and up a flight of stairs. This preoperative assessment can be used to place a patient in risk categories. Again, the history of cardiac or pulmonary disability is useful in assessing the special needs of each patient, especially during the intraoperative and postoperative phases (Table 36-4).

NUTRITIONAL EVALUATION

Malnutrition and an inability to tolerate oral feedings can result in a higher incidence of postoperative complications. Patients with chronic diseases, those with infection or dehiscence after

median sternotomy, and patients at the extremes of age (infancy or elderly) may suffer from the effects of malnutrition. In general, if malnutrition is diagnosed, it is advisable to correct the problem before the surgical procedure.

The *prognostic nutritional index* can be helpful in screening patients suspected of malnutrition. Patients falling into a higher risk category may need preoperative nutritional supplementation. Other parameters that may be useful include body weight, anthropometric measurements, creatinine-height index, serum albumin, serum transferase, total lymphocyte count, and response to antigenic stimuli (delayed hypersensitivity).

If malnutrition is anticipated, it may be prudent to insert a feeding jejunostomy at surgery so that feedings may be begun immediately postoperatively. This may also be done preoperatively if nasogastric feedings are undesirable.

Postoperative cardiac, pulmonary, and nutritional care are discussed later.

INFORMED CONSENT

Unless called to the operating room to assist the surgeon with an unexpected problem related to wound closure, the surgeon may discuss the problems, alternative methods of treatment, and risks with patients and families. As with any operation, it is important to discuss potential complications, such as bleeding, infection, permanent nerve damage (e.g., loss of feeling or ability to control certain muscles), unfavorable scars, treatment failure, and poor tissue healing. Patients and their families accept these possibilities quite well; patients undergoing semiemergent and lifesaving procedures are especially understanding.

In dealing with congenital defects, it is always appropriate, particularly in asymptomatic patients, to emphasize the following:

1. *No treatment* is also an important option.
2. Undertaking surgery is adding elements of uncertainty, risk, and life-threatening complications.

For example, in assessing a child with an asymptomatic pectus excavatum, the parents must be reassured that (1) an operation may be accomplished more safely after attainment of growth, and (2) such procedures may also be delayed until after the patient is old enough to contribute to the decision for surgical correction.

OPERATIONS

One of the earliest successful chest wall reconstructions occurred in 1899, when Parham successfully removed a segment of a chest wall that had been invaded by a tumor. Parham stressed the importance of preserving an intact parietal pleura and maintaining positive-pressure ventilation.[11]

Later, Tansini described the latissimus musculocutaneous flap for reconstruction after mastectomy. Blades, Converse, and Oliveri also made significant contributions to the field of chest wall surgery.[11] Perhaps the most useful contributions have emerged during the past 25 years, as musculocutaneous flaps and omental and prosthetic materials have become more reliable.[9,10,12-14]

FLAP COVERAGE

Although one of the principles of reconstructive surgery is to proceed from the simplest to more complex methods of reconstruction, the unique needs for full-thickness chest wall reconstruction have necessitated a reliance on musculocutaneous flaps because of their excellent blood supply, reliability, and durability for this purpose.

During the planning phase, it is helpful to divide the chest into segments and prioritize selection of coverage, based on the blood supply and range of each flap. Since certain options are more useful for these subunits, subdivisions of these groupings also enhance convenience.

For the anterior thorax, the sternum may be divided into upper, middle, and lower sections; the area lateral to the sternum is divided into upper and lower regions. Prioritization of choices depends primarily on the length of the vascular pedicle and how far it will reach without tension (i.e., range of flap).

The flaps described later are eminently reliable and should not undergo vascular difficulties if mobilized and inset properly and without tension. The guiding principle is to mobilize the vascular pedicles aggressively so that they are completely free. If necessary, the tunnel through which the flap is transferred should be widely opened or divided, rather than risking compression or tension on the pedicle itself.

In the recovery room, if the flap feels cool or appears cyanotic or mottled, it should be explored immediately to relieve any compression of the nutrient vessels or venous drainage. Absolutely no tension must be present at the site of the full-thickness defect in the chest wall. Flaps are literally loose and floppy when placed into the defect, and any tension that may be present must be moved to the donor area from which the flap was harvested. The donor area usually has an intact musculoskeletal layer that can be skin-grafted if primary closure is not possible. If residual tension remains at the farthest point on the defect after flap insertion, another flap should be moved into the defect rather than accept the risk of dehiscence.

Certain conditions also contraindicate the use of specific flaps. For example, a healed right subcostal incision from a previous abdominal procedure and a chevron incision in the upper abdominal wall contraindicate the use of a superiorly based rectus abdominis flap on that side. Such a flap would not survive because (1) the superior epigastric pedicle has been divided and (2) the circulation to the vascular territory of the flap will never reconstitute with time. Also, a previous posterolateral thoracotomy incision would contraindicate the

use of a latissimus dorsi flap derived distal to that incision, since the vascular pedicle was interrupted during the thoracotomy.

IMAGING

The accurate characterization and localization of anatomic irregularities of the chest wall have advanced tremendously over the last two decades with the advent of cross-sectional and three-dimensional imaging techniques. Computed tomography (CT) and magnetic resonance imaging (MRI) precisely delineate chest wall layers and reveal their relationship to the lesion and the intrathoracic viscera.

Conventional chest radiographs are still of value in the determination of the patient's general state of health. Because of its ability to provide contrast resolution in an axial plane, however, CT scanning is more sensitive than standard radiographs in the assessment of soft tissue tumors. Also, MRI appears to offer certain advantages over CT in the assessment of the patient with possible chest wall invasion.[11] Radiologic consultation should be obtained to assess whether CT, MRI, angiography, or ultrasonography (which has had many recent improvements) would be applicable to a specific problem. The CT scan has proved quite useful, particularly in assessing the position or displacement of the heart and great vessels in congenital lesions such as pectus excavatum.

LATISSIMUS DORSI MUSCLE/MUSCULOCUTANEOUS FLAP

The latissimus dorsi musculocutaneous flap, located in such a way as to reach both the anterior (superolateral) and the posterior sectors of the thorax, can provide excellent, well-vascularized coverage for many defects of the upper thorax. It is also quite useful to eliminate intrathoracic defects, such as from an empyema or a pulmonectomy cavity, and to provide coverage for a bronchial stump and exposed pulmonary vessels. The two blood supplies to the latissimus dorsi muscle and its overlying skin are the thoracodorsal artery and the posterior branches of the intercostal arteries from the ninth thoracic (T9) to T11 vertebral segments.

The latissimus dorsi is a thin, broad muscle that originates from the thoracolumbar fascia and the lower six thoracic vertebral regions. This diamond-shaped muscle gains thickness as it approaches the axilla and spirals to insert posterior to the intertubercular groove of the humerus. The muscle adducts, extends, and internally (medially) rotates the humerus. This muscle is largely dispensable, given the normal function of other shoulder girdle musculature.[11]

Vascular Supply

The blood supply to the latissimus dorsi muscle originates from the axillary artery and its large subscapular branch, which then gives off the thoracodorsal artery. Proximal to this is a substantial branch to the serratus anterior muscle (also quite useful, especially for the obliteration of apical pleural spaces). The thoracodorsal artery then divides into two branches: a superior branch that parallels the muscle's superior border and an anterior branch that parallels its anterior border. Both these vessels course along the deep aspect of the muscle and contribute perforators and other branches throughout the muscle. Musculocutaneous branches then arborize into the overlying dermis after traversing the fat layer.

The artery to the serratus anterior muscle is usually divided during mobilization of the latissimus dorsi flap. The vascular territory is quite large, and the overlying skin will survive based on the musculocutaneous perforators and the associated venules and thoracodorsal vein. In order to include these perforators with the flap, the skin island should be at least 8 cm in diameter and 8 cm in length.

When using the secondary perforators to vascularize the flap, the defect is generally located over the lumbar region, and the thoracodorsal pedicle must be divided so that the flap can reach the target area. When the flap is based on this secondary blood supply, however, the blood flow is not as robust as when it emanates from the thoracodorsal vessels. To increase the blood flow, it may be prudent to perform a delay procedure before transferring the flap.

Uses

Areas over the shoulder (Figure 36-1), the upper lateral anterior thorax, the nape of the neck, and the supraclavicular fossa (Figure 36-2) are easily covered by the latissimus dorsi flap. This muscle can also be used to reconstruct congenital absence of the pectoralis major muscle (Poland's syndrome) to augment cardiac output, as well as for use as a free tissue transfer. The latter two uses are beyond the scope of this chapter.

Scars

The presence of surgical scars crossing the area of the vascular pedicle usually contraindicates use of the latissimus dorsi flap. Once an incision has partitioned a blood supply, the vessels never reconstitute fully, and the flap distal to the scar fails because of ischemia. This is of critical importance when planning reconstructive operations. The most common previous incisions are as follows:

1. Right subcostal incision (from cholecystectomy) that divides the superior epigastric artery to the rectus abdominis flap
2. Previous posterolateral thoracotomy incision that divides the pedicle to the lower latissimus dorsi flap

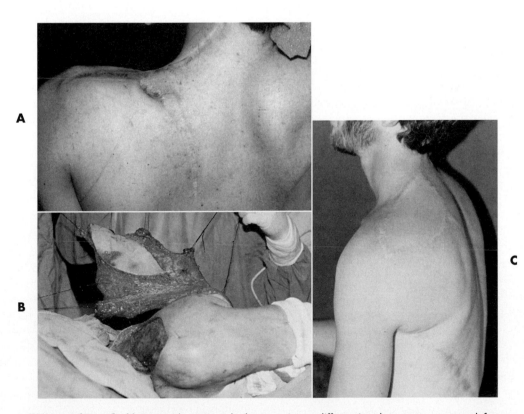

Figure 36-1. **A,** Young male patient had aggressive undifferentiated sarcoma removed from left shoulder region. Wound was large, and flaps were advanced and closed under tension. Dehiscence delayed postoperative radiation therapy. Seroma was beneath caudal flap. **B,** Latissimus dorsi musculocutaneous flap mobilized to resurface area after radical debridement. Because of vascular pedicle length, no tension occurs on incision closure. **C,** Several months after healing of flap. Patient was able to begin radiation therapy shortly after original flap closure and continued to do well.

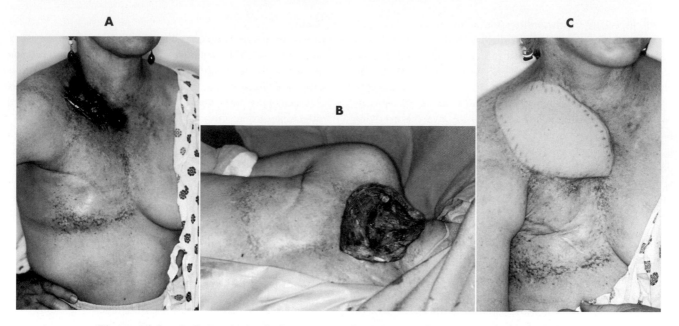

Figure 36-2. **A,** Patient had radical mastectomy for aggressive inflammatory carcinoma of right breast, as well as high-dose radiation therapy and bone marrow transplant. Other than this localized recurrence, she was doing well clinically. Biopsy showed inflammatory carcinoma. **B,** Radical excision of aggressive metastasis. **C,** Coverage with latissimus dorsi musculocutaneous flap, which healed well and sustained radiation therapy.

Technique

The best position for access to the latissimus dorsi muscle is the lateral thoracotomy position. Usually, and especially for anterior defects, patients are supine and after endotracheal anesthesia are placed on their side, and the exposed upper extremity, thorax, neck, hip, and abdomen are prepared. The lateral buttock and thigh are also prepared in anticipation of possible skin grafting of the muscle or the flap donor site. The drapes are stapled to the skin, a double stockinette is placed on the upper extremity, and the patient is then turned to the supine position. The anterior field is then prepared and draped.

After the ablative portion of the operation, the patient is then turned to the lateral position. The margins of the previously planned skin island are again marked after measurement of the defect. The surgeon can use an inelastic cloth, such as a hand towel, to plan specifically for the skin island that will be used with the flap. The proposed skin island is drawn on the cloth, and the mobile end of the cloth "flap" can be rotated over the planned operating defect, keeping the "pedicle" of the cloth on the posterior axillary fold. This will predict the ultimate reach of the flap and how the skin island will conform to the defect on the chest wall. If the latissimus is found to be suitable to the task, the incision is then outlined.

The margins of the skin island are incised to the latissimus fascia. The entire latissimus muscle (or portion to be used) is uncovered, working away from the skin paddle. The anterior edge is located, and the oblique fibers can be seen as distinct from the serratus anterior fibers, which are proceeding in the opposite general direction.

The submuscular dissection begins at the midpoint of the anterior edge and proceeds caudally to the iliolumbar lumbar region as far as possible to the iliac crest. The dissection is then carried medially to the paraspinous muscles and caudally to the iliolumbar lumbar fascia. The latissimus is freed distally until it can be grasped between the thumb and fingers and as far caudally as possible. The caudal border can then be transected using electrocautery.

After hemostasis has been achieved, the muscle's origin is serially divided from the spinal attachments, working cephalad. As the muscle is released, it is gently elevated and retracted with silk sutures. The filmy, submuscular plane over the ribs can be bluntly dissected with the fingertip. The cephalad margin is then sharply freed from any attachments over the inferior angle of the scapula, working carefully toward the axilla. A search is made for the thoracodorsal vascular pedicle along the deep margin of the muscle as the insertion on the humerus is approached. A few inches below the insertion, the arterial pulse can be felt and the muscle lifted for direct visualization of the pedicle. After identification of the pedicle, the muscle is mobilized and the pedicle dissected up to the subscapular artery and its origin from the axillary artery. The circumflex scapular and serratus branches are ligated and divided. The insertion can also be transected if more length on the muscle is necessary.

The subcutaneous fat is dissected off the deep fascia anteriorly so that the ablative defect can be connected to the defect of the axillary region. The tunnel should be widely open so that the flap has a direct route to the defect. The flap can be pushed through the defect, since it is dangerous to pull the flap and possibly disrupt perforating vessels and the pedicle.

The flap should be "loose and floppy" in the defect. The donor site is closed primarily, if possible. Depending on the size of the skin island removed, the donor site gap can be closed by mobilizing the skin and subcutaneous fat at the level of the deep fascia. Segments wider than 9 to 12 cm may require skin grafting. Retention sutures with no. 1 monofilament are helpful in obtaining a safe closure.

In certain patients the muscle alone should be used rather than the composite flap of skin and muscle. For example, in the patient with Poland's syndrome, the muscle can be transposed without the skin paddle and folded to resemble the natural fullness of the medial aspect of the pectoralis major muscle.

Consequences of Latissimus Removal

Forceful coughing, depression of the shoulder, and strong extension and internal rotation of the arm may be impaired in the absence of the latissimus muscle. In an unpublished study, however, 11 patients were measured for weakness with a computed testing system. All recovered from this weakness by 3 months after removal of the latissimus dorsi muscle. One patient described weakness in doing situps with fingers locked behind his head, but this seemed to be related to touching the knees with the elbows, which includes adduction of the humerus, and also improved with time. Some patients had transient complaints of weakness in opening twist-off lids and ironing clothes.

If the shoulder girdle retains the other important muscles, only transient weakness should be associated with transposition of the latissimus dorsi muscle.

PECTORALIS MAJOR MUSCLE FLAP

The pectoralis major muscle is usually used for anterior defects of the chest wall, anterior intrathoracic reconstructions (e.g., bronchopleural or tracheoesophageal fistula) or to provide lining or coverage of head and neck defects. Free tissue transfers have largely supplanted this latter use. The flap can also provide coverage for the external ear, cheek areas, and anterolateral neck. Again, free tissue transfers usually employ the pectoralis major muscle because of the tethering of these areas by the flap connected to the clavicular region.

After measurement of the ablative defect, an appropriately sized skin island is planned (as with other muscle flaps) and drawn over the pectoralis major muscle to reconfirm the preoperative assessment. The skin and subcutaneous tissues around the margin of this island are incised down to the deep fascia, and the muscle is exposed working away from the skin paddle. The inferolateral border is located, and depending on how much will be used, the muscle is either immobilized around the edge or split in the direction of its fibers according to the needs of the ablative defect. Preserving the muscle's edge may help to retain the contour of the axillary fold and avoid a cosmetic deformity caused by total removal of the inferior border. The maneuver usually does not significantly compromise flap size and breadth.

The pectoralis major muscle is then elevated, using finger dissection beneath the muscle. The ribs can be felt, and fascia under the muscle is easily separated from the ribs in this areolar plane, sweeping upward to the clavicle and then caudally along the sternum and down toward the xyphoid process. Muscle thins out in this inferior area and can be torn if dissection is too forceful.

The thick muscular attachments along the sternal body are then divided with scissors or electrocautery. Large perforating branches of the internal thoracic artery can be seen and ligated before transection. The muscle can be elevated to search for the thoracoacromial vascular pedicle. This pedicle arises just medial to the coracoid process of the scapula, and its arterial pulsations can be felt. The course of the arteries is gently traced as the pedicle clings to the deep muscle surface. The dissection is then carried toward the humeral insertion. The muscle near the insertion can be divided at a convenient level, with care taken not to injure the underlying axillary neurovascular structures. The pedicle's position is frequently checked.

After division of the muscle near the insertion, the flap can be turned upward so that the vascular pedicle can be directly visualized. The clavicular attachments are now divided, working toward the pedicle from both medial and lateral directions. The flap is then transposed to the defect (Figure 36-3).

The pectoralis major flap can also be used based on the perforators originating from the internal mammary artery. The dissection remains the same, except the sternal border is preserved and the thoracoacromial vessels are divided near their origin from the axillary artery. The muscle flap is then transposed medially, with consideration of the perforating vessels within the muscle. This flap can be used when middle and lower sternal defects require more bulk for coverage and the internal mammary artery is intact.

OMENTUM

A bowel preparation is usually administered, according to the surgeon's preference. For anterior defects the patient is usually in the supine position. The thoracic defect is packed and covered with a rubber-dam patch cut from a sterile surgeon's glove. A sterile sponge is covered with the patch, which is stapled to the skin around the wound. The sponge absorbs drainage and prevents spread of contamination. An iodine-adherent plastic drape is then placed over the chest, further sealing the ablative defect from the abdominal area. The abdominal area is prepared again. The thighs are also draped for use as donor sites for skin grafts.

The abdomen is then entered through an upper midline incision that extends to just below the umbilical region. A nasogastric tube is inserted and its position routinely checked. After a brief exploration the omentum is assessed gently because the vessels are easily injured. The omentum is then lifted from the colon. Any adhesions are isolated and sharply divided while protecting the viscus from which they are liberated. After the omentum is freed, its filmy attachment to the transverse colon is isolated and serially divided with care

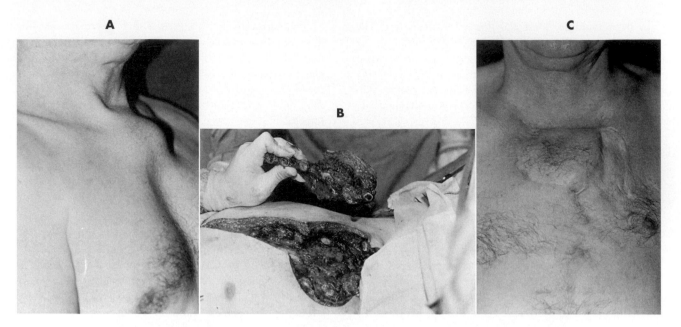

Figure 36-3. A, Patient noted gradually enlarging, firm tumor over base of neck. Imaging and clinical evaluation showed bony tumor consistent with sarcoma of manubrium. **B,** Patient underwent subtotal sternectomy, including medial claviculectomies; xyphoid area was spared. Tumor is shown, with clear interval subjacent to manubrium. Left pectoralis major musculocutaneous flap was rotated into defect, and exposed portions of muscle were covered with split-thickness skin grafts that were meshed 1.5:1. **C,** Patient healed well, with no evidence of recurrence for 5 years, after which he was lost to follow-up. He could accomplish heavy labor using upper extremities, despite absence of clavicles and left pectoralis major muscle.

taken to avoid injury to the middle colic vessels within the transverse mesocolon.

The epiploic appendices are left intact to avoid diverticula. The small blood vessels are individually clamped with hemostats and immediately ligated with fine ties to avoid injuring the blood vessels by the clamps' weight. If this is not accomplished gently, a hematoma may develop and can rapidly spread between the omental leaves, making the tissue difficult to use.

The short vessels between the gastroepiploic arcade and the greater curvature of the stomach are segmentally divided. Both the anterior and the posterior rows are individually ligated immediately close to the serosa. Then the omentum is attached by the left gastroepiploic artery (a terminal branch of the splenic artery) and the right gastroepiploic artery near the pylorus.

Before further dissection the omentum can be gently lifted from the abdomen and over the chest to ascertain its reach. Often it easily covers the defect without further mobilization. If more length is needed, the left gastroepiploic vessels are divided at a convenient point, with care taken to avoid entering the splenic hilum. The omentum usually can reach to the head and neck areas with this additional length.

The omentum should fit loosely into the defect, filling in the cavity without tension on the pedicle. This maintains good circulation within the flap and prevents gastric outlet obstruction by tethering of the right gastroepiploic vessels.

As noted earlier, in many patients, especially if elderly or debilitated, it may be helpful to insert a feeding jejunostomy so that enteral nutrition can be started immediately after the operation.

The omentum is removed from the wound's cephalad portion, draped over the chest wall, and protected with warm, moist laparotomy sponges. The abdomen is closed after the organs and donor sites are assessed for any residual bleeding in the omental dissection region. The cephalad portion of the abdominal wound is left open 3 to 4 fingerbreadths to prevent constriction of the omental vessels as they cross this layer and are brought into the chest. The skin is closed up to the omentum and the chest uncovered. The intact skin between the abdominal and chest defects can be incised, and the omentum is allowed to lie in the open area, with a direct route to the defect.

A skin graft can be used to cover the omentum. Alternatively, a large subcutaneous tunnel can be established to push the omentum through the chest wound; pulling can be harmful to omental tissues. Room should be sufficient to allow the open hand to go through the tunnel with ease. After transposition of the omentum through the tunnel, the skin of the abdominal incision is closed.

The omentum is then placed in the deep cavity around the chest organs. Alternatively, a synthetic mesh is placed in the musculoskeletal layer of the chest wound, and the omentum is placed in the defect and covered with a meshed skin graft. Meshing allows the graft to fit the irregular contours of the flap, and leaving it unexpanded allows the graft to heal as a sheet of durable skin. A few quilting sutures of 4-0 chromic are placed to ensure that every part of the graft is secured to the omentum (Figure 36-4).

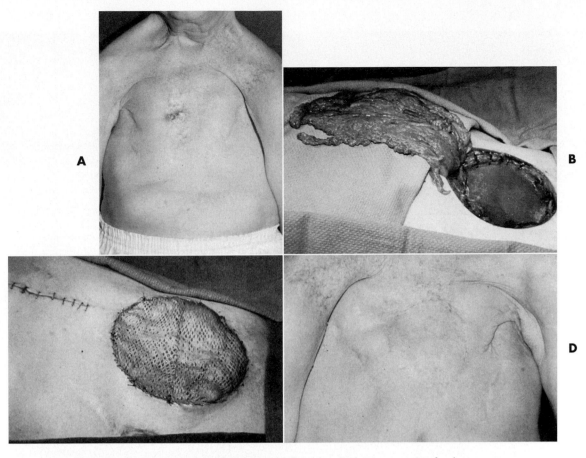

Figure 36-4. **A,** Elderly female had received bilateral radical mastectomies for breast cancer. Latissimus dorsi muscle was defunctionalized, and pressure over sternum resulted in copious drainage of purulent and necrotic material, indicating a necrotic sternum. **B,** Omentum was harvested and brought through subcutaneous tunnel to defect, which has been supported with proline mesh. **C,** Omentum covered by meshed, unexpanded, split-thickness skin graft, with quilting sutures of 4-0 chromic used to stabilize graft. **D,** Area shows excellent healing and durability.

RECTUS ABDOMINIS FLAP

The rectus abdominis is useful as a muscle flap alone or as a combined musculocutaneous flap. It affords thick coverage and a variety of options in tailoring the skin segment to meet specific needs. The areas directly over the muscle and near the umbilicus are safer with regard to blood flow than other regions because of the higher concentration of vessels to the overlying skin in these locations. The flap can have various skin patterns (e.g., transverse, vertical, oblique) to cover a variety of defects. The range of the rectus abdominis flap is its greatest asset.

The composite musculocutaneous flap is used most effectively in patients who have a thick but tight layer of abdominal fat, especially in the region of the umbilicus and hypogastrium. This should not be loose fat that hangs as an apron. Such laxity is a relative contraindication to the use of this flap, since the blood supply to the fat and skin are much attenuated in these patients. Advanced age is also a relative contraindication. Smoking can cause vascular compromise in the flap's periphery and in the abdominal flap used to close the defect.

For sternal defects the surgeon must ensure that the internal thoracic artery, on which the flap is based, is intact. Previous radiation is not a contraindication because the flap can survive this. Sternal resections or sternal retention sutures, however, can interrupt the course of this artery and render the flap unusable from a vascular standpoint. In such cases a free rectus muscle flap may be a reasonable substitute. A previous cholecystectomy incision or any incision that has divided the rectus muscle contraindicates its use distal to this incision. Again, a free tissue transfer based on the inferior pedicle may be a useful substitute. If any question remains about the pedicle, duplex scanning or arteriography should be done.

Mobilization of a vertical musculocutaneous flap is described here because it is more common in chest wall reconstruction. This flap can easily reach the sternal notch and is also reliable for anterolateral defects of the chest wall (Figure 36-5). This option is more reliable than the transverse flap, since it incorporates the rectus with the skin and fat that directly overlies the muscle. Therefore the perforators directly arborize into almost the entire skin segment.

The vertical flap is mobilized the same as the transverse flap (see Chapter 39). The exception is that a vertical ellipse of skin

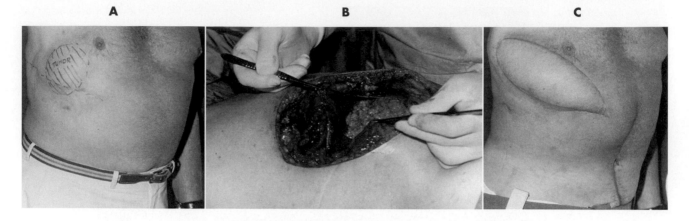

Figure 36-5. **A,** Patient had recurrent chondrosarcoma after excision several years earlier. **B,** Thoracoabdominal excision was performed with right adrenalectomy and removal of portion of diaphragm. Forceps held diaphragm before repair. **C,** Superiorly based rectus abdominis flap provided excellent, durable, well-vascularized coverage.

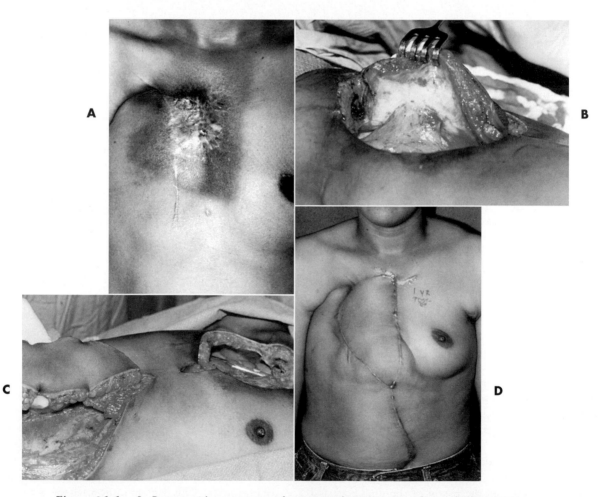

Figure 36-6. **A,** Patient with recurrence of aggressive breast cancer after radical mastectomy and high-dose radiation therapy. Area was tender, and central open region was portion of ulcerated recurrence. **B,** Underlying lung was adherent to cancer in small area. This was removed and excised with chest wall segment involved with tumor. **C,** Superiorly based contralateral rectus abdominis musculocutaneous flap mobilized for placement in defect without tension. **D,** Patient continued to do well 1 year postoperatively. Note improvement in radiation damage to adjacent area of skin over chest wall. This seems to be consistent in patients who have received well-vascularized flaps. This phenomenon seems to bring new, uninjured blood flow into injured regions.

and subcutaneous tissue is left undisturbed over the anterior fascia. In planning this flap, the surgeon determines that a longitudinal flap is desirable in reconstructing the defect. Also, this flap may be useful for sternal defects in which removal of skin and deep tissues has left a sizable cavitary defect. This defect is measured, and a corresponding ellipse or other suitable skin island is marked over the selected rectus abdominis muscle. Again, the internal thoracic artery to the rectus must be confirmed as being intact before use of the flap. The vessel may be ablated if the sternal defect is large, and an alternative flap must be used.

After the arc of rotation is checked and dimensions of the defect are measured, a final pattern is marked, and the skin and soft tissues are incised down to the anterior rectus fascia. The umbilicus is avoided and the incision beveled away from the flap's skin segment. The flap is incised over the suprapubic region and the rectus muscle isolated and divided. The dermis of the skin segment is sutured to the fascia so that the muscle and skin are mobilized as a unit.

The dissection continues in a cephalad direction. The flap is mobilized, leaving a 1-cm cuff of rectus fascia both medially and laterally for later closure. The flap is then fully mobilized, with the vascular pedicle carefully preserved, and is transposed into the defect.

Fascial closure usually incorporates synthetic mesh. The umbilicus is moved slightly to the donor side due to the deficiency of tissue in this region. The flap is then sutured into the recipient bed and should be loose and floppy in the defect. Care is taken to protect the pedicle at all times, with continuous assessment (Figure 36-6).

An incision hernia at the fascial level is possible after this procedure. This is decreased by incorporating a synthetic mesh to reinforce the abdominal fascial closure if any undue tension is noted. Weakness in sitting up has been reported but is usually well compensated after approximately 3 months. This can be a more serious problem in young, active individuals and has not been studied in athletes. It is more debilitating if both muscles are harvested, but this is also transient in most patients.

TRAPEZIUS FLAP

The trapezius muscle flap is most useful for midline defects of the upper posterior thorax and cervical spine. This flap can also reach the posterior aspect of the occipital area. Its most common use may be the posterior neck regions after dehiscence from a previous orthopedic or neurosurgical operation. The trapezius flap can be mobilized effectively without loss of shoulder strength as long as the upper portion of the muscle and the spinal accessory nerve are preserved. This flap can also carry a large segment of the overlying skin.

Functionally and aesthetically, the trapezius muscle can be divided into two portions: an upper region and a lower region. The *upper region* courses as a strip from the base of the neck laterally toward the acromion and constitutes the neck's upper border as it joins the shoulder. This is the muscle's most

functional portion for shoulder elevation and must be preserved. Although this part has been used for reconstructive purposes, problems related to the donor site (e.g., pain, weakness, dysesthesias around shoulder, sensitivity over skin graft) have limited its effectiveness.

The *lower region* of the trapezius muscle, on the other hand, seems to be aesthetically and functionally dispensable. It can provide richly vascularized tissue to compromised regions and is reliable, is easy to mobilize, and readily accepts skin grafts. The arc of coverage is extensive and, as stated, can reach the upper occipital area, opposite the scapular spine, and midline areas cephalad to T12. This flap can also be used for cavitary defects of the upper midline spinal region, which may be it most useful application.

To ensure that the skin island overlies the muscle, the surgeon determines borders of the muscle and notes the blood supply. The pivot point of the flap is the superficial transverse cervical artery (descending branch), which runs along the deep aspect of the muscle and enters approximately 5 to 7 cm lateral to the midline at approximately the level of spinous process C7. In the posterior neck, C7 is palpated and marked; the spinous processes are then counted from the prominent C7 down to T12, which is also marked. The acromion is then marked, and this triangle generally contains the trapezius muscle. An extended flap can be employed that exceeds the border of the muscle. It is recommended, however, that these extended areas be "delayed" before rotating the flap definitively.

Again, and as with other flaps, the skin island overlying the flap should be in the range of 8 cm in width and length to incorporate perforators entering the skin and subcutaneous tissues from the fascia of the muscle itself. The larger the skin segment, the more likely it is to survive because it will contain more skin perforators from the muscle.

After thorough cleansing of the defect recipient bed, the skin island is circumferentially incised down to the deep fascia. The muscle is then uncovered at the plane between the subcutaneous fat and the deep fascia. Dermal/fascial sutures from the skin island to the trapezius fascia are inserted to protect the perforators against shearing. Starting along the muscle's lateral border, the thin fascia separating the trapezius from the underlying latissimus dorsi muscle is entered and a plane established subjacent to the trapezius. Muscle is carefully separated from the paraspinous muscle, proceeding laterally to medially and moving closer to the spinous processes. As the muscle is freed, its origin from the spinous processes is sharply incised and elevated. The surgeon gradually elevates the muscle, working cephalad and searching for the vascular pedicle that will be seen coming from the region of the medial scapular spine.

The sturdy attachments of the trapezius from the lateral scapular spine are sharply divided, allowing the muscle to be easily mobilized in a cephalad direction. The neurovascular pedicle is seen on the flap's underside as the medial aspect of the nape is approached. The defect can be sharply connected to the trapezius region by incising the skin and fat from the recipient bed down to the mobilization area of the trapezius.

The skin is easily closed at the donor defect and the trapezius musculocutaneous flap easily fitted into the defect. As with other flaps, the flap should be loose and floppy in the defect without tension. The defect is then closed in layers.

RECONSTRUCTION OF CONGENITAL DEFECTS

Pectus deformities and Poland's anomalies are amenable to effective reconstruction.

Pectus Excavatum

In pectus excavatum the superior aspect of the manubrium and the first and second ribs are usually normal. The main deformity usually affects the anterior thoracic wall distal to the sternal angle of Louis. Costal cartilages are abnormally curved inward, resulting in a concavity of the sternal body with variable depth. This concavity places abnormal pressure over the mediastinal structures, resulting in cardiac displacement, rotation of the heart, and reduction in the lung space. In later years, this abnormality may cause exercise intolerance, palpitations, or even heart murmurs.

Pectus deformity is often cosmetically unacceptable and embarrassing to patients and their families. The psychosocial implications of these deformities can be compelling. Also, cardiorespiratory disturbances are possible.

CT, routine chest radiography, multigated acquisition scanning, and MRI are often used to evaluate these deformities. In a 5- or 6-year-old child a sternovertebral distance less than 5 cm on a lateral chest radiograph is considered a severe deformity; 5 to 7 cm is considered moderate; and greater than 7 cm is considered mild. Our usual preoperative operation utilizes standard anteroposterior and lateral chest radiographs, 12-lead electrocardiogram, and ultrasonography or CT scanning.

The patient is placed supine on the operating table, and a midline incision is made. Even in females this midline approach seems to be associated with a more cosmetic scar than the standard inframammary approach. The dissection is made with the cautery and bilateral pectoralis muscle flaps, which are developed from the midline to the midclavicular line laterally, up to the second intercostal space, and down to the seventh intercostal space inferiorly. This exposes the abnormal ribs and the xyphoid region. The xyphoid is elevated with a towel clip or Kocher clamp, exposing the posterior surface of the sternum. The pleura is bluntly freed from the posterior sternum and the medial aspect of both sternocostal margins with the fingertip.

The lowermost cartilages are dissected first, incising the perichondrium longitudinally. A dental elevator or perichondrial dissector is used to strip the perichondrium from the cartilage. When the superior and inferior surfaces of the chondral cartilages are exposed, the elevator is advanced beneath the costal cartilage and the cartilage transected at a convenient point. The cartilage is then elevated completely and removed from the sternum all the way to the costochondral junction. This is performed for the lowermost four or five costochondral cartilages bilaterally, resecting the abnormally formed and shaped cartilages but leaving a perichondrial sleeve. The cartilage does regenerate, but not as vigorously as some describe.

Sternal wedge osteotomies are made after placement of a broad, malleable retractor beneath the sternum to protect the great vessels and heart. The sternum is usually divided in two places. A greenstick fracture technique is used for the posterior table in some patients to elevate the sternum into a more natural position. A Washington strut can be fashioned to elevate the sternum, placing the tips of the bar on the lateral surfaces of the bony ribs and wiring them into position. Alternatively, a thin titanium metallic plate can be used to secure the sternum (Figure 36-7).

Pectus Carinatum

Pectus carinatum is a protrusion of the chest wall and is much is less common that the excavatum deformities. The operative technique used for the excavatum deformity is also used to correct the carinatum deformity.

Poland's Anomaly

Poland's syndrome includes a constellation of hypoplastic deformities that are combined unilaterally to the chest wall and upper extremity. It always involves partial or total absence of the pectoralis major muscle and other associated deformities, such as brachysyndactyly. Most patients are diagnosed because of the perception of a cosmetic defect associated with the absence of the pectoralis major muscle and its corresponding soft tissue deficit over the upper chest wall.

The full-blown syndrome may involve extensive deformities of the costochondral cartilages and sternum and ipsilateral absence of portions of the second to fourth ribs. The spectrum of deformities associated with this anomaly vary from a simple absence of the sternocostal head of the pectoralis major muscle to segmental absence of all parietal components of the chest wall except skin and pleurofascial membrane. Brachysyndactyly usually consists of hypoplasia of the musculoskeletal elements of the upper extremity and syndactyly. The syndactyly includes foreshortened fingers and extension contractures of the small digital joints.

Options for reconstruction include anterior transfer of the latissimus dorsi muscle through a transaxillary tunnel and attachment of the muscle to the clavicle and sternum. In the female this is accompanied by submuscular insertion of a mammary prosthesis to ameliorate the soft tissue deformity. In severe defects, reconstruction may also require resection of portions of deformed cartilages and repositioning of the cartilages before latissimus muscle transposition.

I have found that custom-made chest wall prostheses and use of alloplastic or allogeneic materials have been ineffective compared with autogenous tissues, such as muscle transposition, combined with a submuscular mammary prosthesis in the female (Figures 36-8 and 36-9).

Despite the effectiveness of the latissimus transposition, restoration of abnormal-appearing anterior axillary folds continues to be challenging. Detachment of the latissimus insertion with anterior reattachment on the humerus sometimes ameliorates this problem.

The long-term results of chest wall reconstruction for Poland's anomaly have been relatively good using the options described. In males, the latissimus transposition, with folding

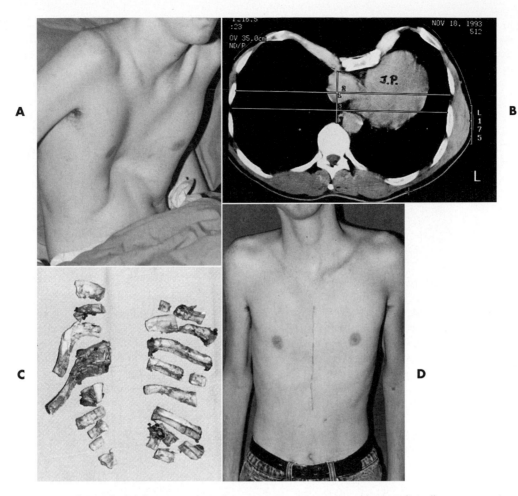

Figure 36-7. A, Adolescent male with severe pectus excavatum. He was clinically symptomatic because of displaced heart and great vessels. **B,** Axial CT scan shows displacement of mediastinal structures that can occur secondary to pectus excavatum. **C,** Cartilage removed. Subperichondrial dissection left envelope of perichondrium. **D,** Excellent healing after repair of pectus excavatum. Clinically, patient's cardiorespiratory endurance improved.

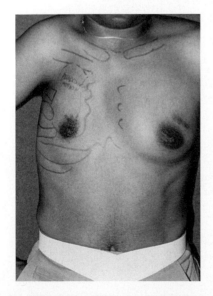

Figure 36-8. Patient with Poland's anomaly has shortening of entire hemothorax, with absence of second to fifth ribs, hypoplasia of nipple/areolar complex, and absence of sternocostal head of pectoralis major muscle. Portion of clavicular head is also absent.

Figure 36-9. Patient had custom-made soft silicone prosthesis inserted to supply fullness for Poland's anomaly. It subsequently was removed because of migration and symptomatic irregularities along edge of prosthesis that interfaced with musculoskeletal elements.

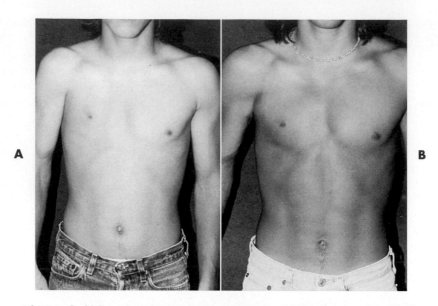

Figure 36-10. **A,** Male patient has most common form of Poland's anomaly, with absence of sternocostal head of pectoralis major muscle. Ipsilateral latissimus dorsi muscle is intact. **B,** Patient underwent transposition of ipsilateral latissimus dorsi muscle. Muscle has been folded along sternal surface and inferior border to resemble natural pectoralis major muscle in fullness and direction of fibers. Humeral insertion has been transposed anteriorly and sutured to periosteum anterior to bicipital groove of humerus.

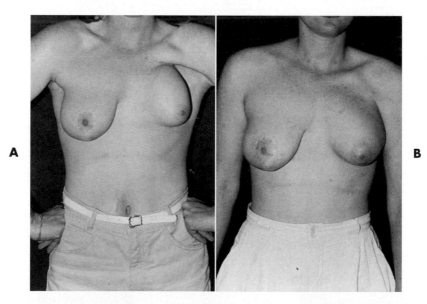

Figure 36-11. **A,** Female patient treated for Poland's anomaly with prosthesis. She is activating clavicular head of pectoralis major muscle, distorting implant and chest wall. Note that ipsilateral latissimus dorsi muscle is intact. **B,** After transposition of latissimus dorsi muscle, with submuscular insertion of mammary prosthesis. This seems to provide excellent contour.

of the distal latissimus to augment the sternal fullness, seems to give the best result. The direction of the fibers is reconstituted in the same direction as a normal pectoralis major muscle. The inferior border can also be folded, and combined with an insertional reattachment, the results have been quite good (Figure 36-10). In females, a latissimus flap augmented by a submuscular implant usually restores the soft tissues effectively (Figure 36-11).

OUTCOMES

It has been quite difficult to obtain long-term data on all the musculocutaneous flaps that have been performed. The author reviewed the musculocutaneous flaps performed for chest wall reconstruction at Walter Reed Army Medical Center and found that 295 flaps had been performed over 11 years. Since that time an additional 32 flaps have been performed. This series involved 13 minor dehiscences that consisted of subcutaneous tissue and skin separations that healed secondarily.

One death was associated with myocardial infarction postoperatively. A contributing factor was pulmonary insufficiency secondary to the total sternectomy defect resulting from treatment for an aggressive basal cell carcinoma that invaded all chest wall layers. The patient had a prolonged period of ventilatory assistance because of the severe instability associated with the total sternectomy.

Infection was rare in this series, but several dehiscences had associated subcutaneous abscesses. Infection was associated with polypropylene mesh in five patients. Treatment included reelevation of the flap, excision of the loose mesh (which had not been incorporated in the healing process), and reclosure. All these individuals healed uneventfully after removal of the foreign material.

With the congenital defects, one patient's sternum was sectioned, elevated, and stabilized with a Steinmann pin. The pin broke at the junction of the sternum and the left rib cage and was removed. The patient healed uneventfully. In another patient, plates were used to stabilize the sternum, and loosening of one screw necessitated its removal. This was associated with a palpable screw beneath the skin, without infection. Again, the patient healed uneventfully.

None of the patients required reoperation for hematoma, but all those with musculocutaneous flaps had seromas develop at the donor site. These seromas reaccumulated after removal of the suction drains and eventually resorbed without intervention.

AESTHETIC RESULTS

Aesthetic results with chest wall reconstruction have been quite good with regard to contour and extremely favorable compared with a large defect in the chest wall. This was especially true for patients with tumor resections and reconstruction.

Musculocutaneous flaps resulted in uniformly good results compared with the previous defect. This was especially true with full-blown Poland's syndrome when the pectoralis major muscle and portions of the anterior ribs were missing before the muscle transfer.

Of 11 patients treated with custom-made chest wall prostheses, 10 had their prostheses removed. The reasons for removal included the following:
1. Migration of the prosthesis
2. Persistent seromas related to alloplastic materials
3. Poor contour
4. Uncomfortable rigidity of prosthetic device

These failures have resulted in abandonment of prosthetic devices to reconstruct the musculoskeletal layer in Poland's syndrome. Mammary prostheses combined with the latissimus muscle flap, however, have achieved excellent aesthetic results in female patients. Likewise, the latissimus dorsi muscle flap alone, which may be folded to achieve a more natural contour, has been uniformly well accepted by male patients.

PHYSICAL FUNCTIONING

Current data on functional outcomes indicate that patients have transient weakness when a muscle is harvested and moved to another location to fulfill reconstructive needs. For example, in an unpublished study of 11 patients who received free flap reconstruction using the latissimus dorsi muscle to close complex lower extremity defects, patients experienced a transient weakness that lasted as long as 8 weeks. Preoperative and postoperative computed muscle testing indicated that as long as the other shoulder girdle musculature was intact, patients regained preoperative strength characteristics between 6 and 8 weeks postoperatively.

A similar decrease in function would be expected for other muscle groups, depending on the patient's health, adjacent compensatory musculature, and which muscle is removed from its normal location. These characteristics are similar to those involved in tendon transfers. Fortunately, certain muscles seem to be dispensable for normal activities of daily living. More precise (e.g., athletic) muscle functioning would be expected to decline after harvesting of a muscle that is critical for that particular activity.

A contour deformity can also develop after use of muscle and musculocutaneous flaps in chest wall reconstruction. For example, the use of the latissimus dorsi muscle leaves a hollowing in the flank and posterior back region after its use in the reconstruction of Poland's anomaly. The results in the anterior thorax seem to outweigh this deficit, however, and patients have been pleased with the outcome.

GENERAL HEALTH STATUS AND QUALITY OF LIFE

The use of muscle and musculocutaneous flaps to close large defects of the chest wall improves quality of life and allows the patient to be discharged earlier. Likewise, achievement of primary healing of an open wound is favorable in terms of the following:
1. Mobilizing the patient
2. Shortening the period of convalescence
3. Achieving protection of intrathoracic viscera
4. Restoring chest wall mechanics

Therefore the patient's health status and quality of life are uniformly improved after these operations, despite the scarring over the donor site and the risks discussed earlier.

Reconstruction of the sternum in pectus excavatum and carinatum patients also has been favorable for quality of life from a social standpoint and allows the patient to wear apparel more easily. My experience also indicates that pulmonary mechanics improve after repair of the pectus excavatum deformity.

COSTS OF CARE

The closure of chest wall defects has allowed patients to be discharged earlier than if the chest wall defect had not been repaired, with decreased expense and costs of care. The patient with a congenital malformations is mobilized the day of surgery and usually discharged after the first postoperative night. Unfortunately, long-term data on costs of pectus excavatum are unavailable. Patients are uniformly pleased with the results, however, and the minor complications discussed earlier have not resulted in extensive hospitalization except in rare patients.

PATIENT SATISFACTION

The nature of chest wall reconstruction is such that the patients are uniformly pleased with the results compared with the previous chest wall tumor or congenital deformity. Preoperative counseling is key to ensuring realistic expectations. As a rule, however, chest wall reconstruction has been very well accepted by patients.

REFERENCES

1. Azarow K, Molloy M, Seyfer AE, Graeber G: Preoperative evaluation and general preparation for chest wall operation, *Surg Clin North Am* 69:899-910, 1989.

2. Farley J, Seyfer AE: Chest wall tumors: experience with 58 patients, *Milit Med* 156:413-415, 1991.

3. Garcia V, Seyfer AE, Graeber G: Reconstruction of congenital chest wall deformities, *Surg Clin North Am* 69:1103-1118, 1989.

4. Graeber G, Seyfer AE, Wind G: Reconstruction of the dehisced median sternotomy, *Surg Rounds* 11:94-99, 1988.

5. Seyfer AE: Correction of the infected mediastinum after cardiac surgery, *Contemp Surg* 38(5), 1991.

6. Seyfer AE: The lower trapezius flap for recalcitrant wounds of the posterior skull and spine, *Ann Plast Surgery* 20:414-419, 1988.

7. Seyfer AE: Management of chest wall deformity in male patients with Poland's syndrome, *Plast Reconstr Surg* 87:674-678, 1991.

8. Seyfer AE: Radiation-associated lesions of the chest wall: longitudinal experience with 31 patients, *Surg Gynecol Obstet* 167:129-131, 1988.

9. Seyfer AE: Use of trapezius muscle for closure of complicated upper spinal defects, *Neurosurgery* 14:341, 1984.

10. Seyfer AE, Graeber G: The use of latissimus dorsi and pectoralis major musculocutaneous flaps in chest wall reconstruction, *Contemp Surg* 22:29, 1983; *Contemp Orthop* 7:30, 1983.

11. Seyfer AE, Graeber G, Wind G: *Atlas of chest wall reconstruction*, Rockville, Md, 1986, Aspen.

12. Seyfer AE, Graeber G, Wind G: Chest wall reconstruction: anterior and axillary defects, *Surg Rounds* 11:99-107, 1988.

13. Seyfer AE, Graeber G, Wind G: Chest wall reconstruction: posterior defects, *Surg Rounds* 11:85-89, 1988.

14. Seyfer AE, Graeber G, Wind G: Current techniques for sternal reconstruction, *Surg Rounds* 11:105-113, 1988.

15. Seyfer AE, Graeber G, Wind G: The radiation-damaged chest wall: reconstruction using a rectus abdominis musculocutaneous flap, *Surg Rounds* 11:69-71, 1988.

16. Seyfer AE, Walsh D, Graeber G, et al: Chest wall implantation of lung cancer after thin-needle aspiration biopsy, *Ann Thorac Surg* 48:284-286, 1989.

17. Stahl R, Seyfer AE: Chest wall reconstruction. In Russell R, editor: *Instructional course lectures, Plastic Surgery Educational Foundation,* St Louis, 1990, Mosby.

18. Waldorf K, Seyfer AE: Poland's syndrome, *Surg Rounds* 16:669-677, 1993.

Abdominal Wall Reconstruction

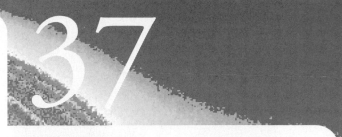

Grant Carlson
John Bostwick

INDICATIONS

Anterior abdominal wall defects may present as a deficiency of the fascia, the overlying skin and soft tissue, or both. The defect can also be characterized as to (1) presence or absence of infection or contamination, (2) location, and (3) size. Final wound evaluation includes any previous abdominal operations and coexisting medical conditions. Each abdominal wall defect should be evaluated individually as to requirements for reconstruction and maintenance of long-term integrity.

TUMOR RESECTION

Desmoid tumors are often found in the abdominal wall and represent an unencapsulated accumulation of fibrous tissue arising from the musculoaponeurotic layers to the torso (Figure 37-1). Females are affected more often than males, usually in the third to fifth decades of life and frequently after pregnancy. These lesions are histologically benign but locally invasive. Treatment consists of full-thickness abdominal wall resection. Despite aggressive surgery, local recurrence has been reported in up to 40% of patients, most within 2 years of initial treatment. Adjuvant radiation therapy may reduce recurrence when wide margins cannot be obtained.

Dermatofibrosarcoma protuberans is a rare cutaneous tumor that presents as a slowly growing, bluish red nodule, located most often on the trunk. The tumor extensively infiltrates the dermis and subcutaneous tissue. Aggressive resection of the skin and underlying subcutaneous tissue is usually adequate treatment.

Primary and secondary malignancies of the abdominal wall occur with equal frequency. Sarcomas are among the most common of the primary malignancies. Histologically high-grade lesions are usually treated with surgery and external beam radiation therapy. Metastatic tumors usually arise from the gastrointestinal or genitourinary tracts. These invariably require full-thickness abdominal wall resection.

INFECTION

Rapidly progressive soft tissue infections are usually caused by mixed aerobic and anaerobic organisms. Treatment generally consists of aggressive surgical debridement and intravenous (IV) antibiotics. Abdominal wall reconstruction is performed when the infection is controlled and the wound has stabilized.

Necrotizing fasciitis presents with toxemia and painful skin erythema. Within 24 hours, dusky purple areas of skin develop with blistering and bullae. Rapid subcutaneous tissue necrosis causes deep undermining superficial to the myofascial layer. Streptococcal gangrene is a type of necrotizing fasciitis caused by β-hemolytic *Streptococcus,* usually combined with *Staphylococcus aureus.* Treatment is based on prompt identification of the problem, IV antibiotics, and early surgical debridement.

Postoperative *clostridial myonecrosis* of the abdominal wall is a rare entity. It is a mixed aerobic and anaerobic infection involving at least one *Clostridium* species. Clostridia produce a number of exotoxins, including lecithinase, collagenase, and hyaluronidase, which play a major role in the infectious process. The infection occurs early in the postoperative period, with wound swelling, tenderness, and serosanguineous discharge. A small amount of gas with crepitation can usually be detected. The patient has tachycardia and hypotension out of proportion to temperature elevation. Clostridial myonecrosis requires prompt diagnosis, IV antibiotics, and wide surgical debridement of all abdominal wall layers.

TRAUMA

Traumatic injuries to the abdominal wall, usually from gunshot wounds, result in extensive soft tissue damage. Abdominal viscera are usually injured, resulting in gross contamination. These injuries require extensive debridement and are associated with a high mortality rate. Abdominal wall reconstruction is often performed in multiple stages to allow the patient's medical condition to improve and the wounds to stabilize.

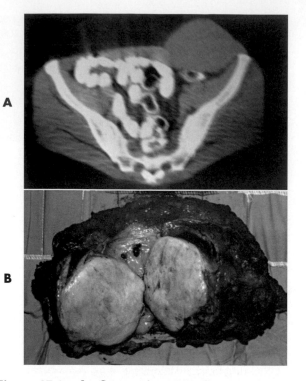

Figure 37-1. A, Computed tomography scan shows large desmoid tumor originating in abdominal wall. **B,** Gross histologic appearance after surgical resection.

INCISIONAL HERNIATION

The rate of hernia associated with abdominal incisions is estimated at 4% to 10%.[29] Postoperative wound infection and dehiscence increase the risk of ventral herniation. Other predisposing factors include patient age, type of incision, obesity, malnutrition, anemia, and steroid dependence.[41]

Transverse incisions run parallel to the natural horizontal lines of force in the abdominal wall, which tends to close the wound. They have the lowest rate of herniation compared with midline and paramedian incisions.

Lateral traction on the rectus abdominis muscles by contraction of the flat abdominal muscles (external oblique, internal oblique, transversus abdominis) promotes visceral protrusion. Incisional hernias tend to progress as the rectus abdominis muscles assume a lateral orientation and the hernia orifice enlarges. Increased intraabdominal pressure plays a minor role in this progression.

ANATOMY AND PHYSIOLOGY

The anterior abdominal wall is a complex anatomic and functional system comprising nine layers: (1) skin, (2) subcutaneous tissue, (3) superficial fascia (Scarpa's fascia), (4) external oblique muscle (EO), (5) internal oblique muscle (IO), (6) transversus abdominis muscle (TA), (7) transverse fascia (TF), (8) extraperitoneal adipose and areolar tissue, and (9) peritoneum.

Scarpa's fascia is a discrete layer that can be demonstrated in the lower abdominal wall. It adds little strength to wound closure, but its approximation assists in a tension-free wound closure, especially in the lower abdomen.

The muscular abdominal wall is composed of three flat muscles with broad origins (EO, IO, TA). Anteriorly, these muscles give way to flat aponeuroses that fuse to form the investing sheath of the rectus abdominis muscles. The function of each muscle results from its balance with the others. The aponeuroses are in continuity across the linea alba and rectus sheath with the tendon fibers from the opposite side. This creates a digastric arrangement, with the linea alba and rectus sheath serving as the linking elements.[3]

The rectus abdominis muscles arise inferiorly from the crest of the pubis. The muscles insert on the cartilages of the fifth, sixth, and seventh ribs. Each muscle is crossed by three fibrous bands called *tendinous intersections.* One is at the level of the umbilicus, one at the level of the xiphoid process, and the third midway between the other two.

The *linea semicircularis* (semicircular line), or *arcuate line,* is found midway between the umbilicus and the pubis. Superior to this line, the IO aponeurosis splits into two layers; one fuses with the EO aponeurosis as it passes in front of the rectus abdominis muscle, and the other blends with the TA aponeurosis to form the posterior layer of the sheath (Figure 37-2). Below the level of the linea semicircularis, the three aponeuroses join to pass in front of the rectus muscle so that the posterior layer of the sheath is composed of only the TF. This layer is considered to be crucial against the development of incisional hernia. The TF is separated from the peritoneum by extraperitoneal fat.

The *linea semilunaris* (semilunar line) forms the lateral boundary of the rectus muscle. It is formed by the union of the aponeuroses of the IO and TA as they join to form the rectus sheath. The EO aponeurosis joins the rectus sheath medial to the linea semilunaris.

The plane between the IO and TA contains the segmental neurovascular structures that supply the abdominal wall. The intercostal nerves of T7 to L1 enter the undersurface of the rectus abdominis muscle at the junction of its lateral and medial third.

Compression of the abdomen is generated by the joint action of the flat muscles; their bilateral contraction is coordinated by the midline aponeurotic structures. Intense electromyographic activity has been recorded from these muscles during the "bearing down" efforts necessary to evacuate the rectum and bladder or to deliver a fetus from the uterus. The lower fibers of the IO and TA show continuous activity during standing.

Normal breathing does not involve abdominal muscle activity. Electrical activity is noted in the flat muscles during forced expiration and coughing. The rectus abdominis muscles are not involved in these functions.

Trunk movements are produced by the abdominal muscles. Trunk flexion is produced by the rectus abdominis muscles, with some participation by the oblique muscles. Unilateral muscle harvest, as with transverse rectus abdominis myocutaneous (TRAM) flap reconstruction, results in loss of the ability to do situps in 17% of patients.[21] Trunk rotation results from the joint contraction of one EO plus the contralateral IO.

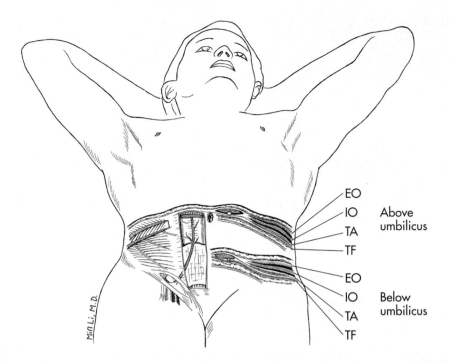

Figure 37-2. Cross-sectional anatomy of abdominal wall. Superior to arcuate line (linea semicircularis), internal oblique muscle *(IO)* aponeurosis splits into two layers. External oblique muscle *(EO)* aponeurosis joins rectus sheath medial to linea semilunaris. *TA,* Transversus abdominis muscle; *TF,* transverse fascia.

The abdominal muscles assist in support the lumbar spine. The IO and TA attach to the lumbodorsal fascia, which attaches to the lumbar spinous processes, ribs, and iliac crest.

Nahai et al[36] divide the abdominal wall into three zones based on vascular anatomy. *Zone I* covers the area between the lateral borders of the rectus sheaths, extending from the xiphoid and costal margin superiorly to the level of a line drawn between the anterosuperior iliac spines. The blood supply to the skin and subcutaneous tissue is derived from the perforating branches of the superior and inferior epigastric vessels. *Zone II* covers the area below a line drawn between the anterior iliac spines to the pubic and inguinal creases. The area is supplied by branches of the circumflex iliac and external pudendal vessels. *Zone III* covers the area lateral to zone I and superior to zone II. The blood supply is derived from the branches of the intercostal and lumbar vessels.

OPERATIONS

PREOPERATIVE PLANNING

Abdominal wall reconstruction should be divided into its component parts: (1) skin, (2) soft tissue, and (3) fascia. Adequate soft tissue can often be obtained by simple advancement of the abdominal skin. For large soft tissue defects, pedicled or free flap closure can be used. In clean wounds, fascial replacement is best accomplished with synthetic mesh provided there is adequate soft tissue coverage. In contaminated fields, autologous tissue or absorbable mesh can be used to provide fascial integrity.

Computed tomography (CT) scanning may be helpful in determining the size of ventral hernias and the retraction of the abdominal muscles. In massive ventral hernias the "right of domain" of the abdominal viscera is lost. Reduction of viscera can compress the inferior vena cava and immobilize the diaphragm. Gradual pneumoperitoneum injected percutaneously or via a Tenckhoff catheter can expand the abdominal cavity to allow reduction of the viscera and abdominal closure without interfering with pulmonary function.[12]

A two-stage reconstruction is often indicated in contaminated fields and in difficult and prolonged operations, such as in trauma and fistula closure.[38] Extensive enterolysis may result in bowel edema and intestinal dilation, which can compromise reconstruction. Primary wound closure would result in prohibitive morbidity. Absorbable mesh is used to close the fascia and skin, and subcutaneous tissue is left open. The mesh is allowed to granulate and then skin grafted. After 6 to 12 months, the skin graft matures and is no longer adherent to the underlying viscera. At the second stage the skin graft can be easily excised and definitive closure performed.

DIRECT APPROXIMATION

In 1990 Ramirez et al[42] described the "components separation" technique to close large fascial defects. The rectus abdominis muscle is separated from the posterior rectus sheath by posterior dissection, and the EO is separated from the IO in an avascular plane (Figure 37-3). A compound flap of rectus muscle, anterior sheath, and attached IO/TA can be advanced toward the midline.

Thomas et al[49] described a modification of this technique

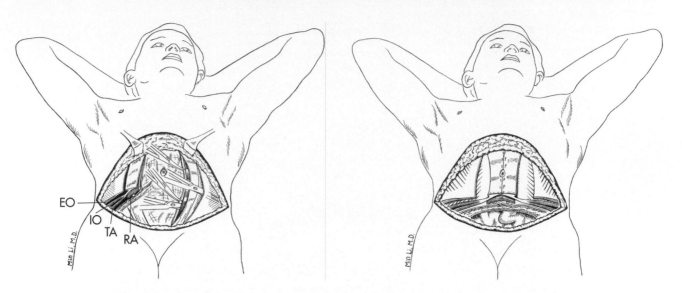

Figure 37-3. "Components separation" technique releases rectus sheath, enabling advancement of myofascial unit.

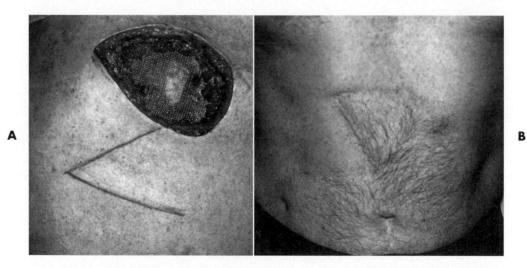

Figure 37-4. **A,** Defect after resection of recurrent dermatofibrosarcoma protuberans of epigastrium. Anterior rectus sheath has been reconstructed with polypropylene mesh. **B,** Appearance after fasciocutaneous flap closure of defect.

by simply making an incision in the EO fascia laterally to allow coadaptation of the linea alba. This method takes advantage of the EO aponeurosis inserting on the rectus sheath medial to the linea semilunaris.

SKIN AND FASCIAL GRAFTS

Skin grafts will take when applied to the abdominal viscera[18] or granulated prosthetic mesh. As mentioned, skin grafts can provide a temporary wound closure in contaminated cases or after extensive intraabdominal surgery. Within 6 to 12 months the skin graft matures and will separate easily from the abdominal viscera.

Autogenous fascia lata grafts have been used successfully to reconstruct the myofascial layer.[20,33] Free fascial grafts survive autotransplantation to maintain their structural integrity.[14] Hamilton[20] reported his experience with 47 ventral hernia repairs in 45 patients using fascia lata free grafts. The overall hernia recurrence rate was 6.4%. Free fascia lata grafts have also been used for static repair of facial paralysis and in various ophthalmologic procedures.[28]

Clinical experience has shown that the exposed fascia lata does not granulate and is therefore not useful in open abdominal wounds. Free fascia lata grafts can supplant pedicled tensor fascia lata myofascial flaps in patients who do not require soft tissue and skin. Circumferential suturing to close the fascial defects interferes with the blood supply of the pedicled myofascial flaps.

FASCIOCUTANEOUS FLAPS

Fasciocutaneous flaps based on the superior or inferior epigastric perforating vessels can sometimes be useful to provide soft tissue coverage of the abdominal wall[24] (Figure 37-4). In most

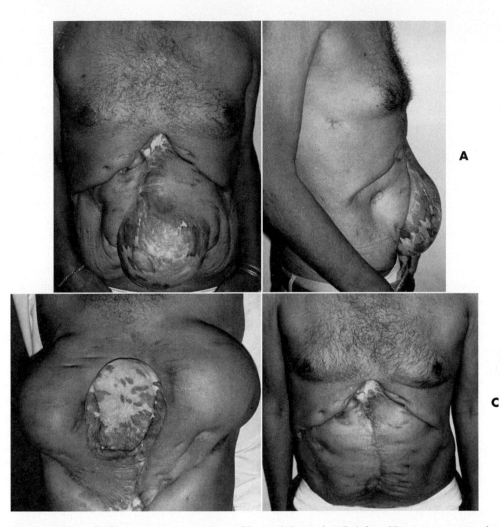

Figure 37-5. **A,** Preoperative appearance of large abdominal wall defect. Viscera are covered with skin graft. **B,** Large tissue expanders have been placed under skin and subcutaneous tissue. **C,** Appearance after expander removal, polypropylene mesh placement, and advancement of expanded flaps.

patients, especially through midline incisions, the abdominal wall skin and soft tissue can be widely undermined to the flanks to permit local tissue advancement for wound closure. In extreme cases, relaxing incisions can be placed in the flanks to allow bipedicled advancement flap closure over synthetic mesh; the resultant flank defects are closed with skin grafts.

TISSUE EXPANSION

Scattered reports have discussed the use of tissue expansion to reconstruct the abdominal wall.[10,22,25,38] This technique can provide good aesthetic results in terms of color match, contour, and minimal donor site morbidity. The disadvantages are that it requires multiple stages and a stable wound (Figure 37-5).

Byrd and Hobar[10] described expanding the myofascial layers in infants to close congenital abdominal wall defects. Hobar et al[22] later described placing tissue expanders in an adult between the IO and TA through an incision in the rectus sheath. They believed this provided autogenous, innervated, contractile tissue for abdominal wall reconstruction. Jacobsen

et al[25] described a similar approach in four patients with massive ventral hernias. The expanders were placed between the EO and IO through remote lateral incisions. All patients were successfully reconstructed without synthetic mesh.

Okunski et al[38] described the use of tissue expansion in staged abdominal wall reconstruction. Four patients with intraabdominal catastrophes and open abdominal wounds were treated initially by skin grafting of granulated abdominal viscera. After the wounds were stable, tissue expanders were inserted between the subcutaneous fat and the anterior rectus sheath. After adequate expansion, the skin grafts were excised, mesh was inserted, and expanded soft tissue closed.

ALLOPLASTIC MATERIAL

Synthetic material predates use of autologous tissue in abdominal wall reconstruction. Silver mesh was used in Germany at the turn of the twentieth century.[4,19,56] Silver mesh had a tendency to oxidize and corrode in tissues, however, and was supplanted by tantalum in the 1940s. Tantalum fell into disfavor because of its tendency to fragment after repeated flexion.[8,9]

In the late 1950s and early 1960s the synthetic polymers were developed, such as polypropylene and polyethylene (Dacron).[50] Current materials used for fascial replacement include polypropylene (Marlex, Prolene), polytetrafluoroethylene (PTFE, Gore-Tex), polyester (Mersilene), and polyglactin 910 (Vicryl, Dexon). Each material has unique properties.

Types

Polypropylene has become the standard synthetic prosthetic material to reestablish musculofascial integrity. Complications (e.g., wound sepsis, bowel fistula, mesh extrusion) have made polypropylene most suitable for clean wounds with adequate soft tissue coverage. Prolene has greater pliability and porosity than Marlex and appears to have a lower fistulization rate.

Polyester mesh (Mersilene) is light and strong, readily conforms to the contours of the abdominal viscera, and provokes a brisk inflammatory response. Stoppa et al[47] and Wantz[53] reported extensive experience using Mersilene in the repair of large ventral hernias. Stoppa[46] reported an 18.5% recurrence rate of 133 polyester mesh repairs of midline hernias, with a mean follow-up of 5½ years. Wantz[53] reported no incisional hernia recurrences in 23 cases using Mersilene mesh. Aldloff and Arnaud[2] reviewed its use for repair of large incisional hernias in 130 patients, with follow-up longer than 3 years in 80% of patients. No obstructive complications occurred, with a 4.5% hernia recurrence rate.

Experimental studies have shown that *polytetrafluoroethylene* (Gore-Tex) has fewer adhesions to abdominal viscera than polypropylene but has poorer tissue ingrowth. Bauer et al[4a] reviewed their experience using expanded PTFE in the repair of large abdominal wall defects in 28 patients. Reherniation occurred in three (10.7%) patients. No complications were related to adhesions or erosion of patch material into viscera or skin. PTFE may have an advantage over polypropylene mesh because of the low foreign body reaction, which may result in separation at the native fascia–mesh interface and seroma formation in the subcutaneous tissue.

Absorbable *polyglactin 910* or *polyglycolic mesh* (Vicryl, Dexon) is a good temporary fascial substitute in contaminated wounds. It dissolves in over several months, which can result in large ventral hernias, especially when covered by skin grafts if secondary placement of permanent mesh is not performed.[7,35]

Techniques

The most common method of using prosthetic material is as an *inlay graft* attached to the fascial edges. This type of repair depends on the integrity of the fascial edges. Abdominal pressure and muscle contraction result in lateral distraction, which can lead to recurrences between the mesh and the native fascia.

The placement of prosthetic material in the space between the rectus abdominis muscles and the peritoneum was devised in Europe by Rives[43] and Stoppa et al.[47] Wantz[53] has described the technique extensively in the American literature. The advantages of the *retrorectus repair* are that it uses the forces of abdominal pressure to push the peritoneum and posterior rectus fascia against the mesh, which is isolated from the abdominal contents (Figure 37-6). The only chance of a midline recurrence is cephalad or caudad to an incompletely reinforced midline. McLanahan et al[32] reported 106 midline ventral hernia repairs using the retrorectus repair and polypropylene mesh, with a recurrence rate of 3.5%.

MUSCULOCUTANEOUS FLAPS

Ach[1] first reported musculocutaneous flaps in abdominal wall reconstruction in 1910 when he used a pedicled fascia lata flap to close the femoral ring. In 1913 Polya[40] reported the use of a compound pedicled flap of skin, fascia, and sartorius muscle in the repair of a large inguinal hernia. MacKenzie[30] made the first report in the English literature in 1924. He described the use of tensor fascia lata (TFL) flap in the repair of a large defect

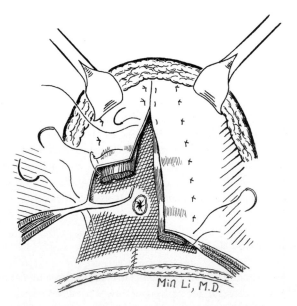

Figure 37-6. Retrorectus placement of mesh above peritoneum.

Table 37-1.
Musculocutaneous Flaps and Abdominal Wall Reconstruction

FLAP	ABDOMINAL DEFECT	USE OF FASCIA
Tensor fascia lata	Lower	Yes
Rectus femoris	Lower	Yes
Rectus abdominis	Upper, lower	No
Latissimus dorsi	Upper	No

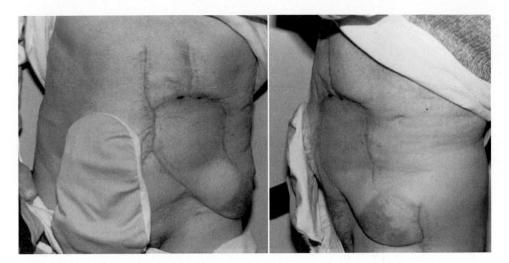

Figure 37-7. Postoperative appearance after tensor fascia lata (TFL) musculocutaneous flap reconstruction of abdominal wall.

in the lower abdomen. Wangensteen[52] popularized by the use of the TFL flap for abdominal wall reconstruction in his report of 14 cases in 1934.

Select musculocutaneous flaps can provide fascial supports as well as soft tissue for abdominal wall reconstruction. They are generally used in contaminated operative fields where nonabsorbable synthetic mesh cannot be safely used. In clean cases, such as those seen after tumor resection, several additional flaps can provide soft tissue coverage of synthetic mesh (Table 37-1).

Tensor Fascia Lata Flap

The TFL musculocutaneous flap is a reliable and versatile method of reconstructing full-thickness defects of the abdominal wall (Figure 37-7). It is supplied by the lateral femoral circumflex vessels, which enter the deep surface of the muscle approximately 10 cm below the anterosuperior iliac spine. The artery divides into several branches before entering the muscle. Inferior branches course superficial to the TFL. These vessels send perforating branches to supply the overlying skin.

The skin territory is supplied by two sensory nerves: (1) the lateral cutaneous branch of T12, which innervates the skin overlying the iliac crest, and (2) the lateral cutaneous branch of L2-3, which innervates the skin of the lateral thigh. Both these nerves are easily identifiable and may be included in a sensory TFL flap.

The skin territory is large, measuring up to 15×40 cm (6×16 inches). The center of the flap is a line from the greater trochanter to the midlateral aspect of the knee. The posterior border is a line from the greater trochanter to the lateral knee at the margin of the biceps femoris muscle. Anteriorly, the flap may include skin over the rectus femoris muscle. The donor site can be closed primarily if the flap width is less than 10 cm (4 inches).

The origin of the TFL muscle is the anterior iliac spine and the greater trochanter of the femur. It is a small muscle with a large fascial extension that inserts on the lateral aspect of the

knee. Occasional knee instability is noted with flap harvest, but suturing the distal cut margin into the fascia of the vastus lateralis muscle may reduce this complication. The rotation arc of the pedicled flap will reach the costal margin if the tensor muscle is completely detached from its origin and raised as an island flap (Figure 37-8).

The problem with using the TFL flap in the upper abdomen is that the distal one third of the skin island has a random blood supply and is unreliable. The blood supply to this area is normally through perforating vessels from the underlying vastus lateralis muscle, which are severed during flap elevation. The parallel fibers of the TFL are at a mechanical disadvantage when placed in a vertical orientation (Figure 37-8).

Rectus Femoris Flap

The rectus femoris musculocutaneous flap can provide muscle, dense fascia, and overlying skin for abdominal wall reconstruction.[6,15,16,39] Many surgeons prefer it over the TFL flap for suprapubic and lower abdominal wall coverage because of proximity, reliability, and ease of elevation. The rectus femoris is not as suitable as the TFL flap for groin coverage and does not reach the upper abdomen unless it is used as a turnover, muscle-only flap.

The rectus femoris flap is supplied by the lateral femoral circumflex vessels, which enter the deep surface of the muscle lateral to the sartorius muscle 6 to 8 cm (about 3 inches) below the pubis. The muscle originates from the anteroinferior iliac spine and inserts on the patellar tendon. The muscle's primary function involves the terminal 15 to 20 degrees of knee extension. This potential loss may be overcome by suturing the vastus medialis and lateralis muscles to the cut rectus femoris tendon.

The cutaneous segment can be expanded to three times the width of the rectus femoris muscle by including the adjacent fascia lata. The fasciocutaneous segment encompasses the majority of the anterior thigh skin.[15] The muscle is approxi-

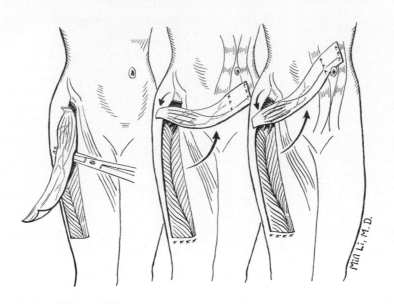

Figure 37-8. Fibers of TFL flap assume vertical orientation when used above umbilicus.

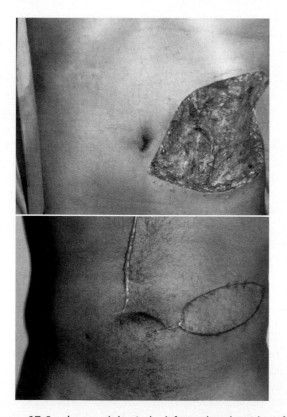

Figure 37-9. Large abdominal defect closed with inferiorly based, vertically oriented rectus abdominis musculocutaneous flap.

mately 6 cm (2½ inches) in width, but the associated fascia is strong enough to reconstruct a defect 15 to 20 cm (6 to 8 inches) in diameter. The pedicle is the limiting factor in upward flap rotation. Dividing the muscle origin does not facilitate flap mobility.

Rectus Abdominis Flap

The rectus abdominis musculocutaneous flap can provide soft tissue coverage for abdominal wall reconstruction.[5,31] This versatile flap can be based on either the inferior or superior epigastric vessels (Figure 37-9). Taylor et al[48] has described the extended deep inferior epigastric (EDIE), flap an oblique form of the inferiorly pedicled rectus abdominis musculocutaneous flap. A bilobed modification can allow closure of large upper abdominal wall defects[13] (Figure 37-10).

Latissimus Dorsi Flap

The latissimus dorsi muscle receives its dominant blood supply from the thoracodorsal vessels originating from the subscapular vessels. This large muscle can be used as a pedicled or free flap; as a pedicled flap, it has been used to reconstruct the breast and upper abdomen. Houston et al[23] described using an extended latissimus dorsi flap to include the lumbar dorsal and pregluteal fascia to increase the arc of rotation. Six patients with successful ventral hernia repair showed no evidence of lumbar hernia formation. This flap may be useful to provide soft tissue in the epigastric area, but the skin overlying the fascial extensions can be unreliable.

FREE FLAPS

Free tissue transfer may overcome the rotation limitations seen with extremity-based flaps. This makes free flaps attractive for reconstruction of the upper abdomen; use of the free TFL flap has been described.[37,55] Recipient vessels include the inferior epigastric and the gastroepiploic.[44] Williams et al[55] reported seven cases without a total flap loss (Figure 37-11). Distal tip necrosis was seen in three cases. The authors thought that the free TFL flap was useful in supraumbilical defects, especially with contaminated wounds.

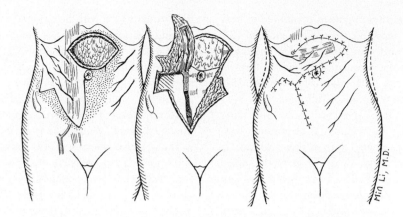

Figure 37-10. Extended deep inferior epigastric (EDIE) flap.

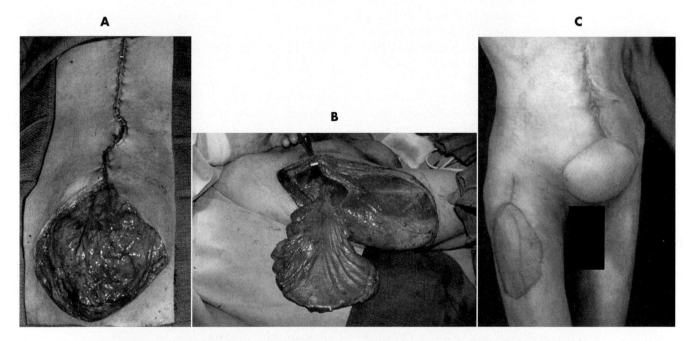

Figure 37-11. A, Lower abdominal wall defect after resection of sarcoma. **B,** TFL musculocutaneous free flap isolated on lateral femoral circumflex vessels. **C,** Postoperative appearance after free TFL flap reconstruction. Donor site was closed with skin graft.

OUTCOMES

Successful abdominal wall reconstruction provides stable soft tissue coverage and restores fascial integrity. The success of various methods is usually expressed in terms of hernia recurrences and flap necrosis rates.

Data are lacking on functional impairments after latissimus dorsi muscle harvest. Clinically, minimal functional impairment of arm adduction has been noted. Rectus abdominis muscle harvest can impact lower back stability. The abdominal muscles support the back through connections with the lumbodorsal fascia. A few patients have had lower back problems after breast reconstruction with bipedicled TRAM flaps. Therefore bilateral rectus muscle harvest or unilateral harvest in patients with lower back problems should be done sparingly.

No studies have assessed the effects of abdominal wall reconstruction on activities of daily living. Cost analyses are also unavailable. These are productive areas for future research.

ALLOPLASTIC MATERIAL

Synthetic mesh requires adequate soft tissue coverage to avoid complications. Voyles et al[51] reviewed their experience with polypropylene mesh for the immediate closure of abdominal defects. Mesh extrusion or enteric fistulization occurred in

93% (14/15) of cases that were skin grafted or allowed to heal secondarily. Stone et al[45] reported their experience in 124 patients with abdominal closure using polypropylene mesh followed by skin grafting over the granulation tissue that formed in the mesh. Of these patients, 40% eventually required mesh removal because of extrusion or enteric fistulization.

Nagy et al[35] reported their experience using Gore-Tex, Dexon, and Marlex mesh in temporary abdominal wall closure. Marlex mesh was associated with a high fistulization rate. The resulting hernias after the use of Dexon mesh tended to be large. Gore-Tex mesh resulted in fewer fistulas and less adhesions, but granulation tissue did not form over it.

Concern about erosion of polypropylene mesh into viscera has lead many to advocate the use of PTFE or Mersilene when intraperitoneal placement is necessary. Experience has shown that this concern may be unwarranted when minimal adhesion lysis is performed. Many authors have reported no problems placing polypropylene mesh in direct contact with viscera. Others believe this leads to dense adhesions and fistula formation. Placing omentum or absorbable mesh over the viscera has been advocated to prevent these complications.

Karakousis et al[26] reported their experience of placing omentum or free peritoneal patches between the abdominal viscera and polypropylene mesh during abdominal wall reconstruction. When mesh was placed directly on abdominal viscera, the incidence of enterocutaneous fistula was 23% (6/26). Placing omentum or peritoneum under the mesh eliminated fistula formation in 30 patients.

MUSCULOCUTANEOUS FLAPS

With its abundant fascia and proximity, the TFL flap would seem to be ideal for abdominal wall reconstruction. Williams et al[54] reviewed 27 cases using the TFL flap, including 12 free grafts, nine pedicled flaps, and six free flaps. The mean follow-up was 23.6 months. One patient had a recurrent hernia (free graft), and donor site complications occurred in

five patients (one with hematoma, two with seroma, two with wound dehiscence). Three of the nine pedicled flaps and three of the six free flaps developed partial flap necrosis. This emphasized the unreliability of the distal skin.

Figure 37-12 shows an algorithm for use of the TFL flap in abdominal wall reconstruction. The TFL graft is used in defects of fascia only with well-vascularized, adequate local soft tissue coverage. Wounds may be clean or contaminated but without active infection. The fascia may also be used as an onlay graft in repairs where the primary fascia may be tenuous. Vascularized tissue is preferable in defects with active infection or relatively ischemic native tissue. The pedicled musculocutaneous flap can be used in lower abdominal wounds of limited size requiring both fascia and soft tissue. If the wound involves the epigastrium or requires two pedicled flaps for coverage, the free flap can be used.

The rectus femoris flap may be more versatile than the TFL flap. The former is easier to dissect, and the overlying skin is more reliable. The dense fascia of the thigh make the rectus femoris useful in reconstruction of the lower abdomen. We have no experience using it as a turnover flap of muscle and fascia to reach the upper abdomen.[17] The donor site may have problems. Caulfield et al[11] used a dynamometer to study leg extension in seven patients after rectus femoris flaps and found an average 25% decrease in leg extension in six patients. As mentioned, this may be overcome by suturing the vastus medialis and lateralis tendons together in the midline.

The rectus abdominis flap can provide abundant soft tissue to reconstruct defects in the upper or lower abdomen. Sacrifice of an entire rectus abdominis muscle appears to be well tolerated by most patients. Kind et al[27] studied abdominal wall function with a dynamometer in 14 patients after breast reconstruction with unipedicled TRAM flaps. At 6 months after surgery, maximum isometric flexion torque was 89% of baseline. Mizgala et al[34] reported that 15.4% of patients could not perform a situp after unipedicled TRAM flap reconstruction. Also, 35% reported decreased abdominal muscle strength on questionnaire evaluation.

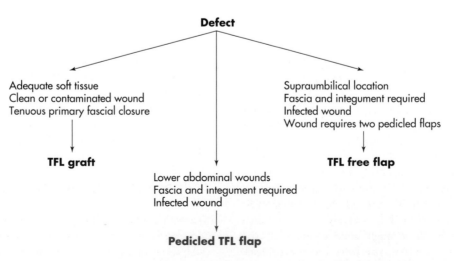

Figure 37-12. Algorithm for use of TFL flap in abdominal wall reconstruction.

The latissimus dorsi flap can provide soft tissue coverage of the upper abdomen to the midline. The muscle can be skin grafted because the skin overlying the lumbodorsal fascia is unreliable.

REFERENCES

1. Ach A: Neue art plastischen bruchpforten verschlusses bei cruralhernlien, *Beitr Z Klin Chir* 70:358, 1910.

2. Adloff M, Arnaud JP: Surgical management of large incisional hernias by an intraperitoneal Mersilene mesh and an aponeurotic graft, *Surg Gynecol Obstet* 165:204, 1987.

3. Askar OM: Surgical anatomy of the aponeurotic expansions of the anterior abdominal wall, *Ann R Coll Surg Engl* 59:313, 1977.

4. Bartlett W: An improved filigree for the repair of large defects in the abdominal wall, *Ann Surg* 38:47, 1903.

4a. Bauer JJ, Salky BA, Gelernt IM, Kreel I: Repair of large abdominal wall defects with expanded polytetrafluoroethylene, *Ann Surg* 206:765-769, 1987.

5. Bostwick J, Hill HL, Nahai F: Repairs in the lower abdomen, groin, or perineum with myocutaneous or omental flaps, *Plast Reconstr Surg* 63:186, 1979.

6. Brown DM: Closure of complex abdominal wall defects with bilateral rectus femoris flaps with fascial extensions, *Surgery* 114:112, 1993.

7. Buck JR, Fath JJ, Chung S, et al: Use of absorbable mesh as an aid in abdominal wall closure in the emergent setting, *Am Surg* 61:655, 1995.

8. Burke GL: The corrosion of metals in the tissues; and an introduction to tantalum, *CMAJ* 43:125, 1940.

9. Burton LC: Fascia lata, cutis, and tantalum grafts in repair of massive abdominal incisional hernias, *Surg Gynecol Obstet* 109:621, 1959.

10. Byrd HS, Hobar PC: Abdominal wall expansion in congenital defects, *Plast Reconstr Surg* 84:347, 1989.

11. Caulfield WH, Curtsinger L, Powell G, et al: Donor leg morbidity after pedicled rectus femoris muscle flap transfer for abdominal wall and pelvic reconstruction, *Ann Plast Surg* 32:377, 1994.

12. Coelho JCU: Progressive preoperative pneumoperitoneum in the repair of large abdominal hernias, *Eur J Surg* 159:339, 1993.

13. Cormack GC, Quaba AA: Bilobe modification of the deep inferior epigastric artery flap for abdominal wall defect reconstruction, *Br J Plast Surg* 44:541, 1991.

14. Crawford JS: Nature of fascial lata and its fate after implantation, *Am J Ophthalmol* 67:900, 1969.

15. Dibbell DG, Mixter RC, Dibbell DGS: Abdominal wall reconstruction (the "mutton chop" flap), *Plast Reconstr Surg* 87:60, 1991.

16. Freedman AM, Gayle LB, Vaughan ED, et al: One-stage repair of the anterior abdominal wall using bilateral rectus femoris myocutaneous flaps, *Ann Plast Surg* 25:299, 1990.

17. Ger R, Duboys E: The prevention and repair of large abdominal-wall defects by muscle transposition: a preliminary communication, *Plast Reconstr Surg* 72:170, 1983.

18. Gervin AS, Fischer RP: The reconstruction of defects of the abdominal wall with split thickness skin grafts, *Surg Gynecol Obstet* 155:413, 1982.

19. Goepel R: Ueber die verschliessung von bruchpforten durch einheilung geflochtener, fertiger silberdrahtnetze (Silberdrahtpelotten), *Verh Dsch Ges Chir* 29:174, 1900.

20. Hamilton JE: The repair of large or difficult hernias with mattressed onlay grafts of fascia lata: a 21-year experience, *Ann Surg* 167:85, 1968.

21. Hartrampf CR, Bennett GK: Autogenous tissue reconstruction in the mastectomy patient: a critical review of 300 patients, *Ann Surg* 205:508, 1987.

22. Hobar PC, Rohrich RJ, Byrd HS: Abdominal-wall reconstruction with expanded musculofascial tissue in a posttraumatic defect, *Plast Reconstr Surg* 94:379, 1994.

23. Houston GC, Drew GS, Vazuez B, et al: The extended latissimus dorsi flap in repair of anterior abdominal wall defects, *Plast Reconstr Surg* 81:917, 1988.

24. Iwahira Y, Maruyama Y, Shiba T: One-stage abdominal wall reconstruction with oblique abdominal fasciocutaneous flaps, *Ann Plast Surg* 19:475, 1987.

25. Jacobsen WM, Petty PM, Bite U, et al: Massive abdominal-wall hernia reconstruction with expanded external/internal oblique and transversalis musculofascia, *Plast Reconstr Surg* 100:326, 1997.

26. Karakousis CP, Volpe C, Tanski J, et al: Use of a mesh for musculoaponeurotic defects of the abdominal wall in cancer surgery and the risk of bowel fistulas, *J Am Coll Surg* 181:11, 1995.

27. Kind GM, Rademaker AW, Mustoe TA: Abdominal-wall recovery following TRAM flap: a functional outcome study, *Plast Reconstr Surg* 99:417, 1997.

28. Kirschner M: Der gegenwartige stand und die nachsten aussichten ser autoplastischen freien fascien-uebertragung, *Beitr Klin Chir* 86:5, 1913.

29. Larson GM, Vandertoll, DJ: Approaches to repair of ventral hernia and full-thickness losses of the abdominal wall, *Surg Clin North Am* 64:335-349, 1984.

30. MacKenzie K: The repair of large abdominal herniae by muscle transposition, *Br J Surg* 12:28, 1924.

31. Mathes SJ, Bostwick J: A rectus abdominis myocutaneous flap to reconstruct abdominal wall defects, *Br J Plast Surg* 30:282, 1977.

32. McLanahan D, King LT, Weems C, et al: Retrorectus prosthetic mesh repair of midline abdominal hernia, *Am J Surg* 173:445, 1997.

33. McPeak CJ, Miller TR: Abdominal wall replacement, *Surgery* 47:944, 1960.

34. Mizgala CL, Hartrampf CR, Bennett GK: Assessment of the abdominal wall after pedicled TRAM flap surgery: 5 to 7 year follow-up of 150 consecutive patients, *Plast Reconstr Surg* 93:988, 1994.

35. Nagy KK, Fildes JJ, Mahr C, et al: Experience with three prosthetic materials in temporary abdominal wall closure, *Am Surg* 62:331, 1996.

36. Nahai F, Brown RG, Vasconez LO: Blood supply to the abdominal wall as related to planning of abdominal incisions, *Am Surg* 42:691, 1976.

37. O'Hare PM, Leonard AG, Brennen MD: Experience with the tensor fasciae latae free flap, *Br J Plast Surg* 36:98, 1983.

38. Okunski WJ, Sonntag BV, Murphy RX: Staged reconstruction of abdominal wall defects after intra-abdominal catastrophes, *Ann Plast Surg* 36:475, 1996.

39. Peters W, Cartotto R, Morris S, et al: The rectus femoris myocutaneous flap for closure of difficult wounds of the abdomen, groin, and trochanteric areas, *Ann Plast Surg* 26:572, 1991.

40. Polya E: Beitrag zum plastischen verschlusz der Leistenbruchpforte, *Arch F Path Anat* 63: 504, 1913.

41. Poole GV: Mechanical factors in abdominal wound closure: the prevention of fascial dehiscence, *Surgery* 97:631, 1985.

42. Ramirez OM, Ruas E, Dellon AL: "Components separation" method for closure of abdominal wall defects: an anatomic and clinical study, *Plast Reconstr Surg* 86:519, 1990.

43. Rives J: Major incisional hernia. In Cherval JP, editor: *Surgery of the abdominal wall,* Paris, 1987, Springer-Verlag.

44. Sekido M, Yamamoto Y, Sugihara T, et al: Microsurgical reconstruction of chest and abdominal wall defects associated with intraperitoneal vessels, *J Reconstr Microsurg* 12:425, 1996.

45. Stone HH, Fabian TC, Turkleson ML: Management of acute full-thickness losses of the abdominal wall, *Ann Surg* 193:612, 1981.

46. Stoppa RE: The treatment of complicated groin and incisional hernias, *World J Surg* 13:545, 1989.

47. Stoppa R, Louis D, Verhaeghe P: Current surgical treatment of postoperative eventrations, *Int Surg* 72:42, 1987.

48. Taylor GI, Corlett RJ, Boyd JB: The extended deep inferior epigastric flap: a clinical technique, *Plast Reconstr Surg* 72:751, 1983.

49. Thomas WOI, Parry SW, Rodning CB: Ventral/incisional abdominal herniorrhaphy by fascial partition/release, *Plast Reconstr Surg* 91:1080, 1993.

50. Usher FC, Ochsner J, Tuttle LLD: Use of Marlex mesh in the repair of incisional hernias, *Am Surg* 24:969, 1958.

51. Voyles CR, Richardson JD, Bland KI, et al: Emergency abdominal wall reconstruction with polypropylene mesh, *Ann Surg* 194:219, 1981.

52. Wangensteen OH: Repair of recurrent and difficult hernias and other large defects of the abdominal wall employing the iliotibial tract of fascia lata as a pedicled flap, *Surg Gynecol Obstet* 59:766, 1934.

53. Wantz GE: Incisional hernioplasty with Mersilene, *Surg Gynecol Obstet* 172:129, 1991.

54. Williams JK, Carlson GW, deChalain T, et al: The role of tensor fascia lata in abdominal wall reconstruction, *Plast Reconstr Surg* 101:713-718, 1998.

55. Williams JK, Carlson GW, Howell RL, et al: The tensor fascia lata free flap in abdominal-wall reconstruction, *J Reconstr Microsurg* 13:83, 1997.

56. Witzel O: Yber den verschluss von bauchwunden und bruchpforten durch versenkte silverdrahtnetze (einheilung von filigranpelotten), *Centralb Chir* 27:257, 1900.

Hip and Pelvic Wall Reconstruction

Daniel Reichner
Robert E. Montroy

Hip and pelvic wall defects result from infection, pressure necrosis, radiation injury, trauma, or residual defects after tumor excision. This chapter only discusses major structural reconstruction of the hip and pelvis; other chapters discuss lower genitourinary system reconstruction and repair of soft tissue defects caused by infection, pressure ulcers, and radiation injury. This discussion includes major indications for hip and pelvic reconstruction, anatomic considerations in planning reconstruction, major types of hip and pelvic wall surgery, and surgical outcomes.

HIP RECONSTRUCTION

Indications

The indications for hip reconstruction usually involve chronic wounds caused by infected orthopedic hardware or infected total hip replacements.[6] Approximately 1% to 2% of all total hip arthroplasties become infected, or 800 to 1600 cases per year in the United States. The standard treatment has been removal of the prosthesis with methylmethacrylate and antibiotic therapy. Then a new prosthesis with antibiotic-impregnated methylmethacrylate is implanted immediately or delayed for 1 to 3 months, depending on the individual circumstances.

Each year approximately 100 to 200 of these patients develop a chronic, nonhealing hip wound. These wounds usually have an open draining sinus with woody induration of the surrounding tissue and polymicrobial cultures that may include yeast and fungus.

Reconstruction is started by debridement of soft tissue, scar tissue, bone, and all methylmethacrylate. The reconstruction will fail if all infected bone and methylmethacrylate are not removed. The reconstruction team must ensure adequate debridement of all infected bone before wound reconstruction.

A rectus femoris transposition muscle flap can be used in small wounds and vastus lateralis or rectus abdominis muscle flaps in larger wounds (Figure 38-1). Free muscle flaps may be necessary if local transposition flaps fail or if the defect is large. If a skin defect remains after the muscle flap reconstruction, a split-thickness skin graft can be used to close the

wound immediately or may be delayed until the infection is controlled.

Operations
RECTUS FEMORIS FLAP

Anatomy. The rectus femoris muscle is one of the quadriceps. The muscle originates at the anteroinferior iliac spine and upper portion of the acetabulum and inserts into the large quadriceps patellar tendon. The major arterial supply is the lateral femoral circumflex branch of the deep femoral artery. This artery enters the rectus femoris muscle approximately 10 cm (4 inches) below the anterosuperior iliac spine. A secondary arterial supply to the muscle is located 2 cm (about 1 inch) below the primary supply (Figure 38-2).

Reconstruction. The rectus femoris muscle can be elevated through a lateral thigh incision. The muscle is transposed to the defect as a pedicle based on the lateral femoral circumflex artery. It is secured above the acetabulum to ensure that the entire defect is filled. The vastus lateralis and vastus medialis muscles are then approximated for about 10 to 15 cm (4 to 6 inches) with permanent sutures, starting at the patellar tendon. The lateral skin is closed primarily.

Deep drains are placed in the defect and donor site and retained for 2 weeks or more depending on the amount of drainage. The knee is immobilized for 2 weeks after surgery. The major morbidity using the rectus femoris muscle for reconstruction involves weakness with knee extension.

VASTUS LATERALIS FLAP

Anatomy. The vastus lateralis muscle originates on the lateral surface of the greater trochanter and the trochanteric line and inserts into the rectus femoris tendon and the upper lateral patella. The blood supply is the lateral femoral circumflex branch of the deep femoral artery, which enters the muscle 10 to 12 cm (4 to 5 inches) below the anterosuperior iliac spine. The distal one third of the muscle is supplied by perforating branches of the superficial femoral artery. Therefore only the proximal two thirds of the muscle can be reliably elevated based on the proximal pedicle, and the distal one third should be resected until adequate bleeding is found.

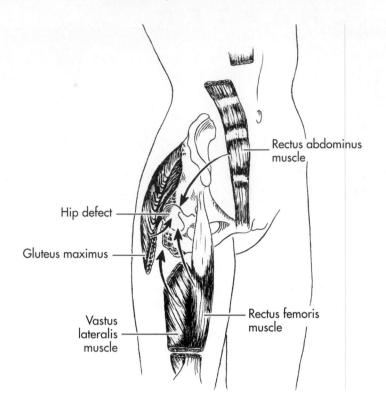

Figure 38-1. Rectus abdominis, gluteus maximus, vastus lateralis, and rectus femoris muscle flaps for hip reconstruction.

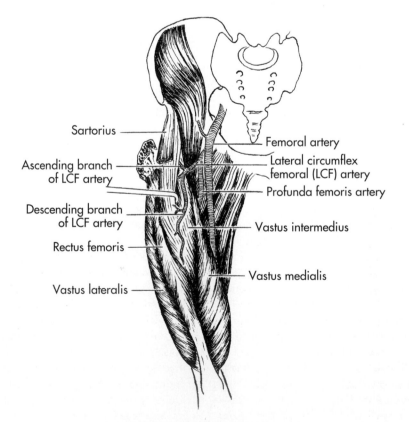

Figure 38-2. Anterior thigh anatomy.

Reconstruction. Vastus lateralis elevation is performed through a lateral incision and is more difficult than elevation of the rectus femoris muscle, particularly the more distal portion. Also, firm vascular attachments to the femur connect to the major vascular pedicle proximally. Care must be taken not to divide the terminal branches of the lateral femoral circumflex artery. The vastus lateralis muscle has been used alone or in combination with the rectus femoris to reconstruct larger tissue defects.

One drawback to using the vastus lateralis muscle is significant weakness related to knee extension and lateral knee instability. Postoperative care is similar to that for the rectus femoris flap.

RECTUS ABDOMINIS FLAP

Anatomy. The rectus abdominis muscle originates from the costal margins of the sixth through ninth ribs and inserts into the pubic tubercles. The two major blood supplies to the rectus abdominis muscle are the inferior and superior epigastric arteries. The inferior epigastric is a branch of the external iliac artery and can supply the entire muscle as an inferior pedicle.

Reconstruction. The rectus abdominis flap is elevated through a midline skin incision, opening the anterior rectus sheath and dividing the muscle superiorly, as well as the superior epigastric artery and vein. The muscle can then be then transposed preperitoneally to the hip region. The acetabular roof is then opened and the muscle transposed into the defect (Figure 38-3). Some reconstructive surgeons prefer using a free rectus flap as a first choice. In either case, the resulting abdominal wall defect may lead to significant abdominal wall weakness and possible hernia formation.

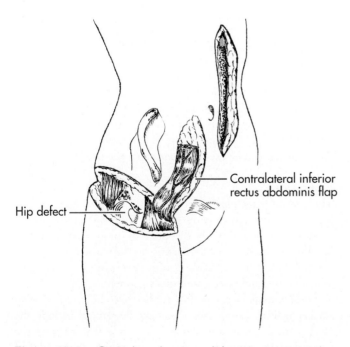

Figure 38-3. Contralateral rectus abdominis reconstruction for lateral pelvic defect.

FREE MUSCLE FLAPS. Free muscle flaps may be necessary to reconstruct large defects or defects in which prior muscle flaps have failed. The latissimus dorsi and rectus abdominis free flaps are typically used for this purpose. The anatomy and elevation of these flaps are discussed in other chapters.

Free flap reconstruction of hip defects may require the addition of an arteriovenous fistula with a saphenous loop. This fistula is made by elevating the saphenous vein and anastomosing it to the femoral artery. The loop is tunneled to the defect under the thigh skin. The latissimus dorsi muscle can then be elevated as a myocutaneous flap to cover most large lateral thigh defects. A microvascular anastomosis it made between the thoracodorsal artery and vein and the divided saphenous arteriovenous fistula. The rectus abdominis muscle is used in a similar way.

Outcomes

Meland[6] reported a series of 31 patients with infected arthroplasty wounds. He used 40 muscle flaps in 30 patients. The rectus femoris was used in 20 patients, vastus lateralis in six, rectus abdominis in three, and tensor fascia latae in one, with a combined latissimus dorsi serratus anterior free flap in five patients. With an average follow-up of 6.4 years, 18 patients could walk with minor pain, five with a cane, seven with a walker, six with crutches, and four unassisted. All wounds healed without complications or drainage after reimplantation of the total hip prosthesis.

PELVIC WALL RECONSTRUCTION

Indications

The indications for pelvic wall reconstructions are large defects usually caused by tumor ablation (with or without radiation injury), infections of pelvic soft tissue and bone, and trauma. Traumatic injuries usually involve avulsions or crushing of the lower extremity and pelvis. The mechanisms of these injuries include the following[5]:

1. Lower extremity or pelvic avulsion by entanglement in machinery
2. Motor vehicle accidents causing sacroiliac joint disruption and pubic symphysis separation
3. Massive crush injuries to the groin, disrupting the vessels, nerves, soft tissue, and pelvic bones

Many of these patients undergo heroic limb-salvage procedures. When these procedures are unsuccessful, an immediate hip disarticulation or hemipelvectomy may save the patient's life. Immediate surgery prevents sepsis and allows wide exposure for hemostasis, debridement, and assessment and management of associated injuries to the lower genitourinary system and rectum.

Trauma is a relatively rare indication for pelvic reconstruction, but the principles for reconstruction are the same as those for large defects resulting from tumor ablation.[7] The surgeon should remember that if thigh musculature is viable, it may be useful in pelvic reconstruction for additional soft tissue coverage.

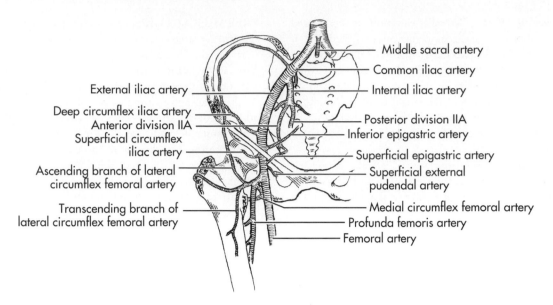

Figure 38-4. Pelvic blood supply.

PELVIC TUMORS. Soft tissue and bony defects resulting from en bloc tumor resection are the most common indications for pelvic reconstruction. Considering primary tumors alone, an estimated 2000 new cases of bone sarcoma and 5700 cases of soft tissue sarcoma are diagnosed annually in the United States. Approximately 5% to 10% involve the pelvis.[3] Chemotherapy and surgical techniques now offer patients with nonmetastatic disease a 50% or greater chance for long-term disease-free survival.

Preoperative radiographic imaging studies have allowed surgeons to define the anatomic extent of these tumors accurately and plan the surgical procedure more precisely. Once the extent and type of tumor have been determined, the surgeon can plan the options for resection and reconstruction.

Hemipelvectomy was considered the standard operation for pelvic sarcomas, but newer limb-sparing procedures (e.g., internal hemipelvectomy) have been designed to achieve local tumor control while maximizing function. Secondary tumors tend to be more invasive into surrounding soft tissues and often require a full or modified hemipelvectomy. These major reconstructive procedures require careful planning and thorough understanding of pelvic anatomy.

ANATOMY. The pelvis is defined as the region above lower extremities and below the abdomen. The iliac crest, pubic symphysis, sacrum, and greater trochanter are the bony landmarks that help define the pelvis.

The major arteries in the pelvis include the common iliac artery, which divides into the external and internal iliac arteries (Figure 38-4). The deep circumflex iliac and inferior epigastric arteries branch off the external iliac before it exits the pelvis under the inguinal ligament to become the femoral artery. The internal iliac artery enters the true pelvis and divides into anterior and posterior divisions. The anterior

division divides into the inferior gluteal, obturator, internal pudendal, umbilical, inferior vesical, middle rectal uterine, and vaginal arteries. The posterior division branches into the superior gluteal, iliolumbar, and lateral sacral arteries.[1]

The bones of the pelvis include the ilium, ischium, and pubis, which form the innominate. The pelvic brim is formed by the sacral promontory, iliopectineal line, and pubic symphysis. The true and false pelvis lines are below and above the brim, respectively (Figure 38-5).

The musculature outside and above the bony pelvis includes the quadratus lumborum, transversus abdominis, internal oblique, external oblique, and rectus abdominis. The muscles outside and below the pelvis include the gluteus maximus/medius/minimus, tensor fascia lata, gemellus, rectus femoris, sartorius, vastus lateralis/medialis, adductor brevis/longus/magnus, gracilis, semitendinosus, and semimembranosus muscles. Inside the bony pelvis, the pelvic diaphragm consists of the levator ani (puborectalis, pubococcygeus, iliococcygeus), coccygeus, and piriformis. The lateral internal wall of the bony pelvis is covered by the obturator, psoas major/minor, and iliacus. Alone or in combination, many of these muscles can be used to reconstruct the pelvis.

Operations

The general principles of reconstructive surgery apply to the pelvis as in other parts of the body. The reconstructive ladder should be followed with the goal of preserving as much function as possible without sacrificing the patient's long-term survival. Soft tissue coverage is often necessary because bone, joints, nerves, and vessels are usually exposed.

Local muscle flaps should be the first choice for closing smaller defects. Local flaps that have been used include the gluteus maximus, rectus abdominis, rectus femoris, and the vastus lateralis muscles. Prosthetic material can be added if

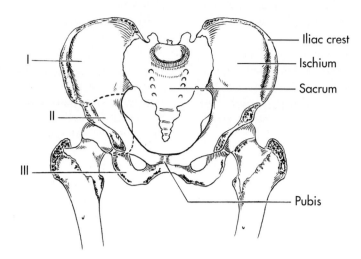

Figure 38-5. Bony pelvis.

necessary to close fascial or bony defects. If the defects are extremely large, a free flap may be used to provide the necessary soft tissue coverage.

As with other major reconstructions, the choice of procedure depends on the defect's size and location. We divide pelvic reconstruction into anterior, lateral, and posterior wall defects.

ANTERIOR DEFECTS. Defects in the anterior pelvic region can be difficult to close primarily because local tissue is lacking due to size of the resection, prior irradiation, and previous procedures.[2] Although resection of the anterior pelvis is stable, abdominoperineal hernias can be a problem without adequate reconstruction.

Several traditional procedures are used to close anterior defects, including local muscle flaps and free flaps. Fascia must be incorporated into these flaps to prevent hernias. The rectus abdominis muscle flaps have been used for anterior defects. Another approach, described by Evans et al,[2] incorporates prosthetic mesh for pelvic bone reconstruction and muscle flaps to cover the mesh. This reestablishes the pelvic floor and bony support by anchoring the nonabsorbable mesh posteriorly to the sacrum, coccyx, and posterior iliac wings, anteriorly to the costal margins, and laterally to the iliac crest and abdominal fascia (Figure 38-6).

Omentum or the rectus abdominis can be used for internal coverage to prevent contact between the mesh and viscera. The muscle is brought inside the mesh through a small opening and fixed to the sacrum and coccyx. The tensor fascia lata or rectus femoris, both based on the lateral circumflex femoral artery can also be used separately or together for internal or external mesh soft tissue coverage. Other options for soft tissue coverage include the gracilis, sartorius, and vastus lateralis muscles.

If necessary, free tissue transfer can also provide internal or external coverage. The recipient vessels include internal and external iliac vessels and their branches.

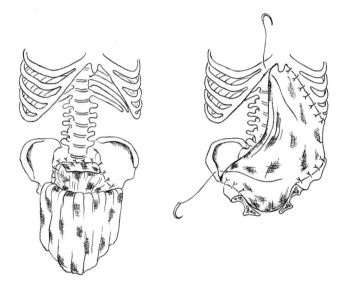

Figure 38-6. Mesh used in reconstruction of anterior defects. Note posterior sacral and costochondral fixation.

LATERAL DEFECTS. Resection of all or part of the hemipelvis is indicated for primary tumors, secondary locally invasive tumors, and metastatic bone disease. The choice for reconstruction of the lateral pelvis depends on the extent and location of tumor resection. Smaller defects with a stable pelvis can be covered with local or free muscle flaps, including the rectus abdominis, external oblique, and rectus femoris. Larger pelvic tumors traditionally have required amputation of lower limb, with more extensive resection of the pelvic bone and soft tissue as well as hemipelvectomy reconstruction.

Again, the current trend is toward limb-sparing procedures or internal hemipelvectomy with limited resection of bone and soft tissue, bone replacement with allograft, and hip joint reconstruction.

Hemipelvectomy. This procedure involves removal of the entire lower extremity and ipsilateral hemipelvis. A *radical* hemipelvectomy involves dividing the bone proximal to the sacroiliac joint. A *conservative* hemipelvectomy involves preservation of part of the iliac bone.

If the tumor is located in the groin or iliac fossa, a posterior flap reconstruction is best. Posterior tumors involving the buttock usually require an anterior flap. If the local soft tissue defect is extensive, transposition muscle flaps or free flaps maybe necessary for immediate reconstruction of the pelvic defect.[3]

Posterior Flap. Major indications for a posterior flap include (1) primary tumors of the innominate bone or femur that have invaded the hip joint and (2) tumors of the upper thigh that extend through the obturator foramen into the pelvis, and (3) anterior pelvic wall tumors.[1] The incisions for the anterior dissection start 5 cm proximal and 2 cm medial to the anterosuperior iliac spine. This incision follows the inguinal ligament to the pubic symphysis (Figure 38-7).

The lateral incision extends to the anterosuperior iliac spine, over the anterior portion of the greater trochanter, then posteriorly, distal and parallel to the gluteal groove to the perineum, and around the proximal thigh to meet the anterior incision at the pubis. The anterior dissection divides the insertion of the rectus abdominis at the pubic tubercle and the external, internal, and transversus muscles, thus freeing the pelvis from the abdominal wall.

The viscera are retracted and the common iliac vessels ligated and divided. The branches of the internal iliac vessels are also divided, preserving the sacral nerve roots to the bladder and rectum. The posterior incision is deepened to the gluteal fascia, gluteus maximus, and muscle. The gluteal fascia is divided at the iliotibial tract and tensor fascia lata, creating a myocutaneous flap based on gluteal arteries (Figure 38-8). This flap is elevated proximally to the iliac crest and posterosuperior and posteroinferior iliac spines. The muscular attachments to the ilium and sacrum are released, and the psoas muscle and nerves to the lower extremity are transected. The pubic symphysis, sacral nerve roots, pelvic diaphragm, and sacroiliac joint are then divided.

The wound is closed by suturing the gluteal fascia to the anterior abdominal wall fascia. The skin and subcutaneous tissues are closed in layers (Figure 38-9). Closed-suction catheters are placed deep in the wound, exiting outside the posterior flap.

Anterior Flap. The primary indications for anterior flap reconstruction are tumors that involve the upper thigh or buttock.[1] The anterior flap uses a myocutaneous flap supplied by perforators of the external iliac and superficial femoral arteries.

The anterior incision begins 2 cm proximal and posterior to the anterosuperior iliac spine and parallels the inguinal

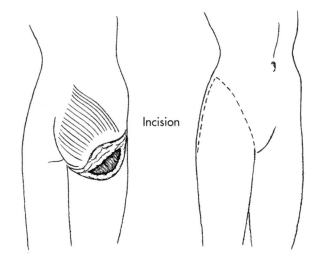

Incision

Figure 38-7. Skin markings for posterior hemipelvectomy flap.

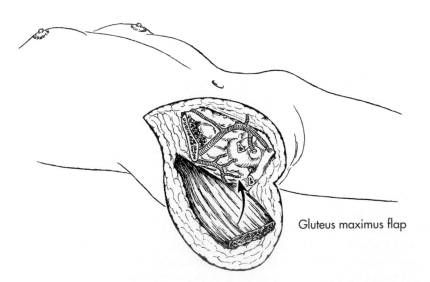

Gluteus maximus flap

Figure 38-8. Elevation of posterior hemipelvectomy flap based on gluteus maximus muscle.

ligament to the pubic tubercle (Figure 38-10). The longitudinal skin incisions on the thigh are on the posterolateral and posteromedial aspects and are joined by a transverse incision proximal to the patella. The lateral incision parallels the iliac wing, then extends distally along the thigh's lateral aspect to the level of the quadriceps muscle's tendinous insertion, superior to the patella.

Releasing all muscular attachments skeletonizes the iliac

crest and sacrum. The anterior incision is deepened, and all quadriceps muscles are exposed. The anterior myocutaneous flap supplied by the vastus lateralis or rectus femoris is based on the superficial femoral vessels (Figure 38-11).

The fascia of the quadriceps is reapproximated with the fascia of the quadratus lumborum, sacral, and levator ani muscles. The skin and subcutaneous tissues are closed in layers with deep drains (Figure 38-12).

In some patients, with both the anterior and the posterior flaps, additional soft tissue must be elevated to cover the defect. Ipsilateral, contralateral, and free flaps have been used for soft tissue reconstruction. The reconstructive surgeon should also consider using soft tissue from the amputated limb.

Internal Hemipelvectomy. This procedure involves partial resection of innominate bone with preservation of the lower extremity. The surgical goal is to obtain wide surgical margins to control tumor recurrence while maximizing function. The standard skin incision for an internal hemipelvectomy follows the iliac crest posteriorly and then posterolaterally down the thigh (Figure 38-13). A variable amount of soft tissue and bone is resected, depending on the tumor's size and location (Figure 38-14).

The reconstruction is the same as for the pelvic defects previously described, except for the use of bone replacement with allograft and hip joint reconstruction. If local muscle flaps are inadequate to cover the reconstruction, transposition muscle flaps or free flaps are used to reconstruct the defect (Figure 38-15).

POSTERIOR DEFECTS. Posterior pelvic wall defects usually result from composite resections of primary or secondary pelvic tumors (e.g., advanced rectal cancers). Primary tumors of the posterior pelvis (sacrum) can usually be resected with preservation of the rectum.[3] The major complications after these operations are injuries of nerves to the rectum, bladder, and lower extremities. Secondary tumors are usually more extensive, and composite resections of soft tissue, bone, and viscera may be necessary.

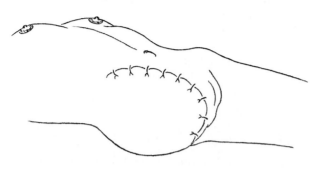

Figure 38-9. Closure of posterior hemipelvectomy flap.

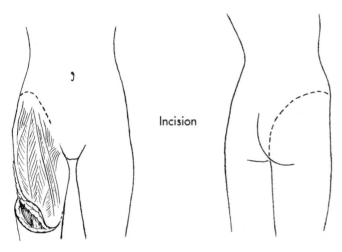

Figure 38-10. Skin markings for anterior hemipelvectomy flap.

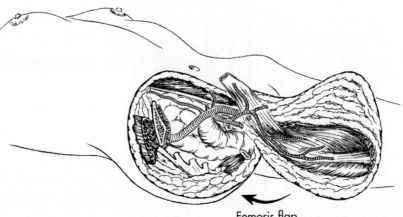

Femoris flap

Figure 38-11. Elevation of anterior hemipelvectomy flap based on rectus femoris muscle.

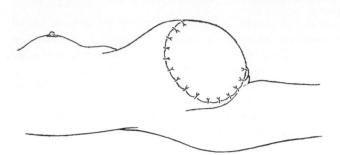
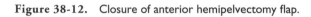

Figure 38-12. Closure of anterior hemipelvectomy flap.

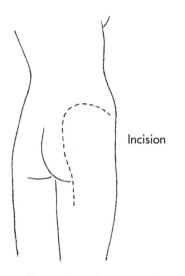

Incision

Figure 38-13. Skin markings for internal hemipelvectomy.

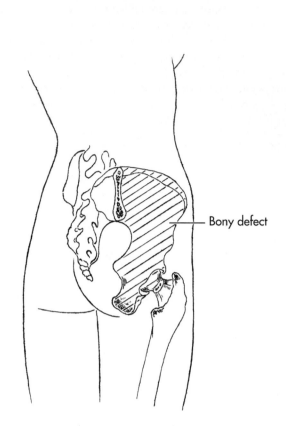

Bony defect

Figure 38-14. Internal hemipelvectomy bony defect.

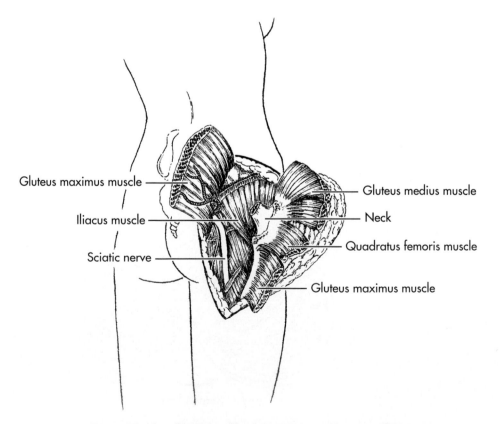
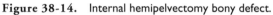

Gluteus maximus muscle

Iliacus muscle

Sciatic nerve

Gluteus medius muscle

Neck

Quadratus femoris muscle

Gluteus maximus muscle

Figure 38-15. Elevation of local internal hemipelvectomy flaps.

As with other pelvic tumors, careful preoperative evaluation of lower extremity neuromuscular function is critical. A careful physical examination to assess the extent of the tumor is also important. Preoperative imaging should include computed tomography or magnetic resonance imaging, chest radiography, bone scanning, and plain films of the lumbosacral spine to determine the extent of resection and presence of distant metastasis. Preoperative planning must include coordination with the oncologist so that radiation and chemotherapy, if necessary, can be scheduled before surgery. If the sacrum is resected at the S3 level or below, urinary continence is maintained. If the resection is at the S1 level, pelvic stability is still maintained. If the S1 or S2 nerve roots are excised, however, bladder function is compromised, and cystectomy may be necessary.

The incision for sacral reconstruction should extend from the defect down the midline and then laterally at the gluteal crease (Figure 38-16). If preserved, the gluteus maximus muscle can be mobilized to the fascial origins and approximated at the midline (Figure 38-17). Greater mobility can be obtained by releasing the muscle on the greater trochanter. The skin and subcutaneous flaps are elevated separately and closed with skin grafting if necessary (Figure 38-18). If the gluteus maximus muscle is insufficient to close the soft tissue defect, rectus abdominis or latissimus dorsi flaps may be necessary.

Outcomes

In one study of 68 patients undergoing hemipelvectomy, 21 required additional soft tissue reconstruction.[8] Of this group, 17 (81%) had internal hemipelvectomy, and four (19%) had standard hemipelvectomy with limb amputation. Twelve patients (57%) underwent immediate soft tissue reconstruction, one had a planned two-stage procedure, and eight (38%)

had delayed reconstruction for complications after pelvic resection and primary closure. Sixteen patients (76%) underwent attempted curative resection of a primary tumor. Four patients (19%) had resection of isolated metastases, with one for osteoradionecrosis.

The 20 patients were reconstructed using a total of 25 flaps. This included 20 pedicled flaps in 15 patients and five free tissue flaps in five patients. Tables 38-1 and 38-2 list the

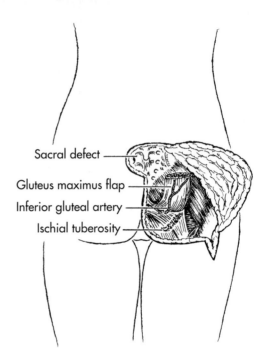

Figure 38-17. Elevation of skin and gluteus maximus muscle flaps.

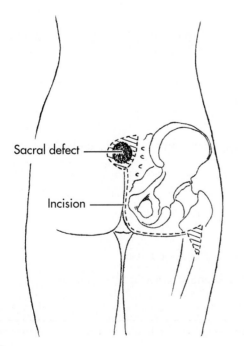

Figure 38-16. Sacral defect with skin markings.

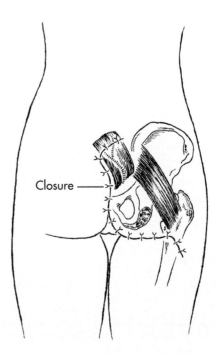

Figure 38-18. Closure of gluteal flap.

Table 38-1.
Flaps Used in Immediate Reconstruction and Associated Complications

FLAP(S)*	COMPLICATION	OUTCOME
PEDICLED		
iVRAM	Total flap loss	Replaced with vastus medialis myocutaneous flap
iVRAM	Seroma, wound infection, wound breakdown	Debridement: additional cTRAM flap required
iVRAM	None	
iRAM	Seroma	Resolved spontaneously
iRAM	Edge necrosis, abscess (3)	Draining of abscess; dressings
cVRAM	None	
cTRAM	None	
LDHB	Wound breakdown	Additional gluteus maximus rotation flap
LDHB	Wound breakdown, infected allograft	Removal of allograft; debridement; primary closure
TFL	None	
FREE		
Thigh fillet	None	
Lower leg fillet	None	

*All single flaps.
iVRAM, Ipsilateral vertical rectus abdominis myocutaneous flap; *cVRAM*, contralateral vertical rectus abdominis myocutaneous flap; *cTRAM*, contralateral transverse rectus abdominis myocutaneous flap; *iRAM*, ipsilateral rectus abdominis muscle flap; *LDHB*, latissimus dorsi myocutaneous hemiback flap; *TFL*, tensor fascia lata flap.

Table 38-2.
Flaps Used in Delayed Reconstruction and Associated Complications

FLAP(S)	COMPLICATION	OUTCOME
PEDICLED		
iVRAM and V-YGMax (1)	Wound breakdown, seroma	Debridement and resuturing under local anesthesia
iVRAM (1)	None	
cVRAM (2)	None	
cTRAM (2)	None	
FREE		
iRAM/STSG (1)	Venous occlusion	Resolved on exploration
cVRAM (1)	Edge necrosis	Debridement under local anesthesia
LDM (1)	None	

See Table 38-1 for abbreviations; *LDM*, latissimus dorsi myocutaneous flap; *V-YGM*, gluteus maximus V-Y myocutaneous advancement flap; *STSG*, split-thickness skin graft.

complications and outcomes for the immediate-reconstruction and delayed-reconstruction groups.

In another study, 62 procedures were performed on 59 patients, with 42 posterior flap hemipelvectomies, five anterior flap hemipelvectomies, and 15 internal hemipelvectomics.[4] Of the internal hemipelvectomies, seven patients had complete resection of the hemipelvis, three had resection of the iliac bone, and five had resection of the pubic bone. Marlex mesh was used in two of the posterior flap hemipelvectomies.

The 5-year survival rate for the 36 patients with curative surgery was 43%. The estimated 2-year survival of the 23 patients with palliative surgery was 25%, with a median survival of 12 months. No wound complications occurred in 38 procedures (61%), with flap necrosis in seven (11%), infection in nine (15%), and flap necrosis and infection in two (3%). The operative mortality was 1%, a death from pulmonary embolism.

REFERENCES

1. Aboulafia AJ, Monson DK: Pelvis. In Wood WC, Skandalakis JE, editors: *Anatomic basis of tumor surgery,* St Louis, 1999, Quality Medical.

2. Evans GR, Goldberg DP, Ames FC: Complex abdominal-perineal reconstruction: options after pelvic bone resection, *Plast Reconstr Surg* 98(4):735-739, 1996.

3. Karakousis CP: Pelvic and sacral saracomas: principles and operative techniques. In Sugarbaker PH, editor: *Pelvic surgery and treatment for cancer,* St Louis, 1994, Mosby.

4. Karakousis CP, Emrich LJ, Driscoll DL: Variants of hemipelvectomy and their complications, *Am J Surg* 158:404-408, 1989.

5. Lawless MW et al: Massive pelvis injuries treated with amputations: case reports and literature review, *J Trauma* 42:1169-1174, 1997.

6. Meland NB: Reconstruction of hip and pelvic defects. In Cohen M, editor: *Mastery of plastic and reconstructive surgery,* volume II, New York, 1994, Little, Brown and Company.

7. Rieger H, Dietl KH: Traumatic hemipelvectomy: an update, *J Trauma* 45:422-426, 1998.

8. Ross DA et al: Soft tissue reconstruction following hemipelvectomy, *Am J Surg* Vol 176:25-28, 1998.

CHAPTER

Breast Reconstruction

Grant W. Carlson
Glyn Jones
John Bostwick

INTRODUCTION

Breast reconstruction has undergone a steady evolution since the introduction of the silicone gel prosthesis in 1963.[10] The original goals of freeing the patient of an external appliance and improving the appearance in clothes have been met. As the experience with breast reconstruction has increased, so have the aesthetic demands to match the remaining breast in dimensions, position, and contour. The improvement in the quality of breast reconstructions can be attributed in part to a refinement in mastectomy technique. There is an increasing emphasis on individualizing skin incisions to allow skin preservation, thus avoiding surgery on the opposite breast to achieve symmetry.[8] In earlier reconstructions the contralateral breast had to be modified in more than half the patients. From an oncologic standpoint, no reconstruction on the opposite side ensures future physical and mammographic evaluation of the remaining breast and facilitates future reconstruction if a contralateral cancer develops.

INDICATIONS

Immediate breast reconstruction after total mastectomy is being increasingly performed. It currently accounts for approximately 40% of breast reconstructions in a recent American Society of Plastic and Reconstructive Surgeons survey. Studies have refuted the claims that immediate reconstruction delays the detection of recurrences and results in poorer survival.[19,21,31] The theory that prolonged operative time and increased blood loss result in tumor enhancement has never been proved.

The potential advantages of immediate reconstruction can be viewed from a technical as well as a psychologic standpoint.

Reconstruction is easier in the immediate setting because of the liability of the native skin envelope and the delineation of the inframammary fold. The psychologic trauma associated with breast loss, including a sense of mutilation, depression, and diminished feelings of femininity, can be greatly reduced by immediate reconstruction.[11,60,63]

METHOD SELECTION

Currently, several options are available to a woman seeking reconstruction after mastectomy (Table 39-1). They vary in degrees of complexity and potential morbidity but generally are separated into those using only autologous tissue and those employing some form of breast implant or expander. The condition of the chest wall skin and muscles, breast size, body habitus, and availability of flap donor sites are considered during preoperative evaluation. Medical factors, including smoking, obesity, diabetes, and history of chest wall irradiation, also influence treatment options. Current restrictions on the use of silicone gel breast implants have increased the reliance on autologous tissue reconstruction.

Trabulsy et al[61] reviewed their 13-year experience with 455 breast reconstructions. The use of autogenous reconstruction increased from 13% during 1979 to 1983 to 37% during 1988 to 1991. The authors noted significant decreases in the use of implants and the latissimus dorsi flap, whereas tissue expansion and TRAM flap use increased significantly during the study period.

Implants and Tissue Expansion

The use of breast implants and tissue expanders is the most common method of breast reconstruction. The simplicity, lack of donor site, and rapid recovery make it an attractive method despite the moratorium on silicone gel breast implants. A subpectoral implant can reconstruct a small, nonptotic breast after a skin-preserving mastectomy with good aesthetic results. The currently available breast implants usually contain saline

Table 39-1.
Methods of Breast Reconstruction*

METHOD	COMPLEXITY	AESTHETIC RESULT
Implant	+	+
Tissue expander/ implant	++	+
Latissimus dorsi flap (+/− implant)	+++	++
TRAM flap	++++	++++
Free flaps (TRAM, gluteal)	++++	++++

TRAM, Transverse rectus abdominis myocutaneous.
*Grading scale, + to ++++, with increasing complexity.

and are selected to match the opposite breast in volume, shape, and contour. A larger, more ptotic breast can be reconstructed with placement of a tissue expander without using distant flaps (Figure 39-1). The patient must understand that symmetry usually cannot be achieved without manipulation of the opposite breast. The method was introduced by Radovan[49] in 1982 as a way of utilizing local tissue to form a breast mound. It is a relatively simple technique that generally is well tolerated.

The procedure involves placement of a saline or biluminal saline and silicone gel reservoir under the skin and chest wall muscles. Saline is gradually injected into the reservoir over weeks or months. The soft tissue is slowly stretched until adequate breast volume is achieved. The reservoir is then filled with additional saline and left for 3 to 6 months to allow the surrounding capsule to mature. Depending on the type of expander used, the volume then can be reduced to achieve symmetry, and the access port can be removed or the expander replaced with a permanent breast implant. Expansion can be performed safely during chemotherapy administration if periods of myelosuppression are avoided.

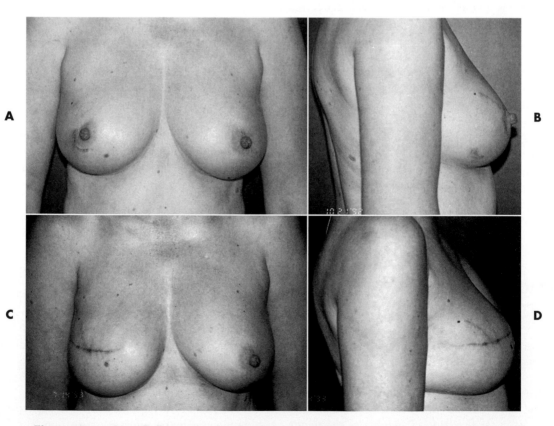

Figure 39-1. **A** and **B,** Preoperative views of 51-year-old woman with diffuse ductal carcinoma in situ of right breast. **C** and **D,** Postoperative views after total mastectomy and tissue expander/implant reconstruction.

Latissimus Dorsi Flap

The use of the latissimus dorsi musculocutaneous flap in breast reconstruction was first described by Schneider et al[53] and Muhlbauer and Olbrisch.[46] It became the standard method of breast reconstruction in the 1970s. At that time, most women had radical mastectomy deformities, and the flap was useful to replace missing skin, muscle, and supply additional autogenous fill. It is a more complex procedure than implant and expander placement, requiring hospitalization and a recovery period of 2 to 4 weeks. A breast implant is usually placed beneath the flap to provide adequate volume. It is useful in patients with thin, contracted, or previously irradiated skin and in those who are not candidates for TRAM flap reconstruction (see next section).

An extended deepithelialized skin island that does not require an implant had been described.[29,53] The large flap size increases surgical morbidity and results in a large back scar. Hokin and Silverskiold[29] reported its use in 55 patients, with a major flap complication rate of 14.5%.

Transverse Rectus Abdominis Myocutaneous (TRAM) Flap

Robbins[50] first reported using a vertically oriented flap of rectus abdominis muscle and skin in breast reconstruction in 1979. Hartrampf et al[28] introduced the transverse rectus abdominis musculocutaneous (TRAM) flap in 1982. The skin island is oriented transversely across the abdomen to camouflage the scar and double as an abdominoplasty (Figure 39-2). It has become the method of choice for

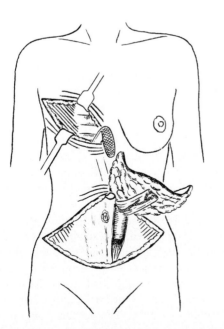

Figure 39-2. Breast reconstruction with transverse rectus abdominis myocutaneous (TRAM) flap, designed as abdominoplasty in lower abdominal area and transferred to chest, pedicled on upper rectus abdominis muscle containing superior epigastric artery.

autologous tissue reconstruction. The ellipse of skin and underlying fat of the lower abdomen are supplied by perforators from the underlying rectus abdominis muscles vascularized by the superior and inferior epigastric vessels. The pedicled flap is tunneled under the remaining abdominal wall and rotated into the mastectomy defect based on one or both muscles. Both rectus muscles typically used in patients at high risk for tissue necrosis: history of chest irradiation, obesity, significant abdominal scarring, and large tissue requirements.[62] This method can produce a soft, large breast without the use of an implant. The concomitant abdominoplasty and lower abdominal incision make this an appealing technique.

Free Flaps

Free tissue transfer is the method of choice when neither local tissues nor pedicled flaps are available. Thin patients and those with abdominal scars that prevent conventional TRAM flaps are ideal candidates. Free TRAM flap breast reconstruction has gained popularity in an attempt to increase flap vascularity and decrease the abdominal wall morbidity seen with the conventional pedicled flap. The free TRAM flap uses the inferior epigastric vessels, which are the main blood supply to the lower rectus muscle and overlying skin (Figure 39-3). Microvascular anastomoses are usually performed to the thoracodorsal vessels. Vein grafts are seldom necessary because of the long pedicle length. The free flap has better vascularity and requires less muscle harvest than the pedicled flap, thus reducing abdominal wall morbidity. A large skin island can be used based on one pedicle and designed lower in the abdomen to hide the incision.

The buttocks area has abundant soft tissue that can be used as a free flap for breast reconstruction. Gluteal free flaps based on the superior gluteal artery were first described by Fujino et al[20] in 1975. The flap was refined by Shaw,[57] who reported 10 successful cases. A portion of the gluteus maximus muscle and the overlying skin are used. The superior gluteal vessels tend to be short, and in thin patients the tissue is insufficient for reconstruction. The short pedicle length dictates that the flap be anastomosed to the internal mammary vessels to avoid vein grafts. The internal mammary vein is frequently insufficient for microvascular anastomoses, necessitating use of neck or axillary veins.

The inferior gluteal flap using a portion of muscle and skin based on the inferior gluteal vessels was first described by LeQuang[36] in 1979. Paletta et al[48] reported its use in three breast reconstructions. This flap has the advantage of a low donor site scar in the inferior gluteal fold and a longer pedicle than the superior gluteal flap. There is concern that removing the inferior portion of the gluteus maximus can interfere with hip extension and external rotation and place the exposed sciatic nerve at risk for injury. Gluteal flaps are used when other reconstructive options are not available. They are technically demanding,

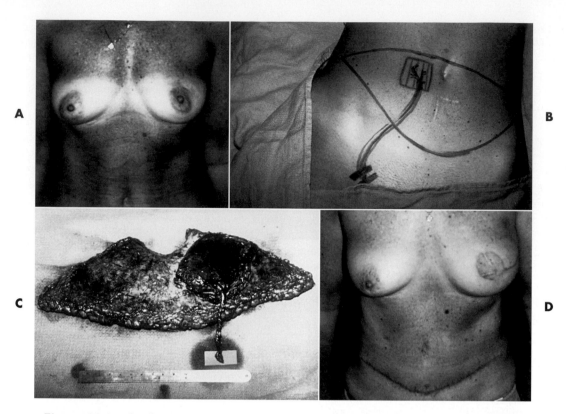

Figure 39-3. A, Preoperative view of 44-year-old woman with cancer of left breast. **B,** Intraoperative markings for free TRAM flap based on right inferior epigastric vessels. **C,** Portion of muscle and overlying skin after flap elevation. Note long inferior epigastric pedicle. **D,** Postoperative view after total mastectomy and free TRAM flap reconstruction.

may result in morbidity at donor sites, but can produce good results.

RECONSTRUCTION AFTER BREAST CONSERVATION

Breast cosmesis after partial mastectomy and radiation depends on patient selection and treatment-related factors. Large resections and radial incisions lead to poor results, especially in small breasts. Resection of large amounts of skin creates contour deformities and nipple distortion. Whole-breast irradiation doses greater than 50 Gy and overlapping treatment fields can result in a constricted, fibrotic skin envelope. Surgical technique influences aesthetic outcomes more than radiation therapy.[39]

Reconstruction after breast conservation is seldom necessary, even in Europe where quandrantectomies are performed. The cosmetic results of breast conservation are judged to be excellent or good by 60% to 90% of patients.[2,25,38] The majority of poor results have a deficiency of parenchymal volume and skin and distortion of the nipple location. A latissimus dorsi flap can be useful in these cases, but close corroboration with the surgical oncologist and mammographer is necessary to follow these patients postoperatively.[4,58]

RECONSTRUCTION AFTER FAILED BREAST CONSERVATION

Lumpectomy with radiation therapy has become the treatment choice for the majority of stage I and II breast cancers. The 10-year local failure rate after breast conservation has been reported as 14% to 19%.[17,18,34] The majority of patients who develop a recurrence require a total mastectomy and many seek breast reconstruction. Surgery in these patients can be compromised by radiation fibrosis and endarteritis, which interfere with the skin's blood supply and impair wound healing.

Tissue expansion is not a good option after failed breast conservation. The radiated skin expands poorly and is prone to breakdown, leading to implant exposure. Dickson and Sharpe,[12] in their review of 75 cases of tissue expansion, identified 10 patients who had chest irradiation before expansion. The complication rate in this subgroup was 70% and the failure rate 30%. The authors questioned whether patients who have received radiation therapy should undergo tissue expansion. Dowden,[13] in his experience with 176 cases of implant and expander reconstruction, concluded that prior radiation increased the risk of failure.

TRAM flap reconstruction is also affected by previous radiation. The blood supply may be affected because the superior epigastric vessels that supply the flap are within the field of radiation. Hartrampf and Bennett[27] found that 17% of 300 patients had received prior radiation. The overall partial flap necrosis rate was 6.3%, 32% of whom had received radiation. The authors thought that the findings were inconclusive regarding the effect on flap loss. Watterson et al[62] reviewed the Emory experience with 556 TRAM flap reconstructions; 91 patients had received previous chest wall irradiation. The overall complication rate for those receiving radiation was 37.4%, versus 21.1% for those with no radiation history. Partial flap loss occurred in 13.2% of the radiation patients, versus 3.4% for those with no radiation. TRAM flap reconstruction in such patients should include both rectus abdominis pedicles or should be performed as a free flap.

OPERATIONS

IMPLANTS AND TISSUE EXPANDERS

An implant alone can reconstruct a small, nonptotic breast in a single stage. This simple method is applicable to a small minority of patients and those who only want freedom from an external prosthesis. Tissue expansion is generally a two-stage procedure, with initial expander placement followed in 3 to 6 months by replacement with an anatomically designed saline implant. Textured expanders appear to have a very low incidence of capsular contraction.[3] The textured surface prevents implant migration, which assists in the development of a well-defined inframammary fold. An integrated fill valve is preferred to reduce deflation and infection.

Expander Placement

The breast base diameter is measured to determine the size of the tissue expander. In delayed reconstruction a subpectoral pocket is formed by releasing the attachments of the pectoralis major muscle from the sternum and costal margin. The textured expander is placed at the level of the opposite inframammary fold. As the expander is inflated, the fold is passively established. The inferior pole of the expander can be safely left in the subcutaneous plane. The cut edge of the pectoralis muscle is sutured to the inferior skin flap to provide coverage over the skin incision.

In immediate reconstruction the surgeon must ensure viability of the skin flaps. If healthy inferior skin flaps are present, providing muscle coverage of the expander's inferior pole is unnecessary. If the skin flaps are thin, it is best to provide complete muscle coverage. The lower half of the pocket consists of subrectus fascia, external oblique muscle, and serratus anterior muscle. The fascia-muscle flap is dissected off the chest wall in a medial to lateral direction to the anterior axillary fold (Figure 39-4). The flap is dissected several centimeters below the opposite breast and the expander placed (Figure 39-5). Alterations of the opposite breast necessary to achieve symmetry are generally done during the first stage of reconstruction.

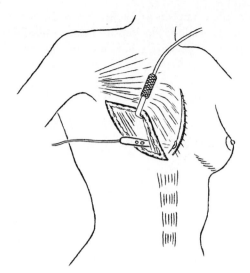

Figure 39-4. Immediate reconstruction with complete submuscular expander/implant. Lower half of pocket consists of subrectus fascia, external oblique muscle, and serratus anterior muscle.

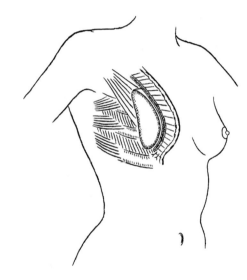

Figure 39-5. Implant/expander is placed under muscle flaps, which are closed with absorbable suture.

Expansion

The expander is filled immediately to a volume that does not jeopardize the circulation to the overlying skin flaps. Expansion proceeds on a weekly basis, with 50 to 100 ml added, depending on the tension of the overlying tissue. Expansion can be performed safely during chemotherapy if the patient's blood counts are normal. Scar contracture of the skin and soft tissue can impede the expansion process if it is delayed. The implant is overfilled based on the ptosis of the opposite breast.

Permanent Implant Placement

Placement of a permanent prosthesis is delayed 3 to 6 months to allow capsule maturation. The expander is removed through the previous mastectomy incision. An inferior pole capsulectomy may be required to lower the inframammary fold. An anatomic saline implant is chosen based on breast width, height, and projection. The implant must be filled to volume specifications to prevent significant rippling and implant failure. Overfilling distorts the implant spherically and may create scalloping at the periphery. Small adjustments to the opposite breast are also made at this stage.

LATISSIMUS DORSI FLAP

Anatomy

The anatomy of the latissimus dorsi muscle contributes to its usefulness in breast reconstruction. It is a large, triangular back muscle whose primary pedicle is the thoracodorsal vessels branching from the subscapular vessels that originate from the axillary vessels. Before sending the terminal branches to the latissimus dorsi muscle, the thoracodorsal vessels give off several collateral vessels to the serratus anterior muscle. These vessels need to be ligated to allow a greater arc of rotation for the flap. Many musculocutaneous perforating vessels over the entire surface of the muscle support the overlying skin.

Flap Elevation

The patient is placed in the lateral decubitus position with the back and anterior chest prepared and draped. Skin islands can be designed in a variety of positions over the latissimus dorsi muscle, depending on the reconstructive demands (Figure 39-6). A low, oblique skin island allows inferolateral inset of the flap and better definition of the inframammary fold. This produces good projection for the mound and maximum fullness in the lower half of the breast (Figure 39-7). To reconstruct a radical mastectomy defect, the skin island is designed high on the muscle to provide fill in the infraclavicular area.

The skin and subcutaneous tissue are dissected off the muscle and overlying skin island. The entire muscle is usually harvested proceeding from distal to proximal by dividing the attachments to the chest wall. The pedicle can be identified on the muscle's undersurface. When the proximal blood supply is confirmed, the collateral vessels to the serratus anterior muscle are divided. The muscle's humeral insertion is divided to provide better definition to the anterior axillary fold. A subcutaneous tunnel is made across the axillary apex to pass the flap from back to front.

The donor site is closed by placing absorbable tacking sutures to hold skin and subcutaneous tissue against the donor chest wall to reduce seroma formation. Closed suction drains are placed for 7 to 10 days. Reduced arm mobility is encouraged to allow adherence of the tissues.

Flap Inset

In delayed reconstruction the mastectomy incision is opened and the mastectomy defect recreated. The latissimus flap is brought through the axillary defect. The muscle is positioned to give satisfactory cover to an appropriately sized implant. Depending on the amount of muscle harvested, the pectoralis major muscle may have to be detached from the sternum and costal margin to provide coverage of the implant's superior pole. The skin is positioned in the opened mastectomy scar when the scar is low and oblique. Placement of the latissimus dorsi skin island in a high incision is unattractive; it should be placed in a separate oblique incision in the lower outer quadrant of the reconstructed breast. This will balance the symmetry and provide ptosis to the breast reconstruction (Figure 39-8).

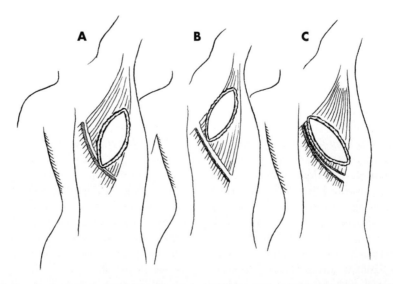

Figure 39-6. **A,** Latissimus dorsi skin island can be designed in various positions over latissimus dorsi muscle. When oriented laterally, transposed flap can reach inframammary fold, and only a portion of muscle is necessary. **B,** When latissimus skin island is oriented beneath brassiere strap in back and is transposed anteriorly, lower portion of muscle can fill infraclavicular area. **C,** When oriented obliquely across back, skin island is in natural skin lines, with most inconspicuous donor scar.

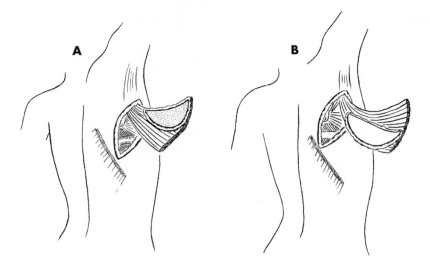

Figure 39-7. **A,** In radical mastectomy defect, latissimus dorsi skin island can be deepithelialized to fill in infraclavicular area. **B,** After modified radical mastectomy, skin island flap can be used to supplement skin in lower outer portion of breast.

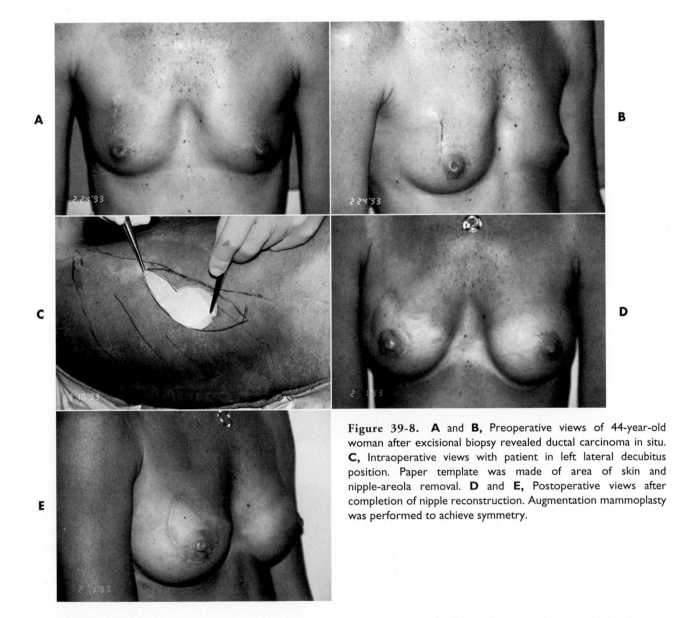

Figure 39-8. **A** and **B,** Preoperative views of 44-year-old woman after excisional biopsy revealed ductal carcinoma in situ. **C,** Intraoperative views with patient in left lateral decubitus position. Paper template was made of area of skin and nipple-areola removal. **D** and **E,** Postoperative views after completion of nipple reconstruction. Augmentation mammoplasty was performed to achieve symmetry.

PEDICLED TRAM FLAP

Anatomy

Scheflan and Dinner[52] describe the vascular anatomy of the TRAM flap. The primary source of circulation to the rectus muscle in the lower abdomen is the deep inferior epigastric artery (DIEA). The skin overlying the muscle at or below the umbilicus (zones I and II) is supplied by a few large musculocutaneous perforators from the DIEA and the superficial inferior epigastric artery (SIEA) (Figure 39-9). At the extremes of the abdominal ellipse (zones III and IV), the skin is nourished through communications between the SIEA and the superficial circumflex iliac artery, with few or no musculocutaneous perforators.

Moon and Taylor[44] studied the anatomy of the deep superior epigastric artery (DSEA) and the DIEA and their influence on TRAM flaps. They found three patterns of connections between these two arteries (Figure 39-10). A type I blood supply was a single DSEA and a single DIEA, occurring in 29% of cases. A type II supply was a double-branched connection between the two systems, present in 57%. A type III pattern involved three or more vessels, occurring 14% of the time.

The superior skin island receives its primary blood supply from the DSEA with little contribution from below. Cutaneous vessels cross the midline as far as the lateral border of the opposite rectus muscle. The middle skin island is centered at the umbilical level. The main blood supply to this flap comes from perforators of the distal DIEA. These perforators fill from the DSEA through "choke" vessels within the muscle above the umbilicus. The subdermal plexus provides vessels over the entire flap almost to the anterior axillary fold. The lower skin island is perfused by the DIEA and contains fewer perforating vessels than the other two flap designs. Moon and Taylor[44] noted no vascular filling in the deep subcutaneous fat below the subdermal plexus across the midline. The skin paddle appeared to be vascularized to the lateral edge of the contralateral rectus (zone II). The lower transverse flap is most vulnerable to vascular compromise. A pedicled TRAM flap necessitates reversal of blood flow through the choke vessels. For this reason, most surgeons center the TRAM flap just below the umbilicus instead of in the suprapubic region.

Carramenha e Costa[9] described two vertical rows of perforators lying along the rectus muscle, one in the lateral third and the other in the medial third. Vascular insufficiency probably occurs when attempts are made to preserve the lateral third of the muscle in a muscle-splitting flap. As noted, Moon and Taylor[44] described a single, centrally placed vessel in only 29% of their specimens. Harris et al[26] studied the effects of occluding the medial and lateral thirds of the rectus muscle. They found a decrease in arterial pressure in 80% of patients and advised against muscle preservation during flap harvest.

A "delay" of the TRAM flap by ligation of the ipsilateral DIEA and SIEA before transfer may improve flap viability.[7,40,44] Ozgentas et al[47] experimentally showed delay to the TRAM flap increases the area of flap survival significantly.

The rectus abdominis muscle receives segmental innervation from the seventh to twelfth thoracic intercostal nerves. The motor branches travel on the undersurface of the muscle

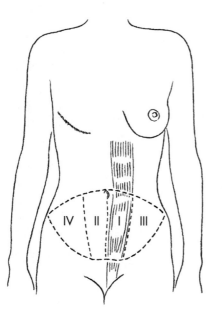

Figure 39-9. Vascular zones of lower TRAM flap (see text).

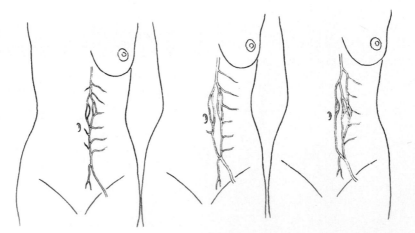

Figure 39-10. Variations in supply to rectus abdominis muscle from deep superior and inferior epigastric arteries (see text).

and penetrate its midportion.[14,35,44] Preservation of a lateral strip of muscle during elevation probably results in denervation of the remaining muscle.

Preoperative Planning

A unipedicle TRAM flap is preferred to reduce abdominal wall morbidity. A bipedicle TRAM flap is indicated in the presence of tobacco smoking, obesity, large volume requirements, history of chest wall irradiation, and abdominal scarring.[62]

A preoperative assessment of breast dimensions must be made to plan TRAM flap positioning (Figure 39-11). A long *vertical* tissue deficiency in a relatively narrow breast requires vertical flap positioning. An *oblique* positioning is a variant of the vertical mound-shaping technique. After the flap is positioned vertically, the lower portion is rotated outward to give additional lower breast fullness. This ensures good fill in the medial upper portion of the breast and restores upper breast cleavage. In patients who have wide breasts with increased fullness in the lower pole and significant ptosis, *horizontal* flap positioning is indicated.

Care is taken to avoid placing zones II and IV medially in unipedicle flap reconstruction. In this approach the flap is rotated 180 degrees, and the umbilicus is placed along the inframammary crease and can be closed vertically to give additional breast projection and contour. A contralateral pedicle is generally used for unilateral breast reconstruction. When a TRAM flap needs to be set in a horizontal position, an ipsilateral pedicle is sometimes used to place zone I in the medial portion of the reconstruction.

Flap Dissection

The patient is marked in a standing position before surgery. A skin ellipse is usually oriented from just above the umbilicus to above the pubis. It may be oriented higher in the abdomen in patients at risk for flap ischemia to improve the blood supply. The lateral limbs are above the inguinal ligament and medial to the anterosuperior iliac spines. In older or heavier patients the ellipse is widened to accommodate lateral redundancy.

The superior abdominal skin apron is elevated off the anterior abdominal wall over the costal margins. The epigastric tunnel is dissected from above and below, in the midline and often under the opposite breast, but not under the breast to be reconstructed (Figure 39-12).

Flap dissection is carried out from the lateral side medially until the lateral vascular perforators are seen exiting the fascia. Once adequate perforators are observed, the flap is elevated from the contralateral side across the midline until the medial row of perforating vessels are encountered. The umbilicus is carefully incised with a small cuff of fibrofatty tissue. In bipedicle flap reconstruction a midline tunnel is made from the umbilicus to the flap's inferior margin. The medial fascial incisions in the rectus sheaths are made after the muscles have been divided and the flap is being elevated.

A sterile Doppler probe is used to trace the course of the DSEA. Methylene blue dye is used to mark out a 1-cm strip of anterior fascia over the vessel course in the upper abdomen. This strip of fascia protects the underlying pedicle during flap elevation, especially at the tendinous inscriptions. The fascia is

carefully incised and mobilized medially and laterally to the markings and around the perforators. The segmental intercostal vessels and nerves are controlled, and the entire muscle is mobilized out of the rectus sheath. Care is taken at the tendinous inscriptions because the sheath is adherent to the muscle and the pedicle can be injured. Below the umbilicus the lateral border of the rectus muscle is retracted medially to expose the DIEA vessels on the muscle's undersurface. These are carefully dissected down to the external iliac vessels in case conversion to a free flap is required. The vessels are individually ligated, and the inferior muscle is divided with cautery.

The muscle is elevated out of the rectus sheath over the costal margin. The lateral third of the muscle is divided above the margin, thus protecting the pedicle from injury. Care is taken to divide the eighth intercostal nerve at the costal margin to reduce postoperative muscle fullness in the epigastrium. The

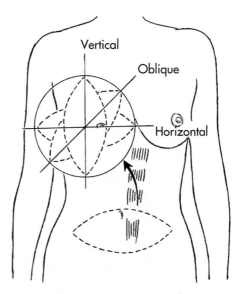

Figure 39-11. TRAM flap positioning depends on preoperative assessment of breast dimensions.

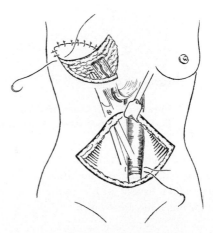

Figure 39-12. Abdominal skin apron has been completely dissected over costal margins. Tunnel is made in midline and under native breast to preserve inframammary fold on operated side. Flap is brought through tunnel and rotated 90 to 180 degrees, depending on situation.

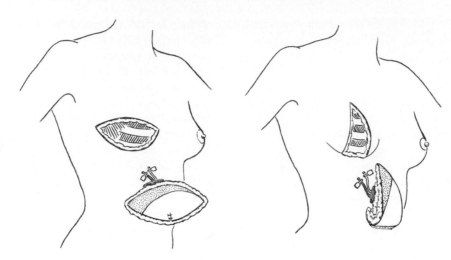

Figure 39-13. Flap can be inset in transverse or vertical orientation, depending on volume of defect and shape of opposite breast.

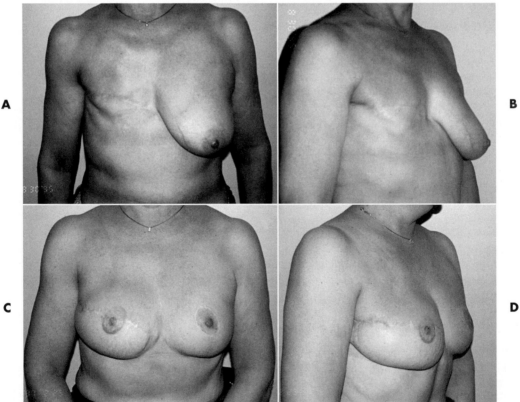

Figure 39-14. **A** and **B,** Preoperative views of patient with modified radical mastectomy. **C** and **D,** Postoperative views after unipedicled TRAM flap reconstruction and contralateral mastopexy.

flap is brought through the subcutaneous tunnel and rotated 90 to 180 degrees, depending on the situation (Figure 39-12). The pedicle should have a gentle twist; folds can lead to vascular compromise and are avoided.

Flap Inset

The flap is positioned according to the dimensions of the native breast, as previously discussed. Portions of the flap are trimmed and deepithelialized as needed (Figure 39-13). The final flap volume can be adjusted with liposuction during

nipple reconstruction in the second stage. Attempts are made to place zone I medially to reduce ischemic complications. The flap's superior portion is sutured to the pectoralis major muscle to prevent the infraclavicular hollow seen with flap settling (Figures 39-14 and 39-15).

Donor Site Closure

Meticulous donor site closure is necessary to prevent complications. In unipedicle reconstruction the fascia can usually be closed primarily. An imbricating running suture

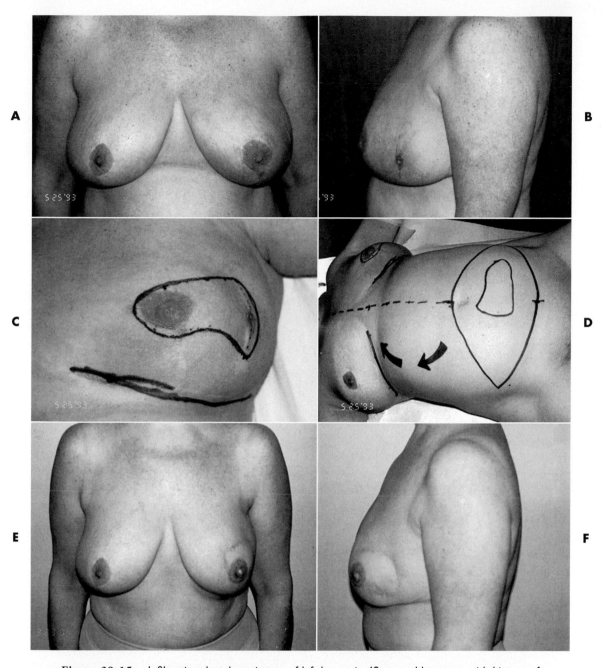

Figure 39-15. Infiltrating ductal carcinoma of left breast in 48-year-old woman with history of bilateral reduction mammoplasty. **A** and **B,** Preoperative views. **C,** Preoperative outline of area of skin removal. Note inclusion of biopsy incision. **D,** Preoperative outline of TRAM flap with area of skin replacement. **E** and **F,** Postoperative views after reconstruction.

is placed in the opposite anterior rectus sheath to provide symmetry and to help bring the umbilicus to the midline. Mesh closure is necessary in most cases of bipedicle flap reconstruction.

The abdominal skin apron is closed after placing the patient in a semiupright position. The position of the umbilicus is marked in the midline, and a Y-incision opening provides hooding to the superior umbilical pole. Midline abdominal fat above the umbilicus is trimmed with the scissors and the abdomen closed in multiple layers. Suction drains are placed through separate suprapubic stab incisions.

FREE TRAM FLAP

Flap Selection

Previous abdominal incisions may dictate which pedicle is used. If the patient requires infraclavicular fill or has a large degree of ptosis, the ipsilateral muscle is used in a vertical orientation by rotating the flap 90 degrees (Figure 39-16, *A*). A slightly oblique orientation allows the re-creation of the anterior axillary fold. A wide breast is best reconstructed using the contralateral muscle in a horizontal orientation by rotating the flap 180 degrees (Figure 39-16, *B*). The infraclavicular fill

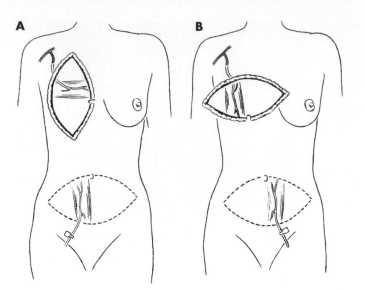

Figure 39-16. **A,** Vertical orientation is achieved by rotating flap 90 degrees. **B,** Horizontal orientation is achieved by rotating flap 180 degrees.

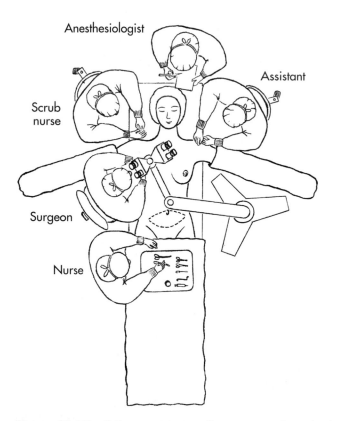

Figure 39-17. Patient positioning allows access above both arms to facilitate microsurgery.

is limited by the flap width. Increased projection is obtained by closing the umbilical defect to form a cone.

Patient Positioning

The free TRAM flap is well suited for immediate reconstruction because of the exposure of the axillary vessels. The patient is positioned with both arms abducted 90 degrees and secured to the arm boards. The draping requires cooperation with the

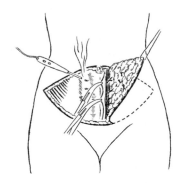

Figure 39-18. Medial row of perforating vessels are encountered after crossing midline.

anesthesiologist to allow free access above both arms. This permits the assistant to be 180 degrees across from the surgeon during microsurgery (Figure 39-17). The operating microscope is brought into the field below the opposite arm. The surgeon can be seated during the microsurgery, but the assistant generally must stand to work over the chest wall and head.

Flap Elevation

The free TRAM flap may be designed lower in the abdomen than the pedicled flap because of the better vascularity. Before flap elevation the surgeon must ensure adequacy of the recipient vessels in the axilla. The initial flap dissection proceeds in a similar manner to the pedicled flap. The flap is initially elevated from the side opposite the pedicle. The lateral and medial rows of perforators are identified and individually ligated. This gives valuable information on the probable vertical location of the ipsilateral perforators. The midline is crossed until the ipsilateral medial perforators are encountered (Figure 39-18).

The flap is then elevated on the ipsilateral side up to the lateral row of perforators. Inferiorly the flap is elevated up to the arcuate line. The vascular territory perforating the anterior rectus sheath is then outlined with methylene blue. An oblique

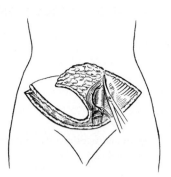

Figure 39-19. Incision inside rectus muscle is continued downward to identify inferior epigastric pedicle.

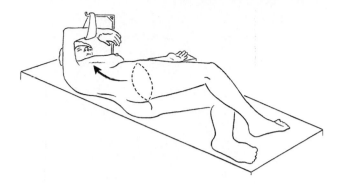

Figure 39-20. Patient position for harvest of inferior gluteal flap and re-creation of mastectomy defect. Ipsilateral arm is left free within surgical field to improve axillary vessel exposure.

incision is made in the anterior sheath below this territory to allow exposure of the inferior epigastric vessels before dividing the muscle. Gentle traction of the muscle medially at the arcuate line allows identification of the vessels entering the undersurface. The muscle can then be divided superiorly to facilitate the pedicle dissection. The course of the vessels generally permits leaving a strip of rectus muscle laterally (Figure 39-19). This facilitates fascial closure and prevents retraction of the cut muscle.

The rectus muscle is then divided inferiorly at the arcuate line to include both medial and lateral rows of perforators. The assistant can then place gentle traction on the pedicle to facilitate the dissection. The DIEA is approximately 2.5 mm in diameter and is accompanied by two venae comitantes, which usually join to form one branch off the external iliac vein. Dissection down to the external iliac vessels can obtain a pedicle of 10 cm (4 inches).

Microsurgery

Adequate preparation is essential for successful microvascular anastomosis. The skin incisions may have to be extended to gain access to the axilla. An Adson-Beckman self-retaining retractor is useful to provide exposure. The operating table is tilted toward the assistant to reduce the depth of the wound and to alleviate the difficulty of working over the lateral chest wall. The thoracodorsal vessels are the recipient vessels of choice, even when an axillary dissection is not performed. These vessels are of large caliber and have adequate length to avoid vein grafting. Use of the circumflex scapular or internal mammary vessels is indicated when the thoracodorsal vessels are unavailable.

The position of the flap during the microvascular anastomoses depends on the flap's size and the exposure in the axilla. Insetting and shaping are done after the microsurgery. Small flaps may be placed medially over the chest wall and not interfere with exposure. Large flaps may be turned over and placed lateral to the axilla to increase exposure. The surgeon must be careful not to twist the vessels. The microvascular anastomoses are performed in an end-to-end-manner with 9-0 suture. Double-approximating clamps can be used if the field is adequately prepared. This reduces the responsibility of the surgical assistant, who is in an awkward position.

INFERIOR GLUTEAL FREE FLAP

Patient Positioning

The patient is positioned to allow simultaneous harvest of the gluteal flap and dissection of the recipient vessels (Figure 39-20). The pelvis and lower extremity are in true lateral position, whereas the upper body is in a semilateral position. The ipsilateral upper extremity is prepared as part of the field to improve exposure of the axillary vessels. The ipsilateral thigh is similarly prepared circumferentially.

Flap Elevation

The flap is harvested from the same side as the reconstruction to facilitate simultaneous donor and recipient area dissection. The horizontally oriented flap is centered 3 to 4 cm above the inferior gluteal crease (Figure 39-21).

The first step in flap elevation is identification of the posterior femoral cutaneous nerve and accompanying vessels. These structures serve as the key landmarks for safe flap elevation. The initial incision is limited to the inferior skin marking and extends from the ischium approximately 5 cm (2 inches) laterally. Once the nerve is identified, the remaining incision can be made. The fat is divided in a beveled manner away from the flap's center to provide maximum volume. This dissection is completed with exposure of the gluteal muscles superiorly and the posterior thigh muscles inferiorly.

The flap is then elevated from lateral to medial off the gluteus maximus muscle. The locations of the posterior cutaneous nerves and vessels are noted as dissection approaches these structures. Gentle traction under the inferior edge of the gluteus maximus muscle exposes the inferior gluteal vessels. The lateral flap elevation stops several centimeters short of these vessels (Figure 39-22).

With the inferior gluteal vessels directly visualized, the muscular portion of the flap may now be elevated. The muscle is divided from its free inferior edge lateral to the gluteal vessels for 5 to 8 cm (2 to 3 inches) superiorly. The muscle is then divided medial to the gluteal vessels, starting at the inferior border. The superior border is divided last. The vascular pedicle is carefully dissected superiorly to the level of the piriformis muscle. A pedicle of 8 to 10 cm (3 to 4 inches) can be consistently dissected. It will consist of the inferior gluteal

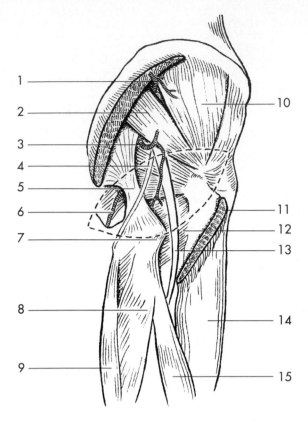

Figure 39-21. Inferior gluteus musculocutaneous flap based on inferior gluteal artery. *1,* Superior gluteal artery; *2,* piriformis muscle; *3,* inferior gluteal artery; *4,* posterior femoral cutaneous nerve; *5,* sacrotuberous ligament; *6,* internal pudendal artery; *7,* ischial tuberosity; *8,* semitendinosus muscle; *9,* semimembranosus muscle; *10,* gluteus medius muscle; *11,* gluteus maximus muscle; *12,* quadratus femoris muscle; *13,* sciatic nerve; *14,* iliotibial tract; *15,* biceps femoris muscle.

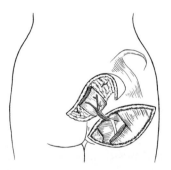

Figure 39-22. Elevation of gluteus maximus muscle. Retraction on muscle allows development of 8- to 10-cm pedicle.

artery and one or two accompanying veins, all measuring at least 2 to 3 mm in diameter.

Donor Site Closure

Meticulous closure of the donor site is important to minimize complications. The closure should be completed with the hip in extension. The remaining gluteus maximus muscle is mobilized to cover the sciatic nerve. The proximal end of the posterior cutaneous nerve is buried with the muscle. The soft tissue is closed over suction drains in multiple layers.

NIPPLE-AREOLAR RECONSTRUCTION

Method Selection

The following factors influence the choice of technique:
1. Length of the contralateral nipple
2. Height of the contralateral nipple
3. Willingness of the patient with a long, projectile nipple to undertake nipple sharing
4. Diameter, texture, and color of the normal areola

The most realistic nipple is one produced by grafting part of the normal nipple to the reconstructed breast mound.[23] This matches the color and texture perfectly and can be combined with an areola tattoo to reduce skin graft morbidity. It requires a relatively long donor nipple to be effective without eliminating too much height at the donor site and can be carried out as either a wedge excision or cap amputation. Psychologically, it should be used with caution in women who place great importance on erotic nipple sensibility during sexual arousal. If the nipple is very broad as well as long, a cap amputation is useful to match the width, as opposed to taking a wedge of nipple for grafting.

When nipple sharing is not feasible, local flaps with or without skin grafting are used. Although many different techniques have been described, the skate flap has proved to be reliable, with the potential for a long, projectile nipple if needed.[37] It does require skin grafting to the donor site. The C-V flap modification is a good alternative to avoid skin grafting.[5] This combines direct donor site closure with areolar tattooing, obviating the need for skin grafts, although early impressions are that this flap does not seem to maintain vertical height as well as the skate procedure.

Nipple-Sharing Technique

The donor nipple is anesthetized locally after determining whether a wedge or cap removal is to be performed. Wedge excision involves removing a quadrant of the nipple vertically as a hemiamputation down to the base of the nipple (Figure 39-23). The residual vertical column of the donor nipple is turned down to the base of the donor site and sutured. The recipient site is then deepithelialized to provide a healthy bed for the graft. The graft is sutured into the proper location and protected from trauma with carefully placed dressings.

If the patient has a long nipple, the tip can be transversely amputated and grafted to the recipient site. The donor site is closed either as a purse-string closure or a direct side-to-side closure.

Skate Flap Technique

The skate flap involves raising from the breast mound a local flap that can be wrapped on itself to produce a projectile nipple (Figure 39-24). It leaves a large raw donor site that requires immediate skin grafting. The exact location of the nipple-areola complex is marked on the breast mound while the patient is in an erect position. A line is drawn horizontally across the areola circle at the level of the uppermost point of the planned nipple base (i.e., the 12 o'clock position). This upper section of the circle is deepithelialized. The lateral wings of the flap are carefully raised superficially beginning in the

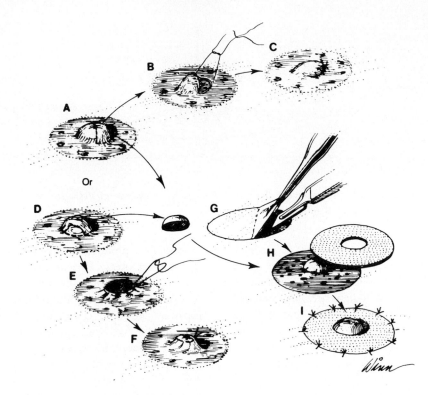

Figure 39-23. Nipple-sharing technique showing cap amputation and wedge excision procedures. (From *Operative techniques in plastic and reconstructive surgery,* Philadelphia, 1994, Saunders.)

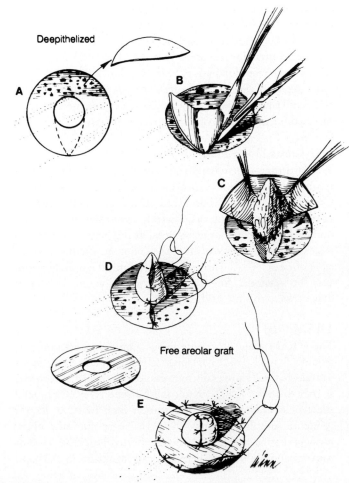

Figure 39-24. Skate flap technique showing elevation of flap margins, dissection of central pedicle, and final flap wraparound to effect closure. Raw donor site is then skin grafted as shown. (From *Operative techniques in plastic and reconstructive surgery,* Philadelphia, 1994, Saunders.)

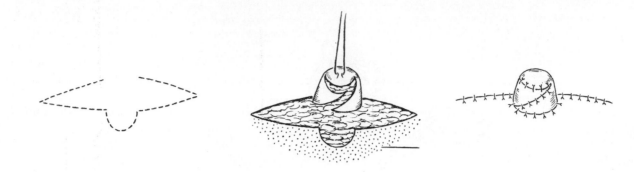

Figure 39-25. C-V flap technique illustrating flap design, elevation of V-shaped and C-shaped flaps, and final wraparound with donor site closure.

subcutaneous plane and peripherally beveling in medially toward the base of the planned nipple. This provides a progressively thicker pedicle for vascularity as one approaches the center of the nipple. The skin flaps are then wrapped around the elevated central skin-fat pedicle that is based superiorly.

A full-thickness skin graft is harvested from the groin or axillary portion of the mastectomy scar. The graft is then secured to the recipient bed.

C-V Flap Procedure

This modification of the skate flap was developed to reduce the need for skin grafting the areola. The concept is to raise bilateral skin flaps from the donor sites that may be closed primarily. The reconstruction should be measured as 25% longer to allow for subsequent settling and height loss. Two long, triangular V flaps extending laterally and medially from the nipple base are drawn with a base width equal to the planned nipple height desired (Figure 39-25). These are raised in a beveled manner similar to the skate procedure, from peripheral to central, leaving a core of fat centrally equal in width to the nipple's desired diameter. From the most inferior ends of these flaps, a semicircular C flap of skin is raised to provide a cap for the new nipple.

The central fat pedicle is carefully released as necessary to allow vertical rotation into the erect position. The lateral and medial flaps are then wrapped around this core and sutured. The semicircular flap is closed over the top of the nipple mound and sutured in place; its donor site is filled with the base of the reconstructed nipple. The triangular flap donor sites are closed primarily with interrupted sutures.

OUTCOMES

COMPLICATIONS

Implants and Expanders

Reconstruction of a large, ptotic breast with tissue expansion is difficult. McCraw et al[43] compared tissue expansion and TRAM flap breast reconstructions, and found that expansion took longer and required more revisions. The TRAM flap was more likely to produce better results and obtain symmetry with the opposite breast. Patient selection is extremely important when considering using this method.

Complications, including infection, implant exposure, and expander deflation, can result in a failure rate of 3% to 40%.[12,13,31,43,49] Obese patients and those with prior chest wall irradiation are especially prone to failure. Capsular contraction is the most common complication, reported in 4.6% to 29% of cases.[43,49] The introduction of textured saline implants and expanders has reduced this complication to less than 5%.[16,24,41]

Spear and Majidian[59] reviewed 171 consecutive patients undergoing immediate breast reconstruction in two stages using textured, integrated-valve tissue expanders and breast implants. There was a 7% method failure rate (one expander deflation, two infections, six impending exposures requiring flap coverage, three unsalvageable reconstructions). Significant capsular contraction occurred in five patients (2.9%), four of whom had received radiation. Seven permanent implants (4%) were replaced because of deflation. A subgroup of 42 consecutive patients were evaluated by questionnaire, and 98% reported being satisfied with their reconstruction.

Latissimus Dorsi Flap

The latissimus dorsi flap is a versatile, reliable method of reconstruction with a flap necrosis rate of less than 5%.[45] Capsular contraction around the implant is the most common complication, occurring in 20% to 56% of cases.[6,42] Information regarding the use of textured saline implants in this setting is lacking. Seroma formation in the donor site occurs in 9% to 33% of cases.[31,45,58] The use of an implant, the back incision, and the potential for shoulder dysfunction are the main drawbacks to this method.

TRAM Flap

The TRAM flap procedure is a complex operation that requires 5 to 7 days of hospitalization and 4 to 6 weeks of convalescence. The overall complication rate has been reported as 16% to 28%.[27,32,43,52] Kroll and Netscher,[32] examining the effect of obesity on the complication rate, found a 15.4% incidence in thin patients versus 41.7% in morbidly obese patients. Partial flap loss has been reported in 6% to 31% of patients and abdominal herniation or weakness in 0.3% to

13%. Smoking predisposes to flap necrosis and is a contraindication to performing the flap in many centers.

Hartrampf and Bennett[27] reviewed 300 TRAM flap reconstructions and found that 17% of patients with unipedicle and 64% those with bipedicle flaps lost the ability to do situps after surgery. Lejour and Dome[35] tested the abdominal wall function of 57 patients after TRAM flap reconstruction and concluded the functional compromise after a unipedicle TRAM flap was acceptable but restricted the use of the bipedicle flap. The free TRAM flap is preferred when improved vascularity is required.

The TRAM flap is the gold standard in breast reconstruction. It produces the most natural-looking and natural-feeling breast. The results must be balanced against the complexity of the procedure and its potential morbidity.

Free TRAM Flap

The main disadvantage of free TRAM flap reconstruction is the dependence on microsurgery, with total flap loss reported as 1% to 6% in a large series.[1,55] Grotting et al[22] compared 44 pedicled and 10 free TRAM flaps and found that the free TRAM procedure took approximately 1 hour longer to perform but with less blood loss. The pedicled flaps had an 18% complication rate, compared with no reported complications for the free TRAM flap. The free TRAM flap appears to have many advantages over the conventional TRAM flap and has gained popularity as experience has increased.

Schusterman et al[54] compared 48 pedicled with 20 free TRAM flaps for immediate reconstruction. Fat necrosis was noted in 11 (23%) and hernia formation in five (10%) of the pedicled flaps. Total flap loss occurred in two (10%) and hernia in two (10%) of the free flaps. No evidence of fat necrosis was reported in the free flap group. Elliot et al[15] reported 128 cases of immediate breast reconstruction, including 48 free TRAM flaps. The operative time for free flap reconstruction, including mastectomy, averaged 6 hours. There was one total flap loss (2%) and one case of fat necrosis.

The reduction in abdominal wall morbidity is an attractive feature of free TRAM flap reconstruction. A small portion of rectus muscle above the arcuate line, but below the periumbilical tendinous inscription, is sacrificed to include the musculocutaneous perforators. Arnez et al[1] preserved the medial perforators, harvesting the medial half of the muscle between the arcuate line and the umbilicus after dividing the lateral row of perforators. Grotting et al[22] and Elliot et al[15] both described leaving both a medial strip and a lateral strip of muscle but including both rows of perforators. Saving a strip of rectus muscle may facilitate fascial closure, but its usefulness has been questioned.

Duchateau et al[14] studied the innervation of the rectus abdominis muscle in six cadavers and found that the intercostal nerves travel on the muscle's undersurface and penetrate its midportion. Removal of the central portion of the muscle in the TRAM flap may denervate the lateral strip. They performed abdominal computed tomography (CT) scans on six patients after TRAM reconstruction with a lateral strip preserved. Four patients had no evidence of muscle more than

6 months after surgery. In two patients, CT scans showed that the residual muscle had become fibrotic 5 months after surgery.

Kind et al[30] studied abdominal wall function with a dynamometer in 25 patients after TRAM flap breast reconstruction (14 unipedicle flaps, nine free flaps, two bilateral free flaps). Six months after surgery the maximum isometric flexion torque increased for both the unipedicle and the free TRAM flap groups, to 89% and 93% of baseline, respectively. The authors concluded that the ultimate clinical effect of sacrificing an entire rectus muscle appears to be well tolerated by most patients.

METHOD COMPARISON

Few reports in the literature have compared the results of various methods of breast reconstruction. McGraw et al[43] found a higher complication rate and lower patient satisfaction after tissue expansion than after TRAM flap reconstruction. Rosen et al[51] found that the complication rates were similar between the two methods but that the aesthetic outcomes were better after TRAM flap reconstruction.

Kroll and Baldwin[31] compared the aesthetic quality and risk of unsuccessful outcome in 325 postmastectomy reconstructions (105 tissue expansions, 47 latissimus dorsi flaps, 173 TRAM flaps). Independent observers found that the aesthetic successes achievable were similar for the three methods but that tissue expansion was not as successful as the other techniques in obese patients. The failure rates for the various methods were tissue expansion, 21%; latissimus flap, 9%; and TRAM flap, 3%.

Serletti and Moran[56] performed a cost-comparison and outcome analysis of free versus pedicled TRAM flap reconstruction. The average operating room time and hospital reimbursement were the same. The length of hospital stay for the free TRAM group was 7 days versus 8 days for the pedicled TRAM flap group. The time to return to work was similar, as was abdominal wall strength. The authors reported no differences in outcome or complications between the two groups but a modest cost increase of $1500 for free TRAM flap reconstruction.

Kroll et al[33] compared resource costs between implant-based and TRAM flap breast reconstruction. They reviewed cases of 86 implant cases and 154 TRAM flap reconstructions. The method failure rate of implant reconstruction was 16.5%. After correcting for patients whose reconstructions were unsuccessful and including the costs of surgery subsequent to the initial reconstruction, the cost of implant reconstruction disappeared.

The psychosocial outcomes of breast reconstruction with TRAM flaps and breast implants were evaluated in the Michigan Breast Reconstruction Outcome Study.[64] Ninety-nine patients at 14 institutions underwent either implant or TRAM flap reconstruction. Quality-of-life questionnaires were administered before and 1 year after surgery. Both groups showed statistically significant gains in psychosocial well-being. TRAM flap patients showed great increases in the "ability to feel like a woman" and in improved body image compared with the implant patients.

REFERENCES

1. Arnez ZM, Bajec J, Bardsley AF, et al: Experience with 50 free TRAM flap breast reconstructions, *Plast Reconstr Surg* 87:470-478, 1991.

2. Beadle G, Silver B, Botnick L: Cosmetic results following primary radiation therapy for early breast cancer, *Cancer* 54:2911, 1984.

3. Beasley ME: Eighty-four consecutive breast reconstructions using a textured silicone tissue expander, *Plast Reconstr Surg* 89:1035, 1992.

4. Berrino P, Campora E, Santi P: Postquandrantectomy breast deformities: classification and techniques of surgical correction, *Plast Reconstr Surg* 79:567-572, 1987.

5. Bostwick J: Creating a nipple. In Berger K, Bostwick J, editors: *A women's decision,* St Louis, 1994, Quality Medical.

6. Bostwick J, Scheflan M: Latissimus dorsi musculocutaneous flap: a one-stage breast reconstruction, *Clin Plast Surg* 7:71, 1980.

7. Boyd JB, Taylor GI, Corlett R: The vascular territories of the superior epigastric and the deep inferior epigastric systems, *Plast Reconstr Surg* 73:1-14, 1984.

8. Carlson GW, Bostwick J, Styblo TM, et al: Skin sparing mastectomy: oncological and reconstructive considerations, *Ann Surg* 225:570-578, 1997.

9. Carramenha e Costa MA: An anatomic study of the venous drainage of the transverse rectus abdominis musculocutaneous flap, *Plast Reconstr Surg* 79:208, 1987.

10. Cronin TD, Gerow FJ: Augmentation mammoplasty: a new natural feel prosthesis. In *Transactions of the Third International Congress of Plastic and Reconstructive Surgery,* Amsterdam, 1963, Excerpta Medica.

11. Dean C, Chetty U, Forrest AP: Effects of immediate breast reconstruction on psychosocial morbidity after mastectomy, *Lancet* 22:459-462, 1983.

12. Dickson MG, Sharpe DT: The complications of tissue expansion in breast reconstruction: a review of 75 cases, *Br J Plast Surg* 40:629-635, 1987.

13. Dowden RV: Selection criteria for successful immediate breast reconstruction, *Plast Reconstr Surg* 88:628-634, 1991.

14. Duchateau J, Declety A, Lejour M: Innervation of the rectus abdominis muscle: implications for rectus flaps, *Plast Reconstr Surg* 82:223-227, 1988.

15. Elliot LF, Eskenazi L, Beegle PH, et al: Immediate TRAM flap breast reconstruction: 128 consecutive cases, *Plast Reconstr Surg* 92:217-227, 1993.

16. Ersek RA: Rate and incidence of capsular contracture: a comparison of smooth and textured silicone double-lumen breast prostheses, *Plast Reconstr Surg* 87:879-884, 1991.

17. Fisher B, Anderson S, Fisher ER, et al: Significance of ipsilateral breast tumour recurrence after lumpectomy, *Lancet* 338:327-331, 1991.

18. Fisher B, Redmond C, Poisson R, et al: Eight-year results of a randomized clinical trial comparing total mastectomy and lumpectomy with or without irradiation in the treatment of breast cancer, *N Engl J Med* 320:822-828, 1989.

19. Frazier TG, Noone RB: An objective analysis of immediate simultaneous reconstruction in the treatment of primary carcinoma of the breast, *Cancer* 55:1202-1205, 1985.

20. Fujino T, Harashina T, Aoyagi F: Reconstruction for aplasia of the breast and pectoral region by microvascular transfer of a free flap from the buttock, *Plast Reconstr Surg* 56:178-181, 1975.

21. Georgiade GS, Riefkohl L, Cox E, et al: Long-term clinical outcome of immediate reconstruction after mastectomy, *Plast Reconstr Surg* 76:415-420, 1985.

22. Grotting JC, Urist MM, Maddox WA, et al: Conventional TRAM flap versus free microsurgical TRAM flap for immediate breast reconstruction, *Plast Reconstr Surg* 83:828-841, 1989.

23. Gruber RP: Nipple-areola reconstruction: a review of techniques, *Clin Plast Surg* 6:71-83, 1979.

24. Hakelius L, Ohlsen L: A clinical comparison of the tendency to capsular contracture between smooth and textured gel-filled silicone mammary implants, *Plast Reconstr Surg* 90:247-254, 1992.

25. Harris J, Levene M, Svensson G, et al: Analysis of cosmetic results following primary radiation therapy for stages I and II carcinoma of the breast, *Int J Radiat Oncol Biol Phys* 5:257, 1979.

26. Harris NR, Webb MS, May JW: Intraoperative physiologic blood flow studies in the TRAM flap, *Plast Reconstr Surg* 90:553-561, 1992.

27. Hartrampf CR, Bennett GK: Autogenous tissue reconstruction in the mastectomy patient: a critical review of 300 patients, *Ann Surg* 205:508-519, 1987.

28. Hartrampf CR, Scheflan M, Black PW: Breast reconstruction with a transverse abdominal island flap, *Plast Reconstr Surg* 69:216-224, 1982.

29. Hokin JAB, Silverskiold KL: Breast reconstruction without an implant: results and complications using an extended latissimus dorsi flap, *Plast Reconstr Surg* 79:58-64, 1987.

30. Kind GM, Rademaker AW, Mustoe TA: Abdominal-wall recovery following TRAM flap: a functional outcome study, *Plast Reconstr Surg* 99:417-428, 1997.

31. Kroll SS, Baldwin B: A comparison of outcomes using three different methods of breast reconstruction, *Plast Reconstr Surg* 90:455-462, 1992.

32. Kroll SS, Netscher DT: Complications of TRAM flap breast reconstruction in obese patients, *Plast Reconstr Surg* 84:886-892, 1989.

33. Kroll SS, Evans GR, Reece GP, et al: Comparison of resource costs between implant-based and TRAM flap breast reconstruction, *Plast Reconstr Surg* 97:364-372, 1996.

34. Kurtz JM, Amalric R, Brandone H, et al: Local recurrence after breast-conserving surgery and radiotherapy, *Cancer* 63:1912-1917, 1989.

35. Lejour M, Dome M: Abdominal wall function after rectus abdominis transfer, *Plast Reconstr Surg* 87:1054-1068, 1991.

36. LeQuang C: Two new free flaps proceeding from aesthetic surgery: the lateral mammary flap and the inferior gluteal flap. In *Transactions of the 7th International Congress of Plastic and Reconstructive Surgery,* Rio de Janeirio, 1979, Excerpta Medica.

37. Little JW, Spear SL: The finishing touches in nipple-areola reconstruction, *Perspect Plast Surg* 2:1-17, 1988.

38. Margolese R: Cosmesis in segmental mastectomy, *Can J Surg* 24:198, 1981.

39. Matory W, Wertheimer M, Fitzgerald T, et al: Aesthetic results following partial mastectomy and radiation therapy, *Plast Reconstr Surg* 85:739-746, 1990.

40. Maxwell GP: Technical alternatives in transverse rectus abdominis breast reconstruction, *Perspect Plast Surg* 1:1, 1987.

41. Maxwell GP, Falcone PA: Eighty-four consecutive breast reconstructions using a textured silicone tissue expander, *Plast Reconstr Surg* 89:1022-1034, 1992.

42. McCraw JB, Maxwell GP: Early and late capsular "deformation" as a cause of unsatisfactory results in the latissimus dorsi breast reconstruction, *Clin Plast Surg* 15:717-726, 1988.

43. McCraw JB, Horton CE, Grossman JAI, et al: An early appraisal of the methods of tissue expansion and transverse rectus abdominis musculocutaneous flap in reconstruction of the breast following mastectomy, *Ann Plast Surg* 18:93-113, 1987.

44. Moon HK, Taylor GI: The vascular anatomy of rectus abdominis musculocutaneous flaps based on the deep superior epigastric system, *Plast Reconstr Surg* 82:815-829, 1988.

45. Moore TS, Farrell LD: Latissimus dorsi myocutaneous flap for breast reconstruction: long-term results, *Plast Reconstr Surg* 89:666-672, 1992.

46. Muhlbauer W, Olbrisch R: The latissimus dorsi myocutaneous flap for breast reconstruction, *Chir Plast* 4:27, 1977.

47. Ozgentas HE, Shenaq S, Spira M: Study of the delay phenomenon in the rat TRAM model, *Plast Reconstr Surg* 94:1018, 1994.

48. Paletta CE, Bostwick J, Nahai F: The inferior gluteal free flap in breast reconstruction, *Plast Reconstr Surg* 84:875-883, 1989.

49. Radovan C: Breast reconstruction after mastectomy using the temporary expander, *Plast Reconstr Surg* 69:195-206, 1982.

50. Robbins TH: Rectus abdominis myocutaneous flap for breast reconstruction, *Aust NZ J Surg* 49:527-530, 1979.

51. Rosen PB, Jabs AD, Kister SJ: Clinical experience with immediate breast reconstruction using tissue expansion or transverse rectus abdominis musculocutaneous flaps, *Ann Plast Surg* 25:249, 1990.

52. Scheflan M, Dinner MI: The transverse abdominal island flap. Part I. Indications, contraindications, results, and complications, *Ann Plast Surg* 10:24-35, 1983.

53. Schneider WJ, Hill HL, Brown RG: Latissimus dorsi myocutaneous flap for breast reconstruction, *Br J Plast Surg* 30:277-281, 1977.

54. Schusterman MA, Kroll SS, Weldon ME: Immediate breast reconstruction: why the free TRAM over the conventional TRAM flap? *Plast Reconstr Surg* 90:255-261, 1992.

55. Schusterman MA, Kroll SS, Miller MJ, et al: The free transverse rectus abdominis musculocutaneous flap for breast reconstruction: one center's experience with 211 consecutive cases, *Ann Plast Surg* 32:234-242, 1994.

56. Serletti JM, Moran SL: Free versus the pedicled TRAM flap: a cost comparison and outcome analysis, *Plast Reconstr Surg* 100:1418-1424, 1997.

57. Shaw WW: Breast reconstruction by superior gluteal microvascular free flaps without silicone implants, *Plast Reconstr Surg* 72:490-499, 1983.

58. Slavin SA, Love SM, Sadowsky NL: Reconstruction of the radiated partial mastectomy defect with autogenous tissues, *Plast Reconstr Surg* 90:854-865, 1992.

59. Spear SL, Majidian A: Immediate breast reconstruction in two stages using textured, integrated-valve tissue expanders and breast implants: a retrospective review of 171 consecutive breast reconstructions from 1989 to 1996, *Plast Reconstr Surg* 101:53-63, 1998.

60. Stevens LA, McGrath MH, Druss RG, et al: The psychological impact of immediate breast reconstruction for women with early breast cancer, *Plast Reconstr Surg* 73:619-628, 1984.

61. Trabulsy PP, Anthony JP, Mathes SJ: Changing trends in postmastectomy breast reconstruction: a 13-year experience, *Plast Reconstr Surg* 93:1418-1427, 1994.

62. Watterson PA, Bostwick J, Hester TR, et al: TRAM flap anatomy correlated with a 10-year clinical experience with 556 patients, *Plast Reconstr Surg* 95:1185-1194, 1995.

63. Wellisch DK, Schain WS, Noone RB, et al: Psychosocial correlates of immediate versus delayed reconstruction of the breast, *Plast Reconstr Surg* 76:713-718, 1985.

64. Wilkins EG: Autogenous tissue breast reconstruction seems to provide better psychological outcomes. In *Oncology,* 1997.

Index

W